Candida and Candidiasis

Edited by
RICHARD A. CALDERONE
Department of Microbiology and Immunology
Georgetown University School of Medicine
Washington, D.C.

ASM PRESS
Washington, D.C.

Candida and Candidiasis

Address editorial correspondence to ASM Press, 1752 N St. NW, Washington, DC 20036-2904, USA

Send orders to ASM Press, P.O. Box 605, Herndon, VA 20172, USA
Phone: (800) 546-2416 or (703) 661-1593
Fax: (703) 661-1501
E-mail: books@asmusa.org
Online: www.asmpress.org

Library of Congress Cataloging-in-Publication Data

Candida and candidiasis / edited by Richard A. Calderone.
p. ; cm.
Includes bibliographical references and index.
ISBN 1-55581-212-0
1. Candidiasis. 2. Candida. I. Calderone, Richard A.
[DNLM: 1. Candida. 2. Candidiasis. QW 180.5.D38 C2173 2002]
QR201.C27 C365 2002
616.9′69—dc21 2001053525

10 9 8 7 6 5 4 3 2 1

Cover photo: Chlamydospores of *Candida dubliniensis* on cornmeal tween agar. Since this species also produces germ tubes, it can be misidentified as *Candida albicans*. Photo courtesy of David Coleman.

CONTENTS

CONTRIBUTORS

Maqsood Bhatti
Division of Infectious Diseases, Department of Medicine, Medical College of Wisconsin, Milwaukee, WI 53226, and Infectious Diseases Section/CC-111N, Consultant Care Division, VA Medical Center, Milwaukee, WI 53295

Jacques Bille
Institute of Microbiology, University Hospital of Lausanne (CHUV), 1011 Lausanne, Switzerland

Dirk P. Bockmühl
Institut fur Mikrobiologie, Heinrich-Heine Universitat, Universitatsstr. 1/26.12, D-40225 Dusseldorf, Germany

Alistair J. P. Brown
Molecular and Cell Biology, Institute of Medical Sciences, University of Aberdeen, Foresterhill, Aberdeen AB25 2ZD, United Kingdom

Richard A. Calderone
Department of Microbiology and Immunology, Georgetown University School of Medicine, 3900 Reservoir Road NW, Washington, DC 20007

Petteri Carlson
Department of Bacteriology, Helsinki University Central Hospital Laboratory Diagnostics, Haartmaninkatu 3, PO Box 400, 00029 HUS, Finland

Neeraj Chauhan
Department of Microbiology and Immunology, Georgetown University School of Medicine, 3900 Reservoir Road NW, Washington, DC 20007

Hiroji Chibana
Research Center for Pathogenic Fungi and Microbial Toxicoses, Chiba University, 1-8-1, Inohana, Chuoku, Chiba 260-8673, Japan

David C. Coleman
Department of Oral Medicine and Pathology, Microbiology Research Unit, School of Dental Science, University of Dublin, Trinity College, Dublin 2, Republic of Ireland

Jim E. Cutler
Department of Microbiology, Montana State University, Bozeman, MT 59717-3520

Joachim F. Ernst
Institut fur Mikrobiologie, Heinrich-Heine Universitat, Universitatsstr. 1/26.12, D-40225 Dusseldorf, Germany

Paul L. Fidel, Jr.
Department of Microbiology, Immunology, and Parasitology, Louisiana State University Medical Center, New Orleans, LA 70112

Scott G. Filler
Harbor-UCLA Medical Center, 1000 W. Carson Street, RB-2, Torrance, CA 90509

Neil A. R. Gow
Department of Molecular and Cell Biology, Institute of Medical Sciences, University of Aberdeen, Foresterhill, Aberdeen AB25 2ZD, United Kingdom

Bruce L. Granger
Department of Microbiology, Montana State University, Bozeman, MT 59717-3520

Yongmoon Han
Department of Microbiology, Montana State University, Bozeman, MT 59717-3520

Bernhard Hube
NG4, Robert Koch-Institut, Nordufer 20, D-13353 Berlin, Germany

Michael Kruppa
Department of Microbiology and Immunology, Georgetown University School of Medicine, 3900 Reservoir Road NW, Washington, DC 20007

Bart Jan Kullberg
Department of Medicine, Nijmegen University Medical Center St Radboud, Geert Grooteplein 8, Mailstop 541, 6525 GA Nijmegen, The Netherlands

Dongmei Li
Department of Microbiology and Immunology, Georgetown University School of Medicine, 3900 Reservoir Road NW, Washington, DC 20007

P. T. Magee
Department of Genetics, Cell Biology, and Genetics, University of Minnesota, St. Paul, MN 55105

Herbert L. Mathews
Department of Microbiology and Immunology, Stritch School of Medicine, Loyola University of Chicago, 2160 South First Avenue, Maywood, IL 60153-3304

Thomas G. Mitchell
Department of Microbiology, Duke University Medical Center, Durham, NC 27710

María D. Moragues
Departamento de Enfermería I, Universidad del País Vasco, Barrio Sarriena s/n, 48940 Leioa, Vizcaya, Spain

Gary P. Moran
Department of Oral Medicine and Pathology, Microbiology Research Unit, School of Dental Science, University of Dublin, Trinity College, Dublin 2, Republic of Ireland

Julian Naglik
Division of Oral Medicine, Pathology, Microbiology, and Immunology, Floor 28, Guy's Tower, Kings College London (Guy's Campus), London Bridge, London SE1 9RT, United Kingdom

Justin M. O'Sullivan
Department of Biosciences, University of Kent, Canterbury, Kent CT2 7NJ, United Kingdom

José Pontón
Departamento de Inmunologia, Microbiologia, y Parasitologia, Facultad de Medicina y Odontologia, Universidad del País Vasco, Barrio Sarriena s/n, 48940 Leioa, Vizcaya, Spain

Guillermo Quindós
Departamento de Inmunologia, Microbiologia, y Parasitologia, Facultad de Medicina y Odontologia, Universidad del País Vasco, Barrio Sarriena s/n, 48940 Leioa, Vizcaya, Spain

Malcolm D. Richardson
Mycology Unit, Department of Bacteriology and Immunology, University of Helsinki, Haartman Institute, P.O. Box 21, Haartmaninkatu 3, 00014 Helsinki, Finland

Luigina Romani
Microbiology Section, Department of Experimental Medicine and Biochemical Sciences, University of Perugia, Via del Giochetto, 06122 Perugia, Italy

Marcus Ruhnke
Department of Medicine, Division of Hematology/Oncology, Charite Campus Mitte der Humboldt-Universitat Berlin, Schumannstr. 20/21, D-10117 Berlin, Germany

Dominique Sanglard
Institute of Microbiology, University Hospital of Lausanne (CHUV), 1011 Lausanne, Switzerland

Manuel A. S. Santos
Department of Biosciences, University of Kent, Canterbury, Kent CT2 7NJ, United Kingdom

Stewart Scherer
3938 Paseo Grande, Moraga, CA 94556

Praveen Singh
Department of Microbiology and Immunology, Georgetown University School of Medicine, 3900 Reservoir Road NW, Washington, DC 20007

Jack D. Sobel
Department of Microbiology, Immunology, and Parasitology, Louisiana State University Medical Center, New Orleans, LA 70112

Peter G. Sohnle
Division of Infectious Diseases, Department of Medicine, Medical College of Wisconsin, Milwaukee, WI 53226, and Infectious Diseases Section/CC-111N, Consultant Care Division, VA Medical Center, Milwaukee, WI 53295

David R. Soll
Department of Biological Sciences, University of Iowa, Iowa City, IA 52242

Derek J. Sullivan
Department of Oral Medicine and Pathology, Microbiology Research Unit, School of Dental Science, University of Dublin, Trinity College, Dublin 2, Republic of Ireland

Shigeo Suzuki
Sendai Research Institute for Mycology, 1-14-34, Toshogu, Aoba-ku, Sendai 981-0908, Miyagi, Japan

Mick F. Tuite
Department of Biosciences, University of Kent, Canterbury, Kent CT2 7NJ, United Kingdom

David K. Wagner
Division of Infectious Diseases, Department of Medicine, Medical College of Wisconsin, Milwaukee, WI 53226, and Infectious Diseases Section/CC-111N, Consultant Care Division, VA Medical Center, Milwaukee, WI 53295

Linda Witek-Janusek
Department of Maternal Child Health Nursing, Niehoff School of Nursing, Loyola University of Chicago, 2160 South First Avenue, Maywood, IL 60153-3304

Jianping Xu
Department of Biology, McMaster University, Hamilton, Ontario L8S 4K1 Canada

PREFACE

The most recent text on *Candida* and candidiasis, which was published in 1988, still stands as a major reference on these organisms. At about the time of its publication, research emphasis with these pathogens was beginning to shift dramatically to molecular approaches in studies of virulence, strain typing and diagnosis, drug discovery and resistance to drugs, and immunity. Much of this research has been supported by the near completion of the genome sequence of *Candida albicans*. Moreover, the more classical approaches of biochemical analysis, immunity, and taxonomy have continued to yield important discoveries. The past 15 years have also witnessed a change in the variety of *Candida* species that are isolated from patients. Thus, while *C. albicans* remains the major focus of study, we now know more about the non-*albicans* species of *Candida*, such as *C. glabrata, C. dubliniensis,* and *C. krusei,* and their importance in disease, especially as drug-resistant species.

For these reasons, the study of *Candida* and candidiasis has expanded tremendously over the past 10 to 15 years. There was a need for a text that would unify concepts and observations, as well as illustrate possible solutions to the problems of drug discovery and diagnosis that exist with these organisms.

The text is divided into seven sections, including history and general properties of *Candida*, virulence properties, cell biology, immunity, genomics, diseases and therapy, and, lastly, laboratory work up of candidiasis. Section editors have contributed chapters and have selected others to write specific chapters. This organizational aspect was necessitated by the inability of anyone (at least as far as I can determine) to be thoroughly familiar with all aspects of *Candida* and candidiasis and to be able to manage the time to write a comprehensive text.

Candida and Candidiasis is meant to be a reference text for all researchers in this area of study or those contemplating such a move. It should also find a strong application in graduate courses in medical mycology, mycology, general microbiology, or infectious diseases and should be extremely useful to technicians, diagnosticians, and scientists in industry.

As much as this volume is a statement about ongoing research, its purpose is also to acknowledge the interesting biology and importance of these organisms.

Richard A. Calderone
July 2001

ACKNOWLEDGMENTS

I am very fortunate to have worked with Paul Fidel, David Coleman, Pete Magee, Neil Gow, and Scott Filler as section editors in the development of this text. I would like to especially acknowledge Paul and David for their encouragement and contributions beyond their assignments. I deeply appreciate the outstanding efforts of all chapter authors and their recognition that this text is an important contribution to the medical mycology and microbiology communities.

Special thanks are also extended to ASM Press (Greg Payne and Pamela Lacey), David Coleman for the cover page photograph, and John P. Utz for his help with the chapter on history and whose seminar at a medical mycology conference in 1973 inspired my entry into this area of study. Much of the research presented has been financially supported by numerous public and private organizations. This support is acknowledged in several of the chapters.

This volume is dedicated to all past and current individuals who have studied *Candida* and candidiasis.

I. HISTORY AND GENERAL PROPERTIES OF *CANDIDA*

Candida and Candidiasis
Edited by Richard A. Calderone

Chapter 1

Introduction and Historical Perspectives

Richard A. Calderone

A historical treatise on the biology of *Candida albicans* and its activities as a human pathogen is presented in this chapter. Other historical accounts by Winner (93), Odds (60), and Rippon (67) are also recommended. The historical section is presented as broad observations that have provided an impetus for more study. In the second part of the chapter, the importance of candidiasis as a cause of morbidity and mortality is described.

HISTORY OF *CANDIDA* AND CANDIDIASIS

Interestingly, approximately 200 years were required before the etiological agent of thrush, the first type of candidiasis that was described, was identified correctly. The first reference to "thrush" (probably derived from the Scandinavian word, "torsk") is from the writings of Pepys in 1665 (quoted in reference 93), although the original description of a case of thrush probably should be credited to Hippocrates, who predates Pepys. However, it was not until 1846, when Berg used a scientific approach to the study of thrush, that the presence and relationship of the fungus to the disease were documented (8). Even then, confusion still existed about the identity of the organism causing the disease, and the nomen conservandum (*C. albicans* [Robin] Berkhout 1923) was not officially approved until 1954.

Why was thrush the type of candidiasis that was studied initially, and why did it take so long to arrive at conclusions about the etiology of the disease? The answers are somewhat obvious. First, oral thrush was easily recognized as an abnormality and even today remains as one of the most easily diagnosed forms of candidiasis. Second, the early descriptions of the disease (usually thrush) predate the concept of a "contagion." Pepys wrote (in his early descriptions of thrush) that "he [a patient] hath a fever, a thrush and a hiccup." This could be interpreted as implying that the malady was of host origin only, an idea that was perpetuated even as recently as the early 1900s when Castellani quoted previous accounts of thrush as "morbid secretions of the oral mucosa" (12). So one of the continuing arguments in defining the etiology of the disease was whether the infection was due exclusively to abnormalities of the host or whether it was caused by a contagion, or both. There were several key individuals who developed the concept that thrush was caused by a contagion and that the disease might not only occur in the oral cavity but could evolve into more serious complications. Foremost among these clinician/scientists was Rosen von Rosenstein (69), who in 1771 indicated that the disease was of significant consequence and who probably should be credited with defining an invasive form of thrush, even though no etiology was described. He believed that the invasive form of the disease could exist in the lungs but did not describe blood-borne spread of an organism. Langenbeck in 1839 is credited with first recognizing a fungus in an oral aphtha (ulcer) of a patient with typhoid fever; his conclusion, however, was that the aphtha was caused by the typhoid bacterium rather than the fungus (47). J. H. Bennett in 1844 criticized Langenbeck's conclusion since Bennett had observed the presence of a cryptogamic plant that he found growing in the sputum and the lungs of the same patient with a pneumothorax (7). He described morphologically the same organism as that indicated by Langenbeck and concluded that the disease was "indicative of great depression of the vital powers and impairment of the nutritive functions of the economy [host?]." Berg in 1846 (8) presented observations that thrush was caused by a fungus; among his conclusions were that healthy children were less prone to thrush, epidemics

Richard A. Calderone • Department of Microbiology and Immunology, Georgetown University School of Medicine, 3900 Reservoir Rd. NW, Washington, DC 20007.

could occur which were associated with communal feeding bottles, and, most important, "descriptions of the disease unsupported by demonstration of the fungus could not substantiate the diagnosis." He was able to reproduce the disease in healthy children (try getting that protocol through the discriminating eye of an institutional review board). His scientific approach to the study of thrush is probably one of the most important of the early contributions. Following Berg's studies, it became clear to others that the disease had several different manifestations in addition to the oral infection. The idea that the organism could cause several forms of the same disease gradually gained support. In 1792, J. P. Frank (quoted in reference 93) and, then in 1849, Wilkinson observed that aphthae also occurred in the sexual organs and that a dimorphic fungus was the probable cause (91). Prior to this time, vaginitis and vaginal discharge were thought to be a consequence of marriage and childbirth. Mayer in 1862 described six cases of vaginal thrush and was able to reproduce the infection experimentally in rabbits (57). Other forms of candidiasis were described, including cutaneous and, less commonly, systemic disease. It is not surprising that systemic disease caused by this fungus was rarely described since diagnosis by blood culture of invasive disease even today is problematic. Imagine the difficulty the early investigators faced without today's modern detection methods. Also, it is very likely that systemic disease was not as common as it is today.

The other major problem associated with defining thrush as caused by a contagion was the confusion in the literature about the identification of the pathogen. As mentioned above, Langenbeck first observed a fungus associated with thrush, but the identity of that organism was incorrect, and its importance to the disease was minimized. In 1842, Gruby studied the organism isolated by Langenbeck but came to the conclusion that it was a species of *Sporotrichum* (34). The same organism was also studied in great detail by Robin in 1847, who reclassified it as *Oidium albicans* (68). This was the first use of the name *albicans* (which means "to whiten") with the fungus of thrush. It should be stated that the incorrect identification of the causative organism of thrush was perpetuated by the insistence of several (at the time) key taxonomists that the thrush fungus should be a species of *Monilia,* a fungus that is mostly noted for its growth in plant materials. Perplexingly, the literature at the time stated that the organism described by Berg and others was clearly morphologically different from *Monilia.* Thus, the generic name *Monilia* came to be diverted from those organisms it had formerly been used to describe and applied incorrectly to the fungus of thrush (93). The controversy was perpetuated until Berkhout among others in 1923 proposed that the organism of thrush lesions was clearly not a species of *Monilia* and, as a consequence, she proposed that the favored generic name should be *Candida* (9). The name is derived from the Latin phrase *toga candida,* which was used to describe a special white robe worn by candidates for the Roman Senate. The derived name is in probable reference to the whitish colonies on agar or the oral lesions of aphthae or thrush. Other investigators attempted to classify the thrush agent by using biochemical and serological assays, even prior to the studies of Berkhout and Robin. Major contributors in this regard are Castellani (12), Bisserie, and Malvoz (quoted in reference 93). Benham (4) focused her research on the use of more rigid criteria in the identification of the fungus, concluding that, of all the yeastlike fungi, only *C. albicans* was pathogenic for laboratory animals. Although certainly not entirely correct in her concept of the limits she imposed on the species that cause candidiasis, nevertheless, her research is noted for its detail and emphasis on mycological accuracy. Eventually, the early investigators arrived at the correct conclusions, and given the lack of sophisticated methodologies, their observations have stood the test of time, especially in regard to the observations on the morphology of *C. albicans* as well as generalizations about the status of immune competence in patients and the severity of candidiasis.

THE RECENT ERA

I have arbitrarily chosen the 1950s as a beginning for the recent era of research for no other reason than 1954 marks the date that the Eighth Botanical Congress officially adopted the binomial *Candida albicans* as the nomen conservandum. During the 1950s to 1990s the early studies were expanded, especially in the areas of taxonomy, biochemistry, and microscopy. Molecular biological approaches to the study of *C. albicans* were first published during the 1980s; the organism was proven to have a diploid genome, and natural heterozygosity was described in isolates (89). This observation in part explained the difficulty in obtaining mutants of *C. albicans* in comparison to *Saccharomyces cerevisiae* for which mutants could be easily made by chemical or irradiation mutagenesis. Methods for transformation, gene isolation and deletion, strain typing, and chromosome analysis (karyotyping) were developed (26, 33, 41, 43, 44, 54, 71, 73). The sequencing of the *C. albicans* genome is nearly completed, and new evidence for mating in *C. albicans* has been obtained (39, 55). Of all the methodologies that have been used during the past 50 years, perhaps those of molecular biology have contributed most to the recent literature. During this same period, the number of new species of *Candida* described increased significantly and currently totals approximately 150. The importance of species other than *C. albicans* in disease is exemplified by the studies of Wingard (92) on *C. tropicalis*. The most recent addition to the list of pathogenic species of *Candida*, *C. dubliniensis*, has been shown to be very similar phenotypically to *C. albicans* and is an important pathogen in AIDS patients (74). *Torulopsis glabrata* has been reclassified as a species of *Candida*, and we have learned that *C. stellatoidea* actually is composed of two different strain types (I and II) and that type II *C. stellatoidea* is sucrose-negative *C. albicans* (see chapter 2) (45, 46). Doubt remains as to whether type I *C. stellatoidea* is sufficiently different to be classified as a separate species.

CELL BIOLOGY

The cell wall of *Candida* species became a major area of study during this same time frame. The impetus was based on pure biological interests as well as the desire to identify new targets that could be exploited for the identification of antifungal agents. As described in chapter 12, the cell wall of the organism contains key biomolecules that are not found in mammalian cells; hence, the specificity of the cell wall components for the fungus is compatible with investigations on the identification of potential targets. Cell wall studies accomplished during the 1950 to 1970 era (or thereabouts) focused on the determination of cell wall organization and the identification of individual components of the cell wall. Thus, chitin, glucan, and mannan as the primary constituents of the cell wall were characterized through the efforts of a number of individuals, including Gooday, Chattaway, Elorza, and Sentandreu (14, 22, 23, 32). Beyond the characterization of cell wall components, ultrastructural and biochemical observations by Cassone (11) and Poulain (64) revealed a layered arrangement of wall components, consisting of an inner wall composed of structural polysaccharides and an outer layer(s) containing primarily mannan, mannoproteins, or nonglycosylated proteins. The outer layer of the cell wall was revealed by lectin studies to be mannan (11); these observations along with parallel studies in *S. cerevisiae* by Ballou (2) led to the dissection and identification of reactive, mannan epitopes of *Candida* spp. Previously, Hasenclever and Mitchell had identified two serological types of *C. albicans* (A and B) and showed that other species may or may not share reactive epitopes (36). Also, a key observation was that serological differences between serotypes A and B resided in the mannan (75). Some of the major contributions to our understanding of serological reactivity of mannan came from investigations by Suzuki and Sunayama (epitope identity, antigenic activity and determinants, immunochemical characterization) (76, 77, 79, 80), Reiss (cross-reactivity, immune properties of specific components such as peptidoglucomannan (65, 66), Nishikawa (serotyping) (59), Tsuchiya (numerical taxonomy) (82), and Fukazawa (immunochemical basis of serologic specificity) (27–29). The outcome of these observations has been the characterization of the major antigens of *Candida* species. As stated above, protocols used in the study of the cell wall of *S. cerevisiae* were applied to similar studies with *C. albicans*, and many of the conclusions drawn from the former organism were equally applicable to *C. albicans*. Nevertheless, differences between these two organisms were found to be profound, and it became necessary to assume that not all things are equal between these two species, an idea clearly compatible with the virulence of *C. albicans* and the comparative avirulence of *S. cerevisiae*.

IMMUNE PROTECTION

While complex analyses of the *C. albicans* cell wall were made, parallel studies on the host response to the organism and the biological characterization of complex or partially purified antigen preparations were reported. The factors thought to be involved in protective immunity were defined both in animal models and in patient populations. The effects of certain types of immune cells on the organism were studied in vitro. Typifying the quality studies of this nature were observations from the laboratory of R. Lehrer who defined several mechanisms of phagocytosis as well as the components of the phagocytic cells (oxidative and nonoxidative) that were responsible for their candidicidal activity (49–52). His observations on neutrophils along with those made by Diamond (19) were critical to understanding the role that these cells play in protection. Equally important, a number of investigations, especially those made in the Cutler and Domer laboratories, established the components of the immune system that are responsible for protection in animal models (17, 20, 21, 30, 53). The role of cell-mediated and humoral immunity in limiting murine candidiasis was described, although the protective effect of antibody has only recently been elucidated. It turns out that there is both good and bad antibody, and the Cutler laboratory has been able to identify those antibodies that are protective (see chapter 17). The Cassone, Domer, Poulain, and Reiss laboratories were also partially responsible for the initial characterization of antigens of the organism that trigger cell-mediated and humoral immune mechanisms. The animal studies took many different forms, but usually protection was monitored following vaccination or naive animals were subjected to immune transfer with either serum (58) or immune cells from previously infected animals. Animals either were inbred, immune competent or were engineered to lack specific host responses such as a deficiency in complement or in T cells (the nude mouse). Vaccines were of different types, including whole cells (either heat-killed or attenuated), crude fractions of cells, and, more recently, purified antigens. The data from these studies indicated that innate, humoral, and cellular immunities were required for protection. Interestingly, many of the observations on immunity in animal models duplicated those observed in humans. Among the most important of the human studies were those related to the host response in patients with chronic mucocutaneous candidiasis. Kirkpatrick et al. demonstrated that inherited T-cell (T-lymphocytes) deficiencies in patients resulted in chronic mucocutaneous candidiasis (42). Even today, the association of AIDS patients with mucosal candidiasis fits the model that T-cell deficiencies trigger mucosal disease. We now know that immunity to *Candida* spp. is even more complex (see chapters 13 to 17), and innate and humoral antibodies contribute to protection against *C. albicans,* an idea first noted by the early scientists when they observed that patients with poor health were often more susceptible to candidiasis. Protection may even be site-specific, i.e., the factors affecting protection in the vaginal canal may be different or only partially similar to the protective mechanisms that exist systemically (25). Nevertheless, the early studies were instrumental in detailing some of the components of protective immunity. The search also began for antigens that could be used in a diagnostic assay for detecting antibody in patients or be used to make antibody that might be useful in antigen detection (see chapter 27). Thus, enolase and several heat shock proteins were evaluated for diagnostic testing by the studies of Matthews and Burnie (56). Although progress has been made, an assay for diagnosing invasive disease by immunological or other means remains elusive.

VIRULENCE

The characterization of virulence factors during this period resulted in many interesting observations that reveal the sophistication of this organism as a pathogen (see chapters 6 to 10). Adherence of the organism to host cells was initially described (48). Since then, genes encoding adherence proteins have been isolated and their role in virulence has been studied (13, 38, 78). It has long been recognized that conversion of yeast forms into a filamentous growth (hypha), a process referred to as morphogenesis, might be important to the invasiveness of *C. albicans* and other *Candida* species. As stated above, the pioneer studies that led to the delineation of the thrush pathogen included descriptions of the multiple growth forms of the organism isolated from patients. Clearly, one of the early arguments (which, in fact, still persists) was the debate as to whether one of the growth forms (yeast or hypha) of the organism contributes more to virulence, an argument that clearly is irrelevant since growth in tissues requires replicative rounds of both yeast and hyphae as well as a third type of growth, the pseudohyphae. Notwithstanding, much has been learned about morphogenesis in *C. albicans*. Differences in cell wall composition and cell wall antigens between the two growth forms have been noted (1, 10, 13, 22, 63, 78). Further, the isolation of an avirulent, spontaneous, agerminative strain of *C. albicans* pointed toward the essential role of morphogenesis in the pathogenicity of the organism. Attempts were made to identify hypha-specific proteins by using a variety of approaches including various forms of electrophoresis and Western blot analyses. Contributions in this regard came from many laboratories, including those of Brown, Chaffin, Fonzi, Jones, Sentandreu, Sypherd, and Sundstrom (1, 10, 22, 63, 78; summarized in reference 13). However, the identification of regulatory and signal genes involved in morphogenesis had to wait until the advent of molecular approaches that could be used to identify gene function. That, in fact, has been accomplished. We know now that there are several signal transduction pathways that are required (at least partially) for morphogenesis. Interestingly, the expression of yeast or hypha-specific genes recently has been shown to be regulated by several transcription factors. Clearly, these studies have implications for understanding the biology of the organism but may also have translational implications. As it turns out, the construction of specific gene-deleted strains (26) and the application of molecular Koch's postulates have resulted in the definition of other virulence factors, including secreted enzymes (aspartyl proteinases and phospholipase B) and adhesin proteins that are important in the recognition of host cells. The laboratories of Arisawa, Berman, Brown, Calderone, Cassone, Chaffin, Cutler, DeBernardis, Edwards, Ernst, Filler, Fink, Fonzi, Ghannoum, Gow, Hostetter, Hoyer, Hube, Johnson, Kwon-Chung, Leberer, Sanglard, Soll, Sundstrom, Thomas, and Whiteway have each made important contributions to the understanding of virulence in this organism as defined by molecular Koch's postulates (see subsequent chapters). Similar studies have also been published with *C. glabrata*. A rediscovery of phenotypic switching in *C. albicans* (and other *Candida* species) has provided thought about the plasticity of these organisms and how this may help their survival in vivo (72).

ANTI-*CANDIDA* DRUGS

The identification of antifungal drugs began in the late 1940s and continues today. In this regard, the isolation and identification of nystatin (the first antifungal agent) by Hazen and Brown in 1950 (37) were of major significance not only in treating this disease but also serving as an impetus to isolate compounds of a similar nature (polyenes). Thus, the discovery of nystatin was followed by the isolation of other polyene antifungal agents, most notably amphotericin B by Vandeputte (85) and Gold (31). This compound still remains the "gold standard" to which all other antifungal agents are compared. In the 1970s, 5-fluorocytosine was suggested as a potential antifungal drug from the studies of Titsworth and Grunberg, Utz, Warner et al., and Bennett (5, 6, 81, 83, 84, 89). It should be noted that although relatively ineffective by itself against *C. albicans,* the drug has been found useful in combination therapy with amphotericin B, especially in certain clinical settings. Probably the most important event that signaled the arrival of drug discovery against the mycoses was the importance placed on fungal diseases by the pharmaceutical industry. Thus, Janssen developed one of the first azoles (miconazole), which was followed over the years by the discovery of the triazoles such as fluconazole (Pfizer) and itraconazole (Janssen Pharmaceuticals, Inc.) that, although fungistatic, have, importantly, less toxicity than amphotericin B.

A CHRONOLOGICAL "WHO'S WHO"

Much of what is described above is indicated in Table 1. The major contributors during the past several hundred years and their observations on candidiasis and *Candida* species are presented in chronological order. The information in Table 1 is intended to include pivotal observations that have been the impetus for further study.

Today's scientists make similar observations as those made by the early *Candida* scientists but do so at a level of sophistication that, in fact, adds more complexity. For example, one of the early conclusions was that oral disease (thrush) must be caused by a variety of different organisms, although no attempt was made early on to specifically identify the variety of species causing these diseases. Today, we use molecular typing experiments to define different species and strains of *Candida* that cause disease. We speak of succession of organisms as occurs in recurrent disease, trace lineages to predict whether the organism is clonal or displays signs of recombination in nature (see chapter 5), and predict whether specific strains are drug resistant. Nevertheless, it is both interesting and informative to reflect on the early observations of candidiasis. Perhaps it puts into perspective where we have come from and strengthens our conclusion that important science is being done that will enable us, perhaps in the short-term future, to learn how to better control disease caused by these organisms. There has been a steady progression of knowledge about candidiasis since the first descriptions. We can properly conclude that *Candida* species are a highly evolved group of pathogens whose diversity constantly surprises us and tests our ability to arrive at conclusions. There is a sense of urgency for *Candida* biologists that, in part, is generated by the competition among laboratories and by the need to develop new approaches to the treatment of these diseases. The competition will speed the discovery of important translational observations on therapy and detection, not only with *C. albicans* but with the other species of *Candida* that are pathogens.

CURRENT INTERESTS IN *CANDIDA* SPECIES

The most recent edition of *Candida and Candidosis* by Odds (60) included an estimate of the number of publications on either the biology of these organisms or the diseases they cause. A reasonable estimate of approximately 750 publications was noted for 1985. More recent estimates that are based on literature searches through Index Medicus are presented in Fig. 1 as numbers of published papers from 1980 through 2000. The data are expressed as the number of publications during 5-year intervals and reflect subject headings on *Candida* and candidiasis, as well as papers with a specific focus, as, for example, antifungal agents, but which include only papers on drug testing, mode of action, resistance, and sensitivity testing of *Candida* species. It is clear that interest not only remains high but, in fact, may not have reached its peak in popularity. Thus, from 1995 to 2000, more than 6,900 papers were published, two times the number of papers published from 1980 to 1985.

It is very likely that these data reflect an interest in *Candida* species as pathogens (see below) that has

Table 1. *Candida* and candidiasis: a partial list of the "who's who" of contributors

Discovery	Contributor(s)	Year
Oral thrush is described	Hippocrates	4th century BC
Description of thrush	Pepys	1665
Prognosis and state of health	Rosen von Rosenstein	1771
Describes aphthae in genitals	Frank, Wilkinson	1790s
First isolation from oral thrush	Langenbeck	1839
Dimorphic fungus isolated	J. H. Bennett	1844
Disease severity and health status	Berg	1846
Experimental reproduction of disease	Berg	
Grows dimorphic fungus from patient	Berg	
Describes esophageal invasion	Virchow	1821
Describes *Oidium albicans*	Robin	1847
Describes first systemic candidiasis	Zenker	1861
Experimental vaginitis model	Mayes	1862
Classifies thrush fungus as *Monilia*	Hansen	1888
Suggests *Candida* as generic name	Berkhout	1923
Defines characteristics of *Candida*	Benham	1931
Bloodstream spread of organism	Joachim, Polayes	1940
Discovery of nystatin	Hazen, Brown	1950
C. albicans—nomen conservandum		1954
Serotyping studies	Hasenclever, Mitchell	1961
Immunochemical studies	Suzuki, Suzuki, Sakaguchi	1967
Cell wall composition	Chattaway	1968
Neutrophil studies	Lehrer	1969
Antigenic determinants	Sunayama, Suzuki	1970
CMI in patients	Kirkpatrick, Rich, Bennett	1971
Cell wall organization	Cassone, Poulain	1973, 1978
Antigen identification	Reiss	1974
Serologic classification	Tsuchiya, Shinoda	1974
Mannan structure of yeast	Ballou	1976
Experimental immunity	Domer	1978
Serotype A determinant	Suzuki, Fukazawa	1982
Diploidy in isolates	Whelan, Magee	1980
	Whelan, Partridge, Magee	1981
Secreted proteinases	Ruchel	1981
Cell wall of growth forms	Elorza, Sentandreu, Jones	1983
Complementation, disruption	Gorman	1985
Transformation system	Kurtz, Kirsh	1986, 1987
One-step gene disruption	Kelly, Kurtz, Kirsch	1987
Chromosome karyotyping	Snell, Wilkins	1986
	B. Magee, P. Magee	1987
DNA typing method	Scherer, Stevens	1987
Drug resistance	Prasad, Sanglard, White	1980s–1990s
Candida and Candidosis text	Odds	1988
Urablaster gene disruption	Fonzi	1993
Mating in *C. albicans*	Hull, Johnson	2000
	B. Magee, P. Magee	2000

been fueled in part by recent advances in molecular techniques. Thus, an outburst of studies on virulence factors, the identification of new targets, immunoprotection, and the development of reagents that are potentially useful in the diagnostic laboratory has been the outgrowth of the development of molecular tools. Other major areas of research include studies on drug resistance (see subsequent chapters) and definitions of the mechanisms of drug resistance (90). In particular, *C. albicans* has been the object of these studies, although, more recently, the emergence of drug-resistant non-*C. albicans* species as pathogens has extended our interests. It is also apparent that the disease potential of these organisms has resulted in the need to develop concepts of new treatments, be they chemotherapeutic or immune.

HOW MUCH CANDIDIASIS IS THERE?

Candidiasis remains an important clinical problem (see chapter 2), primarily in the immunocompro-

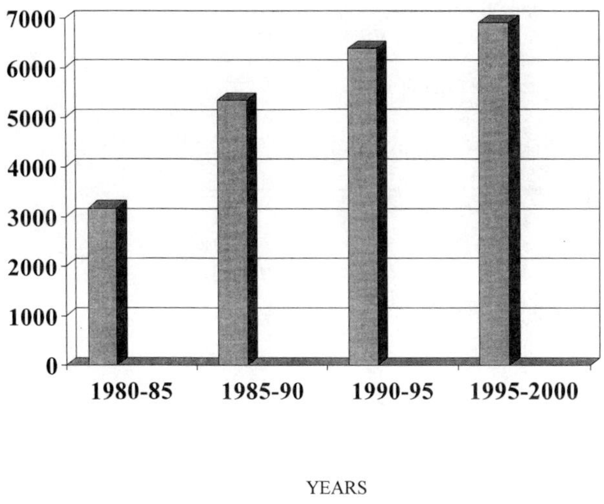

Figure 1. The total number of publications on *Candida* species and candidiasis from 1980 to 2000. The numbers of publications are represented for 5-year intervals.

mised patient population. Not unexpectedly, whereas initially our focus was on *C. albicans* as the most important pathogen, now other species have gained importance clinically, as, for example, *C. glabrata, C. krusei,* and *C. dubliniensis.* In part, this has occurred because of scientific advances. The use of fluconazole, a drug that gained considerable importance as an alternative to amphotericin B, has resulted in the emergence of some of these organisms as pathogens since they either are inherently resistant to fluconazole or develop resistance (summarized in reference 90).

How common is candidiasis, especially in comparison with other infectious diseases, and in what setting does it occur? Are morbidity and mortality data available and are these numbers comparable to those of other types of infectious diseases? First, candidiasis invariably occurs in the setting of the immunocompromised patient, but other predisposing factors can spark disease. Odds (60) listed four types of predisposing factors: natural, dietary, mechanical, and iatrogenic factors. Natural factors include microbial infections (other than fungi), endocrine dysfunctions (diabetes), lymphocyte defects (or reduction in number), phagocyte abnormalities, pregnancy, infancy, and old age. Dietary factors, probably the least studied, include excess (carbohydrate-rich diets) or deficiencies (such as vitamin deficiencies). Mechanical factors include trauma, burns, wounds, occlusion, prosthetic devices (such as dentures), or thumb sucking. Iatrogenic factors include treatment with drugs that eliminate or reduce the bacterial competitors of the gut and other body sites (antibiotics) or alter host defenses (immunosuppressive drugs), surgery, and the insertion of mechanical devices (catheters). One of the more readily identifiable risk factors for the development of candidemias, for example, is the use of a central intravenous catheter, which has increased the risk of blood-borne candidiasis by over threefold (3). This list of predisposing factors has not changed significantly since the publication of the text by Odds (60). Most likely the greatest increase in candidiasis during the past 15 years has occurred as a result of the AIDS epidemic, proving that the clinical settings for candidiasis do change. The significance of this observation is that human pathogens need to be constantly studied so that we will be ready to combat their effects on human suffering. Witness the epidemic of tuberculosis that has accompanied AIDS and the reluctance to study *Mycobacterium tuberculosis* until tuberculosis became a serious disease once again. We should be constantly aware that infectious diseases constitute important problems in regard to human suffering. However, the opportunists, like *Candida* species, pose a special problem. They are so commonly represented in the host (normal flora) or in the environment that they can quickly become causes of morbidity and mortality. This observation is apparent from a recent study of candidiasis following solid organ transplantation in patients (16). Fungal infections occurred in approximately 20% of transplant recipients; of 28 patients who developed candidemias, 20 became blood test positive within the first 1 to 2 weeks posttransplant, underscoring the need to develop sensitive, diagnostic assays.

How common then is candidiasis? Some examples are given below that address this question. The incidence of fungal infections among postoperative infections has steadily increased from 1960 to 1999 (3, 35). Among the most common nosocomial infections reported from four Swiss hospitals were candidemias (35). In this study, *Candida* spp. ranked fourth in frequency (10%), behind the *Enterobacteriaceae* (28%), *Staphylococcus aureus* (13%), and *Pseudomonas* spp. (11%). These numbers corroborate data from a U.S. study that candidemias in the nosocomial patients rank fourth in frequency (3). The U.S. study included surveillance cultures from 115 large or small, teaching or non-teaching hospitals over a period from 1980 to 1990. *Candida* species accounted for 78.3% of all nosocomial fungal infections (30,477 reports). The proportion of *Candida* infections among all nosocomial infections increased from 6% in 1980 to 10.4% in 1990. Among the largest increases were urinary tract infections caused by *Candida* species, which rose from 5.0 in 1980 to 20.5 (rate per 10,000 discharges). Recent data from the National Nosocomial Infections Surveillance system have shown that candidiasis ranks among the most common of the nosocomial diseases (Table 2). Interestingly, *Candida* species rank from fourth (bloodstream infections) to

Table 2. Percent distribution of the top seven nosocomial pathogens isolated from selected major infection sites in coronary care units, 1992–1997

Pathogen	% cases caused by organism				
	Bloodstream	Pneumonia	UTI[a]	Cardiovascular	Eye, ear, nose, throat
Candida spp.	6	9.2	17	6.3	17
Coag. (-) staph.	37	2	3	46	18
S. aureus	24	21	3	20	17
Enterococcus	10	2	14	11	5
Escherichia coli	3	4	28	2	3
Enterobacter spp.	3	9	4	2	6
Pseudomonas aeruginosa	2	14	7	2	8

[a] Urinary tract infection.

second in prevalence (urinary tract infections and eye, ear, nose, and throat infections).

Other studies have addressed candidemias in specific patient populations. For example, a study of nosocomial pneumonias among adult bone marrow transplant recipients revealed that *Candida* species accounted for 5.4% of the pneumonias (61). It should be mentioned that this number reflects only those cases in which a pathogen could be isolated; blood-borne candidiasis is notoriously hard to detect. The most common pathogens among chronic hemodialysis patients were *Candida* spp. and enterococci (18). Blood-borne candidiasis occurred in about 20% of liver transplant recipients (16). Neonatal candidiasis (candidemia) occurs in about 1.2% of all neonatal intensive care unit patients (70), and complications such as meningitis are not an infrequent event. For the extremely low-birth-weight infant, mortality from systemic candidiasis was 37% (24). Postoperative nosocomial candidiasis is among the most common of the opportunistic infections and has been steadily increasing since the 1960s (86). However, data on the frequency of mortality caused by candidiasis are harder to obtain, except for a few surveys that may or may not be used to draw conclusions. For example, the Oklahoma Health Statistics for 1996 and 1997 indicated a mortality rate for candidiasis of 0.3 (deaths per 100,000 population). That rate is very similar to that of other infectious diseases, including tuberculosis and intestinal infectious diseases but lower than that of viral hepatitis (which is 1.3). Pittet and Wenzel (62) have reported on the incidence of all microbial bloodstream infections from 1980 to 1992. This survey included data from 260,834 patients at a 900-bed tertiary care hospital. Nosocomial bloodstream infections during this period increased from 6.7 to 18.4 per 1,000 hospital discharges. Both gram-positive cocci and yeasts (mostly *Candida* species) were at least partially responsible for the increased rates of infections (62). Importantly, the in-hospital population-attributable mortality among infected patients increased from 3.55 deaths in 1981 to 6.22 per 1,000 discharges. Attributable mortality as a consequence of nosocomial candidemia has been estimated to be 35% (88). Of further importance, case-patients who survived candidemia required an additional 30 days of hospital stay, thus indicating that candidemia is both deadly and costly (88).

Data on the frequency of candidiasis in AIDS patients have been published. A United Nations (UNAIDS, October 1998) technical update on the frequency of candidiasis from several countries including Brazil, Mexico, and Thailand indicated frequencies of 13% (Thailand), 11% (Mexico), and 30% (Brazil). A study of the changing spectrum of human immunodeficiency virus infections in Spain has demonstrated that candidal esophagitis (28.6%) ranked third behind tuberculosis (52.3%) and *Pneumocystis carinii* pneumonia (30%) (15). Interestingly, although the frequency of tuberculosis and *P. carinii* pneumonia decreased, candidal esophagitis showed a biphasic pattern from 1985 to 1997, and the authors believe that the second increase in candidiasis is due to the emergence of fluconazole resistance among strains (15). In Taiwan, the five leading human immunodeficiency virus-associated opportunistic infections included oropharyngeal candidiasis as the most common (40). These are a few examples that indicate the importance of candidiasis in today's patient population.

REFERENCES

1. **Bailey, D. A., P. J. F. Feldman, M. Bovey, N. A. R. Gow, and A. J. P. Brown.** 1996. The *Candida albicans HYR1* gene, which is activated in response to hyphal development, belongs to a

gene family of yeast cell wall proteins. *J. Bacteriol.* **178:** 5353–5360.
2. **Ballou, C.** 1976. Structure and biosynthesis of the mannan component of the yeast cell envelope. *Adv. Microbiol. Physiol.* **14:**93–158.
3. **Beck-Sague, C. M., and W. R. Jarvis.** 1993. Secular trends in the epidemiology of nosocomial fungal infections in the United States, 1980–1990. *J. Infect. Dis.* **167:**1247–1251.
4. **Benham, R. W.** 1931. Certain monilias parasitic on man: their identification by morphology and by agglutination. *J. Infect. Dis.* **49:**183–215.
5. **Bennett, J. E.** 1974. Chemotherapy of systemic mycoses. *N. Engl. J. Med.* **289:**30–32.
6. **Bennett, J. E.** 1975. Chemotherapy of systemic mycoses. *N. Engl. J. Med.* **290:**320–324.
7. **Bennett, J. H.** 1844. On the parasitic vegetable structure found growing in living animals. *Trans. R. Soc. Edin.* **15:**277–294.
8. **Berg, F. T.** 1846. *Om Torsk Hos Barn.* L. J. Hjerta, Stockholm, Sweden.
9. **Berkhout, C. M.** 1923. De schimmelgeschlachten *Monilia, Oidium, Oospora,* en *Torula.* Dissertation. University of Utrecht, The Netherlands.
10. **Birse, C. E., M. Y. Irwin, W. A. Fonzi, and P. S. Sypherd.** 1993. Cloning and characterization of *ECE1,* a gene expressed in association with cell elongation of the dimorphic pathogen, *Candida albicans. Infect. Immun.* **61:**3648–3655.
11. **Cassone, A., E. Mattia, and L. Boldrini.** 1978. Agglutination of blastospores of *Candida albicans* by concanavalin A and its relationship with the distribution of mannan polymers and the ultrastructure of the cell wall. *J. Gen. Microbiol.* **105:** 263–273.
12. **Castellani, A.** 1920. The etiology of thrush. *J. Trop. Med. Hyg.* **23:**17–22.
13. **Chaffin, W. L., J. L. Lopez-Ribot, M. Casanova, D. Gozalbo, and J. P. Martinez.** 1998. Cell wall and secreted proteins of *Candida albicans:* identification, function and expression. *Microbiol. Mol. Biol. Rev.* **62:**130–180.
14. **Chattaway, F. W., M. R. Holmes, A. J. E. Barlow.** 1968. Cell wall composition of the mycelial and blastospore forms of *Candida albicans. J. Gen. Microbiol.* **51:**367–376.
15. **Collazos, J., J. Mayo, and E. Martinez.** 1999. Changing spectrum of HIV infection and its associated conditions in Spain: the end of the beginning? *AIDS Patient Care Sex. Trans. Dis.* **13:**347–353.
16. **Collins, L. A., M. H. Samore, M. S. Roberts, R. Luzzati, R. L. Jenkins, W. D. Lewis, and A. W. Karchmer.** 1994. Risk factors for invasive fungal infections complicating orthotopic liver transplantation. *J. Infect. Dis.* **170:**644–652.
17. **Cutler, J. E.** 1976. Acute systemic candidiasis in normal and congenitally thymic deficient (nude) mice. *J. Reticuloendothel. Soc.* **19:**121–124.
18. **D'Agata, E. M., D. B. Mount, V. Thayer, and W. Schaffner.** 2000. Hospital-acquired infections among chronic hemodialysis patients. *Am. J. Kidney Dis.* **35:**1083–1088.
19. **Diamond, R. D., R. A. Clark, and C. C. Haudenschild.** 1980. Damage to *Candida albicans* pseudohyphae by the myeloperoxidase system and oxidative products of neutrophil metabolism in vitro. *J. Clin. Invest.* **66:**908.
20. **Domer, J. E.** 1988. Intragastric colonization of infant mice with *Candida albicans* induces systemic immunity demonstrable upon challenge as adults. *J. Infect. Dis.* **157:**950–958.
21. **Domer, J. E., and R. H. Hector.** 1987. Enhanced immune responses in mice treated with penicillin-tetracycline or trimethoprim-sulfamethoxazole when colonized intragastrically with *Candida albicans. Antimicrob. Agents Chemother.* **31:** 691–696.
22. **Elorza, M. V., H. Rico, D. Gozalbo, and R. Sentandreu.** 1985. Dimorphism in *Candida albicans:* contributions of mannoproteins to the architecture of yeast and mycelial cell walls. *J. Gen. Microbiol.* **131:**2209–2216.
23. **Elorza, M. V., H. Rico, D. Gozalbo, and R. Sentandreu.** 1983. Cell wall composition and protoplast regeneration in *Candida albicans. Ant. Van Leeuwenhoek J.* **49:**457–469.
24. **Friedman, S., S. E. Richardson, S. E. Jacobs, and K. O'Brien.** 2000. Systemic *Candida* infection in extremely low birth weight infants: short-term morbidity and long-term neurodevelopmental outcome. *Pediatr. Infect. Dis.* **19:**499–504.
25. **Fidel, P. L., Jr., M. E. Lynch, D. H. Conway, L. Tait, and J. D. Sobel.** 1995. Mice immunized by primary vaginal *C. albicans* infection develop acquired vaginal mucosal immunity. *Infect. Immun.* **63:**547–553.
26. **Fonzi, W. A., and M. Y. Irwin.** 1993. Isogenic strain construction and gene mapping in *Candida albicans. Genetics* **134:** 717–728.
27. **Fukazawa, Y., T. Shinoda, and T. Tsuchiya.** 1968. Response and specificity of antibodies for *C. albicans. J. Bacteriol.* **95:** 754–763.
28. **Fukazawa, Y., N. P. Elinov, T. Shinoda, and T. Tsuchiya.** 1968. Immunological specificity of soluble polysaccharides of *Candida albicans. Jpn. J. Microbiol.* **12:**283–292.
29. **Fukazawa, Y., A. Nishikawa, M. Suzuki, and T. Shinoda.** 1980. Immunochemical basis of the serologic specificity of the yeast: immunochemical determinants of several antigenic factors of yeast. *Zentralbl. Bakteriol.* 8(Suppl.):127–135.
30. **Giger, D. K., J. E. Domer, S. A. Moser, and J. T. McQuitty, Jr.** 1978. Experimental murine candidiasis: pathological and immune responses in T-lymphocyte depleted mice. *Infect. Immun.* **21:**729–737.
31. **Gold, W., H. A. Stout, J. F. Pagano, and R. Donovick.** 1956. Amphotericins A and B, antifungal antibiotics produced by a streptomycete. I. In vitro studies. *Antibiot. Ann. 1955* **56:** 579–586.
32. **Gooday, G. W., and N. A. R. Gow.** 1983. A model of the hyphal septum of *Candida albicans. Exp. Mycol.* **7:**370–373.
33. **Gorman, J. A., W. Chan, and J. Gorman.** 1991. Repeated use of *GAL1* for gene disruption in *Candida albicans. Genetics* **129:**19–24.
34. **Gruby, M.** 1842. Recherches anatomiques sur ue plant cryptogame qui constitute le vrai muguet des enfants. *C. R. Acad. Sci.* (Paris) **14:**634–636.
35. **Harbarth, S., C. Rued, P. Francioli, A. Widmer, and D. Pittet.** 1999. Nosocomial infections in Swiss university hospitals: a multi-centre survey and review of the published experience. *Schweiz Med. Wochenschr.* **23:**1521–1528.
36. **Hasenclever, H. F., and W. O. Mitchell.** 1961. Antigenic studies of *Candida.* I. Observation of two antigenic groups in *Candida albicans. J. Bacteriol.* **82:**570–573.
37. **Hazen, E. L., and R. Brown.** 1950. Two antifungal agents produced by a soil actinomycete. *Science* **112:**423.
38. **Hoyer, L. L.** 1998. *Candida albicans ALS3* and insights into the nature of the *ALS* gene family. *Curr. Genet.* **33:**451–459.
39. **Hull, C. M., R. M. Raisner, and A. D. Johnson.** 2000. Evidence for mating of the "asexual" yeast *Candida albicans* in a mammalian host. *Science* **289:**307–310.
40. **Hung, C. C., M. Y. Chen, S. M. Hsich, W. H. Sheng, and S. C. Chang.** 2000. Clinical spectrum, morbidity, and mortality of acquired immunodeficiency syndrome in Taiwan: a 5-year prospective study. *J. Acquir. Immune Defic. Syndr.* **24:** 378–385.
41. **Kelly, R., S. M. Miller, and M. B. Kurtz.** 1988. One-step gene disruption by co-transformation to isolate double auxotrophs in *Candida albicans. Mol. Gen. Genet.* **214:**24–31.

42. **Kirkpatrick, C. H., R. R. Rich, and J. E. Bennett.** 1971. Chronic mucocutaneous candidiasis: model building in cellular immunity. *Ann. Intern. Med.* **74:**955–978.

43. **Kurtz, M. B., M. W. Cortelyou, S. M. Miller, M. Lai, and D. R. Kirsch.** 1987. Development of autonomously replicating plasmids for *Candida albicans*. *Mol. Cell. Biol.* **7:**209–217.

44. **Kurtz, M. B., M. W. Cortelyou, and D. R. Kirsch.** 1986. Integrative transformation of *Candida albicans,* using a cloned *Candida ADE2* gene. *Mol. Cell. Biol.* **6:**142–149.

45. **Kwon-Chung, K. J., W. S. Riggsby, R. A. Uphoff, J. B. Hicks, W. L. Whelan, E. Reiss, B. B. Magee, and B. L. Wickes.** 1989. Genetic differences between type I and type II *Candida stellatoidea. Infect. Immun.* **57:**527–532.

46. **Kwon-Chung, K. J., B. L. Wickes, and W. G. Merz.** 1988. Association of electrophoretic karyotype of *Candida stellatoidea* with virulence in mice. *Infect. Immun.* **56:**1814–1819.

47. **Langenbeck, B.** 1839. Auffinggung von Pilzen aus der Schleimhaut der Speiserohne einer Typhus-Leiche. *Neue Not. Geb. Natur-u-Helik (Froriep)* **12:**145–147.

48. **Lee, J. C., and R. D. King.** 1983. Characterization of *Candida albicans* adherence to human vaginal epithelial cells in vitro. *Infect. Immun.* **41:**1024–1030.

49. **Lehrer, R. I., D. Szklarek, T. Ganz, and M. Selsted.** 1986. Synergistic activity of rabbit granulocyte peptides to *Candida albicans. Infect. Immun.* **52:**902–904.

50. **Lehrer, R. I., D. Szklarek, T. Ganz, and M. Selsted.** 1985. Correlation of binding of rabbit granulocyte peptides to *Candida albicans* with candidacidal activity. *Infect. Immun.* **49:** 207–211.

51. **Lehrer, R. I., and M. J. Cline.** 1969. Interaction of *Candida albicans* with human leukocytes and serum. *J. Bacteriol.* **98:** 966–1004.

52. **Lehrer, R. I., and M. J. Cline.** 1969. Leukocyte myeloperoxidase deficiency and disseminated candidiasis: the role of myeloperoxidase in resistance to *Candida* infection. *J. Clin. Invest.* **48:**1478–1488.

53. **Lyon, F., R. F. Hector, and J. E. Domer.** 1986. Innate and acquired immune responses against *Candida albicans* in congenic B10.D2 mice with deficiency of the C5 complement component. *J. Med. Vet. Mycol.* **24:**359–367.

54. **Magee, B. B., Y. Koltin, J. A. Gorman, and P. T. Magee.** 1988. Assignment of cloned genes to the seven electrophoretically separated *Candida albicans* chromosomes. *Mol. Cell. Biol.* **8:** 4721–4726.

55. **Magee, B. B., and P. T. Magee.** 2000. Induction of mating in *Candida albicans* by construction of *MTLa* and *MTLα* strains. *Science* **289:**310–313.

56. **Matthews, R. C., J. P. Burnie, and S. Tabaqchali.** 1984. Isolation of immunodominant antigens from sera of patients with systemic candidiasis and characterization of serological response to *Candida albicans. J. Clin. Microbiol.* **25:**230–237.

57. **Mayer, L.** 1862. Die Pflanzlichen Parasiten der weiblichen Sexualorgane in ihrer praktischen Bedeutung. *Mschr. Geburtsch. Frauenkrank* **20:**2–16.

58. **Mourad, S., and L. Friedman.** 1968. Passive immunization of mice against *Candida albicans. Sabouraudia* **6:**103.

59. **Nishikawa, T., S. Harada, H. Hatano, Y. Fukazawa, and T. Tsuchiya.** 1970. Biological and serological properties of *Candida* isolated from cutaneous candidiasis. *Jpn. J. Med. Mycol.* **11:**120–124.

60. **Odds, F. C.** 1988. History, p. 1–6. *In Candida and Candidosis.* Bailliere Tindall, London, United Kingdom.

61. **Pannuti, C., R. Gingrich, M. Pfaller, and R. Wenzel.** 1991. Nosocomial pneumonias in adult patients undergoing bone marrow transplantation—a 9-year study. *J. Clin. Oncol.* **9:** 77–83.

62. **Pittet, D., and R. P. Wenzel.** 1995. Nosocomial bloodstream infections. Secular trends in rates, mortality, and contribution to total hospital deaths. *Arch. Intern. Med.* **155:**1177–1184.

63. **Ponton, J., and J. M. Jones.** 1986. Identification of two germ-tube specific cell wall antigens of *Candida albicans. Infect. Immun.* **54:**864–868.

64. **Poulain, D., G. Tronchin, J. F. Dubremetz, and J. Biguet.** 1978. Ultrastructure of the cell wall of *Candida albicans* blastospores: study of its constitutive layers by use of a cytochemical technique revealing polysaccharides. *Ann. Inst. Pasteur Microbiol.* **129:**141–153.

65. **Reiss, E.** 1986. *Candida albicans,* p. 191–250. *In* E. Reiss (ed.), *Molecular Immunology of Mycotic and Actinomycotic Infections.* Elsevier, New York, N.Y.

66. **Reiss, E., S. H. Stone, and H. F. Hasenclever.** 1974. Serological and cellular immune activity of peptidoglucomannan fractions of *Candida albicans* cell walls. *Infect. Immun.* **9:**881–890.

67. **Rippon, J. W.** 1974. Candidosis, p. 175–204. *In* J. W. Rippon (ed.), *Medical Mycology: The Pathogenic Fungi and the Pathogenic Actinomycetes.* W.B. Saunders Co., Philadelphia, Pa.

68. **Robin, C. P.** 1853. Histoire naturelle des vegetaux. Parasites qui croissent sur l'homme et sur les animaux vivants. Balliere, Paris, France.

69. **Rosen von Rosenstein, N.** 1771. *Underrattelse om Barms Sjukdomar och Deras Botemedal.* Wenneberg and Nordstrom, Stockholm, Sweden.

70. **Saiman, L., E. Ludington, M. Pfaller, S. Rangel-Frausto, R. T. Wilbin, J. Dawson, H. Blumberg, J. E. Patterson, M. Rinaldi, J. E. Edwards, R. P. Wenzel, and W. Jarvis.** 2000. Risk factors for candidemia in neonatal intensive care unit patients. The National Epidemiology of Mycosis Survey study group. *Pediatr. Infect. Dis.* **19:**319–324.

71. **Scherer, S., and D. A. Stevens.** 1987. Application of DNA typing methods to epidemiology and taxonomy of *Candida* species. *J. Clin. Microbiol.* **25:**675–679.

72. **Slutsky, B., J. Buffo, and D. R. Soll.** 1985. High frequency switching of colony morphology in *Candida albicans. Science* **23:**666–669.

73. **Snell, R. G., I. F. Hermans, R. J. Wilkins, and B. E. Conner.** 1987. Separation of chromosomal DNA molecules from *Candida albicans* by pulsed field gel electrophoresis. *Nucleic Acids Res.* **14:**4401–4406.

74. **Sullivan, D. J., T. J. Westerneng, K. A. Haynes, S. E. Bennett, and D. C. Coleman.** 1995. *Candida dubliniensis* sp. nov.: phenotypic and molecular characterization of a novel species associated with oral candidosis in HIV-infected individuals. *Microbiology* **141:**1507–1521.

75. **Summers, D. F., A. P. Grollman, and H. F. Hasenclever.** 1964. Polysaccharide antigens of the *Candida* cell wall. *J. Immunol.* **92:**491–499.

76. **Sunayama, H.** 1970. Studies on the antigenic activities of yeasts. IV. Analysis of the antigenic determinant groups of the mannan of *Candida albicans* serotype A. *Jpn. J. Microbiol.* **14:** 27–39.

77. **Sunayama, H., and S. Suzuki.** 1970. Studies on the antigenic activities of yeasts. VI. Analysis of the antigenic determinants of the mannan of *Candida albicans* serotype B-792. *Jpn. J. Microbiol.* **14:**371–379.

78. **Sundstrom, P.** 1999. Adhesins in *Candida albicans. Curr. Opin. Microbiol.* **2:**353–357.

79. **Suzuki, S., and Y. Fukazawa.** 1982. Immunochemical characterization of *Candida albicans* cell wall antigens: specific determinant of *Candida albicans* serotype A. *Microbiol. Immunol.* **26:**387–402.

80. **Suzuki, S., M. Suzuki, K. Yokota, H. Sunayama, and O. Sakaguchi.** 1967. On the immunochemical and biochemical studies

of fungi XI. Cross reactions of the polysaccharides of *Aspergillus fumigatus, Candida albicans, Saccharomyces cerevisiae,* and *Trichophyton rubrum* against *Candida albicans* and *Saccharomyces cerevisiae* antisera. *Jpn. J. Microbiol.* **11**:269–273.

81. **Titsworth, E., and E. Grunberg.** 1973. Chemotherapeutic activity of 5-fluorocytosine and amphotericin B against *Candida albicans* in mice. *Antimicrob. Agents Chemother.* **4**:306–308.
82. **Tsuchiya, T., Y. Fuazawa, M. Taguchi, M. Nakase, and T. Shinoda.** 1974. Serologic aspects of yeast classification. *Mycopathology* **53**:77–91.
83. **Utz, J. P.** 1966. Treatment of *Candida* infections, p. 221–224. *In* H. I. Winner and R. Hurley (ed.), *Symposium on Candida Infections.* Livingstone, Edinburgh, United Kingdom.
84. **Utz, J.** 1972. Flucytosine. Editorial. *New Engl. J. Med.* **286**: 777–778.
85. **Vandeputte, J., J. L. Wachtel, and E. T. Stiller.** 1956. Amphotericins A and B, antifungal antibiotics produced by a streptomycete. II. The isolation and properties of the crystalline amphotericins. *Antibiot. Ann. 1955* **56**:587–591.
86. **Wallace, W. C., M. E. Cinat, F. Nastanski, W. B. Gornick, and S. E. Wilson.** 2000. New epidemiology for postoperative nosocomial infections. *Am. Surg.* **66**:874–878.
87. **Warner, J. F., R. F. Magee, R. J. Duma, R. F. McGehee, S. Shadomy, and J. P. Utz.** 1971. 5-Fluorocytosine in human candidiasis. *Antimicrob. Agents Chemother.* **15**:473–475.
88. **Wenzel, R. P.** 1995. Nosocomial candidiasis: risk factors and attributable mortality. *Clin. Infect. Dis.* **20**:1531–1534.
89. **Whelan, W. L., and P. T. Magee.** 1981. Natural heterozygosity in *Candida albicans. J. Bacteriol.* **145**:896–903.
90. **White, T. C., K. A. Marr, and R. A. Bowden.** 1998. Clinical, cellular and molecular factors that contribute to antifungal drug resistance. *Clin. Microbiol. Rev.* **11**:382–402.
91. **Wilkinson, J. S.** 1849. Some remarks upon the development of epiphytes with the description of new vegetable formation found in connection with the human uterus. *Lancet* **2**:448.
92. **Wingard, J. R., W. G. Merz, and R. Saral.** 1979. *Candida troplicalis.* A major pathogen in immunocompromised patients. *Ann. Intern. Med.* **91**:539.
93. **Winner, H. I., and R. Hurley.** 1954. *Candida albicans.* Little, Brown and Company, Boston, Mass.

Candida and Candidiasis
Edited by Richard A. Calderone
© 2002 ASM Press, Washington, D.C.

Chapter 2

Taxonomy and Biology of *Candida*

RICHARD A. CALDERONE

In this chapter, the characteristics of the human pathogenic species of *Candida* will be discussed. Emphasis will be placed upon the biological features that identify and distinguish these organisms; serological differences are described in chapter 3. Also included is a brief discussion of the types of candidiasis caused by each species. Although there are about 150 species of *Candida,* it is well established that only a small number are human pathogens, and, in fact, approximately 65% of *Candida* species are unable to grow at a temperature of 37°C (53), a trait that is certainly a prerequisite for an organism to be a successful pathogen. In establishing an approximate number of pathogenic species, one must realize that surveys of isolates from patients often list specific species, but in numerous studies, an additional category of unnamed "other species" of yeasts is indicated. Thus, we are left to our own imagination as to what and how many of these unnamed species exist in human disease. It should also be pointed out that, on the other hand, this unnamed group accounts for a rather low number of isolates, albeit significant. Another point to be made is that the number of pathogenic *Candida* spp. has increased because of taxonomic changes (*Torulopsis glabrata* is now reclassified, appropriately, as *Candida glabrata*) and because of the addition of a new species (*Candida dubliniensis*) that is closely aligned with *C. albicans* (5, 12, 36–38, 41, 44, 51, 56–58, 61). Further, the close scrutiny of cultures from patients has resulted in the identification of several other species that cause disease, such as *C. famata, C. inconspicua,* and others mentioned below. Although these species are rarely reported, nevertheless, we have become aware of their potential as pathogens in the immunocompromised patient. On the other hand, it is clear that *C. stellatoidea* is synonymous with *C. albicans* and most clinical laboratories do not distinguish it from *C. albicans* (27, 30, 31).

Whereas *Candida* species are ubiquitous organisms, most are not human pathogens but exist as environmental saprophytes as stated above. On the other hand, the pathogens, such as *C. albicans,* are most often reported only as isolates from patients or as commensals of the human host; hence, most candidiasis is believed to be of endogenous origin. However, the acquisition of *Candida* species, such as *C. albicans,* from the environment has not been studied to any great detail but surely occurs. Currently, the belief is that the recovery of *Candida* spp. from the environment reflects contamination from patients or health workers. Of importance, while candidiasis is an endogenous disease (as stated above), lateral transmission from health care workers to patients (especially in certain clinical settings such as the surgical intensive-care unit) occurs. Acquisition of organisms also occurs vertically, as from mother to the neonate. These subjects will be discussed in depth in chapter 28.

GROWTH FORMS OF *CANDIDA*

The pathogenic *Candida* spp. are listed in Table 1 along with the teleomorph (sexual) stage binomial designation, if known. The genus *Candida* is composed of an extremely heterogenous group of organisms that grow as yeasts (Fig. 1A, blastoconidia; see Table 2). Most members of the genus also produce a filamentous type of growth (pseudohyphae, pseudomycelium, Fig. 1C; Table 2), but *C. albicans* and *C. dubliniensis* also form true hyphae (true mycelium) (Fig. 1B) in addition to pseudohyphae (pseudomycelium). Therefore, both species are considered to be polymorphic. The distinction that is made between hyphae and pseudohyphae is related to the way in which they are formed. Pseudohyphae form from

Richard A. Calderone • Department of Microbiology and Immunology, Georgetown University School of Medicine, 3900 Reservoir Rd. NW, Washington, DC 20007.

Table 1. A partial list of pathogenic species of *Candida*

Reported by 1988[a]	Current list	Sexual (teleomorph form)[d]
C. albicans	*C. albicans*	Not described
C. tropicalis	*C. tropicalis*	Not described
C. glabrata	*C. glabrata*	Not described
C. parapsilosis	*C. parapsilosis*	Not described
C. krusei	*C. krusei*	*Issatchenkia orientalis*
C. guilliermondii	*C. guilliermondii*	*Pichia guilliermondii*
C. kefyr[b]	*C. kefyr*	*Kluyveromyces marxianus*
C. viswanathii	*C. viswanathii*	Not described
	C. lusitaniae	*Clavisopora lusitaniae*
	C. dubliniensis	Not described
	C. famata[c]	*Debaryomyces hansenii*
	C. inconspicua	Not described
	C. utilis	*Pichia jadinii*

[a]Reference 40.
[b]Formerly *C. pseudotropicalis*.
[c]Formerly *T. candida*.
[d]Reference 29.

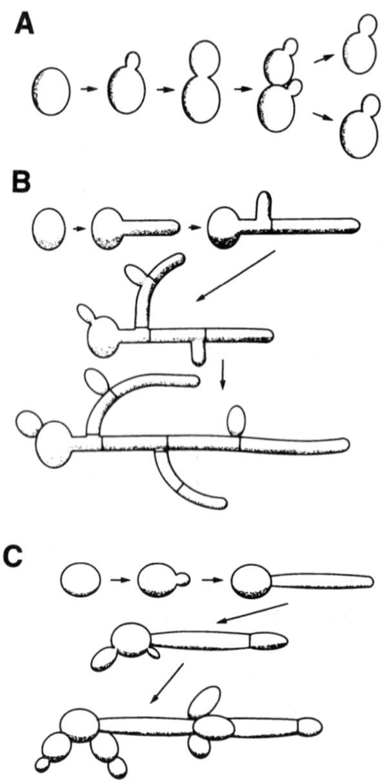

Figure 1. The growth forms of *Candida* species. All species grow as yeasts (A), and most produce some type of pseudohyphae (C). *C. dubliniensis* and *C. albicans* also form true hyphae (B). Budding in *Candida* species occurs at numerous sites on the cell surface. The newly formed bud increases in size, then becomes separated following the final stages of mitosis. Hyphal formation is initiated by an outgrowth (germ tube) followed by apical extension. Septa (cross walls) form, and branching of the hyphae or budding occurs just behind the septa. Reprinted from reference 40 by permission of the publisher, Bailliere Tindall.

yeast cells or from hyphae by budding, but the new cell remains attached to the parent cell and elongates, resulting in filaments with constrictions at the cell-cell junctions of the filaments. In comparison, true hyphae form from yeast cells or as branches of existing hyphae. Outgrowths of the yeast cell (germ tubes) grow by apical extension and cross walls (septa) are formed behind the growing tip of the hyphae. Budding occurs laterally just behind the septa (Fig. 1B), the latter of which are perpendicular to the main axis of the hyphae. The appearance of hyphae differs somewhat when grown in serum, where hyphal branching occurs and budding is delayed. The pseudohypha appears to be an intermediate growth form of yeast and hyphal morphologies. Because *C. albicans* and *C. dubliniensis* produce hyphae from yeast cells, these species are also referred to as being germ tube positive (Table 2).

The germ tube test is commonly employed in the diagnostic mycology laboratory to identify isolates rapidly from patients as either of these two species. Germination can be induced in complex media (peptone broth), chemically defined media, and serum (see chapters 7, 8, and 11). The environmental factors that favor germination include a temperature greater than 35°C and a pH of 6.5 to 7.0 or slightly alkaline. Lower temperatures and an acid pH favor yeast growth. Actually, temperature and pH are only two factors that regulate the growth pattern of *C. albicans*. In fact, Odds has listed numerous other conditions that have been reported by various laboratories as essential for either yeast or hyphal growth (40). Thus, impoverished media, an inoculum of $<10^6$ ml^{-1}, partial anaerobiosis, and stationary-phase cells favor hyphal growth, whereas glucose (as a sole carbon source), a

Table 2. Morphological features of selected pathogenic species of *Candida*

Species	Chlamydospore[a]	Germ tube[a]	Pseudohyphae[a,b]	Size of yeasts (μm)	CHROM-agar reaction[c]
C. albicans	+	+	+	4–6 × 6–10	Blue-green
C. tropicalis[d]	±	–	+	4–8 × 5–11	Dark blue-blue gray
C. glabrata	–	–	–[f]	1–4	White, pink-purple
C. parapsilosis	–	–	+	2.5–4 × 2.5–9	White, pale pink
C. krusei[e]	–	–	+/–[g]	3–5 × 6–20	Pale pink, purple, rough
C. dubliniensis	+	+	+	3–7 × 3–14	Dark green
C. guilliermondii	–	–	Primitive	2–5 × 3–7	Pale pink, purple
C. lusitaniae	–	–	Variable	2–6 × 3–10	Pink, grayish purple
C. kefyr	–	–	+	2.5–5 × 5–10	Pink, purple
C. inconspicua	–	–	Primitive	1.5–3 × 3–5	White, pink
C. famata	–	–	Primitive	3.7–5 × 2.7–4.7	White, light pink, purple

[a]The yeast cell size, production (+) or absence (–) of chlamydospore, germ tube, and pseudohyphal formation are indicated along with the colony color phenotype on CHROMagar.
[b]As reported on Dalmau plates of cornmeal-Tween agar (29).
[c]CHROMagar reactions according to Odds and Bernaerts (41); *C. dubliniensis* reaction on CHROMagar according to Sullivan et al. (58), except that *C. dubliniensis* reactions can be lost following subculture or storage.
[d]*C. tropicalis* also forms a dark halo on CHROMagar and produces chlamydospores under certain conditions.
[e]*C. krusei* and *C. inconspicua* are closely related phenotypically but can be distinguished by randomly amplified polymorphic DNA hybridization with a *C. krusei*-specific probe, and karyotyping (3, 6, 14). *C. famata* is formerly *T. candida.*
[f]Pseudohyphae have been observed in *C. glabrata* when grown on synthetic low-ammonium dextrose agar (9).
[g]+/–, strain dependent.

pH of <6.5 to 7.0, temperature of <35°C, and larger inoculum size favor yeast growth. A number of standard lab media are chosen for propagation of hyphal growth, including Lee's medium (amino acids-salts) and tissue culture media (such as M-199), whereas serum and single amino acids (such as proline) can induce filamentation. Nutritionally minimal media, such as synthetic low-ammonium dextrose or Spider agar, are often used in inducing filamentous growth and have become standard media for evaluating the morphogenesis patterns of gene-deleted strains of *C. albicans*. Certainly, pH and temperature are two environmental parameters that are most often critically maintained when one is manipulating the growth in *C. albicans* as well as other *Candida* species.

C. albicans and *C. dubliniensis* also produce large (8 to 12 μm), refractile, thick-walled cells referred to as chlamydospores (Table 2 and Fig. 2) that are most often observed in vitro on nutrient-poor media, such as cornmeal-Tween agar and other equally nutritionally poor media (13, 29). They have been observed in host tissues, but this event is apparently quite rare.

The medical mycology diagnostic laboratory utilizes both microscopic and growth parameters in identifying *Candida* spp. from clinical specimens. In addition to the germ tube test and chlamydospore formation, growth on CHROMagar (Table 2) (41) and assimilation profiles (Table 3) are often used in identifying *Candida* spp. These subjects will be discussed more completely in chapter 26.

TAXONOMY OF *CANDIDA*

In older taxonomic treatises, species of the genus *Candida* that lacked a sexual stage (teleomorph) were designated Deuteromycetes, the class of fungi that does not reproduce sexually. On the other hand, the teleomorph stages of several pathogenic (Table 1) and nonpathogenic *Candida* species have been described, but for familiarity's sake, those organisms (especially the pathogens) retain their designation as *Candida* species. *C. krusei,* for example, is not routinely referred to as *Issatchenkia orientalis,* in spite of the fact that the teleomorph stage is known for this species. Therefore, the anamorph (asexual stage name) is specified in distinguishing species of *Candida,* even if the sexual stage (teleomorph) is identified as described above. This policy, whether taxonomically correct or not, creates a unity for this group of pathogens (and reduces stress for medical students and clinicians who must learn new names of pathogens). As stated above, the older classification of many species of *Candida* as Deuteromycetes was based on the fact that they lacked a sexual stage. However, for those species of *Candida* for which a teleomorph has been described (Table 1), the sexual stages are ascomycetous (29). Further, comparative sequence data from a number of studies support the idea that both the sexual and nonsexual *Candida* species are related phylogenetically to the Ascomycete rather than to the Basidiomycete class of fungi. For example, parsimony analyses of nucleotides from SSU rDNA sequences of 75 representative Ascomycetes and Basidiomycetes clearly val-

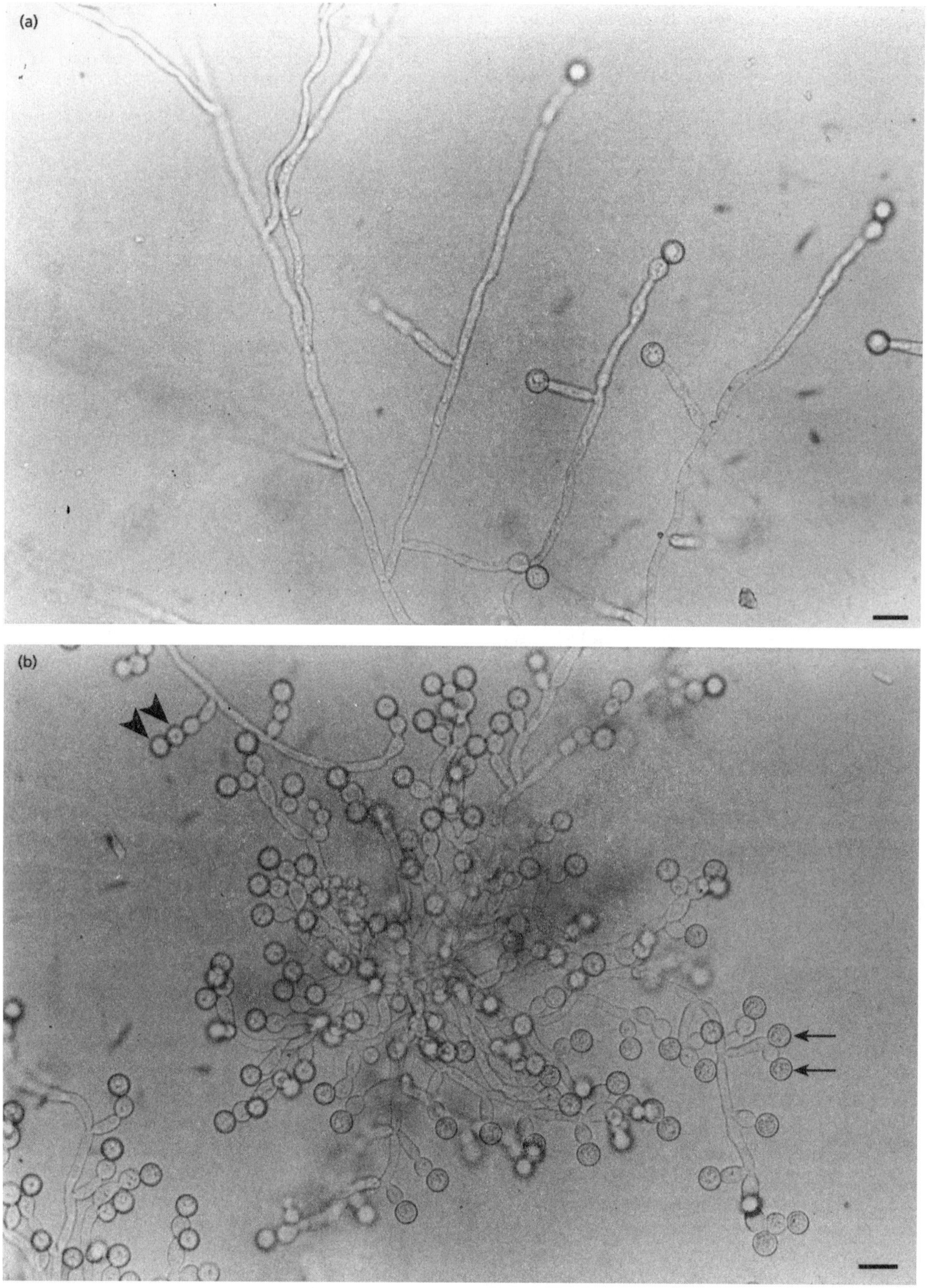

Figure 2. Chlamydospores of *C. albicans* (upper) and *C. dubliniensis* (lower) from cultures grown on cornmeal-Tween agar. Chlamydospores are thick-walled, spherical, refractory cells that are approximately 8 to 12 μm in diameter. The number of chlamydospores and their arrangement differ between the two species. Reprinted from reference 58 by permission of the Society for General Microbiology.

Table 3. Biochemical assimilation profiles (API20C) of selected pathogenic species of *Candida*

Species	% Isolates demonstrating a positive reaction[a]																		
	GLU	GLY	2KG	ARA	XYL	ADO	XLT	GAL	INO	SOR	MDG	NAG	CEL	LAC	MAL	SAC	TRE	MLZ	RAF
C. albicans	100	14	89	2	88	94	90	88	0	84	85	99	0	0	99	97	5	0	0
C. dubliniensis	100	96	99	0	0	99	0	100	3	99	0	40	0	0	100	60	0	0	0
C. famata	100	96	98	60	80	98	75	99	0	100	98	99	29	20	100	100	96	78	75
C. glabrata	100	20	0	0	0	0	0	0	0	0	0	0	0	0	0	0	94	0	0
C. guilliermondii	100	99	97	79	85	97	92	99	0	97	88	99	95	0	94	100	99	90	95
C. kefyr	100	27	0	1	18	1	25	100	0	26	0	0	1	95	1	100	1	1	95
C. krusei	99	73	0	0	0	0	0	6	0	2	0	44	0	0	0	0	0	0	0
C. lusitaniae	100	90	95	1	64	95	20	30	0	93	60	95	80	0	100	99	100	89	0
C. parapsilosis	100	94	88	89	89	93	3	99	0	99	89	99	0	0	100	100	93	99	1
C. tropicalis	100	9	99	1	96	99	12	99	0	99	59	99	17	1	99	72	100	72	1

[a]GLU, glucose; GLY, glycerol; 2KG, 2-keto-D-gluconate; ARA, arabinose; XLY, xylose; ADO, adonitol; XLT, xylitol; GAL, galactose; INO, inositol; SOR, sorbose; MDG, isomethyl-D-glucoside; NAG, *N*-acetyl-D-glucosamine; CEL, cellobiose; LAC, lactose; MAL, maltose; SAC, sucrose; TRE, trehalose; MLZ, melzibiose; RAF, raffinose.

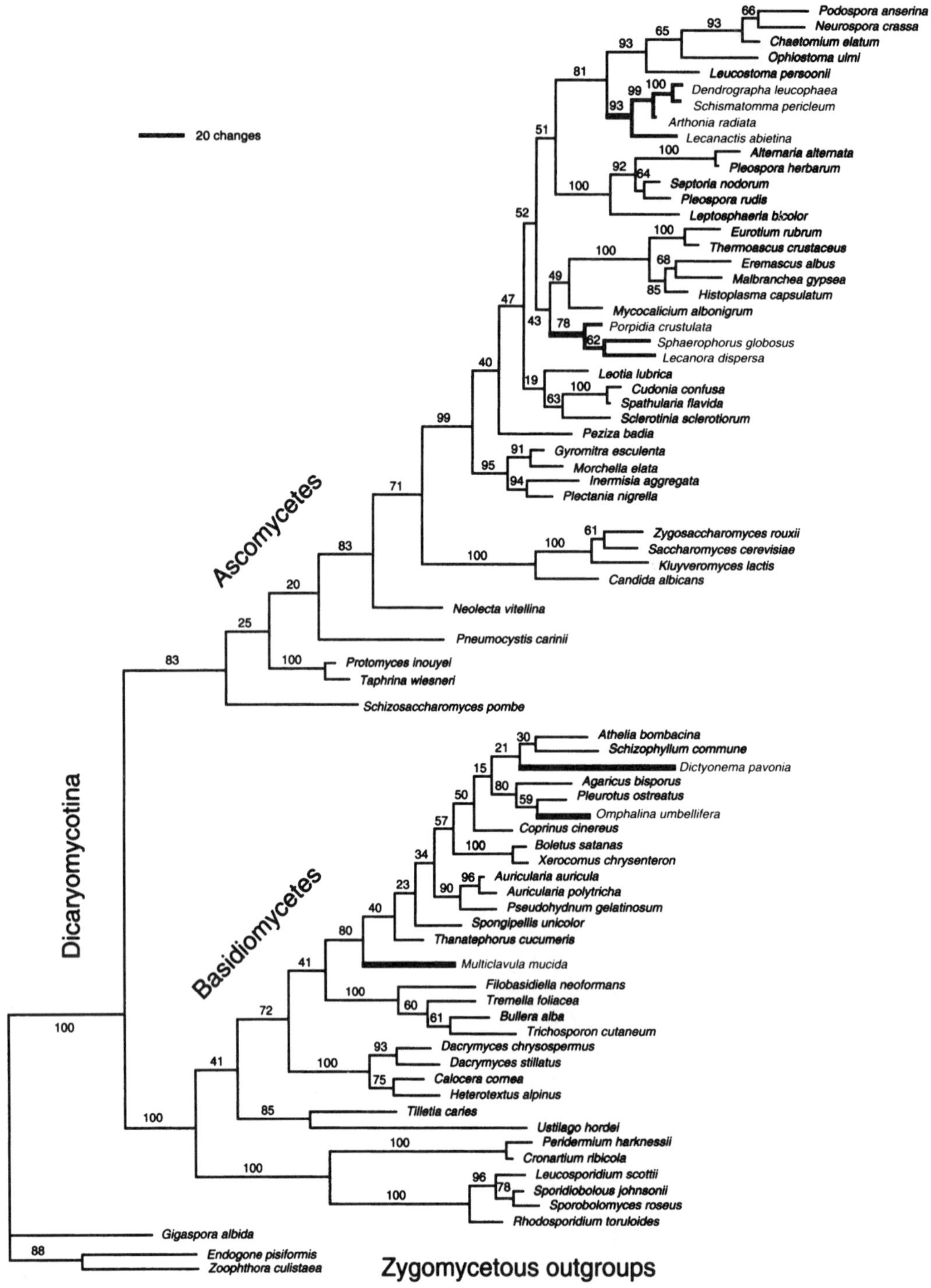

Figure 3. Parsimony analysis of 1,927 nucleotides of SSU rDNA sequences from 75 representative basidiomycetous and ascomycetous fungi. In the upper part of the figure, the alignment of *C. albicans* with the ascomycetous fungi is indicated. Reprinted with permission from reference 18. Copyright 1995 American Association for the Advancement of Science.

idate the taxonomic alignment of species of *Candida* among the Ascomycetes (Fig. 3) (18). Additionally, there are other characteristics that distinguish *Candida* species as an ascomycetous and not a basidiomycetous yeast. For example, they are urease negative, nonencapsulated, fermentative, and noninositol assimilative; make β-glucans in their cell wall; and do not produce starch or carotenoid pigments. Budding in *Candida* species results in one bud per locus, typical of Ascomycetes, whereas in the Basidiomycetes, cells bud repeatedly from a single locus. Also, the molecular structure of the cross walls (septa) differ, being transparent and homogenous in the Ascomycetes (such as *Candida*) while tripartite in the Basidiomycetes (29). In comparison, *Cryptococcus neoformans,* another human pathogen, is a basidiomycetous yeast that is urease positive, encapsulated, and nonfermentative; assimilates inositol; and produces unicellular, budding yeasts only (50).

A scheme that illustrates the current views on the taxonomy of the anamorphic *Candida,* their teleomorphic stages, as well as a close relative of *Candida* (*Saccharomyces*) is presented in Table 4. This scheme is derived from Kurtzman and Fell (29), and most of the description that follows is derived from this source. In some instances, assignments of members of the order Saccharomycetales are uncertain, and those genera are indicated by a question mark. The teleomorph forms of *Candida* species are diverse structurally but tentatively are assigned to two families of Ascomycetes (Table 4). Sexual reproduction (conjugation) is induced on media such as V8 agar, yeast-malt extract agar, or on McClary's acetate medium and occurs between compatible mating types (heterothallic species), an example being *Pichia guilliermondii* (*C. guilliermondii*), but other species are self-sterile (homothallic), as in the case of *Kluyveromyces marxianus* (*C. kefyr*). Interestingly, conjugation in the homothallic species, *Debaryomyces hansenii* (*C. famata* and others), occurs between a cell and its bud. This type of conjugation is referred to as heterogamous (conjugation between cells of different size or shape) versus isogamous conjugation that occurs between cells of similar size and shape. Often sexual reproduction is described as unconjugated, indicating that diploids persist before they eventually undergo meiosis to form sexual spores (ascospores). Both asci and ascospores vary in shape from species to species; asci can be persistent (*Debaryomyces, Issatchenkia*), deliquescent (*Clavispora*), or both (*Pichia*). The number of ascospores that form from a diploid cell following meiosis is also species dependent but usually is from 1 to 4 (29). One of the more interesting of the teleomorphs is *Metschinkowia* species, in which asci can arise from spheroidal chlamydospores (29).

Table 4. The classification of the anamorphic *Candida*, teleomorph stages of *Candida* and *Saccharomyces* (29)

Phylum: Ascomycota
  Class: Hemiascomycetes[a]
    Order: Saccharomycetales[b]
      Family: Metschnikowiaceae
        Genus: *Clavispora*
      Family: Saccharomycetaceae
        Genus: ? *Debaryomyces*[c]
          ? *Issatchenkia*[c]
          ? *Pichia*[c]
          Kluyveromyces
          Saccharomyces
      Family: Candidaceae (Anamorphic)
        Genus: *Candida*

[a] Hemiascomycetes are Ascomycetes whose asci are naked, and no ascogneous hyphae or ascocarps are formed.
[b] Fungi of the Saccharomycetales produce asci from zygotes, and each zygote is derived from the conjugation of two cells or from a single cell.
[c] ?, uncertain affiliation.

MATING IN *C. ALBICANS*

As described in chapter 18, sequencing of the *C. albicans* genome has provided vast amounts of information on genes that are both unique to *C. albicans* as well as homologs (genes that resemble those of other organisms). Among the latter category, a mating-type locus (*MTL*) has been described that resembles the mating type (*MAT*) locus of *Saccharomyces cerevisiae* (22). Given that other genes from *C. albicans* have been identified that are homologs of genes from *S. cerevisiae* that function in mating and meiosis, recent investigations have focused on identifying mating in *C. albicans.* In *S. cerevisiae,* two haploid mating types exist, *MAT***a** and *MAT*α, and when haploid cells of each are mixed together, conjugation occurs, the outcome of which is a diploid cell. The diploid cell can continue to divide in nutritionally rich media but is unable to mate; meiosis can be induced in diploids by growing cells on a medium containing acetate as the sole carbon source. Relevant to this discussion, Hull et al. (22) have shown that the *C. albicans MTL* locus probably encodes proteins similar to the transcriptional regulators encoded by *MAT* in *S. cerevisiae,* including **a***1*, α*1*, and α*2*. This observation indicates that *C. albicans* is heterozygous for *MTL* and that the diploid genome is represented by an **a***1*-like gene carried at one *MTL* locus α*1*-, and α*2*-like genes carried on the other *MTL* locus. Thus, it would appear that *C. albicans* as a diploid is unable to mate since gene products from both *MTL* alleles preclude mating, probably in a fashion much like that described for diploid *S. cerevisiae* (*MAT***a**/*MAT*α). Therefore, if one of either *MTL* alleles was nonfunctional or absent, then mating might occur in *C. albicans* when compatible, single-allele strains (*MTL1*) are mixed together.

Simultaneously, two different approaches have been used to construct mating-type strains in *C. albicans* (22, 34). Hull et al. (22) constructed "a" strains by deleting the entire *MTL*α locus or by deleting only the α1α2 genes of the *MTL*α locus. To construct "α cells," the *MTL***a** locus or the **a***1* gene was deleted. **a** and α cells were also auxotrophic for either adenine (Ade2$^-$ Ura$^+$) or uridine (Ade2$^+$ Ura$^-$) so that successful mating could be detected in minimal medium lacking adenine and uridine (Ade$^+$ Ura$^+$) since only mated cells (conjugants) should grow on minimal medium. Mating was conducted in mice infected via the lateral tail vein with varying ratios of **a** and α cells. Subsequently, at 24 h postinfection, mice were euthanized, and the kidneys of infected animals were homogenized and plated on rich medium. Approximately 10^3 colonies grew on rich medium, whereas 44 colonies grew on minimal medium from animals infected with the **a** + α mix of cells. Results from control mice infected with strains deleted of both **a** and α (*mtl***a**/*mtl*α) produced only a single colony on minimal medium. Other control cell mixtures also verified that mating required both *MTL***a** and *MTL*α cells. Conjugants were confirmed by Southern hybridization; all formed germ tubes and had substantially increased DNA content, as expected if mating occurred. While mating was established in vivo, it is likely to be an extremely rare event in this organism in nature, because strains that are monosomic for *MTL* or a part of a chromosome should be quickly lost from a natural population (22). Nevertheless, the data are provocative.

As another approach to constructing strains that lack either *MTL***a** or *MTL*α, Magee and Magee used the observation (24) that growth of *C. albicans* in sorbose results in monosomy in either homolog of chromosome 5 (34). Conveniently, the *MTL* locus is found on chromosome 5. Thus, *MTL***a** and *MTL*α strains were isolated from media containing sorbose as the sole carbon source, mated in vitro by cross-streaking on rich medium and replica-plated to minimal medium, since each mating type exhibited a different auxotrophy (see Color plate 1). Conjugants, if mating occurred, should arise by complementation of the auxotrophy associated with each mating type. These investigators showed that the frequency of conjugation was greatest at room temperature rather than at 30 or 37°C and when mating pairs were allowed to remain in contact on nonselective medium for 3 to 12 days before replication onto minimal medium. The DNA content of the conjugants was about twice that of parent cells (nearly tetraploid). Thus, the experiments from both laboratories indicate that the first step of sexual reproduction, i.e., mating and the formation of recombinants with the genome of both parents, can occur but with strains that are altered to express only *MTL***a** or *MTL*α. Additional experiments are needed to define the events related to mating (pheromone production, sexual agglutinins, regulation of mating), as well as the mechanisms that regulate reduction division.

PATHOGENIC *CANDIDA* SPECIES AND THEIR PREVALENCE IN PATIENTS

A good starting point for enumerating the species of pathogenic *Candida* is the account of Odds (40), who listed eight. The species listed in Table 1 should probably be expanded as more recent surveillance studies have included *C. famata, C. inconspicua, C. utilis, C. lusitaniae,* and other species from blood and other sites of patients with candidiasis, albeit at much lower frequencies. Also, a new species, *C. dubliniensis,* which is very similar phenotypically to *C. albicans* (produces germ tubes and chlamydospores among other similar traits), has now been identified (51, 56–58) and is included among the list of pathogens.

The phylogenetic relationships among the most common of the *Candida* spp. that are pathogenic, as determined by DNA sequences of the V3 variable region of the large ribosomal subunit gene, are shown in Fig. 4. A bootstrap analysis of the 10 sequences

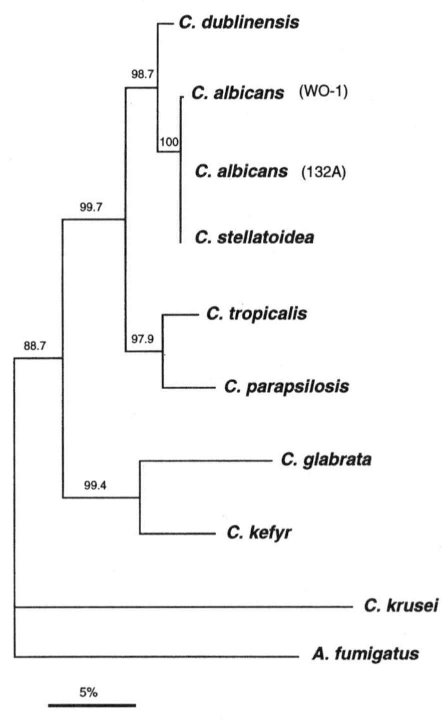

Figure 4. An uprooted phylogenetic neighbor-joining tree generated from the alignment of a 500-bp fragment of the V3 region of the large rDNA genes of *C. dubliniensis* and other *Candida* species. The scale bar represents a 5% difference in nucleotide sequence. Reprinted from reference 58 by permission of the Society for General Microbiology.

Table 5. Surveillance studies of *Candida* species from patients

Type of candidiasis[a]	Predominant species	Location	Reference
Candidemia, cancer	*C. guilliermondii*	U.S.	35
Hemodialysis, nosocomial	*Candida* spp.	U.S.	10
Sepsis, low-birth-weight infants	*Candida* spp.	Canada	17
Meningitis, premature infant	*Candida* spp.	U.S.	15
Oral, solid-tumor patients	*Candida* spp.	Holland	46
HIV, septicemia	*C. albicans* (48%), *C. tropicalis* (19%), *C. glabrata* (11%)	Italy	59
Cancer, septicemia	*C. albicans* (46%), *C. tropicalis* (25%), *C. glabrata* (8%), *C. parapsilosis* (7%), *C. krusei* (4%), *C. lusitianiae* (?), *C. stellatoidea* (1%)	U.S.	62
Oral, HIV-seropositive	*C. dubliniensis* (all)	U.S.	36
Surveillance cultures	*C. dubliniensis*	Holland	37
Esophagitis, HIV patients	*Candida* spp.	Spain	7
Esophageal disease, HIV patients	*Candida* spp. (63%)	Taiwan	23
Bloodstream, surgical ICU	*C. albicans* (48%), *C. glabrata* (24%), *C. tropicalis* (19%), *C. parapsilosis* (7%)	U.S.	47
Bloodstream, neonatal ICU	*C. albicans* (63%), *C. parapsilosis* (29%)	U.S.	47
Candidemia, variety of conditions	*C. albicans* (53%), non-*C. albicans* (47%)	U.S.	25
Bloodstream, variety of services	*C. albicans* (53%), *C. parapsilosis* (21%), *C. glabrata* (12%), *C. tropicalis* (6%), *C. famata* (2%), *C. krusei* (1%), *C. inconspicua* (1%)	Europe	42
Head and neck cancers, oral	*C. albicans* (78%)	U.S.	48
Candidemia	*C. albicans* (53.6%)	Israel	49
Bloodstream	*C. albicans* (54%), *C. glabrata* (16%), *C. parapsilosis* (15%), *C. tropicalis* (8%), *C. krusei* (1.6%)	U.S., Canada, Latin America	43
Peritonitis, dialysis patients	*C. parapsilosis* (17 cases)	China	21
Nosocomial fungemia, GI tract and hemologic diseases	*C. albicans* (50%), *C. parapsilosis* (17%)	Brazil	8

[a]ICU, intensive-care unit; GI, gastrointestinal.

shown indicates that *C. dubliniensis* is grouped separately from the cluster of *C. albicans* and *C. stellatoidea* and that the other species tested are more divergent.

The data in Table 5 and other accounts (1, 2, 4, 8, 10, 15, 17, 19, 23, 25, 42, 43, 46–49, 59, 60, 61) indicate that the predominant human pathogen among species of *Candida* is *C. albicans,* regardless of the clinical setting and location of the study. Thus, *C. albicans* is the most often observed pathogen in the AIDS patient (mucosal disease) as well as from septicemias (fungemias) associated with cancer chemotherapy, transplant patients, premature infants, surgical infections, or other predisposing conditions. Next in frequency among the *Candida* pathogens is *C. tropicalis* (4, 8, 26, 39, 42, 43, 47, 49, 62), *C. parapsilosis* (8, 19, 21, 25, 39, 42, 43, 47, 49, 59, 60, 62, 65), or *C. glabrata* (2, 4, 16, 25, 42, 43, 47, 49, 60, 64), at least in regard to blood isolates. These three species alternate as the second most common pathogen, depending on the source of the data. Of interest, a higher mortality is often reported for septicemias caused by *C. glabrata,* but the reasons for this observation are not well understood (16, 49, 64). Likewise, *C. dubliniensis* has emerged as a new and important pathogenic species (54). Finally, a group of *Candida* species usually reported as infrequent pathogens (*C. inconspicua, C. lusitaniae, C. guilliermondii, C. kefyr, C. famata,* and *C. utilis*) are now added to the list of human pathogens. In chapter 4, descriptions of the major human pathogenic non-*albicans Candida* spp. are presented. Several of these species have recently received attention because they are increasing in frequency among all clinical isolates (4, 7, 19, 26, 62–64). The list of pathogens includes those species whose increase in isolation rate has been associated with their resistance to drugs such as fluconazole (chapter 4).

The Uncommon Human *Candida* Pathogens

The following species of *Candida* are considered as less common causes of disease in humans. This group includes *C. inconspicua, C. krusei, C. famata* (formerly *Torulopsis candida*), *C. guilliermondii, C. viswanathii, C. kefyr* (formerly *C. pseudotropicalis*), *C. utilis,* and *C. lusitaniae.* All of these species grow as yeasts, but the type of pseudohyphae varies from species to species (Table 2). On Dalmau plates of cornmeal agar, for example, *C. krusei, C. kefyr,* and

C. lusitaniae produce "typical" pseudohyphae, whereas strains of *C. guilliermondii, C. famata,* and *C. lusitaniae* produce "primitive" pseudohyphae that are composed of ovoid cells in chains (29). However, strain variability in this property has been reported. For example, in other accounts, *C. guilliermondii* has been reported to produce pseudomycelium that is fine in texture and short (50). *C. krusei* produces flat, dry colonies with a prominent surface film that extends several millimeters up on the inner surface of culture tubes. This phenotype and its elongated yeast (bud) cells provide a fairly easy way to identify *C. krusei* (13). Culture phenotypes of *C. krusei* and *C. inconspicua* are identical, and separation of these two species is obtained only by molecular methodologies, including randomly amplified polymorphic DNA, Southern hybridization using specific probes, or karyotype analyses (3, 6, 14).

As stated above, these species are uncommon pathogens, and probably for that reason, their study has lagged behind those species described above. Nevertheless, there is indication that they cause disease and some of these studies are discussed. For example, the total number of *C. krusei* isolates from bronchial secretions has statistically increased from initial surveillance studies over time from 1987 to 1992 (4). The frequency of isolation of *C. krusei* compared to all *Candida* species from blood cultures of patients has ranged from 1.0 to 5.8% of all *Candida* isolates (42, 43, 63), whereas the frequencies of *C. famata* (2%) and *C. inconspicua* (1 to 4.1%) indicate their low level of recovery from human disease. *C. famata* (*T. candida*) was first reported in 1986 in a case of catheter-induced septicemia (55). In addition to these surveillance studies, *C. guilliermondii* has been reported as a cause of a fungemia in cancer patients (35); *C. kefyr* was the cause of esophagitis (32) and vaginitis (2), *C. utilis* in chronic urinary tract infections (20), *C. viswanathii* in meningitis (52), and *C. famata* from infections in a surgical patient, peritonitis (45), and fungemias (44). *C. inconspicua* has also been reported from patients with human immunodeficiency virus (HIV) infections (3) and in hematological malignancies (11).

Certainly, the list of uncommon pathogens of humans described above is incomplete. Hazen, for example, also has included *C. ciferri* (nails, ear), *C. zeylanoides* (groin, nails), *C. rugosa* (blood, burn wounds, catheter), *C. haemulonii* (toe, nails, blood), *C. norvegensis* (blood, peritoneal fluid), and *C. pulcherrima* (nails) as emerging disease-causing species (19). In addition, *C. chiropterum, C. humicola,* and *C. pintolopesii* are also referenced as isolates from human disease (19). Of this latter group of fungi, the teleomorph stages of *C. ciferrii, C. lipolytica, C. norvegensis, C. pulcherrima,* and *C. pintolopesii* have been described (referenced in reference 19).

Is There an Increase in Non-*C. albicans* Species among Patient Isolates?

As stated above, *C. albicans* still predominates as the most common cause of disease caused by *Candida* species. However, there is widespread belief that non-*C. albicans* species have emerged within the past 15 years as causes of significantly more disease (1, 4, 7, 19, 26, 28, 62, 64). Most often, the species that are mentioned in this regard are *C. glabrata, C. krusei, C. parapsilosis,* and *C. dubliniensis.* In part, the increase in frequency of disease caused by some of these organisms has been associated with their resistance to antifungal drugs such as fluconazole, especially in regard to *C. krusei* and *C. glabrata.* Thus, prophylaxis of patients is thought to select for drug-resistant organisms. In the setting of an immunocompromised host, this selection is thought to be in part responsible for the larger number of cases of candidiasis caused by the non-*C. albicans* species that are part of the normal flora. However, other data may question this interpretation. For example, a shift in species that cause vulvovaginal disease was not observed to any great extent in a recent study of non-HIV-positive women (33). Also, a comparison of non-*C. albicans* species reported from the urines of hospitalized patients before the advent of fluconazole therapy (1962) revealed that approximately 41% of the isolates were non-*C. albicans* and that 29.5% were *C. glabrata* (40). These numbers are not much different from those reported currently in the era of fluconazole resistance. For example, a recent estimate is that approximately 50% of the urinary tract infections are caused by non-*C. albicans* species (*C. glabrata* was the most common non-*C. albicans* species) (16).

On the other hand, there are numerous reports of a shift in the frequency of species of *Candida* that cause disease from *C. albicans* to non-*C. albicans* species, as stated above (1, 4, 7, 25, 61, 63). In a study of the spectra of fungal species that were isolated from respiratory and bronchial secretions as well as urines over a period from 1987 to 1991, the number of *C. albicans* isolates decreased, *C. tropicalis* remained the same but *C. glabrata* isolates doubled, and the numbers of mixed *Candida* species increased significantly. Data on the dynamics of *Candida* isolations from patients during the period from 1992 to 1995 indicated that *Candida* accounted for 50.5% of all mycological cultures. However, the percentage of *C. albicans* isolates decreased from 76% to approximately 54%, whereas *C. glabrata* increased from 11.7 to 28.4%.

The prevailing and justifiable opinion, therefore,

is that the incidence of candidiasis caused by the non-*C. albicans* species is increasing. There is little doubt that drug resistance has contributed at least partially to the increase in frequency of non-*C. albicans* strains in candidiasis (see chapters 4 and 25). Certainly, the resistant strains present management problems for the clinician. So their presence in the patient is significant and very likely to contribute to the survival of the fungus in the host. It is also likely that the awareness of these organisms as pathogens and perhaps the skills (or methods) in identifying these organisms have also increased.

REFERENCES

1. **Abi-Said, D. E., O. Uzon, I. Raad, H. Pinzcowski, and O. Vartivarian.** 1997. The epidemiology of hematogenous candidiasis caused by different *Candida* species. *Clin. Infect. Dis.* **24:**1122–1128.
2. **Abu-Elteen, K. H., A. M. Abdul Malek, and N. A. Abdul Wahid.** 1997. Prevalence and susceptibility of vaginal yeast isolates in Jordan. *Mycoses* **40:**179–185.
3. **Baily, G. G., C. B. Moore, S. M. Essayag, S. de Wit, J. P. Burnie, and D. W. Denning.** 1997. *Candida inconspicua,* a fluconazole-resistant pathogen in patients infected with human immunodeficiency virus. *Clin. Infect. Dis.* **25:**161–163.
4. **Borg-von Zepelin, M., H. Eiffert, M. Kann, and R. Ruchel.** 1993. Changes in the spectrum of fungal isolates: results from clinical specimens gathered in 1987/88 compared with those in 1991/92 in the university hospital Gottingen, Germany. *Mycoses* **36:**247–253.
5. **Boucher, H., S. Mercure, S. Montplaisir, and G. Lemay.** 1996. A novel group I intron in *Candida dubliniensis* is homologous to a *Candida albicans* intron. *Gene* **180:**189–196.
6. **Carlotti, A., A. Couble, J. Domingo, K. Miroy, and J. Villard.** 1996. Species-specific identification of *Candida krusei* by hybridization with the CkF1,2 DNA probe. *J. Clin. Microbiol.* **34:**1726–1731.
7. **Collazos, J., J. Mayo, and E. Martinez.** 1999. Changing spectrum of HIV infection and its associated conditions in Spain: the end of the beginning? *AIDS Patient Care Sex. Transm. Dis.* **13:**347–353.
8. **Costa, S. F., I. Marinho, E. A. Araujo, A. E. Manrique, E. A. Medeiros, and A. S. Levin.** 2000. Nosocomial fungaemia: a 2-year prospective study. *J. Hosp. Infect.* **45:**69–72.
9. **Csank, C., and K. Haynes.** 2000. *Candida glabrata* displays pseudohyphal growth. *FEMS Microbiol. Lett.* **189:**115–120.
10. **D'Agata, E. M., D. B. Mount, V. Thayer, and W. Schaffner.** 2000. Hospital-acquired infections among chronic hemodialysis patients. *Am. J. Kidney Dis.* **35:**1083–1088.
11. **D'Antonio, D., B. Violante, A. Mazzoni, T. Bonfini, M. A. Capuani, F. D'Aloia, A. Iacone, F. Schioppa, and F. Romano.** 1998. A nosocomial cluster of *Candida inconspicua* infections in patients with hematological malignancies. *J. Clin. Microbiol.* **36:**792–795.
12. **Donnelly, S. M., D. J. Sullivan, D. B. Shanley, and D. C. Coleman.** 1999. Phylogenetic analysis and rapid identification of *Candida dubliniensis* based upon analysis of *ACT1* intron and exon sequences. *Microbiology* **145:**1871–1882.
13. **Emmons, C. W., C. H. Binford, J. P. Utz, and K. J. Kwon-Chung.** 1977. Candidiasis, p. 185–210. *In Medical Mycology,* 3rd ed. Lea and Febiger, Philadelphia, Pa.
14. **Essayag, S. M., G. G. Baily, D. W. Denning, and J. P. Burnie.** 1996. Karyotyping of fluconazole-resistant yeasts with a phenotype reported as *Candida krusei* or *Candida inconspicua. J. Clin. Microbiol.* **46:**35–40.
15. **Fernandez, M., E. H. Moylett, D. E. Noyola, and C. J. Baker.** 2000. Candidal meningitis in neonates: a 10-year review. *Clin. Infect. Dis.* **31:**458–463.
16. **Fidel, P. L., J. A. Vazquez, and J. D. Sobel.** 1999. *Candida glabrata:* review of epidemiology, pathogenesis, and clinical disease with comparison to *C. albicans. Clin. Microbiol. Rev.* **12:**80–96.
17. **Friedman, S., S. E. Richardson, S. E. Jacobs, and K. O'Brien.** 2000. Systemic *Candida* infection in extremely low birth weight infants: short term morbidity and long-term neurodevelopmental outcome. *Pediatr. Infect. Dis.* **19:**499–504.
18. **Gargas, A., P. T. DePriest, M. Grube, and A. Tehler.** 1995. Multiple origins of lichen symbioses in fungi suggested by SSU rDNA phylogeny. *Science* **268:**1492–1495.
19. **Hazen, K. C.** 1995. New and emerging yeast infections. *Clin. Microbiol. Rev.* **8:**462–478.
20. **Hazen, K. C., G. W. Theisz, and S. A. Howell.** 1991. Chronic urinary tract infection due to *Candida utilis. J. Clin. Microbiol.* **37:**824–827.
21. **Huang, Y. C., T. Y. Lin, H. S. Leu, H. L. Peng, J. H. Wu, and H. Y. Chang.** 1999. Outbreak of *Candida parapsilosis* fungemia in neonatal intensive care units: clinical implications and genotyping analysis. *Infection* **27:**97–102.
22. **Hull, C. M., R. M. Raisner, and A. D. Johnson.** 2000. Evidence for mating of the "asexual" yeast *Candida albicans* in a mammalian host. *Science* **289:**307–310.
23. **Hung, C. C., M. Y. Chen, S. M. Hsieh, W. H. Sheng, and S. C. Chang.** 2000. Clinical spectrum, morbidity, and mortality of acquired immunodeficiency syndrome in Taiwan: a 5-year prospective study. *J. Acquir. Immune Defic. Syndr.* **24:** 378–385.
24. **Janbon, G., F. Sherman, and E. Rustchenko.** 1998. Monosomy of a specific chromosome determines L-sorbose utilization: a novel regulatory mechanism in *Candida albicans. Proc. Natl. Acad. Sci. USA* **95:**5150–5155.
25. **Kao, A. S., M. E. Brandt, W. R. Pruitt, L. A. Conn, B. A. Perkins, D. S. Stephens, W. S. Baughman, A. L. Reingold, G. A. Rothrock, M. A. Pfaller, R. W. Pinner, and R. A. Hajjeh.** 1999. The epidemiology of candidemia in two United States cities: results of population-based active surveillance. *Clin. Infect. Dis.* **29:**1164–1170.
26. **Knoke, M., K. Schulz, and H. Bernhardt.** 1997. Dynamics of *Candida* isolations from humans from 1992–1995 in Greifswald, Germany. *Mycoses* **40:**105–110.
27. **Kobayashi, H., M. Takaku, Y. Nishidate, S. Takahashi, N. Shibata, and S. Suzuki.** 1992. Structure of the D-mannan of the pathogenic yeast, *Candida stellatoidea* ATCC 20408 (type II) strain, in comparison with that of *C. stellatoidea* ATCC 36232 (type I) strain. *Carbohydr. Res.* **231:**105–116.
28. **Kremery, V., Jr., and G. Kovacicova.** 2000. Longitudinal 10-year prospective survey of fungaemia in Slovak Republic: trends in etiology in 310 episodes. Slovak Fungaemia Group. *Diagn. Microbiol. Infect. Dis.* **36:**7–11.
29. **Kurtzman, C. P., and J. W. Fell.** 1998. *The Yeasts, a Taxonomic Study,* 4th ed. Elsevier Science, BV, Amsterdam, The Netherlands.
30. **Kwon-Chung, K. J., W. S. Riggsby, R. A. Uphoff, J. B. Hicks, W. L. Whelan, E. Reiss, B. B. Magee, and B. L. Wickes.** 1989. Genetic differences between type I and type II *Candida stellatoidea. Infect. Immun.* **57:**527–532.
31. **Kwon-Chung, K. J., B. L. Wickes, and W. G. Merz.** 1988. Association of electrophoretic karyotype of *Candida stella-*

toidea with virulence of mice. *Infect. Immun.* **56:**1814–1819.

32. **Listemann, H., K. D. Schulz, R. Wasmuth, F. Begemann, and W. Meigel.** 1998. Oesophagitis caused by *Candida kefyr. Mycoses* **41:**343–344.
33. **Lynch, M. E., J. D. Sobel, and P. L. Fidel, Jr.** 1996. Role of antifungal drug resistance in the pathogenesis of recurrent vulvovaginal candidiasis. *J. Med. Vet. Mycol.* **34:**337–339.
34. **Magee, B. B., and P. T. Magee.** 2000. Induction of mating in *Candida albicans* by construction of *MTL*a and *MTL*α strains. *Science* **289:**310–313.
35. **Mardani, M., H. A. Hanna, E. Gregory, and I. Raad.** Nosocomial *Candida guilliermondii* fungemia in cancer patients. *Infect. Con. Hosp. Epidemiol.* **21:**336–337.
36. **Meiller, T. F., M. A. Jabra-Rizk, A. Baqui, J. I. Kelley, V. I. Meeks, W. G. Merz, and W. A. Falker.** 1999. Oral *Candida dubliniensis* as a clinically important species in HIV-seropositive patients in the US. *Oral Surg. Oral Med. Oral Pathol. Oral Radiol.* **88:**573–580.
37. **Meis, J. F., F. M. Lunel, P. E. Vermeij, and A. Voss.** 2000. One-year prevalence of *Candida dubliniensis* in a Dutch university hospital. *J. Clin. Microbiol.* **38:**3139–3140.
38. **Moran, G. P., D. J. Sullivan, M. C. Henman, C. E. McCreary, B. J. Harrington, D. B. Shanley, and D. C. Coleman.** 1997. Antifungal drug susceptibilities of oral *Candida dubliniensis* isolates from human immunodeficiency virus (HIV)-infected and non-HIV infected subjects and generation of stable fluconazole-resistant derivatives in vitro. *Antimicrob. Agents Chemother.* **41:**617–623.
39. **Nucci, M., M. Silveira, N. Spector, F. Silveira, E. Velasco, C. Martins, A. Derossi, A. Columbo, and W. Pulcheri.** 1998. Fungemia in cancer patients in Brazil: predominance of non-albicans species. *Mycopathologia* **141:**65–68.
40. **Odds, F. C.** 1988. Biological aspects of pathogenic *Candida* spp., p. 7–15. *In Candida and Candidosis.* Bailliere Tindall, London, United Kingdom.
41. **Odds, F. C., and R. Bernaerts.** 1994. CHROMagar Candida, a new differential isolation medium for presumptive identification of clinically important *Candida* species. *J. Clin. Microbiol.* **32:**1923–1929.
42. **Pfaller, M. A., R. N. Jones, G. V. Doern, A. C. Fluit, J. Verhoef, H. S. Sader, S. A. Messer, A. Houston, S. Coffman, and R. J. Hollis.** 1999. International surveillance of blood stream infections due to *Candida* species in the European SENTRY program: species distribution and antifungal susceptibility including the investigational triazole and echinocandin agents. SENTRY Participant Group (Europe). *Diagn. Microbiol. Infect. Dis.* **35:**19–25.
43. **Pfaller, M. A., R. N. Jones, G. V. Doern, H. S. Sader, S. A. Messer, A. Houston, S. Coffman, and R. J. Hollis.** 2000. Bloodstream infections due to *Candida* species: SENTRY antimicrobial surveillance program in North America and Latin America, 1997–1998. *Antimicrob. Agents Chemother.* **44:**747–751.
44. **Polacheck, I., J. Strahilevitz, D. Sullivan, S. Donnelly, I. F. Salkin, and D. C. Coleman.** 2000. Recovery of *Candida dubliniensis* from non-human immunodeficiency virus-infected patients in Israel. *J. Clin. Microbiol.* **38:**170–174.
45. **Quindos, G., F. Cabrera, M. Arilla, A. Burgos, R. Ortiz-Vigon, J. Canon, and J. Ponton.** 1994. Fatal *Candida famata* peritonitis in a patient undergoing continuous ambulatory peritoneal dialysis who was treated with fluconazole. *Clin. Infect. Dis.* **18:**658–660.
46. **Raber-Durlacher, J. E., N. I. Weijl, M. Abu Saris, B. deKoning, A. H. Zwinderman, and S. Osanto.** 2000. Oral mucositis in patients with chemotherapy for solid tumors: a retrospective analysis of 150 cases. *Support Care Cancer* **8:**366–371.
47. **Rangel-Frausto, M. S., T. Wilbin, H. M. Blumberg, L. Saiman, J. Patterson, M. Rinaldi, M. Pfaller, J. E. Edwards, W. Jarvis, Jr., J. Dawson, and R. P. Wenzel.** 1999. National epidemiology of mycoses (NEMIS): variations in rates of bloodstream infections due to *Candida* species in seven surgical intensive care units and six neonatal intensive care units. *Clin. Infect. Dis.* **29:**253–258.
48. **Redding, S. W., R. C. Zellars, W. R. Kirkpatrick, R. K. McAtee, M. A. Caceres, A. W. Fothergill, J. L. Lopez-Ribot, C. W. Bailey, M. G. Rinaldi, and T. F. Patterson.** 1999. Epidemiology of oropharyngeal *Candida* colonization and infection in patients receiving radiation for head and neck cancer. *J. Clin. Microbiol.* **37:**3896–3900.
49. **Rennert, G., H. S. Rennert, S. Pitlik, R. Finkelstein, and R. Kitzes-Cohen.** 2000. Epidemiology of candidiemia—a nationwide survey in Israel. *Infection* **28:**26–29.
50. **Rippon, J. W.** 1974. Candidosis, p. 175–204. *In* J. W. Rippon (ed.), *Medical Mycology: The Pathogenic Fungi and the Pathogenic Actinomycetes.* W. B. Saunders Co., Philadelphia, Pa.
51. **Salkin, I. F., W. R. Pruitt, A. A. Padhye, D. Sullivan, D. Coleman, and D. H. Pincus.** 1998. Distinctive carbohydrate assimilation profiles used to identify the first clinical isolates of *Candida dubliniensis* recovered in the United States. *J. Clin. Microbiol.* **36:**1467–1468.
52. **Sandhu, D. K., R. S. Sandhu, and V. C. Misra.** 1976. Isolation of *Candida viswanathii* from cerebrospinal fluid. *Sabouraudia* **14:**251–254.
53. **Schauer, F., and R. Hanschke.** 1999. Taxonomy and ecology of the genus *Candida. Mycoses* **42**(Suppl. 1)**:**12–21.
54. **Schorling, S. R., H. C. Kortinga, M. Froschb, and F. A. Muhlschegel.** 2000. The role of *Candida dubliniensis* in oral candidiasis in human immunodeficiency virus-infected individuals. *Crit. Rev. Microbiol.* **26:**59–68.
55. **St.-Germain, G., and M. Laverdiere.** 1986. *Torulopsis candida,* a new opportunistic pathogen. *J. Clin. Microbiol.* **24:**884–885.
56. **Sullivan, D., and D. Coleman.** 1998. *Candida dubliniensis:* characteristics and identification. *J. Clin. Microbiol.* **36:**329–334.
57. **Sullivan, D., K. Haynes, J. Bille, P. Boerlin, L. Rodero, S. Lloyd, M. Henman, and D. Coleman.** 1997. Widespread geographic distribution of oral *Candida dubliniensis* in human immunodeficiency virus-infected individuals. *J. Clin. Microbiol.* **35:**960–964.
58. **Sullivan, D. J., T. J. Westerneng, K. A. Haynes, S. E. Bennett, and D. C. Coleman.** 1995. *Candida dubliniensis* sp. nov.: phenotypic and molecular characterization of a novel species associated with oral candidosis in HIV-infected individuals. *Microbiology* **141:**1507–1521.
59. **Tumbarello, M., E. Tacconelli, K. deGaetano Donati, G. Morace, G. Fadda, and R. Cauda.** 1999. Candidemia in HIV-infected patients. *Eur. J. Clin. Microbiol. Infect. Dis.* **18:**478–483.
60. **Viscoli, C., C. Girmenia, A. Marinus, L. Collette, P. Martino, B. Vandercam, C. Doyen, B. Lebeau, D. Spence, V. Kremery, B. De Pauw, and F. Meunier.** 1999. Candidemia in cancer patients: a prospective, multicenter surveillance study by the Invasive Fungal Infection Group (IFIG) of the European Organization for Research and Treatment of Cancer (EORTC). *Clin. Infect. Dis.* **28:**1071–1079.
61. **Willis, A. M., W. A. Coulter, D. J. Sullivan, D. C. Coleman, J. R. Hayes, P. M. Bell, and P. J. Lamey.** Isolation of *Candida dubliniensis* from insulin-using diabetes mellitus patients. *J. Oral Pathol. Med.* **29:**86–90.
62. **Wingard, J. R.** 1995. Importance of *Candida* species other than

C. albicans as pathogens in oncology patients. *Clin. Infect. Dis.* **20:**115–125.

63. **Wingard, J. R., W. G. Merz, M. G. Rinaldi, T. R. Johnson, J. E. Karp, and R. Saral.** 1991. Increase in *Candida krusei* infection among patients with bone marrow transplantation and neutropenia treated prophylactically with fluconazole. *N. Engl. J. Med.* **18:**1274–1277.
64. **Wingard, J. R., W. G. Merz, M. G. Rinaldi, C. B. Miller, J. E. Karp, and R. Saral.** 1993. Association of *Torulopsis glabrata* infections with fluconazole prophylaxis in neutropenic bone marrow transplant patients. *Antimicrob. Agents Chemother.* **37:**1847–1849.
65. **Wong, P., S. Mak, K. Lo, G. Tong, and A. Wong.** 2000. A retrospective study of seven cases of *Candida parapsilosis* peritonitis in CAPD patients: the therapeutic implications. *Perit. Dial. Int.* **20:**76–79.

Candida and Candidiasis
Edited by Richard A. Calderone

Chapter 3

Serological Differences among the Pathogenic *Candida* spp.

SHIGEO SUZUKI

This chapter focuses on the recent findings of the serological investigations of the pathogenic *Candida* species with the intent to develop a serological classification and procedures that might be used in the identification of species of *Candida*. Because of the increased number of cases of candidiasis in immunocompromised patients caused by the comparatively less pathogenic non-*C. albicans* species of *Candida* such as *C. dubliniensis, C. glabrata, C. inconspicua, C. lusitaniae,* and *C. utilis,* as described in chapter 2 classical serological analysis should be extended to include these newly recognized pathogenic species. In this chapter, I will attempt to correlate phenotypic properties (chemical structure of the antigenic polysaccharide mannans) with genotypic data (18S rRNA evolutionary and 18S rDNA phylogenetic trees) to provide a novel concept for predicting serological specificities by phylogenetic alignments of the emerging *Candida* spp.

MANNAN AS THE MAJOR ANTIGEN OF *CANDIDA* SPECIES

Serological diversity in *Candida* spp. and especially *C. albicans* was first described by Hasenclever and Mitchell in 1961 (5). This species was classified into two serotypes, A and B, based on cross-agglutination reactions of the serotypes by using heterologous antisera. Thereafter, Summers et al. (28) revealed that mannan, one of the cell wall polysaccharides of *Candida* spp., rather than β-glucan or chitin, contributes to the serological specificity of each *Candida* sp.

ESTABLISHMENT OF AN ANTIGENIC FORMULA FOR THE MEDICALLY RELEVANT *CANDIDA* SPECIES

During the early 1950s, Tsuchiya and his coworkers (35) also began an intensive serological study of yeasts, and in 1968, Fukazawa et al. (3) described the antigenic formula of seven medically important *Candida* spp. that included 10 antigenic factors or epitopes. Subsequently, these workers developed 10 polyclonal rabbit factor sera, designated 1, 4, 5, 6, 8, 9, 11, 13, 13b, and 34, for identifying the seven *Candida* spp., i.e., *C. albicans* type A, *C. albicans* type B (including *C. stellatoidea*), *C. tropicalis, C. guilliermondii, C. krusei, C. parapsilosis, C. kefyr* (formerly *C. pseudotropicalis*), and *C. glabrata* (*Torulopsis glabrata*). "Candida Check" IgG fractions of the 10 factor sera have been available commercially from Iatron, Tokyo, Japan, since the early 1970s. The manual of Candida Check describes the antigenic formula of medically relevant *Candida* spp. as shown in Table 1, slightly modified from the original data described by Tsuchiya et al. (35a) in 1984. Shinoda et al. (27) published a comparative study of Candida Check and API 20C for the identification of medically important *Candida* spp., including a table of the formula of the major pathogenic fungi *Candida* spp. Among the 10 antigenic factors from 1 to 34, the first former one corresponds to α-1,2-linked oligomannosyl residues that range in size from a biose to tetraose, Mα1-2M to Mα1-2Mα1-2Mα1-2M. Antigenic factor 1 is common to all *Candida* spp., whereas the other sera (anti-4 to anti-34) correspond to each of the other specific epitopes. In practical operations, therefore, serum factor 1 can be used for the identification of all *Candida* spp. from a mixture of different yeasts, whereas the other sera can be used to differentiate *Candida* spp. by serial agglutination procedures, as also described in the manual of Candida Check (chart not shown). However, reproducibility of this procedure is problematic because of the polyclonal nature of the factor sera. Therefore, development of a large-scale production of the 10 monoclonal factor antibodies and a microscale flow-cytometry system for fractionation of the *Candida* cell mixture should be initiated.

Shigeo Suzuki • Sendai Research Institute for Mycology, 1-14-34, Toshogu, Aoba-ku, Sendai 981-0908, Miyagi, Japan.

Table 1. Antigenic formula of medically important *Candida* species[a]

Strain (serotype)	Antigenic factor									
C. albicans (A)	1	4	5	6						
C. albicans (B)[d]	1	4	5						13b[c]	
C. tropicalis	1	4	5	6[b]						
C. guilliermondii	1	4				9				
C. krusei	1						11			
C. parapsilosis	1							13	13b	
C. kefyr (*C. pseudotropicalis*)	1				8					
C. glabrata (*Torulopsis glabrata*)	1	4		6						34

[a]This table is based on the description by Tsuchiya et al. (35a) and was cited from the *Candida Check* manual (6). For more details, see also Fukazawa et al. (3), Shinoda et al. (27), and Tsuchiya et al. (35).
[b]A part of strains lacks this factor.
[c]A part of strains possesses this factor.
[d]Including *C. stellatoidea.*

SEROLOGICAL PROPERTIES OF MANNANS OF *CANDIDA* SPECIES

The general structure of the antigenic mannans of the major medically relevant *Candida* spp. (Table 2) provided by Suzuki (33) indicates that all mannans, except that of *C. krusei,* possess a highly branched structure and that these branches correspond to each specific epitope, i.e., antigenic factors. These findings were obtained by a series of degradation reactions of the mannans, such as partial acid hydrolysis, alkali degradation, acetolysis, and α-mannosidase digestion, to give various elimination (degradation) products that can be compared by proton magnetic resonance (PMR) spectra to the intact mannans. Among these procedures, acetolysis under mild conditions, developed by Kobayashi et al. (14), is indispensable in providing important structural information related to the serological specificities of the parent yeast cells as shown in Table 2 (33). Antigenicity of each mannan and its degradation products can be analyzed by an enzyme-linked immunosorbent assay using both polyclonal and monoclonal anti-*Candida* sera, as reviewed by Mathews (18). It is noteworthy that yeast mannans (mannoproteins) are readily adsorbed on the surface of polystyrene microtiter plates by hydrophobic bond formation via their protein moiety as reported by Tojo et al. (34). Furthermore, each polyclonal rabbit factor serum in Candida Check can also be used for serological investigation of *Candida* mannans by an enzyme-linked immunosorbent assay, although extreme care should be taken in interpreting results. For example, Shibata et al. (26) and Kobayashi et al. (12) reported a cross-reaction between the mannans of *C. guilliermondii* and *C. famata* with factor 9 serum that recognizes two entirely different structures.

The growth conditions for *Candida* spp., especially temperature, are important, e.g., *C. albicans* serotype A does not form β-1,2 linkages in the mannan of cells grown in yeast extract-glucose-peptone medium at 37°C, as reported by Okawa et al. (22). For structural investigations, the method of isolating mannan from cells of *Candida* is important, i.e., conditions should not be drastic to avoid cleavage of labile sugar residues by exposing the mannan to high concentrations of acid and/or alkali. By far, the best method is a combination of hot water extraction of the yeast cells according to Peat et al. (23), followed by the fractional precipitation of the crude extract with cetyltrimethylammonium bromide (Cetavlon) as described by Lloyd (17). These extractions can be done on a small scale, i.e., cultivation of *Candida* cells in 1 liter of a glucose-peptone medium, and extraction of mannan as an aqueous suspension in an autoclave. Fractional precipitation of the mannan can be done in a 50-ml centrifuge tube. Another fractionation procedure using Fehling's solution and then removing the copper ion by a cation-exchange resin is more facile for most serological investigations (33).

Because mannans are found in the cell wall as mannoprotein, it is desirable to isolate the intact molecule. Recent findings by Watanabe et al. (37) on the isolation of a mannoprotein from the culture filtrate of a *C. albicans* type A strain grown in RPMI 1640 medium at 37°C that causes hemolysis (hemolytic factor) are of interest because a PMR spectrum of this mannoprotein exhibited the presence of antigenic factors 5 and 6.

SEROLOGICAL CHARACTERIZATION OF THE EMERGING NON-*C. ALBICANS* SPECIES

Since the early 1980s, several non-*C. albicans* species, *C. dubliniensis, C. famata, C. glabrata* (*T.

Table 2. General structure for two groups of mannans of *C. albicans, C. tropicalis, C. stellatoidea, C. glabrata, C. guilliermondii,* and *C. kefyr* possessing different lengths of branches corresponding to α-1,2-linked mannotetraosyl and α-1,2-linked mannotriosyl moieties, respectively[a]

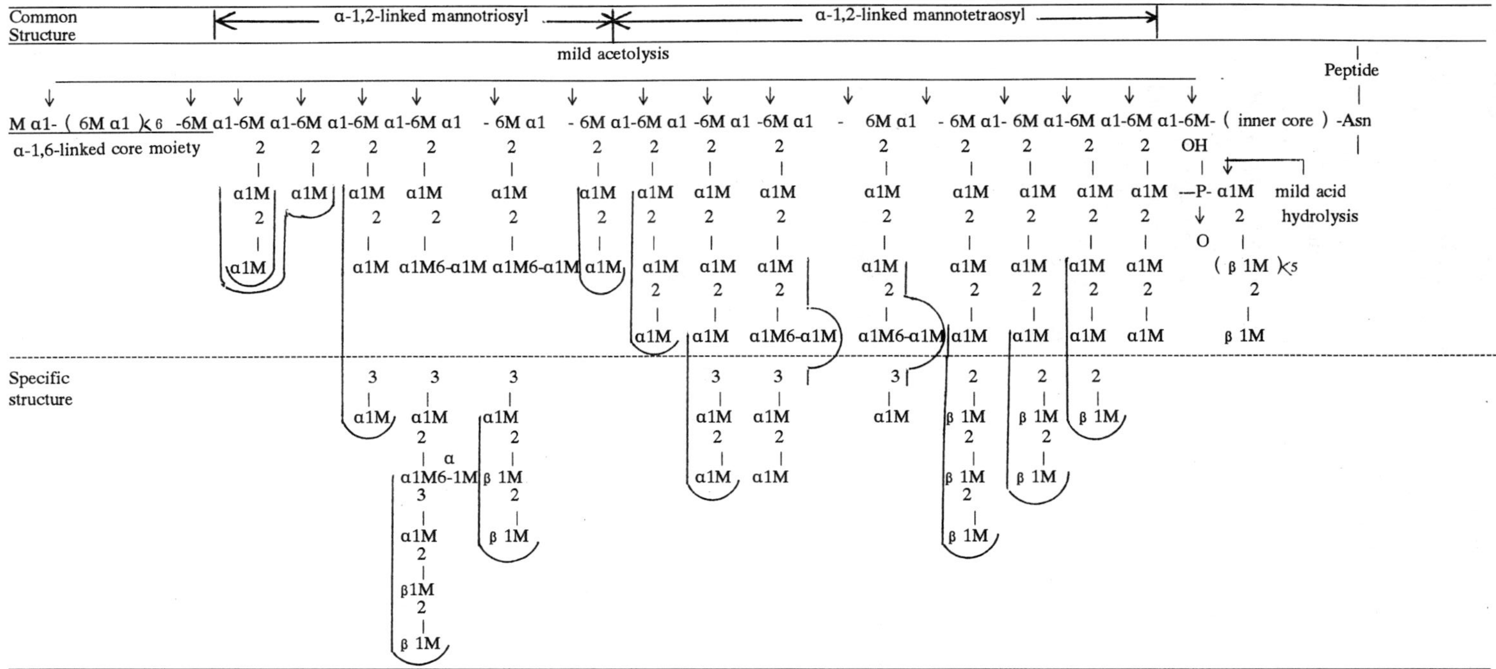

Antigenic factor	9'	8/1	34	9	9	1	1	13b	4	4	6/5	6/5	6	5
Species	*Cf* *C.sa* *C.gu*	*C.k*	*C.gl*	*C.gu*	*C.gu*	All species	All species	*C.a* (A) *C.p*	*C.a* (A) *C.a* (B) *C.s* *C.p* *C.t*	*C.a* *C.a* (B) *C.s* *C.t*	*C.a* (A)	*C.a* (A)	*C.a* (A)	*C.a* (A) *C.a* (B) *C.s* *C.t* *C.g*

[a]Mild acetolysis and mild acid-hydrolysis indicate the labile bonds, consecutive α-1,6 linkages in the backbone moiety of mannan and 1-O-α-phosphorylated mannose unit, respectively. O-Linked sugar residues on the peptide moiety were not depicted because of the negligible extent of their participation in antibody-binding effect of the parent mannans due to low densities. M denotes a mannopyranose unit. The sequence of branches or antigenic factors was not specified. *C.a, C. albicans; C.f, C. famata; C.s, C. stellatoiodea; C.sa, C. saitoana; C.t, C. tropicalis; C.gl, C. glabrata; C.gu, C. guilliermondii; C.k, C. krusei; C.p, C. parapsilosis.* Reprinted from reference 33 with permission of Prous Science.

glabrata), *C. inconspicua, C. kefyr* (*C. pseudotropicalis*), *C. lusitaniae, C. parapsilosis, C. utilis,* and *C. viswanathii,* have been isolated from immunocompromised patients as discussed in chapter 2. Among these *Candida* species, *C. glabrata* and *C. kefyr* have been included in the antigenic formula of medically relevant *Candida* species proposed by Tsuchiya et al. (35a) in 1984 (Table 1). In this section, important serological findings on these *Candida* mannans will be discussed. However, *C. inconspicua* is not included in this discussion because it has not been studied in any great detail.

Candida dubliniensis

Sullivan and coworkers demonstrated the location of *C. dublinensis* in an unrooted evolutionary tree and its phylogenetic relationship to other *Candida* spp. (29). Such data indicate that *C. dubliniensis* is quite close phylogenetically to *C. albicans*. It should be noted that antigenic factor 6 is common to both *C. dubliniensis* and *C. albicans,* as pointed out by Sullivan (29) and Kamei et al. (8); this common feature correlates well with the phylogenetic proximity of both species. However, structural investigations of the *C. dubliniensis* mannan using degradation procedures have not yet been done.

Candida famata

Shibata et al. compared the mannan of a *C. famata* strain with those of *C. guilliermondii* and *C. saitoi* (26). They proposed that these species have a common reactivity with factor serum 9, in spite of the existence of a large structural difference between the mannans of *C. famata* and those of *C. guiiliermondii* and *C. saitoi*. For example, *C. famata* lacks a β-1,2-linked mannose residue in its mannan whereas the other two species have the residue. Kobayashi et al. (12) have shown that an α-1,6-linked oligomannosyl residue, Mα1-(6Mα1)n-6Mα1-, is able to react with factor 9 serum, demonstrating the existence of each of the two factor 9 epitopes in the mannan and of antibodies in the factor 9 serum (see Table 2). In the same year, Nishikawa et al. (20) published a taxonomic study of five clinical isolates of *C. famata,* showing that two isolates were identified as *Debaryomyces hansenii* var. *hansenii* whereas two other isolates were *D. hansenii* var. *fabryi,* and the fifth was *C. guilliermondii*. Nishikawa et al. (20) also demonstrated PMR spectra of these mannans. Their data indicate a strong chemical shift at 5.07 ppm, corresponding to the α-1,6-linked oligomannosyl residue identified by Shibata et al. (26). These findings strongly suggest the importance of developing monoclonal factor antibodies.

Candida glabrata

As shown in Table 1, yeast cells of *C. glabrata* contain the four antigenic factors, 1, 4, 6, and 34. An investigation by Kobayashi et al. (10) revealed a mannan consisting of the following structural oligosaccharide branches: Antigenic factor 1, Mα1-2M and Mα1-2Mα1-2M; antigenic factor 6, Mβ1-2Mα1-2M and Mβ1-2Mα1-2Mα1-2Mα1-2Mα1-2Mα1-2M; antigenic factor 34, Mα1-3Mα1-2Mα1-2M and Mα1-3Mα1-2Mα1-2Mα1-2Mα1-2Mα1-2M. Kobayashi et al. (13) further defined the positive reactivity of this mannan with factor 4 serum in spite of the absence of antigenic factor 4, Mα1-3(Mα1-6)Mα1-2M. However, factor 4 serum contains small amounts of factor 6 antibody, which cross-reacts with the antigenic factor 6 epitope, Mβ1-2Mα1-2M. This finding again strongly suggests the need to develop monoclonal antifactor antibodies.

Candida kefyr (*pseudotropicalis*)

According to Tsuchiya et al. (35a) (Table 1), yeast cells of this species possess only two antigenic factors, 1 and 8. The results of a structural analysis of the mannan from *C. kefyr* IFO 0586 strain conducted by Kobayashi et al. (9) yielded a relatively simple structure as shown in Table 2. These workers identified antigenic factor 8 as one of the branched pentaose structures, Mα1-2Mα1-2(Mα1-2Mα1-6)M (12).

Candida lusitaniae

Little information is available on the mannan structure of this species, except for preliminary studies by Shibata et al. (described in a review by Suzuki [32] in 1996). It was demonstrated that the mannan contains branches corresponding to antigenic factor 6, Mβ1-2Mβ1-2Mβ1-2Mα1-2Mα1-2M, Mβ1-2Mβ1-2Mα1-2Mα1-2M, and Mβ1-2Mβ1-2Mα1-2M. Because the maximum length of an α-1,2-linked mannose residue is limited to a triose, Mα1-2Mα1-2M, it is possible to group this species in the non-*C. albicans* group.

Candida parapsilosis

Yeast cells of this species possess antigenic factors 1, 13, and 13b (Table 1). In 1995, Shibata et al. (24) published the structural determination of the mannans of a *C. parapsilosis* strain in comparison to that of a *C. albicans* serotype B strain that contains antigenic factors 1, 4, and 5. Interestingly, antigenic factor 4 possesses a pentaose structure common to antigenic factor 13b, Mα1-2Mα1-3Mα1-2Mα1-2M, which can be converted into an antigen common to factor 4 by introducing one 6-O-linked mannose residue at the 3-O-substituted mannose residue to give a branched hexaose structure, Mα1-2Mα1-3(Mα1-6)Mα1-2Mα1-2M. To develop a modified serodiagnostic procedure for *C. parapsilosis,* therefore, preparation of the two monoclonal antibodies corresponding to antigenic factors 4 and 13b is desirable. It is also noteworthy that the minimum common structure of the mannans of both *C. albicans* serotype B and *C. parapsilosis* is an α-1,2-linked mannotetraosyl residue, Mα1-2Mα1-2Mα1-2M, indicating that *C. parapsilosis* belongs to the *C. albicans* group. This view is supported by the data of Gorin and Spencer on chemotaxonomy of yeasts by PMR spectrometry of the mannose-containing polysaccharides (4) and by the observation on the 18S rRNA evolutionary and 18S rDNA phylogenetic trees proposed by Barns et al. (1) and Suzuki et al. (31), respectively. Because of the latter observation, *C. parapsilosis* is phylogenetically aligned closely to *C. albicans* on the basis of these three taxonomic procedures. Recently, De Bernardis et al. (2) described the biotyping and virulence of skin isolates of *C. parapsilosis.*

Candida utilis

The cell wall of *C. utilis* was shown to contain a glucomannan. To determine the structure, the glucomannan was investigated by acetolysis, methylation, and PMR spectrometry. According to the findings by Ogawa et al. (21) in 1990 on a *C. utilis* strain, the structure of the glucomannan resembled that of the other *Candida* spp. except that the longer tetra- and pentasaccharide side chains are terminated with a glucosyl residue as follows: Gα1-6Mα1-2Mα1-2M and Gα1-6Mα1-2Mα1-2Mα1-2M. On the other hand, Kogan et al. (15) published a different structure for a *C. utilis* mannan, i.e., the longer side chain has an α-1,2-linked glucosyl residue at the nonreducing terminals as follows: Gα1-2Mα1-2Mα1-2Mα1-2M and Gα1-2(Mα1-3)Mα1-2Mα1-2Mα1-2M. Therefore, depending on the strain used for study, structural differences that accompany serological diversity can be seen in the glucomannans of this species.

Candida viswanathii

Gorin and Spencer (4) showed by PMR spectrometry that the mannan of *C. viswanathii* could be classified in the *Pichia robertsii–Candida tropicalis* group, in which a *C. albicans* serotype A strain was included. However, subsequently, there have been only a few descriptions on the serological and pathological properties of this *Candida* sp., except for a report by Vecchiarelli et al. (36). These investigators compared in vitro killing of *Candida* species by murine immunoeffector cells and demonstrated almost the same resistance to killing as that of *C. albicans,* whereas *C. parapsilosis* cells were killed much more quickly. Therefore, *C. viswanathii* can be regarded as one of the emerging *Candida* pathogens. Furthermore, both 18S rRNA evolutionary and 18S rDNA phylogenetic findings on *C. viswanathii* provided by Barns et al. (1) and Suzuki et al. (31), respectively, substantiate its close proximity to *C. albicans* species. This assumption can be confirmed by characterization of an α-1,2-linked mannotetraosyl residue, Mα1-2Mα1-2Mα1-2M in the mannan oligosacchrides obtained by acetolysis of this mannan.

CORRELATION AMONG CHEMICAL STRUCTURE OF MANNANS AND 18S rRNA—AN EVOLUTIONARY TREE OF MEDICALLY RELEVANT *CANDIDA* SPECIES

As shown in Table 2, Suzuki and coworkers (33) have conducted a series of structural investigations of mannans of the major pathogenic *Candida* spp. that provide a general structure of these mannans. The data indicate that the mannans of *C. albicans* group possess α-1,2-linked mannotetraosyl residues, Mα1-2Mα1-2Mα1-2M, which is the longest branch of a common structure, whereas those of the non-*C. albicans* group contain α-1,2-linked mannotriosyl residues, Mα1-2Mα1-2M. Subsequently, we have attempted to correlate the structural differences of mannans and with phylogenetic data of *Candida* spp. An 18S rRNA evolutionary tree of major *Candida* spp. and their relatives, proposed by Barns et al. (1) (Fig. 1A), can be divided into three clusters, *C. albicans* or "top," non-*C. albicans* or "middle," and galactomannan or "bottom." These data, apparently, correlate with the results of structural investigation of mannans as revealed by Kobayashi et al. in a preliminary communication (11). The study by Barns et al. (1) is noteworthy because it is the first description of the relationship between evolution and structural differences in mannan. These workers state that PMR studies by Gorin and Spencer (4) published in 1970 also group *C. albicans, C. tropicalis, C. viswanathii, C. guilliermondii,* and *C. lusitaniae.* With *C. lusitaniae,* Melo et al. (19) demonstrated a significant change of location of this species in an evolutionary tree obtained by randomly amplified polymorphic DNA

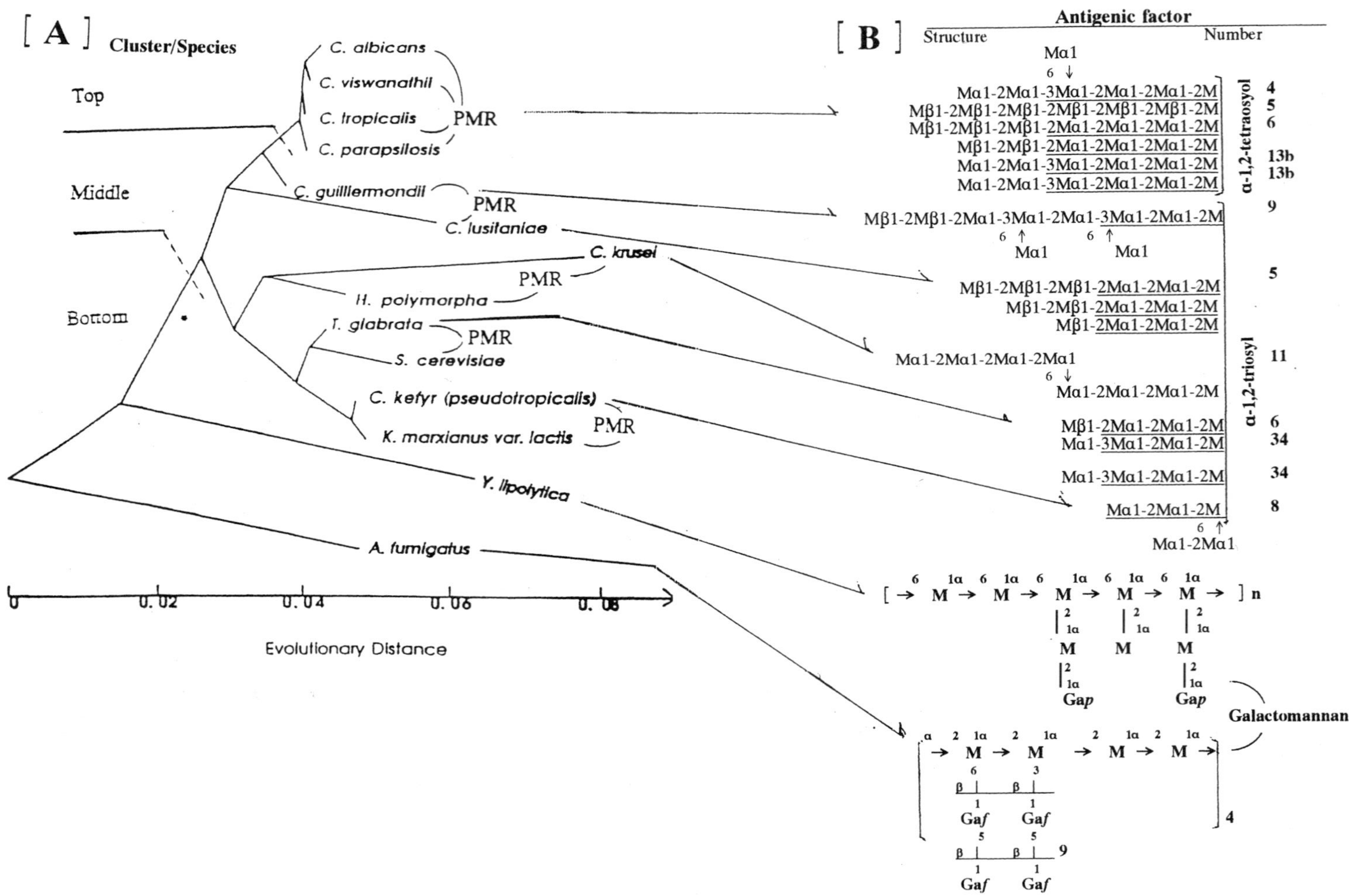

Figure 1. Correlation of the 18S rRNA evolutionary tree (A) proposed by Barns et al. (1) with the chemical structures of antigenic factors (B) of medically relevant *Candida* species summarized by Suzuki (33). Note that antigenic factors 4, 6, and 13b in *C. albicans* group of "top" cluster in common contain α-1,2-linked mannotetraosyl residue, Mα1-2Mα1-2M-2M, α-1,2-tetraosyl, while those of non-*C. albicans Candida* and non-*Candida* groups of "middle" cluster are α-1,2-linked mannotriosyl residue, Mα1-2Mα1-2M, α-1,2-tiosyl. These common residues in the structures are underlined (B). The structures of galactomannans of *C. lipolytica* (7) and *A. fumigatus* (16), "bottom" cluster, are also included. M, Ga*f*, and Ga*p*, denote mannosyl, galactofuranosyl, and galactopyranosyl, respectively. PRM indicates yeast species possessing mannans of resembled PMR spectra stated by Golin and Spencer (4) in 1970. Reprinted from Kobayashi et al. (11) with permission.

method in comparison with the location in the 18S rRNA evolutionary tree by Barns et al. (1).

These findings indicate that 18S rRNA contains the base sequences corresponding to mannosyl and/or galactosyl transferases for the synthesis of cell wall mannans and galactomannans. This view can be applied as a key concept for the classification of many fungi possessing mannose-containing polysaccharides.

On the basis of the suggestion by Barns et al. (1), more extensive data, including analytical data on the carbohydrate composition of cell wall, PMR spectra of mannose-containing polysaccharides, and coenzyme Q analysis, have been published by several workers during the past decade, as summarized by Suzuki and Nakase (30) in 1999. Therefore, the structural findings of manose-containing polysaccharides are important in solving the general evolutionary status of fungi as suggested by Gorin and Spencer (4). Because the structural difference of mannans between the two clusters, *C. albicans* and non-*C. albicans,* is attributable to only one α-1,2-linked mannose residue, further studies should be done on the identification of base sequences corresponding to the other mannosyl residues, α-1,3-, α-1,6-, and β-1,2-linked ones, composing antigenic factors 4, 5, 6, 9, 13, 13b, and 34.

Differences between the two clusters, middle and bottom, in Fig. 1A are quite clear, because *Yarrowia (C.) lipolytica* in the "bottom" cluster contains a galactomannan as reported by Ikuta et al. (7). A fisson yeast, *Schizosaccharomyces pombe,* which is grouped in the lower cluster of an 18S rDNA phylogenatic tree together with several of the *Candida* spp., as proposed by Suzuki and Nakase (30), also contains a galactomannan.

Furthermore, a euascomycetous fungus, *Aspergillus fumigatus,* which is placed in the bottom cluster of the evolutionary tree, was found to possess a galactomannan containing a β-galactofuranosyl residue, as reported by Latgé et al. (16). Therefore, the bottom cluster consists of fungi producing galactomannans, which have entirely different epitopes from those of many *Candida* and related genera in the top and middle clusters (Fig. 1B). It is therefore possible to state that the suggestion by Barns et al. (1) on the existence of a close relationship between 18S rRNA evolutionary tree and structural difference of mannans, shown in Fig. 1A and 1B, respectively, is now confirmed by providing structural data of mannans and galactomannans. This view is consistent with that implied by the finding that the 18S rDNA phylogenetic data correlate with a variety of *Candida* spp. as proposed by Suzuki and Nakase (30). As one of the applications of this concept, it is possible to predict that *C. dubliniensis,* closely related to *C. albicans,* will locate in the "top" cluster of the 18S rRNA evolutionary tree, if the α-1,2-linked mannotetraosyl residue is retained in the *C. dubliniensis* mannan.

CONCLUSIONS

This chapter summarizes the recent serological findings on the emerging *Candida* spp. in comparison to those species that have been previously described. The major points are as follows:

1. Presently, data on the serological properties of both whole cells and antigenic mannans of emerging *Candida* spp. seem to be insufficient to assemble an authentic identification procedure.
2. To develop a highly reproducible characterization procedure for any emerging *Candida* spp., improving the present serological procedures, especially the use of monoclonal factor sera corresponding to Candida Check, is desirable.
3. The chemotaxonomy of yeasts based on PMR spectrometry of mannan published by Gorin and Spencer in 1970 should be revised to include those of the novel *Candida* spp.
4. Correlation of the mannan chemical structure of *Candida* spp. with their alignment in the 18S rRNA evolutionary and 18S rDNA phylogenetic trees seems to be important as one of the identification procedures of *Candida* spp.
5. In the near future, it will be possible to identify any clinical isolate of *Candida* spp. by the improved procedures described above.

REFERENCES

1. **Barns, S. M., D. J. Lane, M. L. Sogin, C. Bibeau, and W. G. Weisburg.** 1991. Evolutionary relationships among pathogenic *Candida* species and relatives. *J. Bacteriol.* **173:**2250–2255.
2. **De Bernardis, F., F. Mondello, R. San Millan, J. Pouton, and A. Cassone.** 1999. Biotyping and virulence properties of skin isolates of *Candida parapsilosis. J. Clin. Microbiol.* **37:** 3481–3486.
3. **Fukazawa, Y., T. Shinoda, and T. Tsuchiya.** 1968. Response and specificity of antibodies for *Candida albicans. J. Bacteriol.* **95:**754–763.
4. **Gorin, P. A. J., and J. F. T. Spencer.** 1970. Proton magnetic resonance spectroscopy—an aid in identification and chemotaxonomy of yeasts. *Adv. Appl. Microbiol.* **13:**25–89.
5. **Hasenclever, H. R., and W. O. Mitchell.** 1961. Antigenic studies of *Candida.* I. Observation of two antigenic groups in *Candida albicans. J. Bacteriol.* **82:**570–573.
6. **Iatron Co. Ltd.** *Candida Check Manual.* Iatron Co. Ltd., Tokyo, Japan.
7. **Ikuta, K., N. Shibata, K. Hisamichi, H. Kobayashi, S. Suzuki, and Y. Okawa.** 1997. NMR assignment of the galactomannan of *Candida lipolytica. FEBS Lett.* **414:**338–342.

8. **Kamei, K., M. J. McCullough, and D. A. Stevens.** 2000. Initial case of *Candida dubliniensis* infection from Asia: non-mucosal infection. *Med. Mycol.* **38:**81–83.
9. **Kobayashi, H., M. Komido, M. Watanabe, K. Matsuda, M. Suzuki, T. Ikeda, H. Oyamada, N. Shibata, and S. Suzuki.** 1994. Structure of cell wall mannan of *Candida kefyr* IFO 0586. *Infect. Immun.* **62:**4425–4431.
10. **Kobayashi, H., H. Mitobe, K. Takahashi, T. Yamamoto, N. Shibata, and S. Suzuki.** 1992. Structural study of a cell wall mannan-protein complex of the pathogenic yeast *Candida glabrata* IFO 0622 strain. *Arch. Biochem. Biophys.* **294:** 662–669.
11. **Kobayashi, H., H. Oyamada, N. Shibata, Y. Okawa, and S. Suzuki.** 2000. Relationship between 18S rRNA evolutionary tree and chemical structures of mannan of medically relevant *Candida* species, p. 21–22. *In* J. P. van Dijken and W. A. Scheffers (ed.), *10th International Symposium on Yeasts.* Delft University Press, Delft, The Netherlands.
12. **Kobayashi, H., H. Oyamada, A. Suzuki, N. Shibata, S. Suzuki, and Y. Okawa.** 1996. Identification of the antigenic determinants of factors 8, 9, and 34 of genus *Candida. FEBS Lett.* **395:**109–112.
13. **Kobayashi, H., H. Oyamada, N. Iwadate, H. Suzuki, H. Motobe, K. Takahashi, N. Shibata, S. Suzuki, and Y. Okawa.** 1998. Structural and immunochemical characterization of β-1,2-linked mannobiosyl phosphate residue in the cell wall mannan of *Candida glabrata. Arch. Microbiol.* **169:**188–194.
14. **Kobayashi, H., N. Shibata, T. Yonezu, and S. Suzuki.** 1987. Structural study of phosphomannan-protein complex of *Citeromyces matritensis* containing a β-1,2 linkage: application of partial acid degradation and acetolysis techniques under mild conditions. *Arch. Biochem. Biophys.* **256:**381–396.
15. **Kogan, G., J. Ŝandula, and V. Ŝimkovicová.** 1993. Glucomannan from *Candida utilis.* Structural investigation. *Folia Microbiol.* **38:**219–224.
16. **Latgé, J.-P., H. Kobayashi, J.-P. Debeaupuis, M. Diaquin, J. Sarfati, J.-M. Wieruszeski, E. Parra, J.-P. Bouchara, and B. Fournet.** 1994. Chemical and immunological characterization of the extracellular galactomannan of *Aspergillus fumigatus. Infect. Immun.* **62:**5424–5433.
17. **Lloyd, K. O.** 1970. Isolation, characterization, and partial structure of peptide galactomannans from the yeast form of *Cladosporium werneckii. Biochemistry* **9:**3446–3453.
18. **Mathews, R. C.** 1996. Comparative assessment of the detection of candidal antigens as a diagnostic tool. *J. Med. Vet. Mycol.* **34:**1–10.
19. **Melo, A. S. A., L. P. de Almeida, A. L. Colombo, and M. R. S. Briones.** 1998. Evolutionary distances and identification of *Candida* species in clinical isolated by randomly amplified polymorphic DNA(RAPD). *Mycopathologia* **142:**57–66.
20. **Nishikawa, A., H. Tomomatsu, T. Suzuki, R. Ikeda, and T. Shinoda.** 1996. Taxonomic position of clinical isolates of *Candida famata. J. Med. Vet. Mycol.* **34:**411–419.
21. **Ogawa, K., K. Matsuda, K. Tamari, and S. Kiyooka.** 1990. Immunochemical analysis of the glucomannan from *Candida utilis. Agric. Biol. Chem.* **54:**596–597.
22. **Okawa, Y., T. Takahashi, M. Kawamata, M. Miyauchi, N. Shibata, A. Suzuki, H. Kobayashi, and S. Suzuki.** 1994. Temperature-dependent change of serological specificity of *Candida albicans* NIH A-207 cells cultured in yeast extract-added Sabouraud liquid medium: disappearance of surface antigenic factors 4, 5, and 6 at high temperature. *FEBS Lett.* **345:** 167–171.
23. **Peat, S., W. J. Whelan, and T. E. Edwards.** 1961. Polysaccharides of baker's yeast IV. Mannans. *J. Chem. Soc.* (London) **1:**29–34.
24. **Shibata, N., R. Akagi, T. Hosoya, K. Kawahara, A. Suzuki, K. Ikuta, H. Kobayashi, K. Hisamichi, Y. Okawa, and S. Suzuki.** 1995. Existence of novel branched side chains containing β-1,2 and α-1,6 linkages corresponding to antigenic factor 9 in the mannan of *Candida guilliermondii. J. Biol. Chem.* **271:** 9259–9266.
25. **Shibata, N., I. Ikuta, T. Imai, Y. Satoh, R. Satoh, A. Suzuki, C. Kojima, H. Kobayashi, K. Hisamichi, and S. Suzuki.** 1995. Existence of branched side chains in the cell wall mannan of pathogenic yeast, *Candida albicans. J. Biol. Chem.* **270:** 1113–1122.
26. **Shibata, N., M. Onozawa, N. Tadano, Y. Hinosawa, A. Suzuki, K. Ikuta, H. Kobayashi, S. Suzuki, and Y. Okawa.** 1996. Structure and antigenicity of the mannans of *Candida famata* and *Candida saitoi:* comparative study with the mannan of *Candida guilliermondii. Arch. Biochem. Biophys.* **336:**49–58.
27. **Shinoda, T., L. Kaufman, and A. A. Padye.** 1981. Comparative evaluation of the Iatron serological Candida Check kit and the API 20C kit for identification of medically important *Candida* species. *J. Clin. Microbiol.* **13:**513–517.
28. **Summers, D. F., A. P. Gollman, and H. F. Hasenclever.** 1964. Polysaccharide antigens of the *Candida* cell wall. *J. Immunol.* **92:**491–499.
29. **Sullivan, D., and D. Coleman.** 1997. *Candida dubliniensis:* an emerging opportunistic pathogen. *Curr. Top. Med. Mycol.* **8**(1–2):15–25.
30. **Suzuki, M., and T. Nakase.** 1999. A phylogenetic study of ubiquinone Q-8 species of the genera *Candida, Pichia,* and *Citeromyces* based on 18S ribosomal DNA sequence divergence. *J. Gen. Appl. Microbiol.* **45:**239–246.
31. **Suzuki, M., S. Q. Suh, T. Sugita, and T. Nakase.** 1999. A phylogenetic study of galactose-containing *Candida* species based on 18S ribosomal DNA sequences. *J. Gen. Appl. Microbiol.* **45:**229–238.
32. **Suzuki, S.** 1996. Structural investigation of mannans of medically relevant *Candida* species: determination of chemical structures of antigenic factors, 1, 4, 5, 6, 7, and 13b, p. 1–15. *In* S. Suzuki and M. Suzuki (ed.), *Fungal Cells in Biodefense Mechanism.* Saikon Publishing, Tokyo, Japan.
33. **Suzuki, S.** 1997. Immunochemical study on mannans of genus *Candida.* I. Structural investigation of antigenic factors 1, 4, 5, 6, 8, 9, 11, 13, 13b and 34. *Curr. Top. Med. Mycol.* **8**(1–2): 57–70.
34. **Tojo, M., N. Shibata, T. Mikami, M. Suzuki, and S. Suzuki.** 1987. Participation of peptide moieties in adhesive behavior of antigenic mannans of *Candida albicans* to the plastic microtiter plate in enzyme-linked immunosorbent assay. *Clin. Chem.* **33:** 1925–1928.
35. **Tsuchiya, T., S. Iwahara, F. Miyazaki, and Y. Fukazawa.** 1954. Studies on the classification of genus *Candida* antigenic analysis of seven species of genus *Candida. Jpn. J. Exp. Med.* **24:**95–103.

35a. **Tsuchiya, T., M. Taguchi, Y. Fukazawa, and T. Shinoda.** 1984. Serological characterization of yeasts as an aid in identification and classification. *Methods Microbiol.* **16:**75–126.

36. **Vecchiarelli, A., F. Bistoni, E. Cenci, S. Perito, and A. Cassone.** 1985. In-vitro killing of *Candida* species by murine immunoeffectors; its relationship to the experimental pathogenicity. *Sabouraudia* **25:**377–387.
37. **Watanabe, T., M. Takano, M. Murakami, H. Tanaka, A. Matsuhisa, N. Nakao, T. Mikami, M. Suzuki, and T. Matsumoto.** 1999. Characterization of a haemolytic factor from *Candida albicans. Microbiology* **145:**689–694.

Candida and Candidiasis
Edited by Richard A. Calderone
© 2002 ASM Press, Washington, D.C.

Chapter 4

Emergence of Non-*Candida albicans Candida* Species as Pathogens

GARY P. MORAN, DEREK J. SULLIVAN, AND DAVID C. COLEMAN

Over the past two decades many non-*Candida albicans Candida* (NCAC) species have emerged as significant pathogens of clinical importance (30, 38, 77, 80). As the genus *Candida* is a form genus, the NCAC species are a very heterogeneous group of organisms that are fundamentally different from each other and from *C. albicans* at the biological level (9, 23). This diversity in the range of *Candida* species now associated with human infection has provided new challenges in the diagnosis and treatment of candidiasis and in the study of their virulence and biology. Although close to 200 *Candida* species have been described, relatively few of these are of medical significance (9, 23, 72, 73) (Table 1). In the early 20th century, *C. albicans* was considered the only *Candida* species of real medical importance, although *C. stellatoidea* (now considered synonymous with *C. albicans*), *C. parapsilosis, C. tropicalis,* and *C. guilliermondii* were considered occasional pathogens (38, 72). However, during the 1980s and 1990s, the frequency with which these organisms were recovered from sites of infection increased and species that were previously considered nonpathogenic, such as *C. glabrata, C. krusei,* and *C. lusitaniae,* emerged as pathogens (77, 79, 80). In addition in 1995, a novel *Candida* species, termed *C. dubliniensis,* was identified for the first time (109). The reasons for this shift in the epidemiology of *Candida* infections may be linked to the general increase in the incidence of mycoses that occurred from the 1960s onward (6, 45, 117). The advent of new medical therapies and procedures to treat cancer, the increase in invasive medical procedures, and the widespread use of broad-spectrum antibiotics have all been linked with this increase in fungal infections. The emergence of human immunodeficiency virus (HIV) and AIDS has also increased the incidence of mucosal candidiasis caused by *Candida* species (19, 29). Many of these organisms are commensals, or at least transient commensals, of the human alimentary canal. *C. albicans,* the most common human commensal of the genus *Candida,* is generally regarded as the most virulent of the *Candida* species (72). The NCAC species are generally regarded as being less pathogenic or nonpathogenic, and accordingly, infections caused by these species are usually seen only in severely immunocompromised hosts or in individuals with serious underlying disease (2, 79, 114). Hence, the increased longevity of severely immunologically compromised individuals in modern hospitals has allowed many of these species to emerge and cause disease. This chapter summarizes the current state of the epidemiology of candidiasis caused by NCAC species and traces the shifts in the epidemiology of both superficial and systemic candidiasis that occurred during the 1980s and 1990s. In addition, the major biological differences among the medically significant *Candida* species will be highlighted, with particular attention to virulence and antifungal drug susceptibility.

CLASSIFICATION AND BIOLOGY OF *CANDIDA* SPECIES

Taxonomy and Evolutionary Relationships

The genus *Candida* is a form genus consisting of yeasts that do not possess a known natural sexual cycle (9). Most of the medically important species within the genus possess the ability to produce pseudomycelium and are otherwise morphologically very similar, usually appearing as spherical to ovoid budding yeast cells or blastospores (9, 23, 72). Tradition-

Gary P. Moran, Derek J. Sullivan, and David C. Coleman • Microbiology Research Unit, Department of Oral Medicine and Pathology, School of Dental Science, University of Dublin, Trinity College, Dublin 2, Republic of Ireland.

Table 1. The most commonly encountered NCAC species of medical importance

Species	Sites infected or affected	Underlying disease/risk factors[a]	References
C. dubliniensis	Oral mucosa, blood	HIV infection, BMT	20, 64, 105, 109
C. glabrata	Urinary tract, mucosal, blood, disseminated infection	HIV infection, solid tumors, leukemia, BMT	28, 52, 70, 89
C. krusei	Oral mucosa, blood, disseminated infection	HIV infection, BMT, leukemia	1, 60, 98, 122
C. parapsilosis	Blood, endocarditis, bone/joint infection	Premature birth, parenteral nutrition, intravenous catheter	34, 58, 72, 126
C. tropicalis	Oral mucosa, blood, disseminated infection, bone/joint infection	HIV infection, solid tumors, BMT, leukemia	52, 72, 104, 120

[a]BMT, bone marrow transplantation.

ally, species within the genus have been classified and identified on the basis of a limited number of morphological features and biochemical properties such as the ability to produce true hyphae or chlamydospores (both features associated with *C. albicans*) and the ability to assimilate a range of compounds as the sole source of carbon or nitrogen. Many investigators have expressed dissatisfaction with these methods of classification as different species can share a range of specific phenotypic properties (107). It has also been noted that phenotypic properties can also vary greatly between strains of the same species, making classification of isolates by these criteria alone problematic. In addition, the application of molecular phylogenetics to the taxonomy of *Candida* species has provided many new insights into the evolutionary relationships between these organisms, which challenge many of the conventional taxonomic classifications (10, 53). For example, genetic analysis of several medically important yeasts currently classified within the genus *Candida*, including *C. krusei, C. guilliermondii, C. lusitaniae*, and *C. kefyr*, has demonstrated that these organisms are in fact asexual (anamorphic) forms of sexually reproductive (teleomorphic) yeasts (10, 72). Controversy has also surrounded the traditional taxonomic classification of *C. stellatoidea* as a species distinct from *C. albicans* (55–57). *C. stellatoidea* is unable to utilize sucrose as the sole source of carbon but is otherwise phenotypically very similar to *C. albicans* and has been subdivided into two subtypes, termed type I and type II (55). Type II *C. stellatoidea* isolates have been shown to be variants of *C. albicans* that have lost the ability to utilize sucrose as the sole source of carbon, whereas type I *C. stellatoidea* isolates are somewhat different, being less virulent than *C. albicans* and possessing karyotypes that are distinct from those of *C. albicans* (55–57, 119). However, further analysis has suggested that type I *C. stellatoidea* should be considered a synonym of *C. albicans* based on the close homology of the nucleotide sequences encoding the V3 region of the large-subunit ribosomal RNA (rRNA) genes of these organisms (109). Recently, molecular genetic and phylogentic studies were instrumental in the identification of a novel species of *Candida* associated with human disease, termed *C. dubliniensis*, which previously had been misidentified as *C. albicans* by classical phenotypic tests in a number of studies (19, 109) (see "Epidemiology of Candidiasis Caused by Different NCAC Species" below). Due to the anomalies in the traditional classification of yeasts within the genus *Candida*, several investigators have begun to use molecular techniques to classify and identify medically important yeast species.

Many different techniques have been employed to investigate genetic relatedness among yeast species, including nuclear DNA reassociation analysis, restriction fragment length polymorphism (RFLP) analysis, and hybridization analysis with species-specific DNA sequences (53, 56, 107). However, the technique that has been most useful in determining the precise phylogenetic relationships between *Candida* species involves comparison of nucleotide sequences encoding rRNA genes. Studies involving comparative sequence analysis of the 5′ end of the large-subunit rRNA genes and the small-subunit rRNA genes of several *Candida* species have demonstrated that *C. albicans, C. dubliniensis, C. parapsilosis*, and *C. tropicalis* form a closely related clade in phylogenetic trees (Fig. 1) (10, 33, 53, 109). Comparative sequence analysis has also demonstrated that *C. guilliermondii, C. lusitaniae, C. krusei*, and *C. glabrata* are progressively less related to the members of this clade (10). A number of phylogenetic studies have also shown that, in evolutionary terms, *C. glabrata* (formerly *Torulopsis glabrata*) falls into a distinct subgroup and is more closely related to *Saccharomyces cerevisiae* and *C. kefyr* (formerly *C. pseudotropicalis*) than to other *Candida* species (10, 53). Further comprehensive analyses of the genetic structure of the medically important *Candida* species (perhaps involving the relatively new science

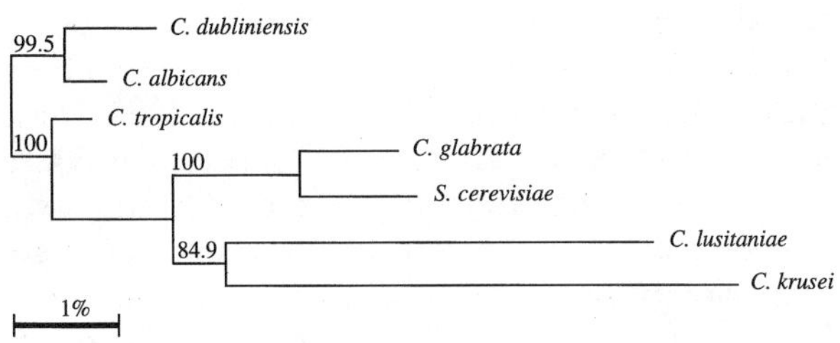

Figure 1. An unrooted phylogenetic neighbor joining tree generated from the alignment of the sequences encoding the small rRNA genes from *C. albicans* and different NCAC species and *S. cerevisiae*. The scale bar represents a 1% difference in nucleotide sequence. The numbers at each node were generated by bootstrap analysis and represent the percentage of times the arrangement occurred in 1,000 randomly generated trees. Reprinted from *Microbiology* (33) with the permission of the publisher.

of genomics) is required to provide a fuller understanding of the evolutionary relationships between these organisms.

Biology and Virulence

Because of the genetic diversity of organisms within the form genus *Candida* demonstrated by phylogenetic studies, it is not surprising that the basic biology and virulence of these species can vary considerably. The NCAC species have received limited specific attention at this level; however, due to their increasing clinical importance, many investigators have begun to study the biology and virulence of these organisms in detail. Morphologically, most *Candida* species exist as spherical to ovoid blastospores or yeast cells, typically 4 to 6 μm in diameter (23). Most *Candida* species are capable, to various degrees, of producing chains of elongated blastospores termed pseudohyphae, both in vivo, and under certain conditions, in vitro (Fig. 2). With the exception of *C. dubliniensis* and rare isolates of *C. tropicalis,* none of the NCAC species can produce the true unconstricted hyphae or thick-walled chlamydospores typical of *C. albicans* (72, 109). *C. glabrata* grows exclusively as small (1 to 4 μm diameter) blastospores and only produces hyphae under very specific conditions in vitro. Blastospores of *C. krusei* and *C. kefyr* are distinctive among the *Candida* species in that they are usually elongated in shape, measuring 2 to 5 by 4 to 15 μm (72, 98).

The virulence of different NCAC species in humans and in animal models of infection varies considerably (3, 22, 42, 73, 121). *C. albicans* is known to be the most virulent of the medically important *Candida* species, and this may be due to its ability to adhere strongly to host surfaces and its ability to produce hydrolytic enzymes such as lipases and a family of related secreted aspartyl proteinases (SAPs) (43, 73).

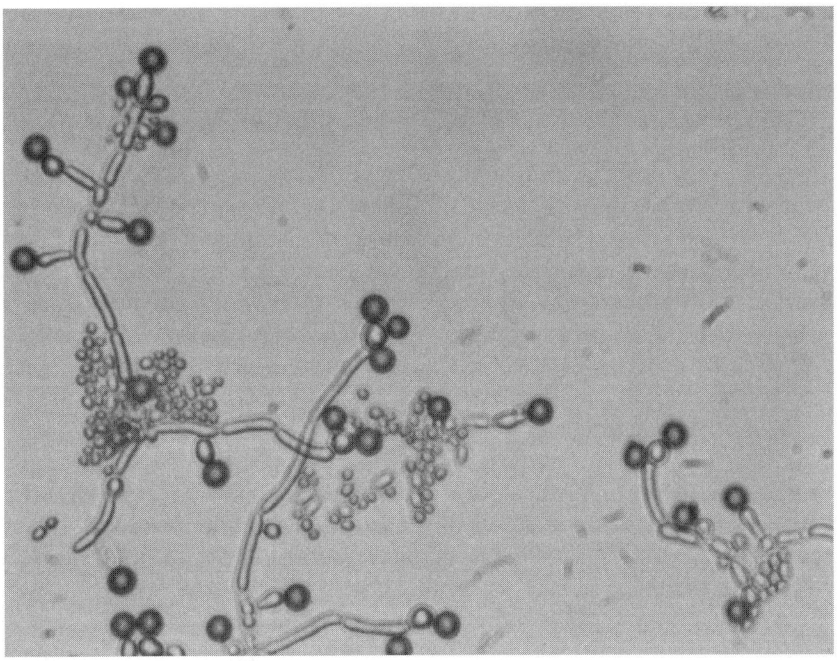

Figure 2. Light micrograph showing the production of pseudohyphae and chlamydospores by *C. dubliniensis* on Rice agar Tween (RAT) agar incubated at 25°C for 72 h. Chlamydospores are stained with lactophenol cotton blue. Reprinted from *Microbiology* (109) with the permission of the publisher.

Other putative virulence factors, such as the ability to produce hyphae and the ability to rapidly change its expressed phenotype (termed phenotypic switching), may also play a role in pathogenesis. It has become clear that the less virulent NCAC species are less able or are unable to produce many of these factors. In vitro studies have shown that specific NCAC species are less adherent to buccal epithelial and vascular endothelial cells and secrete less proteinases than *C. albicans,* which may account, at least in part, for their reduced virulence (43, 48, 51). *C. tropicalis* appears to be the most virulent of the NCAC species and has been shown to be capable of colonization and penetration of the gastrointestinal mucosa in mice (31, 121). This virulence may in part be due to its greater ability to adhere to epithelial cells in vitro and its ability to secrete moderate amounts of proteinase relative to the other NCAC species (48, 127). Several genes encoding SAPs have been isolated from *C. tropicalis* (*SAPT1* through *SAPT4*), and an integrin-like protein, similar to that found in *C. albicans,* has also been characterized that may be important for adherence to host surfaces (41, 127). Proteinase secretion and genes encoding SAPs have also been characterized in *C. parapsilosis* (22, 24). High levels of proteinase production have been associated with *C. parapsilosis* isolates recovered from human skin, which seems to be the primary niche for this species in humans (22, 72). However, although *C. parapsilosis* is less virulent than *C. albicans* and *C. tropicalis* in mouse systemic models of candidiasis, isolates from blood culture produce an extracellular polysaccharide, or slime, which may aid adherence and biofilm formation on plastic surfaces. This characteristic may explain why *C. parapsilosis* infections are often associated with indwelling catheters and prosthetic devices (16, 34, 126). Biochemical analysis of the proteinases from *C. albicans, C. tropicalis,* and *C. parapsilosis* has revealed differences in substrate specificity and activities at neutral pH, which may suggest different roles for these enzymes in vivo (32, 115). Adherence and proteinase secretion have not yet been examined in detail in *C. dubliniensis,* the *Candida* species most closely related to *C. albicans.* Two studies have suggested that *C. dubliniensis* may be more adherent to buccal epithelial cells than *C. albicans,* and one study indicated that *C. dubliniensis* may also be highly proteolytic (33, 62). However, only a single study to date has examined the in vivo virulence of *C. dubliniensis,* which demonstrated that this organism is less virulent than *C. albicans* in a mouse systemic candidiasis model (33).

The remaining *Candida* species of medical importance, including *C. glabrata, C. krusei,* and *C. lusitaniae,* are considered less pathogenic, particularly in animal models of infection, although they may be associated with virulent infection in severely immunocompromised individuals (1, 3, 4, 28, 98, 114). These organisms adhere poorly to host surfaces and produce less proteinase than *C. tropicalis* and *C. parapsilosis.* Several studies have shown that these organisms are capable of causing systemic disease in mice; however, the animal host must be immunosuppressed or infected with a very high inoculum of cells before significant infection can develop (3, 4). *C. glabrata* is also unable to produce hyphae in vivo, which, along with its poor proteinase production, may account for its reduced virulence (28).

Antifungal Drug Susceptibility

The biological diversity of the organisms classified in the genus *Candida* has other implications for the management of infections caused by these species and for the development of antifungal agents. The ideal antifungal agents need to be effective against a broad spectrum of organisms, including all of the medically important yeasts of the genus *Candida* (36). Developing such agents has become increasingly challenging due to the multitude of fungi that are now recognized to cause human disease. The most important classes of antifungal agents effective against *Candida* species are the azole and the polyene antifungal agents (13, 21, 50). The first generation of drugs in these classes was introduced between the 1950s and the 1970s, when *C. albicans* was responsible for most fungal infections. Although most of the medically significant NCAC species are susceptible to these agents in vitro, concern has arisen due to the emergence of organisms with intrinsic (primary) resistance and to the emergence of organisms that have a tendency to develop (secondary) resistance to these agents (112, 118). In recent years, the widespread use of antifungal drugs has increased both therapeutically and prophylactically, due mainly to the general increased incidence of candidiasis. Evidence has been produced that suggests that this has led to changes in the epidemiology of candidiasis and the emergence of *Candida* species that are less susceptible to these agents (70, 90, 123).

Fluconazole is now one of the most commonly used azole antifungal agents and has proven efficacious in the treatment of both superficial and systemic fungal disease (21, 40). However, a number of NCAC species are now recognized to exhibit intrinsic resistance to this drug. It is now generally accepted that *C. krusei* is intrinsically resistant to fluconazole in vitro and that fluconazole therapy is totally inappropriate for treatment of infections caused by this species (93, 94). In addition, *C. inconspicua* and *C. nor-*

vegensis, two species that have only recently been associated with human disease, also exhibit intrinsic resistance to fluconazole (5, 100). In contrast, *C. glabrata* possesses the ability to rapidly develop resistance to fluconazole (28, 116). In comparison with most *Candida* species, which are diploid, *C. glabrata* is haploid and this may partly explain why mutations that lead to the development of fluconazole resistance arise at high frequency in this organism. Developed resistance to azole drugs has been described in other NCAC species including isolates of *C. dubliniensis, C. guilliermondii,* and *C. tropicalis,* usually recovered from HIV-infected patients following prolonged azole therapy (15, 46, 68). Both *C. dubliniensis* and *C. tropicalis* have been shown to acquire resistance to fluconazole following exposure to this drug in vitro (7, 67, 68). Since the introduction and widespread use of fluconazole in the 1990s there have been changes in the epidemiology of candidiasis, with many studies reporting an increase in the incidence of *C. glabrata* infection and the emergence of *C. krusei* (85, 122, 123). Although not proven conclusively, many studies have suggested that the introduction and widespread use of the newer azole drugs itraconazole and fluconazole may have contributed significantly to the selection and emergence of strains and species of *Candida* with reduced susceptibility to these agents (90, 122, 123).

The polyene agent amphotericin B has been in use since the 1950s and has a low incidence of developed resistance in the clinical setting (13). *C. albicans* isolates that exhibit resistance to amphotericin B have been described only rarely (112, 118). However, recent evidence suggests that a significant proportion of *C. glabrata* and *C. krusei* isolates may exhibit resistance to this agent (12, 47, 69). Resistance to amphotericin B is most often associated with *C. lusitaniae,* a relatively uncommon pathogen. Although this organism is usually susceptible to amphotericin B, several reports have described the recovery of amphotericin B-resistant isolates from blood culture (37, 76).

EPIDEMIOLOGY OF CANDIDIASIS CAUSED BY NCAC SPECIES

The NCAC species are associated with a similar spectrum of infections as *C. albicans,* including superficial infections of the oral and vaginal mucosae and life-threatening systemic and deep-seated infections (19, 79, 103). Although the study of specific predisposing factors that lead to candidiasis caused by NCAC species has received relatively little attention, they appear to be similar to those associated with *C. albicans* infection (45, 79, 117). However, it appears that candidiasis due to NCAC species is usually associated with more severe immunosuppression, such as that seen in neutropenic patients and patients in the advanced stages of AIDS (2, 104, 114). This may be related to the reduced virulence of these organisms relative to *C. albicans* and/or to their increased susceptibility to the antimicrobial mechanisms of the immune system. Carriage of NCAC species in the oral cavity, the vagina, and gastrointestinal tract is well documented in healthy individuals (72). Prior colonization is known to be a risk factor for infection with most of the NCAC species, suggesting that most infections are endogenous in origin (79). *C. glabrata* and *C. tropicalis* appear to be the NCAC species recovered most frequently from the vagina, the oral cavity, and gastrointestinal tract, whereas *C. guilliermondii* and *C. parapsilosis* have a propensity for colonization of the skin (39, 72). Few factors have been identified that specifically predispose individuals to carriage of NCAC species. However, in one study, HIV-infected individuals were reported to be almost twice as likely to be colonized by NCAC species (30.7 versus 15.9%) (102). In the same study, cigarette smoking was also associated with increased carriage of NCAC species, both in HIV-positive and HIV-negative individuals (102).

NCAC species colonizing the oral cavity and vaginal mucosa are commonly isolated in mixed culture, usually in combination with *C. albicans* (19, 102, 103). Colonies of different *Candida* species are often morphologically indistinguishable upon primary isolation using conventional mycological media such as Sabouraud's agar (19). The homogenous appearance of colony types of different *Candida* species may in the past have led to an underestimation of the prevalence of colonization with NCAC species. However, in recent years, the use of differential culture medium such as Sabouraud's agar supplemented with triphenyltetrazolium chloride and the recently introduced chromogenic agar medium, CHROMagar Candida, has greatly facilitated the identification of multiple *Candida* species present in the same clinical sample (Color plate 2) (19, 74).

Superficial Candidiasis Caused by NCAC Species

The most common superficial infections caused by *Candida* species occur in the oral and vaginal mucosae (72, 97, 103). Oral infections with *Candida* species are most commonly seen in denture wearers, diabetics, and HIV-infected and AIDS patients. Oral candidiasis is particularly common in patients with HIV infection and can be predictive of the future development of AIDS (19, 97). Although *C. albicans* is the most commonly recovered yeast from the oral cavities of HIV-infected patients, other yeasts are also frequently isolated, including *C. dubliniensis, C. glabrata, C. krusei, C. tropicalis,* and *S. cerevisiae* (15, 46, 61, 101, 102). Other *Candida* species such as *C. guilliermondii, C. parapsilosis,* and *C. kefyr* are occasionally isolated. Given that NCAC species are often co-isolated with *C. albicans* in the oral cavities of healthy individuals, it is not surprising that mixed cultures have also been recovered from HIV-infected individuals, both in the presence and absence of symptoms of oral candidiasis. *C. albicans* is usually the most abundant organism recovered, raising questions concerning the significance of co-isolated NCAC species in the etiology of mixed oropharyngeal infections (27). Some investigators have reported that clinical symptoms of oral thrush (pseudomembranous candidiasis) are not seen in HIV-infected patients harboring NCAC species in the absence of *C. albicans*. In a study involving 100 AIDS patients, Maenza et al. (61) reported that approximately 50% of patients who were culture-positive for oral *C. albicans* presented with clinical symptoms of thrush, yet none of 10 patients harboring only oral NCAC species had oral thrush. Similarly, Sangeorzan et al. (101) analyzed 82 episodes of thrush in 92 HIV-infected patients, and although *C. glabrata* was commonly recovered from these individuals, clinical symptoms of pseudomembranous candidiasis were never observed in patients who yielded this species only. However, in both of the above studies, oral candidiasis was defined as thrush (pseudomembranous candidiasis), and unusual clinical presentations of oral candidiasis such as erythematous candidiasis or hyperplastic candidiasis may not have been diagnosed. In this regard, it is important to note that erythematous candidiasis is the most common manifestation of oral candidiasis observed in HIV-infected individuals (19, 20). In contrast, however, several studies have documented the occurrence of clinical symptoms of oral thrush or erythematous candidiasis in patients in whom NCAC species were the only organisms recovered from the site of infection (15, 17, 60). Powderly (89) described eight cases of oropharyngeal candidiasis in HIV-infected individuals in whom NCAC species, including *C. glabrata, C. krusei,* and *C. tropicalis,* were the only species recovered from the oral cavity. Sullivan et al. (104) also reported that 10 of 25 HIV-infected intravenous drug users, most of whom had developed AIDS, who had clinical symptoms of oral erythematous candidiasis harbored a single NCAC species. Although in most HIV-infected individuals, NCAC species are less abundant than *C. albicans* in the oral cavity, evidence has accumulated that treatment with azole antifungals for protracted periods may lead to the selection of NCAC species, some of which have been shown to be less susceptible than *C. albicans* to these agents (17, 95, 102, 111). In particular, long-term fluconazole therapy for suppression of recurrent oral candidiasis in HIV-infected patients has been associated with the selection of *C. glabrata* and *C. krusei*. Johnson et al. (46) reported a higher prevalence of *C. glabrata* and *C. krusei* isolates recovered from the oral cavities of HIV-infected patients who had received long-term azole therapy compared to a group of patients who had not received therapy. In several of these patients, NCAC species were the only *Candida* species recovered following culture. Schoofs et al. (102) have shown that prior azole therapy was a risk factor for carriage of NCAC species in HIV-infected patients, although most of the NCAC isolates were recovered in mixed culture with *C. albicans*. These studies suggest that azole therapy may be responsible, at least in part, for the selection of organisms with reduced azole susceptibility, which, prior to therapy, may have formed only a minor constituent of the oral flora. In addition to reports of azole resistance in isolates of *C. glabrata* and *C. krusei,* resistance to azole antifungals has also been described in isolates of *C. dubliniensis, C. tropicalis, C. parapsilosis,* and *C. guilliermondii* recovered from HIV-infected patients, although there is little evidence to suggest that azole therapy has led to any increased prevalence of these species in this patient cohort (15, 17, 61, 67).

NCAC species have also been associated with *Candida* vaginitis, a common disease that can occur in otherwise apparently healthy women (72, 103). Approximately 10% of patients with vaginitis present with chronic symptoms or suffer from recurrent infection. Although NCAC species are commonly recovered from the vagina in healthy women, the reported incidence of vaginitis caused by NCAC species is low. *C. albicans* is responsible for approximately 90% of cases of *Candida* vaginitis (72). In the remaining 10% of cases, *C. glabrata* is the most commonly recovered organism (28, 103). Relatively few studies have investigated whether azole therapy is any less effective in the treatment of *C. glabrata* vaginitis compared to vaginitis caused by *C. albicans*. There is also little evidence to suggest that widespread use of azole drugs to treat vaginitis has led to any increased incidence of vaginitis caused by NCAC species that exhibit reduced susceptibility to these agents in vitro.

Nosocomial Candidemia Caused by NCAC Species

Candida species are important agents of nosocomial infection, and candidemia accounts for 10 to 15% of all hospital-acquired bloodstream infections (45, 78, 79). It has been well documented that the rate of nosocomial candidemia increased steadily throughout the 1980s and into the 1990s (30, 77). Banerjee et al. (6) noted a 75 to 487% increase in the rate of candidemia during the 1980s in hospitals participating in the National Nosocomial Infection Surveillance system in the United States. This increase has been associated with recent advances in medical technology that have resulted in very significant increases in the numbers and types of patients at risk from nosocomial candidiasis (117). Patients most at risk of infection are those with indwelling catheters, those receiving broad-spectrum antibiotics, and patients with neutropenia due to therapy with anticancer agents or immunosuppressive drugs. *C. albicans* is still the most common etiological agent of nosocomial candidemia, accounting for 50 to 60% of infections (Table 2) (47, 72, 85). However, since the late 1980s there has been an increase in the number of studies describing nosocomial infections with NCAC species, and some institutions have reported changes in the distribution of *Candida* species recovered from blood culture and urine (2, 11, 71, 90). In particular, several institutions reported a decrease in the relative rate of infection caused by *C. albicans* compared to NCAC species. In one study Nguyen et al. (70) noted a steady increase in candidemia caused by NCAC species at four institutions over a 3.5-year period in the early 1990s, where the recovery of NCAC species from patients with candidemia rose from 40 to 53% of patients overall. In a separate study Price et al. (90) noted a dramatic decrease in the rate of candidemia caused by *C. albicans* at one institution, where the rate of *C. albicans* recovery from blood cultures decreased from 87 to 31% between 1987 and 1992. Investigators have suggested that the introduction and widespread use of fluconazole have led to the selection of NCAC species, as many of these organisms are less susceptible to these agents (2, 70, 90, 123). In one recent prospective study of candidemia in cancer patients, antifungal prophylaxis (not only with fluconazole) in hematology patients was significantly associated with candidemia caused by NCAC species (114). However, the results of large multicenter epidemiological studies in the United States do not support the notion that the rate of systemic infection caused by NCAC species has increased nationwide relative to *C. albicans* (82, 83, 85, 86). Several multicenter studies have reported that NCAC species are responsible for 44 to 48% of cases of candidemia in the United States, which is similar to the incidence reported pre-1980 (72, 120). Why some institutions appear to have experienced increased rates of infection caused by NCAC species is unclear, but it may be related to the patient populations of individual hospitals, differences in antifungal agent use, and infection control practices. Interestingly, some studies have shown that infection with NCAC species may be more common in certain patient groups. Viscoli et al. (114) noted, in a prospective multicenter European study, that hematology patients were more often infected with NCAC species than patients with solid tumors (66 versus 30%). Other studies have demonstrated that low neutrophil counts, whatever the underlying disease, were associated with candidemia caused by NCAC species (1, 2, 70).

Although it is still unclear whether the overall rate of candidemia caused by NCAC species has increased, epidemiological studies have revealed shifts in the relative incidence of individual NCAC species recovered from blood culture. During the late 1990s in the United States there was a decrease in the relative rate of recovery of *C. tropicalis* from blood culture and an increase in the rate of recovery of *C. glabrata* and *C. parapsilosis* (Table 2) (85, 86). *C. glabrata* is now consistently reported as the most commonly recovered NCAC species from blood cultures in the United States, accounting for approximately 20% of all *Candida* isolates, including *C. albicans* (11, 85). *C. parapsilosis* is the second most commonly recovered species overall; however, a recent study by the National Epidemiology of Mycoses Survey demonstrated that the incidence of infection caused by *C. parapsilosis* was almost five times that of *C. glabrata* in neonatal intensive care units (91). *C. tropicalis* has been reported to be responsible for 7 to 11% of infections, with the remaining blood culture isolates consisting of *C. famata, C. guilliermondii, C. krusei, C. kefyr,* and *C. lusitaniae* (81, 85, 86).

International studies have demonstrated similar rates of recovery of NCAC species from blood culture in disparate geographic locations, although the distri-

Table 2. Distribution of *Candida* species recovered from blood culture in Europe, Canada, Latin America, and the United States, reported by the SENTRY antimicrobial surveillance program, 1997[a]

Species	Distribution of *Candida* spp. (% of all isolates)			
	United States ($n = 203$)	Europe ($n = 170$)	Canada ($n = 61$)	Latin America ($n = 42$)
C. albicans	56	53	53	41
C. parapsilosis	9	21	23	38
C. glabrata	19	12	11	2
C. tropicalis	7	6	8	12
C. guilliermondii	1	4	—	2
C. krusei	2	1	2	—
Candida spp.[b]	6	3	3	5

[a]Data taken from references 80 and 81.
[b]Includes three isolates of *C. famata*, two isolates of *C. inconspicua*, and 17 isolates of other *Candida* spp.

bution of NCAC species differs considerably (Table 2) (80, 81, 114). The highest prevalence of candidemia due to NCAC species has been reported in Latin America, where *C. albicans* was responsible for only 40% of infections. In contrast to the situation in the United States, *C. parapsilosis* is the NCAC species most commonly recovered from blood culture in Latin America, Europe, and Canada. *C. krusei* was recovered from 2% of *Candida* blood cultures in the United States and Canada but was not reported among any isolates from Latin America.

EPIDEMIOLOGY OF CANDIDIASIS CAUSED BY DIFFERENT NCAC SPECIES

Although many of the risk factors associated with candidiasis caused by NCAC species are similar to those identified for infections caused by *C. albicans,* some differences in patterns of colonization, types of infection, and clinical outcome have been noted for some NCAC species (79). For this reason, some of the features of infection associated with the commonly encountered NCAC species are outlined below.

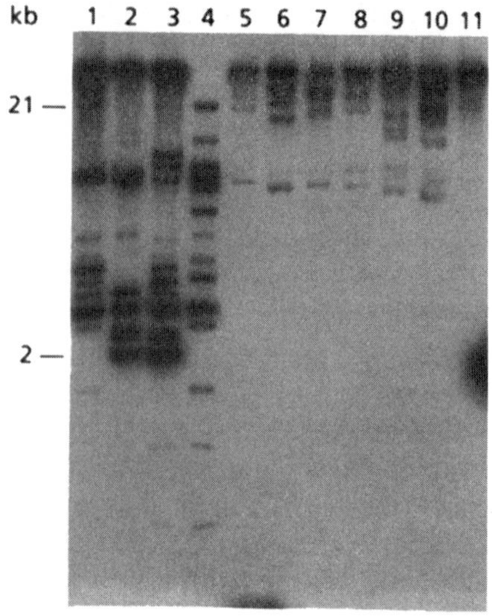

Figure 3. Southern blot analysis of *Eco*RI-digested total genomic DNA from *C. albicans, C. stellatoidea,* and *C. dubliniensis* isolates probed with the *C. albicans*-specific probe 27A. The fingerprints shown correspond to *C. albicans* (lanes 1 and 2), *C. stellatoidea* type II (lane 3), *C. stellatoidea* type I (lane 4), and *C. dubliniensis* (lanes 5 to 11). Size reference markers are indicated in kilobases on the left of the figure. Reprinted from *Microbiology* (109) with the permission of the publisher.

C. dubliniensis

In 1995, a novel species of *Candida, C. dubliniensis,* which is primarily associated with oral carriage and infection in HIV-infected and AIDS patients, was identified and first described (109). During the early 1990s a number of authors reported the recovery of unusual or atypical isolates of *C. albicans* from HIV-infected individuals (19, 20, 62, 104). Although these isolates possessed many of the features characteristic of *C. albicans,* they also exhibited a number of atypical properties. These atypical isolates possessed the ability to produce germ tubes and often produced abundant chlamydospores (109). However, unlike *C. albicans,* these isolates grew poorly or not at all at temperatures of 42°C or higher and could not be definitively identified with commonly used commercially available yeast identification systems based on substrate assimilation profiles, including the API 20C AUX and ID 32C systems (104, 109). Molecular studies demonstrated that DNA from these atypical isolates hybridized very poorly with *C. albicans*-specific DNA fingerprinting probes such as 27A (Fig. 3) (109). In 1995, Sullivan et al. (109) investigated a group of these atypical isolates recovered from the oral cavities of HIV-infected patients in Ireland and Australia and carried out an extensive analysis of their phenotypic and genotypic characteristics. The atypical isolates were found to form a genetically homogeneous group of organisms that possessed a unique genomic organization compared to *C. albicans* and other *Candida* species. The most conclusive evidence demonstrating that these isolates were distinct from other *Candida* species was generated by phylogenetic analysis of nucleotide sequences encoding the V3 region of the large rRNA subunit gene. Nucleotide sequences from atypical isolates from disparate geographical sources were 100% identical but significantly different from those of other *Candida* species, including *C. albicans* (106, 109). It was proposed that these atypical isolates constituted a novel species of *Candida* that Sullivan et al. (109) designated *C. dubliniensis.* A number of subsequent molecular studies have since confirmed this novel taxonomic designation by comparison of nucleotide sequences encoding the small-subunit rRNA genes, the 5′ end of the large rRNA subunit genes, and the *ACT1* genes of *C. albicans* and *C. dubliniensis* (26, 33, 53).

C. dubliniensis is commonly recovered from the oral cavities of HIV-infected and AIDS patients (20, 102, 105). The recovery of *C. dubliniensis* from these patient groups has been reported worldwide, with most studies describing a prevalence rate of 15 to 30% (49, 63, 102, 106). The most comprehensive data on the prevalence of this organism in the oral cavity come from studies of Irish individuals (20, 88, 105, 108).

Table 3. Recovery of *C. dubliniensis* isolates from different cohorts of Irish individuals[a]

Group	No. of subjects	Clinical symptoms of candidiasis	No. (%) of subjects yielding *C. dubliniensis*	Other *Candida* species co-isolated[b]
AIDS	82	Oral candidiasis	26 (31.7)	8 *C. dubliniensis* only 18 *C. dubliniensis* and other *Candida* species
AIDS	36	Asymptomatic	9 (25)	3 *C. dubliniensis* only 6 *C. dubliniensis* and other *Candida* species
HIV-positive	185	Oral candidiasis	48 (26)	12 *C. dubliniensis* only 36 *C. dubliniensis* and other *Candida* species
HIV-positive	216	Asymptomatic	39 (18)	7 *C. dubliniensis* only 32 *C. dubliniensis* and other *Candida* species
HIV-negative[c]	72	Oral candidiasis	10 (13.9)	3 *C. dubliniensis* only 7 *C. dubliniensis* and other *Candida* species
HIV-negative[d]	56	Oral candidiasis	6 (10.7)	2 *C. dubliniensis* only 4 *C. dubliniensis* and other *Candida* species
HIV-negative[e]	202	Asymptomatic	7 (3.5)	1 *C. dubliniensis* only 6 *C. dubliniensis* and other *Candida* species
HIV-negative[f]	414	NA	58 (14)	13 *C. dubliniensis* only 45 *C. dubliniensis* and other *Candida* species
HIV-negative	110	Vaginitis	3 (2.72)	1 *C. dubliniensis* only 2 *C. dubliniensis* and other *Candida* species

[a]Reprinted from reference 88 with permission. Data from references 20, 108, and 119a.
[b]*C. albicans* was the species most commonly co-isolated with *C. dubliniensis*, followed by (in decreasing order of frequency) *C. glabrata*, *C. tropicalis*, *C. krusei*, and, infrequently, several other NCAC species and other yeast species.
[c]HIV-negative subjects with denture-associated oral candidiasis.
[d]HIV-negative subjects with non-denture-associated oral candidiasis.
[e]Normal healthy oral *Candida* carriers.
[f]HIV-negative diabetics. The overall incidence of oral candidiasis was not reported. However, of the 58 diabetics who yielded *C. dubliniensis*, 17 (29.3%) had clinical symptoms of oral candidiasis and 41 (70.7%) did not. Of the 17 symptomatic diabetic patients, 6 (35.3%) yielded *C. dubliniensis* only and 11 (64.7%) yielded *C. dubliniensis* and other *Candida* species. In contrast, of the 41 asymptomatic diabetic patients, 7 (17.1%) yielded *C. dubliniensis* only and 34 (82.9%) yielded *C. dubliniensis* and other *Candida* species.

C. dubliniensis has been recovered from 32% of Irish AIDS patients with clinical symptoms of oral candidiasis ($n = 82$) and from 25% of asymptomatic Irish AIDS patients ($n = 36$) (Table 3). Schoofs et al. (102) recently reported that *C. dubliniensis* was the second most commonly isolated NCAC species from the oral cavities of a group of 130 Belgian HIV-infected individuals. *C. dubliniensis* is most commonly recovered from the oral cavity in mixed culture with other *Candida* species, particularly *C. albicans* (20). However, pure cultures have been recovered from individuals with symptoms of oral candidiasis, indicating that this species is capable of causing oral disease in the absence of other *Candida* species (20, 67). In addition to the oral cavity, *C. dubliniensis* has been recovered from fecal, sputum, vaginal, and blood cultures (65, 75, 87). Two independent studies have reported seven cases of *C. dubliniensis* fungemia, the first study describing three cases in Europe and the second detailing four cases in the United States (14, 64). All of the patients in these studies had severe underlying medical conditions, but only one patient was infected with HIV. Because *C. dubliniensis* has previously been isolated from the gastrointestinal tract of HIV-negative individuals and from fecal surveillance cultures in hematological patients, it is likely that these infections had an endogenous source. The true incidence of fungemia caused by this organism is unknown; however, a recent study of the prevalence of *C. dubliniensis* in a Dutch hospital demonstrated that this organism was present in 0.8% of fungal surveillance cultures (65).

A number of studies have shown that misidentification of *C. dubliniensis* as *C. albicans* has occurred in the past, and it is likely that this species has been an unrecognized constituent of the oral flora for many years (20, 75). The data on the prevalence of *C. dubliniensis* indicate that this species has come to prominence due to the advent of HIV infection and AIDS, and its relatively high prevalence in this cohort group facilitated its recent discovery. The reasons for the emergence of this species in this patient population are presently unclear. As *C. dubliniensis* is only rarely recovered from the oral cavities of healthy individuals (Table 3), its prevalence in HIV-infected and AIDS patients indicates that due to severe immunodeficiency this organism can emerge as an opportunistic pathogen, probably from the patients' own microbial flora. In this environment, the ability of *C. dubliniensis* to adhere strongly to oral epithelial cells may provide it with a competitive advantage over other, less adherent, NCAC species (33, 62). Unlike *C. krusei* and *C. glabrata, C. dubliniensis* is not inherently less susceptible to antifungal drugs such as fluconazole (67, 84). However, *C. dubliniensis* isolates resistant to fluconazole have been recovered from fluconazole-treated HIV-infected individuals (49, 67, 68, 96). Furthermore, susceptible isolates can readily develop resistance to fluconazole in vitro when exposed to this agent (67). This ability may confer *C. dubliniensis* with a further selective advantage in HIV-infected individuals receiving long-term maintenance therapy for suppression of oral candidiasis.

The true prevalence of this organism as an agent of candidiasis will only be ascertained when more reliable and rapid diagnostic tests that allow it to be easily distinguished from *C. albicans* are developed. Currently, PCR tests are the most reliable and the least time-consuming methods for the identification of *C. dubliniensis* (26, 54, 110). The most extensively evaluated PCR test for the identification of *C. dubliniensis* involves amplification of a species-specific genomic DNA fragment using primers specific for *C. dubliniensis ACT1* gene-associated intron sequences (26).

C. glabrata

The incidence of systemic infections caused by *C. glabrata* increased dramatically throughout the 1990s (11, 28, 85). In the United States, *C. glabrata* is second only to *C. albicans* as a cause of systemic candidiasis and candiduria (71, 85). *C. glabrata* is also the NCAC species most commonly recovered from the oral cavities of HIV-infected individuals (61, 101, 102). The increase in *C. glabrata* systemic infections is a subject of considerable concern due to the tendency of this species to rapidly develop resistance to azole antifungal agents and due to the high mortality rate associated with *C. glabrata* fungemia (28). *C. glabrata* is considered a pathogen of low virulence, and infection is usually associated with severely debilitated patients, which may explain why some studies have shown that *C. glabrata* candidemia is associated with a high mortality rate (52, 114). A number of medical centers that have reported increases in *C. glabrata* infection rates have associated this phenomenon with fluconazole use (11, 123). Several studies have noted that a significant proportion of *C. glabrata* isolates are resistant to fluconazole (approximately 9%) and itraconazole (37 to 40%) (8, 81, 90, 92). In addition, this organism can rapidly develop fluconazole resistance in the clinical setting. Warnock et al. (116) noted a 30-fold rise in fluconazole MIC for an isolate of *C. glabrata* recovered from a patient with funguria following 9 days of oral therapy with fluconazole. This evidence suggests that fluconazole use may contribute to the selection and emergence of *C. glabrata* in the hospital setting (11). In one institution, Wingard et al. (123) noted that *C. glabrata* was responsible for fungemia in six of eight bone marrow transplant patients receiving fluconazole therapy. In a retrospective analysis of the distribution of *Candida* species isolated from blood cultures over a 5-year period in a single institution, Price et al. (90) noted that *C. glabrata* rose in incidence from 1% of isolates in 1987 to 26% in 1992. The authors suggested a link between this increase in incidence of *C. glabrata* infection with the introduction of fluconazole. Abi-Said et al. (2), in a multivariate analysis of risk factors for candidemia, noted that *C. glabrata* infection was strongly associated with fluconazole prophylaxis, while, in contrast, Nguyen et al. (70) noted that *C. glabrata* infection was more commonly seen following amphotericin B therapy. Although by no means indisputable, this body of evidence suggests that fluconazole prophylaxis and therapy for fungal infections may have played a significant role in the recent emergence of *C. glabrata.*

Few studies have analyzed the epidemiology of nosocomial *C. glabrata* acquisition. Vazquez et al. (113) investigated *C. glabrata* colonization at multiple sites in 98 patients and found that 24.5% of patients were culture positive for *C. glabrata* at some point during their period of hospitalization. Sixteen of these patients (17%) acquired *C. glabrata* following admission to hospital. Nosocomial acquisition of *C. glabrata* was significantly associated with a longer duration of hospitalization and prior antibacterial therapy. RFLP analysis demonstrated the recovery of an identical strain of *C. glabrata* from three environmental sources and five patients, suggesting the possibility of exogenous acquisition of *C. glabrata* from the hospital environment. A study by Pfaller et al. (86) also suggested the possibility of patient-to-patient transmission of *C. glabrata* strains in the hospital setting. Karyotype analysis has been used to differentiate strains of *C. glabrata* responsible for mucosal infections. Barchiesi et al. (8) showed that recurrent oral candidiasis in HIV-infected patients and recurrent vaginitis in HIV-negative women due to *C. glabrata* were the result of persistent infection with the same strain of *C. glabrata.*

C. krusei

C. krusei is a relatively uncommon pathogen accounting for 2 to 4% of cases of candidemia (82, 85, 86, 98). *C. krusei* fungemia generally occurs in hematology patients with severe neutropenia due to bone marrow transplantation or leukemia (1, 79). Mortality rates due to *C. krusei* fungemia in these patients are high (60 to 80%), and infection is often disseminated (1, 66, 70). In the early 1990s, a number of reports described an increased prevalence of infections caused by *C. krusei* in patients receiving prophylactic fluconazole therapy. It is now generally accepted that *C. krusei* is inherently resistant to fluconazole, and selection of *C. krusei* in fluconazole-treated patients may account for this association (94). Longitudinal studies have also described the replacement of *C. albicans* with *C. krusei* in the oral cavities of HIV-infected patients following azole therapy (17, 18, 60, 95). Lischewski et al. (60) described a patient suffering from oral candidiasis who was infected with the same strain of *C. albicans* through recurrent episodes of oral candidiasis. However, following prolonged fluconazole therapy and subsequent episodes of chronic recurrent candidiasis, only an azole-resistant *C. krusei* was isolated during recurrent episodes of infection.

Several institutions have reported increased rates of recovery of *C. krusei* from blood culture since the introduction of fluconazole (2, 90). Wingard et al. (122) in 1991 reported an association between fluconazole prophylaxis and *C. krusei* colonization among bone marrow transplant patients. *C. krusei* colonization was found in 40.5% of fluconazole-treated patients but only in 16.5% of untreated patients. The rate of *C. krusei* infection was found to be sevenfold higher in the fluconazole-treated group. However, 5 years prior to this study, a report by Merz et al. (66) described an increased rate of *C. krusei* colonization at the same institution, before the introduction of fluconazole therapy. However, in this study the overall frequency of *C. krusei* colonization was lower (12.5%). Although some reports have implicated fluconazole as an important predisposing factor for *C. krusei* infection (2, 70), others have not found similar associations, indicating that institution-specific factors may be involved (44). However, placebo-controlled, prospective studies of the efficacy of fluconazole in the prevention of fungal infections in bone marrow transplant patients have not noted any increased rate of *C. krusei* infection in fluconazole-treated patients (35, 124).

Infecting strains of *C. krusei* usually originate from the gastrointestinal tract (79). Prior colonization with *C. krusei* rather than the presence of indwelling catheters has been reported to be a risk factor for infection, suggesting an endogenous source of infection (1, 66). Due to the inherent resistance of *C. krusei* to fluconazole, fluconazole prophylaxis may promote the proliferation of this organism in the gastrointestinal tract, which in neutropenic patients, may lead to dissemination of the organism into the bloodstream. DNA typing of *C. krusei* isolates from blood culture has shown that patients are normally infected with their own unique strain, confirming the notion that infections arise from the patients' own endogenous flora (12). By using DNA typing techniques, one study demonstrated that two patients and three health care workers in a surgical intensive care unit were colonized by the same strain of *C. krusei*, suggesting nosocomial transmission can occur (86). As already mentioned, *C. krusei* is inherently resistant to fluconazole. However, some investigators have noted reduced susceptibility to other antifungal drugs among isolates of *C. krusei*, leading some to refer to *C. krusei* as a multidrug-resistant pathogen (12, 47, 69). Itraconazole resistance has also been documented in isolates of *C. krusei* (81). In addition, several reports have described cases of breakthrough fungemia in patients receiving amphotericin B and the recovery of isolates for which the in vitro amphotericin B MICs were elevated (1, 70, 94). However, amphotericin B still remains the drug of choice in the treatment of *C. krusei* fungemia (94).

C. parapsilosis

C. parapsilosis has now become the second most frequently recovered *Candida* species from blood culture in Europe, Canada, and Latin America and ranks third in the United States (82, 85). *C. parapsilosis* is a common agent of fungemia and also has a predilection to cause endocarditis in cardiac surgery patients and in intravenous drug users and is also an agent of bone and joint infections (72). The epidemiology of *C. parapsilosis* in the hospital environment is unique among *Candida* species. *C. parapsilosis* is commonly recovered from human skin and can adhere strongly to the surfaces of intravascular catheters and prosthetic devices and has a propensity for proliferation in glucose-containing hyperalimentation solutions (2, 22, 58, 79).

C. parapsilosis has also been shown to be the *Candida* species most commonly recovered from the hands of health care workers, and this may explain why catheters and other devices are readily contaminated (39). The ability to produce an extracellular polysaccharide (often referred to as slime) in vitro has been noted in most *C. parapsilosis* bloodstream isolates, and this property is believed to aid adherence and biofilm formation on artificial surfaces (34, 58). Catheter-related *C. parapsilosis* infections have been described in a wide range of patient groups, and resolution of fungemia generally requires catheter removal, despite antifungal chemotherapy (34, 79). *C. parapsilosis* has also become associated with infection in neonatal intensive-care units. Rangel-Frausto et al. (91) demonstrated that, unlike surgical intensive-care units, where *C. glabrata* was the most commonly recovered NCAC species, *C. parapsilosis* was the NCAC species most commonly recovered in neonatal intensive-care units and was responsible for 29% of candidemias. Levy et al. (59), in a retrospective study of 81 episodes of candidemia, found that *C. parapsilosis* was responsible for 49% of episodes in neonates and was significantly associated with premature birth, the presence of a central venous catheter, and the use of total parenteral nutrition. A number of studies have applied molecular epidemiological techniques to trace the sources of *C. parapsilosis* infection (58, 86, 126). In one study, analysis of the electrophoretic karyotypes of *C. parapsilosis* isolates recovered from patients with fungemia demonstrated that three patients were infected with the same strain of *C. parapsilosis,* which was identical to a strain recovered from a common batch of hyperalimentation infusion (126). However, the source of the contaminating strain was not identified. Levin et al. (58) described a cluster of six cases of *C. parapsilosis* fungemia that were associated with the presence of intravenous catheters. The electrophoretic karyotypes of the isolates recovered from these patients were compared to determine strain relatedness, and two of the patients were found to be infected with the same strain of *C. parapsilosis.* An identical strain of *C. parapsilosis* was also recovered from the hands of health care workers with whom the patients were in regular contact. Although indirect, these data suggest that transmission of *C. parapsilosis* strains from the hands of health care workers to patients, possibly via intravenous catheters, does occur. *C. parapsilosis* is generally susceptible to all of the major antifungal drugs. However, in one study Nguyen et al. (70) reported that *C. parapsilosis* infection was associated with prior fluconazole therapy and was responsible for a number of cases of breakthrough candidemia in patients receiving fluconazole. In addition, reduced susceptibility to amphotericin B has been noted in isolates from patients who failed to respond to amphotericin B therapy (69).

C. tropicalis

Traditionally, *C. tropicalis* has been considered second only to *C. albicans* in virulence and clinical importance in the hospital setting (79, 120). *C. tropicalis* has been consistently reported as the NCAC species most commonly recovered from blood culture in patients with cancer (52, 114, 120). In particular, *C. tropicalis* is associated with patients with leukemia (52, 120). However, studies have shown that during the recent shifts in the epidemiology of candidiasis, *C. tropicalis* has now been superseded by *C. glabrata* and *C. parapsilosis* in overall importance in many institutions (3, 11, 82, 85, 90). *C. tropicalis* has the potential to cause severe invasive disease with multiorgan involvement in neutropenic patients, and hematogenous infection has been associated with a high mortality rate (52, 120). Analogous to infections caused by *C. albicans,* molecular typing suggests that *C. tropicalis* infection originates from the patients' own endogenous flora and that patients are colonized with their own unique strain, often throughout prolonged periods of hospitalization (79, 128). However, some studies using DNA fingerprinting have suggested that in some patients, strains of *C. tropicalis* may be acquired from exogenous sources. Doebbeling et al. (25) used DNA typing techniques to confirm an epidemiological link between isolates of *C. tropicalis* from a surgical scrub nurse and eight patients with *C. tropicalis* sternal wound infection. Two additional studies have used DNA fingerprinting to identify clusters of *C. tropicalis* isolates possessing the same DNA type that was recovered from patients in the same institution, suggesting patient-to-patient transmission of strains (86, 128). The antifungal susceptibility profile of *C. tropicalis* is unremarkable, and isolates recovered from blood culture are generally susceptible to amphotericin B, fluconazole, and itraconazole (83, 94).

C. lusitaniae

C. lusitaniae is considered an extremely rare pathogen that has been shown to be responsible for cases of candidemia in immunocompromised hosts (79). Despite the relative rarity of isolation of this species from cases of infection, considerable interest has been shown in the ability of this organism to develop resistance to amphotericin B. As mentioned earlier in this chapter, although *C. lusitaniae* is normally susceptible to amphotericin B, several studies have detailed the development of amphotericin B resistance in *C. lusitaniae* isolates recovered from patients treated with this drug (37, 76). *C. lusitaniae* isolates can also rapidly develop resistance to amphotericin B in vitro when exposed to this agent (125). However, the widespread use of amphotericin B has not been associated with any increased incidence of infection caused by this species (82, 86). Infection with *C. lusitaniae* is thought to arise endogenously, although no specific risk factors for *C. lusitaniae* colonization have been identified (79). Sanchez et al. (99) demonstrated a relatively high rate of *C. lusitaniae* colonization (7%) among 98 patients in bone marrow transplant and medical intensive-care units. Using RFLP analysis of genomic DNA, the authors identified a cluster of similar *C. lusitaniae* strains shared by five patients and an environmental source, indicating possible exogenous acquisition.

CONCLUDING REMARKS

The increasing clinical importance of NCAC species warrants detailed investigation. The recent shifts in *Candida* epidemiology and the emergence of novel species highlight the need for constant surveillance of *Candida* population dynamics and species distribution. Due to the growth of the immunosuppressed patient population and continued advances in medical technology, the clinical significance of these organisms is likely to grow. Continued surveillance of antifungal drug susceptibilities to existing and new antifungal agents will be critical to identify possible selective pressures for the emergence of particular *Candida* species. In addition, improved practice of basic infection control procedures should help prevent the nosocomial spread of these organisms. The growing interest in the molecular biology of the NCAC species is to be welcomed. In the future, this knowledge should aid in the development of effective, broad-spectrum antifungal agents and should help improve current methods of diagnosis and of investigating the epidemiology of these organisms.

REFERENCES

1. **Abbas, J., G. P. Bodey, H. A. Hanna, M. Mardani, E. Girgawy, D. Abi-Said, E. Whimbey, R. Hachem, and I. Raad.** 2000. *Candida krusei* fungemia: an escalating serious infection in immunocompromised hosts. *Arch. Intern. Med.* **160:** 2659–2664.
2. **Abi-Said, D., E. Anaissie, O. Uzun, I. Raad, H. Pinzcowski, and S. Vartivarian.** 1997. The epidemiology of hematogenous candidiasis caused by different *Candida* species. *Clin. Infect. Dis.* **24:**1122–1128.
3. **Anaissie, E., R. Hachem, C. K.-Tin-U., L. C. Stephens, and G. P. Bodey.** 1993. Experimental hematogenous candidiasis caused by *Candida krusei* and *Candida albicans*: species differences in pathogenicity. *Infect. Immun.* **61:**1268–1271.
4. **Anaissie, E. J., N. C. Karyotakis, R. Hachmen, M. C. Dignani, J. H. Rex, and V. Paetznick.** 1994. Correlation between in vitro and in vivo activity of antifungal agents against *Candida* species. *J. Infect. Dis.* **170:**384–389.
5. **Baily, G. G., C. B. Moore, S. M. Essayag, S. de Wit, J. P. Burnie, and D. W. Denning.** 1997. *Candida inconspicua,* a fluconazole-resistant pathogen in patients infected with human immunodeficiency virus. *Clin. Infect. Dis.* **25:** 161–163.
6. **Banerjee, S. N., T. G. Emori, D. H. Culver, R. P. Gaynes, W. R. Jarvis, T. Horan, J. R. Edwards, J. Tolson, T. Henderson, W. J. Martone, and the National Nosocomial Infections Surveillance System.** 1991. Secular trends in nosocomial primary bloodstream infections in the United States, 1980–1989. *Am. J. Med.* **91**(Suppl. 3B):86S–89S.
7. **Barchiesi, F., D. Calabrese, D. Sanglard, L. Falconi Di Francesco, F. Caselli, D. Giannini, A. Giacometti, S. Gavaudan, and G. Scalise.** 2000. Experimental induction of fluconazole resistance in *Candida tropicalis* ATCC 750. *Antimicrob. Agents Chemother.* **44:**1578–1584.
8. **Barchiesi, F., L. Falconi Di Francesco, D. Arzeni, F. Caselli, D. Gallo, and G. Scalise.** 1999. Electrophoretic karyotyping and triazole susceptibility of *Candida glabrata* clinical isolates. *Eur. J. Clin. Microbiol. Infect. Dis.* **18:**184–187.
9. **Barnett, J. A., R. W. Payne, and D. Yarrow.** 2000. *Yeasts: Characteristics and Identification,* 3rd ed. Cambridge University Press, Cambridge, United Kingdom.
10. **Barns, S. M., D. J. Lane, M. L. Sogin, C. Bibeau, and W. G. Weisburg.** 1991. Evolutionary relationships among pathogenic *Candida* species and relatives. *J. Bacteriol.* **173:** 2250–2255.
11. **Berrouane, Y. F., L. A. Herwaldt, and M. A. Pfaller.** 1999. Trends in antifungal use and epidemiology of nosocomial yeast infections in a university hospital. *J. Clin. Microbiol.* **37:**531–537.
12. **Berrouane, Y. F., R. J. Hollis, and M. A. Pfaller.** 1996. Strain variation among and antifungal susceptibilities of isolates of *Candida krusei. J. Clin. Microbiol.* **34:**1856–1858.
13. **Brajtburg, J., W. G. Powderly, G. S. Kobayashi, and G. Medoff.** 1990. Amphotericin B: current understanding of mechanisms of action. *Antimicrob. Agents Chemother.* **34:** 183–188.
14. **Brandt, M. E., L. H. Harrison, M. Pass, A. N. Sofair, S. Huie, R.-K. Li, C. J. Morrison, D. W. Warnock, and R. A. Hajjeh.** 2000. *Candida dubliniensis* fungemia: the first four cases in North America. *Emerg. Infect. Dis.* **6:**46–49.
15. **Cartledge, J. D., J. Midgley, and B. G. Gazzard.** 1999. Non-*albicans* oral candidosis in HIV-positive patients. *J. Antimicrob. Chemother.* **43:**419–422.
16. **Cassone, A., F. De Bernardis, E. Pontieri, G. Carruba, C. Girmenia, P. Martino, M. Fernandez-Rodriguez, G. Quindos, and J. Ponton.** 1995. Biotype diversity of *Candida parapsilosis* and its relationship to the clinical source and experimental pathogenicity. *J. Infect. Dis.* **171:**967–975.
17. **Chavanet, P., J. Lopez, M. Grappin, A. Bonnin, M. Duong, A. Waldner, M. Buisson, P. Camerlynck, and H. Portier.** 1994. Cross-sectional study of the susceptibility of *Candida* isolates to antifungal drugs and in vitro-in vivo correlation in HIV-infected patients. *AIDS* **8:**945–950.
18. **Coleman, D. C., D. E. Bennett, P. J. Gallagher, S. R. Flint, A. Nolan, F. M. Mulcahy, D. J. Sullivan, M. C. Henman, R. J. Russell, and D. B. Shanley.** 1995. Oral candidiasis and HIV infection: antifungal drug resistance and changes in *Candida* population dynamics, p. 112–118. *In* J. S. Greenspan and D. Greenspan (ed.), *Oral Manifestations of HIV Infection.* Quintessence Publishing Co., Ltd., Chicago, Ill.
19. **Coleman, D. C., D. E. Bennett, D. J. Sullivan, P. J. Gallagher, M. C. Henman, D. B. Shanley, and R. J. Russell.** 1993. Oral *Candida* in HIV infection and AIDS: new perspectives/new approaches. *Crit. Rev. Microbiol.* **19:**61–82.
20. **Coleman, D. C., D. J. Sullivan, D. E. Bennett, G. P. Moran, H. J. Barry, and D. B. Shanley.** 1997. Candidiasis: the emergence of a novel species, *Candida dubliniensis. AIDS* **11:** 557–567.
21. **Como, J. A., and W. E. Dismukes.** 1994. Oral azole drugs as systemic antifungal therapy. *N. Engl. J. Med* 330:263–272.
22. **De Bernardis, F., F. Mondello, R. San Millàn, J. Pontòn, and A. Cassone.** 1999. Biotyping and virulence properties of skin isolates of *Candida parapsilosis. J. Clin. Microbiol.* **37:** 3481–3486.
23. **De Hoog, G. S., and J. Guarra.** 1995. *Atlas of Clinical Fungi.*

Centraalbureau voor Schimmelcultures, Barn and Delft, the Netherlands, and Universitat Rovira i Virgili, Reus, Spain.

24. **De Viragh, P. A., D. Sangard, G. Togni, R. Falchetto, and M. Monod.** 1993. Cloning and sequencing of two *Candida parapsilosis* genes encoding acid proteases. *J. Gen. Microbiol.* **139:**335–342.
25. **Doebbeling, B. N., R. J. Hollis, H. D. Isenberg, R. P. Wenzel, and M. A. Pfaller.** 1991. Restriction fragment analysis of a *Candida tropicalis* outbreak of sternal wound infections. *J. Clin. Microbiol.* **29:**1268–1270.
26. **Donnelly, S. M., D. J. Sullivan, D. B. Shanley, and D. C. Coleman.** 1999. Phylogenetic analysis and rapid identification of *Candida dubliniensis* based on analysis of *ACT1* intron and exon sequences. *Microbiology* **145:**1871–1882.
27. **Dronda, F., M. Alonso-Sanz, F. Laguna, F. Chaves, J. V. Martínez-Suárez, J. L. Rodríguez-Tudella, A. González-López, and E. Valencia.** 1996. Mixed oropharyngeal candidiasis due to *Candida albicans* and non-*albicans Candida* strains in HIV-infected patients. *Eur. J. Clin. Microbiol. Infect. Dis.* **15:**446–452.
28. **Fidel, P. L., J. A. Vazquez, and J. D. Sobel.** 1999. *Candida glabrata*: review of epidemiology, pathogenesis, and clinical disease with comparison to *C. albicans*. *Clin. Microbiol. Rev.* **12:**80–96.
29. **Fischer-Hoch, S. P., and L. Hutwagner.** 1995. Opportunistic candidiasis: an epidemic of the 1980s. *Clin. Infect. Dis.* **21:** 897–904.
30. **Fridkin, S. K., and W. R. Jarvis.** 1996. Epidemiology of nosocomial fungal infections. *Clin. Microbiol. Rev.* **9:**499–511.
31. **Fromtling, R. A., G. K. Abruzzo, and D. M. Giltinan.** 1987. *Candida tropicalis* infection in normal, diabetic, and neutropenic mice. *J. Clin. Microbiol.* **25:**1416–1420.
32. **Fusek, M., E. A. Smith, M. Monod, B. M. Dunn, and S. I. Foundling.** 1994. Extracellular aspartic proteinases from *Candida albicans, Candida tropicalis,* and *Candida parapsilosis* yeasts differ substantially in their specificities. *Biochemistry* **33:**9791–9799.
33. **Gilfillan, G. D., D. J. Sullivan, K. Haynes, T. Parkinson, D. C. Coleman, and N. A. R. Gow.** 1998. *Candida dubliniensis*: phylogeny and putative virulence factors. *Microbiology* **144:** 829–838.
34. **Girmenia, C., P. Martino, F. De Bernardis, G. Gentile, M. Boccanera, M. Monaco, G. Antonnuci, and A. Cassone.** 1996. Rising incidence of *Candida parapsilosis* fungemia in patients with hematologic malignancies: clinical aspects, predisposing factors, and differential pathogenicity of the causative strains. *Clin. Infect. Dis.* **23:**506–514.
35. **Goodman, J. L., D. J. Winston, R. A. Greenfield, P. H. Chandrasekar, B. Fox, H. Kaizer, R. K. Shadduck, T. C. Shea, P. Stiff, and D. J. Friedman.** 1992. A controlled trial of fluconazole to prevent fungal infections in patients undergoing bone marrow transplantation. *N. Engl. J. Med.* **326:**845–851.
36. **Groll, A. H., A. J. De Lucca, and T. J. Walsh.** 1998. Emerging targets for the development of novel antifungal therapeutics. *Trends Microbiol.* **6:**117–124.
37. **Guinet, R., J. Chanas, A. Goullier, G. Bonnefoy, and P. Ambrose-Thomas.** 1983. Fatal septicemia due to amphotericin B-resistant *Candida lusitaniae*. *J. Clin. Microbiol.* **18:** 443–444.
38. **Hazen, K. C.** 1995. New and emerging yeast pathogens. *Clin. Microbiol. Rev.* **8:**462–478.
39. **Hedderwick, S. A., M. J. Lyons, M. Liu, J. A. Vazquez, and C. A. Kauffman.** 2000. Epidemiology of yeast colonisation in the intensive care unit. *Eur. J. Clin. Microbiol. Infect. Dis.* **19:**663–670.
40. **Hood, S., and D. W. Denning.** 1996. Treatment of fungal infection in AIDS. *J. Antimicrob. Chemother.* **37**(Suppl. B): 71–85.
41. **Hostetter, M. K.** 1999. Integrin-like proteins in *Candida* spp. and other microorganisms. *Fungal Genet. Biol.* **28:**135–145.
42. **Howlett, J. A.** 1976. The infection of rat tongue mucosa in vitro with five species of *Candida*. *J. Med. Microbiol.* **9:** 309–316.
43. **Hube, B.** 1996. *Candida albicans* secreted aspartyl proteinases. *Curr. Top. Med. Mycol.* **7:**55–69.
44. **Iwen, P. C., D. M. Kelly, E. C. Reed, and S. H. Hinrichs.** 1995. Invasive infection due to *Candida krusei* in immunocompromised patients not treated with fluconazole. *Clin. Infect. Dis.* **20:**342–347.
45. **Jarvis, W. R.** 1995. Epidemiology of nosocomial fungal infections, with emphasis on *Candida* species. *Clin. Infect. Dis.* **20:**1526–1530.
46. **Johnson, E. M., D. W. Warnock, J. Luker, S. R. Porter, and C. Scully.** 1995. Emergence of azole drug resistance in *Candida* species from HIV-infected patients receiving prolonged fluconazole therapy for oral candidosis. *J. Antimicrob. Chemother.* **35:**103–114.
47. **Kao, A. S., M. E. Brandt, W. R. Pruitt, L. A. Conn, B. A. Perkins, D. S. Stephens, W. S. Baughman, A. L. Reingold, G. A. Rothrock, M. A. Pfaller, R. W. Pinner, and R. A. Hajjeh.** 1999. The epidemiology of candidemia in two United States cities: results of a population-based active surveillance. *Clin. Infect. Dis.* **29:**1164–1170.
48. **King, R. D., J. C. Lee, and A. L. Morris.** 1980. Adherence of *Candida albicans* and other *Candida* species to mucosal epithelial cells. *Infect. Immun.* **27:**667–674.
49. **Kirkpatrick, W. R., S. G. Revankar, R. K. McAtee, J. L. Lopez-Ribot, A. W. Fothergill, D. I. McCarthy, S. E. Sanche, R. A. Cantu, M. G. Rinaldi, and T. F. Patterson.** 1998. Dectection of *Candida dubliniensis* in oropharyngeal samples from human immunodeficiency virus-infected patients in North America by primary CHROMagar Candida screening and susceptibility testing of isolates. *J. Clin. Microbiol.* **36:** 3007–3012.
50. **Klepser, M. E., E. J. Wolfe, R. N. Jones, C. H. Nightingale, and M. A. Pfaller.** 1997. Antifungal pharmacodynamic characteristics of fluconazole and amphotericin B tested against *Candida albicans*. *Antimicrob. Agents Chemother.* **41:** 1392–1395.
51. **Klotz, S. A., D. J. Drutz, J. L. Harrison, and M. Huppert.** 1983. Adherence and penetration of vascular endothelium by *Candida* yeasts. *Infect. Immun.* **42:**374–384.
52. **Komshian, S. V., A. K. Uwaydah, J. D. Sobel, and L. R. Crane.** 1989. Fungemia caused by *Candida* species and *Torulopsis glabrata* in the hospitalized patient: frequency, characteristics, and evaluation of factors influencing outcome. *Rev. Infect. Dis.* **11:**379–390.
53. **Kurtzman, C. P., and C. J. Robnett.** 1997. Identification of clinically important ascomycetous yeasts based on nucleotide divergence in the 5′ end of the large-subunit (26S) ribosomal DNA gene. *J. Clin. Microbiol.* **35:**1216–1223.
54. **Kurzai, O., W. J. Heinz, D. J. Sullivan, D. C. Coleman, M. Frosch, and F. A. Muhlschlegel.** 1999. Rapid PCR test for discriminating between *Candida albicans* and *Candida dubliniensis* isolates using primers derived from the pH-regulated *PHR1* and *PHR2* genes of *C. albicans*. *J. Clin. Microbiol.* **37:**1587–1590.
55. **Kwon-Chung, K. J., J. B. Hicks, and P. N. Lipke.** 1990. Evidence that *Candida stellatoidea* type II is a mutant of *Candida albicans* that does not express sucrose-inhibitable α-glucosidase. *Infect. Immun.* **58:**2804–2808.
56. **Kwon-Chung, K. J., W. S. Riggsby, R. A. Uphoff, J. B. Hicks,**

W. L. Whelan, E. Reiss, B. B. Magee, and B. L. Wickes. 1989. Genetic differences between type I and type II *Candida stellatoidea. Infect. Immun.* **57:**527–532.

57. **Kwon-Chung, K. J., B. L. Wickes, and W. G. Merz.** 1988. Association of electrophoretic karyotype of *Candida stellatoidea* with virulence for mice. *Infect. Immun.* **56:**1814–1819.
58. **Levin, A. S., S. F. Costa, N. S. Mussi, M. Basso, S. I. Sinto, C. Machado, D. C. Geiger, M. C. B. Villares, A. Z. Schreiber, A. A. Barone, and M. L. M. Branchini.** 1998. *Candida parapsilosis* fungemia associated with implantable and semi-implantable central venous catheters and the hands of healthcare workers. *Diagn. Microbiol. Infect. Dis.* **30:**243–249.
59. **Levy, I., L. G. Rubin, S. Vasishtha, V. Tucci, and S. K. Sood.** 1998. Emergence of *Candida parapsilosis* as the predominant species causing candidemia in children. *Clin. Infect. Dis.* **26:**1086–1088.
60. **Lischewski, A., M. Ruhnke, I. Tennagen, G. Schönian, J. Morschhäuser, and J. Hacker.** 1995. Molecular epidemiology of *Candida* isolates from AIDS patients showing different fluconazole resistance profiles. *J. Clin. Microbiol.* **33:**769–771.
61. **Maenza, J. R., W. G. Merz, M. J. Romagnoli, J. C. Keruly, R. D. Moore, and J. E. Gallant.** 1997. Infection due to fluconazole-resistant *Candida* in patients with AIDS: prevalence and microbiology. *Clin. Infect. Dis.* **24:**28–34.
62. **McCullough, M., B. Ross, and P. Reade.** 1995. Characterization of genetically distinct subgroup of *Candida albicans* strains from oral cavities of patients infected with human immunodeficiency virus. *J. Clin. Microbiol.* **33:**696–700.
63. **Meiller, T. F., M. A. Jabra-Rizk, A. Baqui, J. I. Kelley, V. I. Meeks, W. G. Merz, and W. A. Falkler.** 1999. Oral *Candida dubliniensis* as a clinically important species in HIV-seropositive patients in the United States. *Oral Surg. Oral Med. Oral Pathol. Oral Radiol. Endod.* **88:**573–580.
64. **Meis, J. F. G. M., M. Ruhnke, B. E. De Pauw, F. C. Odds, W. Siegert, and P. E. Verweij.** 1999. *Candida dubliniensis* candidemia in patients with chemotherapy-induced neutropenia and bone marrow transplantation. *Emerg. Infect. Dis.* **5:**150–153.
65. **Meis, J. F. G. M., F. M. V. Lunel, P. E. Verweij, and A. Voss.** 2000. One-year prevalence of *Candida dubliniensis* in a Dutch university hospital. *J. Clin. Microbiol.* **38:**3139–3140.
66. **Merz, W. G., J. E. Karp, D. Schron, and R. Saral.** 1986. Increased incidence of fungemia caused by *Candida krusei. J. Clin. Microbiol.* **24:**581–584.
67. **Moran, G. P., D. Sanglard, S. M. Donnelly, D. B. Shanley, D. J. Sullivan, and D. C. Coleman.** 1998. Identification and expression of multidrug transporters responsible for fluconazole resistance in *Candida dubliniensis. Antimicrob. Agents Chemother.* **42:**1819–1830.
68. **Moran, G. P., D. J. Sullivan, M. C. Henman, C. E. McCreary, B. J. Harrington, D. B. Shanley, and D. C. Coleman.** 1997. Antifungal drug susceptibilities of oral *Candida dubliniensis* isolates from human immunodeficiency virus (HIV)-infected and non-HIV-infected subjects and generation of stable fluconazole-resistant derivatives in vitro. *Antimicrob. Agents Chemother.* **41:**617–623.
69. **Nguyen, H. M., C. J. Clancy, V. L. Yu, Y. C. Yu, A. J. Morris, D. R. Snydman, D. A. Sutton, and M. G. Rinaldi.** 1998. Do in vitro susceptibility data predict the microbiologic response to amphotericin B? Results of a prospective study of patients with *Candida* fungemia. *J. Infect. Dis.* **177:**425–430.
70. **Nguyen, M. H., J. E. Peacock, A. J. Morris, D. C. Tanner, M. L. Nguyen, D. R. Snydman, M. M. Wagener, M. G. Rinaldi, and V. L. Yu.** 1996. The changing face of candidemia: emergence of non-*Candida albicans* species and antifungal resistance. *Am. J. Med.* **100:**617–623.
71. **Occhipinti, D. J., P. O. Gubbins, P. Schreckenberger, and L. H. Danziger.** 1994. Frequency, pathogenicity and microbiologic outcome of non-*Candida albicans* candiduria. *Eur. J. Clin. Microbiol. Infect. Dis.* **13:**459–467.
72. **Odds, F. C.** 1988. *Candida and Candidosis: a Review and Bibliography,* 2nd ed. Baillière Tindall, London, United Kingdom.
73. **Odds, F. C.** 1987. *Candida* infections: an overview. *Crit. Rev. Microbiol.* **15:**1–5.
74. **Odds, F. C., and R. Bernaerts.** 1994. CHROMagar Candida, a new differential isolation medium for presumptive identification of clinically important *Candida* species. *J. Clin. Microbiol.* **32:**1923–1929.
75. **Odds, F. C., L. Van Nuffel, and G. Dams.** 1998. Prevalence of *Candida dubliniensis* isolates in a yeast stock collection. *J. Clin. Microbiol.* **36:**2869–2873.
76. **Pappagianis, D., M. S. Collins, R. Hector, and J. Remington.** 1979. Development of resistance to amphotericin B in *Candida lusitaniae* infecting a human. *Antimicrob. Agents Chemother.* **16:**123–126.
77. **Pfaller, M., and R. Wenzel.** 1992. Impact of the changing epidemiology of fungal infections in the 1990s. *Eur. J. Clin. Microbiol. Infect. Dis.* **11:**287–291.
78. **Pfaller, M. A.** 1994. Epidemiology and control of fungal infections. *Clin. Infect. Dis.* **19**(Suppl. 1):S8–S13.
79. **Pfaller, M. A.** 1996. Nosocomial candidiasis: emerging species, reservoirs, and modes of transmission. *Clin. Infect. Dis.* **22**(Suppl. 2):S89–S94.
80. **Pfaller, M. A., R. N. Jones, G. V. Doern, A. C. Fluit, J. Verhoef, H. S. Sader, S. A. Messer, A. Houston, S. Coffman, R. J. Hollis, and the SENTRY Participant Group (Europe).** 1999. International surveillance of blood stream infections due to *Candida* species in the European SENTRY program: species distribution and antifungal susceptibility including the investigational triazole and echinocandin agents. *Diagn. Microbiol. Infect. Dis.* **35:**19–25.
81. **Pfaller, M. A., R. N. Jones, G. V. Doern, H. S. Sader, R. J. Hollis, S. A. Messer, and the SENTRY Participant Group.** 1998. International surveillance of bloodstream infections due to *Candida* species: frequency of occurrence and antifungal susceptibilities of isolates collected in 1997 in the United States, Canada, and South America for the SENTRY program. *J. Clin. Microbiol.* **36:**1886–1889.
82. **Pfaller, M. A., R. N. Jones, G. V. Doern, H. S. Sader, S. A. Messer, A. Houston, S. Coffman, and R. J. Hollis.** 2000. Bloodstream infections due to *Candida* species: SENTRY antimicrobial surveillance program in North America and Latin America, 1997–1998. *Antimicrob. Agents Chemother.* **44:**747–751.
83. **Pfaller, M. A., R. N. Jones, S. A. Messer, M. B. Edmond, R. P. Wenzel, and the SCOPE Participant Group.** 1998. National surveillance of nosocomial blood stream infection due to species of *Candida* other than *Candida albicans:* frequency of occurrence and antifungal susceptibility in the SCOPE program. *Diagn. Microbiol. Infect. Dis.* **30:**121–129.
84. **Pfaller, M. A., S. A. Messer, S. Gee, S. Joly, C. Pujol, D. J. Sullivan, D. C. Coleman, and D. R. Soll.** 1999. In vitro susceptibilities of *Candida dubliniensis* isolates tested against the new triazole and echinocandin antifungal agents. *J. Clin. Microbiol.* **37:**870–872.
85. **Pfaller, M. A., S. A. Messer, R. J. Hollis, R. N. Jones, G. V. Doern, M. E. Brandt, and R. A. Hajjeh.** 1999. Trends in

species distribution and susceptibility to fluconazole among blood stream isolates of *Candida* species in the United States. *Diagn. Microbiol. Infect. Dis.* 33:217–222.

86. **Pfaller, M. A., S. A. Messer, A. Houston, M. S. Rangel-Frausto, T. Wiblin, H. M. Blumberg, J. E. Edwards, W. Jarvis, M. A. Martin, H. C. Neu, L. Saiman, J. E. Patterson, J. C. Dibb, C. M. Roldan, M. G. Rinaldi, and R. P. Wenzel.** 1998. National epidemiology of mycoses survey: a multicenter study of strain variation and antifungal susceptibility among isolates of *Candida* species. *Diagn. Microbiol. Infect. Dis.* **31**:289–296.
87. **Polacheck, I., J. Strahilevitz, D. Sullivan, S. Donnelly, I. F. Salkin, and D. C. Coleman.** 2000. Recovery of *Candida dubliniensis* from non-human immunodeficiency virus-infected patients in Israel. *J. Clin. Microbiol.* **38**:170–174.
88. **Ponton, J., R. Rüchel, K. V. Clemons, D. C. Coleman, R. Grillot, J. Guarro, D. Aldebert, P. Ambroise-Thomas, J. Cano, A. J. Carillo-Muñoz, J. Gené, C. Pinel, D. A. Stevens, and D. J. Sullivan.** 2000. Emerging pathogens. *Med. Mycol.* **38**(Suppl. 1):225–236.
89. **Powderly, W. G.** 1992. Mucosal candidiasis caused by non-*albicans* species of *Candida* in HIV-positive patients. *AIDS* **6**:604–605.
90. **Price, M. F., M. T. La Rocco, and L. O. Gentry.** 1994. Fluconazole susceptibilities of *Candida* species and distribution of species recovered from blood cultures over a 5-year period. *Antimicrob. Agents Chemother.* **38**:1422–1424.
91. **Rangel-Frausto, M. S., T. Wiblin, H. M. Blumberg, L. Saiman, J. Patterson, M. Rinaldi, M. Pfaller, J. E. Edwards, W. Jarvis, J. Dawson, R. P. Wenzel, and the NEMIS Study Group.** 1999. National epidemiology of mycoses survey (NEMIS): variations in rates of bloodstream infections due to *Candida* species in seven surgical intensive care units and six neonatal intensive care units. *Clin. Infect. Dis.* **29**: 253–258.
92. **Rex, J. H., M. A. Pfaller, A. L. Barry, P. W. Nelson, C. D. Webb, the NIAD MSG, and the Candidemia Study Group.** 1995. Antifungal susceptibility testing of isolates from a randomized multicenter trial of fluconazole versus amphotericin B as treatment of nonneutropenic patients with candidemia. *Antimicrob. Agents Chemother.* **39**:40–44.
93. **Rex, J. H., M. A. Pfaller, J. N. Galgiani, M. S. Bartlett, A. Espinel-Ingroff, M. A. Ghannoum, M. Lancaster, F. C. Odds, M. G. Rinaldi, T. J. Walsh, and A. L. Barry.** 1997. Development of interpretive breakpoints for antifungal susceptibility testing: conceptual framework and analysis of in vitro-in vivo correlation data for fluconazole, itraconazole, and *Candida* infections. *Clin. Infect. Dis.* **24**:235–247.
94. **Rex, J. H., T. J. Walsh, J. D. Sobel, S. G. Filler, P. G. Pappas, W. E. Dismukes, and J. E. Edwards.** 2000. Practice guidelines for the treatment of candidiasis. *Clin. Infect. Dis.* **30**: 662–678.
95. **Ruhnke, M., A. Eigler, E. Engelmann, B. Geiseler, and M. Trautmann.** 1994. Correlation between antifungal susceptibility testing of *Candida* isolates from patients with HIV infection and clinical results after treatment with fluconazole. *Infection* **22**:72–76.
96. **Ruhnke, M., A. Schmidt-Westhausen, and J. Morschhäuser.** 2000. Development of simultaneous resistance to fluconazole in *Candida albicans* and *Candida dubliniensis* in patients with AIDS. *J. Antimicrob. Chemother.* **46**:291–295.
97. **Samaranayake, L. P.** 1990. Oral candidosis: an old disease in new guises. *Dental Update* **17**:36–38.
98. **Samaranayake, Y. H., and L. P. Samaranayake.** 1994. *Candida krusei:* biology, epidemiology, pathogenicity and clinical manifestations of an emerging pathogen. *J. Med. Microbiol.* **41**:295–310.
99. **Sanchez, V., J. A. Vazquez, D. Barth-Jones, L. Dembry, J. D. Sobel, and M. J. Zervos.** 1992. Epidemiology of nosocomial acquisition of *Candida lusitaniae. J. Clin. Microbiol.* **30**: 3005–3008.
100. **Sandven, P., K. Nilsen, A. Digranes, T. Tjade, and J. Lassen.** 1997. *Candida norvegensis:* a fluconazole-resistant species. *Antimicrob. Agents Chemother.* **41**:1375–1376.
101. **Sangeorzan, J. A., S. F. Bradley, X. He, L. T. Zarins, G. L. Ridenour, R. N. Tiballi, and C. A. Kauffman.** 1994. Epidemiology of oral candidiasis in HIV-infected patients: colonization, infection, treatment, and emergence of fluconazole-resistance. *Am. J. Med.* **97**:339–346.
102. **Schoofs, A. G., F. C. Odds, R. Colebunders, M. Ieven, and H. Goossens.** 1998. Cross-sectional study of oral *Candida* carriage in a human immunodeficiency virus (HIV)-seropositive population: predisposing factors, epidemiology and antifungal susceptibility. *Mycoses* **41**:203–211.
103. **Sobel, J. D.** 1998. Vulvovaginitis due to *Candida glabrata.* An emerging problem. *Mycoses* **41**(Suppl. 2):18–22.
104. **Sullivan, D., D. Bennett, M. Henman, P. Harwood, S. Flint, F. Mulcahy, D. Shanley, and D. Coleman.** 1993. Oligonucleotide fingerprinting of isolates of *Candida* species other than *C. albicans* and of atypical *Candida* species from human immunodeficiency virus-positive and AIDS patients. *J. Clin. Microbiol.* **31**:2124–2133.
105. **Sullivan, D., and D. Coleman.** 1998. *Candida dubliniensis:* characteristics and identification. *J. Clin. Microbiol.* **36**: 329–334.
106. **Sullivan, D., K. Haynes, J. Bille, P. Boerlin, L. Rodero, S. Lloyd, M. Henman, and D. Coleman.** 1997. Widespread geographic distribution of oral *Candida dubliniensis* strains in human immunodeficiency virus-infected individuals. *J. Clin. Microbiol.* **35**:960–964.
107. **Sullivan, D. J., M. C. Henman, G. P. Moran, L. C. O'Neill, D. E. Bennett, D. B. Shanley, and D. C. Coleman.** 1996. Molecular genetic approaches to identification, epidemiology and taxonomy of non-*albicans Candida* species. *J. Med. Microbiol.* **44**:399–408.
108. **Sullivan, D. J., G. Moran, S. Donnelly, S. Gee, E. Pinjon, B. McCartan, D. B. Shanley, and D. C. Coleman.** 1999. *Candida dubliniensis:* an update. *Rev. Iberoam. Micol.* **16**:72–76.
109. **Sullivan, D. J., T. J. Westerneng, K. A. Haynes, D. E. Bennett, and D. C. Coleman.** 1995. *Candida dubliniensis* sp. nov.: phenotypic and molecular characterization of a novel species associated with oral candidosis in HIV-infected individuals. *Microbiology* **141**:1507–1521.
110. **Tamura, M., K. Watanabe, T. Imai, Y. Mikami, and K. Nishimura.** 2000. New PCR primer pairs specific for *Candida dubliniensis* and detection of the fungi from the *Candida albicans* clinical isolates in Japan. *Clin. Lab.* **46**:33–40.
111. **Tumbarello, M., G. Caldarola, E. Tacconelli, G. Morace, B. Posteraro, R. Cauda, and L. Ortona.** 1996. Analysis of risk factors associated with the emergence of azole resistant oral candidosis in the course of HIV infection. *J. Antimicrob. Chemother.* **38**:691–699.
112. **Vanden Bossche, H., P. Marichal, and F. C. Odds.** 1994. Molecular mechanisms of drug resistance in fungi. *Trends Microbiol.* **2**:393–400.
113. **Vazquez, J. A., L. M. Dembry, V. Sanchez, M. A. Vazquez, J. D. Sobel, C. Dmuchowski, and M. J. Zervos.** 1998. Nosocomial *Candida glabrata* colonization: an epidemiologic study. *J. Clin. Microbiol.* **36**:421–426.
114. **Viscoli, C., C. Girmenia, A. Marinus, L. Collette, P. Martino, B. Vandercam, C. Doyen, B. Lebeau, D. Spence, V. Kremery,**

B. De Pauw, F. Meunier, and the IFIC of the EORTC. 1999. Candidemia in cancer patients: a prospective, multicentre surveillance study by the invasive fungal infection group (IFIG) of the European organization for research and treatment of cancer (EORTC). *Clin. Infect. Dis.* **28:**1071–1079.

115. **Wagner, T., M. Borg-von Zepelin, and R. Ruchel.** 1995. pH-dependant denaturation of extracellular aspartic proteinases from *Candida* species. *J. Med. Vet. Mycol.* **33:**275–278.

116. **Warnock, D. W., J. Burke, N. J. Cope, E. M. Johnson, N. A. Von Fraunhofer, and E. W. Williams.** 1988. Fluconazole resistance in *Candida glabrata. Lancet* **2:**1310.

117. **Wenzel, R. P.** 1995. Nosocomial candidemia: risk factors and attributable mortality. *Clin. Infect. Dis.* **20:**1531–1534.

118. **White, T. C., K. A. Marr, and R. A. Bowden.** 1998. Clinical, cellular, and molecular factors that contribute to antifungal drug resistance. *Clin. Microbiol. Rev.* **11:**382–402.

119. **Wickes, B. L., J. E. Golin, and K. J. Kwon-Chung.** 1991. Chromosomal rearrangement in *Candida stellatoidea* results in a positive effect on phenotype. *Infect. Immun.* **59:** 1762–1771.

119a. **Willis, A. M., W. A. Coulter, D. J. Sullivan, et al.** 2000. Isolation of *C. dubliniensis* from insulin-using diabetes mellitus patients. *J. Oral Pathol. Med.* **29:**86–90.

120. **Wingard, J. R.** 1995. Importance of *Candida* species other than *C. albicans* as pathogens in oncology patients. *Clin. Infect. Dis.* **20:**115–125.

121. **Wingard, J. R., J. D. Dick, W. G. Merz, G. R. Sandford, R. Saral, and W. H. Burns.** 1980. Pathogenicity of *Candida tropicalis* and *Candida albicans* after gastrointestinal inoculation in mice. *Infect. Immun.* **29:**808–813.

122. **Wingard, J. R., W. G. Merz, M. G. Rinaldi, T. R. Johnson, J. E. Karp, and R. Saral.** 1991. Increase in *Candida krusei* infection among patients with bone marrow transplantation and neutropenia treated prophylactically with fluconazole. *N. Engl. J. Med.* **325:**1274–1277.

123. **Wingard, J. R., W. G. Merz, M. G. Rinaldi, C. B. Miller, J. E. Karp, and R. Saral.** 1993. Association of *Torulopsis glabrata* infections with fluconazole prophylaxis in neutropenic bone marrow transplant patients. *Antimicrob. Agents Chemother.* **37:**1847–1849.

124. **Winston, D. J., P. H. Chandrasekar, H. M. Lazarus, J. L. Goodman, J. L. Silber, H. Horowitz, R. K. Shadduck, C. S. Rosenfeld, W. G. Ho, and M. Z. Islam.** 1993. Fluconazole prophylaxis of fungal infections in patients with acute leukemia. Results of a randomized placebo-controlled, double-blind, multicenter trial. *Ann. Intern. Med.* **118:**495–503.

125. **Yoon, S. A., J. A. Vazquez, P. E. Steffan, J. D. Sobel, and R. A. Akins.** 1999. High-frequency, in vitro reversible switching of *Candida lusitaniae* clinical isolates from amphotericin B susceptibility to resistance. *Antimicrob. Agents Chemother.* **43:**836–845.

126. **Zancopé-Oliveira, R. M., M. J. James, A. P. Derossi, J. L. M. Sampaio, M. M. Muniz, R. K. Li, A. S. A. Nascimento, J. M. Peralta, and E. Reiss.** 2000. Strain characterization of *Candida parapsilosis* fungemia by molecular typing methods. *Eur. J. Clin. Microbiol. Infect. Dis.* **19:**514–520.

127. **Zaugg, C., M. Borg-von Zepelin, U. Reichard, D. Sanglard, and D. Monod.** 2001. Secreted aspartic proteinase family of *Candida tropicalis. Infect. Immun.* **69:**405–412.

128. **Zhang, J., R. J. Hollis, and M. A. Pfaller.** 1997. Variations in DNA subtype and antifungal susceptibility among clinical isolates of *Candida tropicalis. Diagn. Microbiol. Infect. Dis.* **27:**63–67.

Candida and Candidiasis
Edited by Richard A. Calderone

Chapter 5

Population Genetic Analyses of *Candida*

Jianping Xu and Thomas G. Mitchell

INTRODUCTION

In recent years, there has been a vast proliferation of information concerning the molecular epidemiology and population biology of fungi pathogenic for humans and other animals. This increase has been stimulated by the rising incidence of mycotic diseases and the increasing availability of strain typing techniques. Chief among the contributors to the current mycological crisis are species of *Candida*. As a result, knowledge of the epidemiology and population biology of *Candida* and candidiasis has grown considerably. However, the powerful potential and contributions of population genetic studies to understanding the basic biology and pathogenesis of medical fungi are slowly being recognized. These contributions are important and should be emphasized and expanded. For example, understanding the population dynamics of a pathogenic fungus will clarify epidemiological trends and assist researchers to select appropriate strains to investigate for virulence factors and to discover appropriate targets for novel antifungal drugs, vaccines, or diagnostic tests.

Because there are extensive reviews on fingerprinting of *Candida* and other human pathogenic fungi (27, 31, 42, 45, 48), this chapter will review approaches based on population genetic analyses of mostly codominant genetic markers to elucidate the patterns of variation in *Candida* spp. We will introduce basic concepts, issues, and rationales for population genetic studies of medical fungi. The chapter will focus on how codominant genetic markers help resolve issues of ploidy, clonality, and recombination and differentiate among populations within species of *Candida*.

What Is a Population?

There are several definitions of population: a population can be (i) the organisms that inhabit a particular locality, (ii) a group of interbreeding organisms that represents the level of organization at which speciation begins, or (iii) a group of individual persons, objects, or items from which samples are taken for statistical measurement. The first definition is based on geographic locations, although the size and boundaries of individual populations can vary widely and are often arbitrary. This definition fits most population genetic studies of fungi and other organisms. The second definition is based on genetics and is the most restrictive. By this definition, a population refers to a group of individuals that are genetically isolated but still capable of interbreeding with individuals of other populations of the same species. For many species, including human pathogenic fungi, it is usually difficult to establish the precise mating boundaries for groups of individuals. In species of plants and animals, both geographical and ecological factors contribute to determining the boundaries of the breeding population (18, 32). An obvious difficulty with this definition is that many species of pathogenic fungi are not known to engage in sexual mating and meiosis.

The third definition is the most versatile. It allows multidimensional analyses of the distribution of genetic variation within a species. This is an operational definition of a population. For example, a population of *C. albicans* may consist of a collection of individual strains from a particular locality. The locality may be defined as a geographical entity (e.g., continent, country, state or province, county, city, hospital unit) or ecological niche (e.g., isolates from patients with certain diseases or risk factors, patients treated with different drugs, specific body sites, or different body sites of the same person). A population of *C. albicans* isolates could be further delimited by the characteristics of the hosts from which they were derived (e.g., sex, age, race and ethnic background).

The main limitation on the number of defining

Jianping Xu • Department of Biology, McMaster University, Hamilton, Ontario L8S 4K1, Canada. **Thomas G. Mitchell** • Department of Microbiology, Duke University Medical Center, Durham, NC 27710.

criteria is that the sample size of the smallest category must be sufficiently large for statistical analysis. The sample size that is sufficient to detect differences among samples depends on the patterns of genetic variation of the population. The smaller the difference among samples, the larger the sample sizes must be for their reliable detection. Typically, the minimum expected count within a category (allelic or genotypic counts) in statistical tests is five (41).

Genetic Markers

A genetic marker can be defined as a unique form of a gene locus. For purposes of population genetics, a genetic locus may be defined as a sequence of DNA that exhibits (i) a single nucleotide polymorphism, (ii) an endonuclease recognition site that detects restriction fragment length polymorphism (RFLP) (usually involving four to six nucleotides), or (iii) a single nucleotide insertion or deletion. In addition, (iv) any nucleotide sequence difference(s) within a region of continuous DNA of variable length may constitute a distinct allele. A genetic locus may also be represented by (v) an enzymatic staining profile. Because of the large variation in the size of the DNA segment or gene that is recognized as a locus, analytical methods may be different. All analytical methods rely on two basic assumptions: (i) once a locus is defined, recombination within the locus is assumed to occur very rarely or not at all, and (ii) each distinct allele is the result of a unique mutational event that occurred only once in the population. With these assumptions, indistinguishable alleles are considered to be "identical-by-descent."

For the species under investigation, the types of markers amenable to population genetic-based analysis depend on the ploidy and the mating system. Genetic markers must be unambiguously interpretable as alleles of a specific locus, and all alleles at each locus must be identifiable for all isolates. In haploid species, most markers are amenable to analysis by population genetic methods. Since there is only one set of genetic material (n) for each strain in haploid species, alleles at each locus can be inferred for each strain (but see below in "Ploidy—Heterozygosity and Homozygosity"). However, in diploid species ($2n$), determining the number of loci and the number of alleles per locus for many fingerprinting-based genotyping techniques can be tedious and is often prone to error. In a species with a tractable mating system, strains can be crossed and the meiotic progenies can be analyzed to determine the number of loci and the number of alleles per locus for a defined marker system. With diploid species that lack sexual mating and/or meiosis, the interpretation of markers is highly problematic. In general, allelic assignments in such strains are best accomplished with the use of codominant, single-copy genetic markers. These markers include allozymes, single locus RFLP (including PCR-RFLP), and single nucleotide polymorphisms. Because the theoretical bases and practical techniques for generating various molecular markers have been reviewed extensively (27, 31, 42, 45), these methods will not be described in this chapter.

Some markers are better able to address certain questions. Selectively neutral, codominant markers are best suited to investigate recombination and gene flow between populations. Loci that are under selective pressure will have a higher probability of convergent and sometimes diversifying evolution than neutral loci. For example, in a clinical environment, genes involved in drug resistance and responses to the host are under constant selective pressure, and these genes may not be suitable to investigate recombination and genetic differentiation in natural populations.

PLOIDY—HETEROZYGOSITY AND HOMOZYGOSITY

Most earlier studies of ploidy in *Candida* and other yeast species examined DNA content through DNA reassociation kinetics (38), flow cytometry, and/or the segregation of auxotrophic mutations via mitotic recombination (50). Using these techniques, the ploidy of only two species have been independently determined and confirmed: *C. albicans* ($2n$) and *C. glabrata* (*Torulopsis glabrata*) (n). Population genetic analyses of these species using codominant genetic markers are consistent with earlier assessments of their DNA content; marker segregation data revealed abundant heterozygosity in *C. albicans* (17, 23, 37, 57, 59) and the lack of any heterozygosity in *C. glabrata* (23).

In the absence of robust data on the DNA content, the putative ploidy of many *Candida* species can be inferred from population genetic analyses. The principle of this inference is that the existence of extensive heterozygosity indicates diploidy (or higher ploidy, depending on the number of alleles in a given individual). Conversely, the total lack of heterozygosity in large samples indicates haploidy. Using this criterion, the putative ploidy of many common *Candida* species can be inferred and are presented in Table 1. However, these findings are not necessarily conclusive as the lack of heterozygosity could also result from extensive self-fertilization or inbreeding among related individuals in diploid species. In addition, in the absence of allelic information for some isoenzyme

Table 1. Confirmed or putative ploidy of some common *Candida* species inferred from population genetic surveys using codominant genetic markers[a]

Species	Ploidy	Reference(s)
C. albicans	Diploid	16, 17, 23, 37, 57, 59
C. stellatoidea	Diploid	23, 36
C. dubliniensis	Haploid	36
C. tropicalis	Diploid	12, 23
C. parapsilosis	Diploid	23
C. glabrata	Haploid	36
C. krusei	Diploid	36
C. guilliermondii	Diploid	39
C. fermentati	Diploid	39
C. lusitaniae	Haploid	26

[a]See text for cautionary comments in interpreting the isoenzyme data for species of *C. stellatoidea, C. dubliniensis, C. tropicalis, C. parapsilosis, C. krusei, C. guilliermondii, C. fermentati,* and *C. lusitaniae.*

bands, the appearance of multiple bands might not result from diploidy and heterozygosity, but rather from multiple genetic loci encoding different forms of an enzyme in a haploid species.

CLONALITY AND RECOMBINATION

In natural populations, patterns of genetic variation can be observed and documented. One of the most intriguing and relevant questions concerning pathogenic fungi (and other microbes) is deciphering the cause(s) of this genetic variation in populations. All microbes undergo mitosis and are therefore able to reproduce asexually. Consequently, natural and clinical samples of most microbial species invariably manifest evidence of some degree of clonality. Samples from all species of *Candida* that have been examined show some evidence of clonality (see below). A major focus of fungal population genetic studies has been to determine whether recombination contributes to the generation of genetic variation in natural populations (45, 57). For clinical and public health reasons, it is important to determine the extent, if any, that recombination contributes to genetic variation within populations of mycotic fungi.

The amount of recombination that occurs in natural populations of microorganisms affects their evolution. Sexual reproduction and recombination pose an evolutionary paradox (24, 30). An organism that reproduces asexually transmits all its genes to each of its progeny, but an organism that reproduces sexually imparts only half of its genes to each progeny. Therefore, under stable, uniform growth conditions, natural selection favors the organism that reproduces asexually over one that reproduces sexually because with an equal number of progeny, the asexual individual has double the fitness of one that reproduces sexually.

In contrast, sexual reproduction affords microorganisms two possible advantages: panmixia and DNA repair (24, 30). The panmictic argument suggests that without the mixing of genes generated by sexual recombination, adaptive evolution is limited to the accumulation of favorable mutations that occur successively in each independently evolving lineage. Sexual recombination allows favorable mutations that arise in separate lineages to become combined in the same individual, providing an advantage in the adaptation to different environments. The repair argument states that the two haplotypes associated with diploidy during sex provide an error-correction mechanism for repairing genetic damage. Genetic damage can occur spontaneously and continuously during replication and possibly transcription. The intact DNA of one haplotype can serve as a template for correcting the damaged DNA in the other haplotype. Moreover, deleterious mutations in one haplotype can be overcome by compensatory dominant mutations in diploids. Whether one or both of these purported advantages of sexual recombination accounts for the origin and maintenance of sexual reproduction has stimulated considerable debate and investigation.

Another reason to assess the role of recombination in natural populations relates to issues of sampling, research, and treatment strategies. If recombination occurs in natural populations, there may be significant ramifications for the evolution and dissemination of genes related to antibiotic resistance, pathogenicity, and host specificity. A recombining population structure implies that the selected properties reflect distinct genes or nonrecombining genetic elements. (Discrete genes are usually assumed to be nonrecombining units, even though intragenic recombination has been demonstrated in all organisms that have been critically examined.) Conversely, a clonal population structure implies that the selected units are clones or clonal lineages. To study medically relevant traits in a clonal population, representatives of every clonal lineage should be sampled. However, in a recombining population, it would be more productive to focus primarily on individual genes.

To determine whether a microbial population structure is predominantly clonal or recombining, population microbiologists employ genetic tests. The remainder of this section will discuss the tests used to dissect the genetic structure within a population. These tests differ somewhat for haploid and diploid species.

Analysis of Clonality and Recombination in Haploids

Since a haploid genome contains only one set of chromosomes, each isolate has only one allele for each locus. Consequently, tests of recombination in natural, haploid populations involve examining the allelic associations between different loci (4, 13, 25, 46) (Table 2).

In tests for the occurrence of recombination in natural populations, there are two distinct questions. First, is the population panmictic? A panmictic population structure implies that alleles at all loci are randomly associated with each other. If the hypothesis of panmixia is statistically rejected and a clonal population structure is assumed, the second question arises: Can all or part of the genetic variation in natural populations be attributed to recombination? Since all medical fungi are capable of reproducing asexually through mitosis, a clonal component is expected in populations. A common approach is to analyze one representative of each multilocus genotype to distinguish between the null hypothesis of recombination and the alternative hypothesis of clonality (57, 59).

Quite often, a small number of genotypes are dominant or overrepresented within a population. It is common in these analyses to include the genotypes of all isolates in the population as well as only the unique genotypes within the population; this smaller group is the "clone-corrected" sample. The rejection of panmixia for the total sample but acceptance of panmixia for the clone-corrected sample is usually regarded as evidence of clonal expansion but with random mating in the genetic structure (25). However, there are several caveats related to the truncation of a sample by clone-correction before testing. Even though generally assumed, it is usually not confirmed that identical multilocus genotypes are actually clonal in origin. The justification for clonal-correction of the sample should be based on biological and ecological considerations. The decrease in sample size may also decrease the power of the statistical test for rejection of the null hypothesis of random recombination (i.e., panmixia).

Tests for whether a haploid population is panmictic involve comparing the observed allelic associations with those derived under the null hypothesis of random mating. The two most widely used population genetic tests for haploid genomes are tests for allelic association (linkage equilibrium) between pairs of loci (46) and the overall index of association (I_A), which involves alleles at all loci (3, 25). A third test compares the observed genotypic diversity with that expected under the null hypothesis of random mating (44, 57). A fourth test uses phylogenetic analysis of DNA sequence-based characters (1, 4, 20). In this test, incongruences between different gene genealogies for a set of strains are considered to be consistent with the hypothesis of recombination.

Linkage disequilibrium

Linkage disequilibrium (gametic phase disequilibrium or gametic disequilibrium) is a measure of the association between alleles at pairs of loci (44, 55, 58). Random association between alleles at different loci in a population is inferred to reflect recombination between these two loci. The test for random association can be described as follows: If alleles at two loci, A and B, segregate independently, then the expected frequency of the genotype A_iB_i is simply the product of the frequencies of the two alleles A_i and B_i. A chi-square test or Fisher's exact test can be performed to determine whether the observed genotypic counts are significantly different from the expected counts. If the observed and expected counts are not significantly different, then the population under study is assumed to have a recombining structure.

Table 2. Common criteria for distinguishing clonality and recombination in microbial populations with large population size and examined with neutral, genetically unlinked markers

Criteria	Ploidy	Clonality	Recombination
Allelic association within a locus			
HWE	Diploidy or higher	No	Yes
Excess homozygosity	Diploidy or higher	Yes	No
Excess heterozygosity	Diploidy or higher	Yes	No
Allelic association between loci			
Random	All ploidy	No	Yes
Nonrandom	All ploidy	Yes	No
Gene genealogy congruence	All ploidy (but mostly for haploids)	Yes	No
Overrepresentation of certain multilocus genotypes	All ploidy	Yes	No

Conversely, if the observed and expected counts are significantly different, the population is assumed to have a clonal structure as inferred by this pair of loci. With balanced gene frequencies, in a completely panmictic population, less than 5% of locus pairs are expected to have genotypic counts significantly different from those expected.

A crucial factor in this test is the independence of the loci. If the paired loci are linked, they are not completely independent. The degree of linkage between loci affects the association of alleles at these loci. However, it is generally assumed and has been mathematically proven that if the loci under study are selectively neutral, any positive and/or negative allelic association between the loci will be broken down rapidly if sexual mating and meiosis are frequent. If an organism reproduces clonally (through either mitotic division or homothallic mating), the entire genome is effectively linked since there is no segregation and reassortment of alleles. Both linkage and clonal reproduction can cause deviations from the expected (random) genotypic frequencies for any pair of loci.

Index of association (I_A)

To assess the overall allelic associations in haploid organisms, an I_A has been used widely in fungal population genetic analyses. This index was first used by Brown et al. (3) to determine the population structure in *Hordeum spontaneum,* and it was used later to demonstrate nonrandom association of alleles in *Escherichia coli* (13, 51) and other bacteria (25). I_A is a generalized measure of linkage disequilibrium and has an expected value of zero if there is no association between loci. The calculation of I_A has been described in detail elsewhere (3, 25).

Phylogenetic methods

As shown above, both linkage disequilibrium and the association index were tested against the null hypothesis of random mating. However, testing against a null hypothesis of random mating can create a type II error, the probability of accepting a false hypothesis, especially when sample size is small and the allele frequencies are skewed. Furthermore, in a population determined to have a predominantly clonal structure, it is often difficult to determine whether recombination contributes at all to variation.

To overcome these problems associated with testing against the null hypothesis of panmixia, phylogenetic analysis offers tests against the alternative hypothesis of strict clonality. There are two types of phylogenetic tests for clonality and recombination. The first uses population genetic data of allelic information at individual loci for each strain. The premise is that if populations are clonal, the ancestry of isolates will be represented by a phylogenetic tree of good fit. However, for recombining populations, there will be little or no phylogenetic consistency because different loci reflect different patterns of descent among individuals (1, 45). In addition, the length of the tree can be compared with the minimum length expected if the population were strictly clonal.

The second phylogenetic test uses sequences from several genes. By comparing phylogenetic trees constructed for different genes, clonality can be distinguished from recombination. There is strong evidence for clonality if the trees for different genes are concordant, but if the trees are in conflict, recombination is a likely explanation (20). The partition homogeneity test was developed to assess the congruences of gene genealogies. For congruent gene trees, the sum of the lengths of the most parsimonious tree for each gene should not change significantly if the polymorphic nucleotides in each gene are swapped among genes. Conversely, for incongruent gene trees, the sum of the gene trees for the observed data should be shorter than the sum of gene trees constructed after polymorphic nucleotides have been swapped among genes. This is true because recombination is assumed to be correlated with linkage relationships in the genome. Intragenic recombination, if existing at all, would be much rarer than intergenic recombination. The statistical significance of this test is established by making many resampled data sets and comparing the observed sum of tree lengths to the distribution of tree lengths of 1,000 or more resampled data sets.

Analysis of Clonality and Recombination in Diploid Species

Hardy-Weinberg equilibrium test

Since each diploid strain has two alleles at each locus, tests for recombination in diploid organisms are somewhat different from those in haploid species. In diploid species, the association of alleles within a locus is often used as a measure of recombination (17, 54, 57). A chi-square goodness of fit test can be performed to compare the observed and expected genotypic counts at each locus and summed across loci (54, 57). This computation is the test for Hardy-Weinberg equilibrium (HWE). If observed counts of genotypes are not significantly different from expected counts, then the population is in HWE and assumed to have a recombining structure. However, it is essential to know that Hardy-Weinberg frequencies are valid only when populations comply with several common but crucial assumptions: (i) the population size is large,

(ii) there is no selective pressure on the markers being analyzed, (iii) migration and mutation are negligible, and (iv) the population undergoes random mating (46).

It is imprudent to infer population structure from HWE tests alone. First, violation of any of the first three assumptions above may cause significant deviation from the expected frequencies, even if the population is randomly mating. Second, failure to reject the null hypothesis of HWE does not guarantee that the population is indeed randomly mating (type II error). Third, different populations of the same species may exhibit different population structures (e.g., reference 54).

Composite genotypic disequilibrium

In this test, the probability of the set of multilocus genotypes in a sample, based on allelic counts, is calculated from the multinomial theory under the hypothesis of random mating (60). Alleles are then permuted and the conditional probability is calculated for the permuted genotypic array. The proportion of arrays no more probable than the original sample provides the level of significance of the test. This test is not limited by the number of loci. It allows the calculation of the probability of multilocus genotypes based on genotypic counts at individual loci. Separating the allelic association test within a locus from genotypic association among loci can be very useful for diploid species, such as *C. albicans,* because deleterious recessive mutations may be common and genotypic counts at many loci may deviate significantly from Hardy-Weinberg expectations.

Evidence of Clonality in *Candida* Species

Surprisingly, despite their medical significance, the issues of clonality and recombination have not been studied for many pathogenic fungal species. From the reports to date, there is evidence for clonality in almost all species of genus *Candida.* However, the evidence for recombination is very limited among these species. Table 3 presents the current findings of clonality and recombination for some of the common clinical species of *Candida.* These findings are briefly described below.

C. albicans

Many studies have examined the population biology and epidemiology of *C. albicans* infections. However, few publications used codominant genetic markers, which are crucial for assessing clonality and recombination in this important diploid pathogen. Some of these studies are described below.

Pujol et al. (37) used 21 isozyme loci to characterize the genotypes of 55 strains of *C. albicans* isolated from patients infected with the human immunodeficiency virus (HIV). Among these strains, 13 of the 21 enzymatic loci were polymorphic. Six of the 13 polymorphic loci deviated significantly from HWE. The expected counts for some of the multilocus genotypes were also much lower than observed counts. They concluded that *C. albicans* has a clonal population structure (37).

Gräser et al. (17) developed 12 single nucleotide-based markers to characterize a mixed sample of *C. albicans* isolates from Durham, N.C. Among the 52 strains analyzed, 27 unique multilocus genotypes

Table 3. Summary of population genetic evidence for clonality and recombination in *Candida* species[a]

Criterion	Genetic evidence for clonality[b]								
	Ca	Cd	Cgl	Cgu	Ck	Cl	Cp	Cr	Ct
Allelic association within a locus (diploidy or higher)									
Hardy-Weinberg equilibrium	Y	NT	NA	NT	NT	NT	NT	NT	NT
Excess homozygosity	Y	NT	NA	NT	NT	NT	NT	NT	NT
Excess heterozygosity	Y	NT	NA	NT	NT	NT	NT	NT	NT
Allelic association between loci									
Random	Y	NT	Y	NT	NT	NT	NT	NT	NT
Nonrandom	Y	NT	Y	NT	NT	NT	NT	NT	NT
Gene genealogy congruence	NT	NT	NT	NT	NT	NT	NT	NT	NT
Overrepresentation of certain multilocus genotype(s)	Y	Y	Y	Y	Y	Y	Y	Y	Y

[a]Reprinted from reference 56 by courtesy of Marcel Dekker Inc.

[b]RCa, *C. albicans* (7, 11, 16, 17, 37, 53, 57); Cd, *C. dubliniensis* (21); Cgl, *C. glabrata* (15, 40); Cgu, *C. guilliermondii* (39); Ck, *C. krusei* (14); Cl, *C. lusitaniae* (22, 28, 34); Cp, *C. parapsilosis* (2, 5, 9, 19, 23, 35, 43, 49); Cr, *C. rugosa* (10); Ct, *C. tropicalis* (12, 23); NA, not applicable; Y, yes; NT, not tested.

were detected. Similar to the findings of Pujol et al. (37), about half the markers showed significant deviation from HWE (17). However, when they calculated the associations of alleles among loci, more than 70% of the comparisons of pairwise loci were not significantly different from random association. They concluded that the population structure of *C. albicans* included both clonal and recombinational components. Similar patterns have been confirmed among populations of *C. albicans* from different groups of hosts, including HIV-infected patients, non-HIV patients, and healthy persons (57, 59).

More recently, through the use of control samples, a group of 78 strains of *C. albicans* from a single geographic area were examined for the relationship between genetic relatedness and fluconazole resistance (58). Although the analysis revealed little evidence for genotypic clustering according to the HIV status or body site, a small group of fluconazole-resistant strains isolated from patients infected with HIV formed a genetically distinct cluster. Statistical analysis suggested that this cluster most likely represented a single origin of fluconazole resistance and the resistant genotype was subsequently spread among different individuals. In addition, two fluconazole-resistant strains were isolated from individuals who had never taken fluconazole, one from a patient infected with HIV and the other from a healthy person. Therefore, molecular markers and population studies confirmed that both clonal and spontaneous origins of fluconazole resistance existed in *C. albicans* (58). In a comparable study, genotypes of *C. albicans* generated by restriction digests of genomic DNA showed differences in susceptibilities to fluconazole and flucytosine (26). These genotypic groups resembled potentially different species of the *C. albicans* species complex (26).

Other *Candida* species

Preliminary evidence for clonality has been found in *Candida* species other than *C. albicans* (Table 3). For example, various epidemiological surveys found genetically identical or similar strains of *C. glabrata, C. guilliermondii, C. dubliniensis, C. krusei, C. lusitaniae, C. parapsilosis, C. rugosa,* and *C. tropicalis* (Table 3). Evidence of clonality for these species is mostly derived from analysis of DNA fingerprints; various fingerprinting techniques were recently reviewed by Soll (42). Whereas these results are consistent with the clonal spread of certain genotypes, the small sample size and the lack of information on a genetically defined set of loci preclude the more stringent statistical analysis for evidence of clonality and recombination. More critical tests are required to demonstrate clearly the contributions of clonality and recombination in these species.

Epidemic Clones—Calculations and Implications

Analyzing the genetic structure of populations to determine the extent of clonality versus recombination is a critical step toward understanding population history and the evolution of pathogenicity. This knowledge will help explain why certain populations maintain a particular genetic structure. Many factors contribute to the genetic structure of a population, including the history of the population, the mutation rate, the mutation spectrum (i.e., the distribution of mutations that are lethal, deleterious, neutral, and advantageous), genetic drift, population size, the mating system (or lack of mating), and the selection pressure from the natural environment and the host. It is often difficult to examine simultaneously the relative contribution of each factor to the genetic structure of natural populations.

One approach is to investigate whether and why certain genotypes are more prevalent than expected. This information can be obtained by inspecting the relative frequencies of different multilocus genotypes or by calculating the expected frequencies of individual genotypes based on allelic frequencies under the hypothesis of random mating (i.e., random associations of alleles within and among loci) (44, 57). When predominant genotypes are identified, the medically important traits of those isolates can be compared with less common genotypes in the population to explore possible associations between the genotype and clinically relevant phenotypes.

In a recent analysis of different samples of *C. albicans* using codominant, single-copy PCR-RFLP markers, one multilocus genotype preponderated in each of the four samples that were investigated (59). One sample was obtained from HIV-infected patients in Vitória, Brazil, and three samples came from the United States (Durham, N.C.). The preponderate genotype was much more prevalent in all four samples than would be expected under random mating. This genotype might be selectively more advantageous in human populations than other genotypes of *C. albicans*. The pathogenicity, transmission pattern, and antifungal drug susceptibility profiles of isolates with this genotype warrant further investigation.

GENETIC DIFFERENTIATION—ANALYSIS OF GENETIC VARIATION BETWEEN POPULATIONS

Issues and Analytical Methods

Depending on the questions of interest, there are multiple methods to compare genetic variation among populations. The first general approach is to compare the genetic parameters calculated for each population. These parameters include gene diversity (32), heterozygosity, genotypic diversity (44), relative percentage of polymorphic loci, and number of alleles per locus. The extent of recombination and clonality might differ among natural populations of the same species because population histories, environmental conditions, and selective pressure can all vary among populations. Any associations between specific environmental factors and genetic elements can be evaluated through general statistical analysis.

The second approach is the more traditional analysis of the population genetics. Calculations can determine the extent of subdivision within the population, genetic differentiation, and gene flow among populations based on differences in the gene and genotype frequency and measures of inbreeding coefficients (6, 8, 47). The effects of population subdivision are measured by a quantity called the fixation index (symbolized F_{ST}), which is the reduction in heterozygosity of a subpopulation due to genetic drift (47).

The statistical test of whether pairs of populations are significantly different is usually achieved by a direct comparison of gene frequencies (54, 55, 57, 59). This assessment may be accomplished with chi-square contingency table tests. Alternatively, Fisher's exact test is used when the sample sizes are small or when the lowest expected allele count is less than five. Population genetic relationships are also frequently described in UPGMA phenograms (32, 54, 55). These phenograms are based on population genetic distances. There are several measures of genetic distances, all based on population gene frequencies and inbreeding coefficients. The most widely used is Nei's genetic distance D (32). After pairwise population genetic distances are calculated, the similarities among populations can be described on a UPGMA phenogram (32). Genetic distances are often compared to geographic distances. Assuming that the rate of migration is rather constant, pairs of populations that are situated farther apart geographically would be expected to demonstrate greater genetic distance. This comparison is known as isolation by distance (52).

Sample Comparison of Populations of *C. albicans*

Many researchers have compared geographically disparate samples of *Candida* species (e.g., references 7, 42). However, few studies used rigorous and genetically informative, codominant single-copy markers to analyze *C. albicans,* which is diploid. One of the most surprising results is that geographically separated populations of the *C. albicans* from HIV-infected patients in Vitória, Brazil, and Durham, N.C., were genetically indistinguishable (59). The overall F_{ST} estimates between these two samples were 0.017 and 0.002 for comparisons of all the isolates from each sample or the clone-corrected samples, respectively. The number of migrants estimated from F_{ST} values ranged from 6.9 to 4 per generation between the two geographic populations. Sixteen loci were examined in this study, and both samples shared the same most common multilocus genotype (59).

CONCLUSIONS AND PERSPECTIVES

This chapter reviewed the contributions of population genetic analysis using codominant markers to an understanding of ploidy, clonality and recombination, and genetic differentiation in some common species of *Candida.* Whereas codominant genetic markers are ideal for addressing these issues, most reports of molecular epidemiology of *Candida* and candidiasis have used dominant, DNA fingerprinting markers (42). Fingerprinting techniques often prove to be excellent for identifying species and strains (e.g., reference 29). However, when these dominant markers are applied to population studies, the results are frequently difficult to interpret. First, there is a lack of standardization among these techniques. Without standardization, comparing results from different laboratories can be highly problematic. Second, many publications do not include the genotypic data, which prevents other researchers from independently comparing and analyzing the data with additional or alternative tests. Third, many studies use inadequate control samples or insufficient sample sizes, and consequently, statistical analyses are compromised or infeasible. To draw tenable conclusions, it is imperative to control for variables, such as the location of the patients from whom the population sample was obtained, body site, underlying condition, demographic information, and so forth. Eliminating confounding factors in the analysis is necessary to identify the contributions of separate ecological and epidemiological factors to the overall patterns of genetic variation. Properly controlled population studies using rigorous methods of genotypic analysis will clarify the population dynamics of *Candida* species and lead to predictive information about the epidemiology, prognosis, diagnosis, treatment, and prevention of candidiasis.

REFERENCES

1. **Archie, J. W.** 1989. A randomization test for phylogenetic information in systematic data. *Syst. Zool.* **38:**239–252.
2. **Branchini, M. L. M., M. A. Pfaller, J. Rhine-Chalberg, T.**

Frempong, and H. D. Isenberg. 1994. Genotypic variation and slime production among blood and catheter isolates of *Candida parapsilosis. J. Clin. Microbiol.* **32:**452–456.

3. **Brown, A. H. D., M. W. Feldman, and E. Nevo.** 1980. Multilocus structure of natural populations of *Hordeum spontaneum. Genetics* **96:**523–536.
4. **Burt, A., D. A. Carter, G. L. Koenig, T. J. White, and J. W. Taylor.** 1996. Molecular markers reveal cryptic sex in the human pathogen *Coccidioides immitis. Proc. Natl. Acad. Sci. USA* **93:**770–773.
5. **Carruba, G., E. Pontieri, F. De Bernardis, P. Martino, and A. Cassone.** 1991. DNA fingerprinting and electrophoretic karyotype of environmental and clinical isolates of *Candida parapsilosis. J. Clin. Microbiol.* **29:**916–922.
6. **Chakraborty, R., and O. Leimar.** 1987. Genetic variation within a subdivided population, p. 90–120. *In* N. Ryman and F. Utter (ed.), *Population Genetics and Fisheries Management.* University of Washington Press, Seattle, Wash.
7. **Clemons, K. V., F. Feroze, K. Holmberg, and D. A. Stevens.** 1997. Comparative analysis of genetic variability among *Candida albicans* isolates from different geographic locales by three genotypic methods. *J. Clin. Microbiol.* **35:**1332–1336.
8. **Cockerham, C. C., and B. S. Weir.** 1993. Estimation of gene flow from F-statistics. *Evolution* **47:**855–863.
9. **Dassanayake, R. S., and L. P. Samaranayake.** 2000. Characterization of the genetic diversity in superficial and systemic human isolates of *Candida parapsilosis* by randomly amplified polymorphic DNA (RAPD). *Acta Pathol. Microbiol. Immunol. Scand.* **108:**153–160.
10. **Dib, J. C., M. Dube, C. Kelly, M. G. Rinaldi, and J. E. Patterson.** 1996. Evaluation of pulsed-field gel electrophoresis as a typing system for *Candida rugosa:* comparison of karyotype and restriction fragment length polymorphisms. *J. Clin. Microbiol.* **34:**1494–1496.
11. **Díaz-Guerra, T. M., J. V. Martínez-Suárez, F. Labuna, and J. L. Rodríguez-Tudela.** 1997. Comparison of four molecular typing methods for evaluating genetic diversity among *Candida albicans* isolates from human immunodeficiency virus-positive patients with oral candidiasis. *J. Clin. Microbiol.* **35:** 856–861.
12. **Doebbeling, B. N., P. F. Lehmann, R. J. Hollis, L.-C. Wu, A. F. Widmer, A. Voss, and M. A. Pfaller.** 1993. Comparison of pulsed-field gel electrophoresis with isoenzyme profiles as a typing system for *Candida tropicalis. Clin. Infect. Dis.* **16:** 377–383.
13. **Dykhuizen, D. E., and L. Green.** 1991. Recombination in *Escherichia coli* and the definition of biological species. *J. Bacteriol.* **173:**7257–7268.
14. **Essayag, S. M., G. G. Baily, D. W. Denning, and J. P. Burnie.** 1996. Karyotyping of fluconazole-resistant yeasts with phenotype reported as *Candida krusei* or *Candida inconspicua. Int. J. Syst. Bacteriol.* **46:**35–40.
15. **Fidel, P. L., Jr., J. A. Vazquez, and J. D. Sobel.** 1999. *Candida glabrata:* review of epidemiology, pathogenesis, and clinical disease with comparison to *C. albicans. Clin. Microbiol. Rev.* **12:**80–96.
16. **Forche, A., G. Schönian, Y. Gräser, R. J. Vilgalys, and T. G. Mitchell.** 1999. Genetic structure of typical and atypical populations of *Candida albicans* from Africa. *Fungal Genet. Biol.* **28:**107–125.
17. **Gräser, Y., M. Volovsek, J. Arrington, G. Schönian, W. Presber, T. G. Mitchell, and R. J. Vilgalys.** 1996. Molecular markers reveal that population structure of the human pathogen *Candida albicans* exhibits both clonality and recombination. *Proc. Natl. Acad. Sci. USA* **93:**12473–12477.
18. **Hartl, D. L., and A. G. Clark.** 1989. *Principles of Population Genetics.* Sinauer Associates, Sunderland, Mass.
19. **Huang, Y. C., T. Y. Lin, H. S. Leu, H. L. Peng, J. H. Wu, and H. Y. Chang.** 1999. Outbreak of *Candida parapsilosis* fungemia in neonatal intensive care units: clinical implications and genotyping analysis. *Infection* **27:**97–102.
20. **Huelsenbeck, J. P.** 1996. Combining data in phylogenetic analysis. *TREE* **11:**152–158.
21. **Joly, S., C. Pujol, M. Rysz, K. Vargas, and D. R. Soll.** 1999. Development and characterization of complex DNA fingerprinting probes for the infectious yeast *Candida dubliniensis. J. Clin. Microbiol.* **37:**1035–1044.
22. **King, D., J. Rhine-Chalberg, M. A. Pfaller, S. A. Moser, and W. G. Merz.** 1995. Comparison of four DNA-based methods for strain delineation of *Candida lusitaniae. J. Clin. Microbiol.* **33:**1467–1470.
23. **Lehmann, P. F., B. J. Kemker, C.-B. Hsiao, and S. Dev.** 1989. Isoenzyme biotypes of *Candida* species. *J. Clin. Microbiol.* **27:** 2514–2521.
24. **Maynard Smith, J. M.** 1978. *The Evolution of Sex.* Cambridge University Press, Cambridge, United Kingdom.
25. **Maynard Smith, J. M., N. H. Smith, M. O'Rourke, and B. G. Spratt.** 1993. How clonal are bacteria? *Proc. Natl. Acad. Sci. USA* **90:**4384–4388.
26. **McCullough, M. J., K. V. Clemons, and D. A. Stevens.** 1999. Molecular and phenotypic characterization of genotypic *Candida albicans* subgroups and comparison with *Candida dubliniensis* and *Candida stellatoidea. J. Clin. Microbiol.* **37:** 417–421.
27. **McEwen, J. G., J. W. Taylor, D. A. Carter, J. Xu, M. S. S. Felipe, R. J. Vilgalys, T. G. Mitchell, T. Kasuga, T. J. White, T. Bui, and C. M. A. Soares.** 2000. Molecular typing of pathogenic fungi. *Med. Mycol.* **38**(Suppl. 1):189–197.
28. **Merz, W. G., U. Khazan, M. A. Jabra-Rizk, L.-C. Wu, G. J. Osterhout, and P. F. Lehmann.** 1992. Strain delineation and epidemiology of *Candida (Clavispora) lusitaniae. J. Clin. Microbiol.* **30:**449–454.
29. **Meyer, W., G. N. Latouche, H.-M. Daniel, M. Thanos, T. G. Mitchell, D. Yarrow, G. Schönian, and T. C. Sorrell.** 1997. Identification of pathogenic yeasts of the imperfect genus *Candida* by polymerase chain reaction fingerprinting. *Electrophoresis* **18:**1548–1559.
30. **Michod, R. E., and B. R. Levin.** 1987. *The Evolution of Sex: An Examination of Current Ideas.* Sinauer Associates, Sunderland, Mass.
31. **Mitchell, T. G., and J. Xu.** Molecular methods to identify pathogenic fungi. *In* D. H. Howard (ed.), *Fungi Pathogenic for Humans and Animals,* in press. Marcel Dekker, New York, N.Y.
32. **Nei, M.** 1975. *Molecular Population Genetics and Evolution.* American Elsevier, New York, N.Y.
33. **Odds, F. C.** 1988. *Candida and Candidosis.* Bailliere Tindall, London, United Kingdom.
34. **Pfaller, M. A., S. A. Messer, and R. J. Hollis.** 1994. Strain delineation and antifungal susceptibilities of epidemiologically related and unrelated isolates of *Candida lusitaniae. Diagn. Microbiol. Infect. Dis.* **20:**127–133.
35. **Pfaller, M. A., S. A. Messer, and R. J. Hollis.** 1995. Variations in DNA subtype, antifungal susceptibility, and slime production among clinical isolates of *Candida parapsilosis. Diagn. Microbiol. Infect. Dis.* **21:**9–14.
36. **Pujol, C., F. Renaud, M. Mallié, T. de Meeûs, and J.-M. Bastide.** 1997. Atypical strains of *Candida albicans* recovered from AIDS patients. *J. Med. Vet. Mycol.* **35:**115–121.
37. **Pujol, C., J. Reynes, F. Renaud, M. Raymond, M. Tibayrenc,**

F. J. Ayala, F. Janbon, M. Mallié, and J.-M. Bastide. 1993. The yeast *Candida albicans* has a clonal mode of reproduction in a population of infected human immunodeficiency virus-positive patients. *Proc. Natl. Acad. Sci. USA* **90:**9456–9459.
38. **Riggsby, W. S., L. J. Torres-Bauza, J. W. Wills, and T. M. Townes.** 1982. DNA content, kinetic complexity, and the ploidy question in *Candida albicans. Mol. Cell. Biol.* **2:** 853–862.
39. **San-Millán, R. M., L. C. Wu, I. F. Salkin, and P. F. Lehmann.** 1997. Clinical isolates of *Candida guilliermondii* include *Candida fermentati. Int. J. Syst. Bacteriol.* **47:**385–393.
40. **Schwab, U., F. Chernomas, L. Larcom, and J. J. Weems, Jr.** 1997. Molecular typing and fluconazole susceptibility of urinary *Candida glabrata* isolates from hospitalized patients. *Diagn. Microbiol. Infect. Dis.* **28:**11–17.
41. **Sokal, R. R., and F. J. Rohlf.** 1988. *Biometry.* W.H. Freeman, New York, N.Y.
42. **Soll, D. R.** 2000. The ins and outs of DNA fingerprinting the infectious fungi. *Clin. Microbiol. Rev.* **13:**332–370.
43. **Solomon, S. L., R. F. Khabbaz, R. H. Parker, R. L. Anderson, M. A. Geraghty, R. M. Furman, and W. J. Martone.** 1984. An outbreak of *Candida parapsilosis* bloodstream infections in patients receiving parenteral nutrition. *J. Infect. Dis.* **149:** 98–102.
44. **Stoddart, J. A.** 1983. A genotypic diversity measure. *J. Heredity* **74:**489–490.
45. **Taylor, J. W., D. M. Geiser, A. Burt, and V. Koufopanou.** 1999. The evolutionary biology and population genetics underlying fungal strain typing. *Clin. Microbiol. Rev.* **12:** 126–146.
46. **Weir, B. S.** 1996. *Genetic Data Analysis.* Sinauer Associates, Sunderland, Mass.
47. **Weir, B. S., and C. C. Cockerham.** 1984. Estimating F-statistics for the analysis of population structure. *Evolution* **38:** 1358–1370.
48. **Weising, K., H. Nybom, K. Wolff, and W. Meyer.** 1995. *DNA Fingerprinting in Plants and Fungi.* CRC Press, Boca Raton, Fla.
49. **Welbel, S. F., M. M. McNeil, R. J. Kuykendall, T. J. Lott, A. Pramanik, R. Silberman, A. D. Oberle, L. A. Bland, S. Aguero, M. Arduino, S. Crow, and W. R. Jarvis.** 1996. *Candida parapsilosis* bloodstream infections in neonatal intensive care unit patients: epidemiologic and laboratory confirmation of a common source outbreak. *Pediatr. Infect. Dis. J.* **15:**998–1002.
50. **Whelan, W. L., R. M. Partridge, and P. T. Magee.** 1980. Heterozygosity and segregation in *Candida albicans. Mol. Gen. Genet.* **180:**107–113.
51. **Whittam, T. S., H. Ochman, and R. K. Selander.** 1983. Multilocus genetic structure in natural populations of *Escherichia coli. Proc. Natl. Acad. Sci. USA* **80:**1751–1755.
52. **Wright, S.** 1943. Isolation by distance. *Genetics* **28:**114–138.
53. **Xu, J., C. M. Boyd, E. Livingston, W. Meyer, J. F. Madden, and T. G. Mitchell.** 1999. Species and genotypic diversities and similarities of pathogenic yeasts colonizing women. *J. Clin. Microbiol.* **37:**3835–3843.
54. **Xu, J., R. W. Kerrigan, P. Callac, P. A. Horgen, and J. B. Anderson.** 1997. Genetic structure of natural populations of *Agaricus bisporus,* the commercial button mushroom. *J. Heredity* **88:**482–488.
55. **Xu, J., R. W. Kerrigan, A. S. Sonnenberg, P. Callac, P. A. Horgen, and J. B. Anderson.** 1998. Mitochondrial DNA variation in natural populations of the mushroom *Agaricus bisporus. Mol. Ecol.* **7:**19–33.
56. **Xu, J., and T. G. Mitchell.** Strain variation and clonality in species of *Candida* and *Cryptococcus neoformans. In* R. L. Cihlar and R. A. Calderone (ed.), *Fungal Pathogenesis: Principles and Clinical Applications,* in press. Marcel Dekker, New York, N.Y.
57. **Xu, J., T. G. Mitchell, and R. J. Vilgalys.** 1999. PCR-restriction fragment length polymorphism (RFLP) analyses reveal both extensive clonality and local genetic differences in *Candida albicans. Mol. Ecol.* **8:**59–73.
58. **Xu, J., A. R. Ramos, R. J. Vilgalys, and T. G. Mitchell.** 2000. Clonal and spontaneous origins of fluconazole resistance in *Candida albicans. J. Clin. Microbiol.* **38:**1214–1220.
59. **Xu, J., R. J. Vilgalys, and T. G. Mitchell.** 1999. Lack of genetic differentiation between two geographically diverse samples of *Candida albicans* isolated from patients infected with human immunodeficiency virus. *J. Bacteriol.* **181:**1369–1373.
60. **Zaykin, D., L. Zhivotovsky, and B. S. Weir.** 1995. Exact tests for association between alleles at arbitrary numbers of loci. *Genetica* **96:**169–178.

II. VIRULENCE PROPERTIES

Candida and Candidiasis
Edited by Richard A. Calderone

Chapter 6

Host Recognition by *Candida* Species

RICHARD CALDERONE AND NEIL A. R. GOW

Candida spp. rank as the fourth most common cause of nosocomial disease in the United States, and their importance worldwide in similar clinical settings is well established (31, 113, 138, 139). It has been shown that attributable mortality due to bloodstream infections caused by *Candida* spp. approaches 35% (113). Approximately 5 to 10 per 10,000 admissions to hospitals (10% of all bloodstream infections) will develop candidemias. In some settings, such as urinary tract infections, candidiasis is second in frequency among all microbial infections at this site. In comparison to invasive diseases, *Candida* spp. are also responsible for a significant amount of mucosal disease in several patient populations, most notably in the human immunodeficiency virus (HIV)-positive patient who may develop oropharyngeal candidiasis, vaginitis, and/or esophagitis. In fact, candidiasis is an AIDS-defining disease. The most common species that causes candidiasis is *C. albicans,* but others, such as *C. glabrata, C. parapsilosis,* and *C. dubliniensis,* also cause significant amounts of disease. The latter group is considered to be part of the emerging species of fungal pathogens (see chapters 2 and 4). In its usual setting, candidiasis occurs as infections of the immunocompromised host, and a number of predisposing factors act to increase host susceptibility (see chapters 1, 22–24).

The fact that candidiasis develops in the immunocompromised patient might indicate that the contribution of virulence factors by these organisms to disease development is minimal. In fact, data from infection models argue against this hypothesis. Thus, in the case of *C. albicans,* specific gene deletions result in avirulence of the organism in both mucosal and invasive animal models. Also, recently, reverse transcriptase-PCR studies have demonstrated that several of the secretory aspartyl proteinases (SAPs) of *C. albicans* are expressed during human disease (120). These enzymes are believed to be virulence factors (see chapter 9). Thus, candidiasis is a consequence of both the abrogation of host defenses and the invasiveness of the organisms that cause this disease. Much of the data supporting this idea have been established with *C. albicans,* whereas for other *Candida* spp. such data are not yet available. Another point to be made is the adaptability of this group of pathogens. *Candida* spp. are commensals of the human host and must be able to compete with other microorganisms at sites such as the oral, vaginal, and gastrointestinal mucosa. That they are not eliminated from the host speaks to their success as commensals. Thus, *Candida* spp., and especially *C. albicans,* might be considered a highly evolved group of pathogens that utilize their resources to persist in the normal host and invade when host immune deficiencies occur.

In this chapter and in chapters 7 to 10, virulence factors of *C. albicans* (and other species when possible) will be discussed. However, first, a brief overview of virulence in *Candida* spp. is presented below. Not surprisingly, as a commensal and pathogen, *C. albicans* has evolved to persist on mucosal surfaces of the host. Its inability to do this would surely result in its clearance from the host. The components of the organism that promote host recognition and colonization are referred to as adhesins. The avidity of *Candida* species for host epithelia is a good correlate of relative virulence (see later), and so adhesion must be recognized as a major virulence determinant.

Additionally, it has long been recognized that the interconversion of yeast forms to a filamentous growth (hyphae or pseudohyphae), an event referred to as morphogenesis, is associated with invasiveness of the organism. This idea is supported by histopathological observations of lesions that demonstrate a re-

Richard Calderone • Department of Microbiology and Immunology, Georgetown University Medical Center, SE 312 Med Dent Building, 3900 Reservoir Rd. NW, Washington, DC 20007. **Neil A. R. Gow** • Department of Molecular and Cell Biology, Institute of Medical Sciences, University of Aberdeen, Aberdeen AB25 2ZD, Scotland.

markable proliferation of filamentous forms (both pseudohyphae and true hyphae) in both experimental disease (animal models) and human disease. Before the advent of molecular techniques that are now used to construct strains deleted in specific genes, an agerminative strain (at 37°C) of *C. albicans* isolated in vitro was shown to be avirulent in a vaginitis animal model compared to a wild-type strain (124). Strain B311V6 is a spontaneous mutant, and, therefore, since it was not otherwise isogenic, the direct correlation of morphogenesis with virulence was not absolute. More recently, however, the use of the "ura-blaster" technique of gene deletion (35) has resulted in the construction of numerous signal transduction mutants (and mutants in transcription factors that regulate expression of hyphal growth) that are at least partially defective in their ability to undergo morphogenesis in vitro. Likewise, these strains are either attenuated in their virulence or avirulent (see chapters 7 and 8). Virulence of *C. albicans* also requires the production of digestive enzymes such as the SAPs, a family of approximately nine proteins, and phospholipase B (PLB) (92, 120).

In addition, it is possible that *Candida* species may be able to bind host plasminogen, which, if appropriately activated, would result in local generation of a host-derived proteolytic system capable of augmenting tissue degradation due to secreted fungal hydrolytic enzymes (95a). It seems logical to suppose that enzymes that degrade host tissues should be a prerequisite for invasion.

Finally, the ability of *C. albicans* to change phenotypically, referred to as phenotypic switching, has been studied extensively and postulated as a virulence attribute. Switching may involve changes in the expression of cell surface antigens, tissue affinities of the organism, enzyme production, and even drug sensitivity. Clearly, this phenomenon could have important implications in pathogenesis and is offered as yet another virulence attribute of not only *C. albicans* but other species of *Candida* (see chapter 10). In summary, then, adherence, morphogenesis, the production of key degradative enzymes, and phenotypic switching all may contribute to virulence. These factors and their interactions with the host are shown in Fig. 1. The model depicts the colonization of mucosal surfaces by yeast or hyphal forms of *Candida* spp., conversion to a filamentous growth that occurs sometime during immunocompromising conditions as well as invasion of the bloodstream and tissues, both of which are probably promoted by morphogenesis of the organism and invasive enzymes. However, yeast cells may also cross the mucosal surface by persorption or induced phagocytosis as described by others (22). Phenotypic switching is seen as providing a means for the organism to adapt to specific sites in the body or perhaps develop drug resistance and avoid immune surveillance. Collectively, these factors lead to disease progression. Clearly, this model is an oversimplification. Thus, the fungal factors that are required for disease development at each site (for example, kidney versus vaginal mucosa) are quite different. Adaptation to a tissue-specific environment could involve nonconventional, reversible methods for gene expression, such as aneuploidy (75, 112). Here, chromosomal rearrangements and aneuploidy are believed to provide mechanisms for the utilization of substrates and the development of drug resistance. It is

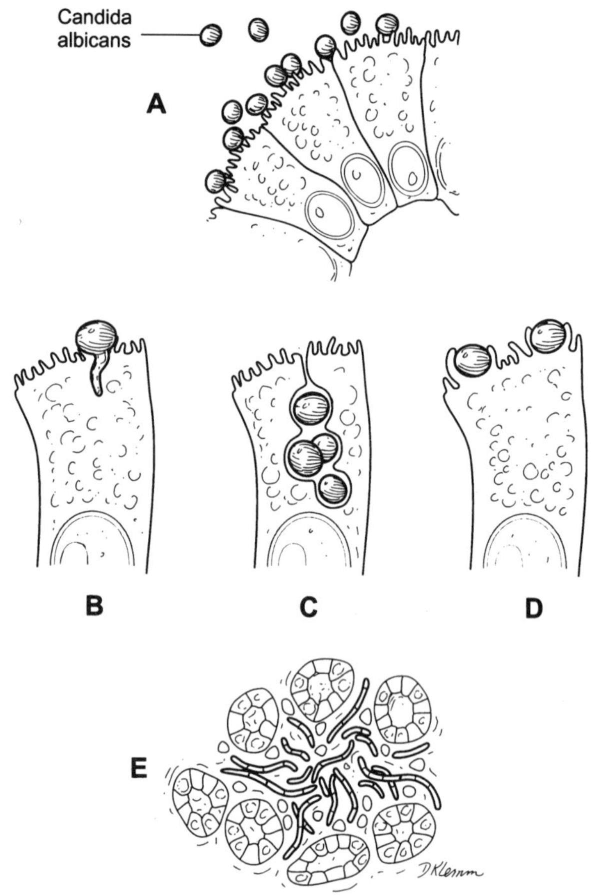

Figure 1. The interaction of *C. albicans* with mucosal surfaces. (A) Yeast cells adhere to mucosal cells. Shedding and recolonization probably occur at the mucosal surface. (B) Phase transition may precede invasion of mucosal cells. (C) However, persorption of yeast cells also promotes ingression of the organism. (D) Induced phagocytosis by esophageal and endothelial cells may contribute to invasion of the mucosal cells. Invasion of the mucosal surface is probably followed by lymphatic and blood-borne spread to tissues such as the kidney where local aggregates of filamentous forms occur. (E) Reseeding of the blood by the organism has been described and may also serve to promote invasion of tissues. The events depicted in A to C have been described by Cole et al. (22).

important to realize that candidiasis occurs in a number of sites in the human host, each with its own set of environmental conditions, such as pH, nutrient availability, etc. It is safe to conclude that virulence in these organisms is multifactoral, and invasion will depend on the sum of the attributes of the fungus, host environmental influences, and the loss/depletion of host defenses.

Many of the studies described here and in many other chapters on virulence and pathogenesis predate the era in which targeted mutagenesis has been possible in *C. albicans*. Appropriate gene inactivation studies can provide stable mutants that can provide the most convincing evidence that specific proteins, adhesins, or virulence factors are important in host interactions and pathogenesis. Such studies usually involve creation of one or more isogenic mutants by gene deletion. Also, complementary strains are commonly created in which the deleted gene is reintroduced into the null mutant to validate the hypothesis that the primary deletion led to the phenotype of the null. This approach is often said to enable the satisfaction of the molecular biological version of Koch's postulates that relate the etiology of a phenotype to the effect of a specific mutation. In addition, certain *C. albicans* genes encoding putative adhesins have been expressed heterologously in *Saccharomyces cerevisiae* to demonstrate that transformation with a cloned gene is sufficient to confer adhesive properties to a poorly adherent, nonpathogenic species, such as brewer's yeast. Below, we discuss the adhesins of *C. albicans* and, when possible, studies of other species. Subsequent chapters focus on morphogenesis, enzymes (SAPs and PLB), and phenotypic switching.

ADHERENCE AS A VIRULENCE FACTOR OF *C. ALBICANS*

The idea that host recognition by *C. albicans* could be required for disease development may have been initially suggested by parallel studies that were published at the time on numerous bacterial pathogens. That is, if pathogenic bacteria that colonized tissues and mucosal surfaces utilized their cell surface biomolecules to adhere to host cells, then surely *C. albicans* also expresses adhesins. Whereas the active biomolecules should be different for yeasts versus bacteria, because of differences in their cell surface composition, nevertheless, this type of reasoning certainly provided impetus to study host recognition in *C. albicans*. The previous statement regarding the dissimilarity of *Candida* versus bacterial adhesins is partially incorrect, since one of the *C. albicans* adhesins (at least the host recognition domain) is homologous to an adhesin of *Pseudomonas aeruginosa* (discussed below and in references 90, 145–148). As a commensal of mucosal surfaces, *C. albicans* has adapted mechanisms to persist at these sites, either through interactions with colonizing bacteria or with the host mucosa, or both.

An observation that adherence could be important for virulence came from the studies described by King et al., which probably represent the first of this nature for *C. albicans* (82). These investigators developed an assay for measuring adherence that utilized radiolabeled yeast cells, which were added (at specific densities) to either human buccal or vaginal exfoliated epithelial cells (HBEC or HVEC) in suspension. Subsequently, nonadhering yeasts were removed by filtration through 10 μm filters, and adherence was then measured as the amount of radiolabeled organism adhering to the epithelial cells that were retained on the filters. Importantly, visual assays were also employed to verify the radiometric assays. The important observation made by this group was that of seven species of *Candida* tested, *C. albicans* adhered to the greatest extent, followed by *C. tropicalis* and *C. stellatoidea*. These data added credence to the hypothesis that adherence could be important to virulence since *C. albicans* was (and still is) considered the most virulent of *Candida* spp. and also adhered more extensively in this assay. Adherence was best at a pH of 7.3 and at 37°C when using yeast cells for inoculum that had been cultivated for 12 to 48 h (late-log phase to stationary phase). Further, these data also established at least tentatively that adherence assays could be used as an expression of virulence even though they are in vitro assays. In a second paper by the same group, adherence of *C. albicans* was shown only to be inhibited when yeast cells were treated with reducing agents or with several proteolytic enzymes whereas viability was not critical to adherence (89). These authors also established that heat-treated extracts of *C. albicans* but not *C. krusei* (a relative nonpathogen) partially blocked adherence of the organism to vaginal epithelial cells, again demonstrating that the more pathogenic species expressed factor(s) that were different from the more nonpathogenic species.

Another contribution to the hypothesis that adherence contributes to virulence of the organism came from a series of observations with spontaneous, cerulenin-resistant strains of *C. albicans* (15, 17, 58, 91). These strains were thought to be altered in their cell surface properties since cerulenin is a drug that inhibits fatty acid synthesis and, perhaps, the effect of the resistance to the drug might be due to alterations in activities of cell wall biosynthetic enzymes that are membrane-associated. In fact, alterations in cell wall proteins and polysaccharides were observed (17, 58).

Two of the cerulenin-resistant mutants were also less able to adhere to human buccal epithelial cells; these strains were subsequently shown to be avirulent in animal models of endocarditis and vaginitis (15, 91). Thus, there appeared to be a correlation between a reduced adherence in vitro with reduced virulence of strains, again suggesting that adherence may be critical to disease development. Similarly, other studies on the adherence of spontaneous or induced mutants have been reported (38). Clotrimazole-resistant strains of *C. albicans* adhered significantly less to HBEC than clotrimazole-sensitive strains (36). Finally, clones of *C. albicans,* isolated by panning with anti-*C. albicans* rabbit serum, had abnormal adherence properties in regard to their binding to complement ligands (140). These clones had been initially mutagenized, and then consecutively reacted with antiserum until they no longer were agglutinated by the antiserum; among the changes observed was a loss of reactivity with cells treated with antibodies to the cell surface mannan, changes in mannan profiles, and a loss of complement receptor activity, establishing the lack of certain reactive, cell surface epitopes.

The undeniable problem with each of these observations is that the mutants were spontaneous (or mutagenized) and, therefore, not otherwise isogenic in regard to their genetic background compared to wild-type cells, i.e., a number of silent mutations probably exist for each of the mutants. Therefore, an absolute correlation of adherence with a virulence phenotype was not possible. As stated above, it is important to realize that methods were not at that time available to construct single-gene deleted strains. Nevertheless, the observations described above provided an impetus for extensive investigations on adherence by a number of laboratories.

ADHERENCE ASSAYS

Before proceeding with some of the observations on the specific adhesins of *C. albicans* and other *Candida* spp., examples of adherence assays will be discussed, summarized in Table 1. In general, the cell-cell adherence assays using *Candida* spp. and host cells are either done in suspension or host cells are grown (or attached) in monolayers to which *Candida* spp. are added. The general requirements for preparation of inoculum are that yeast cells should be in late-log or stationary phase, although variation in this theme does exist in the literature and growth phase is known to affect cell adhesiveness quite markedly (82). Adherence of filamentous growth forms has also been reported, but the inherent clumping of hyphae and pseudohyphae necessitates mild sonication to disrupt aggregated cells. Indeed, a visible indicator that a liquid culture of yeast cells is converting efficiently to hyphae is manifest as a change from a turbid emulsified cell culture to a clarified medium with small pellets of aggregated filamentous cells. A variety of media have been used to propagate the inoculum, including complex (glucose-phytone peptone) yeast nitrogen base (with supplements), or synthetic (Lee's medium); Douglas et al. have found that cells are more adherent when grown in high amounts of sugar (500 mM), for example, galactose or sucrose (101, 102), that are surprisingly similar to physiological concentrations in saliva. Measurements of adherence are done visually, counting the number of epithelial cells with adhering yeasts, or by radiometric analysis. In the latter situation, yeast cells of the organism are labeled with ^{14}C-glucose or amino acids (^{3}H-substrate, ^{35}S-methionine, and ^{125}I are also suitable) for a designated time, washed, recounted, standardized to radioactivity/cell,

Table 1. Conditions for adherence assays of *Candida* sp. and mammalian cells or their ligands

Age (h) of culture[a]	Growth medium	Ligand or host cells	Assay time	Type of assay[b]	Suspension or monolayer[c]	Reference
6–7	YPD	ECM	30 min	Visible	S	42
18	PPG	HBEC	1 h	Visible	S	56
2.5	M199	HBEC	1 h	cpm	S	125
Mid-ex	SD	HeLa	1 h	cpm	M	41
20–48	YNB	FN	3 h	cpm	S	143
24	PPG	HBEC	30 min	cpm	S	82
24	PPG	HVEC	30 min	cpm	S	89
48	SA	HBEC	3 h	Visible	S	136
Mid-ex	YNB-Gal	Mucin	18 h	cpm	Bound	59
24	Lee's	HBEC	1 h	Visible	S	38
ON	SA	HBEC	1 h	Biotin	S	148

[a]Mid-ex, mid-exponential phase; ON, overnight.
[b]Biotin, fimbriae of *C. albicans* were biotin labeled prior to mixing with host cells or ligand.
[c]S, adherence done in a suspension assay; M, monolayer of host cells; Bound, bound substrate.

and added to cell suspensions or monolayers of host cells as mentioned above. If cell suspension assays are used, the entire suspension can be passed through a standard filter that retains cells that are 10 to 12 μm in size (epithelial cells, for example) while eliminating nonadhering *Candida* cells that pass directly through the filter. Following extensive washing, the filters can be stained directly or placed face down on glass slides. The face-down filters are then removed, leaving an impression of the adherent cells that is stained with any one of several dyes (crystal violet, periodic acid-Schiff stain, Congo red) and used to measure adherence. If a radiometric assay is to be used, then the washed filters are counted directly in a scintillation counter and the number of adhering *Candida* cells determined by knowing the specific activity of the radiolabeled organism (cpm/cell). In Table 1, the specifications of several cell-cell adherence assays are presented.

On the other hand, the adherence of *Candida* species to semipurified or purified ligands may be measured (122) (Table 1). Or, in a variation of this theme, binding of semipurified candidal adhesin to host cells or ligands of host cells has been reported (Table 1). Most of these types of assays have been elegantly described in a series of papers from the Irvin and Roberts laboratories (90, 142–148). For example, Yu et al. measured the adherence (binding) of biotinylated cell surface fimbriae preparations or whole cells of *C. albicans* to HBEC or to the glycosphingolipid asialo-GM1 ligand of HBEC (90, 145–148). To accomplish biotinylation, yeast cells were grown overnight on Sabouraud agar, washed extensively, and resuspended in 100 mM phosphate buffer (pH 8.5). Washed cells were then incubated in biotinamido-caproate *N*-hydroxysuccimidyl ester, and after a designated time, washed, and then added to immobilized ligand or HBEC. Following incubation, nonadhering yeast or fimbriae were washed away, and binding of biotinylated whole cells or fimbriae was quantitated using a Streptavidin-alkaline phosphatase conjugate. In another approach, the ligand can be tagged, as in the studies described by Yan et al. (142–144). These investigators were interested in measuring the induction of binding of *C. albicans* to the fibronectin (FN) ligand, one of the extracellular matrix (ECM) proteins of mammalian cells (see below). In this study, rather than label the organism, FN was labeled by iodination. Subsequently, the binding of ^{125}I-FN was measured in a suspension culture of *C. albicans*.

Adherence of *C. albicans* has also been characterized in ligand overlay assays (76). In experiments using this approach, yeasts were radiolabeled with Na^{125}I. To measure binding of the labeled cells, various glycosphingolipids were chromatogramed on aluminum-backed silica gel high-performance thin-layer plates. Then, the separated compounds were either treated to determine the mobility of each sphinogolipid on the gel or overlaid with radiolabeled organisms to identify specific ligands. In this manner, *C. albicans* was shown to bind to lactosylceramide. In a variation of this scheme, candidal proteins have been electrophoresed (sodium dodecyl sulfate-polyacrylamide gel electrophoresis [SDS-PAGE]), transferred to nitrocellulose paper, and then reacted in Western blots with antibodies to cell integrins (20, 44, 63, 64, 100). Binding of the primary antibody to a *Candida* protein was visualized by treatment with a secondary antibody conjugate. In this way, proteins of *Candida* species with some degree of homology to mammalian cell proteins can be identified.

Coaggregation assays of *C. albicans* or *C. dubliniensis* with oral bacteria have been described (73, 74). The *Candida* organisms were grown in Sabouraud agar, adjusted to 10^7 cells per ml, and mixed with 10^8 bacteria (growth conditions vary per bacterium). Cocultures were incubated in suspension for 12 h at room temperature, and mixtures were viewed by dark-field microscopy. Coaggregation of *C. dubliniensis* or *C. albicans* with the oral bacterium *Fusobacterium nucleatum* (as well as other oral bacteria) was followed in suspension cultures (74). *F. nucleatum* was chosen for study since it is reported to be the most frequently isolated microbe from the subgingival plaque of periodontal lesions and because it coaggregates with a number of other oral microorganisms. The organisms were mixed together in a total volume of 300 μl (100 μl of *Candida* [10% suspension] and 200 μl of bacteria [1% suspension]), incubated in CoAg buffer for a total of 5 min, and measured visually for coaggregation on a scale from 0 to +4. The visual assay was compared to a turbidometric assay such that a decrease in turbidity indicated coaggregation; the extent of coaggregation varied between the two *Candida* species, but for both, coaggregation was inhibited by mannose or α-methyl mannoside. The *Candida* receptor appeared to be heat stable while that of *F. nucleatum* was heat labile. These types of study should be extremely informative in regard to identifying microorganisms to which *Candida* spp. interact not only in the oral cavity but elsewhere. Finally, in vitro assays are often used to isolate adhesins by blocking adherence with extracted proteins from cells of *C. albicans* (33).

THE ADHESINS OF *C. ALBICANS* AND THEIR LIGANDS

In this section, we will discuss the major adhesins of *C. albicans* and other species of *Candida* for which data are available. The reader is also directed to excellent reviews on cell wall biomolecules and putative adhesins of *Candida* spp. (13, 16, 18, 21, 29, 50, 63, 64, 66, 128, 129). Adhesins of *C. albicans* are usually polysaccharide or glycoprotein. Of these two types, by far most are glycoprotein in nature. Ligands can be either cell-associated or found in serum. In the former category, one can also distinguish between epithelial ligands and endothelial ligands, although several are found on both types of cells. The *C. albicans* adhesin literature that emphasizes their biochemical nature most often predates the molecular studies. In some cases, links between the less recent, biochemical studies of specific adhesins have been made with the current molecular studies, as, for example, with the isolation of genes encoding proteins that bind to extracellular matrix proteins, such as FN. However, in several situations, the identification of both interesting and novel putative adhesins through biochemical analysis has not been extended to studies on the isolation of genes encoding these proteins in *C. albicans*. Table 2 represents an attempt to list the adhesins of *C. albicans* and *C. glabrata,* the only other *Candida* spp. from which an adhesin-encoding gene has been identified (23). The reader should keep in mind that when the encoding gene is not known and knockout strains are unavailable, one only can speculate as to the function of a protein as an adhesin in vitro and in vivo. For example, a specific protein (or glycoprotein) may have features of an adhesin (binds a ligand or ligands in a saturable fashion, found on the cell surface), but the proof of its identity as an adhesin must also include an evaluation of mutants deleted in the encoding gene. Thus, a loss of adherence function in mutants (as demonstrated by in vitro assays) more firmly establishes that the protein under investigation is an adhesin. Even better, avirulence in an animal model demonstrates that the gene is essential for virulence. Most of the current literature that describes the phenotypic properties of strains deleted in genes encoding putative adhesins fulfills both of these criteria. However, the loss of colonizing (adherence) properties by mutants in vivo is rarely reported. Nevertheless, the list of adhesins in Table 2 is divided into two groups, those for which their encoding genes are known and those for which no encoding gene has been demonstrated.

We have formulated a more conservative definition of an adhesin and propose that deletion of a gene encoding a putative adhesin and the accompanying loss or reduction in adherence are essential to establishing an adhesin function (as stated previously). However, with several of the proposed adhesins, this has not yet been accomplished. Thus, we have modified this restrictive definition to include *C. albicans* biomolecules that have homology to known adhesins from other organisms. For example, the fimbrial protein of *C. albicans* has obvious homology to the *Pseudomonas aeruginosa* PAK pilin adhesin, which has been associated with virulence (see below). Further, we include the heme-inducible fibronectin-binding protein and the lectin adhesin because of their saturable binding kinetics and strain specificity, respectively. The following sections of this chapter discuss each of the adhesins listed in Table 2.

Receptors

The *Candida* literature contains many examples of surface molecules that have been accorded the sta-

Table 2. Adhesin-ligand interactions of *C. albicans* and mammalian cells

Adhesin	Ligand	Cells	Gene-deleted strain		Reference
			In vitro phenotype	Virulence	
MP66[a]	Asialoglycosphingolipid	HBEC	ND[b]	ND	146
MP-lectin[c]	Fucosyl glycoprotein or lipid	HBEC	ND	ND	132
MP-heme[d]	Fibronectin	ND	ND	ND	142
Int1p	ECM	Epi, endothelial	Reduced[e]	Avir.[f]	41
Hwp1p	T-glutaminase substrate	HBEC	Reduced	Avir.	125
Ala1p	Fibronectin	Endothelial	ND	ND	43[g]
Mnt1p	ND	HBEC	Reduced	Avir.	12
Als1p	ND	Endo, epi	ND?	ND	37[g]

[a]MP66 mannoprotein of 66 kDa.
[b]ND, not determined since the encoding gene has not been isolated; consequently, gene-deleted strains are not constructed.
[c]MP-lectin as described in reference 132.
[d]MP-heme, expression of this MP is induced when 0.1% hemoglobin is included in the growth medium.
[e]Reduced, in comparison to parental (and single gene copy constructs), adherence is reduced.
[f]Avir., reduced virulence in a systemic murine model or guinea and mouse models (for Mnt1p).
[g]Heterologous expression of gene-promoted adherence in *S. cerevisiae*.

tus of "receptors" of host ligands and therefore implicated in cell-cell interactions or in modulating host responses. It must be recognized that the K_d of such receptor-ligand interactions has not always been defined and in some cases it is more likely that the affinities of the molecules are well below that generally accepted of true receptors. The hydrophobicity and charge of the cell surface of *C. albicans* are such that many proteins may form weak hydrophobic or ionic associations with it, and such weak adventitious associations with host proteins can be misleadingly likened to receptor-coupled events. At one level it could be argued that it would be surprising if pathogenic *Candida* species evolved true receptors for components of the bloodstream or endothelia since such interactions happen only rarely in the setting of immunocompromised individuals. Also, systemic candidiasis most often kills the host and would be expected to be heavily selected against during the course of host-fungus evolution. Nonetheless, *C. albicans* and other species apparently do bind and interact not only with human epithelial surfaces but also with human proteins of the blood and internal tissues, and the importance of such interactions is now being examined.

The Hemoglobin-Inducible FN Adhesin

An FN-binding mannoprotein of *C. albicans* is induced when cells are grown in a medium that contains 0.1% hemoglobin (142, 143). Actually, *C. albicans* can bind to several domains of the FN molecule, including the RGD (arginine-glycine-aspartic acid), collagen-, and fibrin-binding and cell-binding domains. Whether a single adhesin protein can bind to multiple domains or individual proteins recognize each is uncertain. To understand the nature of the interactions between *C. albicans* and FN, expression of FN binding was followed in a defined medium to which supplements of proteins were added. In preliminary experiments, Yan et al. had shown that yeast cells grown in Sabouraud broth for 20 to 48 h produced the highest ^{125}I-FN binding activity (142). However, the complex nature of Sabouraud broth and the variation from batch to batch of the medium precluded precise analysis of specific components that might induce expression of FN binding. Interestingly, a complex peptamin fraction (peptamin is a proteolytic digest of animal tissues) of the broth medium could substitute for Sabouraud medium in the induction of FN binding. To avoid the use of the peptamin fraction that is still very complex, the authors tried various host cell proteins that the organism might encounter during disease. They found that hemoglobin but not a variety of other heme-proteins could induce FN expression. Hemoglobin must be included in the growth medium for the effect to be seen, for if the compound was added just prior to binding assays, no FN binding was observed. Binding of whole cells to immobilized FN and bovine corneal endothelial cells was also enhanced when cells were grown in hemoglobin. Increased expression was not associated with a change in growth to a hyphal morphology. FN binding to cells was due to an interaction with a single class of receptor (K_d = [2.7 ± 0.1] × 10^{-8} M; R = [2.7 ± 0.4] × 10^5 molecules per cell) (144). In subsequent studies, recombinant and proteolytic fragments of FN were used to map the domain recognized by the *C. albicans* FN-binding protein. As stated above, at least three domains of FN have been reported to bind to this organism. Using competitive inhibition assays, these authors established that hemoglobin-induced binding of yeast cells occurred through the cell-binding domain (located at the carboxy-terminus of FN) but not the RGD domain (144). Further, hemoglobin did not induce cell adhesion to the collagen or fibrin I domains. Finally, a 55-kDa protein of *C. albicans* was determined to have FN-binding activity when a ligand (FN) protection assay was utilized.

Apparently, hemoglobin also induces the binding of yeast cells to a variety of other ECM proteins, such as laminin, fibrinogen, and type IV collagen but not type I collagen or thrombospondin-1 (143). A single receptor (adhesin) was postulated for each ligand since similar 50% inhibitory concentrations (IC_{50}) were obtained during competitive binding assays, whereas a second class of receptor was identified that binds specifically to laminin. Therefore, FN induces the expression of both promiscuous and specific receptors for ECM proteins. Since the studies on FN binding were done in vitro, the function of this protein in growth and virulence awaits the isolation of the encoding gene and the construction of gene-deleted strains.

Other investigators have studied the interactions of proteins of *C. albicans* with FN. Klotz and Smith (85) used gelatin as a source of peptides to block adherence of the organism to a variety of ECM proteins, including type I and IV collagen, fibronectin, laminin, and gelatin. Gelatin was used as a source of the peptides since it is plentiful and structurally is primarily the denatured form of type I collagen. Unfractionated trypsin digests of gelatin blocked adherence of yeast cells to each of the ECM proteins mentioned in the previous sentence. A further study revealed that a 47-mer (known as CB4) from type I collagen blocked adherence of yeast cells to immobilized gelatin, whereas other peptides were inactive except for Pep-Tite-2000, a commercially prepared peptide. The 47-mer inhibitory peptide did not contain an RGD sequence while PepTite 2000 (a 23-mer hydrophobic fibronectin peptide) has an RGD sequence. Interestingly, PepTite 2000 blocked adherence of yeast cells to type I and type IV collagen, laminin, and fibronectin in vitro and significantly inhibited hematogenous candidiasis in rabbits as CFU/g of tissues was significantly lower than that in buffer-treated animals (87). The mechanism of action of the PepTite 2000 was uncertain as the compound did not block adherence of the organism to perfused rabbit aortic endothelium. Additional studies by Penn and Klotz (111) identified the cell-binding domain of FN as that with the greatest avidity for yeast cells of *C. albicans.*

An FN adhesin has been characterized by the Klotz laboratory (84, 86). Yeast cells were extracted with octylglucopyranoside, the extract was passed through an FN-affinity column, and then fractionated by reverse-phase high-pressure liquid chromatography (HPLC). Two proteins were eluted from the FN-affinity column using EDTA, PepTite 2000, or an *N*-terminal peptide from the α-1 chain of type I collagen. SDS-PAGE of eluted material revealed two proteins (unreduced state) of 60 and 105 kDa, whereas reduced samples yielded two proteins of 62 and 72 kDa. The 105-kDa protein was thought to be dimer or represent an aggregate of a lower molecular mass species. Analysis of the 60- and 105-kDa proteins revealed that each was approximately 75% carbohydrate and 25% protein. Both proteins could be eluted from whole cells by dithiothreitol treatment, indicating their probable association with the cell wall.

As mentioned above, a 55-kDa mannoprotein was presumed to be an FN adhesin (receptor) of *C. albicans* (144). The relationship of this protein to that described above by Klotz et al. is unknown, but these proteins appear to be different. Although both recognize the cell-binding domain of FN, the latter protein seems to at least partially require an RGD sequence whereas the protein described by Roberts et al. does not. If this interpretation is correct, it appears that *C. albicans* has at least two FN-binding adhesins and a third that recognizes only laminin (see above). An estimate of the number of ECM-binding adhesins becomes even more complex as we survey the complement receptors of *C. albicans* that also recognize ECM proteins.

Complement Receptors

Nearly simultaneously, four laboratories reported that *C. albicans* hyphae recognize the iC3b (i = inactive) ligand of the alternative complement fixation pathway (1, 16, 32, 34, 44, 55, 65). This "dead end" branch of the alternative pathway results in the deposition of iC3b on the surface of microorganisms and their subsequent phagocytosis via the complement receptor 3 (CR3) of phagocytes. CR3 belongs to a family of mammalian cell integrin proteins. This observation along with those mentioned above in regard to the binding of ECM proteins (ligands of integrins) indicates that, indeed, *C. albicans* expresses an "integrin-like" protein. Along with iC3b, a degradation product of iC3b (C3d) was also recognized by hyphae of the organism. C3d is a ligand of CR2 (complement receptor type 2 of B lymphocytes). Different approaches were used to identify and characterize the *C. albicans* iC3b-binding protein(s) (summarized in reference 63), which was shown to be heat labile, trypsin sensitive, and apparently requiring divalent cations, like the mammalian integrin protein. *C. albicans* pseudohyphae and yeasts are reactive with mammalian anti-integrin antibodies as determined by fluorescent antibody analysis (see below); however, the similarities between the *C. albicans* and mammalian integrins must be minimal based on the concentration of antibody needed to observe reactivity with growth forms of *C. albicans.* Alaei et al. isolated a 42-kDa protein that binds to iC3b (1). Antibody raised against this protein blocked adherence of pseudohyphae to sheep erythrocytes conjugated with iC3b. The 42-kDa protein cross-reacted with OKM-1, a monoclonal antibody (MAb) directed against the human complement receptor type 3 protein. Affinity purification of pseudohyphal extracts also resulted in the isolation of 66- and 55-kDa proteins along with the 42-kDa proteins that apparently represent glycosylated forms of the 42-kDa protein. Previously, proteins of 130, 100, and 50 kDa were observed in OKM-1 immunoprecipitates of ^{125}I-labeled whole-cell antigens of the organism (34). In another approach to identifying integrin-like proteins, Western blotting of cytoplasmic candidal extracts with OKM-1 was used, and a protein of 165 ± 15 kDa was visualized (63). The relationship of this protein to others described above is unknown.

Binding of a series of MAbs that react with epitopes within the human CR3 and other leukocyte antigens to *C. albicans* has been investigated (100). Of a total of 10 such MAbs, only three, Mo1, M1/70HL, and 7C3, reacted with hyphae; the authors postulate that these data suggest a limited identity between the *C. albicans* CR3-like protein and the human CR3. Determinations of the homology of the *C. albicans* integrin-like protein to that of the mammalian cell integrins have been gleaned through studies of the cross-reactivity of MAbs to the mammalian integrin to *C. albicans,* similar to the approach described above. MAbs to either the α- and β-chains of the mammalian cell integrin have been used in screens against *C. albicans.* Of those tested, all of the MAbs to the αm and αx react with the organism as determined by fluorescent antibody assays (100), while both of the MAbs to the β2 chain were not reactive with cells of the organism. These data, therefore, indicate that homology of the *C. albicans* integrin-like protein is more closely related to the α-polypeptide chain of mammalian integrins (see below).

The C3d-binding protein was identified by ligand affinity chromatography as a 60- to 62-kDa mannoprotein, although an additional protein of 70 kDa was also eluted from a C3d-affinity column (16, 95). A monoclonal antibody (CA-A) that blocked binding of C3d to the organism was used in SDS-PAGE-Western blotting of candidal extracts. Several proteins were observed in Western blots, but only the 60-kDa protein, when purified, blocked binding of the organism to C3d-conjugated erythrocytes (95). The 60-kDa C3d-binding protein is glycosylated, based on its reactivity with concanavalin A, its susceptibility to endoglycosidase F, and the identification of mannose in HPLC profiles of the purified protein. Finally, using a combination of immunofluorescence and immunoelectron microscopy, Kanbe et al. (81) as well as Ollert and Calderone (106) demonstrated that the C3d-binding protein is located on the surface of hyphal forms of the organism but is subsurface in yeast forms.

Several functions of the CR-like proteins of *C. albicans* have been suggested, including host recognition and providing an escape mechanism for the organism based on molecular mimicry of host proteins (46). The latter idea is intriguing, but evidence is lacking at this time for such a function. On the other hand, an association of a CR activity and virulence was demonstrated with the cerulenin-resistant, avirulent mutant mentioned above (15, 91). Avirulent strain m-10 lacks an iC3b activity but has normal levels of C3d-binding activity (107); however, the problems associated with obtaining a direct correlation between its phenotype and a lack of virulence have been addressed earlier in this chapter. Other investigators have noted that iC3b expression is augmented (four- to sixfold) when cells are grown in high glucose and, likewise, their adherence to human umbilical cord endothelium is increased and their phagocytosis by neutrophils is reduced (65). Since a large number of patients with various types of candidiasis are hyperglycemic, the observation on glucose augmentation of receptor expression may be important to disease progression (65). A direct association of an integrin-like protein with virulence will be discussed below when the *INT1* gene is discussed.

The MP58 Fibrinogen-Binding Protein

There are, additionally, numerous other accounts of proteins from *C. albicans* that bind serum proteins such as fibrinogen, as well as other ECM proteins, such as laminin, vitronectin, and entactin (8, 9, 20, 21, 117, 128, 134). Binding to yeast and/or hyphae appears to be strain dependent. Tronchin et al. have shown that proteins of 68 and 60 to 62 kDa bind fibrinogen as well as laminin, C3d, and plastic surfaces (134). The authors suggest that these proteins may be related to the mammalian integrin family of proteins. On the other hand, Casanova and Chaffin identified a protein of 58-kDa molecular mass by ligand affinity blotting with fibrinogen and antifibrinogen antibody (20) but not with a number of other ligands such as laminin, fibronectin, type IV collagen, and C3d. This protein should be distinct from the protein identified by Tronchin et al., which, instead, appears to be somewhat related to the C3d-binding protein (CR2-like protein) described by the Calderone laboratory (95). The gene encoding the MP58-binding protein has been isolated (3). *FBP1* (fibrinogen-binding protein) expression occurs in minimal medium; the function of the gene has not been established since knockout strains have not been constructed. Mp58 contains about 25% carbohydrate and has several unusual features, including a type IV collagen-like domain, and the protein is ubiquitinated. Other features of the putative protein include its cell surface location and expression in patients with confirmed systemic and mucocutaneous candidiasis.

The MP66, *P. aeruginosa*-like Adhesin

An intriguing observation has been made that a putative adhesin of *C. albicans* has a host cell recognition domain that is homologous to the *P. aeruginosa* PAK pilus adhesin (90, 142, 145–148). The *P. aeruginosa* PAK pilus consists of a polymer of a single protein subunit termed pilin. The receptor-binding domain of PAK resides in the carboxy-terminal disulfide-looped region (PAK [residues 128 to 144]). Further, the ligand that is recognized by PAK is a glycosphingolipid asialo-GM_1 of epithelial cells. That a similar type of adhesin might be expressed by two dissimilar pathogens was suggested by the discovery that *C. albicans* produced cell surface structures that resembled bacterial cellular appendages referred to as fimbriae. This term is not intended to imply that *C. albicans* fimbriae represent self-assembling structures similar to the fimbriae of bacteria. Initial studies focused on the characterization of the *C. albicans* fimbriae (145). Fimbriae were purified from the yeast phase of the organism grown on Sabouraud agar. Washed cells were subjected to gentle homogenization to shear fimbriae from the cell surface. Subsequently, the supernatant (containing the fimbriae) was concentrated, dialyzed (crude fimbriae, CF), fractionated by HPLC and then rechromatographed to yield a fraction termed the enriched fimbriae (EF). By SDS-PAGE, several proteins ranging in molecular mass from 30 to 97 kDa were observed in the CF fraction, including a protein of 66-kDa molecular mass. However, in the EF fraction, only the 66-kDa protein was observed. A monoclonal antibody (FM 16) raised against the 66-kDa protein agglutinated cells, demonstrating that the fimbriae were located on the cell surface of the organism. FM16 was also used in an enzyme-linked immunosorbent assay (ELISA) to demonstrate that EF could bind to HBEC. A half-maximal binding of 10 μg/ml corresponded to high-avidity binding to HBEC. Further, adherence of yeast cells to HBEC was inhibited by EF (IC_{50} of <7.5 μg/ml). The 66-kDa protein was highly glycosylated (85% carbohydrate, 15% protein), and the amino acid content was heavily hydrophobic (50%).

Thin-layer chromatography was used to separate various glycolipids, and then overlaid with EF. Binding of EF to asialo-GM1 and asialo-GM2 was determined using the Fm16 antibody in an ELISA type of assay (146–148). Binding was specific only for those lipids. Binding to immobilized asialo-GM1 as well as its disaccharide βGa1NAc(1–4)βGa1 was saturable and concentration dependent and was blocked by homologous inhibitors, indicating the specificity of the binding. The disaccharide thus represents the minimal receptor structural requirement for this ligand, and, in fact, the same disaccharide inhibited binding of fimbriae to HBEC. Because of the similarity in the ligand for both *P. aeruginosa* and *C. albicans,* competitive binding experiments were performed using a series of MAbs to the PAK pilus adhesin. MAbs to the PAK pilin as well as to the PAK pilin peptides (anti-PAK [residues 128 to 144]) and anti-PAK (residues 134 to 140) agglutinated whole cells of *C. albicans,* whereas control antibodies to other peptide domains had no effect on agglutination of the organism. It should be stated that the MAbs that agglutinated *C. albicans* are also reactive with the ligand-binding domain of the PAK pilus protein. The *C. albicans* MAb (Fm16) likewise agglutinated *P. aeruginosa* cells. The interactions between the homologous antibody and antigens were inhibited by the heterologous antigens, indicating that both adhesins share a common antigenic determinant(s). These results suggest conserved cell surface receptors for host ligands among two highly divergent microorganisms.

In more recent studies, binding of biotinylated PAK pili to immobilized asialo-GM1 or HBEC was inhibited by the anti-PAK residues (128 to 144) or the anti-PAK residues (134 to 140) MAbs but not with anti-PAk (75 to 84), which corresponds to a peptide domain of PAK, which is not part of the ligand recognition domain. Similar results were obtained in inhibition assays with the *C. albicans* biotinylated fimbriae and the same MAbs. Likewise, synthetic peptides corresponding to the two ligand recognition domains mentioned above also inhibited fimbrial binding to asialo-GM1 and HBEC (147) and inhibited whole-cell binding to HBEC. These data clearly demonstrate the adherence function of the fimbriae protein of *C. albicans.* However, as with the hemoglobin-inducible adhesin described above, the role of the 66-kDa mannoprotein in disease development is not known since gene-deleted strains have not been reported.

The Fucosyl-Lectin Adhesin

Strains of *C. albicans* from patients fell into two categories when reacted with HBEC in adherence assays (25, 103). Depending on the strain, adherence was partially blocked by either fucose or *N*-acetyl-D-glucosamine or by lectins that recognize either of these two sugars. Thus, adherence of strain GDH 2346 was inhibited by fucose or by the winged pea lectin that binds fucose. On the other hand, adherence of strain GDH 2023 was inhibited by *N*-acetyl-D-glucosamine or the wheat germ agglutinin that binds to *N*-acetyl-D-glucosamine (103). In the case of both strains, inhibition of adherence only occurred when yeast cells were preincubated with the sugar or when the HBEC were preincubated with each lectin. The conclusion from this observation is that strains of *C. albicans* express either of two classes of lectins and that adherence is mediated through fucosyl- or *N*-acetyl-D-glucosamine-containing glycolipids or glycoproteins of HBEC. Partial purification of the fucosyl-binding lectin (which was identified as a mannoprotein) was accomplished from dialyzed culture supernatants (26, 102, 132) using affinity adsorbents containing fucosyl-containing blood group determinants. Activity of the lectin was associated with the protein domain of the molecule since removal of carbohydrate by *N*-glycanase and alkali digestion prior to affinity adsorption still yielded a biologically active molecule that blocked binding of strain GDH 2346 to HBEC. Similarly, Brassart et al. have demonstrated that fucosyl-containing oligosaccharides from human milk blocked the attachment of radiolabeled yeast cells of *C. albicans* to HBEC (11). The minimal structural requirement for the active compounds was found to be the Fucα1-2Ga1β determinant, which also happens to be the H sugar sequence found on all blood group substances of the ABO (H) system.

The Hydrophobic Proteins

Approximately 50% of the amino acid content of the *C. albicans* fimbrial mannoprotein (66 kDa), as discussed previously, is composed of hydrophobic residues. Although this protein has not been shown to be hydrophobic, it reminds us that the charge of a protein (or a lack of charge) can have profound influence on function. In this regard, considerable effort has been directed at understanding the contribution of hydrophobic proteins and glycoproteins to the structural and functional activities of the cell wall of *C. albicans*. Hydrophobicity is believed to provide adherence functions in the recognition of both epithelial and endothelial cells, binding to ECM proteins and plastic devices (catheters), and hydrophobicity is thought to confer greater virulence to cells than hydrophilicity (4, 45, 50–54, 97–99, 104). Masuoka et al. (99) have recently shown that antibodies to hydrophobic cell wall proteins of germ tubes blocked adherence of the organism to immobilized extracellular matrix proteins. There are several methods available for the isolation of hydrophobic proteins. In general, reagents such as β-mercaptoethanol can be used to extract total proteins, and this complex fraction is then passed through polystyrene beads that are hydrophobic, resulting in a binding of hydrophobic proteins to the beads. Subsequently, the hydrophobic proteins can be eluted and studied. Or hydrophobic interaction chromatography-HPLC can be used during the purification procedure to enrich for these proteins. Extraction of whole cells with β1–3 glucanase also yields complex preparations that can be partially purified, exploiting the hydrophobic properties of these proteins. Analysis of the proteins that result from the extraction/characterization approaches mentioned above has yielded several interesting observations. First, it appears that there is a greater abundance of hydrophobic proteins in germ tubes compared to yeast forms. Second, most of the hydrophobic proteins appear to be in the 20- to 67-kDa molecular mass range, compared to the hydrophilic proteins that are generally larger than 90 kDa. Third, the hydrophobic proteins are exposed on the cell surface and, in fact, are expressed during human disease. Fourth, the cell surface of hydrophobic cells is quite different in appearance from those of hydrophilic cells. Fifth, of interest, proteins that have been assigned an adhesin function fall into the molecular mass range typical of the hydrophobic proteins. Thus, the MP58 fibrinogen-binding protein and the 60- and 68-kDa proteins mentioned above that promote the binding of the organism to plastic are all in the suggested molecular mass range of hydrophobic proteins. Further, the MP58 appears to have exposed hydrophobic domains. Finally, the acid-labile oligosaccharides of bulk mannan from hydrophobic cells are longer and perhaps in greater abundance than the bulk mannan from hydrophilic cells (97). The latter observation should be potentially interesting in regard to differences in synthesis and assembly between the two forms of the organism, i.e., hydrophobic versus hydrophilic. Further characterization of these proteins and the function of their hydrophobic domains needs to be pursued.

Mannan Adhesins

C. albicans serotype A is known to possess a specific antigen, antigen 6, that is found in cell wall mannan. Although this antigen is associated with serological specificity, its role in specific cell functions was not revealed until mutants lacking antigen 6 were isolated by reason of their nonagglutination with anti-antigen 6 antibody (105). The mutants were generated by treatment with nitrosoguanidine. Nuclear magnetic resonance spectra indicated a loss of signal related to the β-linked side chains and a decreased amount of mannohexaose and mannopentaose in the mutant. Adherence of wild type and mutants to HBEC and a squamous carcinoma cell line (HSC-2) was measured. By visual assays, adherence of the mutant strain to HBEC was approximately 15% of parental cells, whereas for the HSC-2 cells, adherence was also considerably reduced but not as much as that observed with the HBEC. Thus, mutations in the structure of the mannan polysaccharide confer a reduced adherence phenotype. The question that still remains to be answered in regard to this observation is whether silent mutations exist (since the strain was mutagenized) that might be associated with reduced adherence. Or the functional activity of an adhesin may have been lost through spatial rearrangements that occur as a result of abnormal mannan biosynthesis.

Interestingly, a strain deleted in a gene encoding a protein mannosyltransferase (*PMT1*), the first step in protein O-glycosylation, was shown to have reduced adherence to a Caco-2 epithelial cell line, among several abnormal phenotypes (131) (to be discussed later in this chapter).

In addition, deletion of the α-1,2 mannosyltransferase *MNT1*, which is responsible for addition of the second mannose sugar to the O-linked mannan oligosaccharide, was also less adherent to buccal epithelial cells and was attenuated in virulence in rat vaginitis and systemic models of disease (12, 130). This supports the view that O-linked mannan plays a direct role in adhesion to buccal epithelia and possibly other cell types. Other carbohydrate epitopes have been shown to be important for adhesion (93). For example, the acid labile β-1,2-linked tetramannose, which is part of the phosphomannan of the outer *N*-linked carbohydrate, has been implicated as the adhesin for binding to mouse splenic marginal zone macrophages (27, 77–80) and the acid-stable component is responsible for yeast cell binding to the splenic marginal zone (77). Mild acid treatment can break the phosphodiester link that couples the β-1,2-oligomannan to the outer chain of *N*-linked mannan. Hence, this acid-labile fraction is readily removed and isolated and was shown to inhibit recognition and uptake of *C. albicans* yeast cells by macrophages. Also, a complex Zymolyase extract blocked adherence of the organism to mouse spleen marginal zone macrophages. The activity was inhibited by periodate but not protease treatment, indicating that the specificity of the reactivity was associated with a carbohydrate domain. Thus, these observations indicate that mannan is a likely candidate for promoting *Candida*-host cell interactions. Therefore, both the protein and carbohydrate components of *C. albicans* cell wall mannoproteins are important for interaction and adhesion to host surfaces (39). Not all these studies benefit from the availability of stable mutants in isogenic strain backgrounds to evaluate the importance of such epitopes in pathogenesis although significant strides are now being made in this direction.

Sialic Acids

In bacteria sialic acids (*N*-acetyl, *N*-glycolyl, and 5,9-*N*-diacetyl neuramic acids) commonly act as ligands in host-bacteria interactions. The presence of sialic acids on the surface of *C. albicans* has been suggested indirectly by showing that sialidase treatment decreased the apparent molecular mass of certain cell wall glycoproteins (1) and reduced the affinity of an antibody for *C. albicans* complement receptor (138). More recently surface sialic acids have been demonstrated directly on the *C. albicans* cell wall (123). The role of these residues in host-interaction, however, is not yet clear, but their presence suggests that bacterial-like sialic acid-dependent recognition of host surfaces is possible.

SPECIFIC CELL WALL PROTEINS

The structure of the *Candida* cell wall is dealt with elsewhere (chapter 12). In brief, it consists of a fibrous skeletal component consisting of chitin and β,1-3 glucan around which a matrix of a gel-like, branched β,1-6 glucan and heavily glycosylated cell wall mannoproteins are covalently attached via GPI linkages or possibly via ether linkages (PIR-proteins). Mannoproteins account for as much as 50% of the mass of the wall, and since they are greatly enriched on the outer wall surface, they are dominant antigens and are presumed to play key roles in adhesion and other aspects of the interaction with the host. Interestingly, most of the genes that encode proteins whose expression is strictly correlated with hypha formation encode cell wall mannoproteins (see chapter 7 for a detailed examination of their regulation). However, of these, several deserve specific mention in relation to host recognition and interaction.

The Als Protein Family

C. albicans has a family of at least nine *ALS* (agglutinin-like sequence) genes that encode cell surface glycoproteins. These gene products were named after the sexual agglutinin proteins in *S. cerevisiae* that mediate adhesion of mating haploid partners (94). The *ALS* gene family has largely been characterized by Hoyer's group, who have demonstrated the gene structure, pattern of expression, and presence of some of the encoded proteins on the surface of *C. albicans* cells (66–72). In *C. albicans* and other related species, these proteins are thought to play roles in adhesion with the host (and possibly also with itself and other microorganisms). Each gene consists of a central domain with a shorter or longer tandem repeat of a 108-bp motif and a more or less conserved 5′ domain. Some of the proteins are highly conserved at the 5′ regions (e.g., *ALS1*, *ALS3*/*ALS8*, and *ALS5*), perhaps suggesting that they arose by duplication and expansion of specific progenitor genes. The *ALS3* and *ALS8* (and possibly *ALS1*) genes are only expressed during hyphal growth (see chapter 7). When the *C. albicans* *ALS* genes (*ALS1* and *ALA1* for agglutinin-like adhesin) were expressed in *S. cerevisiae*, the transformants were able to stick to epithelial and endothelial cells (37, 42, 43). This suggests that Als proteins are likely to be important adhesins. However, the genes have not yet been deleted systematically to dissect their individual functional roles.

Hwp1

Another hypha cell wall-specific protein is the Hwp1 protein isolated by Staab et al. This protein is encoded by a gene that was initially isolated as a cDNA that encoded a hypha-specific antigen (126, 127). The structure of the protein suggests that it is linked via a GPI-anchor to cell wall β-glucan (127). The importance of this protein in host recognition came from a study by the same group, which demonstrated that the NH_2-terminus of the protein was a substrate for mammalian transglutaminase, a cross-linking enzyme found in the epithelia and endothelia of human tissues (125). This enzyme is capable of cross-linking small proline-rich proteins, such as that found in the *N*-terminus of *C. albicans* Hwp1 to human proteins in keratinized epithelia. This would provide a novel mechanism for host-mediated attachment of *Candida* cells to human epithelia. Consistent with this idea, deletion mutants lacking Hwp1 were no longer a substrate for human transglutaminase, were less adherent to HBEC, and were attenuated in virulence in a mouse systemic model of candidiasis (125, 135).

Int1

The *C. albicans* integrin-like protein Int1 has been shown to have a role in adhesion and in morphogenesis. The *INT1* gene was originally isolated by hybridization of human leukocyte αM integrin (40). This is a CR3 complement receptor, which is known to be a member of the integrin superfamily now known as αMβ2, Mac1, or CD11b/CD18. The *C. albicans* Int1p has only 18% identity with the ligand binding I domain, but various binding experiments preceding the isolation of the gene suggested that *C. albicans* did have integrin-like binding of the complement protein iC3b, including the fact that RGD peptides characteristically inhibited adhesion of *C. albicans* to HeLa cells and other human cell types (63, 64). *C. albicans* Int1p is a transmembrane protein that also has an external EF-hand domain indicative or divalent cation binding and a cytoplasmic talin-interacting domain, which may interact with actin of the cytoskeleton. Deletion of the gene caused multiple phenotypes, including partial reduction in adhesion to epithelia, loss of virulence, and inhibition of hypha formation (41). Heterologous expression of the *INT1* gene in *S. cerevisiae* conferred increased adhesiveness to these yeast cells and induced filamentous growth. These multiple effects of disrupting or heterologously expressing Int1 may reflect the role of the various external and cytoplasmic domains of the protein. In any case, Int1 seems at least to contribute to the adhesive properties of *C. albicans* under some conditions.

Int1 also has some homology to the yeast Bud4 protein, which is required for proper septin assembly and cytokinesis. Bud4 is, however, not required for Int1-induced morphogenesis in *S. cerevisiae* (see chapter 11). Thus, although the sequence similarity to Bud4 suggests that Int1 may affect morphogenesis by regulating cytokinesis, recent observations have demonstrated that the mouse talin-binding C terminus of the protein interacted with the talin-like protein S1a2 and that this interaction was necessary for the Int1-dependent morphogenesis defects in *S. cerevisiae* (2). This suggests that Int1-S1a2 interactions may mediate morphogenesis by modulating the actin cytoskeleton.

ADHERENCE OF NON-*C. ALBICANS* SPECIES

One of the observations mentioned previously is the greater adherence of *C. albicans* to host cells in vitro among all *Candida* species (82). With the emergence of non-*C. albicans* species as important pathogens, investigations more recently have focused on the adherence of non-*C. albicans* species. For example, deRepentigny et al. examined the binding of *Candida* spp. to rabbit intestinal mucin (28). Mucin is considered to be an important target since the organism must traverse this layer to adhere to the underlying mucosal epithelial cells. *Candida* spp. were classified into three adherence groups, with *C. tropicalis, C. albicans,* and *C. dubliniensis* among the highest adhering species, whereas *C. parapsilosis* and *C. lusitaniae* exhibited moderate adherence, and *C. glabrata* and *C. krusei* weak adherence. Adherence of *C. albicans* to mucin was associated with hydrophobic properties of the organism; also, adherence to HBEC was inhibited by mucin, but the inhibition was reversed by treatment of the mucin with Sap2p (28). Presumably, the differences in adherence to mucin were associated with differences in the expression of hydrophobic proteins by the high, moderate, and weakly adherent species.

Adherence of *Candida* spp. to platelets in vivo has also been studied (116). Following the inoculation of mice, platelets were fixed equally to either *C. albicans* or *C. glabrata* after <1, 5, or 30 min postinfection. However, the binding of platelets to each species differed in regard to the nature of the interaction, being cation-dependent in the case of *C. albicans* but different for *C. glabrata.* This observation indicates differences in the surface properties between these two species. Other studies that have compared *Candida* spp. indicate that *C. albicans* exhibited greater adherence than the other *Candida* spp. to porcine blood vessels (83), human epidermal corneocytes (115), human endothelial cells (118), human epidermal keratinocytes (108), HBEC (119), and rabbit bladder mucosa (96). However, interestingly, *C. tropicalis, C. glabrata,* and *C. krusei* have greater cell-surface hydrophobicity than *C. albicans* (104). *C. tropicalis* binding to lysophospholipids has been investigated (114). These investigators utilized an overlay assay using a lipid library that had been separated by chromatography to which radiolabeled yeast cells were added. Binding of the organism to lysophospholipids but not glycolipids or phospholipids was observed. Binding was also observed to lysophospholipids immobilized on microtiter plates. The organism was also capable of catabolizing the ligand once binding occurred. Of interest, *C. albicans* and *C. tropicalis* may use different mechanisms to adhere to host cells (7). Cormack et al. used a genetic screen to isolate nonadherent and hyperadherent mutants of *C. glabrata* (23). They used a modified protocol of the signature-tagged mutagenesis technology devised by Holden (57) for bacterial pathogens. Selection of tagged adhesion mutants was achieved by screening for transformants from a random pool of 4,800 mutants that were less or more adherent to human Hep2 epithelial cells. Most of the mutants with reduced adhesion had mutations in the promoter region of a single gene, *EPA1,* that encoded a lectin that recognized asialo-lactosyl-containing carbohydrates on the epithelial cell surface. Expression of *EPA1* in *S. cerevisiae* was sufficient to enable the transformants to adhere to Hep2 cell lines. This provides strong evidence that Epa1 is a major adhesin in *C. glabrata* and demonstrates how genetic screens can be used to isolate factors concerned with adhesion and virulence in haploid fungal species.

In summary, there are several studies that demonstrate greater adherence of *C. albicans* to host cells than the non-*C. albicans* species. Although the adhesins of most of the non-*C. albicans* species have not been studied, on the other hand, the identification of an adhesin has been accomplished with *C. glabrata,* as mentioned above (23).

THE ADDED COMPLEXITIES OF HOST RECOGNITION

In vitro assays of adherence with yeasts and some types of host cell or host cell ligand have a number of inherent problems compared to in vivo situations. The limitations include determining the contributions (stimulatory or inhibitory) of soluble host proteins to adherence, much of which has not been evaluated. In this section, we will address such issues. An obvious starting point is to summarize the literature on the adherence of *Candida* spp. to the diverse niches of the oral cavity (60, 121), as summarized by Cannon and Chaffin (18). Adherence of various microorganisms to the tooth surface can be modeled in vitro using hydroxyapatite (HA). *C. albicans* does not bind extremely well to HA unless the HA is preincubated with either whole or parotid saliva (14, 18, 19, 109, 110). Oppositely, sIgA reportedly prevents adherence of the organism (136). Previously, the adherence of various *Candida* spp. to HBEC was discussed, although the role of saliva in this binding was not mentioned. More recent evidence has been presented that whole or parotid saliva increases the attachment of *C. albicans* to HBEC (14) and also promotes coaggregation of the organism with certain oral streptococci, indicating that saliva may contain important proteins (or other biomolecules) that promote adherence of the organism in the oral cavity (10, 18). The active components of saliva that promote binding of the organism have been partially characterized. Salivary proteins were separated by SDS-PAGE to which radiolabeled *C. albicans* yeasts were added (109). Binding was observed to several proteins, and of these, two were isolated. End-terminal sequencing revealed that both proteins were basic proline rich proteins (bPRPs). Binding of the organism to bPRP only occurred when the proteins were immobilized but not in solution. When the bPRP was adsorbed to the surface of *Streptococcus gordonii,* an oral bacterium, coaggregation occurred. That *C. albicans* binds to the same protein from saliva on HA that binds to *S. gordonii* was proven since adherence to HA was reduced by >50% when the saliva was first adsorbed with the bacterial cells (14). The receptor on *S. gordonii* that appears to bind the bPRP is believed to be a polysaccharide (61), although cell surface proteins may also be contributory (62). In this study, mutants of *S. gordonii,* deleted in either of two genes that encode high molecular mass proteins (*cshA* and *cshB*), bound from 40 to approximately 80% less of the *C. albicans* cells. However, deletion of another gene encoding a surface lipoprotein (*scaA*) had no effect on the binding of *C. albicans,* indicating the specificity of the mutations of the surface proteins on cell-cell adherence.

The discussion of *Candida* spp. interactions in the oral cavity above is not meant to minimize the importance of other coaggregation reactions involving oral *Candida* spp. and oral bacteria that result in the colonization of the oral cavity. Some of the other coaggregation reactions have been described above (see adherence assays). Likewise, it should be emphasized that colonization of the oral cavity by *Candida* spp. probably requires other salivary constituents in addition to bPRPs. In fact, Hoffman and Haidaris have shown that *C. albicans* yeasts bind to a low molecular weight mucin (MG2) from human saliva and a rat submandibular gland (RSMG) mucin (59). The RSMG active material was partially purified. Recall that the data of deRepetigny et al. indicated that mucins are a suitable substrate for the adherence of *Candida* spp. (28).

Histatins

One of the key classes of antifungal proteins of the saliva in the oral cavity is the histatins. These basic proteins include histatin 1 (Hst1), Hst3, and Hst5 and can be present in concentrations of 50 to 425 μg/ml in human saliva (30). Hst5 seems to be the most potent of these salivary proteins and is produced at concentrations that can kill both yeast and hyphal cells of *C. albicans* in vitro. Hst5 is known to be targeted to the energized fungal mitochondrion where it binds to a target protein with a K_d around 1 μM. Binding leads to induced ATP efflux from the fungus and in mitochondrial membrane depolarization (30, 56, 141). Petite respiratory mutants and wild-type cells treated with respiratory inhibitors were less sensitive to Hst5 killing, demonstrating that only energized mitochondria act as a target for Hst5 (47). The effluxed extracellular ATP may ultimately result in cell death since purinergic angonists reduced viability of *C. albicans* and purinergic antagonists prevented Hst5 killing (88). Hence, some salivary proteins promote *Candida* adhesion whereas others are actively fungicidal.

BIOFILMS

Previously, we discussed the in vitro binding of *C. albicans* to plastic (134). More recently, the study of adherence to surfaces such as catheters has intensified because of the importance of this type of colonization in disease progression. Systemic candidiasis is often initiated by contamination of indwelling catheters in a variety of patient populations. Thus, an understanding of the mechanism(s) that promote colonization of medical devices should be important in controlling disease progression. Equally important, it appears that biofilms confer drug resistance to their inhabitants, most likely because the drugs have poor penetration to cells within the biofilm. The extent of resistance varies depending on the organism and the nature of the material to which the biofilm has formed. Also, it is rather easy to see how a constant seeding of the bloodstream by cells on or from within the biofilm could occur. Thus, for these reasons study of biofilm formation by *Candida* spp. has gained considerable recent interest.

Adherence of *C. albicans* to small discs of catheter material was studied (49). Quantitation of *C. albicans* in the biofilm was measured by radiometric methods, i.e., radiolabeled substrate was added at designated time points to the biofilm that formed on catheters, or by a reduction of a tetrazolium salt (MTT) by organisms in the biofilm. Both assays correlated with dry weight determinations of the biofilm. *C. albicans* cells grown in galactose (high molarity) versus glucose formed biofilms at equal rates, but paradoxically, recent isolates from implant infections formed less biofilm. Unfortunately, this observation may mean that the assay does not reflect the in vivo formation of biofilm. On the other hand, one of the strains that was unable to form hyphae also was less able to form comparable biomass on the catheters, indicating the importance of this growth form in biofilm formation. Of the species of *Candida* tested, *C. albicans* formed the most biofilm mass; *C. parapsilosis, C. glabrata,* and *C. kefyr* formed significantly less biofilm. Different catheter materials were evaluated for promoting biofilm formation by *C. albicans*; those results indicated that latex slightly exceeded polyvinyl catheters (PVC) for supporting biofilm formation whereas biofilm development on polyurethane was the least well developed. More recently, these same investigators showed that biofilm formation on PVC central venous catheters was increased when cultures (in 24-well tissue culture plates) were incubated in shake culture (2 to 60 rpm) instead of statically (48). In the latter experiments, static or shake cultures were incubated for 1 h at 37°C, then washed to remove nonadherent cells and incubated for 48 h in growth medium. Quantitation of biofilm was then measured by dry weight determinations or by using the assays described above (MTT or isotopic). With the shake cultures only, by scanning electron microscopy, cells of the biofilm appeared to be enveloped in extracellular polymer.

The cellular composition during development of the biofilm was determined by microscopy (6). Yeast cells were observed to adhere and form a thin, basal layer followed by the development of a thicker but more open hyphal layer. Biofilm formation by strains unable to produce hyphae or yeast was also followed. As might be expected, depending on which strain was used, only the inner or outer layers formed, but interestingly, the strain capable of only forming the inner, yeast layer was more easily detached from the surface of the catheter. However, biofilm formation differed when cellulose filters were used instead of catheter cylinders in that wild-type strains formed only biofilms consisting of yeast cells. As stated above, the use of shake cultures resulted in the formation of biofilm in which cells appeared to be imbedded in extracellular polymeric (EP) material. The EP has recently been analyzed and compared to the EP of culture supernatants of planktonically (suspended) cultures (5). The results indicate that the biofilm EP had significantly less total carbohydrate and protein, but a higher proportion of glucose, and also contained galactose, suggesting that the composition of the EP biofilm might be unique.

As stated above, it is believed that the organisms embedded in biofilms might be more resistant to antifungal drugs. In fact, the correlation is not absolute, since the amount of resistance depends on the source of the PVC catheter rather than the formation of a biofilm (5). On the other hand, others have shown that organisms of biofilms have increased resistance to amphotericin B (6). Additional experimentation is required to establish firmly the relative susceptibility or resistance of organisms associated with biofilms to antifungal drugs.

SUMMARY

In this chapter, emphasis has been on the proof that adhesins are important in disease progression. This correlate has been achieved through a number of methodologies, the most important of which is the construction of gene-deleted strains of *Candida* spp. and the demonstration of their reduced adherence properties and avirulence. This area of study continues to expand, and in the coming years, other specific adhesins will be sought. Perhaps the greatest need to more mimic host-fungus recognition is to establish assays that include components of the host (for example, saliva) and competing organisms. For example, very little is known about colonization of the gut and vaginal mucosa. In perhaps the most comprehensive study of *Candida*-gut interactions, Cole et al. demonstrated the colonization of the intestine and stomach by *C. albicans* using neonatal murine model (22). Those data indicated that yeast cells adhere to the mucosa and invade through an apparent "persorption" of the organism across the bowel wall and into the bloodstream. Subsequently, a commensal relationship on the mucosal surfaces was established following clearance of the organism from the systemic system. This model could be extremely useful in establishing the role of virulence factors in the establishment of *Candida* in the host. Most of the "action" (survival of the fungus, competition) occurs at mucosal surfaces, as for example, in the gut, vagina, and oral cavity. We need to understand how colonization occurs and how the organism persists. This emphasis of study will naturally include biofilm formation, since binding of *Candida* spp. (or for that matter any pathogen) hardly ever occurs on a one-to-one (fungus-host cell) situation, unless the organism has gained access to the cardiovascular system of the host.

The ultimate objective (aside from the biological curiosity) will be to develop reagents that inhibit adherence of the organism to tissues. It is clear that treatment of fungal diseases has to include new approaches in addition to the usual antifungal drugs, each with their inherent problems.

REFERENCES

1. **Alaei, S., C. Larcher, C. Ebenbichler, W. M. Prodinger, J. Janatova, and M. P. Dierich.** 1993. Isolation and biochemical characterization of the iC3b receptor of *Candida albicans*. *Infect. Immun.* **61:**1395–1399.
2. **Alleson, C. M., E. S. Bensen, C. A. Gale, A.-S. Mlems, C. Kurischko, and J. Berman.** 2001. *Candida albicans INT1*-induced filamentation in *Saccharomyces cerevisiae* depends on Sla2p. *Mol. Cell. Biol.* **21:**1272–1284.
3. **Alloush, H. M., J. L. Lopez-Ribot, and W. L. Chaffin.** 1996. Dynamic expression of cell wall proteins of *Candida albicans* revealed by probes from cDNA clones. *J. Med. Vet. Mycol.* **34:**91–97.
4. **Antley, P. P., and K. C. Hazen.** 1988. Role of yeast cell growth temperature on *Candida albicans* virulence in mice. *Infect. Immun.* **56:**2884–2890.
5. **Baillie, G. S., and L. J. Douglas.** 2000. Matrix polymers of *Candida* biofilms and their possible role in biofilm resistance to antifungal agents. *J. Antimicrob. Chemother.* **46:**397–403.
6. **Baillie, G. S., and L. J. Douglas.** 1999. Role of dimorphism in the development of *Candida albicans* biofilms. *J. Med. Microbiol.* **48:**671–679.
7. **Bendel, C. M., and M. K. Hostetter.** 1993. Distinct mechanisms of epithelial adhesion for *Candida albicans* and *Candida tropicalis*. *J. Invest.* **92:**1840–1849.
8. **Bouali, A., R. Robert, G. Tronchin, and J.-M. Senet.** 1987. Characterization of binding of human fibrinogen to the surface of germ tubes and mycelium of *Candida albicans*. *J. Gen. Microbiol.* **133:**545–551.
9. **Bouchara, J., G. Tronchin, V. Annaix, R. Robert, and J.-M. Senet.** 1990. Presence of laminin receptors on *Candida albicans*. *Infect. Immun.* **58:**48–54.
10. **Branting, C., M. L. Sund, and L. E. Linder.** 1989. The influence of *Streptococcus mutans* on adhesion of *Candida albicans* to acrylic surfaces in vitro. *Arch. Oral Biol.* **34:**347–353.
11. **Brassart, D., A. Woltz, M. Golliard, and J.-R. Nesser.** 1991. In vitro inhibition of adhesion of *Candida albicans* clinical isolates to human buccal epithelial cells by Fucα1-2Gal-bearing complex carbohydrates. *Infect. Immun.* **59:**1605–1613.
12. **Buurman, E. T., C. Westwater, B. Hube, A. Brown, F. C. Odds, and N. A. R. Gow.** 1998. Molecular analysis of CaMnt1p, a mannosyl transferase important for adhesion and virulence of *Candida albicans*. *Proc. Natl. Acad. Sci. USA* **95:**7670–7675.
13. **Calderone, R., and P. C. Braun.** 1991. Adherence and receptor relationships of *Candida albicans*. *Microbiol. Rev.* **55:** 1–20.
14. **Calderone, R., S. Suzuki, R. Cannon, T. Cho, et al.** 2000. *Candida albicans* adherence, signaling and virulence. *Med. Mycology* **38**(Suppl. 1):125–137.
15. **Calderone, R. A., R. Cihlar, D. Lee, K. Hoberg, and W. M. Scheld.** 1985. Yeast adhesion in the pathogenesis of endocarditis due to *Candida albicans:* studies with adherence-negative mutants. *J. Infect. Dis.* **152:**710–715.
16. **Calderone, R. A., L. Linehan, E. Wadsworth, and A. Sandberg.** 1988. Identification of C3d receptors on *Candida albicans*. *Infect. Immun.* **56:**252–258.
17. **Calderone, R. A., and E. Wadsworth.** 1985. Characterization of mannoproteins from a virulent *Candida albicans* strain, and its derived avirulent strain. *Proc. Soc. Exp. Biol. Med.* **185:**325–334.
18. **Cannon, R. D., and W. L. Chaffin.** 1999. Oral colonization by *Candida albicans*. *Crit. Rev. Oral Biol.* **34:**359–383.
19. **Cannon, R. D., A. K. Nand, and H. F. Jenkinson.** 1995. Adherence of *Candida albicans* to human salivary components adsorbed to hydroxylapatite. *Microbiology* **141:**213–219.
20. **Casanova, M., J. L. Lopez-Ribot, C. Monteagudo, A. Llombart-Bosch, R. Sentandreu, and J. Martinez.** 1992. Identification of a 58-kilodalton cell surface fibrinogen-binding man-

noprotein from *Candida albicans. Infect. Immun.* **60:** 4221–4229.

21. **Chaffin, W. L., J. L. Lopez-Ribot, M. Cassanova, D. Gozalbo, and J. P. Martinez.** 1998. Cell wall and secreted proteins of *Candida albicans:* identification, function, and expression. *Microbiol. Mol. Biol. Rev.* **62:**130–180.
22. **Cole, G. T., K. R. Seshan, K. T. Lynn, and M. Franco.** 1993. Gastrointestinal candidiasis: histopathology of *Candida*-host interactions in a murine model. *Mycol. Res.* **97:**385–408.
23. **Cormack, B. P., N. Ghori, and S. Falkow.** 1999. An adhesin of the yeast pathogen *Candida glabrata* mediating adherence to human epithelial cells. *Science* **285:**578–582.
24. Deleted in proof.
25. **Critchley, I. A., and L. J. Douglas.** 1987. Role of glycosides as epithelial cell receptors for *Candida albicans. J. Gen. Microbiol.* **133:**637–643.
26. **Critchley, I. A., and L. J. Douglas.** 1987. Isolation and partial characterization of an adhesin from *Candida albicans. J. Gen. Microbiol.* **133:**629–636.
27. **Cutler, J. E.** 1998. The *Candida albicans* phosphomannan complex in *Candida*-host interactions. *Res. Immun.* **149:** 299–308.
28. **deRepentigny, L., F. Aumont, K. Bernard, and P. Belhumer.** 2000. Characterization of binding of *Candida albicans* to small intestinal mucin and its role in adherence to mucosal cells. *Infect. Immun.* **68:**3172–3179.
29. **Douglas, L. J.** 1987. Adhesion of *Candida* species to epithelial surfaces. *Crit. Rev. Microbiol.* **15:**27–43.
30. **Edgerton, M., S. E. Koshlukova, T. E. Lo, B. G. Chrzan, R. M. Straubinger, and P. A. Raj.** 1998. Candidacidal activity of salivary proteins. Identification of a histatin-5 binding protein on *Candida albicans. J. Biol. Chem.* **273:**20438–20447.
31. **Edmond, M. B., S. E. Wallace, D. K. McClish, M. A. Pfaller, R. N. Jones, and R. P. Wenzel.** 1999. Nosocomial blood stream infections in United States hospitals: a three-year analysis. *Clin. Infect. Dis.* **29:**239–244.
32. **Edwards, J. E., T. A. Gaither, J. J. O'Shea, D. Rotrosen, T. J. Lawley, S. A. Wright, F. F. Frank, and I. Green.** 1986. Expression of specific binding sites on *Candida albicans* with functional and antigenic characteristics of human complement receptors. *J. Immunol.* **137:**3577–3583.
33. **Edwards, J. E., C. L. Mayer, S. G. Filler, E. Wadsworth, and R. A. Calderone.** 1992. Cell extracts of *Candida albicans* block adherence of the organisms to endothelial cells. *Infect. Immun.* **60:**3087–3091.
34. **Eigentler, A., T. F. Schulz, C. Larcher, E. M. Breitwieser, B. Myones, A. I. Petzer, and M. P. Dierich.** 1989. iC3b binding protein on *Candida albicans:* temperature-dependent expression and relationship to human complement receptor type 3. *Infect. Immun.* **57:**616–622.
35. **Fonzi, W. A., and M. Y. Irwin.** 1993. Isogenic strain construction and gene mapping in *Candida albicans. Genetics* **134:** 717–728.
36. **Franzke, S., R. A. Calderone, and K. Schaller.** 1993. Isolation of avirulent clones of *Candida albicans* with reduced ability to recognize the CR2 ligand, C3d. *Infect. Immun.* **61:** 2662–2669.
37. **Fu, Y., G. Rieg, W. A. Fonzi, P. H. Belanger, J. E. Edwards, and S. G. Filler.** 1998. Expression of the *Candida albicans ALS1* in *Saccharomyces cerevisiae* induces adherence to endothelial and epithelial cells. *Infect. Immun.* **66:**1783–1786.
38. **Fukayama, M., and R. Calderone.** 1991. Adherence of cell surface mutants of *Candida albicans* to buccal epithelial cells and analyses of the cell surface proteins of the mutants. *Infect. Immun.* **59:**1341–1345.
39. **Fukazawa, T., and K. Kagaya.** 1997. Molecular basis of adhesion of *Candida albicans. J. Med. Vet. Mycol.* **35:**87–99.
40. **Gale, C., D. Finkel, N. Tao, M. Meinke, M. McClellan, J. Olson, K. Kendrick, and M. Hostetter.** 1996. Cloning and expression of a gene encoding an integrin-like protein in *Candida albicans. Proc. Natl. Acad. Sci. USA* **93:**357–361.
41. **Gale, C. A., C. M. Bendel, M. McClellan, M. Hauser, J. M. Becker, J. Berman, and M. K. Hostetter.** 1998. Linkage of adhesion, filamentous growth, and virulence in *Candida albicans* to a single gene, *INT1. Science* **279:**1355–1357.
42. **Gaur, N. K., and S. A. Klotz.** 1997. Expression, cloning and characterization of a *Candida albicans* gene *ALA1,* that confers adherence properties upon *Saccharomyces cerevisiae* for extracellular matrix proteins. *Infect. Immun.* **65:**5289–5294.
43. **Gaur, N. K., S. A. Klotz, and R. L. Henderson.** 1999. Overexpression of the *Candida albicans ALA1* gene in *Saccharomyces cerevisiae* results in aggregation following attachment of yeast cells to extracellular matrix proteins, adherence properties similar to those of *Candida albicans. Infect. Immun.* **67:**6040–6047.
44. **Gilmore, B. J., E. M. Retsinas, J. S. Lorenz, and M. K. Hostetter.** 1988. An iC3b receptor on *Candida albicans:* structure, function and correlates for pathogenicity. *J. Infect. Dis.* **157:** 38–46.
45. **Glee, P. M., P. Sundstrom, and K. C. Hazen.** 1995. Expression of surface hydrophobic proteins by *Candida albicans* in vivo. *Infect. Immun.* **63:**1373–1379.
46. **Gustafson, K. S., G. M. Vercelloti, J. S. Lorenz, and M. K. Hostetter.** 1991. Molecular mimicry in *Candida albicans.* Role of an integrin in adhesion of the yeast to human endothelium. *J. Clin. Invest.* **87:**1896–1902.
47. **Gyurko, S., U. Lendenmann, R. F. Troxler, and F. G. Oppenheim.** 2000. *Candida albicans* mutants deficient in respiration are resistant to the small cationic salivary gland antomicrobial peptide histatin 5. *Antimicrob. Agents Chemother.* **44:** 348–354.
48. **Hawser, S. P., G. S. Baillie, and L. J. Douglas.** 1998. Production of extracellular matrix by *Candida albicans* biofilms. *J. Med. Microbiol.* **47:**253–256.
49. **Hawser, S. P., and L. J. Douglas.** 1994. Biofilm formation by *Candida* species on the surface of catheter materials in vitro. *Infect. Immun.* **62:**915–921.
50. **Hazen, K. C.** 1990. Cell surface hydrophobicity of medically important fungi, especially *Candida* species, p. 249–295. *In* R. J. Doyle and M. Rosenberg (ed.), *Microbial Cell Surface Hydrophobicity.* American Society for Microbiology, Washington, D.C.
51. **Hazen, K. C., and B. W. Hazen.** 1987. A polystyrene microsphere assay for detecting surface hydrophobicity variations within *Candida albicans* populations. *J. Microbiol. Methods* **6:**289–299.
52. **Hazen, K. C., and B. W. Hazen.** 1992. Hydrophobic surface protein masking by the opportunistic fungal pathogen *Candida albicans. Infect. Immun.* **60:**1499–1508.
53. **Hazen, K. C., and B. W. Hazen.** 1993. Surface hydrophobic and hydrophilic protein alterations in *Candida albicans. FEMS Microbiol. Lett.* **107:**83–88.
54. **Hazen, K. C., J. G. Lay, B. W. Hazen, R. C. G. Fu, and S. Murthy.** 1990. Partial biochemical characterization of cell surface hydrophobicity and hydrophilicity of *Candida albicans. Infect. Immun.* **58:**3469–3476.
55. **Heidenreich, F., and M. P. Dierich.** 1985. *Candida albicans* and *Candida stellatoidea,* in contrast to other *Candida* species, bind iC3b and C3d but not C3b. *Infect. Immun.* **50:** 598–600.
56. **Helmerhorst, E. J., P. Breenwer, W. van't Hof, E. Walgreen-**

Weterings, L. C. J. M. Oomen, E. C. I. Veerman, A. V. N. Amerongen, and T. Abee. 1999. The cellular target of histatin 5 on *Candida albicans* is the energized mitochondrion. *J. Biol. Chem.* **274**:7286–7291.

57. **Hensel, M., J. E. Shea, C. Gleeson, M. D. Jones, E. Dalton, and D. W. Holden.** 1995. Simultaneous identification of bacterial virulence genes by negative selection. *Science* **269**: 400–403.
58. **Hoberg, K. A., R. L. Cihlar, and R. Calderone.** 1986. Characterization of cerulenin-resistant mutants of *Candida albicans*. *Infect. Immun.* **51**:102–109.
59. **Hoffman, M. P., and C. G. Haidaris.** 1993. Analysis of *Candida albicans* adhesion to salivary mucin. *Infect. Immun.* **61**: 1940–1949.
60. **Holmes, A. R., R. D. Cannon, and H. F. Jenkinson.** 1995. Interactions of *Candida albicans* with bacteria and salivary molecules in oral biofilms. *J. Indust. Microbiol.* **15**:208–213.
61. **Holmes, A. R., P. K. Gopal, and H. F. Jenkinson.** 1995. Adherence of *Candida albicans* to a cell surface polysaccharide on *Streptococcus gordonii*. *Infect. Immun.* **63**:1827–1834.
62. **Holmes, A. R., R. McNab, and H. F. Jenkinson.** 1996. *Candida albicans* binding to the oral bacterium *Streptococcus gordonii* involves multiple adhesin-receptor interactions. *Infect. Immun.* **64**:4680–4685.
63. **Hostetter, M. K.** 1994. Adhesins and ligands involved in the interaction of *Candida* spp. with epithelial and endothelial surfaces. *Clin. Microbiol. Rev.* **7**:29–42.
64. **Hostetter, M. K.** 1999. Integrin-like protein in *Candida* spp. and other microorganisms. *Fung. Genet. Biol.* **28**:135–145.
65. **Hostetter, M. K., J. S. Lorenz, L. Preus, and K. K. Kendrick.** 1990. The iC3b receptor on *Candida albicans:* subcellular localization and modulation of receptor expression by glucose. *J. Infect. Dis.* **161**:761–768.
66. **Hoyer, L. L.** 2001. The ALS gene family of *Candida albicans*. *Trends Microbiol.* **9**:176–180.
67. **Hoyer, L. L., J. Clevenger, J. E. Hecht, E. J. Ehrhart, and F. M. Poulet.** 1999. Detection of A1s proteins on the cell wall of *Candida albicans* in murine tissues. *Infect. Immun.* **67**: 4251–4255.
68. **Hoyer, L. L., and J. E. Hecht.** 2000. The *ALS6* and *ALS7* genes of *Candida albicans*. *Yeast* **16**:847–855.
69. **Hoyer, L. L., and J. E. Hecht.** 2000. The *ALS5* gene of *Candida albicans* and analysis of the Als5p N-terminal domain. *Yeast* **18**:49–60.
70. **Hoyer, L. L., T. L. Payne, M. Bell, A. M. Myers, and S. Scherer.** 1998. *Candida albicans ALS3* and insights into the nature of the ALS family. *Curr. Genet.* **33**:441–449.
71. **Hoyer, L. L., T. L. Payne, and J. E. Hecht.** 1998. Identification of *Candida albicans ALS2* and *ALS4* and localization of Als proteins to the fungal cell surface. *J. Bacteriol.* **180**: 5334–5343.
72. **Hoyer, L. L., S. Scherer, A. R. Shatzman, and G. P. Livi.** 1995. *Candida albicans ALS1:* domains related to a *Saccharomyces cerevisiae* sexual agglutinin separated by a repeating motif. *Mol. Microbiol.* **15**:39–54.
73. **Hsu, L. Y., G. E. Minah, D. E. Peterson, J. R. Wingard, W. G. Merz, V. Altomonte, and C. A. Tylenda.** 1990. Coaggregation of oral *Candida* isolates with bacteria from bone marrow transplant recipients. *J. Clin. Microbiol.* **28**:2621–2626.
74. **Jabra-Rizk, M. A., W. A. Flaker, Jr., W. G. Merz, J. I. Kelley, A. A. M. A. Baqui, and T. F. Meiller.** 1999. Coaggregation of *Candida dubliniensis* with *Fusobacterium nucleatum*. *J. Clin. Microbiol.* **37**:1464–1468.
75. **Janbon, G., F. Sherman, and E. Rustchenko.** 1998. Monosomy of a specific chromosome determines L-sorbose utilization: a novel regulatory mechanism in *Candida albicans*. *Proc. Natl. Acad. Sci. USA* **95**:5150–5155.
76. **Jimenez-Lucho, V., V. Ginsburg, and H. C. Krivan.** 1990. *Cryptococcus neoformans, Candida albicans,* and other fungi bind specifically to the glycosphingolipid lactosylceraminde (Galβ1-4Glcβ1-1Cer), a possible adhesion receptor for yeasts. *Infect. Immun.* **58**:2085–2090.
77. **Kanbe, T., and J. E. Cutler.** 1994. Evidence for adhesin activity in the acid-stable moiety of the phosphomannoprotein cell wall complex of *Candida albicans*. *Infect. Immun.* **62**: 1662–1668.
78. **Kanbe, T., and J. E. Cutler.** 1998. Minimum chemical requirements for adhesin activity of the acid-stable part of *Candida albicans* cell wall phosphomannoprotein complex. *Infect. Immun.* **66**:5812–5818.
79. **Kanbe, T., B. Han, M. H. Redgrave, M. H. Riesselman, and J. E. Cutler.** 1993. Evidence that mannans of *Candida albicans* are responsible for adherence of yeast forms to spleen and lymph node tissue. *Infect. Immun.* **61**:2578–2584.
80. **Kanbe, T., M. A. Jutila, and J. E. Cutler.** 1992. Evidence that *Candida albicans* binds via a unique system on phagocytic cells in the marginal zone of the mouse spleen. *Infect. Immun.* **60**:1972–1978.
81. **Kanbe, T., R.-K. Li, E. Wadsworth, R. Calderone, and J. E. Cutler.** 1991. Evidence for expression of the C3d receptor of *Candida albicans* in vitro and in vivo obtained by immunofluorescent and immunoelectron microscopy. *Infect. Immun.* **59**:1832–1838.
82. **King, R. D., J. C. Lee, and A. L. Morris.** 1980. Adherence of *Candida albicans* and other *Candida* species to mucosal epithelium. *Infect. Immun.* **27**:667–674.
83. **Klotz, S. A., D. J. Drutz, J. L. Harrison, and M. Huppert.** 1983. Adherence and penetration of vascular endothelium by *Candida* yeasts. *Infect. Immun.* **42**:374–384.
84. **Klotz, S. A., R. C. Hein, R. L. Smith, and J. B. Rouse.** 1994. The fibronectin adhesin of *Candida albicans*. *Infect. Immun.* **62**:4679–4681.
85. **Klotz, S. A., and R. L. Smith.** 1995. Gelatin fragments block adherence of *Candida albicans* to extracellular matrix proteins. *Microbiology* **141**:2681–2684.
86. **Klotz, S. A., and R. L. Smith.** 1991. A fibronectin receptor on *Candida albicans* mediates adherence of the fungus to extracellular matrix proteins. *J. Infect. Dis.* **163**:604–610.
87. **Klotz, S. A., R. L. Smith, and B. W. Stewart.** 1992. Effect of an arginine-glycine-aspartic acid containing peptide on hematogenous candidal infections in rabbits. *Antimicrob. Agents Chemother.* **36**:132–136.
88. **Koshlukova, S. E., T. L. Llyod, M. W. B. Araujo, and M. Edgerton.** 1999. Salivary histatin 5 induces non-lytic release of ATP from *Candida albicans* leading to cell death. *J. Biol. Chem.* **274**:18872–18879.
89. **Lee, J. C., and R. D. King.** 1983. Characterization of *Candida albicans* adherence to human vaginal epithelial cells in vitro. *Infect. Immun.* **41**:1024–1030.
90. **Lee, K. K., L. Yu, D. I. MacDonald, W. Paranchych, R. S. Hodges, and R. T. Irvin.** 1996. Anti-adhesin antibodies that recognize a receptor-binding motif (adhesintope) inhibit pilus/fimbrial-mediated adherence of *Pseudomonas aeruginosa* and *Candida albicans* to asialo-GM1 receptors and human buccal epithelial cell surface receptors. *Can. J. Microbiol.* **42**:479–486.
91. **Lehrer, N., E. Segal, R. Cihlar, and R. A. Calderone.** 1986. Pathogenesis of *Candida albicans:* studies with a mutant which has reduced ability to adhere. *J. Med. Vet. Mycol.* **24**: 127–131.
92. **Leidich, S., A. S. Ibrahim, Y. Fu, A. Koul, C. Jessup, J. Vitullo,**

W. Fonzi, F. Mirod, S. Nakashima, Y. Nozawa, and M. A. Ghannoum. 1998. Cloning and disruption of *caPLB1,* a phospholipase B gene involved in the pathogenicity of *Candida albicans. J. Biol. Chem.* **273:**26078–26086.

93. **Li, R.-K., and J. E. Cutler.** 1993. Chemical definition of an epitope/adhesin molecule on *Candida albicans. J. Biol. Chem.* **268:**18293–18299.

94. **Lipke, P. N., D. Wojciechowicz, and J. Kurjan.** 1989. *AGα1* is the structural gene for the *Saccharomyces cerevisiae* α-agglutinin, a cell surface glycoprotein involved in cell-cell interactions during mating. *Mol. Cell. Biol.* **9:**3155–3165.

95. **Linehan, L., E. Wadsworth, and R. A. Calderone.** 1988. *Candida albicans* C3d receptor, isolated by using a monoclonal antibody. *Infect. Immun.* **56:**1981–1986.

95a. **Lottenberg, R., D. Minning-Wenz, and M. D. P. Boyle.** 1994. Capturing host plasmin(ogen): a common mechanism for invasive pathogens? *Trends Microbiol.* **2:**20–24.

96. **Lyman, C. A., E. Navarro, K. F. Garrett, D. D. Roberts, P. A. Pizzo, and T. J. Walsh.** 1999. Adherence of *Candida albicans* to bladder mucosa: development and application of a tissue explant assay. *Mycoses* **42:**255–259.

97. **Masuoka, J., and K. C. Hazen.** 1999. Differences in the acid-labile component of *Candida albicans* mannan from hydrophobic and hydrophilic yeast cells. *Glycobiology* **9:**1281–1286.

98. **Masuoka, J., and K. C. Hazen.** 1997. Cell wall mannosylation determines *Candida albicans* cell surface hydrophobicity. *Microbiology* **143:**3015–3021.

99. **Masuoka, J., G. Wu, P. M. Glee, and K. C. Hazen.** 1999. Inhibition of *Candida albicans* attachment to extracellular matrix by antibodies which recognize hydrophobic cell wall proteins. *FEMS Immunol. Med. Microbiol.* **24:**421–429.

100. **Mayer, C. L., R. D. Diamond, and J. E. Edwards, Jr.** 1990. Recognition of binding sites on *Candida albicans* by monoclonal antibodies to human leukocyte antigens. *Infect. Immun.* **58:**3765–3769.

101. **McCourtie, J., and L. J. Douglas.** 1981. Relationship between cell surface composition of *Candida albicans* and adherence to acrylic after growth on different carbon sources. *Infect. Immun.* **32:**1234–1241.

102. **McCourtie, J., and L. J. Douglas.** 1985. Extracellular polysaccharide of *Candida albicans:* isolation, analysis and role in adhesion. *J. Gen. Microbiol.* **131:**495–503.

103. **McCourtie, J., and L. J. Douglas.** 1985. Unequal distribution of adhesins within populations of *Candida albicans. FEMS Microbiol. Lett.* **27:**111–115.

104. **Minagi, S., Y. Miyake, Y. Fujioka, H. Tsuru, and H. Suginaka.** 1986. Cell-surface hydrophobicity of *Candida* species as determined by the contact-angle and hydrocarbon-adherence methods. *J. Gen. Microbiol.* **132:**1111–1115.

105. **Miyakawa, Y., T. Kuribayashi, K. Kagaya, M. Suzuki, T. Nakase, and Y. Fukazawa.** 1992. Role of specific determinants in mannan of *Candida albicans* serotype A in adherence to human buccal epithelial cells. *Infect. Immun.* **60:**2493–2499.

106. **Ollert, M. K., and R. A. Calderone.** 1990. A monoclonal antibody that defines a surface antigen on *Candida albicans* hyphae cross-reacts with yeast cell protoplasts. *Infect. Immun.* **58:**625–631.

107. **Ollert, M. K., E. Wadsworth, and R. A. Calderone.** 1990. Reduced expression of the functionally active complement receptor for iC3b but not for C3d on an avirulent mutant of *Candida albicans. Infect. Immun.* **58:**909–913.

108. **Ollert, M. W., R. Sohnchen, H. C. Korting, U. Ollert, S. Brautigam, and W. Brautigam.** 1993. Mechanisms of adherence of *Candida albicans* to cultured human epidermal keratinocytes. *Infect. Immun.* **61:**4560–4568.

109. **O'Sullivan, J. M., R. D. Cannon, P. A. Sullivan, and H. F. Jenkinson.** 1997. Identification of salivary basic proline-rich proteins as receptors for *Candida albicans* adhesion. *Microbiology* **143:**341–348.

110. **O'Sullivan, J. M., H. F. Jenkinson, and R. D. Cannon.** 2000. Adhesion of *Candida albicans* to oral streptococci is promoted by selective adsorption of salivary proteins to the streptococcal cell surface. *Microbiology* **146:**41–48.

111. **Penn, C., and S. A. Klotz.** 1994. Binding of plasma fibronectin to *Candida albicans* occurs through the cell binding domain. *Microb. Pathog.* **17:**387–393.

112. **Perepnikhatka, V., F. J. Fischer, M. Niimi, R. A. Baker, R. D. Cannon, Y.-K. Wang, F. Sherman, and E. Rustchenko.** 1999. Specific chromosome alterations in fluconazole-resistant mutants of *Candida albicans. J. Bacteriol.* **181:**4041–4049.

113. **Pittet, D., and R. P. Wenzel.** 1995. Nosocomial blood stream infections. Secular trends in rates, mortality and contribution to total hospital deaths. *Arch. Intern. Med.* **155:**1177–1184.

114. **Prakobphol, A., H. Leffler, and S. J. Fisher.** 1994. Specific adherence of *Candida tropicalis* to lysophospholipids. *Biochemistry* **33:**9496–9503.

115. **Ray, T. L., K. B. Digre, and C. D. Payne.** 1984. Adherence of *Candida* species to human epidermal corneocytes and buccal mucosal cells: correlation with cutaneous pathogenicity. *J. Invest. Dermatol.* **83:**37–41.

116. **Robert, R., A. Marot-Leblond, J. Cotton, M. Miegeville, S. Quenouillere, C. Mahaza, and J.-M. Senet.** 2000. Adherence of platelets to *Candida* species in vivo. *Infect. Immun.* **68:**570–576.

117. **Robert, R., J.-M. Senet, C. Mahaza, V. Annaix, M. Miegeville, J.-P. Bouchara, G. Tronchin, and A. Marot-Leblond.** 1992. Molecular basis of the interactions between *Candida albicans,* fibrinogen and platelets. *J. Mycol Med.* **2:**19–25.

118. **Rotrosen, D., J. E. Edwards, Jr., T. R. Gibson, J. C. Moore, A. H. Cohen, and I. Green.** 1985. Adherence of *Candida* to cultured vascular endothelial cells: mechanisms of attachment and endothelial cell penetration. *J. Infect. Dis.* **152:**1264–1274.

119. **Samaranayake, Y. H., P. C. Wu, L. P. Samaranayake, M. So, and K. Y. Yuen.** 1994. Adhesion and colonization of *Candida krusei* on host surfaces. *J. Med. Microbiol.* **41:**250–258.

120. **Schaller, M., W. Schafer, H. C. Korting, and B. Hube.** 1998. Differential expression of secreted aspartyl proteinases in a model of human oral candidosis and in patient samples from the oral cavity. *Mol. Microbiol.* **29:**605–615.

121. **Schmid, J., P. R. Hunter, G. C. White, A. K. Nand, and R. D. Cannon.** 1995. Physiological traits associated with success of *Candida albicans* strains as commensal colonizers and pathogens. *J. Clin. Microbiol.* **33:**2920–2926.

122. **Skerl, K. G., R. A. Calderone, E. Segal, T. Sreevalsan, and W. M. Scheld.** 1983. In vitro binding of *Candida albicans* yeast cells to human fibronectin. *Can. J. Microbiol.* **30:**221–227.

123. **Soares, R. M., R. M. de A. Soares, D. S. Alviano, J. Angluster, C. S. Alviano, and L. R. Travassos.** 2000. Identification of sialic acids on the cell surface of *Candida albicans. Biochim. Biophys. Acta* **1474:**262–268.

124. **Sobel, J. D., G. Muller, and H. R. Buckley.** 1984. Critical role of germ tube formation in the pathogenesis of candidal vaginitis. *Infect. Immun.* **44:**576–580.

125. **Staab, J. F., S. D. Bradway, P. Fidel, and P. Sundstrom.** 1999. Adhesive and mammalian transglutaminase substrate properties of *Candida albicans HWP1. Science* **283:**1535–1538.

126. **Staab, J. F., C. A. Ferrer, and P. Sundstrom.** 1996. Developmental expression of a tandemly repeated, proline- and glutamine-rich amino acid motif on hyphal surfaces on *Candida albicans*. *J. Biol. Chem.* **271:**6298–6305.

127. **Staab, J. F., and P. Sundstrom.** 1998. Genetic organization and sequence analysis of the hypha-specific cell wall protein gene *HWP1* of *Candida albicans*. *Yeast* **14:**681–686.

128. **Sturtevant, J., and R. Calderone.** 1997. *Candida albicans* adhesins: biochemical aspects and virulence. *Iberoamer. Micologia* **14:**90–97.

129. **Sundstrom, P.** 1999. Adhesins in *Candida albicans*. *Curr. Opin. Microbiol.* **2:**353–357.

130. **Thomson, L. M., S. Bates, S. Yamazaki, M. Arisawa, Y. Aoki, N. A. R. Gow.** 2000. Functional characterization of the *Candida albicans MNT1* mannosyltransferase expressed heterologously in *Pichia pastoris*. *J. Biol. Chem.* **275:**18933–18938.

131. **Timpel, C., S. Strahl-Bolsonger, K. Ziegelbauer, and J. F. Ernst.** 1998. Multiple functions of Pmt1p-mediated protein O-mannosylation in the fungal pathogen *Candida albicans*. *J. Biol. Chem.* **273:**20837–20846.

132. **Tosh, F. D., and L. J. Douglas.** 1992. Characterization of a fucoside-binding adhesin of *Candida albicans*. *Infect. Immun.* **60:**4734–4739.

133. **Tronchin, G., J. P. Bouchara, and R. Robert.** 1989. Dynamic changes of the cell wall surface of *Candida albicans* associated with germination and adherence. *Eur. J. Cell Biol.* **50:** 285–290.

134. **Tronchin, G., J. P. Bouchara, R. Robert, and J.-M. Senet.** 1988. Adherence of *Candida albicans* germ tubes to plastic: ultrastructural and molecular studies of fibrillar adhesins. *Infect. Immun.* **56:**1987–1993.

135. **Tsuchimori, N., L. L. Sharkey, W. A. Fonzi, S. W. French, J. E. Edwards, and S. G. Filler.** 2000. Reduced virulence of *HWP1*-deficient mutants of *Candida albicans* and their interactions with host cells. *Infect. Immun.* **68:**1997–2002.

136. **Vudhichamnong, K., D. M. Walker, and H. C. Ryley.** 1982. The effect of secretory immunoglobulin A on the in vitro adherence of the yeast *Candida albicans* to human oral epithelial cells. *Arch. Oral Biol.* **27:**617–621.

137. **Wadsworth E., S. C. Prasad, and R. Calderone.** 1993. Analysis of mannoproteins from blastoconidia and hyphae of *Candida albicans* with a common epitope recognized by anti-complement receptor type 2 antibodies. *Infect. Immun.* **61:** 4675–4681.

138. **Weems, J. J., Jr.** 1992. *Candida parapsilosis:* epidemiology, pathogenicity, clinical manifestations, and antimicrobial susceptibility. *Clin. Infect. Dis.* **14:**756–766.

139. **Wenzel, R. P.** 1995. Nosocomial candidiasis. *Clin. Infect. Dis.* **20:**1531–1534.

140. **Whelan, W. L., J. M. Delga, E. Wadsworth, T. J. Walsh, K. J. Kwon-Chung, R. Calderone, and P. N. Lipke.** 1990. Isolation and characterization of cell surface mutants of *Candida albicans*. *Infect. Immun.* **58:**1552–1557.

141. **Xu, Y., I. Ambudkar, H. Yamagishi, W. Swaim, T. Walsh, and B. C. O'Connel.** 1999. Histatin 3-mediated killing of *Candida albicans:* effect of extracellular salt concentration on binding and internalization. *Antimicrob. Agents Chemother.* **43:**2256–22262.

142. **Yan, S., E. Negre, J. A. Cashel, N. Guo, C. A. Lyman, T. J. Walsh, and D. D. Roberts.** 1996. Specific induction of fibronectin binding activity by hemoglobin in *Candida albicans* grown in defined media. *Infect. Immun.* **64:**2930–2935.

143. **Yan, S., R. G. Rodrigues, D. Cahn-Hidalgo, T. J. Walsh, and D. D. Roberts.** 1998. Hemoglobin induces binding of several extracellular matrix proteins to *Candida albicans*. *J. Biol. Chem.* **273:**5638–5644.

144. **Yan, S., R. G. Rodrigues, and D. D. Roberts.** 1998. Hemoglobin-induced binding of *Candida albicans* to the cell-binding domain of fibronectin is independent of the Arg-Gly-Asp sequence. *Infect. Immun.* **66:**1904–1909.

145. **Yu, L., K. K. Lee, K. Ens, P. C. Doig, M. R. Carpenter, W. Staddon, R. S. Hodges, W. Paranchych, and R. T. Irvin.** 1994. Partial characterization of a *Candida albicans* fimbrial adhesin. *Infect. Immun.* **62:**2834–2842.

146. **Yu, L., K. K. Lee, R. S. Hodges, W. Paranchych, and R. T. Irvin.** 1994. Adherence of *Pseudomonas aeruginosa* and *Candida albicans* to glycosphingolipid (asialo-GM1) receptors is achieved by a conserved receptor-binding domain present on their adhesins. *Infect. Immun.* **62:**5213–5219.

147. **Yu, L., K. K. Lee, W. Paranchych, R. S. Hodges, and R. T. Irvin.** 1996. Use of synthetic peptides to confirm that the *Pseudomonas aeruginosa* PAK pilus adhesin and the *Candida albicans* fimbrial adhesin possess a homologous receptor-binding domain. *Mol. Microbiol.* **19:**1107–1116.

148. **Yu, L., K. K. Lee, H. B. Sheth, P. Lane-Bell, G. Srivastava, O. Hindsgaul, W. Paranchych, R. S. Hodges, and R. T. Irvin.** 1994. Fimbria-mediated adherence of *Candida albicans* to glycosphingolipid receptors on human buccal epithelial cells. *Infect. Immun.* **62:**2843–2848.

Candida and Candidiasis
Edited by Richard A. Calderone

Chapter 7

Expression of Growth Form-Specific Factors during Morphogenesis in *Candida albicans*

ALISTAIR J. P. BROWN

Microscopic analysis of tissues infected with *Candida albicans* often reveals fungal cells growing in several different morphologies (27). These include budding yeast-like cells, chains of more elongated pseudohyphal cells, and true hyphae. In addition, *C. albicans* can be induced to form spore-like structures (chlamydospores). The growth of these different cellular morphologies can be induced in vitro using a wide variety of different experimental conditions.

The transitions between the various growth morphologies represent simple developmental processes that are of significant academic interest. However, the medical importance of *C. albicans* and the apparent contribution of morphological transitions to the virulence of this fungus have increased the significance of these transitions. The misconception that the virulence of this fungus is dependent on the hyphal growth form has arisen largely from the attractive assumption that hyphae are better able to invade host tissues than yeast cells. Certainly, the thigmotropic nature of *C. albicans* hyphae supports the notion that they might be able to detect and penetrate breaks in epithelial or endothelial surfaces (32). However, although they can only grow in the yeast form, some monomorphic isolates of *C. albicans* have retained their virulence. Also, lesions in infected tissues that only contain *C. albicans* yeast cells have been reported (27). *Candida glabrata* is pathogenic, yet it does not display filamentous growth forms. Furthermore, the virulence of other fungal pathogens such as *Histoplasma capsulatum* and *Coccidioides immitis* is dependent on their growth in the yeast form, not a filamentous form. It is clear that both yeast and hyphal forms of *C. albicans* are pathogenic, and both may contribute to different stages in disease establishment and progression (28). For example, hyphal cells may indeed promote tissue invasion, whereas yeast cells may promote dissemination.

In an effort to understand the mechanisms that regulate cellular morphogenesis in *C. albicans* and the contribution it makes to virulence, a number of groups have searched for growth form-specific factors (i.e., proteins that are expressed exclusively in one particular growth form). This chapter describes the identification of growth form-specific factors and their possible roles in *C. albicans*. The main focus is on hypha-specific factors, because this growth form has received more attention than the other growth forms. Interest in these factors was stimulated specifically because of their morphogenetic expression patterns, and hence their regulation is discussed briefly. However, a more detailed discussion of the signal transduction pathways and transcription factors that control their expression can be found in chapter 8.

CELLULAR MORPHOLOGIES IN *C. ALBICANS*

C. albicans undergoes reversible morphological transitions between ovoid, unicellular budding cells (yeast cells, or blastospores) and chains of filamentous cells. The latter cells display different degrees of filamentation, ranging from slightly elongated ovoid cells to significantly extended tube-like cells. Filamentous cells are classified either as pseudohyphae or hyphae depending on their morphology. Although the degree of elongation of pseudohyphal cells can vary considerably, from relatively short to significantly extended cells, they always display constrictions at their septa between individual cellular compartments (Fig. 1). In contrast, true hyphae and their progenitors (germ tubes) show no such constrictions, having parallel walls at their septa.

Alistair J. P. Brown • Molecular and Cell Biology, Institute of Medical Sciences, University of Aberdeen, Foresterhill, Aberdeen AB25 2ZD, United Kingdom.

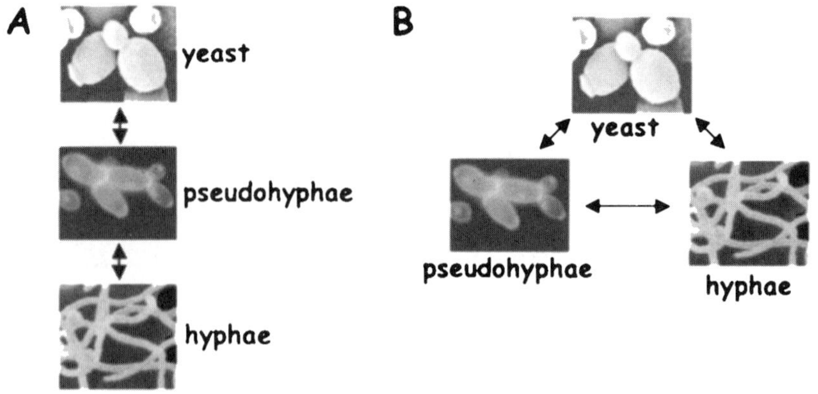

Figure 1. Possible developmental relationships between the yeast, pseudohyphal, and hyphal growth forms of *C. albicans.* (A) According to this model, pseudohyphae represent developmental intermediates between budding and hyphal growth forms. (B) In this model, pseudohyphae are formed via a separate developmental pathway (14). Adapted from reference 9. Copyright Springer-Verlag.

An objective measure of *C. albicans* cell morphology was developed by Merson-Davies and Odds (25). Their "morphology index" is based on three cellular dimensions: the length (l) and maximum diameter (d) of a compartment combined with the diameter at the septal junction (s). The morphology index, which is calculated using the equation ls/d^2, is usually 1.0 to 1.5 for yeast cells, 2.5 to 3.4 for pseudohyphae, and greater than 3.4 for hyphae. This index provides an objective measure of the morphological phenotypes of *C. albicans* mutants, as opposed to the subjective and sometimes misleading descriptions of morphological phenotypes that are often reported. More accurate phenotypic analysis would facilitate the dissection of morphogenetic regulatory mechanisms.

Morphological changes between the yeast and the various filamentous forms occur in response to alterations in the growth conditions. Odds (27) reviewed the wide variety of parameters that have been shown to affect the morphology of *C. albicans.* Parameters that promote hyphal development in vitro include a growth temperature above 35°C, a pH greater than 6.5, nitrogen and/or carbon starvation, nonfermentable carbon sources, low oxygen concentrations, and a wide range of chemicals including *N*-acetylglucosamine, proline (and other amino acids), and alcohols. Serum is one of the most potent inducers of hyphal development, and interestingly, some human hormones, including leutinizing hormone, chorionic gonadotrophin, progesterone, and estradiol, can stimulate hyphal growth (5, 13, 20, 45). It is important to note that a combination of conditions is required to activate hyphal development. For example, serum addition alone is not sufficient to stimulate hyphal development if the growth temperature is below 30°C. Growth of cells in the yeast form is promoted by an inoculum above 10^6 cells ml^{-1}, a growth temperature below 35°C, a pH of less than 6.5, glucose, and ammonium salts (reviewed by Odds [27]). Presumably, some of these treatments reflect the signals that regulate cell morphology during establishment and progression of candidiasis (8).

The situation is further complicated by the high degree of variability displayed by different isolates of *C. albicans.* Some clinical isolates are particularly sensitive to particular morphological stimuli and display vigorous hyphal growth, whereas others form hyphae less well (25). The genetic dissection of loci that account for these strain differences would be particularly revealing. This is yet another aspect of *C. albicans* biology that would benefit from access to an exploitable sexual cycle.

The developmental relationship between yeast, pseudohyphal, and hyphal cells would seem to be intuitively obvious. Based on their degree of elongation and their morphology indices, yeast and hyphal cells would seem to be the morphological extremes, with pseudohyphal cells representing intermediate forms (Fig. 1A) (9). This remains a distinct possibility. However, several observations suggest an alternative view, where pseudohyphal and hyphal growth forms represent distinct developmental stages (Fig. 1B) (9, 14). The diameters of hyphal and pseudohyphal compartments differ significantly, hyphal cells being narrower (25). The position of the first septum differs when a mother yeast cell is generating a new hypha or pseudohypha. This septum occurs at the neck between mother and a daughter pseudohyphal cell, whereas the septum is laid down within the germ tube during hyphal development. Also, the position of the first mitosis differs, occurring at the mother cell neck in pseudohyphae but entirely within the germ tube in hyphae (40). Further differences in cell cycle progression support the notion that pseudohyphae and hyphae represent distinct developmental states (see chapter 11). Also, the phenotypes of some regulatory mutants suggest that pseudohyphal and hyphal growth forms are distinct. For example, the depletion or the overexpression of the regulator, Efg1, forces *C. albicans* into a pseudohyphal morphology (39). Also, a *C. albicans tup1* mutant appears to be fixed in a pseudohyphal morphology in the presence or absence of hypha-inducing signals (6), suggesting that Tup1 might be required for yeast or hyphal growth but not pseudohyphal growth. However, the phenotypes of other regulatory mutants appear to favor the first model (Fig. 1A). For example, *C. albicans nrg1/nrg1* mutants grow as pseudohyphae under noninducing conditions but can develop hyphae in response to hypha-inducing conditions (26). A critical test that would distinguish between these models would be the identification of a *C. albicans* mutant that is unable to form pseudohyphae but can undergo yeast-hypha morphogenesis. The developmental relationship between yeast, pseudohyphal, and hyphal cells remains to be resolved.

Another question that remains to be answered concerns the developmental relationship between these morphological transitions and phenotypic switching in *C. albicans*. Phenotypic switching refers to the spontaneous, and in some cases reversible, interchange between different phenotypic states. Although phenotypic switching is often recognized by changes in colony morphology, it is often accompanied by changes in cell morphology from ovoid to more elongated, rod-like forms (33). Although the relationship between phenotypic switching and yeast-hypha morphogenesis has not been studied in depth, several observations suggest that these phenomena might be related. First, both involve changes in cell morphology. Second, the morphological regulator, Efg1, influences some of the phenotypes associated with the white-opaque switch (34, 36). Third, the white phase-specific *WH11* promoter appears to respond to yeast-hypha morphogenesis and phenotypic switching through similar mechanisms (35). Therefore, similar or overlapping regulatory circuits may control phenotypic switching and morphogenesis.

IDENTIFICATION OF GROWTH FORM-SPECIFIC FACTORS

It is generally assumed that changes in cell morphology in *C. albicans* are associated with changes in the expression of specific factors that are expressed exclusively in a particular growth form. This was confirmed by an early proteomics-based comparison of yeast and hyphal cells that revealed the presence of at least two new proteins in the hyphal cells (15). This stimulated a search for *C. albicans* genes that are expressed in a growth form-specific manner. The rationale was that the analysis of these genes should reveal insights into morphogenetic regulation and the construction of a yeast or hyphal cell.

Little work has been done on hypha-yeast morphogenesis, and the search for growth form-specific genes has focused mainly on hyphal cells. This has been complicated by the fact that the expression levels of most genes fluctuate during the yeast-hypha transition as a result of the major physiological changes that accompany the transition (10, 41, 42). This led to a strict operational definition of what constitutes a hypha-specific gene. These are genes that are expressed specifically during hyphal development but are not expressed in response to the individual conditions that induce hyphal growth (41). On the basis of these criteria, several hypha-specific *C. albicans* genes have now been isolated. *ECE1* was the first hypha-specific gene to be identified (4). This gene was isolated by screening a *C. albicans* library by differential hybridization with probes from yeast and hyphal cells. The level of *ECE1* mRNA correlated with the extent of cell elongation, regardless of the means of induction (4), suggesting that Ecel plays a role in hyphal development. However, a *C. albicans ece1/ece1* mutant was still able to make hyphae, indicating that Ece1 is not required for hyphal development (Table 1). Ece1 is probably an intracellular protein, based on the lack of an obvious signal sequence, but its function remains obscure (4).

The screen that yielded *ECE1* was performed using cDNA from hyphae induced by raising the pH of the culture (4). Not surprisingly, therefore, a number of pH-regulated genes were also identified in this screen, including *PHR1* (pH responsive gene) (30). Although Phr1 plays a role in maintaining cell morphology in *C. albicans,* probably by cross-linking structural components of the cell wall (16, 30), it is not a true hypha-specific factor. *PHR1* responds to pH, being expressed at neutral pH but inactive at acidic pH (30). At the time, this observation confirmed the need for the strict operational definition of hypha-specific genes.

ALS1 was isolated in another differential screen that exploited hybridization probes from yeast and hyphal cells. This time the hyphal probe was generated from cultures induced with the tissue culture medium RPMI, and *ALS1* was isolated on the basis that it was expressed in an RPMI-dependent fashion (17). Sequencing of *ALS1* revealed that it encodes a protein with strong sequence similarity to *Saccharomyces cer-*

Table 1. Hypha-specific genes in *C. albicans*

Gene	Phenotype of null mutant	Function	Reference(s)
ALS3	Normal hyphal development Double *als3 als8* null displays reduced adhesion	Hypha-specific cell surface adhesin	18
ALS8	Normal hyphal development Double *als3 als8* null displays reduced adhesion	Hypha-specific cell surface adhesin	22
ECE1	Normal hyphal development	Unknown; probably intracellular	4
HWP1	Normal hyphal development under serum induction	Hypha-specific cell surface adhesin	31, 38
HYR1	Normal hyphal development	Putative hypha-specific cell surface glycoprotein	3

evisiae AGα1, which is a cell surface agglutinin involved in the mating of haploid cells. Further analysis revealed that *ALS1* is not expressed when hyphal cells are induced using pH-stimulation (18), and hence, strictly speaking, Als1 is not a true hypha-specific factor. However, Als1 could be described as a "conditional hypha-specific gene" in that it appears to be expressed in subset of hypha-inducing conditions (Table 2).

ALS1 proved to be the founder member of a *C. albicans* family of agglutinin-like sequences (*ALS* genes), some of which are hypha-specific. Hoyer and coworkers (18) isolated further members of the *ALS* gene family on the basis of their sequence similarity to *ALS1*. *ALS3*, which displays 81% identity to *ALS1*, proved to be hypha specific, being activated under serum-, *N*-acetylglucosamine-, and proline-inducing conditions (18). More recently, the *ALS8* gene was also shown to encode a hypha-specific cell surface agglutinin (22). Although *ALS8* was isolated by a serendipitous route, as a false positive in a screen for an unrelated transcription factor, a routine Northern analysis revealed that it was hyphally regulated (Table 1). More detailed analyses then confirmed that *ALS8* is expressed under serum-, *N*-acetylglucosamine-, and pH-inducing conditions, and hence that Als8 is a hypha-specific factor (22). Cross-hybridization to other closely related sequences on these Northern blots indicated differential expression of *ALS* gene family members and suggested that some *ALS* genes might be yeast specific. These authors went on to demonstrate that a *C. albicans als3/als3 als8/als8* double mutant can form hyphae, albeit with reduced adhesive properties. Hence, neither Als3 nor Als8 is required for the formation of a viable hypha.

C. albicans secreted aspartyl proteinases are also encoded by a large family of differentially expressed genes. A subset of these *SAP* genes are expressed in a hypha-specific fashion, but only at neutral pH under serum-inducing conditions (*SAP4* through 6) (19). Therefore, like *ALS1*, the *SAP4* through 6 genes could be described as conditional hypha-specific genes (Table 2). Interestingly, these genes are required for normal virulence in systemic infections (29).

The *HWP1* (hyphal wall protein) gene was isolated on the basis that it encodes a hypha-specific antigen (Table 1) (37). Immunological analyses placed Hwp1 at the surface of *C. albicans* hyphae and confirmed that Hwp1 is expressed during infections. Northern analyses confirmed that *HWP1* is a hypha-specific gene, its mRNA being expressed during pH- and cell culture medium-inducing conditions (37). Interestingly, Sundstrum's group showed that Hwp1 acts as a substrate for mammalian transglutaminases that cross-link *C. albicans* cells to most cells and that *hwp1/hwp1* mutant cells are less adhesive (38). Not surprisingly, this null mutant was less virulent in a systemic model of infection. However, a *hwp1/hwp1* null mutant still formed normal hyphae under serum-

Table 2. Conditional hypha-specific genes in *C. albicans*

Gene	Phenotype of null mutant	Function	Reference(s)
ALS1	Not tested	Putative hypha-specific cell surface adhesin Expressed following RPMI-induction	17
SAP4 through 6	No morphological defects Reduced virulence in systemic infections Reduced growth on media containing protein as sole N-source	Hypha-specific secreted aspartyl proteinases Expressed following serum-induction at neutral pH	19, 29

inducing conditions (31), and hence, Hwp1 is not essential for hypha formation.

The *HYR1* (hyphally regulated) gene was isolated serendipitously as a false positive in an immunological screen for signal transduction factors (Table 1). Once again, routine screens involving Northern analysis picked up that *HYR1* is induced specifically during hyphal development during serum-, pH-, or *N*-acetylglucosamine-induction (3). On the basis of its sequence, Hyr1 appears to be a cell wall glycoprotein, but several attempts to confirm this by epitope tagging have proved unsuccessful. An *hyr1*/*hyr1* null mutant displayed normal levels of adhesion and made normal hyphae (3). Therefore, Hyr1p is not required for the development of a hypha.

So far, a total of five true hypha-specific genes have been identified. All appear to encode structural proteins, as opposed to regulatory proteins, and four of the five appear to encode cell surface proteins (Table 1).

Regulation of Hypha-Specific Genes

The identification of a small subset of hypha-specific genes will facilitate the identification of regulatory circuits that mediate their developmental expression patterns. Presumably these hypha-specific genes are subject to common regulatory mechanisms. The signal transduction pathways and *trans*-acting factors that control the expression of hypha-specific genes are discussed in detail in chapter 8. Briefly, during hyphal development the activation of *ALS8, ECE1, HWP1,* and *HYR1* depends upon the Efg1 signaling pathway, whereas the role of the Cph1 signaling pathway is less important (7, 10, 22, 31). Tup1 and Nrg1 repress the transcription of these genes during growth in the yeast form (7, 10, 26).

Limited progress has been made in the identification of the *cis*-acting elements within the *ALS3, ALS8, ECE1, HWP1,* and *HYR1* promoters that control their hypha-specific expression patterns. Promoter dissection is under way, but, to date, the only published reports describe in silico analyses of hypha-specific promoters (10). Interestingly, the *ALS3, ALS8, ECE1, HWP1,* and *HYR1* promoter regions all contain E-boxes (CANNTG) (21), which are binding sites for bHLH transcription factors (24) such as Efg1 (21, 39). Hence, Efg1p might bind to these E-boxes to regulate hypha-specific expression. However, Ernst (14) has pointed out that not all targets of bHLH transcription factors contain E-boxes, implying that other sequences may bind Efg1.

The hypha-specific promoters also contain STRE-like (C_4T), YRE-like (RRTGACTC), and GCRE-like (TGACTC) sequences (10, 22), which mediate transcriptional responses to stresses and amino acid starvation in *S. cerevisiae* (2, 23, 43). Many conditions that promote hyphal development impose stresses and/or nitrogen starvation upon the *C. albicans* cell. Also, *C. albicans* homolog of *S. cerevisiae* transcription factors that interact with these sequence elements have been identified in *C. albicans* (1, 22, 44). These observations have led to the suggestion that hypha-specific promoters coordinate the morphogenetic and environmental signals to activate transcription of *ALS3, ALS8, ECE1, HWP1,* and *HYR1* when an appropriate combination of signals is received (10).

How Relevant Are Growth Form-Specific Factors?

As described above, the search for growth form-specific factors was based on the rationale that an analysis of these genes would provide important insights into morphogenetic regulation. Is this the case? The molecular characterization of morphogenetic regulatory circuits is in its infancy. Nevertheless, growth form-specific genes are already proving useful tools for the dissection of signaling pathways and regulatory components (7, 10, 31) (see chapter 8).

It is often assumed that that all hyphae are equivalent, irrespective of the induction conditions. Clearly, hyphae that form in response to nutrient limitation in defined media may differ significantly from those that form in complex media containing serum or in vivo. Hence, the criteria used to define hypha-specific genes may be too strict, and the assumption that all hypha-specific genes are regulated in a similar fashion may be incorrect. Indeed, Johnson's group has revealed subtle differences in the regulation of *HWP1* and *HYR1,* for example (7). Therefore, so called "hypha-specific" genes may not all respond to an identical set of regulators, a view reinforced by the expression patterns of the "conditional" hypha-specific genes (Table 2).

Has the identification of hypha-specific factors revealed important insights into the construction of a yeast or hyphal cell? Not so far. Of the five hypha-specific genes identified to date (Table 1), none are essential for hypha formation. There are several possible explanations for this. Clearly, none of these genes encodes an essential structural component of the hyphal cell wall. However, they might still contribute to an essential structural component. *ALS3, ALS8,* and *HYR1* are all members of multigene families, and a second *ECE* locus appears to exist in *C. albicans* (11, 12). Hence, functional redundancy might mask the loss of a specific hypha-specific factor.

Alternatively, the hypha-specific factors identified to date may not contribute to the architecture of a hypha. Instead, they may encode hypha-associated functions that contribute to the properties of a hypha, such as increased adhesion or invasiveness, for example, rather than the construction of a hypha. It is conceivable that the actual construction of a new hypha depends on the reorganization of components already present in the yeast cell, rather than the synthesis of new hypha-specific components. If this is the case, the isolation of hypha-specific factors may be leading us toward peripheral properties of this structure, rather than central structural components. More comprehensive screens for hypha-specific factors are required to establish whether there is such a thing in *C. albicans* as a hypha-specific factor that is essential for hyphal development. Such screens might exploit promoter trapping or transcript profiling (26) (see chapters 18 and 19).

FUTURE PROSPECTS

A limited set of growth form-specific factors have been identified in *C. albicans* to date, most of which are specific to the hyphal form. These are providing the basis for the molecular dissection of hypha-specific expression patterns. The identification of yeast-specific and pseudohypha-specific factors (if such factors exist) will provide important insights into morphogenetic processes and also the developmental relationships between hyphal, pseudohyphal, and yeast growth forms. Given the reversibility of morphogenetic transitions in *C. albicans,* such studies would also help to cure us of the unhealthy predilection for the yeast-to-hypha transition.

The identification of more growth form-specific factors would be useful in several ways. Obviously, this would facilitate the analysis of growth form-specific gene regulation. More importantly, the functional analysis of these factors would reveal how they contribute to the construction or properties of the different cell types. Such functional studies should examine the cellular location of these factors as well as their biochemical or structural activities. In this way, analyses of growth form-specific factors will complement parallel studies of cell polarization and growth (chapter 11).

Acknowledgments. I thank numerous colleagues for their stimulating discussion, in particular Neil Gow, Frank Odds, Joachim Ernst, and Bill Fonzi. Work in my laboratory is funded by the U.K. Biotechnology and Biological Sciences Research Council (1/P11585, 1/P10256), The Wellcome Trust (055015, 063204), and the European Commission (QLK2CT 2000-00795). Sequence data for *Candida albicans* were obtained from the Stanford DNA Sequencing and Technology Center website at http://www-sequence.stanford.edu/group/candida.

REFERENCES

1. **Alarco, A. M., and Raymond, M.** 1999. The bZip transcription factor Cap1p is involved in multidrug resistance and oxidative stress response in *Candida albicans. J. Bacteriol.* **181:** 700–708.
2. **Arndt, K., and G. R. Fink.** 1986. *GCN4* protein, a positive transcription factor in yeast, binds general control promoters at all 5′ TGACTC 3′ sequences. *Proc. Natl. Acad. Sci. USA* **83:**8516–8520.
3. **Bailey, D. A., P. J. F. Feldmann, M. Bovey, N. A. R. Gow, and A. J. P. Brown.** 1996. The *Candida albicans HYR1* gene, which is activated in response to hyphal development, belongs to a gene family encoding yeast cell wall proteins. *J. Bacteriol.* **178:**5353–5360.
4. **Birse, C. E., M. Y. Irwin, W. A. Fonzi, and P. S. Sypherd.** 1993. Cloning and characterisation of *ECE1,* a gene expressed in association with cell elongation of the dimorphic pathogen *Candida albicans. Infect. Immun.* **61:**3648–3655.
5. **Bramley, T. A., G. S. Menzies, R. J. Williams, O. S. Kinsman, and D. J. Adams.** 1991. Binding sites for LH in *Candida albicans*: comparison with the mammalian corpus luteum LH receptor. *J. Endocrinol.* **130:**177–190.
6. **Braun, B. R., and A. D. Johnson.** 1997. Control of filament formation in *Candida albicans* by the transcriptional repressor TUP1. *Science* **277:**105–109.
7. **Braun, B. R., and A. D. Johnson.** 2000. *TUP1, CPH1* and *EFG1* make independent contributions to filamentation in *Candida albicans. Genetics* **155:**57–67.
8. **Brown, A. J. P., and N. A. R. Gow.** 1999. Regulatory networks controlling *Candida albicans* morphogenesis. *Trends Microbiol.* **7:**333–338.
9. **Brown, A. J. P., and N. A. R. Gow.** Signal transduction and morphogenesis in *Candida albicans. In* K. Esser and J. W. Bennet (ed.), *The Mycota,* in press. Springer, Berlin, Germany.
10. **Brown, A. J. P., C. J. Barelle, S. Budge, J. Duncan, S. Harris, P. R. Lee, P. Leng, S. Macaskill, A. M. Abdul Murad, M. Ramsdale, C. Wiltshire, J. A. Wishart, and N. A. R. Gow.** 2000. Gene regulation during morphogenesis in *Candida albicans. Contrib. Microbiol.* **5:**112–125.
11. ***Candida albicans* genome sequencing website:** http://www-sequence.stanford.edu/group/candida/search.html.
12. ***Candida albicans* list of sequences genes:** http://alces.med.umn.edu:80/bin/genelist?seqs.
13. **Caticha, O., S. Grover, D. Winge, and W. D. Odell.** 1992. Stimulation of *Candida albicans* transition by human chorionic gonadotrophin and a bacterial protein. *Endocrine Res.* **18:**133–143.
14. **Ernst, J. F.** 2000. Transcription factors in *Candida albicans*—environmental control of morphogenesis. *Microbiology* **146:**1763–1774.
15. **Finney, R., C. J. Langtimm, and D. R. Soll.** 1985. The programs of protein synthesis accompanying the establishment of alternative phenotypes in *Candida albicans. Mycopathologia* **91:**3–15.
16. **Fonzi, W. A.** 1999. *PHR1* and *PHR2* of *Candida albicans* encode putative glycosidases required for proper cross-linking of β-1,3- and β-1,6-glucans. *J. Bacteriol.* **181:**7070–7079.
17. **Hoyer, L. L., S. Scherer, A. R. Shatzman, and G. P. Livi.** 1995. *Candida albicans ALS1:* domains related to a *Saccharomyces cerevisiae* sexual agglutinin separated by a repeating motif. *Mol. Microbiol.* **15:**39–54.
18. **Hoyer, L. L., T. L. Payne, M. Bell, A. M. Myers, and S. Scherer.** 1998. *Candida albicans ALS3* and insights into the nature of the ALS gene family. *Curr. Genet.* **33:**441–449.
19. **Hube, B., M. Monod, D. A. Schofield, A. J. P. Brown, and N.**

A. R. Gow. 1994. Transcriptional regulation of six members of the gene family encoding secretory aspartyl proteinases in *Candida albicans. Mol. Microbiol.* **14:**87–99.

20. **Kinsman, O. S., K. Pitblado, and C. J. Coulson.** 1988. Effect of mammalian steroid hormones and luteinizing hormone on the germination of *Candida albicans* and implications for vaginal candidosis. *Mycoses* **31:**617–626.
21. **Leng, P., P. R. Lee, H. Wu, and A. J. P. Brown.** 2001. Efg1, a morphogenetic regulator in *Candida albicans,* is a sequence-specific DNA binding protein. *J. Bacteriol.* **183:**4090–4093.
22. **Leng, P., M. Straffon, G. Tripathi, J. A. Wishart, L. L. Hoyer, J. Ponton, and A. J. P. Brown.** Unpublished data.
23. **Martinez-Pastor, M. T., G. Marchler, C. Schuller, A. Marchler-Bauer, H. Ruis, and F. Estruch.** 1996. The *Saccharomyces cerevisiae* zinc finger proteins Msn2p and Msn4p are required for transcriptional induction through the stress-response element. *EMBO J.* **15:**2227–2235.
24. **Massari, M. E., and C. Murre.** 2000. Helix-loop-helix proteins: regulators of transcription in eucaryotic organisms. *Mol. Cell. Biol.* **20:**429–440.
25. **Merson-Davies, L. A., and F. C. Odds.** 1989. A morphology index for characterization of cell shape in *Candida albicans. J. Gen. Microbiol.* **135:**3143–3152.
26. **Murad, A. M. A., P. Leng, M. Straffon, J. Wishart, S. Macaskill, D. MacCallum, N. Schnell, D. Talibi, D. Marechal, F. Tekia, C. d'Enfert, C. Gaillardin, F. C. Odds, and A. J. P. Brown.** *NRG1* represses yeast-hypha morphogenesis and hypha-specific gene expression in *Candida albicans. EMBO J.,* in press.
27. **Odds, F. C.** 1988. *Candida and Candidosis,* 2nd ed. Bailliere Tindall, London, United Kingdom.
28. **Odds, F. C.** 1994. *Candida* species and virulence. *ASM News* **60:**313–318.
29. **Sanglard, D., B. Hube, M. Monod, F. C. Odds, and N. A. R. Gow.** 1997. A triple deletion of the secreted aspartyl proteinase genes *SAP4, SAP5* and *SAP6* of *Candida albicans* causes attenuated virulence. *Infect. Immun.* **65:**3539–3546.
30. **Saporito-Irwin, S. M., C. E. Birse, P. S. Sypherd, and W. A. Fonzi.** 1995. *PHR1,* a pH-regulated gene of *Candida albicans,* is required for morphogenesis. *Mol. Cell. Biol.* **15:**601–613.
31. **Sharkey, L. L., M. D. McNemar, S. M. Saporito-Irwin, P. S. Sypherd, and W. A. Fonzi.** 1999. *HWP1* functions in the morphological development of *Candida albicans* downstream of *EFG1, TUP1* and *RBF1. J. Bacteriol.* **181:**5273–5279.
32. **Sherwood, J., N. A. R. Gow, G. W. G. Gooday, G. W. Gregory, and D. Marshall.** 1992. Contact sensing in *Candida albicans:* a possible aid to epithelial penetration. *J. Med. Vet. Mycol.* **30:**461–469.
33. **Soll, D. R.** 1997. Gene regulation during high-frequency switching in *Candida albicans. Microbiology* **143:**279–288.
34. **Sonneborn, A., B. Tebarth, and J. Ernst.** 1999. Control of white-opaque phenotypic switching in *Candida albicans* by the Efg1p morphogenetic regulator. *Infect. Immun.* **67:**4655–4660.
35. **Srikantha, T., L. K. Tsai, and D. R. Soll.** 1997. The *WH11* gene of *Candida albicans* is regulated in two distinct developmental programs through the same transcription activation sequences. *J. Bacteriol.* **179:**3837–3844.
36. **Srikantha, T., L. K. Tsai, K. Daniels, and D. R. Soll.** 2000. *EFG1* null mutants of *Candida albicans* switch but cannot express the complete phenotype of white-phase budding cells. *J. Bacteriol.* **182:**1580–1591.
37. **Staab, J. F., C. A. Ferrer, and P. Sundstrom.** 1996. Developmental expression of a tandemly repeated, proline and glutamine-rich amino acid motif on hyphal surfaces of *Candida albicans. J. Biol. Chem.* **271:**6298–6305.
38. **Staab, J. F., S. D. Bradway, P. L. Fidel, and P. Sundstrom.** 1999. Adhesive and mammalian transglutaminase substrate properties of *Candida albicans* Hwp1. *Science* **283:**1535–1538.
39. **Stoldt, V. R., A. Sonneborn, C. E. Leuker, and J. Ernst.** 1997. Efg1p, an essential regulator of morphogenesis of the human pathogen *Candida albicans,* is a member of a conserved class of bHLH proteins regulating morphogenetic processes in fungi. *EMBO J.* **16:**1982–1991.
40. **Sudbery, P. E.** 2001. The germ tubes of *Candida albicans* hyphae and pseudohyphae show different patterns of septin ring organisation. *Mol. Microbiol.* **41:**19–31.
41. **Swoboda, R. K., G. Bertram, S. Delbruck, J. F. Ernst, N. A. R. Gow, G. W. Gooday, and A. J. P. Brown.** 1994. Fluctuations in glycolytic mRNA levels during the yeast-to-hyphal transition in *Candida albicans* reflect underlying changes in growth rather than a response to cellular dimorphism. *Mol. Microbiol.* **13:**663–672.
42. **Swoboda, R. K., G. Bertram, D. Colthurst, M. F. Tuite, N. A. R. Gow, G. W. Gooday, and A. J. P. Brown.** 1994. Regulation of the gene encoding translation elongation factor 3 during growth and morphogenesis in *Candida albicans. Microbiology* **140:**2611–2616.
43. **Wemmie, J. A., M. S. Szczypka, D. J. Thiele, and W. S. Moye-Rowley.** 1994. Cadmium tolerance mediated by the yeast AP-1 protein requires the presence of an ATP-binding cassette transporter-encoding gene, *YCF1. J. Biol. Chem.* **269:**32592–32597.
44. **Zhang, X., M. de Micheli, S. Coleman, D. Sanglard, and W. S. Moye-Rowley.** 2000. Analysis of the oxidative stress regulation of the *Candida albicans* transcription factor, Cap1p. *Mol. Microbiol.* **36:**618–629.
45. **Zhao, X., P. J. Malloy, C. M. Ardies, and D. Feldman.** 1995. Oestrogen-binding protein in *Candida albicans:* antibody development and cellular localization by electron immunocytochemistry. *Microbiology* **141:**2685–2692.

Candida and Candidiasis
Edited by Richard A. Calderone
© 2002 ASM Press, Washington, D.C.

Chapter 8

Morphogenetic Signaling Pathways in *Candida albicans*

Alistair J. P. Brown

Morphological transitions between yeast, pseudohyphal, and hyphal forms are thought to contribute to the virulence of *Candida albicans,* promoting several stages of disease establishment and progression (8, 64) (see chapter 7). Therefore, considerable effort is being devoted to studies of morphogenesis, but *C. albicans* is not an ideal organism in which to dissect molecular mechanisms that control this phenomenon. For example, no stable haploid *C. albicans* strains have been identified so far, and an exploitable sexual cycle has not been defined for this fungus (38, 53, 54). Furthermore, it displays noncanonical codon usage, translating CUG codons as serine, rather than leucine (75). The recent development of more efficient molecular tools for functional analysis in this fungus (18, 59, 90) and the *C. albicans* genome sequencing effort at the Stanford Sequencing Center (15) have facilitated the molecular dissection of morphogenesis in recent years. Hence, despite its genetic intransigence, *C. albicans* has emerged as an important model fungal pathogen.

Several approaches have been taken to study morphogenetic regulation in *C. albicans.* One approach has involved the isolation and analysis of growth form-specific factors. This is discussed in chapter 7. The other approach has involved the identification of regulatory factors that contribute to morphogenetic signaling or transcription programs. These are discussed here. This topic has been addressed in some other recent reviews (4, 8, 26, 47, 52, 58, 88). In this chapter, the various signaling pathways that have been associated with morphogenetic regulation in *C. albicans* will be discussed. There is insufficient space in this review to cover all of the papers in this rapidly expanding field, and I apologize to colleagues whose work has not been included here.

COMPLEXITY OF MORPHOGENETIC SIGNALING

Morphogenetic regulation in *C. albicans* appears to be complex. This complexity probably reflects two aspects of *C. albicans* biology. First, this fungus can thrive in divergent microenvironments in its host, and the fungus appears to integrate numerous types of environmental signal to assess whether conditions are most favorable for growth in a particular cellular morphology (8). The nature of these signals has been reviewed by Odds (63) and Ernst (26), and discussed in chapter 7. Briefly, they include cell density, medium pH, carbon starvation, nitrogen starvation, oxygen concentration, and some human hormones. Serum is a potent inducer of hyphal development, possibly because it imposes several types of signal. A number of distinct signaling pathways appear to be responsible for transducing different types of signal. However, most of these stimuli require a growth temperature above 35°C to activate hyphal growth (Fig. 1).

A second reason for the apparent complexity of morphogenetic regulation is because, to execute a morphological transition, *C. albicans* must program appropriate changes in cell metabolism and physiology, as well as in cell division and polarity (chapter 11). Hence, there is a need to distinguish upstream regulatory pathways that receive and respond to morphogenetic signals, from downstream pathways that regulate the cellular processes that must respond to

Alistair J. P. Brown • Molecular and Cell Biology, Institute of Medical Sciences, University of Aberdeen, Foresterhill, Aberdeen AB25 2ZD, United Kingdom.

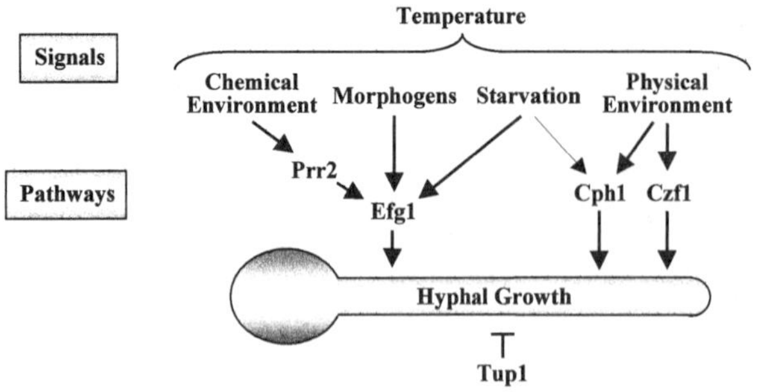

Figure 1. Specific signaling pathways mediate different environmental signals to regulate morphogenesis in *C. albicans.* Signals include chemical parameters (such as ambient pH), morphogens (such as serum or certain human hormones), nutrient starvation (particularly nitrogen and carbon starvation), and physical parameters (such as being embedded in an agar matrix). The efficacy of most, if not all, of these signals is increased by temperature elevation to 37°C. The signaling pathways are defined operationally by a transcription factor that is required for the functionality of that pathway (Efg1, Cph1, Prr2, Czf1, and Tup1). With the exception of ambient pH, the exact nature of the signal(s) that activates each pathway remains to be clarified. Adapted from references 9 and 26.

morphogenetic signaling. This distinction is not particularly clear in the literature at the moment.

Technical issues have also contributed to the apparent complexity of morphogenetic regulation. First, insufficient attention has been paid to the morphological phenotypes of individual *C. albicans* mutants. Initially, pseudohyphae were generally viewed as morphological intermediates between yeast and hyphal growth forms, and this view still prevails. However, more recently it has been suggested that pseudohyphae might represent a developmental form that is distinct from yeast and hyphae (26) (see chapter 7). Therefore, there is a need for more accurate description of the filamentous growth forms of *C. albicans.* A clear picture of morphogenetic regulation is dependent on an understanding of which mutants affect pseudohyphal development and which affect hyphal development.

A second technical issue relates to current assays of *C. albicans* morphology. As pointed out by Ernst (26), assays performed in liquid media generally test the ability of mutant *C. albicans* cells to form germ tubes, the progenitors of hyphae, in the short term (within hours). In contrast, plate assays examine colony morphologies after several days or more. The morphologies of *C. albicans* colonies often reflect the growth forms of their constituent cells, wrinkly colonies being associated frequently with pseudohyphal or hyphal cells (6). However, colonies change the medium they are growing on, and cells on the edge of a colony are exposed to different conditions from those nearer the center of the colony. Therefore, the morphological phenotype of a *C. albicans* colony is complicated by changes in medium composition. In addition, the morphology of *C. albicans* cells may change with time during the period of colony development (26). Therefore, biological and temporal differences exist between morphological assays performed using liquid and solid media. This must be borne in mind when interpreting morphological phenotypes.

Efg1 Signaling Pathway

The factor Efg1 defines an important morphogenetic pathway, which is required for hyphal development in *C. albicans* under a wide range of conditions in vitro and in vivo. Recent data indicate that the Efg1 pathway includes a cAMP signaling module that is conserved in other fungi (26, 28, 47, 82, 85).

The *EFG1* gene was first identified on the basis that it enhances pseudohyphal growth in *Saccharomyces cerevisiae* (85). Inactivation of *EFG1* dramatically reduces hyphal development following induction with serum, pH, *N*-acetylglucosamine, proline, or spider medium (50, 85). Therefore, Efg1 activates hyphal development. However, some *EFG1* phenotypes are more consistent with the behavior of a repressor (85). For example, in the absence of a morphogenetic stimulus, *EFG1* overexpression promotes pseudohyphal growth (as opposed to hyphal development). Also, Efg1 depletion causes the formation of small rod-like cells (as opposed to yeast cells). Furthermore, *EFG1* expression *decreases* transiently following hyphal induction. These observations have led Stoldt et al. (85) to suggest that Efg1 might play a dual role as a morphogenetic activator and as a repressor. They argue that *C. albicans* morphology might depend on the level of activity of Efg1.

Efg1 contains a basic helix-loop-helix (bHLH) motif that is related to bHLH regions in the APSES family of transcription factors, many of which are involved in developmental processes (26, 85). Members of this family include morphogenetic regulators from other fungi such as Sok2 and Phd1 from *S. cerevisiae,* Asm1 from *Neurospora crassa,* and StuA from *Aspergillus nidulans.* Efg1 can bind directly to E-boxes (5′-CANNTG-3′) (45), like other bHLH transcription factors (56, 72). E-boxes have been identified in the promoters of the hypha-specific genes *HYR1, HWP1, ALS3, ALS8,* and *ECE1* (45), and the activation of these genes under hypha-inducing conditions is dependent on *EFG1* (6, 45, 78). Hence, Efg1 appears to be a transcription factor that might act directly on hypha-specific genes to regulate their expression. *EFG1* appears to autoregulate its own expression, but

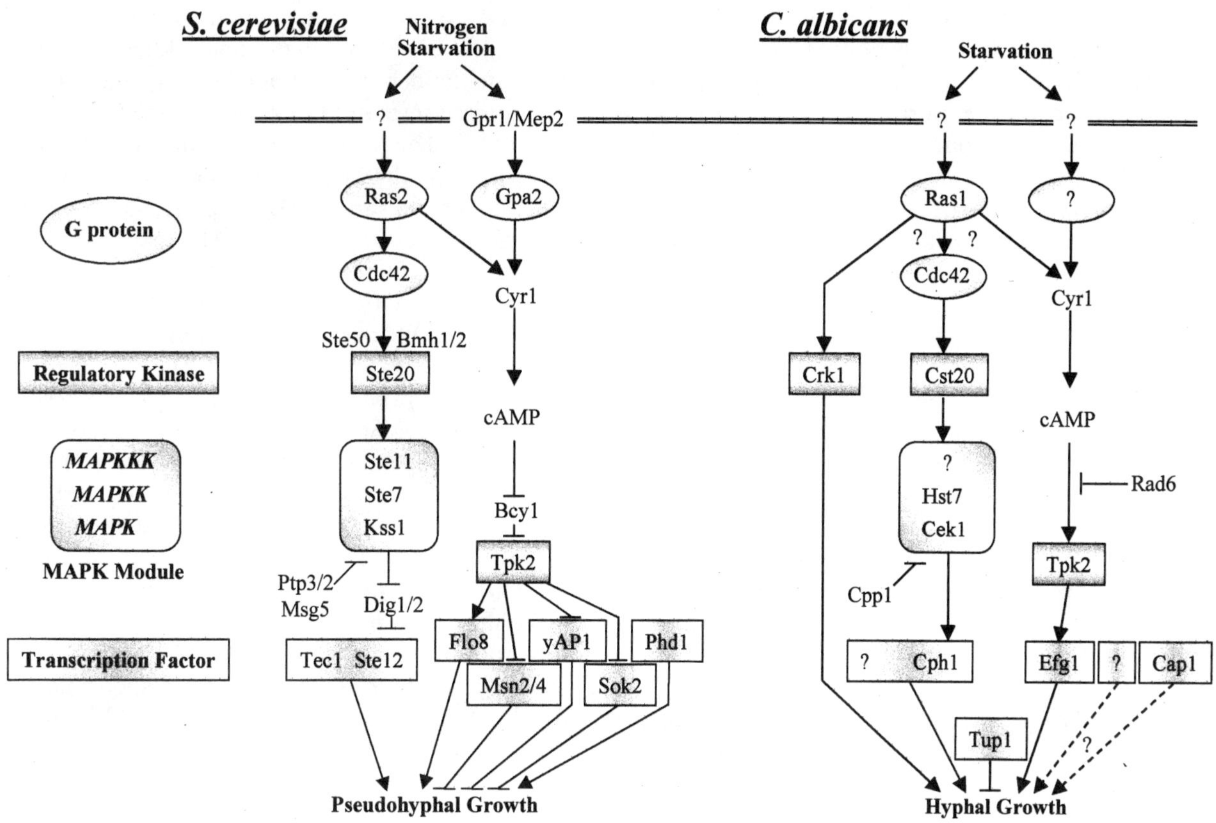

Figure 2. Conserved MAP kinase and Ras-cAMP pathways promote morphogenesis in *S. cerevisiae* and *C. albicans.* In *C. albicans,* the MAP kinase and Ras-cAMP pathways correspond to the Cph1 and Efg1 pathways, respectively. Adapted from reference 9. Copyright Springer-Verlag.

this does not seems to require E-boxes in the *EFG1* promoter (26).

A protein kinase A, encoded by *TPK2,* is thought to lie upstream of Efg1 on this signaling pathway (Fig. 2) (82). In the absence of a morphogenetic stimulus *TPK2* overexpression induces hyphal development in *C. albicans,* but only in the presence of functional Efg1. Efg1 contains a potential Tpk2 phosphorylation site, suggesting that Tpk2 might activate Efg1 directly. Indeed, it has been shown recently that morphogenetic regulation by Efg1 is dependent upon protein kinase A-type phosphorylation site in this protein (3a). Also, a *tpk2/tpk2* mutant displays strong hyphal defects on solid serum or spider media. However, unlike an *efg1/efg1* mutant, *tpk2/tpk2* cells can still form hyphae in response to serum stimulation in liquid culture, although morphogenesis is delayed (82). Hence, Tpk2 is required for hyphal development under some hypha-inducing conditions but is dispensable under other conditions that promote hyphal growth in an Efg1-dependent manner. The existence of another *C. albicans* TPK locus, which encodes a second protein kinase A (Tpk1) that has some functional overlap with Tpk2, probably accounts for these observations (82). Tpk1, Tpk2, and Tpk3 subunits make different contributions to the regulation of pseudohyphal growth in *S. cerevisiae* (65).

By analogy with other fungi (4, 47), Ras and adenylyl cyclase are thought to lie upstream of Tpk2 and Efg1 in this signaling pathway (8, 26). A functional adenylyl cyclase gene, *CYR1,* has been isolated from *C. albicans* (55), but its role in morphogenesis has yet to be published. However, exogenous cAMP stimulates hyphal development (10, 73), and this effect is blocked in an *efg1/efg1* mutant (10). Therefore, cAMP activates *C. albicans* morphogenesis in an Efg1-dependent fashion, consistent with the idea that Efg1 lies downstream from a cAMP signaling module.

S. cerevisiae has two semiredundant *RAS* loci that encode an essential function. In contrast, *C. albicans* might contain a single nonessential *RAS* locus, on the basis of low stringency Southern data and the apparent absence of a second locus in the *C. albicans* genome sequence information (15, 28). A *C. albicans ras1/ras1* mutant is viable, but it shows a strong hyphal defect upon serum stimulation. The expression of a dominant active $RAS1^{V13}$ allele activates hyphal development (28). Clearly, therefore, Ras1 plays an important role in *C. albicans* morphogenesis. In *S. cerevisiae,* Ras2 activates both cAMP and MAPK signaling pathways to promote pseudohyphal growth (47), and, hence, Ras1 might lie upstream of the equivalent cAMP and MAPK signaling pathways in *C. albicans* (Fig. 2) (8). However, $RAS1^{V13}$ can activate hyphal development in an *efg1/efg1 cph1/cph1* double mutant, suggesting that Ras1 acts upstream of a third morphogenetic signaling pathway, in addition to the Efg1 and Cph1 pathways (16).

The Efg1 pathway appears to be down-regulated by Rad6 (46). Rad6 depletion was shown to enhance hyphal development, and Rad6 overexpression inhibited hyphal development. Both effects were dependent on functional Efg1, suggesting that Rad6 might repress Efg1 pathway activity to down-regulate morphogenesis. Since Rad6 is a ubiquitin-conjugating enzyme, this effect might be mediated by targeting an Efg1 pathway component for ubiquitin-mediated protein degradation (46).

The above findings clearly indicate that the Efg1 pathway plays an important role in morphogenetic regulation in response to starvation, pH, and serum stimulation. However, *EFG1* plays additional roles in other developmental transitions in *C. albicans. Efg1/efg1* mutants also show defects in chlamydospore formation and aberrant phenotypic switching (80, 81, 83). Not surprisingly, therefore, Efg1 pathway mutants display strong in vivo phenotypes. *C. albicans efg1/efg1* mutants display significantly attenuated virulence in systemic and oral infections (50, 71).

Cph1 Signaling Pathway

C. albicans contains a MAP kinase pathway capable of activating yeast-hypha morphogenesis. This was the first morphogenetic signaling pathway to be identified in this fungus. Many components on this pathway show a high degree of sequence conservation with components of morphogenetic MAPK signaling pathways in *S. cerevisiae* and other fungi (Fig. 2) (2, 35), and many have been isolated using genetic screens in *S. cerevisiae.*

The MAPK module contains the MAP kinase, Cek1, which was first identified by Whiteway et al. (89) in a screen for *C. albicans* sequences that exert dominant negative effects upon mating pheromone-induced cell cycle arrest in *S. cerevisiae.* Epistasis analyses have placed Cek1 below the MAP kinase kinase, Hst7, which is a functional homolog of *S. cerevisiae* Ste7 (17, 20, 41, 43). Therefore, Cek1 is probably activated directly by Hst7, although this remains to be demonstrated biochemically. Neither *CEK1* nor *HST7* is an essential gene. The final component of this module, the MAP kinase kinase kinase, has not been formally identified, although a sequence homolog of *S. cerevisiae,* Ste11, is present in the *C. albicans* genome (15). This obvious gap in our understanding of the MAPK pathway has existed for about 5 years, which might seem surprising. However, if a Ste11 homolog plays roles in multiple MAPK pathways, like its *S. cerevisiae* counterpart (68), it might be difficult to establish a specific role for this factor in the morphogenetic MAPK pathway in *C. albicans.*

Cst20 appears to lie upstream of this MAK module. Cst20 is a homolog of the *S. cerevisiae* serine/threonine kinase, Ste20, and epistasis experiments have placed Cst20 above Hst7 and Cph1 (41, 43). *S. cerevisiae* contains a second, Ste20-like serine/threonine kinase, called Cla4. Ste20 and Cla4 proteins share an essential function in budding. Although *CST20* and *CaCLA4* can complement the defects of *S. cerevisiae ste20* and *cla4* mutants, respectively (43, 44), it is not yet known whether they share an essential function in *C. albicans.* The factors responsible for activating Cst20 remain to be identified. Although a *CDC42* homolog has been identified in *C. albicans* (57), it is not known whether CaCdc42 acts upstream of Cst20 in the same way as ScCdc42 acts upstream of Ste20 in *S. cerevisiae* (60). Similarly, Ras1 might lie upstream of this MAPK pathway (see above) (Fig. 2).

Cph1 lies downstream of the MAPK module. Cph1 is a functional homolog of the transcription factor Ste12, which lies at the bottom of the pseudohyphal and pheromone signaling pathways in *S. cerevisiae* (49). Epistasis experiments have placed Cph1 below Cst20, Hst7, and Cek1 on the same *C. albicans* signaling pathway (20, 43). In *S. cerevisiae,* Ste12 acts in concert with Tec1 to activate the transcription of genes carrying the filamentous response element (FRE) (51). Recently, a functional homolog of Tec1 has been identified in *C. albicans* (77), but its relationship with Cph1 remains to be confirmed.

The activity of the MAPK pathway appears to be negatively regulated by Cpp1 (19). Cpp1, which is a member of the VH1 family of protein phosphatases, displays tyrosine-specific protein dephosphorylation in vitro. Inactivation of Cpp1 causes hyphal development in *C. albicans* to be derepressed on solid media, and this activity is dependent on the MAP kinase, Cek1 (19, 20). Hence, Cpp1 appears to dephosphorylate Cek1 to modulate the activity of the morphogenetic MAPK signaling pathway.

As one might expect, MAPK pathway null mutants display related phenotypes in vitro. *Cst20/cst20, hst7/hst7, cek1/cek1,* and *cph1/cph1* mutants display relatively weak hyphal defects. These mutations inhibit yeast-hypha morphogenesis only under specific growth conditions. They block hyphal growth in response to nitrogen limitation on solid medium, but not in response to serum, proline, or *N*-acetylglucosamine (27, 41, 43, 49). This suggests that the MAPK pathway responds to nitrogen starvation, but the molecular signals that specifically activate this pathway remain obscure. Also, the activation of hypha-specific genes such as *ALS8, ECE1, HWP1,* and *HYR1* is not significantly inhibited in a *cph1/cph1* mutant (6, 45, 78). Interestingly, MAPK mutants do not display identical virulence phenotypes. In systemic infections, *cst20/cst20* and *cek1/cek1* mutants showed reduced virulence, whereas *hst7/hst7* and *cph1/cph1* mutants did not (20, 43, 50). One way of interpreting these data is to suggest that this MAPK pathway is required for yeast-hypha morphogenesis when nitrogen is limiting on solid medium but that Cst20 and Cek1 have roles in addition to signaling on this pathway.

What is the role of this MAPK pathway? Clearly this pathway is involved in the activation of hyphal development. However, this pathway only appears to be required for morphogenetic activation under a limited set of starvation conditions, and the pathway seems to play a minor role in the progression of systemic disease. Parallel signaling pathway(s) must be responsible for the transduction of most morphogenetic signals in vitro and in vivo. Components of the corresponding MAPK pathway in *S. cerevisiae* play dual roles in the mating and pseudohyphal responses (48). Now that *C. albicans* mating has been demonstrated, albeit between diploid strains rendered homozygous at their *MTL* loci (38, 53), it is conceivable that components of the morphogenetic MAPK pathway might also be involved in a mating response in *C. albicans.*

Czf1 Signaling Pathway

The data of Lo et al. (50) appeared to suggest that Efg1 and Cph1 define the two morphogenetic signaling pathways responsible for triggering hyphal development in *C. albicans.* A double *efg1/efg1 cph1/cph1* mutant was shown to be "avirulent in a mouse model," and "locked in the yeast form" following hypha induction with serum, pH, *N*-acetylglucosamine, proline, or spider medium. However, the existence of an Efg1- and Cph1-independent signaling pathway(s) was highlighted when *efg1/efg1 cph1/cph1* mutants were shown to form hyphae under some conditions in vivo and in vitro. These mutants were filamentous in the tongues of immunosuppressed, germ-free piglets and when plated on rough agar surfaces (71). The gene *CZF1* appears to define one Efg1- and Cph1-independent pathway (Fig. 1).

CZF1 encodes a zinc finger protein that is presumed to act as a transcription factor (12, 89). *CZF1,* which was first identified as an inhibitor of pheromone-induced G1-arrest in *S. cerevisiae* (89), promotes hyphal growth of *C. albicans* cells when embedded in agar (12). Ectopic expression of *CZF1* enhances filamentation in embedded cells, and inactivation of *CZF1* delays filamentation under these conditions. However, a *czf1/czf1* mutant displays normal hyphal responses to serum, pH, *N*-acetylglucosamine, proline, or spider medium, suggesting that Czf1 lies on a separate signaling pathway from the Efg1 and Cph1 pathways. Nevertheless, an interaction between the Czf1 and Cph1 pathways was inferred by the observation that a *cph1/cph1 czf1/czf1* double mutant displays a greater hyphal defect than a *czf1/czf1* single mutant (12).

So far, little is known about the recently discovered Czf1 pathway. However, it is clear that Czf1 promotes hyphal growth under certain specialized conditions (12), and this pathway might account for the hyphal development of *efg1/efg1 cph1/cph1* mutants in some infection models (71). Brown et al. (12) argue that the Czf1 pathway allows *C. albicans* to respond to physical signals, such as a mechanical stress imposed on a fungal cell buried in a matrix. They suggest that this response is independent of the nutrient conditions and is not due to oxygen depletion. However, Ernst (26) has suggested that Czf1 might also contribute to the morphogenesis observed under low oxygen tension (microaerophilic) conditions. He also points out that the different hypha-inducing pathways might stimulate the formation of hyphae with different molecular properties. In other words, the Czf1 pathway might be activated in specific host microenvironments, leading to the development of hyphae expressing specific molecular properties that are required in those microenvironments.

pH Signaling Pathway

Ambient pH strongly influences morphogenesis in *C. albicans:* an acidic pH encourages growth in the yeast form, and neutral pH promotes hyphal development. Early attempts to identify hypha-specific genes in *C. albicans* using pH-stimulated morphogenesis led to the isolation of pH-responsive genes, including *PHR1* (76). *PHR1* and its functional homolog *PHR2* are thought to encode glycosidases that cross-link cell wall glucans, a process required for the maintenance of cell shape and morphology (29, 61). The *PHR1* and *PHR2* genes are differentially regulated by ambient pH, and they contribute to cell morphology in a pH-dependent manner. *PHR1* is expressed at a pH above 5.5, is required for normal morphology at these pH levels, and is required for normal virulence in systematic infections. In contrast, *PHR2* is expressed at an acidic pH, is required for normal cell morphology at an acidic pH, and contributes to virulence in the more acidic vaginal environment (22, 33, 61, 76). These observations suggest that gene expression patterns, cell morphology, and virulence are coordinated by a pH-responsive signaling pathway(s) in *C. albicans,* and this has been borne out by more recent findings.

The identification of pH signaling components in *C. albicans* was facilitated by the conservation of pH signaling pathways in divergent fungi (Fig. 3). In *A. nidulans,* the activity of the transcription factor PacC is regulated by ambient pH (87). At an alkaline pH, the C-terminal region of PacC is cleaved off, releasing the active N-terminal region, which represses the transcription of acid-expressed genes and activates the transcription of alkaline-expressed genes (Fig. 3). The *C. albicans pacC* homolog, *RIM101* (also called *PRR2*), appears to operate in a similar way. Spontaneous mutations that cause C-terminal truncation of Rim101/Prr2 turn it into a dominant activator of alkaline gene expression and a dominant repressor of acidic gene expression. These mutations also promote hyphal development at an acidic pH (25). Interestingly, this activation of hyphal development is dependent on Efg1, indicating the central importance of Efg1 in morphogenetic regulation. Rim101/Prr2 inactivation blocks pH-regulated gene expression and inhibits hyphal development under some conditions (21, 70, 90).

C. albicans rim101/rim101 (prr2/prr2) mutants display a hyphal defect on solid media containing serum or M199 at pH 7.5, and in liquid M119 medium, but they form normal hyphae following serum stimulation in liquid media. Hyphal defects at neutral pH are not suppressed by ectopic expression of *PHR1* (67), indicating that other pH-regulated functions are required for hyphal development under these conditions. The different morphologies of *rim101/rim101 (prr2/prr2)* mutants in liquid and solid media reflect the temporal differences in studying cell and colony morphologies described above, and possibly the effects of colonial growth on the local pH of the medium. Nevertheless, the data clearly indicate the importance of Rim101/Prr2 in the regulation of pH-induced morphogenesis.

A pH signaling pathway regulates PacC activity in *A. nidulans* (Fig. 3) (23, 24). Homologs of some of these signaling components have been identified in *C. albicans,* including Rim8/Prr1 and Rim20 (21, 67). Inactivation of *C. albicans* Rim8/Prr1 or Rim20 causes similar phenotypes to *rim101/rim101 (prr2/prr2)* null mutations, and truncation of Rim101/Prr2 overrides these defects in pH responses and pH-induced morphogenesis. Hence, this pH signaling pathway controls the activity of the transcription factor, Rim101/Prr2.

Davis et al. (21) report that *RIM101/PRR2*

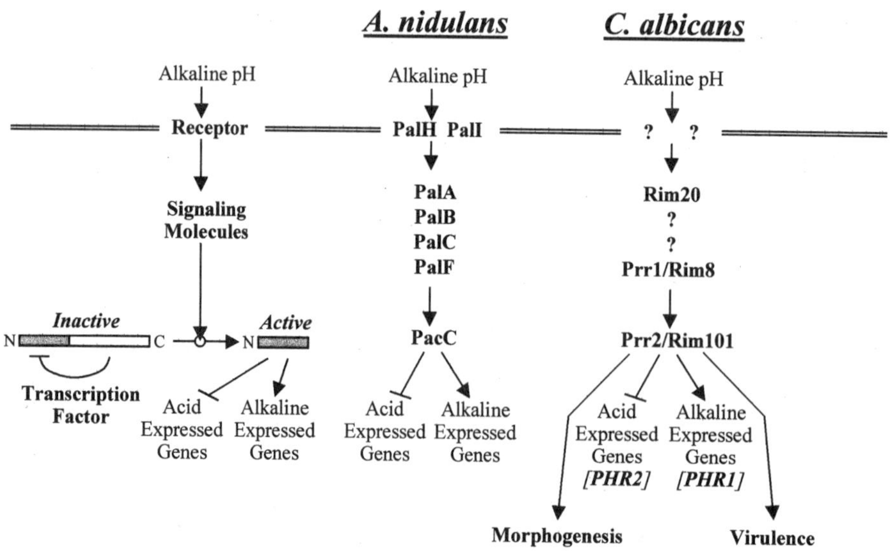

Figure 3. Conserved pH signaling pathways in *A. nidulans* and *C. albicans.* The pH response pathway is illustrated on the left. It involves C-terminal truncation of a critical transcription factor to activate it. In *C. albicans,* this transcription factor is called Prr2 or Rim101. The epistatic relationships between the signaling molecules have not been clarified, and hence, they are ordered alphabetically in the *A. nidulans* pathway. The corresponding *C. albicans* homologs are placed in the equivalent positions to their *A. nidulans* counterparts. Adapted from reference 9. Copyright Springer-Verlag.

expression is itself induced at an alkaline pH. This induction occurred even in the absence of functional Rim8/Prr1 and Rim20, which is consistent with the observation that *RIM8/PRR1* expression decreases at alkaline pH (67). Hence, a Rim-independent pathway might be required for the activation of alkaline expressed genes at alkaline pH values in *C. albicans* (21). Nevertheless, the Rim-dependent pH signaling pathway plays a central role in the control of pH responses, morphogenesis, and niche-specific responses during infections (Fig. 1).

Tup1 Pathway

The Efg1, Cph1, Czf1, and pH signaling pathways all stimulate hyphal development (Fig. 1). It is now clear that negative regulation also plays an important role in the control of *C. albicans* morphogenesis. Johnson's group first identified CaTup1, a repressor of hyphal development (5). Inactivation of *CaTUP1* causes *C. albicans* to grow constitutively in an extended pseudohyphal form. *C. albicans tup1/tup1* mutants grow more slowly than wild-type cells, and they appear unable to form true hyphae or yeast cells (62). Hence, they seem to be fixed in a pseudohyphal form. CaTup1 is a homolog of ScTup1, which interacts with ScSsn6 to form a general corepressor complex that regulates the expression of several different functional classes of gene in *S. cerevisiae.* The ScTup1-ScSsn6 complex is targeted to the promoters of glucose-repressed, cell type-specific, hypoxic, and other genes by sequence-specific DNA binding proteins (79). CaTup1 probably functions in an analogous manner in *C. albicans.*

Recently, a second repressor of hyphal development, CaNrg1, was been identified in *C. albicans* (62). CaNrg1 is a homolog of *S. cerevisiae* Nrg1, which interacts with the ScTup1-ScSsn6 complex to repress the transcription of a glucoamylase gene in response to glucose (66). Pseudohyphal growth is derepressed in a *C. albicans nrg1/nrg1* mutant, but this strain can form true hyphae following serum stimulation. CaNrg1 is a sequence-specific DNA-binding protein that can interact with (C/A)(C/A/G)CCCT (62). Northern analyses have shown that hypha-specific genes are derepressed in *tup1/tup1* and *nrg1/nrg1* strains (6, 7, 62, 78), and this has now been confirmed by transcript profiling (62). Also, repression by CaNrg1 has now been shown to depend upon CaTup1 (7a). Hence, hypha-specific genes are coregulated by CaTup1 and CaNrg1.

Rfg1, a *C. albicans* homolog of *S. cerevisiae* Rox1, might also contribute to CaTup1-mediated repression of hypha-specific functions (40). However, the phenotype of a *rfg1/rfg1* mutant is not as dramatic as that of a *nrg1/nrg1* mutant (40, 62), suggesting that Nrg1 exerts a greater degree of control over hyphal development and hypha-specific gene expression than Rfg1. A homolog of *S. cerevisiae SSN6* has also been identified, and as expected, *ssn6/ssn6* deletion mutants display morphological phenotypes (11). Therefore, CaNrg1 and CaRfg1 probably target a CaTup1-CaSsn6 complex to the promoters of hypha-specific genes to repress their expression and to repress hyphal development, thereby maintaining yeast growth under the appropriate conditions (Fig. 4). Following serum stimulation, this repression appears to be relieved by the down-regulation of *CaNRG1* expression (62).

Other Factors

A number of other factors have been reported to influence yeast-hypha morphogenesis in *C. albicans.* The inactivation of Rbf1, a putative transcription factor, derepresses filamentous growth (39), but the mechanisms by which Rbf1 influences morphogenesis are not clear. *SSK1* is thought to encode a response regulator in a two-component regulatory circuit, possibly involved in responses to osmotic stress (14). *C.*

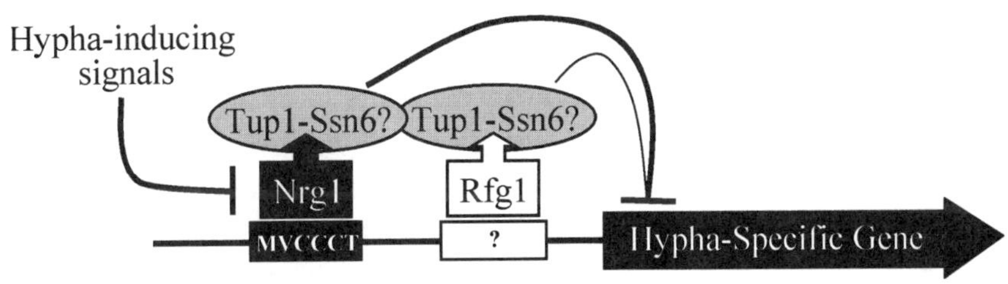

Figure 4. Model illustrating the possible mode of action of CaTup1, CaNrg1, Rfg1, and CaSsn6 in the regulation of hypha-specific genes in *C. albicans.* CaNrg1 and Rfg1 probably bind to different sequences in the promoters of hypha-specific genes. In doing so, they may target a CaTup1-CaSsn6 repressor complex to these promoters (M = A or C; V = G, A, or C). CaNrg1 appears to exert a greater degree of repression than Rfg1. This repression might be relieved by the downregulation of CaNrg1 levels in response to a hypha-inducing signal (40, 62).

albicans ssk1/ssk1 mutants display reduced hyphal growth following serum stimulation. By analogy with *S. cerevisiae* (84), this might reflect an indirect effect of stress responses on morphogenetic regulation in *C. albicans.*

Morphogenesis is dependent on changes in the polarity of growth and the cell cycle (34, 42). A number of genes that may be involved in these processes have now been shown to influence hyphal development. The *C. albicans INT1* gene encodes a cell surface protein with weak sequence similarity to vertebrate integrins that is required for normal rates of hyphal development on solid spider and milk-Tween media, but not in response to serum (31, 32). Expression of *INT1* in *S. cerevisiae* promotes a type of filamentous growth that is dependent on the talin-like protein, Sla2. *ACT1* mutations that disturb the interaction between actin and Sla2 also block this *INT1*-induced filamentous growth (1). These authors also demonstrated that inactivation of *CaSLA2* blocks serum-stimulated hyphal development in *C. albicans,* strongly suggesting that CaSla2 is required for the polarized growth of hyphal cells, possibly by contributing to the organization of actin cables.

Phosphoinositol kinases are involved in numerous cellular processes including the rearrangement of the actin cytoskeleton and intracellular protein and membrane trafficking. Interestingly therefore, the inactivation of the phosphoinositol 3-kinase, CaVps34, blocked hypha formation on solid media and delayed morphogenesis in liquid media (13).

CRK1 is thought to encode a cyclin-dependent protein kinase related to Cdc2 (16). Overexpression of Crk1 stimulates hyphal development in an *efg1/efg1 cph1/cph1* double mutant, and hyphal activation by *RAS1*^{V13} is inhibited in a *crk1/crk1* strain. This might suggest that Crk1 lies on a third Ras1 pathway, parallel to the Efg1 and Cph1 pathways (Fig. 2). Alternatively, Crk1 might execute a common function required for hyphal development that can be activated by Ras1, Efg1, or Cph1. *CaRSR1* is a sequence homolog of *BUD1,* which is involved in polarity and bud site selection in *S. cerevisiae. C. albicans rsr1/rsr1* mutants display reduced hyphal growth and abnormal bud site selection in yeast cells (91).

To summarize, it is becoming apparent that a number of factors involved in cell polarity and division can influence yeast-hypha morphogenesis.

INTEGRATION OF SIGNALING PATHWAYS

Why do multiple signaling pathways regulate *C. albicans* morphogenesis? The current view is that there is some degree of specialization in terms of the environmental signals that each pathway transduces (8, 26). Obviously the pH pathway is responsible for mediating the effects of ambient pH. The Czf1 pathway activates morphogenesis in response to being buried within a solid matrix and possibly to microaerophilic conditions. The Cph1 pathway is thought to play a relatively minor role in transmitting starvation signals compared to Efg1, which seems to play a major role in responses to starvation, morphogens, and pH (Fig. 1). This presumably reflects the complexity and variety of niches this fungus is exposed to within its host (8).

How are these signaling pathways and regulatory components integrated to control yeast-hypha morphogenesis in *C. albicans*? Clearly, the picture is complex, involving a number of distinct pathways (at least five), and the relationships between these pathways are not well defined. Braun and Johnson (6) have pointed out that there are at least two main ways in which these pathways could be organized: via a "central processor" or through "network control." According to their first model, all morphogenetic pathways feeds through a master regulator, the activity of which depends on the inputs from each pathway. This master regulator coordinates the activity of all of the pathways to establish the activity of downstream targets. A prediction of this model is that all hypha-specific genes should respond in a similar manner to this master regulator, and hence to mutations in *EFG1, CPH1,* or *TUP1,* for example. The second network model suggests that morphogenetic pathways make different contributions to the regulation of morphogenetically regulated genes. According to this model, mutations in *EFG1, CPH1,* or *TUP1* might exert different effects on individual hypha-specific genes.

Braun and Johnson (6) tested their predictions by examining the effects of *tup1/tup1, efg1/efg1,* and *cph1/cph1* mutations on the expression of hypha-specific genes. While most hypha-specific genes tested were depressed in *tup1/tup1* strains and inert in *efg1/efg1,* this was not the case for all of these genes. Hence their data support the network model (6). Efg1, Cph1, and Tup1 pathways are thought to make independent contributions to the regulation of hypha-specific functions. Their data also supported previous suggestions that the Cph1 pathway makes a relatively minor contribution to hyphal activation compared to the Efg1 and Tup1 pathways. Phenotypic comparisons of single, double, and triple *tup1/tup1, efg1/efg1,* and *cph1/cph1* mutants indicated that the effects of Efg1, Cph1, and Tup1 upon *C. albicans* morphology are additive. For example, an *efg1/efg1 tup1/tup1* double mutant is less filamentous than a single *tup1/tup1* mutant and is more filamentous than a single *efg1/efg1* mutant

(6). Hence Efg1, Cph1, and Tup1 appear to lie on parallel signaling pathways (Fig. 1).

To what extent are the pH and Czf1 pathways integrated with the Efg1, Cph1, and Tup1 pathways? The pH pathway seems to lie upstream of Efg1, since the hyphal phenotype of a dominant *RIM101/PRR2* mutation is dependent on Efg1 (25). The morphological effects of *czf1/czf1* and *cph1/cph1* mutations appear to be additive (12). Therefore, Czf1 seems to lie on an independent pathway from Cph1, but its relationship to the Efg1 and Tup1 pathways remains unclear (Fig. 1).

The pleiotropic effects of some mutations might complicate the epistatic relationships between morphogenetic signaling components. Transcript profiling of *tup1/tup1* mutants has shown that Tup1 regulates many functions in addition to morphogenetic genes (62), and hence the phenotype of *tup1/tup1* mutants might reflect a number of complex pleiotropic effects. Similarly, Efg1 regulates processes other than yeast-hypha morphogenesis, and *EFG1* expression is subject to autoregulation (26, 80, 81). Hence, the *efg1/efg1* phenotype is complex also. This should be borne in mind when interpreting morphogenetic phenotypes.

The situation is complicated further by possible cross-talk between pathways. For example, the morphogenetic phenotype of a *czf1/czf1* mutant is exacerbated by inactivation of Cph1 (12), suggesting possible cross-talk between the Czf1 and Cph1 pathways. Furthermore, the Tup1 pathway appears to downregulate the activity of the Cph1 pathway, since *CEK1* mRNA levels are derepressed in *nrg1/nrg1* cells (62). The effect of Ras1 on the Efg1 and Cph1 pathways also needs to be clarified (Fig. 2). The regulatory network that controls morphogenesis might be even more complex than the model proposed by Braun and Johnson (6).

The relationship between the Tup1, Efg1, Cph1, Czf1, and pH signaling pathways and other factors that influence morphogenesis is even less clear. These other factors may contribute to cellular processes that execute morphogenetic changes, rather than to the signaling pathways that regulate these changes. For example, morphogenetic transitions are dependent on changes in cell polarity and cell division (34, 42), which presumably are regulated by morphogenetic signaling. Clearly, therefore, mutations that affect genes involved in these downstream processes have the potential to confer hyphal defects. Precedents for this might include *INT1, SLA2, RSR1,* and possibly even *CRK1* (1, 16, 31, 91). In addition, some mutations might affect morphogenesis indirectly, for example, by altering key aspects of cell physiology. Yeast-hypha morphogenesis is accompanied by, and might even depend on, changes in cell physiology (3, 86), and it has been predicted that physiological signals might contribute to the regulation of hypha-specific genes (10). These ideas provide a possible framework with which to classify new factors that influence morphogenesis in *C. albicans.*

COREGULATION OF MORPHOGENESIS WITH OTHER VIRULENCE FACTORS IN *C. ALBICANS*

Evidence is emerging to suggest that yeast-hypha morphogenesis is coregulated with other virulence factors. The *SAP4-6* genes, which are members of a large family of secreted aspartyl proteinase genes that promote the virulence of *C. albicans* (37, 74), are expressed specifically during hyphal development (chapter 7). Similarly, there are hypha-specific members of the agglutinin-like sequence (ALS) family, which are thought to promote adhesion of fungal cells to host tissue (11, 30, 36) (see chapter 7). More recently, transcript profiling in *C. albicans* has extended these observations by showing that, along with hypha-specific genes, *SAP5, ALS3, ALS8, CFL1,* and *FTR1* are all regulated by CaTup1 and CaNrg1 (62). Inactivation of Cfl1 and Ftr1, which are a permease and reductase involved in iron assimilation, attenuates virulence in *C. albicans* (69, 92). Not surprisingly, therefore, inactivation of Tup1 or Nrg1 attenuates virulence significantly (62). Hence, the expression of key virulence attributes, such as yeast-hypha morphogenesis, cell surface adhesins, secreted hydrolases, and iron assimilation, appears to be coregulated in *C. albicans.* Unfortunately, this complicates the interpretation of experiments that examine the relationship between yeast-hypha morphogenesis and virulence, because mutations that impair morphogenesis may also attenuate other virulence attributes. However, this coordinated expression of virulence attributes probably promotes disease establishment and progression.

Acknowledgments. I am grateful to Alexander Johnson and Klaus Schröppel for providing data prior to publication. Also, I thank my colleagues in the Aberdeen Fungal Group for many enjoyable discussions. Work in my laboratory is funded by the U.K. Biotechnology and Biological Sciences Research Council (1/P11585, 1/P10256), The Wellcome Trust (055015, 063204), and the EC (QLK2CT 2000-00795). Sequence data for *C. albicans* were obtained from the Stanford DNA Sequencing and Technology Center website at http://www-sequence.stanford.edu/group/candida.

REFERENCES

1. **Alseson, C. M., E. S. Bensen, C. A. Gale, A.-S. Melms, C. Kurischko, and J. Berman.** 2001. *Candida albicans INT1*-in-

duced filamentation in *Saccharomyces cerevisiae* depends upon Sla2p. *Mol. Cell. Biol.* **21**:1272–1284.

2. **Banuett, F.** 1998. Signalling in the yeasts: an information cascade with links to the filamentous fungi. *Microbiol. Mol. Biol. Rev.* **62**:249–274.
3. **Biswas, S. K., K. Yokoyama, K. Nishimura, and M. Miyaji.** 2000. Effect of pH, carbon source and K+ on the Na+-inhibited germ tube formation of *Candida albicans. Med. Mycol.* **38**:363–369.

3a. **Bockmuhl, D. P., and J. F. Ernst.** 2001. A potential phosphorylation site for an A-type kinase in the Efg1 regulator protein contributes to hyphal morphogenesis of *Candida albicans. Genetics* **157**:1523–1530.

4. **Borges-Walmsley, M. I., and A. R. Walmsley.** 2000. cAMP signalling in pathogenic fungi: control of dimorphic switching and pathogenicity. *Trends Microbiol.* **8**:133–141.
5. **Braun, B. R., and A. D. Johnson.** 1997. Control of filament formation in *Candida albicans* by the transcriptional repressor TUP1. *Science* **277**:105–109.
6. **Braun, B. R., and A. D. Johnson.** 2000. *TUP1, CPH1* and *EFG1* make independent contributions to filamentation in *Candida albicans. Genetics* **155**:57–67.
7. **Braun, B. R., W. S. Head, M. X. Wang, and A. D. Johnson.** 2000. Identification and characterization of *TUP1*-regulated genes in *Candida albicans. Genetics* **156**:31–44.

7a. **Braun, B. R., D. Kadosh, and A. D. Johnson.** 2001. *NRG1*, a *TUP1*-dependent repressor of filamentous growth in *Candida albicans*, is down-regulated during filament induction. *EMBO J.*, in press.

8. **Brown, A. J. P., and N. A. R. Gow.** 1999. Regulatory networks controlling *Candida albicans* morphogenesis. *Trends Microbiol.* **7**:333–338.
9. **Brown, A. J. P., and N. A. R. Gow.** 2001. Signal transduction and morphogenesis in *Candida albicans. In* K. Esser and J. W. Bennet (ed.), *The Mycota*, in press. Springer, Berlin, Germany.
10. **Brown, A. J. P., C. J. Barelle, S. Budge, J. Duncan, S. Harris, P. R. Lee, P. Leng, S. Macaskill, A. M. Abdul Murad, M. Ramsdale, C. Wiltshire, J. A. Wishart, and N. A. R. Gow.** 2000. Gene regulation during morphogenesis in *Candida albicans*, p. 112–115. *In* J. F. Ernst and A. Schmidt (ed.), *Contributions to Microbiology: Dimorphism in Human Pathogenic and Apathogenic Yeasts*, vol. 5. Karger AG, Basel, Switzerland.
11. **Brown, A. J. P., P. Leng, S. Garcia, M. Straffon, G. Tripathi, and J. A. Wishart.** Unpublished data.
12. **Brown, D. H., A. D. Guisani, X. Chen, and C. A. Kumamoto.** 1999. Filamentous growth of *Candida albicans* in response to physical environmental cues and its regulation by the unique *CZF1* gene. *Mol. Microbiol.* **34**:651–662.
13. **Bruckmann, A., W. Kunkel, A. Hartl, R. Wetzker, and R. Eck.** 2000. A phosphatidylinositol 3-kinase of *Candida albicans* influences adhesion, filamentous growth and virulence. *Microbiology* **146**:2755–2764.
14. **Calera, J. A., X. J. Zhao, and R. Calderone.** 2000. Defective hyphal development and avirulence caused by a deletion of the *SSK1* response regulator gene in *Candida albicans. Infect. Immun.* **68**:518–525.
15. ***Candida albicans* genome sequencing website.** http://www-sequence.stanford.edu/group/candida/search.html.
16. **Chen, H., S. Zhou, Q. Wang, X. Chen, T. Pan, and H. Liu.** 2000. Crk1, a novel Cdc2-related protein kinase, is required for hyphal development and virulence in *Candida albicans. Mol. Cell. Biol.* **20**:8696–8708.
17. **Clark, K. L., P. J. F. Feldmann, D. Dignard, R. Larocque, A. J. P. Brown, M. G. Lee, D. Y. Thomas, and M. Whiteway.** 1995. Constitutive activation of the *Saccharomyces cerevisiae* mating response pathway by a MAP kinase kinase from *Candida albicans. Mol. Gen. Genet.* **249**:609–621.
18. **Cormack, B., G. Bertram, M. Egerton, N. A. R. Gow, S. Falkow, and A. J. P. Brown.** 1997. Yeast enhanced green fluorescent protein (yEGFP): a reporter of gene expression in *Candida albicans. Microbiology* **143**:303–311.
19. **Csank, C., C. Makris, S. Meloche, K. Schröppel, M. Rollinghoff, D. Dignard, D. Y. Thomas, and M. Whiteway.** 1997. Derepressed hyphal growth and reduced virulence in a VH1 family-related protein phosphatase mutant of the human pathogen *Candida albicans. Mol. Biol. Cell* **8**:2539–2551.
20. **Csank, C., K. Schröppel, E. Leberer, D. Harcus, O. Mohamed, S. Meloche, D. Y. Thomas, and M. Whiteway.** 1998. Roles of the *Candida albicans* mitogen-activated protein kinase homolog, Cek1p, in hyphal development and systemic candidosis. *Infect. Immun.* **66**:2713–2721.
21. **Davis, D., R. B. Wilson, and A. P. Mitchell.** 2000. *RIM101*-dependent and -independent pathways govern pH responses in *Candida albicans. Mol. Cell. Biol.* **20**:971–978.
22. **De Bernardis, F., F. A. Muhlschlegel, A. Cassone, and W. A. Fonzi.** 1998. The pH of the host niche controls gene expression in and virulence of *Candida albicans. Infect. Immun.* **66**: 3317–3325.
23. **Denison, S. H., M. Orejas, and H. N. Arst, Jr.** 1995. Signalling of ambient pH in *Aspergillus* involves a cysteine protease. *J. Biol. Chem.* **270**:28519–28522.
24. **Denison, S. H., S. Negrete-Urtasun, J. M. Mingot, J. Tilburn, W. A. Mayer, A. Goel, E. A. Espeso, M. A. Penalva, and H. N. Arst, Jr.** 1998. Putative membrane components of signal transduction pathways for ambient pH regulation in *Aspergillus* and meiosis in *Saccharomyces* are homologous. *Mol. Microbiol.* **30**:259–264.
25. **El Barkani, A., O. Kurzai, W. A. Fonzi, A. Ramon, A. Porta, M. Frosch, and F. A. Muhlschlegel.** 2000. Dominant active alleles of *RIM101* (*PRR2*) bypass the pH restriction on filamentation of *Candida albicans. Mol. Cell. Biol.* **20**: 4635–4647.
26. **Ernst, J. F.** 2000. Transcription factors in *Candida albicans*—environmental control of morphogenesis. *Microbiology* **146**:1763–1774.
27. **Ernst, J. F.** 2000. Regulation of dimorphism in *Candida albicans*, p. 98–111. *In* J. F. Ernst and A. Schmidt (ed.), *Contributions to Microbiology: Dimorphism in Human Pathogenic and Apathogenic Yeasts*, vol. 5. Karger AG, Basel, Switzerland.
28. **Feng, Q., E. Summers, B. Guo, and G. Fink.** 1999. Ras signaling is required for serum-induced hyphal differentiation in *Candida albicans. J. Bacteriol.* **181**:6339–6346.
29. **Fonzi, W. A.** 1999. *PHR1* and *PHR2* of *Candida albicans* encode putative glycosidases required for proper cross-linking of β-1,3- and β-1,6-glucans. *J. Bacteriol.* **181**:7070–7079.
30. **Fu, Y., G. Rieg, W. A. Fonzi, P. H. Belanger, J. E. Edwards, Jr., and S. G. Filler.** 1998. Expression of the *Candida albicans* gene *ALS1* in *Saccharomyces cerevisiae* induces adherence to endothelial and epithelial cells. *Infect. Immun.* **66**:1783–1786.
31. **Gale, C. A., C. M. Bendel, M. McClellan, M. Hauser, J. M. Becker, J. Berman, and M. K. Hostetter.** 1998. Linkage of adhesion, filamentous growth, and virulence in *Candida albicans* to a single gene, *INT1. Science* **279**:1355–1358.
32. **Gale, C., D. Finkel, N. Tao, M. Meinke, M. McClellan, J. Olson, K. Kendrick, and M. Hostetter.** 1996. Cloning and expression of a gene encoding an integrin-like protein in *Candida albicans. Proc. Natl. Acad. Sci. USA* **93**:357–361.
33. **Ghannoum, M. A., B. Spellberg, S. M. Saporito-Irwin, and W. A. Fonzi.** 1995. Reduced virulence of *Candida albicans PHR1* mutants. *Infect. Immun.* **63**:4528–4530.

34. **Gow, N. A. R.** 1994. Growth and guidance of the fungal hypha. *Microbiology* **140:**3193–3205.
35. **Gustin, M. C., J. Albertyn, M. Alexander, and K. Davenport.** 1998. MAP kinase pathways in the yeast *Saccharomyces cerevisiae. Microbiol. Mol. Biol. Rev.* **62:**1264–1300.
36. **Hoyer, L. L., T. L. Payne, M. Bell, A. M. Myers, and S. Scherer.** 1998. *Candida albicans ALS3* and insights into the nature of the ALS gene family. *Curr. Genet.* **33:**451–459.
37. **Hube, B., D. Sanglard, F. C. Odds, D. Hess, M. Monod, W. Schafer, A. J. P. Brown, and N. A. R. Gow.** 1997. Gene disruption of each of the secretory aspartyl proteinase genes *SAP1, SAP2* and *SAP3* in *Candida albicans* attenuates virulence. *Infect. Immun.* **65:**3529–3538.
38. **Hull, C. M., R. M. Raisner, and A. D. Johnson.** 2000. Evidence for mating of the "asexual" yeast *Candida albicans* in a mammalian host. *Science* **289:**307–310.
39. **Ishii, N., M. Yamamoto, F. Yoshihara, M. Arisawa, and Y. Aoki.** 1997. Biochemical and genetic characterisation of Rbf1p, a putative transcription factor of *Candida albicans. Microbiology* **143:**429–435.
40. **Kadosh, D., and A. D. Johnson.** 2001. Rfg1, a protein related to the *S. cerevisiae* hypoxic regulator Rox1, controls filamentous growth and virulence in *C. albicans. Mol. Cell. Biol.* **21:** 2496–2505.
41. **Köhler, J. R., and G. R. Fink.** 1996. *Candida albicans* strains heterozygous and homozygous for mutations in mitogen-activated protein kinase signalling components have defects in hyphal development. *Proc. Natl. Acad. Sci. USA* **93:** 13223–13228.
42. **Kron, S. J., and N. A. R. Gow.** 1995. Budding yeast morphogenesis: signalling, cytoskeleton and cell cycle. *Curr. Opin. Cell Biol.* **7:**845–855.
43. **Leberer, E., D. Harcus, I. D. Broadbent, K. L. Clark, D. Dignard, K. Ziegelbauer, A. Schmit, N. A. R. Gow, A. J. P. Brown, and D. Y. Thomas.** 1996. Homologs of the Ste20p and Ste7p protein kinases are involved in hyphal formation of *Candida albicans. Proc. Natl. Acad. Sci. USA* **93:**13217–13222.
44. **Leberer, E., K. Ziegelbauer, A. Schmidt, D. Harcus, D. Dignard, J. Ash, L. Johnson, and D. Y. Thomas.** 1997. Virulence and hyphal formation of *Candida albicans* require the Ste20p-like protein kinase CaCla4p. *Curr. Biol.* **7:**539–546.
45. **Leng, P., P. R. Lee, H. Wu, and A. J. P. Brown.** 2001. Efg1, a morphogenetic regulator in *Candida albicans,* is a sequence-specific DNA binding protein. *J. Bacteriol.* **183:**4090–4093.
46. **Leng, P., P. E. Sudbery, and A. J. P. Brown.** 2000. Rad6p represses yeast-hypha morphogenesis in the human fungal pathogen. *Candida albicans. Mol. Microbiol.* **35:**1264–1275.
47. **Lengeler, K. B., R. C. Davidson, C. D'Souza, T. Harashima, W.-C. Shen, P. Wang, X. Pan, M. Waugh, and J. Heitman.** 2000. Signal transduction cascades regulating fungal development and virulence. *Microbiol. Mol. Biol. Rev.* **64:**746–785.
48. **Liu, H., C. A. Styles, and G. R. Fink.** 1993. Elements of the yeast pheromone response pathway required for filamentous growth of diploids. *Science* **262:**1741–1744.
49. **Liu, H., J. Köhler, and G. R. Fink.** 1994. Suppression of hyphal formation in *Candida albicans* by mutation of a *STE12* homolog. *Science* **266:**1723–1725.
50. **Lo, H. J., J. R. Kohler, B. DiDomenico, D. Loebenberg, A. Cacciapuoti, and G. R. Fink.** 1997. Nonfilamentous *C. albicans* mutants are avirulent. *Cell* **90:**939–949.
51. **Madhani, H. D., and G. R. Fink.** 1997. Combinatorial control required for the specificity of yeast MAPK signaling. *Science* **275:**1314–1317.
52. **Madhani, H. D., and G. R. Fink.** 1998. The control of filamentous differentiation and virulence in fungi. *Trends Cell Biol.* **8:**348–353.
53. **Magee, B. B., and P. T. Magee.** 2000. Induction of mating in *Candida albicans* by construction of *MTLa* and *MTLalpha* strains. *Science* **289:**310–313.
54. **Magee, P. T.** 1998. Analysis of the *Candida albicans* genome. *Methods Microbiol.* **26:**395–415.
55. **Mallet, L., G. Renault, and M. Jacquet.** 2000. Functional cloning of the adenylate cyclase gene of *Candida albicans* in *Saccharomyces cerevisiae* within a genomic fragment containing five other genes, including homologues of *CHS6* and *SAP185*. *Yeast* **16:**959–966.
56. **Massari, M. E., and C. Murre.** 2000. Helix-loop-helix proteins: regulators of transcription in eucaryotic organisms. *Mol. Cell. Biol.* **20:**429–440.
57. **Mirbod, F., S. Nakashima, Y. Kitajima, R. D. Cannon, and Y. Nozawa.** 1997. Molecular cloning of a Rho family, *CDC42Ca* gene from *Candida albicans* and its mRNA expression changes during morphogenesis. *J. Med. Vet. Mycol.* **35:**173–179.
58. **Mitchell, A. P.** 1998. Dimorphism and virulence in *Candida albicans. Curr. Opin. Microbiol.* **1:**687–692.
59. **Morschhauser, J., S. Michel, and P. Staib.** 1999. Sequential gene disruption in *Candida albicans* by FLP-mediated site-specific recombination. *Mol. Microbiol.* **32:**547–556.
60. **Mosch, H.-U., R. L. Roberts, and G. R. Fink.** 1996. Ras2 signals via the Cdc42/Ste20/mitogen-activated protein kinase module to induce filamentous growth in *Saccharomyces cerevisiae. Proc. Natl. Acad. Sci. USA* **93:**5352–5356.
61. **Muhlschlegel, F. A., and W. A. Fonzi.** 1997. *PHR2* of *Candida albicans* encodes a functional homolog of the pH-regulated gene *PHR1* with an inverted pattern of expression. *Mol. Cell. Biol.* **17:**5960–5967.
62. **Murad, A. M. A., P. Leng, M. Straffon, J. Wishart, S. Macaskill, D. MacCallum, N. Schnell, D. Talibi, D. Marechal, F. Tekaia, C. d'Enfert, C. Gaillardin, F. C. Odds, and A. J. P. Brown.** *NRG1* represses yeast-hypha morphogenesis and hypha-specific gene expression in *Candida albicans. EMBO J.,* in press.
63. **Odds, F. C.** 1988. *Candida and Candidosis,* 2nd ed. Bailliere Tindall, London, United Kingdom.
64. **Odds, F. C.** 1994. *Candida* species and virulence. *ASM News* **60:**313–318.
65. **Pan, X, and J. Heitman.** 1999. Cyclic AMP-dependent protein kinase regulates pseudohyphal differentiation in *Saccharomyces cerevisiae. Mol. Cell. Biol.* **19:**4874–4887.
66. **Park, S. H., S. S. Koh, J. H. Chun, H. J. Hwang, and H. S. Kang.** 1999. Nrg1 is a transcriptional repressor for glucose repression of *STA1* gene expression in *Saccharomyces cerevisiae. Mol. Cell. Biol.* **19:**2044–2050.
67. **Porta, A., A. M. Ramon, and W. A. Fonzi.** 1999. *PRR1,* a homolog of *Aspergillus nidulans palF,* controls pH-dependent gene expression and filamentation in *Candida albicans. J. Bacteriol.* **181:**7516–7523.
68. **Posas, F., and H. Saito.** 1997. Osmotic activation of the HOG MAPK pathway via ste11p MAPKKK. *Science* **276:** 1702–1705.
69. **Ramanan, N., and Y. Wang.** 2000. A high-affinity iron permease essential for *Candida albicans* virulence. *Science* **288:** 1062–1064.
70. **Ramon, A. M., A. Porta, and W. A. Fonzi.** 1999. Effect of environmental pH on morphological development of *Candida albicans* is mediated via the PacC-regulated transcription factor encoded by *PRR2*. *J. Bacteriol.* **181:**7524–7530.
71. **Riggle, P. J., K. A. Andrutis, X. Chen, S. R. Tzipori, and C. A. Kumamoto.** 1999. Invasion lesions containing filamentous forms produced by a *Candida albicans* mutant that is defective in filamentous growth in culture. *Infect. Immun.* **67:** 3649–3652.

72. **Robinson, K. A., and J. M. Lopes.** 2000. *Saccharomyces cerevisiae* basic helix-loop-helix proteins regulate diverse biological processes. *Nucleic Acids Res.* **28:**1499–1505.

73. **Sabie, F. T., and G. M. Gadd.** 1992. Effect of nucleosides and nucleotides and the relationship between cellular adenosine 3′:5′-cyclic monophosphate (cyclic AMP) and germ tube formation in *Candida albicans. Mycopathology.* **119:**147–156.

74. **Sanglard, D., B. Hube, M. Monod, F. C. Odds, and N. A. R. Gow.** 1997. A triple deletion of the secreted aspartyl proteinase genes *SAP4, SAP5* and *SAP6* of *Candida albicans* causes attenuated virulence. *Infect. Immun.* **65:**3539–3546.

75. **Santos, M. A. S., G. Keith, and M. F. Tuite.** 1993. Non-standard translational events in *Candida albicans* mediated by an unusual seryl-tRNA with a 5′-CAG-3′ (leucine) anticodon. *EMBO J.* **12:**607–616.

76. **Saporito-Irwin, S. M., C. E. Birse, P. S. Sypherd, and W. A. Fonzi.** 1995. *PHR1,* a pH-regulated gene of *Candida albicans,* is required for morphogenesis. *Mol. Cell. Biol.* **15:**601–613.

77. **Schweizer, A., S. Rupp, B. N. Taylor, M. Rollinghoff, and K. Schröppel.** 2001. The TEA/ATTS transcription factor CaTec1p regulates hyphal development and virulence in *Candida albicans. Mol. Microbiol.* **38:**435–445.

78. **Sharkey, L. L., M. D. McNemar, S. M. Saporito-Irwin, P. S. Sypherd, and W. A. Fonzi.** 1999. *HWP1* functions in the morphological development of *Candida albicans* downstream of *EFG1, TUP1* and *RBF1. J. Bacteriol.* **181:**5273–5279.

79. **Smith, R. L., and A. D. Johnson.** 2000. Turning off genes by Ssn6-Tup1: a conserved system of transcriptional repression in eukaryotes. *Trends Biochem. Sci.* **25:**325–330.

80. **Sonneborn, A., B. Tebarth, and J. F. Ernst.** 1999. Control of white-opaque phenotypic switching in *Candida albicans* by the Efg1 morphogenetic regulator. *Infect. Immun.* **67:**4655–4660.

81. **Sonneborn, A., D. Bockmuhl, and J. F. Ernst.** 1999. Chlamydospore formation in *Candida albicans* requires the Efg1 morphogenetic regulator. *Infect. Immun.* **67:**5514–5517.

82. **Sonneborn, A., D. P. Bockmuhl, M. Gerads, K. Kurpanek, D. Sanglard, and J. F. Ernst.** 2000. Protein kinase A encoded by *TPK2* regulates dimorphism of *Candida albicans. Mol. Microbiol.* **35:**386–396.

83. **Srikantha, T., L. K. Tsai, K. Daniels, and D. R. Soll.** 2000. *EFG1* null mutants of *Candida albicans* switch but cannot express the complete phenotype of white-phase budding cells. *J. Bacteriol.* **182:**1580–1591.

84. **Stanhill, A., N. Schick, and D. Engelberg.** 1999. The yeast Ras/cyclic AMP pathway induces invasive growth by suppressing the cellular stress response. *Mol. Cell. Biol.* **19:**7529–7538.

85. **Stoldt, V. R., A. Sonneborn, C. E. Leuker, and J. Ernst.** 1997. Efg1p, an essential regulator of morphogenesis of the human pathogen *Candida albicans,* is a member of a conserved class of bHLH proteins regulating morphogenetic processes in fungi. *EMBO J.* **16:**1982–1991.

86. **Swoboda, R. K., G. Bertram, S. Delbruck, J. F. Ernst, N. A. R. Gow, G. W. Gooday, and A. J. P. Brown.** 1994. Fluctuations in glycolytic mRNA levels during the yeast-to-hyphal transition in *Candida albicans* reflect underlying changes in growth rather than a response to cellular dimorphism. *Mol. Microbiol.* **13:**663–672.

87. **Tilburn, J., S. Sarkar, D. A. Widdick, E. A. Espeso, M. Orejas, J. Mungroo, M. A. Penelva, and H. N. Arst, Jr.** 1995. The *Aspergillus* PacC zinc finger transcription factor mediates regulation of bot acidic- and alkaline-expressed genes by ambient pH. *EMBO J.* **14:**779–790.

88. **Whiteway, M.** 2000. Transcriptional control of cell type and morphogenesis in *Candida albicans. Curr. Opin. Microbiol.* **3:**582–588.

89. **Whiteway, M., D. Dignard, and D. Y. Thomas.** 1992. Dominant negative selection of heterologous genes: isolation of *Candida albicans* genes that interfere with *Saccharomyces cerevisiae* mating factor-induced cell cycle arrest. *Proc. Natl. Acad. Sci. USA* **89:**9410–9414.

90. **Wilson, R. B., D. Davis, and A. P. Mitchell.** 1999. Rapid hypothesis testing with *Candida albicans* through gene disruption with short homology regions. *J. Bacteriol.* **181:**1868–1874.

91. **Yaar, L., M. Mevarech, and Y. Koltin.** 1997. A *Candida albicans* RAS-related gene (*CaRSRS1*) is involved in budding, cell morphogenesis and hypha development. *Microbiology* **143:** 3033–3044.

92. **Yamada-Okabe, T., O. Shimmi, R. Doi, K. Mizumoto, M. Arisawa, and H. Yamada-Okabe.** 1996. Isolation of the mRNA-capping enzyme and ferric-reductase-related genes from *Candida albicans. Microbiology* **142:**2515–2523.

Candida and Candidiasis
Edited by Richard A. Calderone

Chapter 9

Extracellular Hydrolases

Bernhard Hube and Julian Naglik

All pathogenic microorganisms have developed virulence mechanisms that confer the ability to colonize a host surface, to penetrate into deeper host tissue, or to evade host defenses. One factor that contributes to the process of virulence is hydrolase production, which is known to play a central role in the pathogenicity of bacteria, protozoa, and pathogenic fungi. The production of hydrolytic enzymes may fulfill a number of possible functions in addition to the simple role of digesting molecules for nutrient acquisition, as in the case of saprophytic microorganisms. Secreted hydrolases may have more direct virulence properties and can contribute to host tissue invasion by digesting or distorting host cell membranes, degrading host surface molecules to enhance adhesion, or digesting cells and molecules of the host immune system to avoid or resist antimicrobial attack. The role and function of extracellular hydrolytic enzymes in microbial pathogenesis of many bacterial diseases have served as a base on which to identify comparable virulence traits of *Candida albicans*. *Candida* species, and most notably *C. albicans*, tend to produce hydrolytic enzymes with broad substrate specificities, which is in contrast to the highly substrate-specific enzymes produced by certain bacteria. The three most significant hydrolytic enzymes produced by *C. albicans* are secreted aspartic proteinases, phospholipases, and lipases, although others have been identified, such as glucanases and chitinases, but these are not linked to virulence. Therefore, this chapter will summarize the history of the investigation of secreted proteinases, phospholipases, and lipases of *Candida* species and will emphasize the more recent data. For further details, the reader is referred to a number of reviews dealing with hydrolytic enzymes of *Candida* (36, 38, 45, 85).

SECRETED ASPARTIC PROTEINASES OF *CANDIDA*

Since the discovery of proteolytic activity in *C. albicans* in 1965 (96), a range of terms has been given to describe these proteinases, but the term secreted aspartic proteinase (Sap) (E.C. 3.4.23.6) is now generally accepted by most groups working in the field, with *SAP* symbolizing the gene and Sap, the protein. The Sap family is responsible for the proteolytic activity of *C. albicans*, and the name describes the two most important characteristics of the enzymes: that they are aspartic proteinases that act extracellularly. Biochemically, aspartic proteinases are characterized by (i) having an optimum pH activity in the acid range (Table 1) and (ii) their inhibition by pepstatin A, a hexapeptide from *Streptomyces* species (18).

Among the putative virulence factors of *C. albicans*, the Saps have been one of the most comprehensively studied. However, *C. albicans* is not the only *Candida* species known to produce extracellular proteinases. Many of the pathogenic *Candida* species are known to possess *SAP* genes, including *C. dubliniensis* (37), *C. tropicalis* (67, 103, 116), and *C. parapsilosis* (25, 67), all of which produce active extracellular proteinases in vitro. Although Sap activity was considered to be a virulence factor for *C. tropicalis* (7), its role as a virulence factor for *C. parapsilosis*

Bernhard Hube • NG4, Robert Koch-Institut, Nordufer 20, D-13353 Berlin, Germany. **Julian Naglik** • Division of Oral Medicine, Pathology, Microbiology and Immunology, Floor 28, Guy's Tower, Kings College London (Guy's Campus), London Bridge, London SE1 9RT, United Kingdom.

Table 1. Properties of purified *C. albicans* proteinases

Proteinase	Molecular mass[a] (kDa)	pH range	Optimal pH activity	pI	Reference(s)
Sap1	38, 40, 40	2.5–5.5	3.2–4.5	4.0	8, 95, 113
Sap2	40, 41, 43, 45, 48, 49	2.5–5.5	3.2–3.5	4.25, 4.4	8, 71, 95, 113
Sap3	41, 42	2.0–5.0	3.2–3.5	5.7	8, 95, 113
Sap4	40[a]	4.0–7.0	5.0	ND	8
Sap5	37[a]	3.0–7.0	5.0	ND	8
Sap6	40[a]	3.0–7.0	5.0	ND	8
Sap8	41	ND[b]	ND[b]	ND[b]	71
Sap7, Sap9, Sap10	ND[b]	ND[b]	ND[b]	ND[b]	

[a]Molecular mass values estimated from SDS-PAGE gels.
[b]No information regarding the properties of Sap7, -8, -9, and -10 proteins are presently available. ND, not determined.

remains uncertain (85). Little published information is available with regard to the importance of Saps in the virulence of *C. dubliniensis*. However, as *C. dubliniensis* possesses a similar number of *SAP* genes to *C. albicans* (37), it is probable that proteinase production contributes to the virulence of this fungus. Less or nonpathogenic *Candida* species do not appear to produce significant amounts of proteinase, which has led to the general conclusion that pathogenicity is directly correlated with the level of Sap production (85). Most interestingly, all secreted *Candida* proteinases belong to the same class of aspartic proteinase. Neither extracellular serine-, metallo-, nor cysteine proteinases have been identified in pathogenic *Candida* species.

STRUCTURE OF THE *C. ALBICANS* SECRETED ASPARTIC PROTEINASES

The primary structure of the proteinases deduced from their corresponding genes is shown in Fig. 1. All 10 *SAP* genes encode preproenzymes approximately 60 amino acids longer than the mature enzyme (Table 2). The N-terminal secretion signal is cleaved by the signal peptidase in the endoplasmic reticulum (ER) (Fig. 1). The propeptide is removed to activate the proteinases either by the Kex2 proteinase or other alternative proteinases or by autocatalysis (see below). The mature enzyme contains sequence motifs typical for all aspartic proteinases, including the two conserved aspartate residues of the active site and conserved cysteine residues implicated in the maintenance of the three-dimensional structure. Most Saps contain putative *N*-glycosylation sites (Table 2), but it remains to be determined which Saps are glycosylated. Although Sap2 is not thought to be glycosylated (72), recombinant Sap9 and Sap10 were found to be glycosylated (70).

Structural studies of the *C. albicans* proteinase family have concentrated on Sap2, which is the most abundant secreted protein in vitro when grown in the presence of protein as the sole source of nitrogen (48). The overall structure of Sap2, as determined by Cutfield et al. (16) and Abad-Zapatero et al. (1), conforms to the classical aspartic proteinase fold typified by pepsin. However, comparisons of Sap2 with pepsin have revealed a number of major differences, which make the *C. albicans* proteinase family unique among the aspartic proteinases and probably contribute to the broad substrate specificity of Sap2. At present, only the structure of Sap2 has been determined, but Stewart et al. (99) undertook a comparative structural study by molecular modeling using the sequences of *SAP1* through *SAP6*. Although the structure of Sap1 through Sap6 and their active sites were generally similar, sufficient differences existed to probably allow for different substrate specificity, with the dichotomy

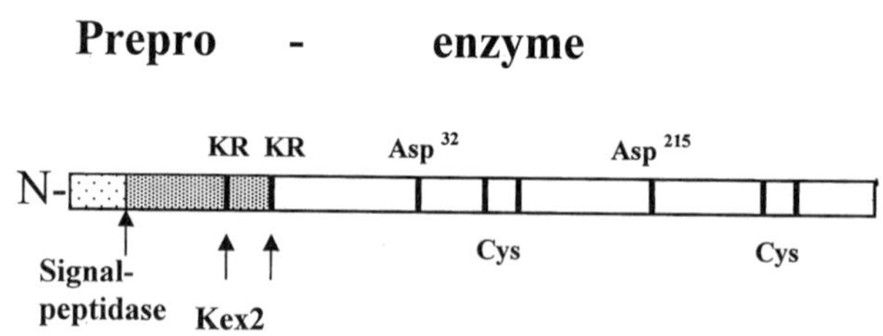

Figure 1. Structure of the deduced Sap1 proteinase with elements and motifs found in all Saps. The *SAP1* gene is translated into a preproprotein. The first 18 amino acids (signal peptide) are processed by the signal peptidase (arrow) in the endoplasmatic reticulum (ER). The propeptide contains two Lys-Arg processing sites (KR), which are targeted by the proteinase Kex2 (arrows) in the Golgi apparatus or by alternative activation processes (see text). Four conserved cysteine residues (Cys) are probably responsible for two conserved disulfide bridges, and the two aspartate residues (Asp^{32} and Asp^{215}), corresponding to the location in the mature Sap1 protein, are common to the active sites of all aspartic proteinases.

Table 2. The *SAP* genes and deduced proteins of *C. albicans*[a]

Gene	Prepropeptide (aa)	KR/KK sites	ORF (bp)	Mature enzyme (aa)	*N*-glycosylation sites (propeptide)	Chromosome	Reference
SAP1	50	2 KR	1,173	341	1 (0)	6	47
SAP2	56	2 KR	1,194	342	0 (2)	R	114
SAP3	58	1 KR	1,194	340	1 (1)	3	113
SAP4	75	4 KR	1,254	342	0 (1)	6	66
SAP5	76	4 KR	1,254	342	0 (0)	6	67
SAP6	76	4 KR	1,254	342	0 (1)	6	67
SAP7	211	1 KK	1,764	377	1 (4)	1	67
SAP8	73	2 KR	1,215	405	1 (1)	3	68
SAP9	50	1 KR 1 KK	1,632	544	4 (0)	3	68
SAP10	38	1 KR	1,326	403	8 (0)	4	28

[a]All Saps contain Lys/Arg (KR)- or Lys/Lys (KK)-processing sites and four conserved cysteine residues. The size of the prepropeptide (signal peptide and propeptide) and the mature enzyme is shown in amino acids (aa), the size of the open reading frame (ORF) in base pairs (bp); also, the number of potential *N*-glycosylation sites, including those located in the propeptide (in parentheses), and the chromosomal location of the gene are shown. Sap9 and -10 have structural elements typical for glycosylphosphatidylinositol (GPI)-proteins (12).

between Sap1 through Sap3 and Sap4 through Sap6 being clearly evident. Furthermore, a potentially significant trend was observed in the total electrostatic charge of the Sap1 through Sap6 enzymes, which might account for the different pH optima of each enzyme, and opens up the exciting possibility that different Saps may target different tissue-specific proteins during the infectious process.

PROCESSING, ACTIVATION, AND REGULATION OF THE *C. ALBICANS* PROTEINASES

All *SAP* genes are translated into preproenzymes, which are processed when transported via the secretory pathway. The N-terminal signal peptide is removed in the ER by a signal peptidase (Fig. 1) and the proenzyme transferred to the Golgi apparatus where it is further processed after Lys-Arg sequences by a Kex2 proteinase (105). To determine the importance of the Kex2 proteinase in Sap secretion, the *KEX2* gene was cloned and disrupted (79). The Kex2-deficient mutants were still capable of secreting active Sap2, but the enzyme was abnormally processed and secreted at reduced levels. Unexpectedly, null mutants were incapable of forming hyphae, instead differentiating into aberrantly shaped cells, indicating that Kex2 may have multiple targets (79). Furthermore, alternative but less efficient processing pathways for Saps are thought to exist (105), as autoactivation was shown to occur extracellularly for Sap1 through Sap3 and Sap6 at certain pH values (56). Intracellular removal of the propeptide not only regulates the activation of the proteinases but also seems to play an essential role for secretion. Beggah et al. (6) showed that a Sap1 protein lacking the propeptide region accumulated within the cell and was not secreted. Further studies using recombinant Sap1 protein and propeptides from other Saps demonstrated that maturation of Sap1 is directed by propeptides through a combination of intra- and intermolecular events.

As the *SAP* gene family encodes preproenzymes, the regulation of proteinase expression can be controlled either at the mRNA or protein level. Comparisons of Sap protein and mRNA levels at identical time points (112) and kinetic studies of proteinase secretion by protein labeling and immunoprecipitation (pulse chase experiments) (43) suggested that proteinase synthesis and secretion were tightly coupled, strongly implying that regulation of Sap activity occurred predominantly at the mRNA level. Studies using the proteinase inhibitor pepstatin A demonstrated that *SAP2* expression in *C. albicans* was also regulated via a positive feedback mechanism, since the proteolytic products of Sap2 and peptides of eight or more amino acid residues induced this gene (48, 63).

PURIFICATION, ACTIVITY, AND PROPERTIES OF *CANDIDA* PROTEINASES

The first observation of extracellular proteolytic activity in *C. albicans* was demonstrated by Staib (96). Since then and up until the early 1990s, a plethora of studies on the purification and biochemical properties of extracellular proteinases from *Candida* species have been reported. The Sap proteinases have been purified and characterized either by direct purification from *Candida* culture supernatants (33, 34, 95, 113) or by expression in recombinant *Pichia pastoris* (8, 116) or *Escherichia coli* (56). This has provided a more detailed insight into the characteristics of the Sap isoenzymes, the general biochemical properties of which are described in Table 1.

In most of the early studies, proteinase activity was induced using culture conditions that were subsequently shown to favor *SAP2* expression (48, 112). As a result, the early biochemical studies of proteinases purified from many different *C. albicans* strains reflected the characteristics of Sap2 (Table 1). Sap2 was shown to act mainly at acidic pH values, a common feature of all aspartic proteinases, and seemed to have broad substrate specificity, being able to degrade many human proteins such as albumin, collagen, hemoglobin, keratin, salivary lactoferrin, lactoperoxidase, mucin, secretory IgA, α-macroglobulin, and cystatin A (reviewed in reference 45). It is possible that these same substrates are degraded in vivo for nutritional purposes, to aid penetration and invasion, or for immune evasion.

The purification and determination of various proteolytic properties of other Sap isoenzymes were subsequently determined by further studies (Table 1). White et al. (113) showed that the white-opaque switching strain WO-1 secreted three distinct Sap isoenzymes (Sap 1 through -3) with different isoelectric points under standard proteinase-inducing conditions. Smolenski et al. (95) also purified and analyzed the biochemical properties of Sap1, Sap2, and Sap3 by comparing optimum pH activity, substrate specificity, and thermal stability. Borg von-Zepelin et al. (8) purified heterologously expressed Sap1 through Sap6 isoenzymes and showed that all six were able to hydrolyze casein. However, distinct differences in pH optima were found among the six proteinases, with Sap1 through -3 having the highest activity at lower pH values and Sap4 through -6 at higher pH values. In addition to different pH optima, the *Candida* Saps may also have different preferential amino acid cleavage sites, a feature already shown for Sap2 (33, 34, 38). Koelsch et al. (56) investigated the functional aspects and substrate specificities of Sap1, Sap2, Sap3, and Sap6. All four Saps cleaved peptide bonds between larger hydrophobic amino acids but had preferences at the P_1 and P'_1 sites. For example, Sap1, Sap2, and Sap6 preferred phenylalanine whereas Sap3 preferred leucine at the P_1 site. These differences may provide useful information for the future design of Sap-specific inhibitors. The biochemical and proteolytic properties of Sap7 through Sap10 enzymes are not presently known. However, sequence analysis of Sap9 and Sap10 suggested that both proteinases appear to be glycosylphosphatidylinositol (GPI)-anchored proteins (28, 68).

A recurring notion in the literature is that Sap2 is only active at acidic pH and undergoes irreversible alkaline denaturation at higher pH values (85), creating a minor dilemma regarding in vivo functions (17). However, it has been demonstrated that Sap2 is stable at neutral pH and is still active under these conditions (11, 109). This relative stability of Sap2 at higher pH values may assist *C. albicans* to colonize and/or infect the host in neutral pH environments such as the oral cavity. In addition, Sap4 through Sap6 are known to be significantly active at physiological pH (8) (Table 1). On the other hand, Sap3 is still active at pH 2.0, providing *C. albicans* with a range of proteolytic activity from pH 2.0 to 7.0. This property may prove vital to the success of *C. albicans* as an opportunistic pathogen, which is able to survive and cause infections on a variety of host tissues, including the oral cavity and vaginal mucosa.

THE *SAP* GENE FAMILY OF *C. ALBICANS*

Ten *SAP* genes have been identified in *C. albicans* over the past decade. The first *Candida SAP* gene (*SAP1*) was cloned using a PCR strategy, which was based on the knowledge of N-terminal sequences from purified proteinases and sequences conserved in all aspartic proteinases (47). The cDNA of *SAP1* was identified a year later in an attempt to isolate switching-specific genes in the *C. albicans* strain WO-1 (73) and was the first study to provide evidence for the switching-regulated expression of the *SAP* genes. A similar PCR-based cloning strategy was used by Wright et al. (114) to isolate *SAP2,* the second secreted aspartic proteinase gene to be identified in *C. albicans.* The remaining eight *SAP* genes were identified by using *SAP1* as a probe (*SAP3, SAP5* through *SAP9*) (67, 68, 113), by sequencing the promoter region of *SAP1* (*SAP4*) (66), or by blast searches and sequence alignments in the *Candida* genome databases (*SAP10*) (http://www-sequence.stanford.edu/group/*Candida*) (28). The open reading frames (ORF) of the genes are between 1,173 and 1,764 bp in length and located on five different chromosomes (Table 2). Only two members of the *SAP* gene family (*SAP1* and *SAP4*) were found to be clustered in tandem (66). Tables 1 and 2 represent the main characteristics of

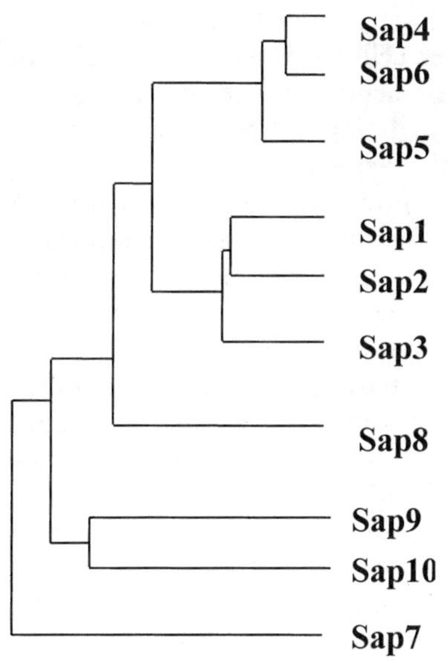

Figure 2. Dendrogram of the *C. albicans* Sap isoenzyme family. Three distinct groups are clustered within the family. Sap1 through -3 are up to 67% identical, and Sap4 through -6 are up to 89% identical, while Sap7 is only 20 to 27% identical to other Saps. Sap9 and Sap10 both have C-terminal consensus sequences typical for GPI proteins. Similar families exist in *C. dubliniensis* and *C. tropicalis*.

the *C. albicans SAP* gene family, and Fig. 2 denotes a dendogram illustrating the deduced amino acid sequence homology between the *C. albicans* Sap isoenzyme family.

IN VITRO EXPRESSION OF THE *SAP* GENE FAMILY

The primary focus of the *SAP* gene expression studies was to understand the regulation of *SAP* genes that resulted from changes in growth environment, morphogenesis between yeast and hyphal forms, and expression of alternative switch phenotypes. Detailed analysis of the in vitro expression of *SAP* genes revealed that proteolytic activity of *C. albicans* at 30 to 37°C in media containing protein as the sole source of nitrogen was primarily due to the *SAP2* gene product (48, 112). Only small amounts of *SAP3* transcripts and Sap3 protein (48, 95) or *SAP8* transcripts (68) were detected under these same growth conditions. However at 25°C, levels of Sap8 protein (71) and *SAP8* transcripts (68) increased, suggesting the expression of this gene was temperature regulated. Expression of *SAP9* and *SAP10* appeared to be independent of external protein, and they were constitutively expressed under most environmental conditions in both yeast and hyphal forms (29). Furthermore, it was discovered that expression of *SAP1* (73) and *SAP3* (113) was controlled during phenotypic switching and was only expressed in the "opaque" but not in the "white" form of strain WO-1. Switching-regulated expression of *SAP1* was also found in *C. albicans* strain 3153A (74). *SAP7* expression has so far not been detected in vitro and, as such, its biological function is completely unknown.

Transcripts of *SAP4* through -6 have been observed during the yeast-to-hyphae transition at neutral pH in the presence of serum or in Lee's medium (48, 112), which indicates that hyphal induction alone is sufficient for the induction of these genes and that protein components in the serum are not necessary. Sequence analysis of the 5′ ends of the three hypha-associated proteinase genes revealed that all three promoter regions contained consensus sequences for the TEA/ATTS transcription factor Tec1 (93). *C. albicans* mutants lacking *TEC1* were not able to express *SAP4* through -6 and failed to produce hyphal cells in vitro, suggesting the existence of joint or coordinated regulatory pathways for hyphal production and proteinase expression. This is supported by the observation that *SAP4* through -6 expression increased in strains lacking a MAP kinase phosphatase (Cpp1), which normally suppresses hyphal formation, and was absent in a strain lacking a key transcriptional regulator of dimorphism (Efg1), which has a reduced ability to form hyphae (92). However, the Efg1-deficient mutant was still able to express *SAP4* through -6 during infection (30), confirming that the environmental milieu present in vivo may have quite different effects on *SAP* gene expression than conditions tested in the laboratory.

SECRETED ASPARTIC PROTEINASES AND *C. ALBICANS* VIRULENCE

The existence of 10 *SAP* genes in *C. albicans* and the demonstration of their controlled expression and tight regulation led to the hypothesis that this enzyme family may have a variety of functions during the infectious process and may be a crucial attribute in *C. albicans* virulence (46, 80). In fact, a number of reports have demonstrated the expression of *C. albicans* proteinases in human infections, but the consequence of Sap secretion in vivo is not precisely known. However, the roles and functions of the proteinases can be deduced from in vitro experimental infection and in vivo animal model data.

In Vivo Detection of Sap Antigen and Antibody

Antigen-antibody studies have provided strong evidence to suggest that Saps are expressed in vivo.

High titers of anti-Sap antibodies in sera of patients with candidiasis indicated the presence of Sap antigen during infection (85). Rüchel et al. (84) also found evidence for the presence of Sap antigen in all organs of immunocompromised patients who had died of systemic *C. albicans* infections, such as the mucosa, central nervous system, lung, heart, liver, pancreas, and kidney. In all cases, the antigen was found within the cell wall of yeast and hyphal cells. In the infected kidney, amorphous deposits of proteinase antigen were found to form a ring around fungal colonies, which may reflect the secretion and subsequent pH-mediated denaturation of the fungal enzymes. The observation that most Sap antigens were present within the *Candida* cell wall and not in the surrounding area was later confirmed (88–91, 100). Using specific antibodies raised against Sap1 through Sap6 (8), a more detailed picture of the location of Sap antigen during infection was possible, which demonstrated that Sap1 through -3 antigens were detected on both yeast and hyphal cells whereas Sap4 through -6 antigens were only found on hyphal cells (88, 90) (Fig. 3). Furthermore, the expression of Sap4 through -6 of *C. albicans* cells was highest after phagocytosis by macrophages (8) or when cells were in close contact with host cells, particularly neutrophils (87).

Although Sap antibodies were useful in demonstrating the expression and localization of the enzymes, the protective effects of Sap antibodies produced by the infected host remain unclear. Ghadjari et al. (35) found that human recombinant antibodies against two Sap2 B-cell epitopes from a patient who had recovered from disseminated candidiasis had no protective activity in a lethal mouse model of candidal infection. In contrast, De Bernardis et al. (21) showed a protective effect of anti-Sap2 antibodies in experimental vaginitis in rats. Unfortunately, the Sap2 epitopes responsible for inducing this protective antibody response were not identified, and thus far, the specific interactions between *Candida* proteinases and the host immune response remain to be investigated.

Expression of Proteinases during *Candida* Infections

The discovery that *C. albicans* possesses a multitude of proteinase genes that are differentially ex-

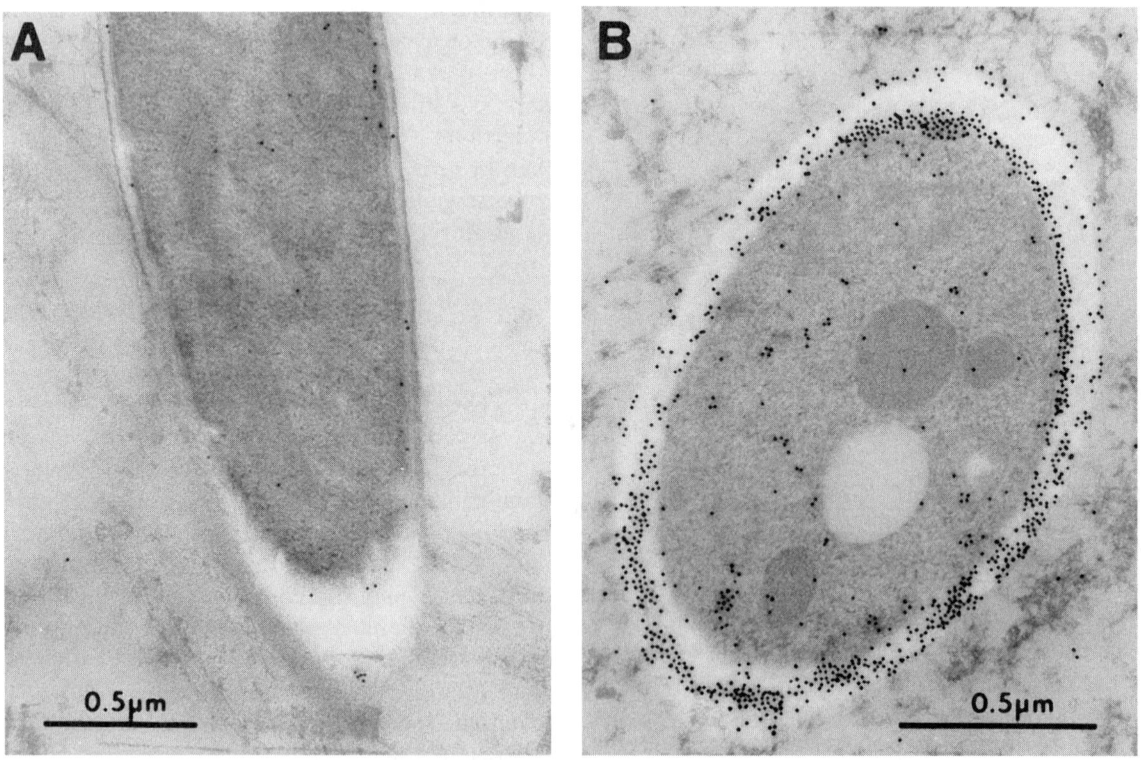

Figure 3. Sap1 through -3 antigen expression on the surface of yeast (B) and Sap4 through -6 antigen expression on hyphal cells (A) during experimental oral infections. Sap1 through -3 antigen was detected in large amounts on the cell surface of yeast and hyphal cells, while Sap4 through -6 antigen was detected on hyphal cells only. Increasing amounts of Sap4 through -6 antigen were found when cells were in close contact to host cells, particularly neutrophils (not shown). Photograph by courtesy of M. Schaller.

pressed under many different conditions in vitro may indicate that this enzyme family makes a significant contribution to the pathogenicity of *C. albicans.* This resulted in a number of studies that have convincingly established a role for Saps in many aspects of *C. albicans* virulence. In an in vitro model of oral candidiasis Schaller et al. (88) showed a distinct order of *SAP* gene expression (*SAP1* and *SAP3* > *SAP6* > *SAP2* and *SAP8*) during the course of infection. In this model, Sap 1 through -3 but not Sap 4 through -6 contributed significantly to tissue damage (89). This may also be the case during in vivo oral infections in humans since a similar expression pattern was observed in patients suffering from oral candidiasis (76, 88, 90). In a detailed study comparing the expression of *SAP1* through *-7* in oral candidiasis patients with *C. albicans* carriers, Naglik et al. (76, 77) demonstrated that *SAP1, SAP3,* and *SAP7* transcripts were predominantly expressed in infected patients as opposed to *Candida* carriers. Interestingly, *SAP2* and *SAP4* through *-6* expression was observed in nearly all patient and carrier subjects tested ($n = 70$), possibly indicating a more housekeeping role or a permanent interaction of these proteinases with host factors in the oral cavity. During experimental in vivo and in vitro vaginal infections, *SAP1* and *SAP2* or *SAP1, SAP2,* and *SAP8* expression was observed, respectively (19, 87). Similarly, expression of *SAP* genes in the order *SAP1* and *SAP2* > *SAP8* > *SAP6* > *SAP3* was also demonstrated in an in vitro model of cutaneous candidiasis when *Candida* cells penetrated the corneal layer of the artificial skin (91). Using a clever gene misexpression strategy in the switching strain WO-1 in which white-phase cells misexpressed the opaque-specific gene *SAP1,* Kvaal et al. (60) demonstrated that *SAP1* caused a dramatic increase in cutaneous infection, probably as a result of increased adherence to and "cavitation" of the skin.

The differential expression of *SAP* genes was also observed during systemic infections. In a model of intraperitoneal (i.p.) infection, expression of *SAP2, SAP4* through *-6,* and *SAP9* was greatest when cells invaded parenchymal organs such as the liver and kidney (30). Using in vivo expression technology (IVET), Staib et al. (98) reported that *SAP5* was the most dominant transcript in this model. When *C. albicans* disseminated via the bloodstream and established infections in internal organs, either during late stages of the i.p. model or after intravenous (i.v.) infection, higher levels of *SAP1* through *-3* transcripts were observed (30, 97, 98). This pattern of *SAP* expression during systemic infections suggested a role for *SAP4* through *-6* during the initial phase of organ invasion and *SAP1* through *-3* in later phases when infection in organs had already been established. The contribution of the proteinases to *C. albicans* virulence was also supported by the observation that *C. albicans* strains from human immunodeficiency virus (HIV)-infected patients had heightened proteinase production compared with isolates from non-HIV-infected individuals (20, 64, 82). Selection and adaptation in these patients are likely to be responsible for the enhanced proteinase activity; however, it cannot be excluded that direct binding of HIV proteins to *Candida* cells (39) or the treatment with antifungal drugs (115) may also influence the proteolytic activities of *Candida* cells in vivo.

Contribution of Sap Proteinases to *C. albicans* Infections: Use of Proteinase Inhibitors and Virulence of Proteinase-Deficient Mutants

In vitro and animal model studies have compellingly shown that Saps are expressed and secreted during different stages and types of *Candida* infections. Recent studies using proteinase inhibitors and *C. albicans* strains lacking distinct proteinase genes suggest that these expressed proteinases indeed contribute to the virulence of this fungus. Fallon et al. (27) used the aspartic proteinase inhibitor pepstatin A to show that inhibition of Saps prevented the initial penetration of *C. albicans* through mucosal surfaces, but not the dissemination of *C. albicans* once the cells had already reached the blood vessels. Pepstatin A also inhibited invasion of oral epithelia and skin by *C. albicans* in models of experimental infections (89, 91). De Bernardis et al. (21, 23) demonstrated similar protective effects in a rat vaginitis model where postinfectious administration of pepstatin A greatly accelerated the clearance of *C. albicans* from the rat vagina.

The interest in discovering new compounds that inhibit Sap activity was also recently given a surprising boost as a result of the evolving HIV epidemic. The observation that AIDS patients on highly active antiretroviral therapy (HAART), a cocktail of HIV aspartic proteinase and reverse transcriptase inhibitors, had reduced prevalence of oral candidiasis led to the hypothesis that HIV aspartic proteinase inhibitors may also act against *Candida* aspartic proteinases in vivo and consequently prevent or reduce the fungal infections (14, 42). In fact, several clinically used HIV proteinase inhibitors were able to inhibit Sap activity (13, 40, 57, 69). Furthermore, pepstatin A and HIV proteinase inhibitors were able to reduce the adherence of *C. albicans* to epithelial cells, suggesting that proteinase activity is involved in the attachment of *Candida* cells to host surfaces, thus providing one possible explanation for the reduction of *Candida* infections in HIV patients treated with HAART (9, 81, 110). These in vitro and in vivo data illustrating the protective effects of pepstatin A and HIV proteinase inhibitors at mucosal surfaces implicate members of the proteinase family in the early stages of *C. albicans* infections.

Studies showing the protective effects of pepstatin A enhanced the efforts to develop novel Sap-specific inhibitors. Sequence analysis, sequence comparison, and crystallization of purified *Candida* proteinases provided new insights into the molecular interactions within the active site, which was essential for the development of new and selective inhibitors such as A-70450 (11).

Although the inhibition of proteolytic activity of medically important *Candida* species demonstrated the general importance of Saps for infection, the defined role and function of the different isoenzymes had to be investigated by molecular approaches, such as the creation of mutants lacking distinct *SAP* genes. These experiments showed that distinct isoenzymes were needed to act at different stages of an infection or during different types of infections, and also that not all *Candida* proteinases were important for virulence per se. For instance, Sapt1 secreted by *C. tropicalis* did not contribute to virulence in a model of i.v. infection, as Sapt1-deficient mutants were only slightly less virulent than the wild type (104). Furthermore, heterologous expression of the *C. albicans* Sap2 in the apathogenic yeast *Saccharomyces cerevisiae* did not make it pathogenic (26). Indeed, the uncontrolled or constitutive expression of Saps may even cause harm to the fungus itself (26).

Schaller et al. (89) demonstrated that *SAP1* through -3 but not *SAP4* through -6 contributed significantly to *C. albicans* infection of artificial oral mucosa (Fig. 4). However, the *SAP*-disrupted mutants were not avirulent, which may be due to the observed up-regulation of alternative *SAP* genes (89) or may implicate other factors in the virulence of *C. albicans* in this model. A major role for *SAP1* through -3 but not *SAP4* through -6 was also demonstrated in experimental vaginal infections using *SAP*-disrupted mutants (22). In contrast, *SAP4* through -6 but not *SAP1* through -3 appeared to be essential for systemic infections, as mutants lacking *SAP4* through -6 were almost avirulent in two rodent models of i.v. infections (49, 86). *SAP4* through -6 also appear to be required for organ invasion after i.p. infection, as mutants lacking *SAP4* through -6 had a significantly reduced ability to cause tissue damage of liver and other parenchymal organs (30, 59). This was most noticeable for *SAP6*-deficient mutants (30). Using the Sap-deficient mutants, Ibrahim et al. (52) showed that although Sap 1 through -3 activity was not necessary for the adherence of *C. albicans* to endothelial cells, Sap2 activity was required for the initial stages of endothelial cell injury. In vivo, this may enable *C. albicans* to escape from blood vessels and cause disseminated infections or to evade immune attack. *SAP4* through -6 may also contribute to *C. albicans* virulence by resisting phagocytic attack, since the corresponding proteinases were mostly expressed by *C. albicans* in phagolysosomes of murine peritoneal macrophages or neutrophils (8, 87). This postulation was indirectly confirmed when a *SAP4* through -6-deficient mutant was shown to be eliminated 53% more effectively after phagocytosis of macrophages (8).

Possible Functions of Secreted Proteinases

Although the *C. albicans* proteinases are known virulence factors, the targets of proteolytic attack are less clear. In vitro experiments show that Saps, generally Sap2, can hydrolyze structural host proteins, proteins of the immune system, proteins of host cascade systems, proteinase inhibitors, or regulatory polypeptides to support colonization, persistence, and invasion. Extracellular matrix and host surface proteins such as laminin, fibronectin, and mucin are also efficiently degraded by Sap2 (15, 75, 85). This degradation of host surface molecules may play a role during the adherence of *Candida* cells to buccal epithelial cells (110). Sap2 can also hydrolyze a number of humoral host defense proteins (55) including secretory IgA, which is normally resistant to most bacterial proteinases (85). The view that *Candida* proteinases may activate host protein precursors is not only supported by the in vitro activation of blood clotting factors (54), the inactivation of the epidermal cysteine proteinase inhibitor cystatin A (108), or the cleavage of human big endothelin-1 (a vasoconstrictive peptide) (107), but also by the in vivo observation that the overall circulating proteolytic activity in traumatized mice challenged with *C. albicans* is enhanced (78). Furthermore, *Candida* proteinases were shown to activate the proinflammatory cytokine interleukin-1β from its precursor, suggesting a role for Saps in the activation and maintenance of the inflammatory response at epithelial surfaces in vivo (5). In summary, the data indicated that *C. albicans* proteinases are likely to have multiple targets and functions in vivo, some of which are illustrated in Table 3.

EXTRACELLULAR PHOSPHOLIPASES OF *C. ALBICANS*

Phospholipases have the ability to hydrolyze one or more ester linkages in glycerophospholipids and have been implicated as putative virulence factors in many bacterial and protozoan infections, such as

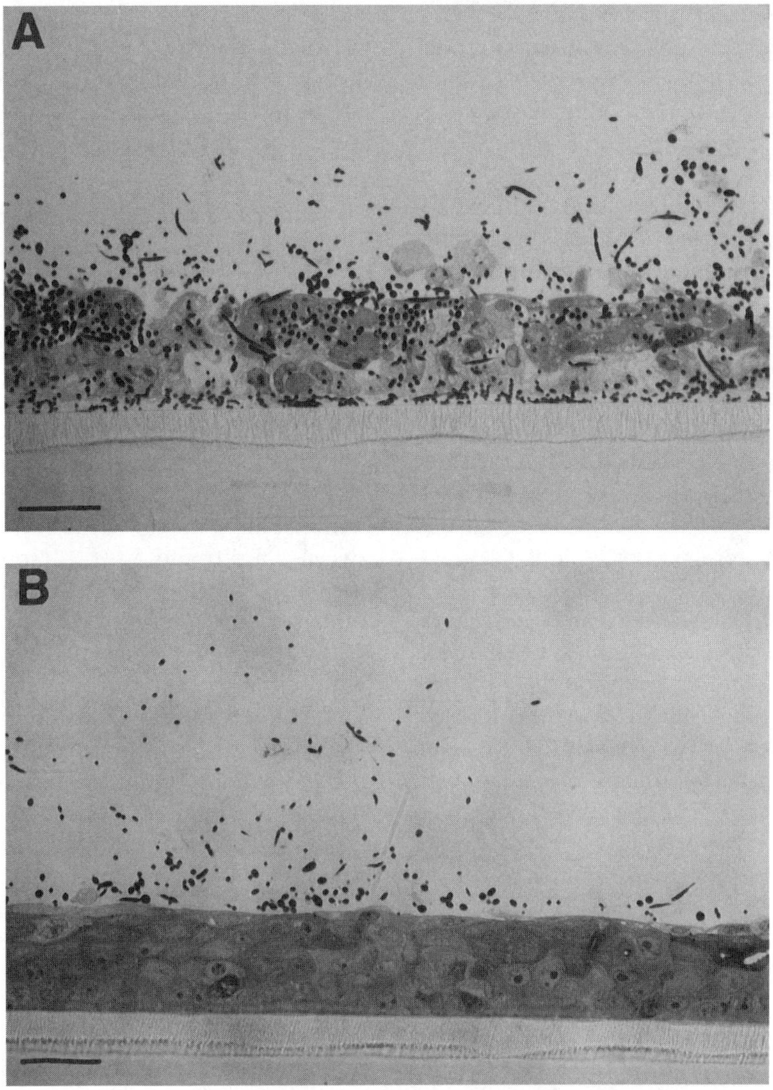

Figure 4. Effect of pepstatin A inhibition of Saps in a model of oral candidiasis based on reconstituted human epithelium (RHE). (A) Light micrograph of untreated RHE 12 h after inoculation with *C. albicans* (strain SC5314). *Candida* cells penetrated into the epithelium and caused severe mucosal erosion with vacuolation, edema, and enlarged intercellular spaces within all keratinocyte layers. (B) In the presence of 15 μM pepstatin A, few *Candida* cells adhered to the superficial keratinocytes and did not cause marked morphological alterations 12 h after inoculation, indicating a strong protective effect of the proteinase inhibitor. (× 400; bars = 10 μm). Photograph by courtesy of M. Schaller.

Table 3. Possible targets of the *C. albicans* proteinases

Target	Possible function	Reference(s)
Host protein	Nutrient acquisition	45
Host tissue, surface proteins	Adhesion	81, 85, 110
Host tissue, surface proteins, extracellular matrix proteins	Penetration and invasion (cell and tissue damage)	15, 75, 85
Immunoglobulins, leukocyte proteins, cytokines, defensins, α-macroglobulin, complement, etc.	Immune evasion or escape	8, 55, 85
Endothelial cell proteins	Cell injury after phagocytosis	52
Coagluation factor, clotting factor, prothrombin, proteins of the kallikrein-kinin system	Activation of blood clotting cascade; enhanced vascular permeability	53, 54

those caused by *Rickettsia prowazekii* and *Rickettsia rickettsii, Listeria monocytogenes, Clostridium perfringens, Staphylococcus aureus, Toxoplasma gondii,* and *Entamoeba histolytica,* and fungal infections, such as those caused by *Aspergillus fumigatus, Cryptococcus neoformans,* and *C. albicans*. Depending on the mode of action and the target within the phospholipid molecule, phospholipases (PLs) are divided into different subclasses: phospholipase A, phospholipase B, lysophospholipase, lysophospholipase-transacylase, phospholipase C, and phospholipase D (36). In *C. albicans,* extracellular phospholipases A (3), B (4), and C (83) have been reported, although extracellular lysophospholipase and lysophospholipase-transacylase activities may also be contained within the same enzymes (51).

Genes Coding for Secreted Phospholipases

Over the years there have been conflicting reports over the number and subclasses of phospholipase enzymes secreted by *C. albicans,* probably due to differences in growth conditions, purification methods, and the type and sensitivity of the assays used. To date, only two extracellular phospholipase B genes, named *PLB1* (44, 62) and *PLB2* (101), have been identified and cloned (Table 4). However, it is likely that more genes encoding extracellular phospholipases will be found.

Since phospholipase B activity was the major phospholipase activity in supernatants of *C. albicans* cultures, PCR approaches were used to clone the corresponding genes (44, 62). The first gene identified (*PLB1*) was located on chromosome 6 and the deduced amino acid sequence was 45% identical to its counterpart in *S. cerevisiae*. *PLB1* contained an N-terminal signal sequence, a conserved Gly-X-Ser-Gly motif found in most lipolytic enzymes, but in contrast to other fungal phospholipase B enzymes, no motifs for a GPI anchor were found (36, 44, 62). Transcripts of *PLB1* were detected in both yeast and hyphal cells (44), but since expression of *PLB1* was increased in *C. albicans* mutants lacking *TUP1*, a repressor of hyphal formation, transcription of *PLB1* may possibly be regulated by factors that also regulate morphology (44). The second phospholipase B gene *PLB2* (101) was 65% identical to *PLB1* and, like PLB1, encoded a preprotein with a signal peptide with no GPI-anchor motifs at the C-terminal end. *PLB2* may account for the remaining PLB activity in *PLB1* null mutants (36).

Purification and Activity of *C. albicans* Phospholipases

The secretion of extracellular phospholipases by *C. albicans* was first reported in the 1960s by Werner (111) after growing *C. albicans* yeast cells on solid media containing lipids. It was not until 1985 that three protein fractions with phospholipase B, lysophospholipase, and lysophospholipase-transacylase activity were purified from *C. albicans* culture supernatants; all were shown to have a pH optimum between pH 4.0 and 5.0 (3). However, another study indicated that the main enzyme in culture supernatants possessed only phospholipase B activity (51). Different forms of lysophospholipase-transacylases with different molecular masses, named LPTA I, LPTA II, and h-LPTA, have been purified (65, 102). The h-LPTA was similar to LPTA I and was a glycoprotein with an estimated molecular mass of 84 kDa with a pH optimum of 6.0 (65).

In earlier studies only *C. albicans* isolates were found to possess phospholipase activity, whereas *C. tropicalis, C. parapsilosis,* and *C. glabrata* did not (61). However, more recently non-*C. albicans* species have also been shown to secrete phospholipases, albeit at lower levels (36). In addition, it had been demonstrated that patient isolates of *C. albicans* produce more phospholipase activity than isolates from *Candida* carriers (51). Furthermore, a correlation between phospholipase activity in vitro and virulence has been demonstrated (4, 58).

In Vivo Expression of *C. albicans* Phospholipases

Using a lecithin-based cytochemical method, Pugh and Cawson (83) demonstrated phospholipase production at the tip of growing hyphae in a chick chorioallantoic membrane model. Leidich et al. (62) later confirmed these early observations by using

Table 4. *C. albicans* phospholipase B genes and deduced proteins

Gene	ORF (bp)	*N*-glycosylation sites	Mature enzyme (aa)	Molecular mass (kDa)	Reference(s)
PLB1	1,815	7	605	66.5[a]	44, 62
PLB2	1,824	6	608	67[a]	101

[a]Predicted from the amino acid sequence. Posttranslational processing and modification may alter molecular weight.

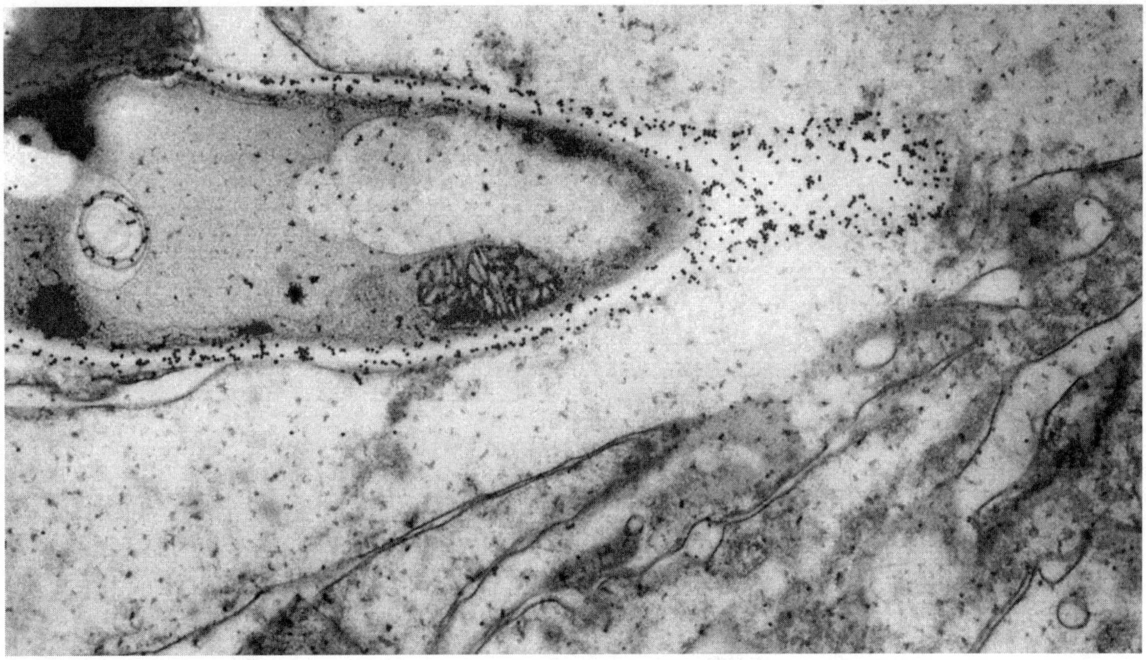

Figure 5. Expression of PLB antigen during invasion of the gastrointestinal mucosa of mice (36). Most immunogold-labeled PLB antigen was detected within the cell wall and at the growing tip in agreement with earlier observations (83). Magnification, ×10,000. Photograph by courtesy of M. Ghannoum. Reprinted from reference 36 with permission.

polyclonal antibodies against purified phospholipase B. The antigen was detected on both yeast and hyphal cells of the wild-type strain and in the surrounding area of *C. albicans* cells, but not on the surface of mutants lacking the major phospholipase B enzyme. The secretion of phospholipase B was also demonstrated during the invasion of the gastrointestinal tract of mice (36) (Fig. 5). Phospholipase B is also produced during human infection, as sera from patients with invasive candidal infection reacted with purified phospholipase B (36).

Contribution of Phospholipases to *C. albicans* Infections

The functions of phospholipases during *C. albicans* infections are not precisely known, but they have been implicated in host cell penetration (36) and may interact with host signal transduction pathways (31). In combination with fluconazole, beta-blocker-like structures, which inhibit phospholipase activity, prevented death in mice inoculated with lethal doses of *C. albicans* (41). Histological examinations indicated these agents acted by inhibiting *C. albicans* tissue penetration. In an i.v. model of murine candidiasis, the virulence of *C. albicans* mutants lacking *PLB1,* which had 1% of the extracellular phospholipase B activity of the wild-type strain, was shown to be significantly attenuated (62). The mouse survival rate increased, the fungal burden in the kidneys was lower, and no candidal foci were detected on renal surfaces (36). Furthermore, the *PLB1*-disrupted mutant was less invasive and caused a reduced inflammatory response in an oral-intragastric infant-mouse model (36). Taken together, these data indicate that candidal phospholipases may be required for the dissemination of *C. albicans* by both the gastrointestinal and hematogenous routes and provide the most convincing evidence to date regarding the contribution of extracellular phospholipases to the pathogenesis of *C. albicans* infections.

EXTRACELLULAR LIPASES OF *C. ALBICANS*

Whereas extracellular proteinases and phospholipases of *C. albicans* have been well characterized, other secreted hydrolytic enzymes such as lipases or esterases have been widely neglected, despite the fact that lipases of nonpathogenic *Candida* species are commonly used in biotechnology. Both types of enzymes are able to catalyze the hydrolysis of ester bonds of triacylglycerols (2). However, esterases and lipases differ in their ability to act on soluble substrates (24). Lipases hydrolyze ester bonds at the interface between the insoluble triacylglycerol phase and the aqueous phase in which the enzyme is dissolved, whereas esterases act on soluble substrates (2).

Extracellular lipase activity of pathogenic *Candida* species was first described by Werner (111), and a secreted esterase has since been characterized by Tsuboi et al. (106). The esterase was induced by lipids, such as Tween 80, and had an optimal activity on α-naphthyl palmitate at pH 5.5. However, it was not able to hydrolyze triolein, tripalmitin, and α-lecithin and was, therefore, defined as monoester hydrolase. Sheridan and Ratledge (94) have observed that *C. albicans* was able to grow in media with triolein as a sole source of carbon, suggesting that other lipolytic enzymes must exist. The substrate specificity of an extracellular lipase from *C. parapsilosis* was studied by Briand et al. (10) for biotechnology purposes. This lipase showed a high acyltransferase activity in the presence of esters with long-chain fatty acids and particularly unsaturated fatty acids.

Genes Coding for Secreted Lipases

The first lipase gene cloned in *C. albicans* was named *LIP1* (32). When the nonlipolytic yeast *S. cerevisiae* was transformed with *LIP1*, transformants produced a secreted lipase that hydrolyzed Tween and triacylglycerols. These same lipids were able to induce *LIP1* expression in *C. albicans* (32). When *LIP1* was used as a probe against genomic DNA from *C. albicans* in a Southern blot analysis, several bands hybridized, suggesting that similar genes existed in this fungus, which may have constituted a lipase gene family (32). Nine further members of this lipase gene family (*LIP2* to *LIP10*) were subsequently cloned and characterized by Hube et al. (50). The open reading frames of all 10 lipase genes were between 1,281 and 1,416 bp in length and encoded highly similar proteins, with up to 80% identical amino acid sequences (Fig. 6). Each deduced lipase sequence had conserved lipase motifs, four conserved cysteine residues, conserved putative *N*-glycosylation sites, and similar hydrophobicity profiles. All *LIP* genes, except *LIP7,* also encoded an N-terminal signal sequence. Sequences similar to *LIP1* through *-10* were also detected in other pathogenic *Candida* species such as *C. tropicalis, C. parapsilosis,* and *C. krusei* but not in *C. glabrata* or *S. cerevisiae* (32, 50).

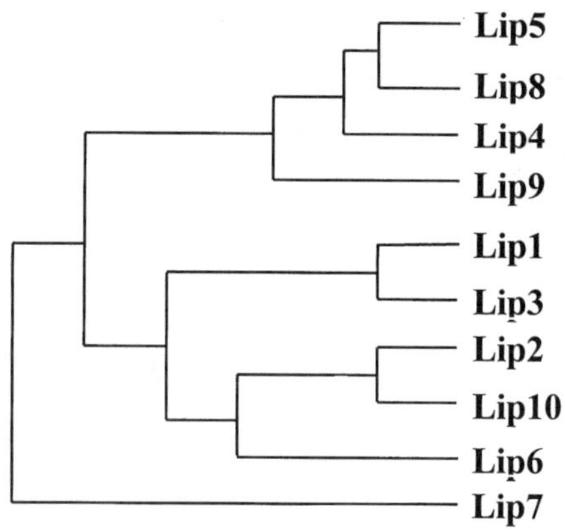

Figure 6. Dendogram of the lipase isoenzyme family of *C. albicans.* All *LIP* genes encode lipases with high similarities to each other and with the same overall structure. Amino acid sequence identities ranged from 33% (between Lip2 and Lip7) to 80% (between Lip5 and Lip8). When clustered, the Lip isoenzyme family could be divided into two subgroups: Lip4, Lip5, Lip8, and Lip9, which were more than 73% identical to each other, and Lip1, Lip2, Lip3, Lip6, and Lip10, which were at least 54% identical to each other. Lip7 was the most divergent lipase in this isoenzyme family. Reprinted from reference 50 with permission of the publisher. Copyright Springer-Verlag.

Expression of *C. albicans* Lipase Genes

The fact that secreted lipases of *C. albicans* are encoded by a family of genes opened the possibility that the lipase genes may be differentially expressed in vitro and in vivo, as has been demonstrated for the *SAP* genes. In vitro expression studies showed that low levels of *LIP3* to *LIP6* were expressed in all media and at all time points of growth tested, independent of the morphological form of the fungus (50). *LIP1, LIP3, LIP4, LIP5, LIP6,* and *LIP8* were expressed in medium with Tween 40 as a sole source of carbon. However, the same genes were also expressed in media without lipids, and two other genes, *LIP2* and *LIP9,* were only expressed in media lacking lipids. This indicates that the transcription of these genes is lipid independent and suggests that lipases may have functions other than solely providing nutrients for the cells. Furthermore, *LIP5, LIP6, LIP8,* and LIP9 were found to be expressed during experimental i.p. infection of mice. Taken together these data indicate lipid-independent, highly flexible in vitro and in vivo expression of a large number of *LIP* genes, possibly reflecting broad lipolytic activity, which may contribute to the persistence and virulence of *C. albicans* in human tissue. However, the roles and functions of lipases during *C. albicans* infections remain to be elucidated.

SUMMARY

The presence of multiple genes encoding extracellular hydrolytic enzymes in *C. albicans* supports the well-accepted viewpoint that candidal pathogenicity is a multifactorial process that is regulated by more than one virulence determinant. The production of a number of hydrolases is a highly regulated and tightly controlled process and suggests that these virulence enzymes are adapted to and contribute to the complex pathogenicity of *Candida* infections. The proteinases in particular appear to be key virulence attributes of *C. albicans* and are known to assist the fungus in the colonization and invasion of host tissues. Although hydrolytic enzymes may contribute to candidal virulence in animal models, their expression, roles, and functions in human infections are not entirely known. Elucidating the complex interaction between hydrolase production and the host during human infections may lead to the development of new prophylactic and therapeutic strategies targeting these virulence enzymes, which would be a valuable addition to the limited repertoire of antifungal agents currently available.

Acknowledgments. We thank Donika Kunze, Robert Koch-Institut, Berlin, and Mahmmoud Ghannoum, University Hospitals of Cleveland and Department of Dermatology, Cleveland, Ohio, for help in preparing this manuscript, and Michel Monod, Centre Hospitalier Universitaire Vaudois, Lausanne, and Martin Schaller, Ludwig Maximilians Universität, München, for making unpublished data available. Our own work is supported by the Deutsche Forschungsgemeinschaft (Hu 528/7 and Hu 525/8), the European Commission ("Galar Fungail"), and the Dunhill Medical Research Trust.

REFERENCES

1. **Abad-Zapatero C., R. Goldman, S. W. Muchmore, C. Hutchins, K. Stewart, J. Navaza, C. D. Payne, and T. L. Ray.** 1996. Structure of a secreted aspartic protease from *C. albicans* complexed with a potent inhibitor: implications for the design of antifungal agents. *Protein Sci.* 5:640–652.
2. **Anthonsen, H. W., A. Baptista, F. Drablos, P. Martel, S. B. Petersen, M. Sebastiao, and L. Vaz.** 1995. Lipases and esterases: a review of their sequences, structure and evolution. *Biotechnol. Annu. Rev.* 1:315–371.
3. **Banno, Y., T. Yamada, and Y. Nozawa.** 1985. Secreted phospholipases of the dimorphic fungus, *Candida albicans*; separation of three enzymes and some biological properties. *Sabouraudia* 23:47–54.
4. **Barrett-Bee, K., Y. Hayes, R. G. Wilson, and J. F. Ryley.** 1985. A comparison of phospholipase activity, cellular adherence and pathogenicity of yeasts. *J. Gen. Microbiol.* 131: 1217–1221.
5. **Beausejour, A., D. Grenier, J. P. Goulet, and N. Deslauriers.** 1998. Proteolytic activation of the interleukin-1beta precursor by *Candida albicans. Infect. Immun.* 66:676–681.
6. **Beggah, S., B. Lechenne, U. Reichard, S. Foundling, and M. Monod.** 2000. Intra- and intermolecular events direct the propeptide-mediated maturation of the *Candida albicans* secreted aspartic proteinase Sap1p. *Microbiology* 146: 2765–2773.
7. **Borg, M., and R. Rüchel.** 1990. Demonstration of fungal proteinase during phagocytosis of *Candida albicans* and *Candida tropicalis. J. Med. Vet. Mycol.* 28:3–14.
8. **Borg-von Zepelin, M., S. Beggah, K. Boggian, D. Sanglard, and M. Monod.** 1998. The expression of the secreted aspartic proteinases Sap4 to Sap6 from *Candida albicans* in murine macrophages. *Mol. Microbiol.* 28:543–554.
9. **Borg-von Zepelin, M., I. Meyer, R. Thomssen, R. Würzner, D. Sanglard, A. Telenti, and M. Monod.** 1999. HIV-protease inhibitors reduce cell adherence of *Candida albicans* strains by inhibition of yeast secreted aspartic proteases. *J. Invest. Dermatol.* 113:747–751.
10. **Briand, D., E. Dubreucq, J. Grimaud, and P. Galzy.** 1995. Substrate specificity of the lipase from *Candida parapsilosis. Lipids* 30:747–754.
11. **Capobianco, J. O., C. G. Lerner, and R. C. Goldman.** 1992. Application of a fluorogenic substrate in the assay of proteolytic activity and in the discovery of a potent inhibitor of *Candida albicans* aspartic proteinase. *Anal. Biochem.* 204: 96–102.
12. **Caro, L. H., H. Tettelin, J. H. Vossen, A. F. Ram, H. van den Ende, and F. M. Klis.** 1997. In silicio identification of glycosyl-phosphatidylinositol-anchored plasma-membrane and cell wall proteins of *Saccharomyces cerevisiae. Yeast* 13: 1477–1489.
13. **Cassone, A., F. De Bernardis, A. Torosantucci, E. Tacconelli, M. Tumbarello, and R. Cauda.** 1999. In vitro and in vivo anticandidal activity of human immunodeficiency virus protease inhibitors. *J. Infect. Dis.* 180:448–453.
14. **Cauda, R., E. Tacconelli, M. Tumbarello, G. Morace, F. De Bernardis, A. Torosantucci, and A. Cassone.** 1999. Role of protease inhibitors in preventing recurrent oral candidiasis in patients with HIV infection: a prospective case-control study. *J. Acquir. Immune Defic. Syndr.* 21:20–25.
15. **Colina, A. R., F. Aumont, N. Deslauriers, P. Belhumeur, and L. de Repentigny.** 1996. Evidence for degradation of gastrointestinal mucin by *Candida albicans* secretory aspartic proteinase. *Infect. Immun.* 64:4514–4519.
16. **Cutfield, S. M., E. J. Dodson, B. F. Anderson, P. C. Moody, C. J. Marshall, P. A. Sullivan, and J. F. Cutfield.** 1995. The crystal structure of a major secreted aspartic proteinase from *Candida albicans* in complexes with two inhibitors. *Structure* 3:1261–1271.
17. **Cutler, J. E.** 1991. Putative virulence factors of *Candida albicans. Annu. Rev. Microbiol.* 45:187–218.
18. **Davies, D. R.** 1990. The structure and function of aspartic proteinases. *Annu. Rev. Biophys. Chem.* 19:189–215.
19. **De Bernardis, F., A. Cassone, J. Sturtevant, and R. Calderone.** 1995. Expression of *Candida albicans SAP1* and *SAP2* in experimental vaginitis. *Infect. Immun.* 63:1887–1892.
20. **De Bernardis, F., P. Chiani, M. Ciccozzi, G. Pellegrini, T. Ceddia, G. D'Offizzi, I. Quinti, P. A. Sullivan, and A. Cassone.** 1996. Elevated aspartic proteinase secretion and experimental pathogenicity of *Candida albicans* isolates from oral cavities of subjects infected with human immunodeficiency virus. *Infect. Immun.* 64:466–471.
21. **De Bernardis, F., M. Boccanera, D. Adriani, E. Spreghini, G. Santoni, and A. Cassone.** 1997. Protective role of antimannan and anti-aspartic proteinase antibodies in an experimental model of *Candida albicans* vaginitis in rats. *Infect. Immun.* 65:3399–3405.
22. **De Bernardis, F., S. Arancia, L. Morelli, B. Hube, D. Sanglard, W. Schäfer, and A. Cassone.** 1999. Evidence that members of the secretory aspartic proteinase gene family, in particular SAP2, are virulence factors for *Candida* vaginitis. *J. Infect. Dis.* 179:201–208.
23. **De Bernardis, F., F. Mondello, G. Scaravelli, A. Pachi, A. Girolamo, L. Agatensi, and A. Cassone.** 1999. High aspartic proteinase production and vaginitis in human immunodeficiency virus-infected women. *J. Clin. Microbiol.* 37: 1376–1380.

24. **Derewenda, Z. S., and A. M. Sharp.** 1993. News from the interface: the molecular structures of triacylglyceride lipases. *Trends Biochem. Sci.* **18:**20–25.
25. **De Viragh, P. A., D. Sanglard, G. Togni, R. Falchetto, and M. Monod.** 1993. Cloning and sequencing of two *Candida parapsilosis* genes encoding acid proteases. *J. Gen. Microbiol.* **139:**335–342.
26. **Dubois, N., A. R. Colina, F. Aumont, P. Belhumeur, and L. de Repentigny.** 1998. Overexpression of *Candida albicans* secretory aspartic proteinase 2 and its expression in *Saccharomyces cerevisiae* do not augment virulence in mice. *Microbiology* **144:**2299–2310.
27. **Fallon, K., K. Bausch, J. Noonan, E. Huguenel, and P. Tamburini.** 1997. Role of aspartic proteases in disseminated *Candida albicans* infection in mice. *Infect. Immun.* **65:**551–556.
28. **Felk, A., W. Schäfer, and B. Hube.** *Candida albicans* secretory aspartic proteinase (*SAP10*) gene. GENbank accession number AF146440.
29. **Felk, A., W. Schäfer, and B. Hube.** Unpublished results.
30. **Felk, A., M. Kretschmar, M. Schaller, T. Nichterlein, D. Sanglard, M. Monod, H. C. Korting, W. Schäfer, and B. Hube.** Unpublished results.
31. **Filler, S. G., B. O. Ibe, P. M. Luckett, J. U. Raj, and J. E. Edwards, Jr.** 1991. *Candida albicans* stimulates endothelial cell eicosanoid production. *J. Infect. Dis.* **164:**928–935.
32. **Fu, Y., A. S. Ibrahim, W. Fonzi, X. Zhou, C. F. Ramos, and M. A. Ghannoum.** 1997. Cloning and characterization of a gene (*LIP1*) which encodes a lipase from the pathogenic yeast *Candida albicans. Microbiology* **143:**331–340.
33. **Fusek, M., E. A. Smith, M. Monod, and S. I. Foundling.** 1993. *Candida parapsilosis* expresses and secretes two aspartic proteinases. *FEBS Lett.* **327:**108–112.
34. **Fusek, M., E. A. Smith, M. Monod, B. M. Dunn, and S. I. Foundling.** 1994. Extracellular aspartic proteinases from *Candida albicans, Candida tropicalis,* and *Candida parapsilosis* yeasts differ substantially in their specificities. *Biochemistry* **33:**9791–9799.
35. **Ghadjari, A., R. C. Matthews, and J. P. Burnie.** 1997. Epitope mapping *Candida albicans* proteinase (SAP2). *FEMS Immunol. Med. Microbiol.* **19:**115–123.
36. **Ghannoum, M. A.** 2000. Potential role of phospholipases in virulence and fungal pathogenesis. *Clin. Microbiol. Rev.* **13:** 122–143.
37. **Gilfillan, G. D., D. J. Sullivan, K. Haynes, T. Parkinson, D. C. Coleman, and N. A. Gow.** 1998. *Candida dubliniensis:* phylogeny and putative virulence factors. *Microbiology* **144:** 829–838.
38. **Goldman, R. C., D. J. Frost, J. O. Capobianco, S. Kadam, R. R. Rasmussen, and C. Abad-Zapatero.** 1995. Antifungal drug targets: *Candida* secreted aspartic protease and fungal wall beta-glucan synthesis. *Infect. Agents Dis.* **4:**228–247.
39. **Gruber, A., E. Lukasser-Vogl, M. Borg-von Zepelin, M. P. Dierich, and R. Würzner.** 1998. Human immunodeficiency virus type 1 gp160 and gp41 binding to *Candida albicans* selectively enhances candidal virulence in vitro. *J. Infect. Dis.* **177:**1057–1063.
40. **Gruber, A., J. Berlit, C. Speth, C. Lass-Florl, G. Kofler, M. Nagl, M. Borg-von Zepelin, M. P. Dierich, and R. Würzner.** 1999. Dissimilar attenuation of *Candida albicans* virulence properties by human immunodeficiency virus type 1 protease inhibitors. *Immunobiology* **201:**133–144.
41. **Hänel, H., R. Kirsch, H. L. Schmidts, and H. Kottmann.** 1995. New systematically active antimycotics from the beta-blocker category. *Mycoses* **38:**251–264.
42. **Hoegl, L., E. Thoma-Greber, M. Rocken, and H. C. Korting.** 1998. HIV protease inhibitors influence the prevalence of oral candidiasis in HIV-infected patients: a 2-year study. *Mycoses* **41:**321–325.
43. **Homma, M., H. Chibana, and K. Tanaka.** 1993. Induction of extracellular proteinase in *Candida albicans. J. Gen. Microbiol.* **139:**1187–1193.
44. **Hoover, C. I., M. J. Jantapour, G. Newport, N. Agabian, and S. J. Fisher.** 1998. Cloning and regulated expression of the *Candida albicans* phospholipase B (*PLB1*) gene. *FEMS Microbiol. Lett.* **167:**163–169.
45. **Hube, B.** 1996. *Candida albicans* secreted aspartic proteinases. *Curr. Top. Med. Mycol.* **7:**55–69.
46. **Hube, B.** 1998. Possible role of proteinases in *Candida* infections. *Rev. Iberoam. Micol.* **15:**68–71.
47. **Hube, B., C. J. Turver, F. C. Odds, H. Eiffert, G. J. Boulnois, H. Köchel, and R. Rüchel.** 1991. Sequence of the *Candida albicans* gene encoding the secretory aspartate proteinase. *J. Med. Vet. Mycol.* **29:**129–132.
48. **Hube, B., M. Monod, D. A. Schofield, A. J. Brown, and N. A. Gow.** 1994. Expression of seven members of the gene family encoding secretory aspartic proteinases in *Candida albicans. Mol. Microbiol.* **14:**87–99.
49. **Hube, B., D. Sanglard, F. C. Odds, D. Hess, M. Monod, W. Schäfer, A. J. Brown, N. A. Gow.** 1997. Disruption of each of the secreted aspartic proteinase genes *SAP1, SAP2,* and *SAP3* of *Candida albicans* attenuates virulence. *Infect. Immun.* **65:**3529–3538.
50. **Hube, B., F. Stehr, M. Bossenz, A. Mazur, M. Kretschmar, and W. Schäfer.** 2000. Secreted lipases of *Candida albicans:* cloning, characterisation and expression analysis of a new gene family with at least ten members. *Arch. Microbiol.* **174:** 362–374.
51. **Ibrahim, A. S., F. Mirbod, S. G. Filler, Y. Banno, G. T. Cole, Y. Kitajima, J. E. Edwards, Jr., Y. Nozawa, and M. A. Ghannoum.** 1995. Evidence implicating phospholipase as a virulence factor of *Candida albicans. Infect. Immun.* **63:** 1993–1998.
52. **Ibrahim, A. S., S. G. Filler, D. Sanglard, J. E. Edwards, Jr., and B. Hube.** 1998. Secreted aspartic proteinases and interactions of *Candida albicans* with human endothelial cells. *Infect. Immun.* **66:**3003–3005.
53. **Kaminishi, H., M. Tanaka, T. Cho, H. Maeda, and Y. Hagihara.** 1990. Activation of the plasma kallikrein-kinin system by *Candida albicans* proteinase. *Infect. Immun.* **58:** 2139–2143.
54. **Kaminishi, H., H. Hamatake, T. Cho, T. Tamaki, N. Suenaga, T. Fujii, Y. Hagihara, and H. Maeda.** 1994. Activation of blood clotting factors by microbial proteinases. *FEMS Microbiol. Lett.* **121:**327–332.
55. **Kaminishi, H., H. Miyaguchi, T. Tamaki, N. Suenaga, M. Hisamatsu, I. Mihashi, H. Matsumoto, H. Maeda, and Y. Hagihara.** 1995. Degradation of humoral host defense by *Candida albicans* proteinase. *Infect. Immun.* **63:**984–988.
56. **Koelsch, G., J. Tang, J. A. Loy, M. Monod, K. Jackson, S. I. Foundling, and X. Lin.** 2000. Enzymic characteristics of secreted aspartic proteases of *Candida albicans. Biochim. Biophys. Acta* **1480:**117–131.
57. **Korting, H. C., M. Schaller, G. Eder, G. Hamm, U. Böhmer, and B. Hube.** 1999. Effects of the human immunodeficiency virus (HIV) proteinase inhibitors saquinavir and indinavir on the in vitro activity of secreted aspartic proteinases of *Candida albicans* isolates from HIV-infected patients. *Antimicrob. Agents Chemother.* **43:**2038–2042.
58. **Kothavade, R. J., and M. H. Panthaki.** 1998. Evaluation of phospholipase activity of *Candida albicans* and its correlation with pathogenicity in mice. *J. Med. Microbiol.* **47:**99–102.
59. **Kretschmar, M., B. Hube, T. Bertsch, D. Sanglard, R.**

Merker, M. Schroder, H. Hof, and T. Nichterlein. 1999. Germ tubes and proteinase activity contribute to virulence of *Candida albicans* in murine peritonitis. *Infect. Immun.* **67:** 6637–6642.

60. **Kvaal, C., S. A. Lachke, T. Srikantha, K. Daniels, J. McCoy, and D. R. Soll.** 1999. Misexpression of the opaque-phase-specific gene *PEP1* (*SAP1*) in the white phase of *Candida albicans* confers increased virulence in a mouse model of cutaneous infection. *Infect. Immun.* **67:**6652–6662.
61. **Lane, T., and J. R. Garcia.** 1991. Phospholipase production in morphological variants of *Candida albicans. Mycoses* **34:** 217–220.
62. **Leidich, S. D., A. S. Ibrahim, Y. Fu, A. Koul, C. Jessup, J. Vitullo, W. Fonzi, F. Mirbod, S. Nakashima, Y. Nozawa, and M. A. Ghannoum.** 1998. Cloning and disruption of caPLB1, a phospholipase B gene involved in the pathogenecity of *Candida albicans. J. Biol. Chem.* **273:**26078–26086.
63. **Lerner, C. G., and R. C. Goldman.** 1993. Stimuli that induce production of *Candida albicans* extracellular aspartyl proteinase. *J. Gen. Microbiol.* **139:**1643–1651.
64. **McCullough, M., B. Ross, and P. Reade.** 1995. Characterization of genetically distinct subgroup of *Candida albicans* strains isolated from oral cavities of patients infected with human immunodeficiency virus. *J. Clin. Microbiol.* **33:** 696–700.
65. **Mirbod, F., Y. Banno, M. A. Ghannoum, A. S. Ibrahim, S. Nakashima, Y. Kitajima, G. T. Cole, and Y. Nozawa.** 1995. Purification and characterization of lysophospholipase-transacylase (h-LPTA) from a highly virulent strain of *Candida albicans. Biochim. Biophys. Acta* **1257:**181–188.
66. **Miyasaki, S. H., T. C. White, and N. Agabian.** 1994. A fourth secreted aspartic proteinase gene (*SAP4*) and a CARE2 repetitive element are located upstream of the *SAP1* gene in *Candida albicans. J. Bacteriol.* **176:**1702–1710.
67. **Monod, M., G. Togni, B. Hube, and D. Sanglard.** 1994. Multiplicity of genes encoding secreted aspartic proteinases in *Candida* species. *Mol. Microbiol.* **13:**357–368.
68. **Monod, M., B. Hube, D. Hess, and D. Sanglard.** 1998. Differential regulation of *SAP8* and *SAP9,* which encode two new members of the secreted aspartic proteinase family in *Candida albicans. Microbiology* **144:**2731–2737.
69. **Monod, M., M. Borg-von Zepelin, A. Telenti, and D. Sanglard.** 1999. The inhibition of *Candida albicans* secreted aspartic proteases by three different HIV protease inhibitors. *Dermatology* **198:**412–414.
70. **Monod, M.** Unpublished results.
71. **Morrison, C. J., S. F. Hurst, S. L. Bragg, R. J. Kuykendall, H. Diaz, J. Pohl, and E. Reiss.** 1993. Heterogeneity of the purified extracellular aspartyl proteinase from *Candida albicans:* characterization with monoclonal antibodies and N-terminal amino acid sequence analysis. *Infect. Immun.* **61:** 2030–2036.
72. **Morrison, C. J., S. F. Hurst, S. L. Bragg, R. J. Kuykendall, H. Diaz, D. W. McLaughlin, and E. Reiss.** 1993. Purification and characterization of the extracellular aspartyl proteinase of *Candida albicans:* removal of extraneous proteins and cell wall mannoprotein and evidence for lack of glycosylation. *J. Gen. Microbiol.* **139:**1177–1186.
73. **Morrow, B., T. Srikantha, and D. R. Soll.** 1992. Transcription of the gene for a pepsinogen, PEP1 is regulated by white-opaque switching in *Candida albicans. Mol. Cell. Biol.* **12:** 2997–3005.
74. **Morrow, B., H. Ramsey, and D. R. Soll.** 1994. Regulation of phase-specific genes in the more general switching system of *Candida albicans* strain 3153A. *J. Med. Vet. Mycol.* **32:** 287–294.
75. **Morschhäuser, J., R. Virkola, T. K. Korhonen, and J. Hacker.** 1997. Degradation of human subendothelial extracellular matrix by proteinase-secreting *Candida albicans. FEMS Microbiol. Lett.* **153:**349–355.
76. **Naglik, J. R., G. Newport, T. C. White, L. L. Fernandes-Naglik, J. S. Greenspan, D. Greenspan, S. P. Sweet, S. J. Challacombe, and N. Agabian.** 1999. In vivo analysis of secreted aspartic proteinase expression in human oral candidiasis. *Infect. Immun.* **67:**2482–2490.
77. **Naglik, J. R., D. Greenspan, J. S. Greenspan, N. Agabian, and S. J. Challacombe.** Unpublished results.
78. **Neely, A. N., R. G. Miller, and I. A. Holder.** 1994. Proteolytic activity and fatal gram-negative sepsis in burned mice: effect of exogenous proteinase inhibition. *Infect. Immun.* **62:** 2158–2164.
79. **Newport, G., and N. Agabian.** 1997. *KEX2* influences *Candida albicans* proteinase secretion and hyphal formation. *J. Biol. Chem.* **272:**28954–28961.
80. **Odds, F. C.** 1994. *Candida* species and virulence. *ASM News* **60:**313–318.
81. **Ollert, M. W., R. Söhnchen, H. C. Korting, U. Ollert, S. Bräutigam, and W. Bräutigam.** 1993. Mechanisms of adherence of *Candida albicans* to cultured human epidermal keratinocytes. *Infect. Immun.* **61:**4560–4568.
82. **Ollert, M. W., C. Wende, M. Gorlich, C. G. McMullan-Vogel, M. Borg-von Zepelin, C. W. Vogel, and H. C. Korting.** 1995. Increased expression of *Candida albicans* secretory proteinase, a putative virulence factor, in isolates from human immunodeficiency virus-positive patients. *J. Clin. Microbiol.* **33:**2543–2549.
83. **Pugh, D., and R. A. Cawson.** 1977. The cytochemical localization of phospholipase in *Candida albicans* infecting the chick chorio-allantoic membrane. *Sabouraudia* **15:**29–35.
84. **Rüchel, R., F. Zimmermann, B. Böning-Stutzer, and U. Helmchen.** 1991. Candidiasis visualized by proteinase-directed immunofluorescence. *Virchows Arch. A Pathol. Anat. Histopathol.* **419:**199–202.
85. **Rüchel, R.** 1992. Proteinase, p. 17–31. *In* J. E. Bennett, R. J. Hay, and P. K. Peterson (ed.), *New Strategies in Fungal Disease.* Churchill Livingstone, Edinburgh, United Kingdom.
86. **Sanglard, D., B. Hube, M. Monod, F. C. Odds, and N. A. Gow.** 1997. A triple deletion of the secreted aspartic proteinase genes *SAP4, SAP5,* and *SAP6* of *Candida albicans* causes attenuated virulence. *Infect. Immun.* **65:**3539–3546.
87. **Schaller, M.** Unpublished results.
88. **Schaller, M., W. Schäfer, H. C. Korting, and B. Hube.** 1998. Differential expression of secreted aspartic proteinases in a model of human oral candidiasis and in patient samples from the oral cavity. *Mol. Microbiol.* **29:**605–615.
89. **Schaller, M., H. C. Korting, W. Schäfer, J. Bastert, W. Chen, and B. Hube.** 1999. Secreted aspartic proteinase (Sap) activity contributes to tissue damage in a model of human oral candidiasis. *Mol. Microbiol.* **34:**169–180.
90. **Schaller, M., B. Hube, M. W. Ollert, W. Schäfer, M. Borg-von Zepelin, E. Thoma-Greber, and H. C. Korting.** 1999. In vivo expression and localization of *Candida albicans* secreted aspartic proteinases during oral candidiasis in HIV-infected patients. *J. Invest. Dermatol.* **112:**383–386.
91. **Schaller, M., C. Schackert, H. C. Korting, E. Januschke, and B. Hube.** 2000. Invasion of *Candida albicans* correlates with expression of secreted aspartic proteinases during experimental infection of human epidermis. *J. Invest. Dermatol.* **114:** 712–717.
92. **Schröppel, K., K. Sprosser, M. Whiteway, D. Y. Thomas, M. Röllinghoff, and C. Csank.** 2000. Repression of hyphal proteinase expression by the mitogen-activated protein

(MAP) kinase phosphatase cpp1p of *Candida albicans* is independent of the MAP kinase cek1p. *Infect. Immun.* **68:** 7159–7161.

93. **Schweizer, A., S. Rupp, B. N. Taylor, M. Röllinghoff, and K. Schröppel.** 2000. The TEA/ATTS transcription factor CaTec1p regulates hyphal development and virulence in *Candida albicans. Mol. Microbiol.* **38:**435–445.
94. **Sheridan, R., and C. Ratledge.** 1996. Changes in cell morphology and carnitine acetyltransferase activity in *Candida albicans* following growth on lipids and serum and after in vivo incubation in mice. *Microbiology* **142:**3171–3180.
95. **Smolenski, G., P. A. Sullivan, S. M. Cutfield, and J. F. Cutfield.** 1997. Analysis of secreted aspartic proteinases from *Candida albicans:* purification and characterization of individual Sap1, Sap2 and Sap3 isoenzymes. *Microbiology* **143:** 349–356.
96. **Staib, F.** 1965. Serum-proteins as nitrogen source for yeastlike fungi. *Sabouraudia* **4:**187–193.
97. **Staib, P., M. Kretschmar, T. Nichterlein, G. Köhler, S. Michel, H. Hof, J. Hacker, and J. Morschhäuser.** 1999. Host-induced, stage-specific virulence gene activation in *Candida albicans* during infection. *Mol. Microbiol.* **32:**533–546.
98. **Staib, P., M. Kretschmar, T. Nichterlein, H. Hof, and J. Morschhäuser.** 2000. Differential activation of a *Candida albicans* virulence gene family during infection. *Proc. Natl. Acad. Sci. USA* **97:**6102–6107.
99. **Stewart, K. W., R. C. Goldman, and C. Abad-Zapatero.** 1999. The secreted proteinases from *Candida:* challenges for structure-aided drug design, p. 117–138. *In* B. M. Dunn (ed.), *Proteases of Infectious Agents.* Academic Press, London, United Kingdom.
100. **Stringaro, A., P. Crateri, G. Pellegrini, G. Arancia, A. Cassone, and F. De Bernardis.** 1997. Ultrastructural localization of the secretory aspartic proteinase in *Candida albicans* cell wall in vitro and in experimentally infected rat vagina. *Mycopathologia* **137:**95–105.
101. **Sugiyama, Y., S. Nakashima, F. Mirbod, H. Kanoh, Y. Kitajima, M. A. Ghannoum, and Y. Nozawa.** 1999. Molecular cloning of a second phospholipase B gene, *caPLB2* from *Candida albicans. Med. Mycol.* **37:**61–67.
102. **Takahashi, M., Y. Banno, and Y. Nozawa.** 1991. Secreted *Candida albicans* phospholipases: purification and characterization of two forms of lysophospholipase-transacylase. *J. Med. Vet. Mycol.* **29:**193–204.
103. **Togni, G., D. Sanglard, R. Falchetto, and M. Monod.** 1991. Isolation and nucleotide sequence of the extracellular acid protease gene (ACP) from the yeast *Candida tropicalis. FEBS Lett.* **286:**181–185.
104. **Togni, G., D. Sanglard, and M. Monod.** 1994. Acid proteinase secreted by *Candida tropicalis:* virulence in mice of a proteinase negative mutant. *J. Med. Vet. Mycol.* **32:**257–265.
105. **Togni, G., D. Sanglard, M. Quadroni, S. I. Foundling, and M. Monod.** 1996. Acid proteinase secreted by *Candida tropicalis:* functional analysis of preproregion cleavages in *C. tropicalis* and *Saccharomyces cerevisiae. Microbiology* **142:** 493–503.
106. **Tsuboi, R., H. Komatsuzaki, and H. Ogawa.** 1996. Induction of an extracellular esterase from *Candida albicans* and some of its properties. *Infect. Immun.* **64:**2936–2940.
107. **Tsushima, H., and H. Mine.** 1995. Cleavage of human big endothelin-1 by *Candida albicans* aspartic proteinase. *FEMS Immunol. Med. Microbiol.* **11:**69–72.
108. **Tsushima, H., H. Mine, Y. Kawakami, F. Hyodoh, and A. Ueki.** 1994. *Candida albicans* aspartic proteinase cleaves and inactivates human epidermal cysteine proteinase inhibitor, cystatin A. *Microbiology* **140:**167–171.
109. **Wagner, T., M. Borg von Zepelin, and R. Rüchel.** 1995. pH-dependent denaturation of extracellular aspartic proteinases from *Candida* species. *J. Med. Vet. Mycol.* **33:**275–278.
110. **Watts, H. J., F. S. Cheah, B. Hube, D. Sanglard, and N. A. Gow.** 1998. Altered adherence in strains of *Candida albicans* harbouring null mutations in secreted aspartic proteinase genes. *FEMS Microbiol. Lett.* **159:**129–135.
111. **Werner, H.** 1966. Studies on the lipase activity in yeasts and yeast-like fungi. *Zentralbl. Bakteriol.* **200:**113–124.
112. **White, T. C., and N. Agabian.** 1995. *Candida albicans* secreted aspartic proteinases: isoenzyme pattern is determined by cell type, and levels are determined by environmental factors. *J. Bacteriol.* **177:**5215–5221.
113. **White, T. C., S. H. Miyasaki, and N. Agabian.** 1993. Three distinct secreted aspartic proteinases in *Candida albicans. J. Bacteriol.* **175:**6126–6133.
114. **Wright, R. J., A. Carne, A. D. Hieber, I. L. Lamont, G. W. Emerson, and P. A. Sullivan.** 1992. A second gene for a secreted aspartate proteinase in *Candida albicans. J. Bacteriol.* **174:**7848–7853.
115. **Wu, T., K. Wright, S. F. Hurst, and C. J. Morrison.** 2000. Enhanced extracellular production of aspartic proteinase, a virulence factor, by *Candida albicans* isolates following growth in subinhibitory concentrations of fluconazole. *Antimicrob. Agents Chemother.* **44:**1200–1208.
116. **Zaugg, C., M. Borg-Von Zepelin, U. Reichard, D. Sanglard, and M. Monod.** 2001. Secreted aspartic proteinase family of *Candida tropicalis. Infect. Immun.* **69:**405–412.

Candida and Candidiasis
Edited by Richard A. Calderone
© 2002 ASM Press, Washington, D.C.

Chapter 10

Phenotypic Switching

DAVID R. SOLL

As the combined chapters in this treatise demonstrate repeatedly, *Candida albicans* and related species are highly successful opportunistic pathogens. They are capable of living as an apparently benign commensal in the oral cavity, vaginal canal, and gastrointestinal tract (75, 87, 128), positioned to increase in density and invade tissue as a pathogen, usually in response to a change in host physiology (27, 73, 79, 87, 110). As opportunistic pathogens, *Candida* species can invade virtually every tissue of the human body, depending on the integrity of the host immune system. Colonization is in many situations persistent even after therapies that radically reduce the level of the pathogen and eradicate symptoms, most notably in yeast vaginitis, where the same strain is usually responsible for recurrent infections following repeated, interspersed periods of therapy (127). Its capacity to live both as a commensal and pathogen, to evade the immune system, to evade drug therapy, to invade a variety of body locations, and to adjust so rapidly to changes in host physiology suggests that it has extraordinary phenotypic plasticity, and can adapt rapidly to environmental changes. Populations of infecting organisms can theoretically attain such phenotypic plasticity in three ways. First, by undergoing fusion, meiosis, and recombination, different combinations of genes lead to offspring with different combinations of alleles and different general phenotypes. This form of phenotypic variability generates strains with different pathogenic capabilities. However, the population structure of *C. albicans* suggests that if recombination does occur, it is a rare event (35, 95, 153), and the recent success in fusing cells by generating homozygous **a** and α cells failed to induce meiosis or recombination (48, 72). The second way in which infecting populations can attain plasticity is through the rapid modulation of gene expression in response to a change in the food source or in response to an environmental change. Most cell types have the capacity to change metabolism in response to available carbon sources and to alter physiology in response to a sudden change in its environment. The third way in which infecting populations can attain phenotypic plasticity is through complex developmental programs. Such programs can occur in response to an alteration in the environment or can occur spontaneously. The "bud-hypha transition," or "dimorphism," has long been known as a mechanism for generating phenotypic variability in a reversible fashion within an infecting population (13, 37, 117) and has been associated with pathogenesis (5, 17, 45, 60, 66, 67, 74, 101, 111, 115). It represents a complex developmental transition between two phenotypic states that can be regulated in vitro by a number of environmental conditions. However, the phenotypic outcome of this program (i.e., two phenotypic states) may not be complex enough to provide the kind of variability necessary to account for the level of phenotypic plasticity that is suggested by the pathogenic success of *Candida* species. "High-frequency phenotypic switching," on the other hand, can generate a variety of general phenotypes, occurs spontaneously, can be affected by environmental changes, and can have a profound effect on pathogenic traits. Switching has been reported in *C. albicans* (93, 112, 113, 120), *Candida glabrata* (64), *Candida tropicalis* (131), *Candida parapsilosis* (28), and *Cryptococcus neoformans* (30, 34). It appears to be a general mechanism for spontaneously generating a variety of phenotypes within a clonal population, and appears to account for at least a portion of the variability within clonal populations (120).

A GENERAL DESCRIPTION OF SWITCHING

Every strain of *C. albicans* so far tested either undergoes high-frequency phenotypic switching or

David R. Soll • Department of Biological Sciences, University of Iowa, Iowa City, IA 52242.

can be stimulated to do so by low doses of UV irradiation (82, 112). Switching leads to colony variants that in turn switch back to the original parental phenotype at high frequency. The frequency of spontaneous phenotypic switching can vary between 10^{-4} and 10^{-1} (i.e., one switch per 10^4 cell divisions to one switch per 10 cell divisions), and different switch phenotypes of a single strain can exhibit very different rates of switching (97, 112). Switching affects a variety of virulence traits, including the bud-hypha transition (2), and for that reason has been considered a "higher order" virulence trait. Switching combinatorially regulates a number of phase-specific genes at the level of transcription (122, 123) and involves phase-regulated *trans*-acting factors (133, 137). Although the mechanism of switching is unknown, there is reason to believe that acetylation/deacetylation and gene silencing through the *SIR* genes play roles in heritable but reversible changes in chromatin state, presumably at specific switch loci (58, 92, 119, 123, 140). A role for switching in pathogenesis is supported by observations that it occurs at sites of commensalism and infection, and that the frequency of switching is elevated, on average, in the latter. All of these points will be reviewed in this chapter.

THE "REDISCOVERY" OF SWITCHING

In 1932, Negroni (86) described a variant rough colony morphology in *Mycotorula albicans,* which was subsequently renamed *C. albicans.* In 1940, Mackinnon (71) followed colony morphology from a smooth to spiky phenotype, a process he referred to as "dissociation." In 1968, Brown-Thomsen (14) described the genesis of aberrant sectors and colony morphologies in stored cultures, and categorized 15 different colony morphologies, or variant phenotypes, in 300 analyzed strains of *C. albicans.* Brown-Thomsen (14) demonstrated differences among the variants in sugar assimilation patterns and the reduction of tetrazolium salts. This brief literature on phenomena that quite likely included high-frequency phenotypic switching received little attention until 1985, when two independent studies were reported of reversible high-frequency phenotypic switching. Pomes et al. (93) described reversible phenotypic switching in *C. albicans* strain 1001, which normally formed smooth colonies. They found that a low dose of UV, which killed 13% of the cell population, stimulated the formation of "rough" colonies at frequencies of $<10^{-4}$ to 3×10^{-3}. Rough variants in turn generated smooth colonies at a frequency $<9 \times 10^{-4}$, but generated rough colonies with smooth sectors at a frequency of 3.5×10^{-3}. At roughly the same time, Slutsky et al. reported that the common laboratory strain 3153A, which normally formed smooth colonies, generated variant colonies spontaneously at a frequency of approximately 10^{-4} (112). Variant phenotypes included "star," "ring," and "irregular wrinkle" (Fig. 1). Slutsky et al. also demonstrated that a low dose of UV that killed approximately 10% of the cell population stimulated the formation of variant colonies at a frequency of 2.5×10^{-2}, which included besides star, ring, and irregular wrinkle, the phenotypes stipple, hat, and fuzzy (Fig. 1) (112). It was demonstrated that cells exhibiting variant phenotypes were able to switch at high frequency to other variant phenotypes, a characteristic referred to as "interconvertability." In both the Pomes et al. (93) and Slutsky et al. (112) studies, it was demonstrated that switching was reversible at high frequency, distinguishing it from conventional genetic mutation. In Fig. 2, an example is presented of a switch from ring to star. In effect, these two studies established spontaneous high-frequency, reversible phenotypic switching as a mechanism for phenotypic variability in *C. albicans.* Both studies clearly demonstrated that the basic spontaneous frequency of variants among the dominant smooth phenotype in a population of freshly cloned cells of strain 1001 or 3153A was approximately 10^{-4}, well above the frequency of point mutation. That means that to see a variant without UV stimulation, one must examine 10,000 colonies, a point not fully appreciated by some who contended early on that strains like 3153A did not switch after examining 10 or so plates each containing 70 colonies, which represented a total of 700 colonies, roughly 14-fold too few. Some have also contended that variants such as those in the 3153A switching system arose as a result of mutation, but the relative high frequencies of reversibility in this system (97, 112) argued against this contention.

Distinction between the Bud-Hypha Transition and High-Frequency Phenotypic Switching

The term switching has also been applied to the bud-hypha transition, and for that reason, there has been some confusion between the latter and high-frequency switching of colony morphology. The bud-hypha transition can be induced en masse by a variety of environmental cues, including pH, temperature, and composition of the supporting medium (87, 116). It involves the cellular transition between a round or ellipsoidal budding cell, which separates from the daughter cell after cytokinesis, and a narrow multi-compartmented hyphal tube that does not undergo cell separation and usually represses cellular division in intermediate (i.e., nonapical) compartments.

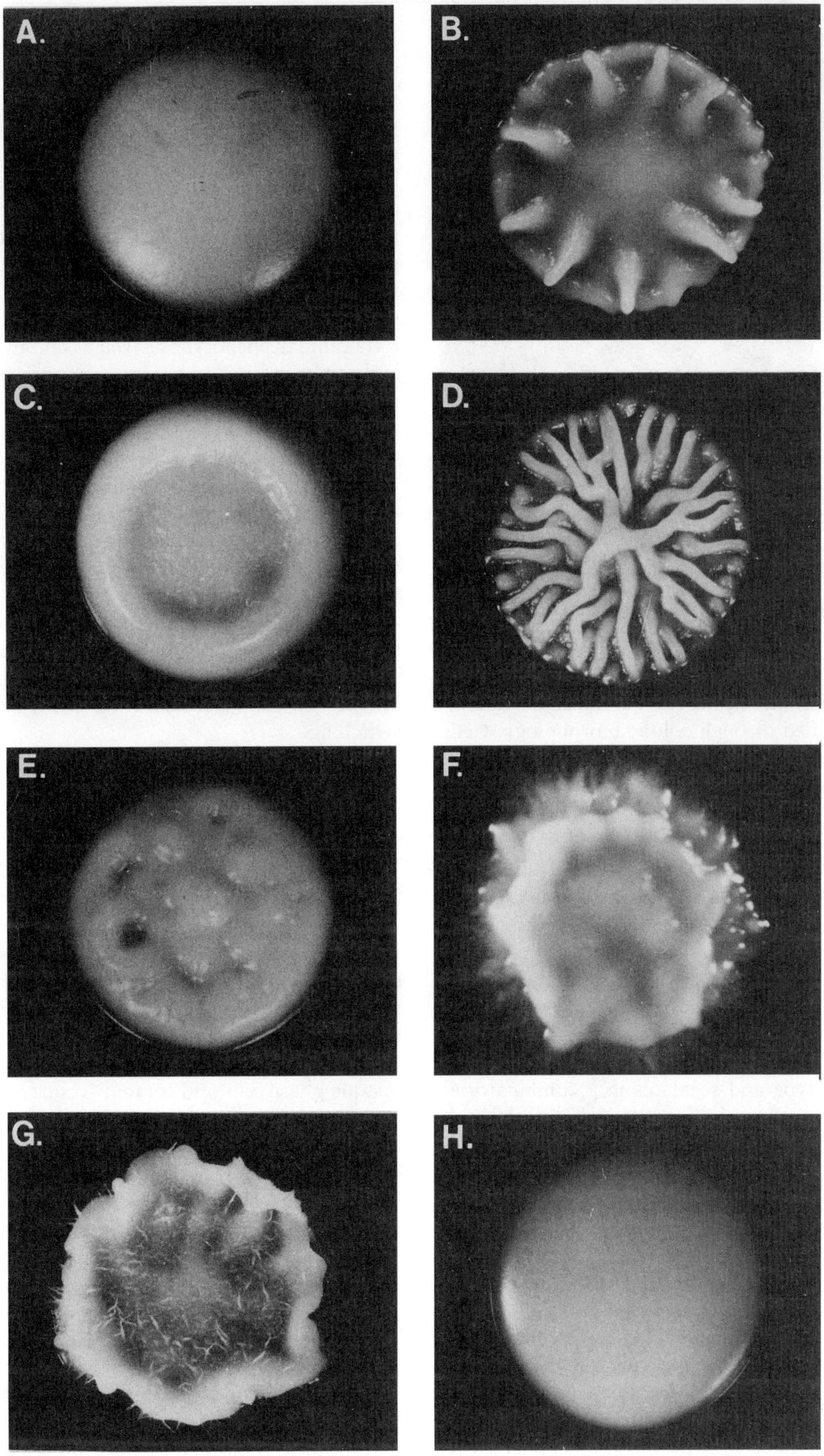

Figure 1. The variant phenotypes in the switching repertoire of *C. albicans* strain 3153A. A, original smooth; B, star; C, ring; D, irregular wrinkle; E, stippled; F, hat; G, fuzzy; H, revertant smooth. Reprinted with permission from reference 112. Copyright 1985 American Association for the Advancement of Science.

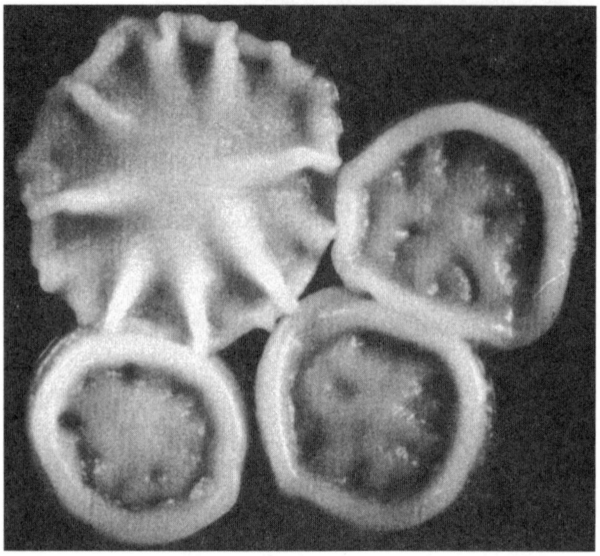

Figure 2. A switch from ring to star in *C. albicans* strain 3153A. Reprinted with permission from reference 112. Copyright 1985 American Association for the Advancement of Science.

Switching, in contrast, occurs spontaneously and is usually identified through colony morphology. Cells in the different switch phenotypes (i.e., different colony morphologies) can be grown in the budding form and induced to generate hyphae without losing their identity based on colony morphology. Except in one case, the opaque to white transition (10, 99, 113), switching cannot be induced en masse, usually involves multiple phenotypes (e.g., seven in the case of strain 3153A), and, as will be described, involves differences in a number of phenotypic characteristics, including the environmental constraints on the bud-hypha transition (2). Therefore, switch phenotypes are maintained whether a cell expresses a budding or hyphal phenotype and regulates in a combinatorial fashion a variety of virulence traits, including the bud-hypha transition.

The White-Opaque Transition: a Model System for Studying Switching

Switching in many strains of *C. albicans* involves multiple phenotypes that sometimes can only be identified on zinc-limiting agar (119). In an analysis of switching in over 100 clinical isolates of *C. albicans* performed in the Soll laboratory between 1985 and 1986, the white-opaque transition was identified in strain WO-1 isolated from the blood of a patient with an ultimately fatal systemic infection (113). Switching in this strain was dominated by a phase transition between a white, hemispherical smooth colony morphology (white phase) and a gray, flat smooth colony morphology (opaque phase). The transition can be recognized on every tested agar, is simple (i.e., involves only two phenotypes), occurs spontaneously at reasonably high frequency in both directions (i.e., one in one thousand cells of a freshly cloned white or opaque phase cell population expresses the opposite phenotype), can be discriminated with the dye phloxine B (i.e., white colonies and white sectors are white or light pink, whereas opaque colonies and sectors stain bright red) (Color plate 3), dramatically affects cellular phenotype as well as colony phenotype, and can be induced to occur en masse in one direction (i.e., opaque to white) by an increase or decrease in temperature (99, 113, 136, 137). It is for these reasons that the white-opaque transition has served as a model for investigating the molecular basis of switching, and has played a prominent role in the discoveries that are described in the following sections. However, it must be kept in mind that the mechanisms that are now being elucidated for the white-opaque transition and the regulation of white and opaque phase-specific genes may or may not be generally applicable to all switching systems in *C. albicans,* as will become clear in the general discussion of the mechanism of switching.

The White-Opaque Transition Impacts Cellular Morphology

The white-opaque transition has a dramatic effect on cellular phenotype as well as colony morphology. Whereas white budding phase cells are round to slightly ellipsoidal and form buds in a fashion similar to that of most other strains of *C. albicans,* opaque phase cells are twice the size of white phase cells, and are elongate or bean shaped, with one end wider than the other (3, 4, 113). A large vacuole is prominent in opaque phase cells and contains vesicles that collapse during fixation and processing for transmission electron microscopy. Perhaps the most unique feature of the opaque phase cell is cell wall architecture. Whereas the wall of white phase cells is smooth when viewed by scanning electron microscopy (SEM), that of opaque phase cells is pimpled. The mean ($\pm$ standard deviation) number of pimples on an opaque phase cell was estimated to be 141 $\pm$ 39, 1.33 pimples per μm^2 (4). In transmission electron microscopy (TEM), channels could be seen traversing the cell wall of the pimple. The blebs observed in SEMs at the apices of pimples appear to be membranous, presumably plasma membrane ballooning through pores. Since these blebs are not observed on living cells under high magnification, there is reason to believe that they are opaque phase-specific SEM artifacts of fixation that reflect opaque phase-specific channels.

GENERAL CHARACTERISTICS OF PHENOTYPIC SWITCHING

Analyses of switching in a variety of *C. albicans* strains and other *Candida* species have provided us with a list of general characteristics of the phenomenon. First, spontaneous switching occurs at frequencies far higher than expected for point mutations (10, 93, 99, 112, 113, 126). Frequencies range from 10^{-4} to 5×10^{-1}. Second, cells can be either in a low-frequency mode or a high-frequency mode of switching, the former in the frequency range of 10^{-4} to 10^{-3}, and the latter in the range of 10^{-2} to 10^{-1}. In several switching systems, the basic smooth phenotype is in a low-frequency mode, while the variants are in high-frequency modes. Third, switching is reversible at high frequency and always generates the original phenotype one started with. Fourth, switching can involve a dominant-phase transition, as in the white-opaque transition (113) or the unmyceliated-myceliated transition (129, 148). Fifth, the switching systems of different *C. albicans* strains may differ in the exact colony phenotypes included in the switching repertoire, but the general characteristics of the switching systems are usually similar (119). Sixth, UV irradiation in all tested cases stimulates switching in strains with very low spontaneous switching frequencies (i.e., 10^{-4} or lower) (82, 93, 97, 112). In addition, temperature (99, 112, 136), the age of a colony (118), and white blood cells and oxidants (59) have been demonstrated to increase the frequency of switching. Seventh, switching can occur without impacting colony phenotype (5, 88). Finally, individual cells can possess more than one switching system (96).

Effects of Switching on Phenotype in General and Virulence Traits in Particular

If switching plays a role in pathogenesis by generating variants in a clonal, infecting population, then variants should differ in the extent to which they express different virulence traits. An analysis of a variety of phenotypic characteristics in the white-opaque transition in strain WO-1 as well as the switching systems of other strains supports this prediction.

Antigenicity

As in bacterial (33) and trypanosome (24) switching systems, switching in *C. albicans* can affect antigenicity (3). A polyclonal rabbit antiserum generated against opaque phase budding cells stained white phase budding cells, white phase hyphae, and opaque phase budding cells (3). When absorbed with white phase budding cells, the antiserum selectively stained hyphae and opaque phase cells, and when additionally absorbed with hyphae, selectively stained opaque phase cells, demonstrating one or more opaque phase-specific antigens were present on the cell wall. Further selective absorption experiments and Western blot analysis demonstrated that the antiserum identified three opaque phase-specific antigens, two intracellular antigens with molecular mass of 21 and 31 kDa, respectively, and one surface antigen with molecular mass of 14.5 kDa. Immuno-gold TEM labeling demonstrated that the 14.5-kDa antigen was localized to the tip of pimples (3).

Adhesion

Switching affects adhesion to human epithelial cells. White phase cells were found to be significantly more adhesive to buccal epithelial cells than opaque phase cells, and opaque phase cells were found to be significantly more hydrophobic than white phase cells (57). In the case of the 3153A switching system, the hierarchy of adhesion to buccal epithelium and stratum corneum was as follows: o-smooth > irregular wrinkle > revertant smooth > star (149).

Hypha formation

Switching affects environmental constraints on the bud-hypha transition. Brown-Thomsen noticed in 1968 that the morphological differences between variants in streaks made on agar were due to differences in the proportions of buds, pseudophyphae, and hyphae (14). The morphologies of variant colonies in the switching system of strain 3153A were also demonstrated to be caused by differences in the proportions and localization of buds, pseudophyphae, and hyphae in the colony domes (118). In the white-opaque transition, Anderson et al. (2) demonstrated that while stationary-phase cultures of white phase budding cells formed hyphae when diluted into fresh medium at pH 4.5 at 37°C, stationary-phase cultures of opaque phase cells treated in the same fashion continued to bud. However, when opaque phase cells were anchored to the chamber wall or to a monolayer of human skin epithelial cells, they formed hyphae. Interestingly, the hyphae formed by opaque phase cells were smooth like those formed by white phase cells when examined by SEM, but formed opaque phase cells when induced to bud (2). These results demonstrate that although both white and opaque phase cells can form hyphae, the environmental constraints and inducing signals differ for the two switch phenotypes.

In the past decade, a variety of genes have been identified that are directly or indirectly involved in hypha formation in *C. albicans*. Mutations in several of these genes led to variant colony morphologies based on the formation of hyphae in the colony dome (e.g., 12, 15, 18). These mutants are not reversible at high frequency, but lead to colony morphologies similar to the switch phenotypes in the 3153A switching system (97, 103, 112) and in the unmyceliated-myceliated transition (129). The similarities suggest that switching in these strains regulates the pathways involved in hypha formation.

Sensitivity to neutrophils

Switching affects the sensitivity of cells to neutrophils and oxidants. Kolotila and Diamond (59) demonstrated that although polymorphonuclear leukocytes phagocytosed white and opaque phase cells equally, white phase cells proved to be more resistant than opaque phase cells to the candidacidal activity of intact polymorphonuclear leukocytes. Similar differences were observed in sensitivities to cell-free oxidants. Perhaps the most interesting observations in these studies, however, were that both polymorphonuclear leukocytes and free oxidants stimulated switching in the white to opaque, but not in the opaque to white direction, a selective effect shared by deletion of the histone deacetylase *HDA1* (58, 140) (see later section on mechanism).

Secretion of proteinase

Switching affects the secretion of proteinase activity (46, 85, 152). Although serum proteins in the supporting medium will stimulate secretion of proteinase activity in white phase cell cultures, this level of stimulation is still 10-fold less than the unstimulated level of secretion in opaque phase cultures (85). Recently, the effects of switching on proteinase secretion in fresh isolates from HIV-positive individuals prior to, during, and after their first episode of oral candidiasis were analyzed (148). In some strains, differences between switch phenotypes differed by as much as 25-fold. As we will discuss in a later section, differences in secretion are due to the activation of opaque phase-specific aspartyl proteinase genes.

Drug susceptibility

Switching affects drug susceptibility. In 1989, Soll et al. (127) presented evidence that switching of a strain responsible for several episodes of recurrent vaginitis changed phenotype and susceptibility to clotrimazole after azole therapy in each successive episode. However, the changes were not in the form of gradual increases in resistance. Rather, the infecting strain switched from smooth to irregular edge to smooth in three sequential episodes, and from low to high to low susceptibility, suggesting that susceptibility was tied more tightly to phenotype than to azole treatment per se. In a recent analysis of drug susceptibility of switch phenotypes in fresh isolates from human immunodeficiency virus-positive individuals, dramatic differences across strains were demonstrated between general switch phenotypes for fluconazole, voricomazole, and 5-FC, but not amphotericin B (148). Within a strain, even more dramatic differences were demonstrated between switch phenotypes. Surprisingly, less dramatic differences were observed between the switch phenotypes of laboratory strains 3153A and WO-1, except in the case of white-opaque phase susceptibility to amphotericin B (148). Both in a study in 1991 (126) and in 2000 (148), opaque phase cells were found to be far more susceptible than white phase cells.

SWITCHING INVOLVES THE REGULATION OF UNLINKED PHASE-SPECIFIC GENES

Switching in *C. albicans*, therefore, differs from that in other pathogens by the pleiotropic effect it exerts on phenotype. The variety of phenotypic characteristics under the regulation of switching in the white-opaque transition suggests that a number of genes must be regulated by switching. Two-dimensional gel electrophoresis of white and opaque phase proteins labeled with ^{35}S-methionine revealed both white and opaque phase-specific proteins (126), and two-dimensional gel electrophoresis of proteins translated from white and opaque phase mRNA in an in vitro translation system (Fig. 3) revealed opaque phase-specific mRNAs (121). Through use of a differential hybridization screen of an opaque phase cDNA library, the first opaque phase-specific gene was cloned in 1992 (85). Sequence analysis revealed that it was a gene encoding an aspartyl proteinase that had been cloned a year earlier by Hube et al. (47). The opaque phase-specific gene cloned from strain WO-1 was named *PEP1* (85) and then renamed *SAP1* (46, 152) when it was discovered that it was a member of a family of secreted aspartyl proteinases. For historical reasons related to switching, therefore, we will refer to this gene as *PEP1(SAP1)* although in the general literature it is referred to simply as *SAP1*. The second cloned opaque phase-specific gene was *OP4*, which has no homology to a known protein (84). This protein contains a hydrophobic region at the amino terminus sufficient to span a plasma membrane. Although *OP4* and *PEP1(SAP1)* are coordinately expressed in the white-opaque transition, they reside

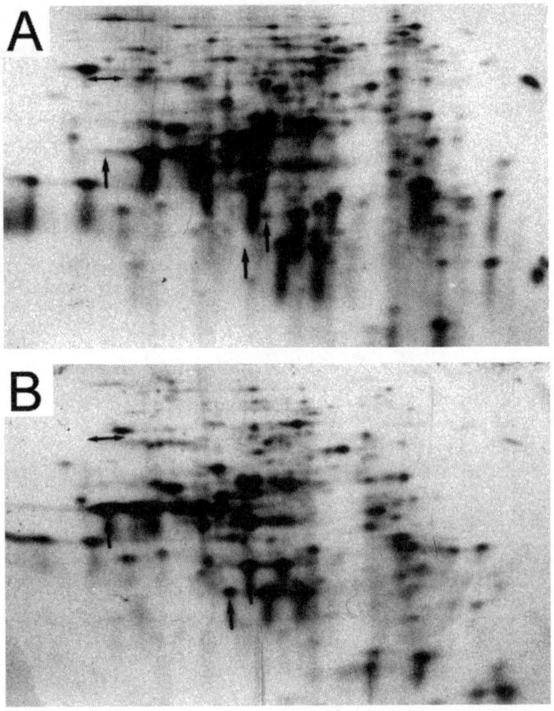

Figure 3. In vitro translation products of mRNA from white (A) and opaque (B) phase cells. Note three proteins (arrows) in opaque not found in white, and charge change (double-headed arrow, upper left of A and B) of one protein.

on different chromosomes (84). The first white phase-specific gene cloned was *WH11* (136). This protein is homologous to the glucose-lipid-regulated protein *GLP1* of *Saccharomyces cerevisiae* (142), which was subsequently identified as a member of a class of low molecular weight heat shock proteins that can serve as chaperones (78). *WH11* is located on a chromosome different from those harboring *SAP1* and *OP4*. The *WH11* protein is distributed throughout the cytoplasm of the opaque phase cell but is excluded from vesicles, nucleus, and plasma membrane (109). A homolog of WH11 was recently cloned from *Aspergillus nidulans,* and has also been found to be developmentally regulated (26). A number of additional white and opaque phase-specific genes have since been identified, including the opaque phase-specific ABC transporter gene *CDR3* (8) and the white phase-specific ABC transporter gene *CDR4* (107), which are members of a family of drug-resistance genes, the white phase-enriched phosphoglycerate mutase gene *GPM1* (67), the opaque phase-specific gene *SAP3* (46), which encodes another aspartyl proteinase, the opaque phase-enriched phosphofructokinase gene *PFK2* (67), the opaque phase-enriched nitric oxide synthase gene *NOS1* (19), and the opaque phase-enriched two component histidine regulator gene, Ca*NIK1* (138). In addition, two genes have been identified that are expressed in both the white and opaque phase, but as different molecular weight transcripts. The transcription factor gene *EFG1* is transcribed as a 3.2-kb transcript in the white phase and a 2.2-kb transcript in the opaque phase (137). The deacetylase gene *HOS3* is transcribed as a 2.5-kb transcript in the white phase and as a 2.3-kb transcript in the opaque phase (140). A more complete list of phase-specific (p-s) and phase-enriched (p-e) genes is presented in Table 1. No doubt, in time, a number of additional phase-specific genes will have been identified, especially when DNA microarrays become available for screening the expression patterns of large numbers of genes.

Although most of what we now know of phase-specific gene regulation has been obtained using the white-opaque transition in strain WO-1 as a model, a limited analysis of the expression of *OP4* and *PEP1-(SAP1)* in the switching system of strain 3153A has revealed important features for complex systems (83). The opaque phase-specific gene *OP4* was expressed in the irregular wrinkle, revertant-smooth, and star phenotypes, but not in the original smooth phenotype. In contrast, *PEP1(SAP1)* was expressed in the star phenotype, but not in either the irregular wrinkle, revertant smooth, or original smooth phenotype. These results demonstrate that expression of these two genes, which are coordinately expressed in the opaque phase of the white-opaque transition, are dissociated in the variant phenotypes of the switching system in strain 3153A. They also lead to a model of combinatorial expression in which different combinations of phase-specific genes are expressed in different variant phenotypes of a complex switching system. Because of the complexity one would expect to be involved in such circuitry, we and others have selected the simpler white-opaque phase transition as a model for analyzing the molecular basis of switching.

Table 1. Genes regulated by the white-opaque transition in *C. albicans* strain WO-1[a]

White phase	Opaque phase
WH11 (p-s)	*OP4* (p-s)
CDR4 (p-s)	*PEP1* (*SAP1*) (p-s)
EFG1-3.2t (p-s)	*SAP3* (p-s)
HOS3-2.5t (p-s)	*CDR3* (p-s)
GPM1 (p-e)	*EFG1*-2.2t (p-s)
	PFK2 (p-e)
	NOS1 (p-e)
	NIK1 (p-e)
	HOS3-2.3t (p-s)

[a]p-s, phase specific; p-e, phase enriched.

CHARACTERIZATION OF PHASE-REGULATED GENE PROMOTERS

To understand how phase-specific genes are regulated, and to begin to generate models of coordinate regulation, the promoters of select white and opaque phase-specific genes have been functionally characterized.

Functional Characterization of the *WH11* Promoter

The first promoter of a phase-specific gene, and for that matter the first promoter of any *C. albicans* gene, functionally characterized was that of *WH11* (133). Because the firefly luciferase gene (*FLUC*), which had been incorporated into the expression vector for characterization, was not translated into a functional protein in *C. albicans* due to altered codon usage, Northern blot analysis was used to quantitate expression of deletion derivatives of the promoter in the white and opaque phases (133). Two *cis*-acting sequences responsible for white phase-specific transcription were identified, a distal activation sequence (DAS) between −475 and −388 bp, and a proximal activation sequence (PAS) between −307 and −230 bp upstream of the transcription start site (133). Deletion of DAS resulted in a sixfold reduction in activity, deletion of PAS resulted in a 15-fold reduction in activity, and deletion of both resulted in the complete loss of activation. Because Northern analysis is time consuming and provides relatively low sensitivity, a chemiluminescent reporter gene was searched for and found that contained no CUG codons, the *Renilla reniformans* luciferase *RLUC* (70). *RLUC* was used to develop a sensitive reporter system for *C. albicans* (134). It was demonstrated that when this reporter construct was integrated at the *ADE2* locus, reporter activity accurately reflected the strength and developmental regulation of the particular promoter that had been inserted upstream at the multiple cloning site (130, 134). With this system, the functional characterization of the *WH11* promoter was repeated (139). Again the two major activation sequences, DAS and PAS, were identified, and in addition, a weaker activation sequence was identified immediately downstream of PAS (Fig. 4). Sequence analysis revealed that the *WH11* promoter contained a number of putative *cis*-acting sequences with affinities to known *trans*-acting factors (e.g., CREB, RAP1, CAAT, and TATA) as well as a binding site for a unique transcription factor, Rbf1p. However, only the binding site for Rbf1p was demonstrated to be within an activation sequence. Ishii (51–53) identified Rbf1p in a *C. albicans* protein extract using the *S. cerevisiae* RPG box of the glycolytic enzyme gene *ENO1* as a trap and demonstrated that recombinant Rbf1p binds directly to PAS.

Functional Characterization of the *OP4* Promoter

The promoter of the opaque phase-specific gene *OP4* was also functionally characterized with the *RLUC* reporter system (68). A deletion that removed the sequence between −854 and −739 bp upstream of the transcription start site of *OP4* reduced opaque phase-specific expression to 50% that of the full-length promoter, and an additional deletion between −469 and −439 bp reduced expression to 20%, but in both cases the reduced level was still opaque phase-specific. Further deletion between −422 and −405 bp resulted in the complete loss of expression. Sequence analysis revealed that the *OP4* promoter contained several sequences homologous to *cis*-acting regulatory sites in other organisms. Two of these, a Ste12p binding site (PRE) and a MADS box protein consensus binding site, fell within the functionally identified proximal enhancer region and the activation region, respectively. In *S. cerevisiae,* Ste12p binds to the pheromone response element (PRE) (23) and Mcm1p binds to a MADS box binding site (91). Ste12p and Mcm1p in turn interact to regulate transcription of pheromone response genes (29). The 14-bp MADS box binding site in the *OP4* promoter was identical to the Mcm1p consensus binding site in *S. cerevisiae* (68). A diagram of the *OP4* promoter is presented in Fig. 5. To test the specificity of the MADS box site in the *OP4* promoter, point mutations were

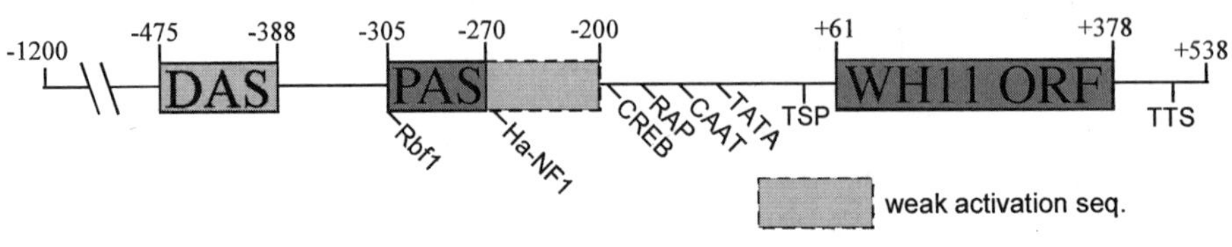

Figure 4. The functionally characterized promoter of the white phase-specific gene *WH11*. DAS, distal activation sequence; PAS, proximal activation sequence; Rbf1, HaNF1, Creb, Rap, CAAT, TATA, sequences with homology to *cis*-acting sequences in other systems; TSP, transcription start site; TTS, transcription termination site; *WH11* ORF, *WH11* open reading frame.

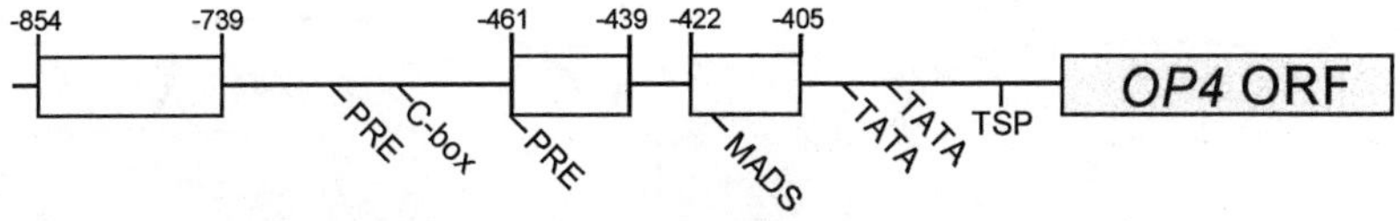

Figure 5. The functionally characterized promoter of the opaque phase-specific gene *OP4*. PRE, pheromone response element; MADS, MADS box binding site; TSP, transcription start site; *OP4* ORF, *OP4* open reading frame.

introduced that result in loss of function in *S. cerevisiae* (1). Phase-specific activation was lost (68). To test directly whether the MADS box site in the *OP4* promoter was necessary for phase-specific activation, the sequence between −416 and −405 bp of the *OP4* promoter was replaced with a polylinker (68). Phase-specific expression was lost. These results, therefore, suggested that the sequences between −854 and −739 bp and between −469 and −439 bp contained enhancers, and the MADS box binding site between −422 and −405 bp was necessary and sufficient for phase-specific activation.

Sequence analysis also revealed that the *OP4* MADS box consensus binding site is bordered upstream by an α2 binding site and downstream by an α1 binding site (Fig. 6). The sites are 78% and 67% identical to the *S. cerevisiae* sites. In *S. cerevisiae,* the Mcm1p binding site of *MAT*a-specific genes is bordered by two α2 sites (108), and *MAT*α-specific genes by one upstream α1 site (54). The *OP4* promoter configuration, with one α2 binding site upstream and one α1 binding site downstream of an Mcm1p binding site, has not been reported in *S. cerevisiae.* Recently, the genes for α1 and α2 as well as **a**1 and **a**2 were identified in *C. albicans* (54). The configuration of the *OP4* promoter (Fig. 7) suggests, therefore, that α1 and α2, in conjunction with Mcm1p, may play roles in the regulation of a subset of opaque phase-specific genes, and raises the possibility that *C. albicans* may have incorporated portions of the mating type regulatory machinery into the machinery for phenotypic switching.

Developing the First Simple Model for Phase-Regulated Gene Expression during Switching

Characterization of the *WH11* and *OP4* promoters demonstrated that white and opaque phase genes are regulated through upstream activation sequences, providing the first simple working model in which white and opaque phase-specific gene expression is controlled by a single white and a single opaque phase-specific activation factor, respectively. In this model, the promoters of genes coordinately expressed in each phase share common *cis*-regulatory sequences. To test this model, promoters were characterized for the additional opaque phase genes *PEP1(SAP1), SAP3,* and the high molecular weight *EFG1* transcript gene, which are coordinately expressed with *OP4* in the opaque phase (46, 85, 152). A preliminary characterization of the *PEP1*(*SAP1*) promoter revealed that although it contains a sequence 60% identical to the MADS box binding site of the *OP4* promoter, this site was outside the activation region (68). More importantly, this site did not substitute for the *OP4* MADS box site in the *OP4* promoter (68). Preliminary characterization of the *SAP3* promoter revealed that a MADS box protein consensus binding site is within the major activation region for opaque phase-specific expression (69). Finally, it was recently demonstrated that the opaque phase promoter of *EFG1* lacks a consensus binding site for any MADS box protein (137). These preliminary results suggest a more complex working model (Fig. 7), one in which a switch from one phase to another leads to the synthe-

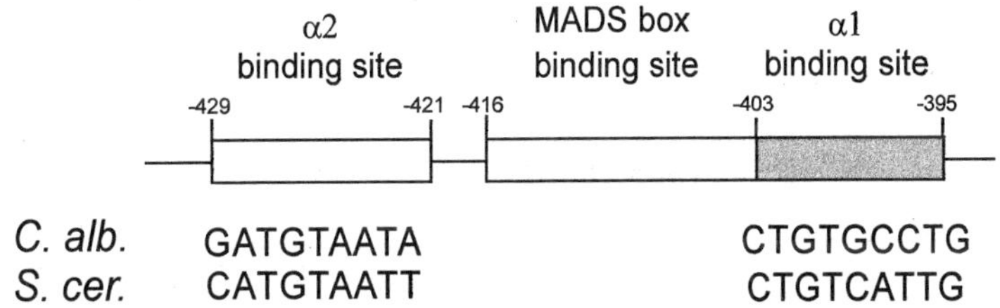

Figure 6. An α1 and α2 binding site border the MADS box binding site in the *OP4* promoter. Sequences are compared to the α1 and α2 binding sites of *S. cerevisiae.*

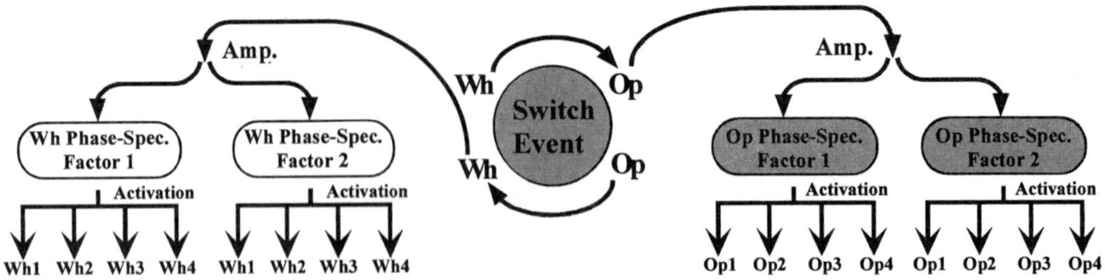

Figure 7. A complex model for the regulation of white and opaque phase genes. Amp., amplification of signal.

sis or activation of multiple phase-specific *trans*-acting factors, each in turn activating a battery of phase-specific genes. This amplification of regulatory complexity predicts that in a "reverse genetic approach" to the elucidation of the switch event (123), in which the circuit from one phase-regulated gene is followed upstream to the switch locus, the most downstream phase-specific gene would be at least three steps away from the switch event.

Gel Mobility Shift Experiments Indicate that *trans*-Acting Factors Interact with Activation Regions of Phase-Specific Gene Promoters

When gel mobility shift experiments were performed with the activation sequences of the *WH11* promoter and with either white or opaque phase cell extract, one white phase-specific complex was identified with DAS, and two with PAS (133). These results suggest that phase-specific factors that interact with DAS and PAS are differentially expressed or activated in the white phase. However, when similar experiments were performed with the activation sequence of the opaque phase-specific gene *OP4*, no phase-specific factors were revealed under the conditions employed (68), suggesting that the same factors interact with the DNA binding sites in the activated and repressed states, and either phase-specific cofactor interactions or factor modifications not revealed by gel retardation experiments are responsible for activation or repression.

Identification of a Phase-Specific *trans*-Acting Factor Downstream of the Switch Event: *EFG1*

EFG1 (66, 132, 137, 141) encodes a protein homologous to transcription factors that are involved in the regulation of cellular morphogenesis in *S. cerevisiae* (32), *A. nidulans* (80), *C. albicans* (see chapter 8), and *N. crassa* (7). Ernst and coworkers reported that *EFG1* was expressed only in the white phase of the white-opaque transition (132). When they deleted *EFG1* in strain CAI8, which undergoes 3153A-like switching (132, 138), the budding cells were elongate like opaque phase cells in strain WO-1, and when they overexpressed *EFG1* in strain WO-1, it stimulated white phase cells to switch to opaque (132). Srikantha et al. also found that transcription of *EFG1* is regulated by the white-opaque transition in strain WO-1 (137), but that regulation was more complex than initially proposed (132). *EFG1* is transcribed as a more abundant 3.2-kb mRNA in the white phase and a far less abundant 2.2-kb mRNA in the opaque phase (137). Using cDNA sequencing and 5′ rapid amplification of cDNA ends, Srikantha et al. further demonstrated that the 1,000-bp difference in molecular size was due to different transcription start sites (137). Finally, using the RLUC reporter system, they demonstrated that although the 1,369-bp region immediately upstream of the ATG transcription start site was sufficient for opaque phase-specific activation of *EFG1*, sequences upstream of −1,369 bp were necessary for white phase-specific activation (137).

To test directly the role of *EFG1* in switching, Srikantha et al. generated null mutants in a *ura3* derivative of strain WO-1 (137). In three independent mutants, cells exhibited an elongate shape, suggesting that the mutant was locked in the opaque phase. However, when cells were shifted from 25 to 42°C, a procedure that induces mass conversion from opaque to white (84, 99, 113, 124, 136), the coordinate activation of the white phase-specific gene *WH11* and the deactivation of opaque phase-specific genes took place concomitantly with the second cell doubling, as in wild-type cells, demonstrating that the fundamental switch event had taken place (137). However, cells did not convert from the elongate to round cell morphology. Scanning electron microscopy revealed that after induction, however, elongate, mutant cells had lost the signature characteristic of opaque phase cells, namely the unique cell wall pimples (137). These results demonstrated that *EFG1* is not essential for the switch event or for the change in cell wall architecture leading to the loss of the opaque phase-specific pimple, but it is essential for generating the round cell morphology of white budding cells, suggesting that *EFG1* regulates expression of one or more genes involved in generating a round cell phenotype. Since *EFG1* transcription is itself regulated by switching, it provides an excellent target in a reverse genetic approach to the basic switch event, since it may be one step closer to the switch event than other phase-regulated genes that encode enzymes (e.g., proteases or ABC transporters) and therefore are positioned at the downstream ends of the regulatory pathways.

REGULATION OF PHASE-SPECIFIC GENES INVOLVES CHANGES IN CHROMATIN STATE

In addition to *trans*-acting factors interacting with *cis*-acting sequences to regulate transcription machinery, the control of eukaryotic gene expression also involves alterations in chromatin state. This is usually achieved by the recruitment of chromatin-modifying activity by both activators and repressors, leading to progressive changes in chromatin along the promoter and gene (143, 144, 151). To test whether the promoters of phase-specific genes undergo changes in chromatin state, Srikantha et al. (135) compared the frequencies of site-specific integration in the expressed and unexpressed phases. In the case of the *WH11* promoter, the frequency of integration at a unique *Spe*I site in the distal activation sequence was sixfold higher in the white phase, and the frequency at a unique *Afl*II site midway between the proximal activation site and the transcription start site was also sixfold higher in the white phase (135). A similar difference was observed at a targeted site in the 3′ end of the *WH11* open reading frame, demonstrating that the entire locus undergoes modification in the switching process. In the case of the opaque phase-specific gene *PEP1*(*SAP1*), the frequency of integration with a fragment containing the *ADE2* gene flanked by 223 bp of the 5′ and 302 bp of the 3′ ends of *PEP1*(*SAP1*) was 30-fold higher in the opaque phase (135). The frequency of integration into *EF1α2*, a constitutively expressed gene, was equal in the two phases (135). These results demonstrate that the regulation of phase-specific genes during switching in *C. albicans* is no exception to the chromatin-modification paradigms that have evolved for eukaryotic gene regulation in general (144). Recent results involving deacetylase knockout strains of *C. albicans*, reviewed in the following section, support this conclusion.

THE BASIC SWITCH EVENT, GENE SILENCING, AND CHROMATIN MODIFICATION

In 1990, Gottschling and coworkers reported that the insertion of the *ADE2* gene in a subtelomeric region of a *S. cerevisiae* chromosome resulted in a cellular phenotype that exhibited spontaneous and reversible switching between an expressed and unexpressed state at frequencies close to 10^{-3}, in effect mimicking switching in *C. albicans* (6, 36). Spontaneous switching in this case proved to be *SIR2* dependent. Because *SIR2* plays a prominent role in silencing not only at subtelomeric regions, but also at the mating type loci and at ribosomal cistrons (31, 35, 41, 65, 100), Soll and coworkers suggested that silencing, and *SIR2* in particular, might also be involved in the regulation of switching in *C. albicans* (119). This suggestion was supported by the discovery that when *C. albicans* strain 3153A entered a high-frequency mode of phenotypic switching, it underwent a concomitant increase in the frequency of recombination between ribosomal cistrons, suggesting that the same mechanism is involved in the suppression of both rDNA recombination and switching (97). In addition to the *SIR* genes, the acetylation and deacetylation of histones H3 and H4 have for a long time been recognized as a mechanism for modulating the state of chromatin in the activation and deactivation of gene expression (43, 143). Recently, a number of acetylases and deacetylases have been cloned and demonstrated to have selective roles in gene regulation (16, 61, 81, 103). Studies have recently been performed to test the roles of gene silencing and the acetylation/deacetylation of histones in high-frequency phenotypic switching.

SIR2

The process of gene silencing has been analyzed in detail at the mating type loci *HML* and *HMR* in *S. cerevisiae* (42). It has been proposed that Sir1p and Sir3p/Sir4p are recruited through an interaction with ORC and Rap1p (11, 25). These complexes in turn recruit Sir2p, initiating nucleation throughout the silenced region. Sir2p possesses both ADP-ribosyltransferase activity and NAD-dependent histone deacetylase activity, but only the latter activity appears to be essential for gene silencing (50). Perez-Martin et al. (92) first deleted a *SIR2* homolog in *C. albicans* strain CAI4 and observed the following three phenotypic effects: an increase in phenotypic switching, spontaneous hypha formation at 30°C in rich medium, and an increase in karyotypic changes. Pujol and Soll (96) cloned the same *SIR2* homolog and generated a null mutant in strain WO-1 by deleting 924 nucleotides encompassing the ADP-ribosyltransferase domain and the NAD-dependent histone deacetylase domain (50, 145). Deletion of *SIR2* in strain WO-1 had no effect on switching in the white to opaque or opaque to white direction. It did, however, have an effect on a "second" switching system in strain WO-1, which includes wrinkled and myceliated phenotypes. There were suggestions of this cryptic switching system in the first description of strain WO-1 (113) and in an analysis of the effects of UV irradiation on switching in strain WO-1 (82). Because switching in this second system normally occurs at low frequency, the variant phenotypes appear as rare sectors primarily at the periphery of aged opaque colonies. The frequency of these variant sectors was two orders of magnitude higher in the *SIR2* mutant than in the parental strain. Variant phenotypes proved heritable when plated, and initially switched at high frequency. These results suggest that strain WO-1 possesses two switching systems, the basic white-opaque transition, which is insensitive to the deletion of *SIR2,* and a second, low-frequency switching system, analogous to the switching systems in strain 3153A and CAI4, that is highly sensitive to *SIR2* deletion (96). These observations suggest that *C. albicans* contains multiple switching systems that involve different regulatory mechanisms.

Deacetylases *HDA1* and *RPD3*

The hypothesis that strain WO-1 contains two distinguishable switching systems was further supported by results obtained in an analysis of the role of deacetylases in switching. Acetylation and deacetylation of histones have been demonstrated to be a critical determinant of the transcriptional state of chromatin at particular gene loci or across entire chromosomes (16, 61, 81, 103). A variety of methods have been used to demonstrate that acetylation primarily of histones H3 and H4 leads to open chromatin structure and deacetylation to closed chromatin structure (20, 21, 76). The two states correlate in most cases with transcriptional activation and deactivation, respectively. In *S. cerevisiae,* Vidal and Gaber (150) first cloned the deacetylase gene *RPD3,* which proved to be a global repressor of transcription. *RPD3* represented the catalytic subunit of the histone deacetylase complex HDB, which includes *SIN3* (56), *SAP3* (156), and *SAP18* (155). Deletion of *RPD3* resulted in hyperacetylation of lysine residues of histones H3 and H4 (103). Rundlett et al. (102) subsequently cloned *HDA1,* the catalytic subunit of the histone deacetylase complex HDA, and the additional deacetylase genes *HOS1, HOS2,* and *HOS3.* Using a PCR strategy, an *HDA1* homolog was first cloned from *C. albicans* (58, 140). Using the same strategy, homologs were subsequently cloned of *RPD3, HOS1, HOS2,* and *HOS3* from *C. albicans* strain WO-1 (140). Northern analysis revealed that *RPD3, HDA1, HOS1,* and *HOS2* were expressed in both the white and opaque phases. Although *HOS3* is expressed in the white and opaque phases, transcript sizes differed between the two phases (Table 1), as in the case of *EFG1* (137).

Deacetylase activity of *S. cerevisiae* is sensitive to trichostatin A (TSA) (39, 154), and TSA has been shown to affect biological functions such as silencing of the *MAT* locus (90). Klar et al. demonstrated that TSA affects switching (58). In repeat experiments on Lee's agar containing phloxine B, TSA stimulated switching in the white to opaque direction, but not in the opaque to white direction (58). The initial pharmacological result suggested that deacetylation was selectively involved in the suppression of switching in the white to opaque transition. However, growth of white phase but not opaque phase cells was slightly depressed in the presence of TSA, suggesting that the observed selective insensitivity of the opaque to white transition may actually reflect lower accessibility of the drug to opaque phase cells. The gene for *HDA1,* which is TSA sensitive (40, 89), was deleted and independent null mutants tested for switching (58, 140). The mutant phenotype supported the conclusion that *HDA1*-mediated deacetylation was involved in selectively suppressing the white to opaque phase transition. When cells from opaque phase colonies were plated, the frequencies of white phase colonies and opaque phase colonies with white phase sectors were similar for wild-type and mutant strains. However, when cells from white phase colonies were plated, the frequency of opaque phase colonies was 22-fold higher and the frequency of white phase colonies with opaque phase sectors was 132-fold higher in mutant cells than wild-type cells. As in the case of TSA treatment, the effect was specifically an increase in the frequency of the transition from white to opaque, supporting the conclusion that deacetylation through Hda1p selectively suppresses the white to opaque phase transition.

Hda1p also plays a role in the selective activation of opaque phase genes (140). In the *HDA1* null mutant, expression of the white phase-enriched gene *EFG1* (32 kb) was down-regulated in the opaque phase. White phase-specific expression of *WH11* in the white phase was normal, as was opaque phase-specific expression of *OP4, PEP1(SAP1),* and *SAP3.* This result seemed contradictory, since deacetylation usually results in a transcriptionally inactive state. However, deletion of the deacetylase *RPD3* in *S. cerevisiae* leads to greater, not less, repression at telomeric loci and increased silencing of HMRa and rDNA loci, presumably through increased expression of silencing genes (22, 102, 114, 146). Therefore, *HDA1* may play a selective role in the repression of silencing genes that in turn suppress *MCM1* expression. *HDA1,* therefore, plays a role not only in the switch event, but also in the regulation of phase-specific genes.

Deletion of the histone deacetylase *RPD3* resulted in increased frequencies of switching in both the white to opaque and the opaque to white directions (140). Deletion of *RPD3* also resulted in down-regulation of the opaque phase-specific genes *OP4*, *SAP1,* and *SAP3.*

The phenotypic effects of deleting *SIR2, HDA1,* and *RPD3* support the suggestion that strain WO-1 possesses two distinguishable, overlapping phenotypic switching systems, the white-opaque transition and a second switching system that includes several additional phenotypes, all differing in the spatial distribution and degree of bud, pseudohypha, and hypha formation in the colony dome. The white-opaque transition involves *HDA1*-mediated suppression of the white to opaque switch and *RPD3*-mediated suppression of switching in both directions whereas the second switching system appears to involve *SIR2*-mediated suppression. The second system preferentially emanates from the opaque phenotype in strain WO-1 and is analogous to the dominant switching system first described in strain 3153A (112) and recently characterized in strain CAI4 (92, 138). It should be noted, however, that in the case of *HDA1, RPD3,* and *SIR2,* it is not clear how direct the effect is on the actual switch event.

CHROMOSOME REORGANIZATION IS NOT INVOLVED IN THE MECHANISM OF REVERSIBLE HIGH-FREQUENCY SWITCHING

Rushenko-Bulgac et al. (104–106) observed that morphological variants isolated from cultures of strain 3153A incubated for extended periods of time in the cold exhibited chromosomal changes identified by pulsed-field gel electrophoresis. However, consistent changes were not demonstrated for specific phenotypes, suggesting that if the morphological variants in fact represented switch phenotypes and not mutants, the chromosomal changes very likely were not causally involved in switching. To test the relationship between chromosomal reorganization and switching, Ramsey et al. (97) stimulated switching in strain 3153A by low UV, and then karyotyped the switching lineages original smooth (osm) → irregular wrinkle (iwr) → iwr → star (st) → revertant smooth (rsm), and osm → iwr → st → rsm → st → rsm. As controls they karyotyped the basic "original smooth" (o-smooth) phenotype through comparable numbers of cell divisions. In the switching lineages, the karyotype changed continuously, but no single karyotype correlated with a particular switch phenotype (97). Changes occurred predominantly in the chromosomes that harbor the ribosomal cistrons. No karyotypic changes were observed in the lineages of o-smooth cells (97). No karyotypic changes have been observed in white-opaque lineages in strain WO-1 (77, 85, 99, 119). These results demonstrate that an increase in the frequency of karyotypic changes can accompany high-frequency phenotypic switching, but these changes are not causally involved. Perez-Martin et al. (92) demonstrated that deletion of *SIR2* resulted both in an increase in switching and an increase in karyotypic change, again primarily in the chromosomes harboring ribosomal cistrons. These results are consistent with those of Gottlieb and Esposito (35), who demonstrated that deletion of *SIR2* in *S. cerevisiae* results in an increase in recombination between ribosomal cistrons.

THE ROLE OF PHASE-SPECIFIC GENES IN ALTERNATIVE MODELS OF PATHOGENESIS

The standard method for testing the role of a gene product in pathogenesis is to delete the gene and compare the virulence of the deletion and parental strains in an animal model. However, if a gene plays a role in general metabolism in the in vivo setting, it will be misconstrued as a virulence trait in the assay. A more definitive strategy, that of gene misexpression, has been used to test the roles of phase-specific genes in virulence. White phase cells are far more virulent than opaque phase cells in the mouse model for systemic infection (62, 63), while, conversely, opaque phase cells are far more virulent than white phase cells in a mouse model for cutaneous infection (62). By placing the ORF of a phase-specific gene under the control of the promoter of a gene differentially expressed in the alternative phase, one can assess whether misexpression confers to cells in the opposite phase any portion of the phenotype or pathogenic advantage specific to the phase in which the gene is normally expressed.

WH11 Misexpression

The white phase gene *WH11* was first misexpressed in the opaque phase by inserting the *WH11* ORF downstream of the promoter of the opaque phase gene *OP4* (63). Misexpression had no effect on the unique morphology of opaque phase cells. It did, however, have dramatic effects on switching frequency and virulence. First, it destabilized cells in the opaque phase, selectively stimulating an increase in the frequency of switching to the white phase that was two orders of magnitude higher than that of wild-type cells (63). Second, it conferred to opaque phase cells the high level of virulence exhibited by white phase cells in the mouse systemic model (63). The increase in virulence was attributed to the increase in the frequency of switching to the white phase, and, therefore, did not necessarily represent a direct role for *WH11* in systemic infections. The increase in switching resulting from misexpression of *WH11* is interesting since *WH11* is restricted to the cytoplasm (109) and shares homology with low-molecular-weight heat shock proteins (94, 147), which can serve as chaperone proteins. Misexpression of *WH11* in the opaque phase, therefore, may result in an abnormal interaction with a factor in the cytoplasm that normally suppresses the opaque to white transition.

PEP1(*SAP1*) Misexpression

The opaque phase-specific gene *PEP1*(*SAP1*) was misexpressed in the white phase by inserting its ORF downstream of the promoter of the white phase-specific gene *WH11* (62). Misexpression had no effect on the white budding cell phenotype, on the frequencies of switching in either the white to opaque or opaque to white direction, or on the virulence of white phase cells in the mouse systemic model. It did, however, have a profound effect on the secretion of aspartyl proteinase and virulence in the model for cutaneous infection. In this model, cells are incubated on mouse skin under a cotton patch for 24 h, and the skin analyzed histologically and by scanning electron microscopy (62). White phase cells in strain WO-1 exhibit extremely low colonization, while opaque phase cells exhibit high levels of colonization, and embed themselves in the skin. Misexpression of *PEP-1*(*SAP1*) resulted in opaque phase levels of aspartyl proteinase secretion in white phase cells and conferred opaque phase levels of colonization and embedding, without affecting cellular morphology (62). This result demonstrates that misexpression of a single phase-specific gene in *C. albicans* can transfer phase-specific virulence.

SWITCHING AND PATHOGENESIS

When switching was first described in 1985, there was a general perception that it was a trivial laboratory artifact since variant colony phenotypes had not been generally described in studies of colonizing populations. There were, however, reasons for this. First, most common agars contained high concentrations of zinc, which suppress many of the phenotypes in the 3153A-type switching system (9). Indeed, Odds and coworkers provided evidence that switching occurred even when variant-colony morphologies did not manifest themselves on agar. Second, most investigators did not monitor colony morphology. Third, when investigators searched for switching, they failed to appreciate that a frequency of 10^{-4}, which is quite high compared to that of a point mutation in a diploid, demands an analysis of over 10,000 colonies in order to observe one variant colony morphology. That represents 200 standard agar plates, each supporting growth of 50 independent colonies. In many cases, researchers would report that they saw no variant colonies on two plates, and in most cases those plates contained nutrient medium high in zinc. When analyzed correctly, switching was demonstrated to occur at sites of commensalism and infection, and that, on average, the frequency of switching was elevated in the latter isolates.

The first study that demonstrated switching at sites of infection involved clonal plating of primary isolates from 11 patients with yeast vaginitis (129). The samples, obtained with sterile swabs, were diluted in buffered salt solution and plated on zinc-limiting agar. Colony morphologies were scored after 7 days of incubation at 25°C. Variant phenotypes were observed in the primary cultures of 4 of the 11 patients. In secondary platings of single primary colonies in which approximately 500 to 5,000 colonies were analyzed for phenotype, 9 out of 11 produced variant phenotypes. In secondary platings the frequencies of variant colonies ranged from 3.7×10^{-1} to 10^{-4}. The median frequency of variant phenotypes in secondary platings was 7×10^{-3}. Switching repertoires identified in these vaginitis samples included the 3153A system, a dominant unmyceliated-heavily myceliated transition and the white-opaque transition. Fingerprinting experiments with the complex Ca3 probe (125) demonstrated that variant phenotypes from individual patients represented the same strains (129). However, the most revealing demonstration of switching at the site of infection was a longitudinal study of a single bloodstream infection patient in 1985 at the University of Iowa Hospitals and Clinics (131). A patient with acute nonlymphoblastic leukemia was diagnosed, within a few weeks after receiving a bone marrow transplant, to be suffering from a bloodstream infection that included two *C. tropicalis* strains, both switching at high frequency between a number of variant colony phenotypes. Again, fingerprinting with the *C. tropicalis*-specific complex probe verified the unrelatedness of the two strains and proved that variants represented phenotypes within the same strains (131). In 1989, a study of recurrence in a single vaginitis patient demonstrated that a single strain could switch phenotypes following drug therapy between each episode of vaginitis (127).

The first controlled comparison of switching between commensal and infecting isolates was performed in 1993 by Hellstein et al. (44). They identified variant phenotypes in 3 out of 19 primary oral isolates from different healthy patients with carriage, and in 9 out of 23 primary oral isolates from different individuals with infections. These results suggested that infecting isolates switched at higher rates, on average, than commensal isolates, and this conclusion was reinforced by two additional studies. First, in 1994 Jones et al. (55) demonstrated that strains isolated from deep mycoses in humans switched on average at frequencies far higher than strains isolated from superficial mycoses. Second, in 2000, Vargas et al. (148) demonstrated that oral isolates from HIV-positive patients switched, on average, at frequencies between one and two orders of magnitude higher than those of healthy controls. More surprisingly, the isolates from HIV-positive individuals were on average in a higher frequency mode of switching prior to the patient's first episode of oral thrush and first therapeutic regimen with antifungal agents. In this study (148) the first convincing data were presented on the extraordinary impact switching has on drug susceptibility. Although the number of reviewed studies is small, they leave little doubt that switching occurs at sites of commensalism and infection and has a very high impact on specific virulence traits, which leads to the concept that virulence represents a higher order virulence trait.

SWITCHING IN SPECIES OTHER THAN *C. ALBICANS*

Although switching was first demonstrated in *C. albicans* and for the most part characterized in detail in that species, switching has been observed in all other *Candida* species tested. *C. tropicalis* strains were demonstrated early on to switch reversibly at frequencies ranging from 10^{-4} to 10^{-2} (131). The phenotypes in the switching repertoire were as diverse as those observed in *C. albicans* and relied heavily on the proportion and topology of hypha formation in the colony dome. Except for brief descriptions of switching, reversibility, and colony variants, there have been no studies published that explore the impact of *C. tropicalis* switching on virulence or gene regulation, and no investigations into mechanism. Variant phenotypes have also been described for *C. parapsilosis* (28), but no studies have been published on switching frequencies, reversibility, impact on virulence, gene expression, or mechanism. Switching has also been observed in *C. lusitaniae* (67), but it has not been characterized. Finally, an elegant switching system was recently identified in *C. glabrata*. Using an indicator agar containing 1 mM $CuSO_4$, Lachke et al. (64) demonstrated that all tested strains of *C. glabrata* switched reversibly and at high frequency between a white, light brown, and dark brown colony phenotype (Color plate 4). As in the case of *C. albicans*, switching in *C. glabrata* was accompanied by the differential expression of genes, in this case the *MT-II* metallothionein gene and a newly identified gene, *HLP*, which encodes a hemolysin-like protein (64). Quantitative slot blot analysis indicated that these genes were expressed in a graded fashion that correlated with the intensity of pigmentation. The fact that one gene is involved in copper detoxification while the other may be involved in red blood cell lysis suggests that just as in the case of *C. albicans*, switching in *C. glabrata* is pleiotropic and again may represent a higher order virulence trait.

SUMMARY

It is probably safe to say that *C. albicans* and related species have evolved relatively sophisticated switching systems for generating a variety of general phenotypes. Switching regulates a number of phase-specific genes in a combinatorial fashion, and a surprisingly high proportion of these genes directly or indirectly impact pathogenesis and virulence. Switching occurs at sites of commensalism and infection, and occurs on average at higher frequencies in the latter. We suggest that switching provides a commensal and infecting population with a variety of minor phenotypes for rapid adaptation to immediate environmental challenges. The regulation of phase-specific genes is mediated at the level of transcription, although other levels of control have not been ruled out. The complexity of the regulatory network is only now emerging, and includes mechanisms that have been employed in gene regulation in other fungi such as the MADS box consensus binding sites and associated MADS box proteins like Mcm1p. There are now hints that mating type regulatory genes such as $\alpha 1$ and $\alpha 2$ may play roles in phase-specific gene expression. Recently, evidence has been presented that single strains can harbor multiple switching systems, that these different switching systems involve different regulatory machinery, and that the mechanism of switching is regulated directly or indirectly by chromatin reorganization that is suppressed by chromatin modulators such as the histone deacetylase Hda1p and the gene for the silencing protein Sir2p. The apparent complexity of the circuitry involved in the regulation of phase specific genes, the possible involvement of mating type regulatory genes, and the emerging involvement of chromatin modulation together suggest that switching is a highly evolved higher order pathogenic trait that deserves our attention.

Acknowledgments. The research performed in the author's laboratory reviewed in this article was funded in part by NIH grant AI2392.

REFERENCES

1. **Acton, T., H. Zhong, and A. Vershon.** 1997. DNA-binding specificity of Mcm1: operator mutations that alter DNA-bending and transcriptional activities by a MADS box protein. *Mol. Cell. Biol.* **17:**1881–1889.
2. **Anderson, J., L. Cundiff, B. Schnars, M. Gao, I. Mackenzie, and D. R. Soll.** 1989. Hypha formation in the white-opaque transition of *Candida albicans. Infect. Immun.* **57:**458–467.
3. **Anderson, J., R. Mihalik, and D. R. Soll.** 1990. Ultrastructure and antigenicity of the unique cell wall "pimple" of the *Candida* opaque phenotype. *J. Bacteriol.* **172:**224–235.
4. **Anderson, J., and D. R. Soll.** 1987. The unique phenotype of opaque cells in the "white-opaque transition" in *Candida albicans. J. Bacteriol.* **169:**5579–5588.
5. **Anderson, M., and F. C. Odds.** 1985. Adherence of *Candida albicans* to vaginal epithelia: significance of morphological form and effect of ketoconazole. *Mykosen* **28:**531–540.
6. **Aparicio, O. M., B. L. Billington, and D. E. Gottschling.** 1991. Modifiers of position effects are shared between telomeric and silent mating-type loci in *S. cerevisiae. Cell* **66:** 1279–1287.
7. **Aramayo, R., Y. Peleg, R. Addison, and R. Mutzenberg.** 1996. *Asm-1*$^{+}$, a *Neurospora crassa* gene related to transcriptional regulators of fungal development. *Genetics* **144:** 991–1003.
8. **Balan, I., A. Alareo, and M. Raymond.** 1997. The *Candida albicans CDR3* gene codes for an opaque-phase ABC transporter. *J. Bacteriol.* **179:**7210–7218.
9. **Bedell, G., and D. R. Soll.** 1979. The effects of low concentrations of zinc on the growth and dimorphism of *Candida albicans:* Evidence for zinc resistant and zinc sensitive pathways for mycelium formation. *Infect. Immun.* **26:**348–354.
10. **Bergen, M., E. Voss, and D. R. Soll.** 1990. Switching at the cellular level in the white-opaque transition of *Candida albicans. J. Gen. Microbiol.* **136:**1925–1936.
11. **Bi, X., M. Braunstein, G. J. Shei, and J. R. Broach.** 1999. The yeast *HMLI* silencer defines heterochromatin domain boundary by directional establishment of silencing. *Proc. Natl. Acad. Sci. USA* **96:**11934–11939.
12. **Braun, B. R., and A. D. Johnson.** 2000. *TUP1, CPH1* and *EFG1* make independent contributions to filamentation in *Candida albicans. Genetics* **155:**57–67.
13. **Brown, A. J., and N. A. Gow.** 1999. Regulatory networks controlling *Candida albicans* morphogenesis. *Trends Microbiol.* **7:**333–338.
14. **Brown-Thomsen, J.** 1968. Variability in *Candida albicans* (Robin) Berkhous. *Hereditas* **60:**335–398.
15. **Bruckmann, A., W. Künkel, A., Härtl, R. Wetzker, and R. Eck.** 2000. A phosphatidylinositol 3-kinase of *Candida albicans* influences adhesion, filamentous growth and virulence. *Microbiology* **146:**2755–2764.
16. **Burgess, S. M., M. Ajimura, and N. Kleckner.** 1999. *GCN5*-dependent histone H3 acetylation and *RPD3*-dependent histone H4 deacetylation have distinct, opposing effects on *IME2* transcription, during meiosis and during vegetative growth, in budding yeast. *Proc. Natl. Acad. Sci. USA* **96:** 6835–6840.
17. **Cawson, R. A., and K. C. Rajasingham.** 1972. Ultrastructural features of the invasive phase of *Candida albicans. Br. J. Dermatol.* **87:**435–443.
18. **Chen, J., S. Zhou, Q. Wang, X. Chen, T. Pan and H. Liu.** 2000. Crk1, a novel Cdc2-related protein kinase, is required for hyphal development and virulence in *Candida albicans. Mol. Cell. Biol.* **20:**8696–8708.
19. **Chinnathambi, S., T. Srikantha, and D. R. Soll.** Manuscript in preparation.
20. **Cosma, M. P., T. Tanaka, and K. Nasmyth.** 1999. Ordered recruitment of transcription and chromatin remodeling factors to a cell cycle- and developmentally regulated promoter. *Cell* **97:**299–311.
21. **Crane-Robinson, C., T. R. Hebbes, A. L. Clayton, and A. W. Thorne.** 1997. Chromosomal mapping of core histone acetylation by immunoselection. *Methods* **12:**48–56.
22. **DeRubertis, F., D. Kadosh, S. Henchoz, D. Pauli, G. Reuter, K. Struhl, and P. Spierer.** 1996. The histone deacetylase *RPD3* counteracts genomic silencing in *Drosophila* and yeast. *Nature* **384:**589–591.
23. **Dolan, J. W., C. Kirkman, and S. Fields.** 1989. The yeast STE12 protein binds to the DNA sequence mediating pheromone induction. *Proc. Natl. Acad. Sci. USA* **86:**5703–5707.
24. **Donelson, J. E.** 1989. DNA rearrangements and antigenic variation in African trypanosomes, p. 763–782. *In* D. E. Berg and M. M. Howe (ed.), *Mobile DNA.* American Society for Microbiology, Washington, D.C.
25. **Donze, D., C. R. Adams, J. Rine, and R. T. Kamakaka.** 1999. The boundaries of the silenced *HMR* domain in *Saccharomyces cerevisiae. Genes Dev.* **13:**698–708.
26. **Dutton, J. R., S. Johns, and B. L. Miller.** 1997. StuAp is a sequence-specific transcription factor that regulates developmental complexity in *Aspergillus nidulans. EMBO J.* **16:** 5710–5721.
27. **Edwards, J. E., Jr., R. Y. Foos, J. Z. Montgomerie, and L. B. Gute.** 1974. Ocular manifestations of *Candida* septicemia: review of seventy-six cases of hematogenous *Candida* endophthalomitis. *Medicine* **53:**47–75.
28. **Enger, L., S. Joly, C. Pujol, P. Simonson, M. Pfaller, and D. R. Soll.** 2001. Cloning and characterization of a complex DNA fingerprinting probe for *Candida parapsilosis. J. Clin. Microbiol.* **39:**658–669.
29. **Errede, B., and G. Ammerer.** 1989. STE12, a protein involved in cell-type-specific transcription and signal transduction in yeast, is part of protein-DNA complexes. *Genes Dev.* **3:** 1349–1361.
30. **Fries, B. C., D. C. Goldman, R. Cherniak, R. Ju, and A. Casadevall.** 1999. Phenotypic switching in *Cryptococcus neoformans* results in changes in cellular morphology and glucuronoxylomannan structure. *Infect. Immun.* **67:**6076–6083.
31. **Gartenberg, M. R.** 2000. The Sir proteins of *Saccharomyces cerevisiae:* mediators of transcriptional silencing and much more. *Curr. Opin. Microbiol.* **3:**132–137.
32. **Gimeno, C. J., and G. R. Fink.** 1994. Induction of pseudohyphal growth by overexpression of *PHD1*, a *Saccharomyces cerevisiae* gene related to transcriptional regulators of fungal development. *Mol. Cell. Biol.* **14:**2100–2112.
33. **Glasgow, A. C., K. T. Hughes, and M. I. Simons.** 1989. Bacterial DNA inversion systems, p. 637–660. *In* D. E. Berg and

M. M. Howe (ed.), *Mobile DNA*. American Society for Microbiology, Washington, D.C.

34. **Goldman, D., B. Fries, S. Franzot, L. Montella, and A. Casadevall.** 1998. Phenotypic switching in the human pathogenic fungus *Cryptococcus neoformans* is associated with changes in virulence and pulmonary inflammatory response in rodents. *Proc. Natl. Acad. Sci USA* **95:**14967–14972.
35. **Gottlieb, S., and S. Esposito.** 1989. A new role for a yeast transcriptional silencer gene, *SIR2*, in regulation of recombination in ribosomal DNA. *Cell* **56:**771–776.
36. **Gottschling, D. E., O. M. Aparicio, B. L. Billington, and V. A. Zakian.** 1990. Position effect at *S. cerevisiae* telomeres: reversible repression of Pol II transcription. *Cell* **63:**751–762.
37. **Gow, N. A.** 1997. Germ tube growth of *Candida albicans*. *Curr. Top. Med. Mycol.* **8:**43–55.
38. **Gräser, Y., M. Volovsek, J. Arrington, J. Schönian, W. Presber, T. G. Mitchell, and R. Vilgalys.** 1996. Molecular markers reveal that population structure of the human pathogen *Candida albicans* exhibits both clonality and recombination. *Proc. Natl. Acad. Sci. USA* **93:**12473–12477.
39. **Grewal, S. I., M. J. Bonaduce, and A. J. Klar.** 1998. Histone deacetylase homologs regulate epigenetic inheritance of transcriptional silencing and chromosome segregation in fission yeast. *Genetics* **150:**563–576.
40. **Grozinger, C. M., C. A. Hassig, and S. L. Schreiber.** 1999. Three proteins define a class of human histone deacetylases related to yeast Hda1p. *Proc. Natl. Acad. Sci. USA* **96:** 4868–4875.
41. **Guarente, L.** 1999. Diverse and dynamic functions of the Sir silencing complex. *Nat. Genet.* **23:**281–285.
42. **Haber, J. E.** 1998. Mating-type gene switching in *Saccharomyces cerevisiae*. *Annu. Rev. Genet.* **32:**561–599.
43. **Hassig, C. A., and S. L. Schreiber.** 1997. Nuclear histone acetylases and deacetylases and transcriptional regulation: HATs off to HDACs. *Curr. Opin. Chem. Biol.* **1:**300–308.
44. **Hellstein, J., H. Vawter-Hugart, P. Fotos, J. Schmid, and D. R. Soll.** 1993. Genetic similarity and phenotypic diversity of commensal and pathogenic strains of *Candida albicans* isolated from the oral cavity. *J. Clin. Microbiol.* **31:**3190–3199.
45. **Howlett, J. A., and C. A. Squier.** 1980. *Candida albicans* ultrastructure: colonization and invasion of oral epithelium. *Infect. Immun.* **29:**252–260.
46. **Hube, B., M. Monod, D. Schofield, A. Brown, and N. Gow.** 1994. Expression of seven members of the gene family encoding aspartyl proteinases in *Candida albicans*. *Mol. Microbiol.* **14:**87–99.
47. **Hube, B., C. J. Turner, F. C. Odds, H. Eiffert, G. J. Boulnois, H. Kochel, and R. Ruchel.** 1991. Sequence of the *Candida albicans* gene encoding the secretory aspartate proteinase. *J. Med. Vet. Mycol.* **29:**129–132.
48. **Hull, C. M., and A. D. Johnson.** 2000. Evidence for mating of the "asexual" yeast *Candida albicans* in a mammalian host. *Science* **289:**307–310.
49. **Hull, C. M., and A. D. Johnson.** 1999. Identification of a mating type-like locus in the asexual pathogenic yeast *Candida albicans*. *Science* **285:**1271–1275.
50. **Imai, S., C. M. Armstrong, M. Kaeberlein, and L. Guarente.** 2000. Transcriptional silencing and longevity protein Sir2 is an NAD-dependent histone deacetylase. *Nature* **403:** 795–800.
51. **Ishii, N., M. Watasabe, S. Fukuchi, M. Arisawa, and Y. Aoki.** 1999. Role of Rbf1 in hyphal formation of *Candida albicans*. *Abstr. Am. Soc. Microbiol. Conf. Candida Candidiasis*, abstr. B25. American Society for Microbiology, Washington, D.C.
52. **Ishii, N., M. Yamanato, H.-W. Lahm, S. Izumi, F. Yoshihara, H. Nakayama, M. Arisawa, and Y. Aoki.** 1997. A DNA-binding protein from *Candida albicans* that binds to the RPG box of *Saccharomyces cerevisiae* and the telomeric repeat sequence of *C. albicans*. *Microbiology* **143:**417–427.
53. **Ishii, N., M. Yamanato, F. Yoshira, M. Arisawa, and Y. Aoki.** 1997. Characterization of Rbf1p, a putative transcription factor of *Candida albicans*. *Microbiology* **143:**429–435.
54. **Jarvis, E. E., D. C. Hagen, and G. F. Sprague.** 1988. Identification of a DNA segment that is necessary and sufficient for α-specific gene control in *Saccharomyces cerevisiae:* implications for regulation of α-specific and a-specific genes. *Mol. Cell. Biol.* **8:**309–320.
55. **Jones, S., G. White, and P. R. Hunter.** 1994. Increased phenotypic switching in strains of *Candida albicans* associated with invasive infections. *J. Clin. Microbiol.* **32:**2869–2870.
56. **Kadosh, D., and K. Struhl.** 1997. Repression by Ume6 involves recruitment of a complex containing Sin3 corepressor and Rpd3 histone deacetylase to target promoters. *Cell* **89:** 365–371.
57. **Kennedy, M. J., A. L. Rogers, L. A. Hanselman, D. R. Soll, and R. J. Yancey.** 1988. Variation in adhesion and cell surface hydrophobicity in *Candida albicans* white and opaque phenotypes. *Mycopathologia* **102:**149–156.
58. **Klar, A., T. Srikantha, and D. R. Soll.** 2001. A histone deacetylase inhibitor and mutant promote colony-type switching of the human pathogen *Candida albicans*. *Genetics* **158:** 919–924.
59. **Kolotila, M. P., and R. D. Diamond.** 1990. Effects of neutrophils and in vitro oxidants on survival and phenotypic switching of *Candida albicans WO-1*. *Infect. Immun.* **58:** 1174–1179.
60. **Kozinn, P. J., and C. L. Taschdjian.** 1962. Enteric candidiasis. Diagnosis and clinical considerations. *Pediatrics* **30:**71–85.
61. **Krebs, J. E., M.-H. Kuo, C. D. Allis, and C. L. Peterson.** 1999. Cell cycle-regulated histone acetylation required for expression of the yeast *HO* gene. *Gen. Dev.* **13:**1412–1421.
62. **Kvaal, C., S. Lachke, T. Srikantha, K. Daniels, J. McCoy, and D. R. Soll.** 1999. Misexpression of the opaque phase-specific gene *PEPI(SAPI)* in the white phase of *Candida albicans* confers increased virulence in a mouse model of cutaneous infection. *Infect. Immun.* **67:**6652–6662.
63. **Kvaal, C. A., T. Srikantha, and D. R. Soll.** 1997. Misexpression of the white phase-specific gene *WH11* in the opaque phase of *Candida albicans* affects switching and virulence. *Infect. Immun.* **65:**4468–4475.
64. **Lachke, S., T. Srikantha, L. Tsai, K. Daniels, and D. R. Soll.** 2000. Phenotypic switching in *Candida glabrata* involves phase-specific regulation of the metallotheionein gene *MT-II* and the newly discovered hemolysin gene *HLP*. *Infect. Immun.* **68:**884–895.
65. **Laurenson, P., and J. Rine.** 1992. Silencers, silencing and heritable transcriptional states. *Microbiol. Rev.* **56:**543–560.
66. **Lo, H. J., J. R. Kohler, B. DiDomenico, D. Loebenberg, A. Cacciapuoti, and G. R. Fink.** 1997. Nonfilamentous *C. albicans* mutants are avirulent. *Cell* **90:**939–949.
67. **Lockhart, S., and D. R. Soll.** Unpublished observations.
68. **Lockhart, S. R., M. Nguyen, T. Srikantha, and D. R. Soll.** 1998. A MADS box protein consensus binding site is necessary and sufficient for activation of the opaque-phase specific gene *OP4* of *Candida albicans*. *J. Bacteriol.* **180:**6607–6616.
69. **Lockhart, S., M. Nguyen, and D. R. Soll.** Functional characterization of the promoters of the opaque phase-specific genes *PEP1(SAP1)* and *SAP3*. In preparation.
70. **Lorenz, W. W., R. O. McCann, M. Longiaru, and M. J. Cormier.** 1991. Isolation and expression of a cDNA encoding *Renilla reniformis* luciferase. *Proc. Natl. Acad. Sci. USA* **88:** 4438–4442.

71. **Mackinnon, J. E.** 1940. Dissociation in *Candida albicans. J. Infect. Dis.* **66/67:**59–77.
72. **Magee, B. B., and P. T. Magee.** 2000. Induction of mating in *Candida albicans* by construction of *MTLa* and *MTLα* strains. *Science* **289:**310–313.
73. **Maksymiuk, A. W., S. Thongpraser, R. Hopfer, M. Luna, V. Fainstein, and G. P. Bodey.** 1984. Systemic candidiasis in cancer patients. *Am. J. Med.* **77:**20–27.
74. **Martin, M. V., G. T. Craig, and D. J. Lamb.** 1984. An investigation of the role of true hypha production in the pathogenesis of experimental oral candidosis. *Sabouraudia J. Med. Vet. Mycol.* **22:**471–476.
75. **Martin, M. V., and G. R. Wilkinson.** 1983. The oral yeast flora of ten year old school children. *Sabouraudia* **21:** 129–135.
76. **Mathis, D. J., P. Oudet, B. Wasylyk, and P. Chambon.** 1978. Effect of histone acetylation on structure and in vitro transcription of chromatin. *Nucleic Acids Res.* **5:**3523–3547.
77. **McEachern, M. J., and J. B. Hicks.** 1991. Dosage of the smallest chromosome affects both the yeast-hyphal transition and the white-opaque transition of *Candida albicans* WO-1. *J. Bacteriol.* **173:**7436–7442.
78. **Merck, K. B., P. J. Groenen, C. E. Voorter, W. A. de Haard-Hockman, J. Horwitz, H. Bloemendal, and W. W. deJong.** 1993. Structural and functional similarities of bovine alpha-crystallin and mouse small heat-shock protein. A family of chaperones. *J. Biol. Chem.* **268:**1046–1052.
79. **Meunier-Carpentier, F., T. E. Kiehn, and D. Armstrong.** 1981. Fungemia in the immunocompromised host. *Am. J. Med.* **71:**363–370.
80. **Miller, K. Y., J. Wu, and B. L. Miller.** 1992. StuA is required for cell pattern formation in *Aspergillus. Genes Dev.* **6:** 1770–1782.
81. **Miska, E. A., C. Karlsson, E. Langley, S. J. Nielson, J. Pines, and T. Kouzarides.** 1999. HDAC4 deacetylase associates with and represses the MEF2 transcription factor. *EMBO J.* **18:**5099–5107.
82. **Morrow, B., J. Anderson, E. Wilson, and D. R. Soll.** 1989. Bidirectional stimulation of the white-opaque transition of *Candida albicans* by ultraviolet irradiation. *J. Gen. Microbiol.* **135:**1201–1208.
83. **Morrow, B., H. Ramey, and D. R. Soll.** 1994. Regulation of phase-specific genes in the more general switching system of *Candida albicans* strain 3153A. *J. Med. Vet. Mycol.* **32:** 287–394.
84. **Morrow, B., T. Srikantha, J. Anderson, and D. R. Soll.** 1993. Coordinate regulation of two opaque-specific genes during white-opaque switching in *Candida albicans. Infect. Immun.* **61:**1823–1828.
85. **Morrow, B., T. Srikantha, and D. R. Soll.** 1992. Transcription of the gene for a pepsinogen, *PEP1,* is regulated by white-opaque switching in *Candida albicans. Mol. Cell. Biol.* **12:** 2997–3005.
86. **Negroni, P.** 1935. Variacion bacia et tipo R de *Mycotorula albicans. Rev. Soc. Argent. Biol.* **11:**449–453.
87. **Odds, F. C.** 1988. *Candida and Candidosis.* Baillière Tindall, London, United Kingdom.
88. **Odds, F. C., and L. A. Mercon-Davies.** 1989. Colony variations in *Candida* species. *Mycoses* **32:**275–282.
89. **Olsson, T. G. S., K. Ekwall, R. C. Allshire, P. Sunnerhagen, J. F. Partridge, and W. A. Richardson.** 1998. Genetic characterization of *hda1*$^+$, a putative fission yeast histone deacetylase gene. *Nucleic Acids Res.* **26:**3247–3254.
90. **Olsson, T. G. S., R. A. Silverstein, K. Ekwall, and P. Sunnerhagen.** 1999. Transient inhibition of histone deacetylase activity overcomes silencing in the mating-type region in fission yeast. *Curr. Genet.* **35:**82–87.
91. **Passmore, S., R. Elble, and B.-K. Tye.** 1989. A protein involved in minichromosome maintenance in yeast binds a transcriptional enhancer conserved in eukaryotes. *Genes Dev.* **3:** 921–935.
92. **Perez-Martin, J., J. A. Uria, and A. D. Johnson.** 1999. Phenotypic switching in *Candida albicans* is controlled by a *SIR2* gene. *EMBO J.* **18:**2580–2592.
93. **Pomes, R., C. Gil, and C. Nombela.** 1985. Genetic analysis of *Candida albicans* morphological mutants. *J. Gen. Microbiol.* **131:**2107–2113.
94. **Praekelt, U. M., and P. A. Meacock.** 1990. *HSP12,* a new small heat shock gene of *Saccharomyces cerevisiae:* analysis of structure, regulation and function. *Mol. Gen. Genet.* **223:** 97–106.
95. **Pujol, C., J. Reynes, F. Renaud, M. Raymond, M. Tibayrenc, F. J. Ayala, F. Jambon, M. Mallie, and J.-M. Bastide.** 1993. The yeast *Candida albicans* has a clonal mode of reproduction in a population of infected human immunodeficiency virus-positive patients. *Proc. Natl. Acad. Sci. USA* **90:** 9456–9459.
96. **Pujol, C., and D. R. Soll.** In preparation.
97. **Ramsey, H., B. Morrow, and D. R. Soll.** 1994. An increase in switching frequency correlates with an increase in recombination of the ribosomal cistrons of *Candida albicans* strain 3153A. *Microbiology* **140:**1525–1531.
98. **Richardson, M. D., and H. Smith.** 1981. Production of germ tubes by virulent and attenuated strains of *Candida albicans. J. Infect. Dis.* **144:**565–569.
99. **Rikkerink, E. H. A., B. B. Magee, and P. T. Magee.** 1988. Opaque-white phenotypic transition: a programmed morphological transition in *Candida albicans. J. Bacteriol.* **170:** 895–899.
100. **Rivier, D. H., and J. Rine.** 1992. Silencing: the establishment and inheritance of stable, repressed transcription states. *Curr. Opin. Gen. Dev.* **2:**286–292.
101. **Rotrosen, D., J. E. Edwards, T. R. Gibson, J. C. Moore, A. H. Cohen, and I. Green.** 1985. Adherence of *Candida* to cultured vascular epithelial cells: mechanism of attachment and endothelial cell penetration. *J. Infect. Dis.* **152:**1264–1274.
102. **Rundlett, S. E., A. A. Carmen, R. Kobayashi, S. Bavykin, B. M. Turner, and M. Grunstein.** 1996. *HDA1* and *RPD3* are members of distinct yeast histone deacetylase complexes that regulate silencing and transcription. *Proc. Natl. Acad. Sci. USA* **93:**14503–14508.
103. **Rundlett, S. E., A. A. Carmen, N. Suka, B. M. Turner, and M. Grunstein.** 1998. Transcriptional repression by *UME6* involves deacetylation of lysine 5 of histone H4 by *RPD3. Nature* **392:**831–835.
104. **Rustchenko-Bulgac, E. P.** 1991. Variations of *Candida albicans* electrophoretic karyotypes. *J. Bacteriol.* **173:** 6586–6596.
105. **Rustchenko-Bulgac, E. P., and D. H. Howard.** 1993. Multiple chromosomal and phenotypic changes in spontaneous mutants of *Candida albicans. J. Gen. Microbiol.* **139:** 1195–1207.
106. **Rustchenko-Bulgac, E. P., F. Sherman, and J. B. Hicks.** 1990. Chromosomal rearrangements associated with morphological mutants provide a means for genetic variation in *Candida albicans. J. Bacteriol.* **172:**1276–1283.
107. **Sanglard, D., F. Ischer, M. Monod, S. Dogra, R. Prasad, and J. Bille.** 1999. Analysis of the ATP-binding cassette (ABC)-transporter gene *CDR4* from *Candida albicans,* abstr. C27. *Abstr. Am. Soc. Microbiol. Conf. Candida Candidiasis.* American Society for Microbiology, Washington, D.C.

108. **Sauer, R. T., D. L. Smith, and A. D. Johnson.** 1988. Flexibility of the yeast alpha 2 repressor enables it to occupy the ends of its operator, leaving the center free. *Genes Dev.* **2:**807–816.
109. **Schröppel, K., T. Srikantha, M. DeCock, D. Wessels, S. Lockhart, and D. R. Soll.** 1996. Cytoplasmic localization of the white phase-specific *WH11* gene product of *Candida albicans. Microbiology* **142:**2245–2254.
110. **Seelig, M. S., C. P. Speth, P. J. Kozinn, C. L. Taschd-Jian, E. F. Toni, and P. Goldberg.** 1974. Patterns of *Candida* endocarditis following cardiac surgery: importance of early diagnosis and therapy. *Prog. Cardiovasc. Dis.* **17:**25–160.
111. **Shepherd, M. G.** 1985. Pathogenicity of morphological and auxotrophic mutants of *Candida albicans* in experimental infections. *Infect. Immun.* **50:**541–544.
112. **Slutsky, B., J. Buffo, and D. R. Soll.** 1985. High frequency "switching" of colony morphology in *Candida albicans. Science* **230:**666–669.
113. **Slutsky, B., M. Staebell, J. Anderson, L. Risen, M. Pfaller, and D. R. Soll.** 1987. "White-opaque transition": a second high-frequency switching system in *Candida albicans. J. Bacteriol.* **169:**189–197.
114. **Smith, J. S., E. Caputo, and J. D. Boeke.** 1999. A genetic screen for ribosomal DNA silencing defects identifies multiple DNA replication and chromatin-modulating factors. *Mol. Cell. Biol.* **19:**3184–3197.
115. **Sobel, J. D., G. Muller, and H. R. Buckley.** 1984. Critical role of germ tube formation in the pathogenesis of candidal vaginitis. *Infect. Immun.* **44:**576–580.
116. **Soll, D. R.** 1984. The cell cycle and commitment to alternative cell fates in *Candida albicans,* p. 143–162. *In* P. Nurse and E. Streiblova (ed.), *The Microbial Cell Cycle.* CRC Press, Boca Raton, Fla.
117. **Soll, D. R.** 1986. The regulation of cellular differentiation in the dimorphic yeast *Candida albicans. Bioessays* **5:**5–11.
118. **Soll, D. R.** 1989. High-frequency switching in *Candida albicans,* p. 791–798. *In* D. E. Berg and M. M. Howe (ed.), *Mobile DNA.* American Society for Microbiology, Washington, D.C.
119. **Soll, D. R.** 1992. High frequency switching in *Candida albicans. Clin. Microbiol. Rev.* **5:**183–203.
120. **Soll, D. R.** 1992. Switching and its possible role in *Candida* pathogenesis, p. 156–172. *In* J. E. Bennett, R. J. Hay, and P. K. Peterson (ed.), *New Fungal Strategies.* Churchill Livingstone, Edinburgh, Scotland.
121. **Soll, D. R.** 1993. Switching and the regulation of gene transcription in *Candida albicans,* p. 73–82. *In* H. V. Bossche, F. C. Odds, and D. Kerridge (ed.), *Dimorphic Fungi in Biology and Medicine.* Plenum Press, New York, N.Y.
122. **Soll, D. R.** 1997. The emerging molecular biology of switching in *Candida albicans. ASM News* **62:**415–420.
123. **Soll, D. R.** 1997. Gene regulation during high frequency switching in *Candida albicans. Microbiology* **143:**279–288.
124. **Soll, D. R.** The molecular biology of switching in *Candida. In* R. Cihlar and R. Chalderone (ed.), *Fungal Pathogenesis: Principles and Clinical Application,* in press. Marcel Dekker, New York, N.Y.
125. **Soll, D. R.** 2000. The ins and outs of DNA fingerprinting the infectious fungi. *Clin. Microbiol. Rev.* **13:**332–370.
126. **Soll, D. R., J. Anderson, and M. Bergen.** 1991. The developmental biology of the white-opaque transition in *Candida albicans,* p. 20–45. *In* R. Prasad (ed.), *Candida albicans: Cellular and Molecular Biology.* Springer Verlag, Berlin, Germany.
127. **Soll, D. R., R. Galask, S. Isley, T. V. G. Rao, D. Stone, J. Hicks, J. Schmid, K. Mac, and C. Hanna.** 1989. "Switching" of *Candida albicans* during successive episodes of recurrent vaginitis. *J. Clin. Microbiol.* **27:**681–690.
128. **Soll, D. R., R. Galask, J. Schmid, C. Hanna, K. Mac, and B. Morrow.** 1991. Genetic dissimilarity of commensal strains carried in different anatomical locations of the same healthy women. *J. Clin. Microbiol.* **29:**1702–1710.
129. **Soll, D. R., C. J. Langtimm, J. McDowell, J. Hicks, and R. Galask.** 1987. High-frequency switching in *Candida* strains isolated from vaginitis patients. *J. Clin. Microbiol.* **25:** 1611–1622.
130. **Soll, D. R., and T. Srikantha.** 1998. Reporters for the analysis of gene regulation in fungi pathogenic to man. *Curr. Opin. Microbiol.* **1:**400–405.
131. **Soll, D. R., M. Staebell, C. J. Langtimm, M. Pfaller, J. Hicks, J. and T. V. G. Rao.** 1988. Multiple *Candida* strains in the course of a single systemic infection. *J. Clin. Microbiol.* **26:** 1448–1459.
132. **Sonneborn, A., B. Tebarth, and J. F. Ernst.** 1999. Control of white-opaque phenotypic switching in *Candida albicans* by the Efg1p morphogenetic regulator. *Infect. Immun.* **67:** 4655–4660.
133. **Srikantha, T., A. Chandrasekhar, and D. R. Soll.** 1995. Functional analysis of the promoter of the phase-specific *WH11* gene of *Candida albicans. Mol. Cell. Biol.* **15:**1797–1805.
134. **Srikantha, T., A. Klapach, W. W. Lorenz, L. K. Tsai, L. A. Laughlin, J. A. Gorman, and D. R. Soll.** 1996. The sea pansey *Renilla reniformis* luciferase serves as a sensitive bioluminescent reporter for differential gene expression in *Candida albicans. J. Bacteriol.* **178:**121–129.
135. **Srikantha, T., B. Morrow K. Schröppel, and D. R. Soll.** 1995. The frequency of integrative transformation correlates with the transcriptional state of phase-specific genes of *Candida albicans. Mol. Gen. Genet.* **246:**342–352.
136. **Srikantha, T., and D. R. Soll.** 1993. A white-specific gene in the white-opaque switching system of *Candida albicans. Gene* **131:**53–60.
137. **Srikantha, T., L. Tsai, K. Daniels, and D. R. Soll.** 2000. *EFGI* null mutants of *Candida albicans* switch, but can not express the complete phenotype of white-phase budding cells. *J. Bacteriol.* **182:**1580–1591.
138. **Srikantha, T., L. Tsai, K. Daniels, L. Enger, K. Highley, and D. R. Soll.** 1998. The two-component hybrid kinase regulator *CaNIK1* of *Candida albicans. Microbiology* **14:**2715–2729.
139. **Srikantha, T., L. Tsai, and D. R. Soll.** 1997. The *WH11* gene of *Candida albicans* is regulated in two distinct development programs through the same transcription activation domains. *J. Bacteriol.* **179:**3837–3844.
140. **Srikantha, T., L. Tsai, K. Daniels, A. Klar, and D. R. Soll.** 2001. The histone deacetylase genes HDA1 and RPD3 play distinct roles in the regulation of high-frequency switching in *Candida albicans. J. Bacteriol.* **183:**4614–4625.
141. **Stoldt, V. R., A. Sonneborn, C. E. Leuker, and J. F. Ernst.** 1997. Efg1p, an essential regulator of morphogenesis of the human pathogen *Candida albicans,* is a member of a conserved class of bHLH proteins regulating morphogenetic processes in fungi. *EMBO J.* **16:**1982–1991.
142. **Stone, R. L., V. Matarese, B. B. Magee, P. T. Magee, and D. A. Bernlorh.** 1990. Cloning, sequencing and chromosomal assignment of a gene from *Saccharomyces cerevisiae* which is negatively regulated by glucose and positively by lipids. *Gene* **96:**171–176.
143. **Struhl, K.** 1998. Histone acetylation and transcriptional regulatory mechanisms. *Gen. Dev.* **12:**599–606.
144. **Struhl, K.** 1999. Fundamentally different logic of gene regulation in eukaryotes and prokaryotes. *Cell* **98:**1–4.

145. **Tanny, J. C., G. J. Dowd, J. Huang, H. Hilz, and D. Moazed.** 1999. An enzymatic activity in the yeast Sir2 protein that is essential for gene silencing. *Cell* **99:**735–745.

146. **Vannier, D., D. Balders, and D. Shore.** 1996. Evidence that the transcription regulators *SIN3* and *RPD3*, and a novel gene (*SDS3*) with similar functions, are involved in transcriptional silencing in *S. cerevisiae. Genetics* **144:**1343–1353.

147. **Varela, J. C., U. M. Praekelt, P. A. Meacock, R. J. Planta, and W. H. Mager.** 1995. The *Saccharomyces cerevisiae HSP12* gene is activated by the high-osmolarity glycerol pathway and negatively regulated by protein kinase A. *Mol. Cell. Biol.* **15:**6232–6245.

148. **Vargas, K., S. A. Messer, M. Pfaller, S. R. Lockhart, J. T. Stapleton, J. Hellstein, and D. R. Soll.** 2000. Elevated phenotypic switching and drug resistance of *Candida albicans* from human immunodeficiency virus-positive individuals prior to first thrush episode. *J. Clin. Microbiol.* **38:**3595–3607.

149. **Vargas, K., P. W. Wertz, D. Drake, B. Morrow, and D. R. Soll.** 1994. Differences in adhesion of *Candida albicans* 3153A cells exhibiting switch phenotypes of buccal epithelium and stratum corneum. *Infect. Immun.* **62:**1328–1335.

150. **Vidal, M., and R. F. Gaber.** 1991. *RPD3* encodes a second factor required to achieve maximum positive and negative transcriptional state in *Saccharomyces cerevisiae. Mol. Cell. Biol.* **11:**6317–6327.

151. **Wahi, M., K. Komachi, and A. D. Johnson.** 1998. Gene regulation by the yeast Ssn6-Tup1 corepressor. *Cold Spring Harbor Symp. Quant. Biol.* **63:**447–457.

152. **White, T. C., S. H. Miyasaki, and N. Agabian.** 1993. Three distinct secreted aspartyl proteinases in *Candida albicans. J. Bacteriol.* **175:**6126–6135.

153. **Xu, J., T. G. Mitchell, and R. Vilgalys.** 1999. PCR-RFLP analyses reveal extensive clonality and local genetic differentiation in *Candida albicans. Ecology* **8:**59–74.

154. **Yoshida, M., S. Horinouchi, and T. Beppu.** 1995. Trichostatin A and trapoxin: novel chemical probes for the role of histone acetylation in chromatin structure and function. *Bioessays* **17:**423–430.

155. **Zhang, Y., R. Iratni, H. Erdjument-Bromage, P. Tempst, and D. Reinberg.** 1997. Histone deacetylases and *SAP18*, a novel polypeptide, are components of a human Sin3 complex. *Cell* **89:**357–364.

156. **Zhang, Y., Z.-W. Sun, R. Iratni, H. Erdjument-Bromage, P. Tempst, M. Hampsey, and D. Reinberg.** 1998. *SAP3*, a novel protein conserved between human and yeast, is a component of a histone deacetylase complex. *Mol. Cell* **1:**1021–1031.

III. CELL BIOLOGY

Candida and Candidiasis
Edited by Richard A. Calderone

Chapter 11

Cell Biology and Cell Cycle of *Candida*

Neil A. R. Gow

When Odds wrote the second edition of *Candida and Candidosis* in 1988 (76), he summarized the work of nearly 6,000 references. This volume was written at a time when the ploidy of this fungus was not known, no genes had been cloned, and no transformation system was available. The principal organism of the text, *Candida albicans,* seemed a very poor model fungus in comparison to those in which rapid progress in fungal cell biology was being made through the application of traditional genetics, mutant analysis, and molecular genetics. Nonetheless, this volume had a strong focus on the cell biology of pathogenic *Candida* species and how, for example, prevailing environmental conditions stimulated the transition from yeast cells (often called blastospores or blastoconidia) to filamentous forms.

In the modern era of molecular genetics, and at a time when the *C. albicans* genome database nears completion, it is easy to lose sight of the work in the premolecular era. There are, however, some important insights to be noted from early work, and Odds's book should be seen as an essential companion to the current volume. This chapter aims to summarize the literature and pre- and postmolecular genetics to provide a guide to our current understanding of the cell biology and morphogenesis of *C. albicans.* A description of the signaling pathways that orchestrate the yeast-hypha transition is covered in chapter 8, and the regulation of cell morphology and regulated gene expression are described in chapter 7. Here the focus is on the shape and form of the various cell types of *C. albicans,* structural organization, and the cell cycle.

STRUCTURAL DIMORPHISM

C. albicans is one of many hundreds of species that are said to exhibit structural dimorphism. This term is taken to mean that vegetative growth of the fungus can occur in either a yeast form, reproducing by budding or by binary fission, or alternatively in a filamentous form in which elongated cells are elaborated and cells fail to separate after cytokinesis, thereby forming filaments of pseudohyphae or hyphae (see Fig. 1, chapter 7). Yeast development by budding is typical of most dimorphic yeast species (e.g., *C. albicans, Saccharomyces cerevisiae* [34, 62], *Histoplasma capsulatum* [64], *Paracoccidioides brasiliensis* [83]. Some produce single buds whereas others, like *H. capsulatum* and *P. brasiliensis,* produce multiple buds simultaneously from the mother cell. Other fungal pathogens, such as *Penicillium marneffii,* produce yeast cells that divide by binary fission (104) in a manner reminiscent of *Schizosaccharomyces pombe.* The formal distinction between pseudohyphae and true hyphae is discussed below.

It is, however, worth stating that there is nothing special about the phenomenon of dimorphism in fungi. Indeed, the vast majority of fungi exhibit at least some capacity to form both spherical cells (spores, phialides, sporangium vesicles, arbuscules, sclerotia, appressoria, etc.) and tubular cells (hyphae, sporangiophores, mating projections, chords, rhizoids, etc.). The regulation of fungal morphogenesis can, for the most part, be reduced to the ability to regulate polarized and nonpolarized (isotropic) cell expansion. It is also highly likely that the basic principles underlying the ability of cells to grow in these two fundamentally contrasting ways are conserved, and that the shape and form of all fungi can be modeled and understood through a knowledge of how cells regulate directional growth. The study of dimorphism in *C. albicans* has now become reasonably amenable to molecular analysis and has a legitimate place among the fungi with accessible sexual genetics as a valued model in the dissection of the ways fungi regulate their shape.

Neil A. R. Gow • Department of Molecular and Cell Biology, Institute of Molecular and Cell Biology, University of Aberdeen, Aberdeen AB25 2ZD, Scotland.

GROWTH FORMS OF *C. ALBICANS*

"Yeast cell" is a straightforward term that is generally understood by all mycologists. It is, in my view, unfortunate that medical mycologists have used the term "blastospores and blastoconidia" as synonyms and the resulting confusion is evident in my experience of inquiries from eminent yeast laboratories asking how yeast cells differ from blastospores and how such spores can be generated in culture! The blastospore has none of the properties of true spores with adaptation for survival, dormancy, or dispersal, and it would be helpful if this term were formally abandoned. Yeast cells of *C. albicans* look very much like those of *S. cerevisiae* but are marginally smaller and less rounded. The budding pattern of *C. albicans* yeast cells is described below.

Pseudohyphae are chains of more or less elongated yeast cells joined end to end. The established formal distinction between pseudohypha cells and true hyphae is that pseudohyphae have visible constrictions at the sites of septa (Table 1). *C. albicans* and its close relative *Candida dubliniensis* are alone among the pathogenic *Candida* species in forming true, nonconstricted hyphae (35, 49), but all *Candida* species seem to be able to form pseudohyphae. Germ tubes are usually taken to mean true hyphae in the first few cell cycles of growth. The formation of unconstricted germ tubes in whole or diluted sera has long been a rapid test used to diagnose *C. albicans* isolates (49). It has been suggested that hyphae may either represent the extreme form of more or less elongated pseudohyphal cells or, alternatively, that hyphae are a separate morphological form (14, 39, 67, 75). There are several aspects of the growth, structure, and regulation of pseudohyphae and true hyphae that differentiate them (Table 1). For example, the buds and mother cells within a pseudomycelium divide synchronously while many of the cells or compartments within a true hypha are arrested in growth (see later). Mitosis in the first cell cycle occurs at the bud neck, as it does in yeast cells, but in germ tubes mitosis occurs about 3 to 15 μm into the germ tube (40, 71, 84, 93, 99). Also, true hyphae form two septin rings during the first cell cycle, one at the site of cell evagination and a second at the eventual site of cytokinesis (see later), whereas pseudohyphae and yeast cells form a single septin ring that is associated with cytokinesis (99). In addition, null mutants of the morphogenesis repressor Tup1 were constitutively pseudohyphal in most laboratory media and could not be induced to form true hyphae by serum (13). Although the *tup1/tup1* mutant can still produce hyphae under other conditions, this implies that Tup1 is required for serum-induction of hyphae but represses serum-induction of pseudohyphae (Table 1).

Chlamydospores are rounded cells formed on the ends of differentiated suspensor cells that develop in media containing complex carbohydrates (3, 69, 72). They are larger, more refractile, and more rounded than yeast cells. The physiological status of the chlamydospore is not certain. There have been no credible reports of the germination of chlamydospores. Few reports exist of chlamydospores in clinical specimens (76). *C. dubliniensis* can be distinguished from *C. albicans* in vitro by the production of more abundant, unilateral or bilateral chlamydospores occurring in pairs or triplets from the suspensor cells (95, 100).

Table 1. Some distinguishing features between pseudohyphae and true hyphae/germ tubes of *C. albicans*

Property	Pseudohyphae	Hyphae	Reference
Morphology of lateral wall at site of septa	Visible constriction	Nonconstricted	41, 47
Growth kinetics	Synchronous development of mother cells and daughter buds	Asynchronous development of secondary germ tubes and branches	52, 53
Growth of cells within compartments of mycelium	All compartments undergoing vegetative growth	Subapical compartments showing growth arrest	40, 41, 52, 53
Site of mitosis	Mother-bud neck	3–15 μm within germ tube	38, 68, 81, 90
Cell cycle regulation of actin	Probably determines cell morphology as in *S. cerevisiae*	Polarization of actin regulated independently of cell cycle	44
Septins	Single septin ring at bud neck	Two septin rings in first cell cycle—the first at the site of germ tube evagination and the second at the site of cytokinesis	95
Vacuoles	Constant vacuole: total cell ratio	Vacuoles mainly in distal compartments	37, 39, 40, 41
Requirement for Tup 1	No	Yes (in serum medium)	13

The chlamydospore is a fragile cell structure compared to yeast cells and can be crushed under a coverslip (37). Therefore, they seem to have no properties to suggest they are robust and adapted for survival or dormancy.

It has been argued that because *C. albicans* forms yeast cells, pseudohyphae, hyphae, chlamydospores (and associated suspensor cells) it should be classified as polymorphic and not dimorphic. Pedantically this is true, but the term dimorphism is usually taken to mean that mitotic reproduction can occur in either a unicellular or multicellular filamentous form. Accordingly, there is no problem with either definition.

EXOGENOUS AND ENDOGENOUS ASPECTS OF HYPHA INDUCTION

The hypha of *C. albicans* has a diameter of around 2.0 μm and extends at a rate of between 15 and 22 μm/h under most conditions in vitro (40, 84). Under optimal conditions in serum-containing medium, almost 100% of yeast cells can produce a germ tube within an hour although the rate of induction is decreased when cells are inoculated into media at higher cell densities or into defined media such as Lee's or *N*-acetyl glucosamine-containing medium. Germ tube formation is also rapid in vivo, for example, after experimental inoculation in animal models of infection, although the precise kinetics of growth is difficult to assess under these conditions. Yeast cells of *C. albicans* can growth in rich media at 37°C with a doubling time of around an hour. Interseptation times of hyphae are not much slower that this (40). This makes the growth rates of both yeast and hyphal forms of *C. albicans* close to the record for any eukaryote, which, to my knowledge, is held by the oomcyete *Achlya ambisexualis* at 51 min (44). The dimorphic transition of some dimorphic fungi such as *P. brasiliensis* is regulated simply by temperature, so that yeast cells are produced at 37°C in the same media that encourage mycelial development at 25°C (83). However, in *C. albicans,* there is a more complex relationship between environmental conditions and the stimulation of the yeast to hypha transition, which is discussed below.

Chapter 7 summarizes information regarding how morphology of *C. albicans* responds to changes in specific environmental conditions. Much of the work done to date has necessarily focused on stimulation of hypha development in vitro, and it is still far from clear what morphogenetic triggers are relevant in vivo. Neutral pH, a temperature of around 37°C, and the presence of specific nutrients are all implicated in dimorphic regulation (see chapter 7 and reference 76 for summaries). It is, however, unlikely that many of the growth conditions used to stimulate hypha induction in vitro are relevant in vivo. For example, changes in pH and temperature, addition of *N*-acetyl glucosamine or serum diluted in amino acids and glucose, the use of Spider medium containing high mannitol concentrations, etc., are unlikely to represent prevailing physiological conditions on the surfaces of mucosa and endothelium or in the bloodstream.

It is also not clear whether hypha induction responds to the presence of specific environmental morphogens. There is no direct evidence for a specific chemical morphogen that would be present at sufficient concentration in situ to stimulate morphogenesis. Attempts have been made to determine the most active hypha-inducing fractions of serum and seminal plasma in vitro (8, 18, 19, 29), and recent evidence showed that a filtrate of serum, with a molecular cutoff below 1 kDa, was most active in hypha induction (29). In an early study, *N*-acetyl mannosamine was shown to act as a gratuitous inducer of hypha development since it could not be transported by *C. albicans* (101). This suggests that at least some signals can be perceived at the cell surface and supports a morphogen-based model for dimorphic regulation. However, it is also possible that many media formulations cause hypha development by inducing a common metabolic condition, for example, one of nitrogen starvation, and this view places less emphasis on the need for environmental morphogens. This seems to offer an explanation for the relative paucity of genes in the *C. albicans* genome database encoding transmembrane receptors and α-subunits for trimeric G-proteins that may be required to perceive morphogen-based signals. Several authors have suggested that a common feature of those media inducing hypha development is that they induce a stress response in the fungus (14). This view has the merit of presenting testable hypotheses at the molecular level.

One specific example of this is the hypothesis that the response to serum proteins may represent a nitrogen starvation response (see chapter 8). Although serum is composed mainly of proteins, these are inaccessible to the fungus until proteolysis takes place. Serum-containing media sustain hyphal growth more efficiently and for longer than other media where reversion to budding occurs rapidly. This may be because serum hydrolysis occurs slowly and cells sustain a starvation response until the serum medium is enriched via hydrolysis by secreted proteases.

Previous work also demonstrated the presence of autoregulatory compounds in growth media such as MARS (for morphogenetic autoregulatory substance) (47, 48). Although the nature of such compounds has proved elusive, it is clear that hypha formation is suppressed when cultures are induced into media at high initial cell densities (76). The recognition that homoserinelactone-mediated density-dependent signaling is an important aspect of the physiology of bacteria provides impetus to revisit this phenomenon in *C. albicans* using new molecular approaches.

PATTERNS OF WALL GROWTH

Bud Site Selection

The shape of a bud or a hypha reflects the way in which the cell wall is laid down. Both growth forms start as polarized evaginations from the cell surface. In *S. cerevisiae* the bud site selection pattern in both haploid and diploid cells is now well established (for a review see reference 17) and is regulated by bud site tags encoded by *BUD* and septin genes (see below). Haploid *S. cerevisiae* strains have an axial budding pattern in which buds form next to the site of the previous bud, whereas diploid cells exhibit bipolar budding in which the buds are formed at both poles of the cell (17, 82). The first bud is usually formed opposite the birth scar and then subsequent buds are formed adjacent to the previous bud. Since all *C. albicans* strains examined to date are diploid and the diploid budding pattern is a prerequisite for pseudohyphal growth of *S. cerevisiae* (55), it would be expected that *C. albicans* yeast cells also exhibit a bipolar budding pattern. Bud scars of *S. cerevisiae* are readily visualized by fluorescence microscopy after Calcofluor staining but are somewhat less clear in Calcofluor-stained yeast cells of *C. albicans*. However, studies to date suggest that the budding pattern of *C. albicans* resembles the bipolar budding of *S. cerevisiae*; this is influenced by temperature so that buds form predominantly by axial growth at 23 to 28°C but form nonadjacent buds and germ tubes at 37°C (16).

Wall Expansion and the Cell Cycle of Buds and Hyphae

After a site of evagination is established, continued expansion of the cell surface is also highly regulated. Polylysine-coated microspores have been used to map out where cell wall expansion in yeast cells and hyphae of *C. albicans* takes place (68, 71, 94). This showed that hyphae were characterized by continuous apical growth. During the bud cell cycle the first two-thirds of the cycle was due to apical growth and in the final phase apical growth was shut down and replaced by isotropic expansion of the entire surface (71). These observations have now been extended and placed in the context of cell cycle regulation (see below).

CYTOSKELETON AND CELL GROWTH

Actin and Polarized Growth

Polarized and isotropic growth of cells is related ultimately to the way in which the secretory vesicles are targeted to the cell membrane. These vesicles carry the biosynthetic enzymes, such as chitin synthase and β-1,3 glucan synthase that give shape to the cell wall and provide new membrane for surface expansion. Vectorial secretion of secretory vesicles is regulated by actin and its associated motor protein myosin, which deliver these vesicles to sites of exocytosis (97). Actin is concentrated as spots (also called patches or plaques) at sites of polarized growth and at the position of developing septa (1). Actin and a variety of proteins that function as molecular markers of future growth at the peripheral cortex and various cell cycle factors act together to promote polarized apical extension. Rhodamine-phalloidin and immunofluorescence staining of F-actin showed that all sites of active cell expansion of *C. albicans* were associated with localized actin patches (2, 4, 46, 108, 109). Such patches have been shown in *S. cerevisiae* to be membrane invaginations stabilized by actin and acting as points of vesicle exocytosis (73). In this yeast *act1* mutants fail to exhibit polarized growth, expand isotropically, and fail to localized chitin synthesis (1). As in other fungi, there is evidence in *C. albicans* that actin microfilaments are essential for polarized growth. The actin inhibitors cytochalasin A (2) and cloropropham (109) dispersed filamentous actin in the cell, prevented germ tube extension, and caused loss of the normal cylindrical shape of the hypha (2). In contrast, the microtubule inhibitor nocodazole did not affect germ tube extension but inhibited nuclear division and migration (104). The microtubule inhibitor benomyl has been shown to inhibit germ tube growth, but it also caused redistribution of the normally asymmetrical tip-high concentration of actin patches, which presumably accounts for the effect of benomyl on germ tube growth (2).

Early in the cell cycle, actin patches have been shown to accumulate at the future bud site (Fig. 1). These patches persisted after bud emergence. Actin also formed a faint ring at the neck of mother and bud, and patches are formed on both sides of the septum (4, 46). A similar pattern of actin staining was seen in hyphae, although the apical actin persisted throughout the cell cycle. The first appearance of polarized cortical actin patches occurred only 30 min after hy-

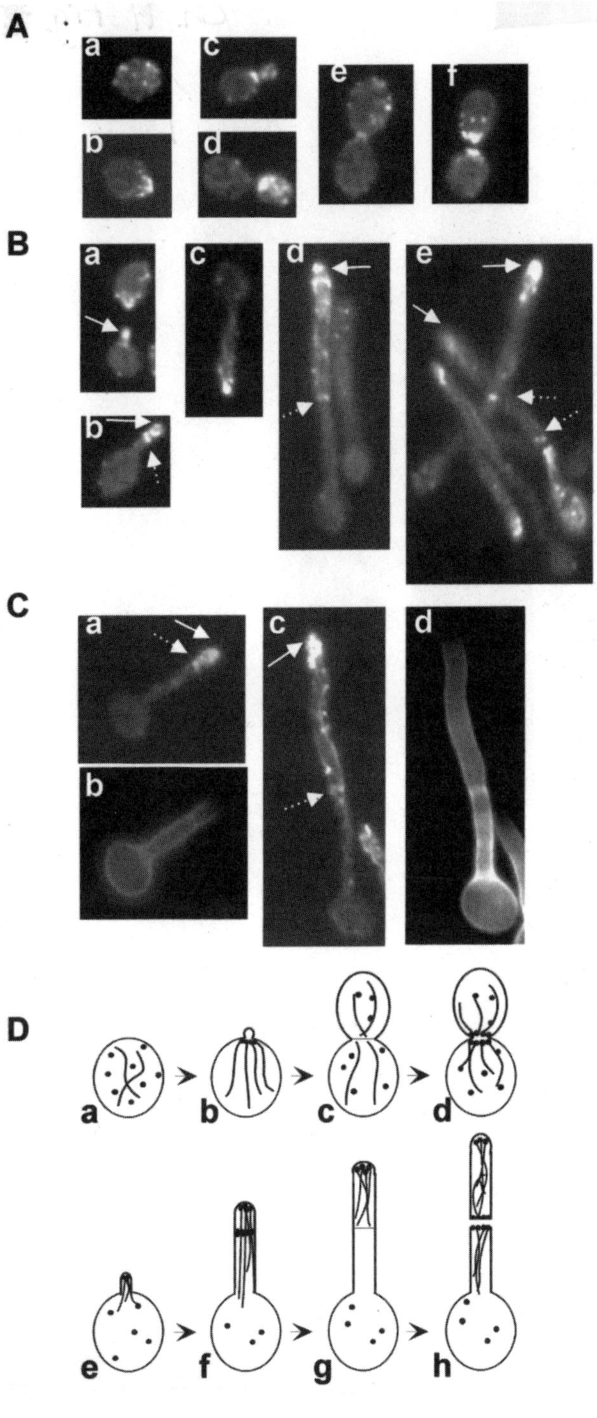

Figure 1. The pattern of actin staining in yeast and hyphal cells of *C. albicans* as described in the text. The actin distribution in yeast cells (A, a–f) and hyphae (B, a–e) is shown after staining with rhodamine-phalloidin. In some specimens, counterstaining with Calcofluor is used to show the cell wall (C, a–d). Cartoon (D, a–h) is based on the microscopical analysis. Actin is shown at the presumptive site of cell growth (A, b) and at future sites of septa (A, c; B, b; and C, a) colocalizing with chitin ring (C, b, d). Dashed arrows indicate actin regulated by cell cycle, and solid arrows indicate actin associated with hypha morphogenesis. Modified from reference 46 with permission.

phal induction in serum, a full 70 min (on average) before the spindle poles duplicated and DNA replication occurred (46). The time of appearance of the ring of actin patches at future sites of septation coincided with the appearance of a duplicated spindle pole body for mitosis in both yeast and hyphae (46).

Actin generates contractile force, for example for cytokinesis, or is able to with work motor proteins to translocate secretory vesicles and organelles, such as the vacuole. Little information is available about these proteins in *C. albicans*. By analogy with *S. cerevisiae*, it may be predicted that vesicle transport, vacuole inheritance, and exocytosis will involve class V myosin (like the *S. cerevisiae* Myo2p), that endocytosis may employ type I myosin (like Myo3 and Myo5 of *S. cerevisiae*), and that cell cytokinesis will involve class II myosins (for reviews see references 96, 97). In *S. cerevisiae* Myo4 is involved in transporting the mRNA of *ASH1*, which is important for bud-specific gene expression (12, 51, 88). Because the hypha cell cycle is highly asymmetric (see later), this motor protein may be important for hyphal morphogenesis in *C. albicans*. Apical growth and cytokinesis are regulated differently in *S. cerevisiae* and *C. albicans* (see below), and filamentous fungi sometimes use alternative motor systems for organelle transport (96). Therefore, the regulation of actin and microtubule motors may be an interesting area for future research in *C. albicans*.

Microtubules and Spindle Pole Bodies

In yeast-like fungi, microtubules are concerned mostly with the positioning, movement, and division of the nucleus (93). Both immunofluorescence (9) and β-tubulin-green fluorescent protein (GFP) fusions (46) using the GFP codon optimized for *C. albicans* (22) have been used to examine microtubule dynamics during the budding and hyphal phases. These studies showed that the global pattern of microtubule organization in yeast cells was similar to that in *S. cerevisiae* (9, 46). The spindle pole body (SPB) is only faintly visible by fluorescence prior to duplication (46) when it was seen either as a brighter spot or rod (Fig. 2). The mitotic spindle is longer in hyphae (12 to 20 μm) compared to yeast (7 to 8 μm) and the hyphae have more prominent microtubules (9, 46). In hyphae and yeasts, SPB duplication occurred around the time of DNA synthesis and the formation of the chitin ring such that SPB and SPB duplication correspond to the G_1 and S/G_2 phases of the cell cycle (46). The presence of elongated, duplicated SPBs coincided with the time of mitosis. Subapical cells of hyphae often maintained single nuclei with unduplicated SPB indicative of growth arrest in these compartments (see later). Fluo-

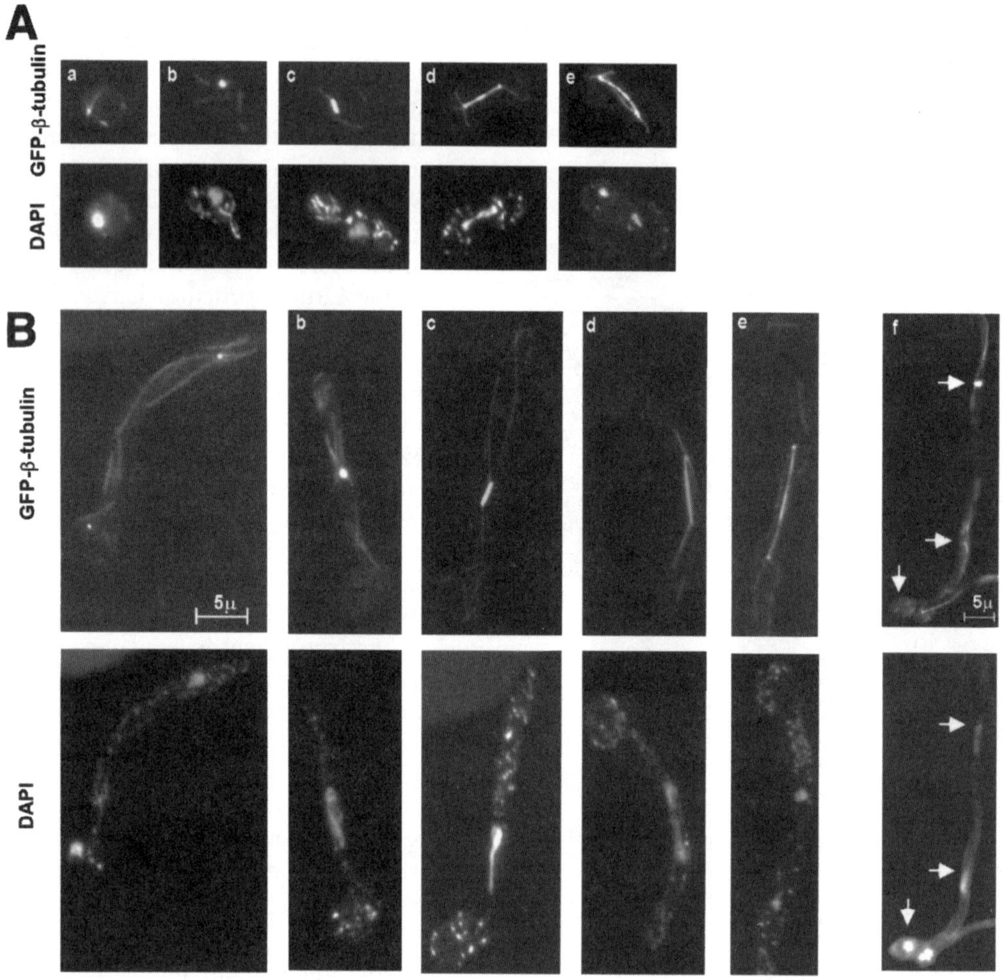

Figure 2. Morphology of the SPB configuration during (A) budding and (B) hypha development in relation to the cell cycle. The microtubules are revealed using a GFP-tubulin protein fusion (upper panels), and the nuclear morphologies of the same cells are shown using 4′, 6′-diamidino-2-phenylinsole (DAPI) staining (lower panels). In both A and B, the SPB is (a) unduplicated, (b) unseparated but duplicated, (c) separated and duplicated, and (d, e) elongated during mitosis. In hyphae, longer spindles are observed (d, e) and cytoplasmic microtubules are more obvious (f). Modified from reference 46 with permission.

rescence in situ hybridization of RPS repetitive sequences has been used to study the segregation of chromosomes during spindle elongation and the anaphase A and B phases of mitosis (21). This study again describes a similar organization of the *C. albicans* and *S. cerevisiae* chromosomes in mitosis. The microtubule motor proteins of *C. albicans* remain to be defined but probably will include homologs of the kinesins Kar3, Kip1, Kip3, and dynein of *S. cerevisiae* (97).

Septins

Septins are encoded by a family of genes including *CDC3, CDC10, CDC11,* and *CDC12,* which were originally discovered in a screen for cell division cycle mutants in *S. cerevisiae* (45), and three more recently identified genes that are important for yeast sporulation (25, 28). Septins are found widely in nature from fungi to mammals and are universally important for cytokinesis (61). They assemble as 10 nm diameter filaments as a double ring at the bud neck of *S. cerevisiae* closely adjacent to the plasma membrane. This ring is formed just prior to the time the actin ring is assembled, which brings about cytokinesis (31). Actin is not required for septin localization since Latrunculin A, an actin depolymerizing drug, did not inhibit their cell cycle-dependent localization. However, septins are required for the formation of an actin-myosin ring (11, 31). Septins may, therefore, form a scaffold upon which actin is assembled at sites of cytokinesis. After cytokinesis the double ring splits, each cell inheriting one ring.

Septins of *C. albicans* were first observed as filament rings at the future sites of septa in thin sections of yeast and hyphal cells by transmission electron microscopy (92). The *C. albicans CDC3* and *CDC10* genes have been isolated by functional complementation in *S. cerevisiae* (26). The localization of the *C. albicans* Cdc11p septin in pseudohyphae and hyphae was studied by immunofluorescence using an anti-*S. cerevisiae* antiserum (99). In pseudohyphae the pattern of Cdc11p localization was similar to that in yeast cells of *S. cerevisiae* with a double ring forming at the mother cell-bud neck. However, a novel organization was seen in true hyphae. A septin ring was first formed at the neck of the germ tube and mother yeast cell, but this disorganized and a second ring formed later in the first cell cycle within the germ tube at the future plane of cytokinesis (Fig. 3) (99). This provides a clear distinction between the cytology of pseudohyphae and true hyphae of *C. albicans* (Table 1).

The *C. albicans* integrin-like protein Int1p has

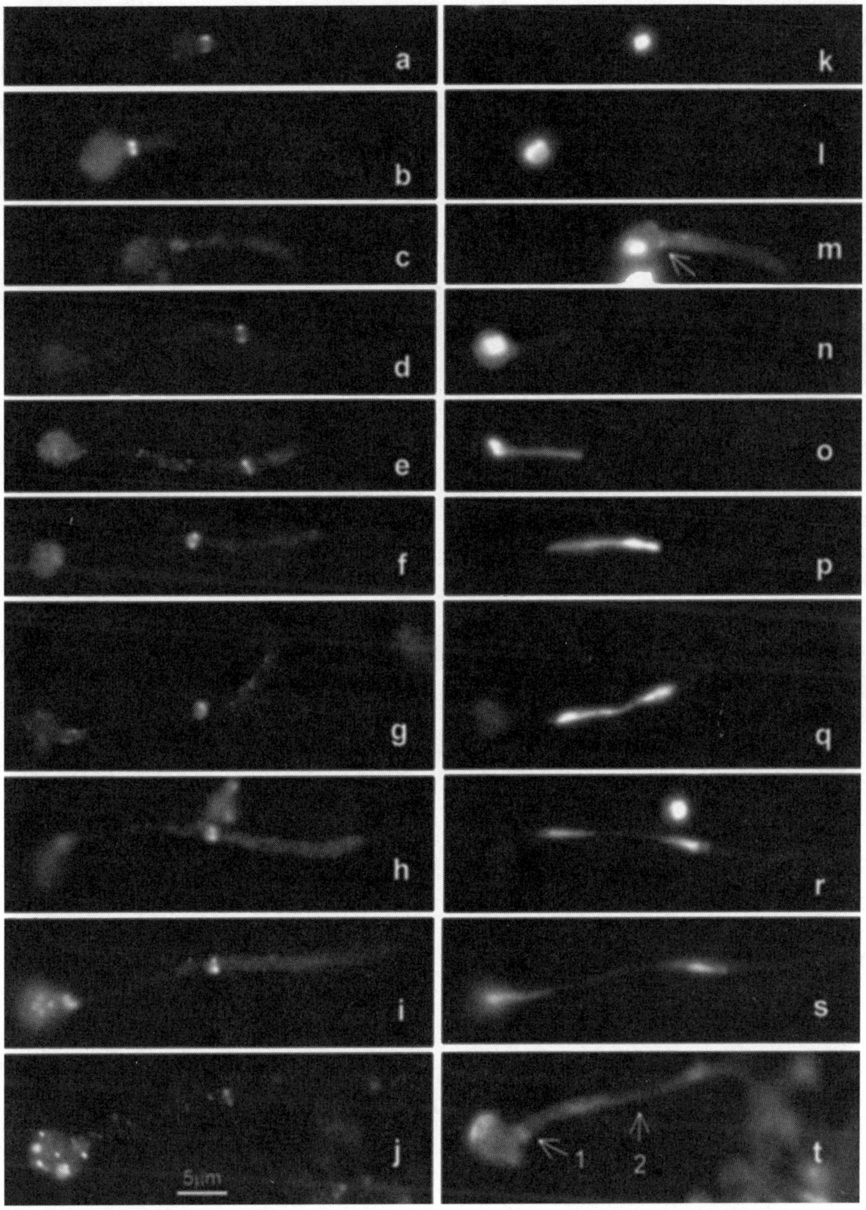

Figure 3. Septin-organization during germ tube growth of *C. albicans* in relation to the nuclear cycle. Images are from cells after 40 min (a, k), 50 min (b, c, 1, m), and 75 min (d–f, n–p). Cells in panels m and t were also stained with Calcofluor. Early germ tubes (a–c) show the first septin ring at the base of the germ tube, whereas longer germ tubes, later in the cell cycle, show the second septin ring (d–j) at the future site of cytokinesis. From reference 99 with permission from Blackwell Science.

some homology to the *S. cerevisiae* Bud4 protein, which affects septin assembly (32, 33). Heterologous expression of *CaINT1* in *S. cerevisiae* induced filamentation (7) and interfered with normal septin architecture (Berman, personal communication), perhaps by preventing septum formation and cytokinesis. This *CaINT1*-dependent morphogenesis also led to sustained polarized actin distribution during the cell cycle (6). Therefore, septins play a key role in organizing actin-mediated dimorphic regulation in *C. albicans*.

CELL CYCLE AND DIMORPHIC REGULATION

In *S. cerevisiae, C. albicans,* and other eukaryotes there is now strong evidence that cell shape changes are regulated by the cyclin-dependent kinase (CDK), encoded by *CDC28/2* (24, 66, 85). The initiation of polarized growth and cell evagination is triggered by the CDK at START in the G_1/S phase of the cell cycle (57). This results in the assembly of actin at the incipient site of evagination. As described above, buds initially exhibit apical growth, then switch to isotropic expansion later in the cell cycle (94). The time of the transition from polarized to apical expansion coincides with the G_2/M transition of the cell cycle. The switch to isotropic growth is again regulated by the CDK. Evidence for this model proposed by Lew and Reed (57, 58) comes from experiments in *S. cerevisiae* in which the expression of G_1 and G_2 cyclins is regulated by mutation or overexpression. For example, pseudohyphae were formed in *grr* mutants that resulted in stabilization of G_1 cyclins. Deletion of the G_2 cyclin Clb2, which acts to promote early onset isotropic growth, also led to bud elongation. On the other hand, overexpression of *CLB1* or *CLB2* resulted in an earlier transition to isotropic growth and consequently rounder cells (57). These mutations therefore affected cell shape by influencing when the active mitosis promoting cyclin-Cdc28/2 complex was assembled during the cell cycle (59). Therefore, in pseudohyphal cells of *C. albicans* it is presumed that the phase of apical expansion may be extended in the cell cycle so that buds become more or less elongated. A *C. albicans cdc13/CLB1/CLB2* B-type cyclin that was able to complement the *S. pombe* cdc13 genes has been isolated (24) that may be involved in pseudohyphal morphogenesis. Pseudohyphae of *S. cerevisiae* have a naturally extended G_2 phase compared to yeast cells (55).

Recent work has shown that this elegant model may be relevant to both the development of *C. albicans* yeast cells and pseudohyphae, but it may not fully account for the regulation of cell shape in true hyphae. In *C. albicans* deletion of the G_1 *CaCLN1* resulted in slower cell cycle progression and the inability to form hyphae or to express certain hypha-specific genes in Lee's synthetic medium (56, 60). However, the *cln1/cln1* mutant did not affect cell shape but formed true hyphae that reverted more rapidly to the yeast form. This suggested that the *C. albicans* Cln1 cyclin is required for the maintenance of hyphal development and prevention of the reversion to the yeast phase but not for hypha development per se (60). Recently, Haoping Liu's group extended their analysis of the *Candida* cell cycle to show that actin polarization occurs before the start of the cell cycle at the G_1/S transition and is therefore regulated independently from the cell cycle (46). The early induction of polarized growth prior to DNA replication is a noticeable departure from the regulation of evagination in *S. cerevisiae.* They also measured the level of total CaCcd28 kinase and the active phosphorylated form Cdc28Tyr19. No evidence was found for alterations in the Tyr19 phosphorylation state of Cdc28 during hypha induction, supporting the view that in *C. albicans* the cell cycle program is not dramatically altered from that in yeast cells and that morphogenesis was regulated in parallel with the cell cycle (46). They also showed that cells at any stage of the cell cycle could be induced to form hyphae, but the shape of the tube depended on the morphology of the cell at the time of induction. Hence, a cell that was induced to form hyphae from an established bud formed a wider protuberance than the normal, narrow 2-μm hyphae formed from nonevaginated mother cells (46). As a consequence, the position of the first septum in the hypha relative to the mother cell was proposed to vary because individual cells will vary in the time elapsing between perception of the induction signal and the onset of the first cell cycle. These results contrast with previous reports that hyphae could only be formed at certain stages of the cell cycle (71). This evidence supports the view that in true hyphae the shape of the cell is not directly coupled to regulation by the CDK but instead that actin-mediated apical expansion is regulated in parallel to cell cycle-coupled events such as cytokinesis and septation (Fig. 4) (46). Uncoupling of CDK regulation of actin-mediated morphogenesis may be necessary to enable tip expansion to be sustained continually throughout the cell cycle, unlike in pseudohyphae and yeasts where isotropic growth must be initiated in the later stage of the cycle.

Asynchronous, Asymmetric Cell Cycle of *C. albicans* Hyphae

Another distinction between the cell cycles of pseudohyphae and true hyphae is that subapical com-

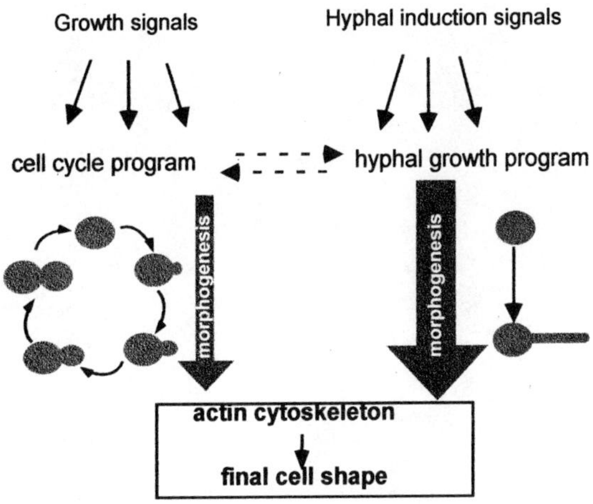

Figure 4. Model proposed by H. Liu and coworkers for independent, parallel regulation of hypha development by the cell cycle and a hypha morphogenesis program. Both programs contribute to the overall shape of the hyphal cell, which is determined ultimately by actin-directed vesicle exocytosis and cell wall assembly. Modified from reference 46 with permission.

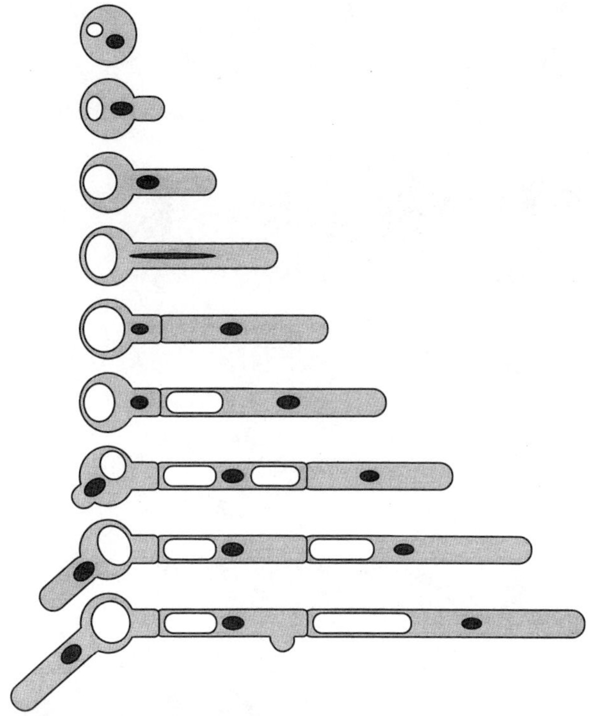

Figure 5. Model summarizing the relationship between germ tube growth, the cell cycle, and extensive subapical vacuolation of *C. albicans*. Vacuolated compartments are G_1 arrested, while the cytoplasm-rich apical cells reenter the cell cycle. Vacuolated compartments regenerated cytoplasm prior to reentering the cell cycle. Adapted from reference 39 with permission from Prous Science.

partments of hyphae often are cell cycle arrested (38, 39, 41–43). These cells are apparently arrested in the G_1 phase of the cycle (54, 56) and are extensively vacuolated. During the first hyphal cell cycle the mother yeast cell becomes extensively vacuolated and the cytoplasm remains with the extending apical cell, as if cytoplasm was migrating into the developing hyphal tube. This results in asymmetric partitioning of cytoplasm by the first cytokinesis event (Fig. 5 and 6a, c). Consequently, the mother cell is depleted of cytoplasm and does not immediately reenter the cell cycle. Similarly, apical cells of hyphae are cytoplasm-rich, but subapical compartments inherit less cytoplasm, are extensively vacuolated, have unduplicated SPBs, and become arrested in the cell cycle (43, 46, 54). Such vacuolated compartments do not reenter the cell cycle or form branches or lateral buds until they have resynthesized cytoplasm. Yeast and hyphal cells of *C. albicans* contain a single giant branched mitochondrion (103), but the vacuolated subapical cells of hyphae have small peripheral mitochondria with a lower energy charge (Fig. 6a, b) (6).

A model for the hyphal cell cycle as influenced by this pattern of subapical vacuolation has been presented (42, 54) which argues that arrested compartments have insufficient active cell cytoplasm to execute the size-dependent START function. In pseudohyphae mother and daughter cells are the same size and have similar total vacuole volume (107). As a consequence, and in contrast to the growth of true hyphae, pseudohyphae exhibit symmetrical, synchronous development of buds and mother cells (55) (Table 1).

The pattern of germ tube extension associated with little de novo cytoplasm synthesis and extensive subapical vacuolation may explain certain aspects of the physiology of germ tube growth in *C. albicans* (40, 65). For example, germ tubes of most filamentous fungi extend with exponential kinetics because the extension of a single apex is supported by an increasing biosynthetic potential, proportional to the length of the germ tube (79). However, in *C. albicans* the active cytoplasm is close to a constant volume and linear hyphal extension results. This result also explains the observed increasing carbon/nitrogen ratio of biomass as hyphal growth proceeds (65). *C. albicans* is not the only fungus that mobilizes and translocates cytoplasm as the hypha extends. A similar model for growth in the dimorphic fungus *Schizosaccharomyces japonicus* has been proposed (89–91). Plant pathogens such as *Uromyces maydis* (98), *Basidiobolus ranarum,* and others all have migratory cytoplasm and subapical vacuolation (43). This pattern of growth seems well adapted for cells growing in nutrient-deleted areas under nitrogen stress—precisely the types of environ-

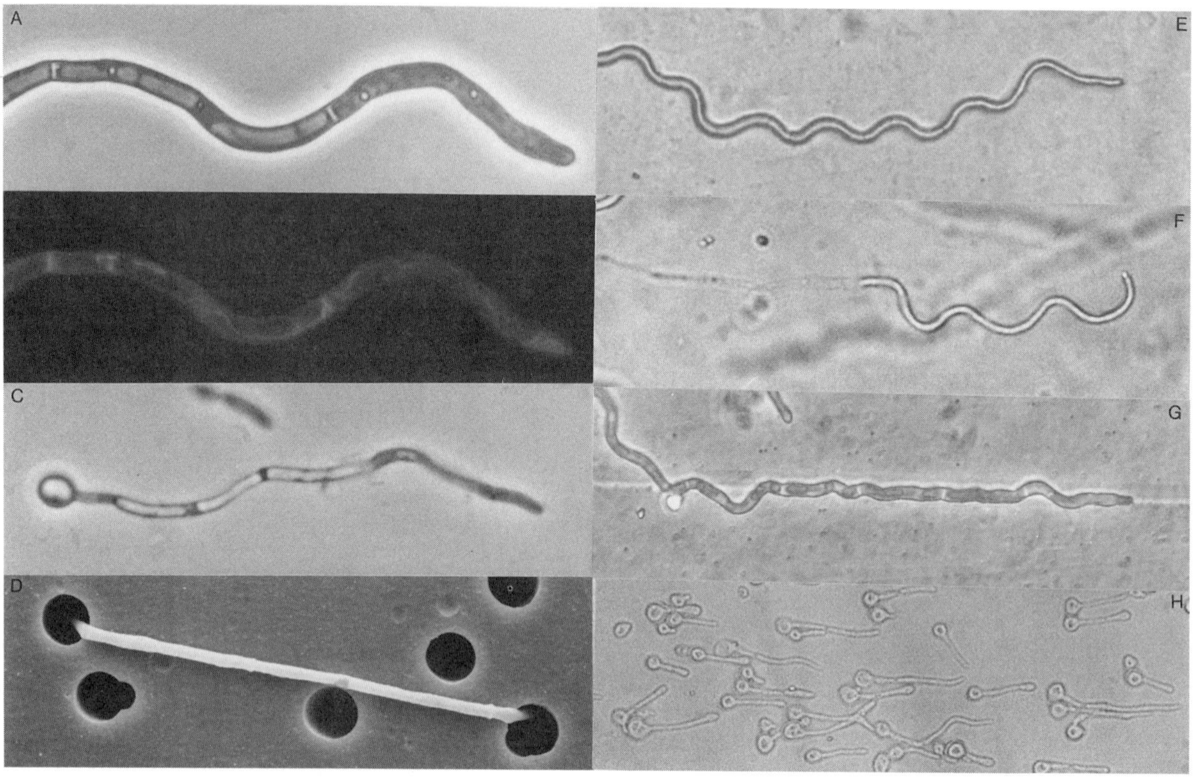

Figure 6. Morphology of and behavior of germ tubes and true hyphae of *C. albicans* (a, b). Phase contrast image of hypha with subapical vacuoles (a, c). Same hypha as (a) stained with DASPMI (b) to reveal giant apical mitochondria. Thigmotropic growth of hypha entering the pores of a Nuclepore membrane (d), and growing along a scratch on a cellophane membrane (e). Helical morphology of a hypha on a firm agar surface (f) and a hypha growing straight while embedded within agar, then exhibiting helical growth upon emerging on the surface (g). Galvanotropism toward the cathode in an electrical field of 28 mV/cm (h). Panels A and B are from reference 6, panel C is from reference 41, panel D is from reference 86, panel F is from reference 87, and panel H is from reference 23.

mental conditions that favor hyphal growth of *C. albicans*.

REGULATION OF POLARITY

As already discussed, polarized growth results from actin-dependent direction of the secretory vesicle traffic to the cell surface. In *S. cerevisiae* the analysis of the molecular genetics of cell polarity is a highly active field, and many regulatory proteins are now known to be located specifically at the site of cell growth. This is a much less developed field in *C. albicans* although there is a clear rationale for studies in this area. Several classes of GTPases play prominent roles in the regulation of polarity in *S. cerevisiae*. The Rho-type GTPase Cdc42 is a key protein of the so-called "polarosome," which also includes the guanine-exchange factor and calcium-binding protein Cdc24, a guanine dissociation factor Rdi, and the GTPase-activating proteins Bem3, Rgal, and Rga2 (20, 52). This Cdc42-dependent module, and in particular Cdc42, Cdc24, and Bem1, has a central role in organizing actin, septins, and other proteins that are involved in establishing polarized growth (52, 70). The Cdc42 GTPase is also involved in regulating cytokinesis, again by interacting with actin (52). Transcription of the *C. albicans CDC42* gene was shown to increase at the onset of budding and germ tube formation (70). Another GTPase, Sec4, of the rab family, is also involved in actin-dependent polarized vesicle secretion (74) whereas Sec3 may act as a molecular tag for the docking process of secretory vesicles at the sites of cell expansion (30). Another family of Rho GTPases in *S. cerevisiae* includes Rho1 through 4, several of which are localized to polarized growth sites (103, 105). Rho1 is involved not in the establishment, but rather in the maintenance of polarized growth and for β-1,3 glucan synthesis (80). Homologs of most or all of these proteins exist in *C. albicans* and other *Candida* species and presumably play vital roles in dimorphic regulation.

GROWTH AND GUIDANCE OF THE *CANDIDA* HYPHA

C. albicans is related to ascomycetous fungi for which there is no evidence for any chemotropic behavior other than the response to sex hormones (36). However, hyphae of *C. albicans* exhibit a number of in vitro tropic responses to oxygen (aerotropism), topography of the substrate (thigmotropism and thigmodifferentiation), and applied electrical fields (galvanotropism).

Hyphae of *C. albicans* grown on solid cornmeal agar exhibited aerotropism to oxygen gradients that were established under a coverslip placed over the culture (5). Yeast production lateral to hyphae was suppressed in the most oxygen-depleted zones in these culture preparations. This might be relevant to the growth of *C. albicans* hyphae in anoxic necrotic lesions.

When hyphae of *C. albicans* were grown on Nuclepore membranes, they entered the pores, emerged on the underside of the membrane, then grew along the underside of the membrane until they encountered another pore (Fig. 6d). This response to topographical signals is called "contact guidance" or thigmotropism and is a well-recognized phenomenon in plant pathogenic fungi (50) as well as in neurites (10), plant roots, and many other biological cell types. On scratched membranes hyphae grew along the scratch (86, 87) in a similar way to the growth of germ tubes of many phytopathogens on leaf and stem surfaces (Fig. 6d, e). It has been suggested that such thigmotropic behavior of *C. albicans* may facilitate tissue infiltration through epithelial invaginations and points of weakened surface integrity (39, 77), although evidence that thigmotropism is a true virulence factor is still lacking. It has been shown that thigmotropic hyphal reorientation is attenuated by gadolinium ions and verapamil, which block stretch-activated and L-type calcium channel blockers in the cell membrane (106). Thigmotropism in other cell types is also calcium dependent (63, 78). Stretch-activated channels have been demonstrated to exist in both hypha and yeast cells by using patch-clamp electrode recordings of isolated protoplasts (101).

Another response of *C. albicans* hyphae to touch is in the generation of helical hyphae (53, 87) (Fig. 6f, g). Helical hyphae are seen when *C. albicans* is grown on the surface of agars that are stiffened with a higher than normal percentage of agar, but they do not form if hyphae are embedded in agar or sandwiched between agar and a coverslip. The helix has a wavelength corresponding to one cell compartment, and it has been speculated that the helical form reflects hyphal turning during extension, with one complete turn occurring per hyphal cell cycle (87).

It has also been shown that hypha formation can be induced by growing cells on rough agar surfaces (81) and embedded in agar (15) (see chapter 8). This has been shown to be mediated via a zinc-finger-containing transcription factor, Cfz1 (15, 81), which may allow the fungus to respond to physical cues in its environment, and possibly in environments with low oxygen tension (27). It remains to be tested whether Cfz1 is required for thigmotropic responses.

The polarized response of germ tubes of *C. albicans* to applied electrical fields is not likely to be a physiological phenomenon, but it is dramatic and can result in near perfect parallel alignment of hyphae (25) (Fig. 6h). This response can therefore be used as an assay for hyphal alignment responses. Thus, both thigmotropism and galvanotropism are calcium-dependent phenomena.

SUMMARY

This chapter argues that the growth of the hyphal form of *C. albicans* is distinct from the growth of both the yeast form and pseudohyphal form in a number of critical respects. In particular, there are clear departures in the way the cell cycle is regulated that suggest that the true hyphal form is a distinct morphological phase that cannot be precisely modeled through the analysis of pseudohyphal growth in *S. cerevisiae*. Although a great deal of progress has been made since Odds's seminal summary in 1988 (76), it is still far from clear how the environment tilts the balance from unicellular to filamentous growth and what the nature of the signals are that are seen by *C. albicans* cells in vitro and in vivo. Finally, it is now becoming apparent that the regulation of dimorphism is linked intimately with the cell cycle and with other events that control how actin-mediated cell expansion is controlled in the various growth forms of *C. albicans*.

Acknowledgments. I thank Haoping Liu and Pete Sudbery for sharing information prior to publication and for donating figures and Frank Odds, Alistair Brown, Graham Gooday, and members of the Aberdeen Fungal Group for discussions and comments on the manuscript. I thank the Wellcome Trust and BBSRC for financial support of my laboratory.

REFERENCES

1. **Adams, A. E. M., and J. R. Pringle.** 1981. Relationship of actin and tubulin distribution to bud growth in wild-type and morphogenetic mutant *Saccharomyces cerevisiae*. *J. Cell Biol.* 98:934–945.
2. **Akashi, T., T. Kanbe, and K. Tanaka.** 1994. The role of

the cytoskeleton in the polarized growth of the germ tube in *Candida albicans. Microbiology* **140**:271–280.

3. **Akisada, T., K. Harada, M. Niimi, and A. Kamaguchi.** 1983. Production of contiguously arranged chlamydospores in *Candida albicans. J. Gen. Microbiol.* **129**:2327–2330.
4. **Anderson, J., and D. R. Soll.** 1986. Differences in actin localization during bud and hypha formation in the yeast *Candida albicans. J. Gen. Microbiol.* **132**:2035–2047.
5. **Aoki, S., S. Ito-Kuwa, K. Nakamura, V. Videtto, and K. Takeo.** 1998. Oxygen as a possible tropic factor in hyphal growth of *Candida albicans. Mycoscience* **39**:231–238.
6. **Aoki, S., S. Ito-Kuwa, Y. Nakamura, and T. Msuhara.** 1989. Mitochondrial behaviour during the yeast-hypha transition of *Candida albicans. Microbios* **60**:79–86.
7. **Asleson, C. M., E. S. Bensen, C. A. Gale, A.-S. Melms, C. Kurischko, and J. Berman.** 2001. *Candida albicans INT1*-induced filamentation in *Saccharomyces cerevisiae* depends on Sla2p. *Mol. Cell. Biol.* **21**:1272–1284.
8. **Barlow, A. J. E., T. Aldersley, and F. W. Chattaway.** 1974. Factors in serum and seminal plasma which promote germ tube formation and mycelial growth of *Candida albicans. J. Gen. Microbiol.* **82**:261–272.
9. **Barton, R., and K. Gull.** 1988. Variation in cytoplasmic microtubule organization and spindle length in the two forms of the dimorphic fungus *Candida albicans. J. Cell Sci.* **91**: 211–220.
10. **Bedlack, R. S., M.-D. Wei, and L. M. Loew.** 1992. Localized membrane depolarizations and localized calcium influx during electric field-guided neurite growth. *Neuron* **9**:393–403.
11. **Bi, E., P. Maddox, D. L. Lew, A. Schmidt, and M. N. Hall.** 1998. Involvement of an actomyosin contractile ring in *Saccharomyces cerevisiae* cytokinesis. *J. Cell Biol.* **142**: 1301–1312.
12. **Bobola, N., R.-P. Jansen, T. H. Shin, and K. Nasmyth.** 1996. Asymmetric accumulation of Ash1p in post-anaphase nuclei depends on a myosin and restricts yeast mating-type switching to mother cells. *Cell* **84**:699–710.
13. **Braun, B. R., and A. D. Johnson.** 1997. Control of filament formation in *Candida albicans* by the transcriptional repressor *TUP1. Science* **277**:105–109.
14. **Brown, A. J. P., and N. A. R. Gow.** 1999. Regulatory networks controlling *Candida albicans* morphogenesis. *Trends Microbiol.* **7**:333–338.
15. **Brown, D. H., Jr., A. D. Giusani, X. Chen, and C. A. Kumamoto.** 1999. Filamentous growth of *Candida albicans* in response to physical environmental cues and its regulation by the *CZF1* gene. *Mol. Microbiol.* **34**:651–662.
16. **Chaffin, W. L.** 1984. Site selection for bud and germ tube emergence in *Candida albicans. J. Gen. Microbiol.* **130**: 431–440.
17. **Chant, J.** 1994. Cell polarity in yeast. *Trends Genet.* **10**: 328–333.
18. **Chattawy, F. W., J. O'Reilly, A. J. E. Barlow, and T. Aldersley.** 1976. Induction of mycelial form of *Candida albicans* by hydrolysates of peptides from seminal plasma. *J. Gen. Microbiol.* **96**:317–322.
19. **Chattaway, F. W., P. R. Wheeler, and J. O'Reilly.** 1980. Purification and properties of peptides which induce germination of blastospores of *Candida albicans. J. Gen. Microbiol.* **120**: 431–437.
20. **Chen, G. C., L. Zhang, and C. S. Chan.** 1996. The LIM domain-containing Dbm1 GTPase-activating protein is required for normal polarized morphogenesis in *Saccharomyces cerevisiae. Mol. Cell. Biol.* **16**:1376–1390.
21. **Chibana H., and K. Tanaka.** 1996. Analysis of the cell cycle of the budding yeast *Candida albicans* by positioning of chromosomes by fluorescence in situ hybridization (FISH) with repetitive sequences. *Genes Cells* **1**:727–740.
22. **Cormack, B. P., G. Bertram, M. Egerton, N. A. R. Gow, S. Falkow, and A. J. P. Brown.** 1997. Yeast-enhanced green fluorescent protein (yEGFP): a reporter of gene expression in *Candida albicans. Microbiology* **143**:303–311.
23. **Crombie, T., N. A. R. Gow, and G. W. Gooday.** 1990. Influence of applied electrical fields on yeast and hyphal growth of *Candida albicans. J. Gen. Microbiol.* **136**:311–317.
24. **Damagnez, V., and G. Cottarel.** 1996. *Candida albicans CDK1* and *CYB1:* cDNA homologues of the *cdcc/CDC28* and *cdc13/CLB1/CLB2* cell cycle control genes. *Gene* **172**: 137–141.
25. **De Virgilio, C., D. J. DeMarini, and J. R. Pringle.** 1996. SPR28, a sixth member of the sptin gene family in *Saccharomyces cerevisiae* that is expressed specifically in sporulating cells. *Microbiology* **142**:2897–2905.
26. **DiDomenico, B. J., N. H. Brown, J. Lupisella, J. R. Greene, M. Yanko, and Y. Kolton.** 1994. Homologs of the neck-filament associated genes—isolation and sequence analysis of *Candida albicans CDC3* and *CDC10. Mol. Gen. Genet.* **242**: 689–698.
27. **Ernst, J. F.** 2000. Transcriptional factors in *Candida albicans*—environmental control of morphogenesis. *Microbiology* **146**:1763–1774.
28. **Fares, H., L. Goetsch, and J. R. Pringle.** 1995. Identification of a developmentally regulated septin and involvement of the septins in spore formation in *Saccharomyces cerevisiae. J. Cell Biol.* **132**:399–411.
29. **Feng, O., E. Summers, B. Guo, and G. R. Fink.** 1999. Ras signaling is required for serum-induced hyphal differentiation in *Candida albicans. J. Bacteriol.* **181**:6339–6346.
30. **Finger, F. P., T. E. Hughes, and P. Novick.** 1998. Sec3p is a spatial landmark for polarized secretion in budding yeast. *Cell* **92**:559–571.
31. **Ford, S., and J. R. Pringle.** 1991. Cellular morphogenesis in the *Saccharomyces cerevisiae* cell cycle: location of *CDC11* gene product and the timing of events at the budding site. *Dev. Genet.* **12**:281–292.
32. **Gale, C., D. Finkel, N. Tao, M. Meinke, M. McClellan, J. Olson, K. Kendrick, and M. Hostetter.** 1996. Cloning and expression of a gene encoding an integrin-like protein in *Candida albicans. Proc. Natl. Acad. Sci. USA* **93**:357–361.
33. **Gale, C. A., C. M. Bendel, M. McClellan, M. Hauser, J. M. Becker, J. Berman, and M. K. Hostetter.** 1998. Linkage of adhesion, filamentous growth, and virulence in *Candida albicans* to a single gene, *INT1. Science* **279**:1355–1357.
34. **Gancedo, J. M.** 2000. Control of pseudohyphae formation in *Saccharomyces cerevisiae. FEMS Microbiol. Rev.* **707**:1–17.
35. **Gilfillan, G. D., D. J. Sullivan, K. Haynes, T. Parkinson, D. C. Coleman, and N. A. R. Gow.** 1998. *Candida dubliniensis:* phylogeny and putative virulence factors. *Microbiology* **144**: 829–838.
36. **Gooday, G. W., and D. J. Adams.** 1993. Sex hormones and fungi. *Adv. Microb. Physiol.* **34**:69–145.
37. **Gooday, G. W., and M. Ferguson.** Unpublished observations.
38. **Gow, N. A. R.** 1994. Growth and guidance of the fungal hypha. *Microbiology* **140**:3193–3205.
39. **Gow, N. A. R.** 1997. Germ tube growth of *Candida albicans. Curr. Top. Med. Mycol.* **8**:43–55.
40. **Gow, N. A. R., and G. W. Gooday.** 1982. Growth kinetics and morphology of colonies of the filamentous form of *Candida albicans. J. Gen. Microbiol.* **128**:2187–2194.
41. **Gow, N. A. R., and G. W. Gooday.** 1982. Vacuolation, branch production and linear growth of germ tubes in *Candida albicans. J. Gen. Microbiol.* **128**:2195–2198.

42. **Gow, N. A. R., and G. W. Gooday.** 1984. A model for the germ tube formation and mycelial growth form of *Candida albicans*. *Sabouraudia* **22:**137–144.
43. **Gow, N. A. R., and G. W. Gooday.** 1987. Cytological aspects of dimorphism in *Candida albicans*. *Crit. Rev. Microbiol.* **15:** 73–78.
44. **Griffin, D. H., W. E. Timberlake, and J. C. Cheney.** 1974. Regulation of macromolecular synthesis, colony development, and specific growth rate of *Achlya bisexualis* during balanced growth. *J. Gen. Microbiol.* **80:**381–388.
45. **Hartwell, L. H.** 1971. Genetic control of the cell division cycle in yeast. IV. Genes controlling bud emergence and cytokinesis. *Exp. Cell Res.* **69:**265–276.
46. **Hazan, I., K. Sepulveda-Becerra, and H. Liu.** Hyphal morphogenesis is independent of cell cycle in *Candida albicans*. Submitted for publication.
47. **Hazen, K. C., and J. E. Cutler.** 1979. Autoregulation of germ tube formation by *Candida albicans*. *Infect. Immun.* **24:** 661–666.
48. **Hazen, K. C., and J. E. Cutler.** 1983. The effect of cobalt and morphogenetic autoregulatory substance (MARS) on morphogenesis of *Candida albicans*. *Exp. Mycol.* **7:**182–187.
49. **Hedden, D. M., and J. D. Buck.** 1980. A re-emphasis—germ tubes diagnostic for *Candida albicans* have no constrictions. *Mycopathologia* **70:**95–101.
50. **Hoch, H. C., R. C. Staples, B. Whitehead, J. Comeau, and E. D. Wolf.** 1987. Signalling for growth orientation and cell differentiation by surface topography in *Uromyces*. *Science* **235:**1659–1662.
51. **Jansen, R.-P., C. Dowser, C. Michaelis, M. Galova, and K. Naysmyth.** 1996. Mother cell specific *HO* expression in budding yeast depends on the unconventional myosin Myo4p and other cytoplasmic proteins. *Cell* **84:**687–698.
52. **Johnson, D. I.** 1999. Cdc42: an essential Rho-type GTPase controlling eukaryotic cell polarity. *Microbiol. Mol. Biol. Rev.* **63:**54–105.
53. **Kaminishi, H., A. Iwata, T. Tamaki, T. Cho, and Y. Hagihara.** 1994. Spiral hyphae of *Candida albicans* formed in anaerobic culture. *Mycoses* **37:**349–352.
54. **Kron, S. J., and N. A. R. Gow.** 1995. Budding yeast morphogenesis: signalling, cytoskeleton and cell cycle. *Curr. Opin. Cell Biol.* **7:**845–855.
55. **Kron, S. J., C. A. Styles, and G. R. Fink.** 1994. Symmetric cell division in pseudohyphae of the yeast *Saccharomyces cerevisiae*. *Mol. Biol. Cell.* **5:**1003–1022.
56. **Lee, K. L., H. R. Buckley, and C. C. Campbell.** 1975. An amino acid liquid synthetic medium for the development of mycelial and yeast forms of *Candida albicans*. *Sabouraudia* **13:**148–153.
57. **Lew, D. J., and S. I. Reed.** 1993. Morphogenesis in the yeast cell cycle: regulation by Cdc28 and cyclins. *J. Cell Biol.* **120:** 1305–1320.
58. **Lew, D. J., and S. I. Reed.** 1995. Cell cycle control of morphogenesis in budding yeast. *Curr. Opin. Gen. Devel.* **5:**17–23.
59. **Lew, D. J., and S. I. Reed.** 1995. A cell cycle checkpoint monitors cell morphogenesis in budding yeast. *J. Cell Biol.* **129:**739–749.
60. **Loeb, J. D. J., M. Sepulveda-Becerra, I. Hazan, and H. Liu.** 1999. A G_1 cyclin is necessary for maintenance of filamentous growth in *Candida albicans*. *Mol. Cell. Biol.* **19:**4019–4027.
61. **Longtine, M. S., C. L. Theesfeld, J. N. McMillan, E. Weaver, J. R. Pringle, and D. J. Lew.** 2000. Septin-dependent assembly of a cell cycle-regulatory module in *Saccharomyces cerevisiae*. *Mol. Cell. Biol.* **20:**4049–4061.
62. **Lorenz, M. C., N. S. Cutler, and J. Heitman.** 2000. Characterization of alcohol-induced filamentous growth in *Saccharomyces cerevisiae*. *Mol. Biol. Cell* **11:**183–199.
63. **Malhó, R., N. D. Read, M. S. Pais, and A. J. Trewavas.** 1994. Role of cytosolic free calcium in the reorientation of pollen tube growth. *Plant J.* **5:**331–341.
64. **Maresca, B., and G. S. Kobayashi.** 1989. Dimorphism in *Histoplasma capsulatum*: a model for the study of cell differentiation in pathogenic fungi. *Microbiol. Rev.* **53:**186–209.
65. **Mattia, E., G. Carruba, L. Angiolella, and A. Cassone.** 1982. Induction of germ tube formation by *N*-acetyl-D-glucosamine in *Candida albicans*: uptake of inducer and germinative response. *J. Bacteriol.* **152:**555–562.
66. **Mendenhall, M. D., and A. E. Hodge.** 1998. The regulation of Cdc28 cyclin-dependent protein kinase activity during the cell cycle of the yeast *Saccharomyces cerevisiae*. *Microbiol. Mol. Biol. Rev.* **62:**1191–1243.
67. **Merson-Davies, L. A., and F. C. Odds.** 1989. A morphology index for characterization of cell shape in *Candida albicans*. *J. Gen. Microbiol.* **135:**3143–3152.
68. **Merson-Davies, L. A., and F. C. Odds.** 1992. Expansion of the *Candida albicans* cell envelope in different morphological forms of the fungus. *J. Gen. Microbiol.* **138:**461–466.
69. **Miller, S. E., and W. R. Finnerty.** 1979. Age-related physiological studies comparing *Candida albicans* chlamydospores to yeasts. *Can. J. Microbiol.* **25:**765–772.
70. **Mirbod, F., S. Nakashima, Y. Kitajima, R. D. Cannon, and Y. Nozawa.** 1996. Molecular cloning of a Rho family, *CDC42a* gene from *Candida albicans* and its mRNA expression changes during morphogenesis. *J. Med. Vet. Mycol.* **35:** 173–179.
71. **Mitchell, L. H., and D. R. Soll.** 1979. Temporal and spatial differences in septation during synthronous mycelium and bud formation by *Candida albicans*. *Exp. Mycol.* **3:**298–309.
72. **Montazeri, M., and H. G. Hedrick.** 1984. Factors affecting spore formation of a *Candida albicans* strain. *Appl. Environ. Microbiol.* **47:**1341–1342.
73. **Mulholland, J., D. Preuss, A. Moon, A. Wong, D. Drubin, and D. Botstein.** 1994. Ultrastructure of the yeast actin cytoskeleton and its association with the plasma membrane. *J. Cell Biol.* **125:**381–391.
74. **Novick, P., and P. Brennwald.** 1993. Friends and family: the role of the Rab GTPases in vesicular traffic. *Cell* **75:**597–601.
75. **Odds, F. C.** 1985. Morphogenesis in *Candida albicans*. *Crit. Rev. Microbiol.* **12:**45–93.
76. **Odds, F. C.** 1988. *Candida and Candidosis*. Ballière Tindall, London, United Kingdom.
77. **Odds, F. C.** 1994. *Candida* species and virulence. *ASM News* **60:**313–318.
78. **Onuma, E. K., and S.-W. Hui.** 1988. Electric field-directed cell shape changes, displacement, and cytoskeletal reorganization are calcium dependent. *J. Cell Biol.* **106:**2067–2075.
79. **Prosser, J. I., and A. J. Taylor.** 1991. Growth mechanisms and growth kinetics of filamentous microorganisms. *Crit. Rev. Biotechnol.* **10:**253–274.
80. **Qadota, H., C. P. Python, S. B. Inoue, M. Arisawa, Y. Anraku, Y. Zheng, T. Watanabe, D. E. Levin, and Y. Ohya.** 1996. Identification of Rho1pGTPase as a regulatory subunit of 1,3-β-glucan synthase. *Science* **272:**279–281.
81. **Riggle, P. J., K. A. Andrutis, X. Chen, S. R. Tzipori, and C. A. Kumamoto.** 1999. Invasive lesions containing filamentous forms produced by a *Candida albicans* mutant that is defective in filamentous growth in culture. *Infect. Immun.* **67:** 3649–3652.
82. **Roemer, T., L. G. Vallier, and M. Snyder.** 1996. Selection of polarized growth sites in yeast. *Trends Cell Biol.* **6:**434–441.
83. **San-Blas, G.** 1986. *Paracoccidioides brasliensis*: cell wall glu-

cans, pathogenicity and dimorphism. *Adv. Med. Mycol.* **1:** 235–257.

84. **Sevilla, M.-J., and F. C. Odds.** 1986. Development of *Candida albicans* hyphae in different growth media—variations in growth rates, cell dimensions and timing of morphogenetic events. *J. Gen. Microbiol.* **132:**3083–3088.
85. **Sherlock, G., A. M. Bahman, A. Mahal, J. C. Shieh, M. Ferriera, and J. Rosamond.** 1994. Molecular cloning and analysis of *CDC28* and cyclin homologues from the fungal pathogen *Candida albicans. Mol. Gen. Genet.* **245:**716–724.
86. **Sherwood, J., N. A. R. Gow, G. W. Gooday, G. W. Gregory, and D. Marshall.** 1992. Contact sensing in *Candida albicans*: a possible aid to epithelial penetration. *J. Med. Vet. Mycol.* **30:**461–469.
87. **Sherwood Higham, J., W.-Y. Zhu, C. A. Devine, G. W. Gooday, N. A. R. Gow, and G. W. Gregory.** 1995. Helical growth of hyphae of *Candida albicans. J. Med. Vet. Mycol.* **32:** 437–445.
88. **Sil, A., and I. Herskowitz.** 1996. Identification of an asymmetrically localized determinant, Ash1p required for lineage-specific transcription of the yeast *HO* gene. *Cell* **64:**711–722.
89. **Sipicki, M., Grallert, and I. Miklos.** 1993. Mycelial and syncytial growth in *Schizosaccharomyces pombe* induced by novel septation mutants. *J. Cell Sci.* **104:**485–493.
90. **Sipicki, M., K. Takeo, M. Yamaguchi, S. Yoshida, and I. Miklos.** 1998. Environmentally controlled dimorphic cycle in a fission yeast. *Microbiology* **144:**1319–1330.
91. **Sipicki, M., K. Takeo, and B. Grallert.** 1998. Growth polarity transitions in a dimorphic fission yeast. *Microbiology* **144:** 3475–3485.
92. **Soll, D. R., and L. H. Mitchell.** 1983. Filament ring formation in the dimorphic yeast *Candida albicans. J. Cell Biol.* **96:** 486–493.
93. **Soll, D. R., G. Bedell, J. Theil, and M. Brummel.** 1981. The dependency of nuclear division on volume in the dimorphic yeast *Candida albicans. Exp. Cell Res.* **133:**55–62.
94. **Staebell, M., and D. R. Soll.** 1985. Temporal and spatial differences in cell wall expansion during bud and mycelium formation in *Candida albicans. J. Gen. Microbiol.* **131:** 1467–1480.
95. **Staib, P., and L. Morschhäuser.** 1999. Chlamydospore formation on Staib agar as a species-specific characteristic of *Candida dubliniensis. Mycoses* **42:**453–459.
96. **Steinberg, G.** 1998. Organelle transport and molecular motors in fungi. *Fung. Genet. Biol.* **24:**161–177.
97. **Steinberg, G.** 2000. The cellular roles of molecular motors in fungi. *Trends Microbiol* **8:**162–168.
98. **Steinberg, G., M. Schliwa, L. Christiane, M. Bölker, R. Kahmann, and J. R. McIntosh.** 1998. Kinesin from the plant pathogenic fungus *Ustilago maydis* is involved in vacuole formation and cytoplasmic migration. *J. Cell Sci.* **111:**2235–2246.
99. **Sudbery, P. E.** The germ tubes of *Candida albicans* hyphae and pseudohyphae show different patterns of septin ring localization. *Mol. Microbiol.* **41:**19–31.
100. **Sullivan, D., and D. Coleman.** 1997. *Candida dubliniensis*: an emerging opportunistic pathogen. *Curr. Top. Med. Mycol.* **8:**15–25.
101. **Sullivan, P. A., and M. G. Shepherd.** 1982. Gratuitous induction by *N*-acetylmannosamine of germ tube formation and enzymes of *N*-acetylglucosamine utilization in *Candida albicans. J. Bacteriol.* **151:**1118–1122.
102. **Tanaka, K., T. Kanbe, and T. Kuroiwa.** 1985. Three-dimensional behaviour of mitochondria during cell division and germ tube formation in the dimorphic yeast *Candida albicans. J. Cell Sci.* **73:**207–220.
103. **Tanaka, K., and Y. Takai.** 1998. Control of reorganization of the actin cytoskeleton by Rho family small GTP-binding proteins in yeast. *Curr. Opin. Cell Biol.* **10:**112–116.
104. **Vannittanakom, N., and T. Sirisanthana.** 1997. *Penicillium marneffei* infection in patients infection with human immunodeficiency virus. *Curr. Top. Med. Mycol.* **8:**35–42.
105. **Wang, T., and A. Bretscher.** 1995. The rho-GAP encoded by *BEM2* regulates cytoskeletal structure in budding yeast. *Mol. Biol. Cell* **6:**1011–1024.
106. **Watts, H. J., A.-A. Véry, T. H. S. Perera, J. M. Davies, and N. A. R. Gow.** 1998. Thigmotropism and stretch-activated channels in the pathogenic fungus *Candida albicans. Microbiology* **144:**689–695.
107. **Yokoyama, K., and K. Takeo.** 1983. Differences of asymmetrical division between the pseudomycelial and yeast forms of *Candida albicans* and their effect on multiplication. *Arch. Microbiol.* **134:**251–253.
108. **Yokoyama, K., H. Kaji, K. Nishimura, and M. Miyaji.** 1994. The role of microfilaments and microtubules during pH-regulated morphological transition in *Candida albicans. Microbiology* **140:**281–287.
109. **Yokoyama, K., H. Kaji, K. Nishimura, and M. Miyaji.** 1990. The role of microfilaments and microtubules in apical growth and dimorphism of *Candida albicans. J. Gen Microbiol.* **136:** 1067–1075.

Candida and Candidiasis
Edited by Richard A. Calderone

Chapter 12

The Cell Wall of *Candida* spp.

NEERAJ CHAUHAN, DONGMEI LI, PRAVEEN SINGH, RICHARD CALDERONE, AND MICHAEL KRUPPA

The cell walls of fungi, plants, and bacteria provide a number of essential functions, including protection against osmotic pressure as a permeability barrier and providing shape for the cell. Importantly, the cell wall of pathogens is critical to their interactions with host cells. Since most human pathogens are acquired from the environment, the cell wall is probably a protective device that increases their chance of survival away from the human or animal host. For *Candida* spp. and probably most microorganisms, the cell wall is viewed as a dynamic structure whose composition changes during cell growth. Adding to the complexity of wall composition in *Candida* spp. is the observation that changes also occur during transitional growth. Thus, the transition of yeast and hyphal growth is accompanied by significant increases in the content of chitin as well as differentially regulated expression of proteins. The subject of yeast and hypha-specific proteins is covered extensively in chapters 7 and 22 and will not be discussed in this chapter. For pathogenic fungi such as *Candida albicans,* the cell wall represents the primary way in which the organism interacts with its host, as stated above. An extensive literature exists on this subject (10, 11), and a number of cell wall mannoproteins as well as mannan have been shown to promote binding of the organism to ligands of host cells in vitro. Of these biomolecules, a smaller number have achieved status as adhesins, which are defined as cell surface glycans, proteins, or glycoproteins that both promote the binding of the organism to host cells and are required for virulence (also covered in chapter 6). The focus of this chapter is on the composition, biosynthesis, and arrangement of the *Candida* spp. cell wall biomolecules and includes sections on β-1,6 glucans, β-1,3 glucans, mannoproteins, chitin, and cell wall lipids. When data exist, the non-*C. albicans* species also will be discussed. Information is drawn from the literature on *Saccharomyces cerevisiae,* and in many situations comparisons are possible. However, differences between the two organisms will also be pointed out.

COMPOSITION OF THE CELL WALL

Of the *Candida* spp., the composition of the cell wall has been mostly studied in *C. albicans,* and a variety of approaches have been utilized, most of which have relied on biochemical analysis. The latter approach is considerably useful, especially in regard to the characterization of glucose polymers on the basis of their extraction in alkali and/or acid. In addition, the identification of solubilized mannoproteins requires further fractionation and analysis such as sodium dodecyl sulfate-polyacrylamide gel electrophoresis and Western blotting to distinguish specific molecules. Thus, determinations of total mannose or mannan and protein provide useful information but do not distinguish differences in specific mannoproteins as a function of growth media, temperature, or even between yeast and mycelial forms of the organism.

Perhaps one of the most complete biochemical analyses of the cell wall was reported by Chattaway et al. in their studies of yeast and hyphal forms of *C. albicans* (13). The gross constituents from the cell wall of each of the two growth forms were characterized from cells propagated in different media and at different temperatures. Among the observations, the yeast cell wall remained relatively constant in composition when cells were grown on different media and at different temperatures. A similar observation was made for mycelial forms except for the content of glucose and mannose that did vary according to the growth conditions. Yeast and hyphal cell walls were similar qualitatively but differed quantitatively in specific

Neeraj Chauhan, Dongmei Li, Praveen Singh, Richard Calderone, and Michael Kruppa • Department of Microbiology and Immunology, Georgetown University Medical Center, 3900 Reservoir Rd., NW, Washington, DC 20007.

components, as, for example, chitin (as measured by the amount of glucosamine). Thus, the mycelial cell wall exhibited an approximate four- to fivefold higher level of chitin. Differences in chitin content of yeast and hyphal cell walls of *C. albicans* have also been demonstrated with chitin synthase assays of crude extracts (5). The observation on similarities between the two growth forms in regard to wall content made by Chattaway et al. was thought to reflect a variation in the activity of common enzymes that produce cell wall components rather than newly expressed, growth-specific components. The molecular interpretation of that statement is that genes common to both growth forms encode cell wall biosynthetic/catabolic enzymes, but no new gene expression occurs during phase transition. Although not entirely correct, it is also unfair to be overly critical of this supposition since methodologies now permit us to distinguish differences at both the level of the gene and protein. Sullivan et al. indicated that the ratio of β-1,3 to β-1,6 glucan in the insoluble fraction of cell walls is similar in both yeast and filamentous growth forms, but the insoluble glucan in the early stages of germination contains many more β-1,3 linkages (114). Thus, it is certain that there are temporal changes in the cell wall composition during filamentous growth. Interestingly, pronase and glucanase susceptibility is reported to be higher in yeast forms of the organism than mycelial forms, again signifying fundamental differences in the cell wall of both growth forms.

The cell wall of *C. albicans* is approximately 80 to 90% carbohydrate, and the majority of this carbohydrate is found in branched polymers of glucose (β-1,3 and β-1,6 glucose polymers [β-glucan]), unbranched polymers of β-1,4 *N*-acetyl-D (chitin) and polymers of mannose (mannan) with or without glucose covalently bound to proteins (11).

Cell wall composition studies are generally based on chemical fractionation utilizing differences in solubility among constituents upon treatment with alkali and acid (14). Such treatment yields mannoproteins and two types of glucan, the latter of which is distributed among three fractions, including an amorphous fraction that is alkali soluble, consisting primarily of glucose chains in β-1,3-O-glycosidic bonds, an alkali-insoluble-acetic acid-soluble fraction that is composed primarily of glucose polymers bound by β-1,6-O-glycosidic linkages, and an alkali-acetic acid-insoluble fraction of β-1,3 glucan that has probably become insoluble in acid and alkali due to the addition of chitin that is in β-1,4 linkage between the terminal reducing residue of a chitin chain and the nonreducing end of the β-1,3 glucan chain.

The relative amounts of each of the three fractions of β-glucan are approximately 25% (alkali-soluble), 5% (alkali-insoluble, acid-soluble), and 35% (alkali- and acid-insoluble). Chitin accounts for approximately 0.6 to 3% and is considered to be a minor (albeit significant) component of the cell wall (103). The numbers given above are expressed as the % weight of the cell wall. Another method for expressing the relative contribution of these components to the cell wall has been suggested by Lipke and Ovalle for *S. cerevisiae* (71). These investigators have calculated molar ratios based on the size (mass) as well as the number of chains of each type of polymer. The molar ratios of the four major polymers mentioned above are 1.0:2.0:0.1–0.3:1.2–2.4 (β-1,3 glucan:β-1,6 glucan:chitin:mannoprotein).

Mannoproteins comprise an important component of the cell wall, accounting for approximately 40% of the total cell wall polysaccharide (β-glucans account for 47 to 60% by weight of the cell wall; chitin and lipid represent the remaining components of the wall) (11). Mannose polymers are found covalently associated with proteins and are designated as mannoproteins. As discussed in chapter 3, mannan confers immunodominant properties to the cell. Compositional studies of mannoprotein have indicated that they are homopolymers in *N*- and *O*-glycosidic covalent linkages with polypeptide residues of asparagine (N-linked via two residues of acetylchitobiose) and threonine/serine (O-linked) (see below). The N-linked mannan is the more complex of the two and is composed of mannopyranosyl residues in an α-1,6-linked backbone to which side chains of mannopyranosyl residues are attached in α-1,2, α-1,3, β-1,2, β-1,6, and phosphodiester linkages. The O-glycosidic mannan is composed of short, unbranched mannose oligosaccharides. As stated above, alkali and acid extraction of cell walls yields complex polymers of glucose (glucan) and chitin-glucan. Alkali extraction of mannoproteins has likewise been described (89, 90, 97); extracts are then precipitated with Fehling's solution to form a copper-mannan complex that can be easily solubilized and studied further. Mannan has also been isolated by autoclaving cells in citrate buffer and then precipitating with copper or with Cetavalon (cetyltrimethylammonium bromide) (86). Obviously, the procedures just described are harsh and result in a loss of much of the protein covalently associated with mannan. Thus, mannoproteins are better extracted with detergents (sodium dodecyl sulfate, *n*-octylglucoside), reducing agents (most often β-mercaptoethanol), or enzymes (proteases, Zymolyase, chitinase). The advantages or disadvantages of using a specific extraction procedure should be evaluated according to the needs of the experiment. Thus, enzyme-digested cells (Zymolyase) are thought to release higher molecular weight mannoproteins most often associated with glucan. Reducing agents, on the other hand, release primarily medium to smaller molecular mass mannoproteins, although this is only a "rule-of-thumb" concept and is disputed by other investigators who have identified larger mannoproteins in extracts obtained with reducing agents (11). Growth conditions are as important as the method chosen to extract mannoproteins. For example, Brawner et al. compared the expression of two cell surface mannoprotein antigens in yeast and hyphal forms of *C. albicans* (6). One of these antigens (C6) was shown to be yeast-cell specific regardless of the nutritional conditions, but the other mannoprotein antigen (H9) was variably expressed so that it appeared to be hyphal specific in one of the media tested and at a specific time of incubation but otherwise was most often associated with yeast-cell growth. The authors state that misinterpretations of expression of cell surface mannoproteins (or any cell surface antigen) can result unless experiments are designed to include growth in both complex and chemically defined media. Also, a variety of assays (agglutination, immunofluorescence, enzyme-linked immunosorbent assay) should be included to establish the cell surface nature of a specific mannoprotein. These rules certainly still apply in today's laboratory that utilizes molecular biology to isolate genes encoding cell wall-specific proteins and construct gene-deleted strains that are compared to parental cells. The concept is that cell surface expression of mannoproteins is dynamic and that many parameters of growth need to be fully explored before statements of expression and gene function can be made.

MOLECULAR ORGANIZATION OF THE CELL WALL

The cell wall polymers in *Candida* spp. are linked by covalent bonds, in addition to hydrogen and hydrophobic bonds. Covalent linkages have been reported between glucan and chitin and between mannoproteins and β-glucans (49, 50, 98, 99, 115). Further, β-1,3 and β-1,6 glucans are also linked to proteins by phosphodiester linkages. It is believed that the cell wall is composed of building blocks of mannoprotein, which are associated through glycosylphosphatidylinositol (GPI) anchor remnants with β-1,6 glucan, which in turn is linked to β-1,3 glucan and chitin. The covalent associations involving these polymers might also be represented in the cell wall as modules, at least for *S. cerevisiae* (71). The prototypical module includes a β-1,3 glucan chain consisting of about 40 to 50 branch points and one or two β-1,6 glucan chains as well as mannoprotein (Color plate 5A). Chitin would be associated with a minority of these modules via covalent linkages to the β-1,3 or β-1,6 glucan chains. It was postulated that macromolecular complexes consisting of these modules are associated by noncovalent interactions in the glucan-chitin layer as well as covalent linkages with mannoprotein (Color plate 5B). These observations are interesting conceptually and mimic, to some extent, the concept of the repeat units of the bacterial peptidoglycan. This cell wall module has only been proposed for *S. cerevisiae,* but this module concept provides a framework for our understanding of the molecular architecture of the cell wall. Mannoproteins are viewed as either secreted or covalently linked to the plasma membrane through GPI anchors; subsequently, transfer of the mannoprotein to β-1,6 or β-1,3 glucan occurs. This observation may partially explain the appearance of mannoproteins within the cell wall of the organism and also their distribution at the outer surface of the cell wall. Mannoprotein biosynthesis follows the secretory pathway whereas the structural polysaccharides (β-1,6 glucan, chitin, and β-1,3 glucan) are synthesized at the level of the plasma membrane and extruded from the cell where final assembly and synthesis occur. In the case of β-1,6 glucan, there is some thought that this polymer may also follow the secretory pathway (see discussion below).

The cell wall of *C. albicans* when viewed by transmission electron microscopy appears layered. The number of these layers has been suggested to be from three to eight, but the actual number may be related to strain variability, morphology (yeast or filaments), media, and the method of preservation used to fix cells (11). The inner layer adjacent to the plasma membrane is microfibrillar in appearance and is most likely more heavily composed of the polysaccharides glucan and chitin. This layer by virtue of its components provides a rigid structure that protects the cell against osmotic and other environmental insults. On the other hand, the outer layer of wall is amorphous and is primarily composed of mannoprotein and proteins that, nevertheless, can also be found throughout the cell wall, albeit in smaller amounts. Under high-resolution microscopy, the outer layer appears to be densely fibrillar or floccular in appearance. The outer surface often can be seen as having appendages that extend beyond the cell wall proper, and for that reason, these appendages have been occasionally referred to as fimbria, a term derived from similar structures observed in several species of bacteria (see chapter 6). The fimbriae are composed of a single, heavily mannosylated protein of about 66 kDa (125).

A second model depicting the molecular architec-

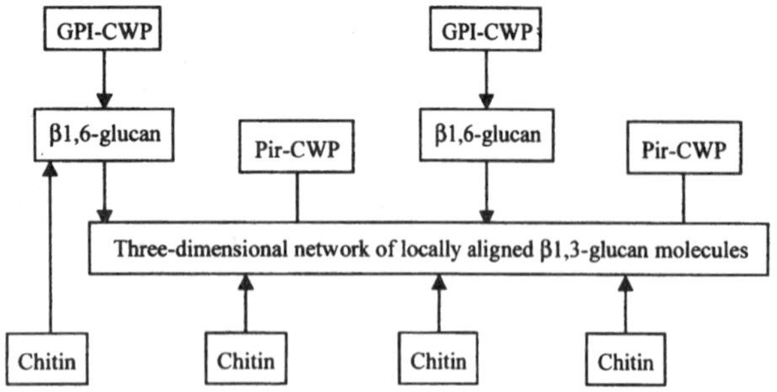

Figure 1. A molecular model depicting the arrangement of cell wall polymers of *S. cerevisiae* and *C. albicans*. The arrows indicate the orientation of each polysaccharide (chitin, β-1,6 glucan). β-1,3 glucan forms a three-dimensional network that surrounds the cell to which most other cell wall components are attached. Reprinted from reference 48 with permission.

ture of the cell wall is shown in Fig. 1 and is discussed in detail below in the section on β-1,3 glucan. In this model the β-1,3 glucan is thought to form a three-dimensional matrix that surrounds the cell (50, 71, 108). Cell wall proteins (CWP) are linked to the multiple, nonreducing ends of the branched β-1,3 molecules through GPI-dependent and through Pir covalent bonds. In the case of the Pir-CWP, direct association with the β-1,3 glucan is thought to occur, but the GPI-CWP are probably linked to the β-1,3 glucan through β-1,6 glucan. The nature of the Pir linkage to the β-1,3 glucan is not known but is alkali labile (54). Recently, Pir-like proteins in *C. albicans* have been suggested on the basis of hybridization signals observed by Southern and Northern analyses with the *S. cerevisiae HSP/PIR2* gene as a probe (46). Chitin has been shown to be linked to both types of β-glucan but at specific times after cytokinesis in what is believed to result in a strengthening of the cell wall.

β-1,6 GLUCAN

The β-1,6 glucans of fungi such as *Candida* spp. and *S. cerevisiae* play an important role in wall structure since they act as an interconnector for most other wall components (Fig. 1) (48, 101). Genetic and structural/biochemical approaches have been used to characterize the function and biosynthesis of β-1,6 glucan. It appears that in *S. cerevisiae,* although much is known about the interactions of each of the wall polymers with β-1,6 glucan, the biosynthesis of this polymer is only partially established. Several genes have been proposed to function in biosynthesis, but fewer gene products (two) are known, and their activities may not contribute directly to polymer synthesis (101).

β-1,6 glucan synthesis has been thought to proceed along the secretory pathway, although controversy exists in regard to this point (81). Thus, the initial reactions of biosynthesis are thought to occur in the endoplasmic reticulum (ER) where a protein-bound primer molecule becomes extended through glucose additions in the Golgi complex. The latter reactions are thought to be catalyzed by two putative glucosyltransferases (Kre6p and Skn1p). Subsequently, maturation of the complex and coupling to other cell wall macromolecules occur at the cell surface. Details of these reactions are as follows: a precursor protein is GPI-*N*- and -*O*-modified. The initial reactions in the ER are thought to involve glucosylation of an N-chain of the protein as well as glucosylation at the carboxy terminus containing the GPI modification. GPI modification occurs as a posttranslational attachment of an ethanolamine-phosphate-Man_5GlcNH_2-inositol phospholipid to the C terminus of the protein; simultaneously, a C-terminal 20- to 30-amino-acid segment of the same protein is displaced by the GPI attachment. The GPI-modified protein remains membrane bound as the protein is processed through the secretory pathway (101). Most of these observations were obtained using the *S. cerevisiae* α-agglutinin as a model glycosylated protein, but the same general rules appear to apply to at least the Als1p and Als5p proteins of *C. albicans* (48) (and see chapter 6 for a description of the Als proteins). Thus, in the ER, glucosylation occurs at the N-chain (at the N terminus) as well as within the GPI anchor. Subsequently, the modified protein undergoes further glucosylation at both sites of the protein within the Golgi complex. The protein is further processed at the cell surface; some of the reactions that are thought to occur at the plasma membrane and cell surface are the loss of the inositol phosphate-GlcNH2 and then subsequent transfer of the newly modified protein to the cell wall network.

The controversy accompanying this model is based on the presumed functions of Kre6p and Skn1p, indicated to be glucosyltransferases as mentioned above. However, data that oppose this model are based on the observation that these two proteins are, in fact, glucosyl hydrolases (based on other sequence analysis) and not glucosyltransferases (81). Further, immunogold staining of cells with an antiserum that was made against β-1,6 glucan oligosaccharides (15 glucose residues on average) revealed staining only at the cell surface and not intracellularly as, for example, within the post-Golgi secretory vesicles. It seems, therefore, that in *S. cerevisiae,* β-1,6 glucan is synthesized at the cell surface, similarly to β-1,3 glucan and chitin.

GPI proteins are either directed to the β-1,6 glu-

Table 1. *C. albicans* putative genes involved in β-glucan synthesis

Gene	Method of isolation	Null phenotype	Reference
KRE9	Complementation	Essential gene fails to form germ tubes; β-1,6 glucan reduced; total β-glucan-like wt cells	75
KRE1	Complementation	Not done	4
KRE6	Plaque hybridization	80% less β-1,6 glucan; no null recovered	80
SKN1	Plaque hybridization	No apparent phenotype	80
BGL2	PCR	Loss of cell wall-associated Bgl2p glucosyltransferase activity	100
GSC1/FKS1	Cross-hybridization	Not done	78
RHO1	PCR/cross-hybridization	Not done	69

can or remain attached to the lipid of the plasma membrane via the GPI anchor. What determines the fate of each GPI protein is apparently determined by a dibasic motif just terminal to the GPI attachment site. Those GPI proteins that lack this motif are directed to the cell wall network. As stated above, β-1,6-anchored cell wall proteins in other fungi such as *C. albicans* have been identified (47, 49, 50).

In *S. cerevisiae,* the genes that are thought to function in β-1,6 glucan synthesis have been identified through two genetic approaches, one of which relies on the resistance of mutants to the K1 killer toxin. Since the toxin binds to the β-1,6 glucan-associated component in the cell wall, cells with lower amounts of β-1,6 glucan develop resistance to the toxin. Oppositely, mutants with general cell wall defects, not just those with defects in β-1,6 glucan, are also hypersensitive to the stain calcofluor white. With these types of screens, the identification of several *KRE* (killer toxin resistant), *CWH* (calcofluor white hypersensitive), and *ECM* (extracellular mutant) genes has been reported.

Homologs of some of these genes have been identified from *C. albicans* (4, 75, 80) (Table 1). The Kre9p of *C. albicans* exhibited a 43% overall homology to that of the *S. cerevisiae* Kre9p with unique sequences associated with the N terminus of each protein (75). Kre1p was 46% identical to the *S. cerevisiae* Kre1p, but disrupted strains were not described so gene function could not be assessed (4). However, the *KRE1* of *C. albicans* complemented the *kre1* mutant of *S. cerevisiae* and restored sensitivity to killer toxin, indicating that the *C. albicans* Kre1p could be a functional homolog. β-1,6 glucan biosynthesis was significantly reduced in strains of *C. albicans* deleted in *KRE9* and *KRE6*. Disrupted strains were unable to grow in the presence of glucose but could produce some growth in other carbon sources such as galactose. In the case of *KRE9*, the *C. albicans* single gene disrupted strain produced 28% less β-1,6 glucan, but interestingly, the total β-glucan was similar to that of the wild-type cells. The *kre9/kre9* null strain could not grow in the presence of glucose, but when grown in galactose, total β-glucan was similar to that of wild-type cells; however, the null strain did not produce germ tubes in a galactose-serum medium compared to the wild-type and heterozygote that could produce germ tubes. An explanation for the absence of growth in glucose was uncertain but was thought to be due to a compensatory mechanism that was galactose-inducible or a lethality associated with aberrant cell wall formation when cells were grown on glucose (75).

β-1,3-GLUCANS

More than half the cell wall is made up of β-1,3 glucan, accounting for 50 to 60% by weight of fungal cell wall. Together with chitin it is responsible for the rigidity of the cell wall, thus determining its shape and strength. β-1,3 glucan has multiple nonreducing ends, allowing it to function as an acceptor for both β-1,6-glucan and chitin (Color plate 5A); when chitin is attached to β-1,3 glucan, it becomes insoluble in alkali, explaining the presence of alkali-soluble and alkali-insoluble β-1,3 glucan (35, 67).

Smits et al. proposed a model of the molecular organization of the *S. cerevisiae* cell wall (108). According to the cell wall model (described earlier in the chapter), β-1,3 glucan molecules form a three-dimensional matrix surrounding the entire cell. Since β-1,3 glucan molecules are branched, they may have multiple nonreducing ends, which may function as attachment sites for CWPs. Cell wall mannoproteins are extractable with β-1,3 glucanase, suggesting that these proteins are linked to the β-1,3 glucan skeleton of the cell wall (46). However, the exact nature of the bonds between these mannoproteins and the β-1,3 glucan skeleton is unknown. It has been shown that the glucanase-extractable mannoproteins of *C. albicans* and *S. cerevisiae* contain a side chain, carrying β-1,6-linked glucose residues, proposed to be involved in cell wall anchorage (49, 72). The alkali-soluble glucan of *C. albicans* cell walls consists of a β-1,6 glucan and β-1,3 glucan heteropolymer. GPI-dependent CWPs and Pir-CWPs are the two main types of covalently linked CWPs that have been identified (53). The GPI-CWPs are attached via β-1,6 glucan to a nonreducing end of a β-1,3 glucan molecule (Fig. 1) (48, 51, 54, 68). The Pir-related CWPs are directly attached through an alkali-labile linkage (Fig. 1) (54). Chitin molecules also join the nonreducing ends of the β-1,3 glucan molecules and, less frequently, to β-1,6 glucan molecules (67, 68). Yeast cells have been shown to be able to compensate for defects in the β-1,3 glucan synthesis and/or assembly by altering the molecular organization of the wall, characterized by a severalfold increase in chitin content (92). As a result of this reaction, a 20-fold increase has been observed in the level of GPI-CWPs that were resistant to β-1,3 glucanase extraction (52).

β-1,3 Glucan Synthesis and Structure

Glucan is the most abundant structural polymer of the cell wall of all yeasts and fungi. Yeast glucan is composed of glucose oligomers having (1,3)-β and (1,6)-β configuration (15). In filamentous fungi and yeast, β-1,3 glucans are synthesized by a plasma membrane-bound glucan synthase complex, which uses UDP-glucose as a substrate. The β-1,3 glucan chains generated by the β-1,3 glucan synthase complex remain unorganized and alkali soluble until covalent linkages occur between β-1,3 glucans and other cell wall components (82) following their extrusion from the plasma membrane to the cell wall proper.

β-1,3 glucan synthase (UDP-glucose: 1,3-β-D-glucan 3-β-D-glucosyltransferase; EC 2.4.1.34) has been purified (40), and the gene encoding its putative catalytic subunit has also been cloned (78). 1,3-β-D-glucan synthase is a multisubunit membrane enzyme complex, which is activated by GTP. The complex has been fractionated into soluble (GTP-binding) and membrane-bound (catalytic) components. To gain further insight into the physiologically relevant mechanisms involved in *C. albicans* β-1,3 glucan biosynthesis, several genetic approaches have recently been developed. Different strategies have been used to isolate mutants and the genes involved in β-1,3 glucan synthesis. A list of genes involved in β-glucan synthesis is presented in Table 1. The *S. cerevisiae* β-1,3 glucan synthase catalytic subunit is encoded by the two isogenes *GSC1* and *GSC2* (also known as *FKS1* and *FKS2*, respectively), which, when disrupted, cause a synthetic lethality (69).

RHO1 (which stands for Ras homologs) from *C. albicans* has been cloned and shown to be a regulator of β-1,3 glucan synthase (69). These molecular switches or regulators are "on" in the GTP-bound form and "off" in the GDP-bound form (119). Rho1p is one of the components of the active complex of β-1,3 glucan synthase of *C. albicans. RHO1* encodes a small Rho-type GTPase. Rho GTPases were shown to be posttranslationally modified at their C terminus, and this modification facilitates the association of Rho GTPases with the membrane. Sarthy et al. reported that *BGL2* encodes a 1,3-β-glucosyltransferase (Bgl2p) present in the cell wall of *C. albicans* (100). Disruption of *BGL2* leads to the loss of cell wall-associated Bgl2p glucosyltransferase activity that is responsible for the elongation of 1,3-β glucans. However, residual non-Bg12p transferase activity was detected, suggesting the presence of another transferase in *C. albicans*.

Glucan Metabolism/Processing

β-glucans are synthesized as linear polymers in vitro whereas the 1,3-β glucans are branched polymers, suggesting that β-glucan chains are modified during or shortly after synthesis. However, technical constraints pose a major hurdle in understanding glucan metabolism in vivo. Following the initial synthesis of glucan there are likely postsynthetic processing/restructuring events, which occur at various points within the cell cycle. Such events are likely to occur during bud emergence, hyphal branching, wall expansion, cell separation, spore formation, and germination but are poorly understood. So far, a set of 1,3-β-glucan-modifying enzymes, with glucanase activity, has been identified. Goldman et al. proposed a model of glucan metabolism (31). This model is based on the fact that β-1,3-glucosyltransferase requires free reducing and free nonreducing termini as substrates. Another gene, *GEL1* (for glucan elongating glucanosyltransferase), encoding a 1,3-β-glucanosyltransferase from *Aspergillus fumigatus* (82), shares significant homology with *GAS1* (from *S. cerevisiae*), *PHR*1 and -2 (from *C. albicans*), and *EPD* (from *C. maltosa*), genes that encode a family of GPI-anchored proteins. Mouyna et al. have also shown that Gel1p, Phr1p, Phr2p, and Gas1p display 1,3-β-glucanosyltransferase activity (82). On the basis of previous studies done on the cell wall of *S. cerevisiae* and *A. fumigatus,* Mouyna et al. (82) have shown the sequential events involved in the synthesis and postsynthetic modifications of the cell wall β-1,3 glucans (Fig. 2) are as follows: (i) biosynthesis of linear β-1,3 glucans; (ii) branching of β-1,3 glucans through β-1,6 linkages; (iii) elongation of β-1,3 glucan side chains; and (iv) cross-linking of other polymers (chitin and pro-

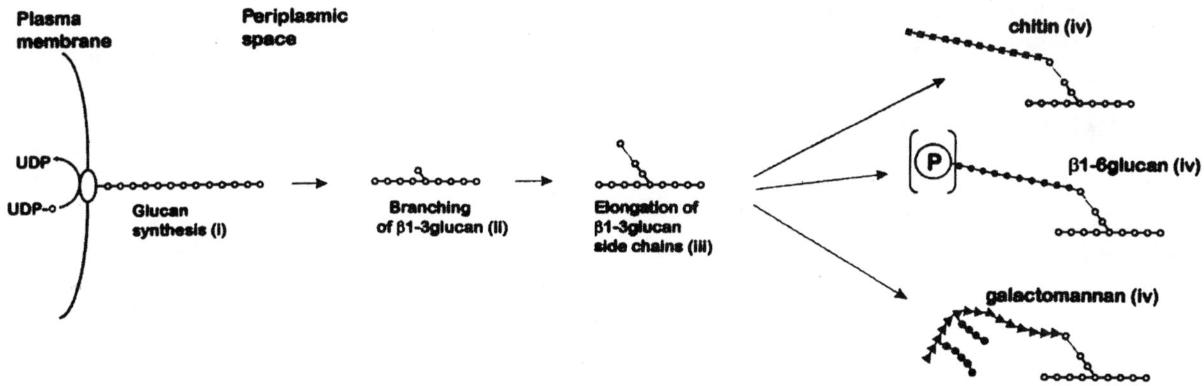

Figure 2. β-1,3 glucan synthesis (I), branching (II), elongation (III), and cross-linking to other wall polymers (IV, protein, chitin and β-1,6 glucan) are indicated. This model has been suggested for *S. cerevisiae* but probably also exists for *C. albicans*. Reprinted from reference 82 with permission.

teins) onto the nonreducing ends of β-1,3 glucan side chains.

Exo-β-(1,3)-Glucanases

Secretory exo-β-glucanases are enzymes that are reported to be involved in the metabolism of β-glucans. In *C. albicans,* exo-β-(1,3)-glucanase activity was found to be secreted mainly during germ tube formation (11). A cell wall exoglucanase from *C. albicans* with specificity for β-1,3 linkages has been crystallized by the hanging drop method in the presence of polyethylene glycol 8000 (18). Gonzalez et al. reported the disruption of the *XOG1* (now *EXG1*) gene of *C. albicans* that encodes a protein with exoglucanase activity (32). Enzymatic analysis of either cell extracts or culture supernatants of disrupted strains revealed that this gene is responsible for the major exoglucanase activity in *C. albicans,* although residual exoglucanase activity could still be detected. *xog1* (null) mutants demonstrate similar growth rates in both rich and minimal liquid medium as compared to the wild-type strain, suggesting that the enzyme is not essential for *C. albicans* growth. However, minor differences were found between the null mutant and wild type with respect to susceptibility to chitin and glucan synthesis inhibitors. Exo-β-(1,3)-glucanase from *C. albicans* (Exg1p/Xog1p) is the product of the *EXG1* gene, which codes for a preproenzyme of 438 amino acids (12). The mature protein of 400 residues is involved in the metabolism of cell wall glucan by catalyzing the hydrolytic removal of a glucose residue at the nonreducing end of β-1,3 glucan and to a much lesser extent, β-1,6 glucan (111). Exg1p is an abundant secreted enzyme possessing both hydrolase and transferase activity with a defined role in cell wall glucan metabolism and possibly in morphogenesis. The structures of Exg1p in both free and inhibited form have been determined to a 1.9 Å resolution (19).

PHR1 and *PHR2*

These genes encode putative GPI-anchored proteins in *C. albicans* (25). Both proteins are functionally related, and expression is pH dependent, as *PHR1* is expressed at neutral/alkaline pH whereas *PHR2* expression occurs at an acid pH range (25). Deletion of either gene results in pH-conditional defects in filamentous growth and avirulence. Homologs of the Phr1p and Phr2p in *S. cerevisiae* (Gas1p), *C. maltosa* (Epd1p), and *A. fumigatus* (Gel1p) have also been described (83). In *A. fumigatus,* Gel1p splits internally β-1,3 glucan and as a result of that enzymatic cleavage transfers the newly formed reducing end to the nonreducing end of another β-1,3 glucan while forming a new β-1,3 linkage. The product of this enzymatic activity is the elongation of the chain. It is believed that Phr1p, Phr2p, and Gas1p also have a similar activity, referred to as 1,3-β-glucanosyltransferase. Mutants in *PHR1* of *C. albicans* have a sixfold increase in chitin content and are hypersensitive to Calcofluor white (93).

MANNAN

The topic of this section is the cell wall mannan or phosphomannan of *Candida* species. This section is divided into essentially three parts, detailing the structure of the carbohydrate component of mannan, the biosynthetic pathway for N- and O-linked mannosylation, and those genes so far identified in *C. albicans* that are responsible for synthesis of the mannan.

Mannan Structure of *Candida* Species

A great amount of work has been done to elucidate the structure of the mannan component of the *Candida* cell surface. Mannan by itself does not exist on the surface of the cell but is covalently bound to protein as either an N-glycosidic bond through two GlcNAc (di-*N*-acetylchitobiose) units to an asparagine residue of a wall protein or O-linked to either a serine or a threonine residue of a wall protein. The general structure of *C. albicans* N-linked mannan is best described as having a backbone of α-1,6-linked D-mannosylpyranose residues with branches containing α-1,2, α-1,3, β-1,2, and β-1,6 and single α-1,6-linked mannose units and phosphodiester bonds (59, 60, 63, 65, 104, 106). Conversely, the O-linked mannan is composed of either a single mannose or short unbranched mannose oligosaccharides (91).

N-linked mannan among the different *Candida* spp. can be categorized into three different groupings, a complex mannan structure, an intermediate structure, and a simple structure, with variations among each group (Fig. 3). The complex mannan structure is found among *C. albicans,* serotypes A and B (formerly), *C. stellatoidea* types I and II, *C. glabrata,* and *C. tropicalis.* This type of mannan features an α-1,6-mannan backbone with α-1,2-linked side branches as well as a phosphodiester-linked branch of predominantly β-1,2-linked mannose residues (Fig. 3A). Other modifications include the substitution of β-1,2-linkages to the α-1,2-linked side chains.

C. albicans serotype A and *C. stellatoidea* contain mannan with side chain branches corresponding to pentaose, hexaose, and heptaose, Mβ1-2Mα1-2Mα1-2Mα1-2M, Mβ1-2Mβ1-2Mα1-2Mα1-

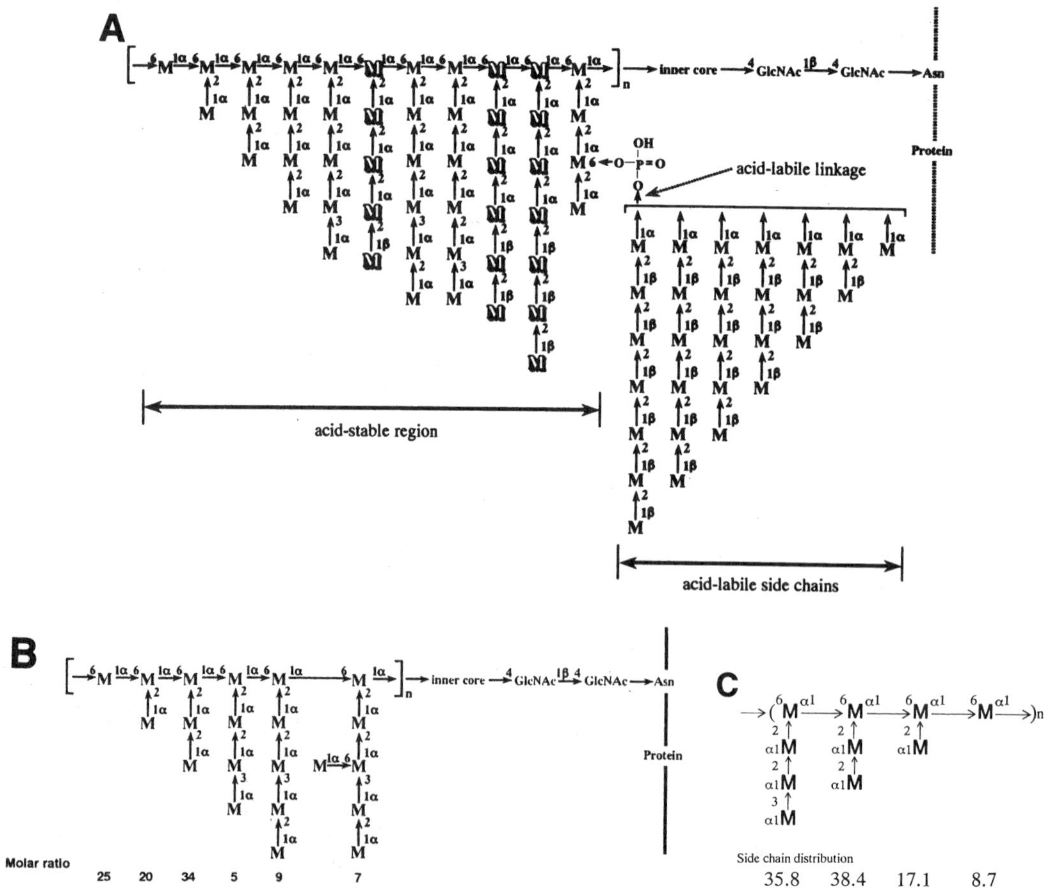

Figure 3. Mannan structures for species of *Candida,* illustrating complex (A), intermediate (B), and simple varieties (C) of the central theme. Consult the text for details. Reprinted from references 104 (A), 107 (B), and 62 (C) with permission.

2Mα1-2M, and Mβ1-2Mβ1-2Mβ1-2Mα1-2Mα1-2Mα1-2M (60, 64). In addition, *C. albicans* has also been shown to have side chain branches as long as 14 mannose residues, depending on growth conditions (123). *C. tropicalis* mannan also shares structural similarity with *C. albicans* A and B serotypes, but it lacks the α-1,3-linked side chains, Mα1-3Mα1-2Mα1-2Mα1-2M and Mα1-2Mα1-3Mα1-2Mα1-2Mα1-2M, when the strain is grown at a pH of 5.9 (57). However, when *C. tropicalis* is grown under more acidic conditions, Kobayashi et al. have reported the detection of α-1,3-linked structures (61). *C. glabrata* also has a semicomplex mannan structure but has shorter phosphate-linked β-1,2-oligomannopyranose side chains than what is seen with *C. albicans*. Additionally, Kobayashi et al. have indicated that the structure of *C. glabrata* mannan is more closely related to that of *S. cerevisiae* mannan (58).

C. famata, C. saitoana, and *C. kefyr* express an intermediate form of N-linked mannan (Fig. 3B). This structure shares many of the features seen with complex mannan, but these strains lack the phosphate-linked β-1,2-mannose side chains. *C. famata* also completely lacks any β-1,2-linked residues, whereas *C. saitoana* has two types of β-1,2-linked mannose side chains that can be released by treatment of the mannan by acetolysis, Mβ1-2Mβ1-2Mα1-3Mα1 and Mβ1-2Mα1-3Mα1 (107). In addition to the α-1,2-linked side chains, a secondary α-1,6 single mannose can be attached to these branches. *C. kefyr* mannan has short side chains of α-1,2-linked mannopyranose residues and completely lacks the β-1,2 and α-1,3 mannopyranose residues (56).

C. catenulata manufactures a very simple N-linked mannan formed along a standard α-1,6-linked backbone, with short α-1,2-linked side chains of no more than two residues, but can have substitution of an α-1,3-end-linked mannose (Fig. 3C) (62). In addition, *C. catenulata* lacks any β-1,2-linked mannopyranose. The mannan of *C. lipolytica* is different from other mannans so far discussed in that it contains galactose in addition to mannose. This galactomannan has the same basic structure of an α-1,6-linked backbone with a short α-1,2-mannose-α-1,2-galactose side chain (38). The last example of a simple N-linked mannan structure is found in *C. krusei,* which has a backbone containing both α-1,6-linked and α-1,2-linked mannose residues, with short side chains of α-1,2-linked mannose (66). The ratio of α-1,2- and α-1,6-linked mannose residues is 3:1, respectively.

Biosynthesis of Mannan

N-linked mannosylation

Biosynthesis of N-linked mannan has not been well characterized in *Candida* spp. whereas in *S. cerevisiae* the synthesis of N-linked mannan has been well studied and dissected, through both biochemical and genetic analyses. There are a number of reviews on this subject in yeast to which the reader is referred (8, 20, 43).

So far only three genes have been identified in *C. albicans* that are involved in N-linked mannan synthesis. Thus far, only *MNN9* has been characterized. Mnn9p is a member of a family of proteins including Van1p and Anp1p (109). Mnn9p is required for synthesis of the outer chain mannan in *S. cerevisiae* and probably performs the same function in *C. albicans.* A strain lacking *MNN9* has a number of defects, including impairment of yeast to hyphae transition, lower amounts of mannan in the cell wall, and increased sensitivity to hygromycin and glucanase (109).

Slightly more has been learned with regard to *Candida* sp. mannan side chain biosynthesis. So far three enzyme activities have been biochemically characterized; however, the genes encoding these enzymes have not been identified. Suzuki et al. have characterized an α-1,6 mannosyltransferase from *C. albicans* that is involved in branch chain synthesis. This transferase catalyzes the attachment of a branch through an α-1,6 linkage to an α-1,3-linked residue within an α-1,2-linked side chain (117). They have also characterized a β-1,2 mannosyltransferase from *C. guilliermondii,* which they determined to be involved in synthesis of antigen 9 (discussed in chapter 3) (116). This enzyme has been shown to catalyze the addition of a β-1,2 mannose to a nonreducing end of an α-1,3 terminal residue of an Mα1-3(Mα1-6)-Mα1-2Mα1-2M mannosylpentoase resulting in an Mβ1-2Mα1-3(Mα1-6)-Mα1-2Mα1-2M mannosylhexaose. Another β-1,2 mannosyltransferase has been described from *C. albicans* that plays a role in synthesis of the serotype A antigen (118). This transferase acts on an Mβ1-2Mα1-2Mα1-2Mα1-2M pentaose and adds another β-1,2-linked mannose to yield Mβ1-2Mβ1-2Mα1-2Mα1-2Mα1-2M hexaose.

O-linked mannosylation

Protein O-mannosylation has been well studied using the model yeast *S. cerevisiae.* Many of the proteins and their genes that play a role in O-mannosylation have been identified in this system. In recent years, a few homologs of these genes have been identified in *C. albicans,* and they have been shown to have analogous functions to their *Saccharomyces* counterparts. To describe what has been learned about O-mannosylation in *C. albicans,* we must first look at the pathway as defined from study in *S. cerevisiae.*

O-linked mannosylation is initiated with the

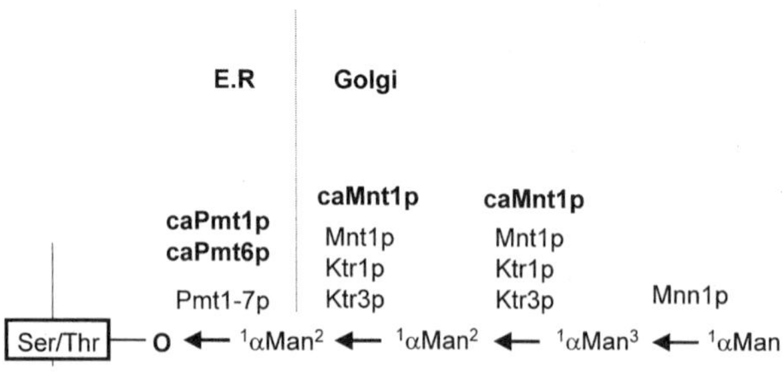

Figure 4. O-glycosylation reactions in *S. cerevisiae*. The *C. albicans* homologs are bolded. Consult the text for details. Modified from reference 9 with permission. Copyright 1998 National Academy of Sciences, U.S.A.

transfer of a mannose to a serine or threonine residue using, as a donor, dolicyl-phosphate-mannose (Dol-P-β-D-mannose) catalyzed by Dol-P-β-D-Man:protein O-α-D-mannosyltransferase, a reaction that takes place within the endoplasmic reticulum (Fig. 4). In *Saccharomyces* sp. this reaction is catalyzed by any of the proteins coded by *PMT1* through *PMT7*, a family of α-mannosyltransferases (27–29, 39, 73, 110). The reason that *S. cerevisiae* has a number of these *PMT* genes is that it appears that each of these proteins has different protein specificities (30, 73). The transfer of this mannose also results in the inversion of the beta-configuration to an α-D-mannosyl linkage. After this initial step, the protein is then translocated to the Golgi complex where further additions are made. Proteins responsible for the addition of the second α-1,2-linked mannosyl residue are encoded by the *KTR1, KTR3,* and *MNT1* genes (74). Mnt1p has also been shown to be responsible for addition of the third α-1,2-linked mannose. The addition of a fourth and sometimes fifth mannose residue linked by an α-1,3-linkage is catalyzed by Mnn1p, a protein that has also been reported to play a role in N-linked glycosylation as well (16, 41, 85).

With regard to O-mannosylation in *C. albicans,* the majority of O-linked carbohydrate is no more than three residues in length, but this can be extended to as long as seven residues (36). The initial step of O-linked addition is essentially the same as that in *S. cerevisiae.* Timpel et al. identified the *C. albicans PMT1* gene using a low stringency hybridization with the *ScPMT1* through *ScPMT7* genes as probes (121). A protein showing 49% amino acid identity to *S. cerevisiae* Pmt1p was designated *CaPMT1. CaPMT1* can complement a *S. cerevisiae pmt1* null strain. This observation indicates that Pmt1p may play the same role in *Candida* sp. as it does in *Saccharomyces* sp. Interestingly, when the *CaPMT1* was deleted, the resulting null mutant exhibits an inability to form hyphae on spider medium. This defect is apparently due to the lack of a signaling component that is required for hypha formation since expression of CaPmt1p is not connected to hypha development. Timpel et al. also demonstrated that *CaPMT1* is required for adhesion to tissue and virulence in a mouse model.

In addition to *PMT1,* Timpel et al. have identified another *PMT* family member in *C. albicans* called *PMT6* (122). A strain lacking *PMT6* still maintains an ability to form hyphae in the presence of serum or GlcNAc but has a significant reduction in the ability to form hyphae on spider medium, although the phenotype is not as dramatic as seen in a *pmt1* null mutant. In fact, a *pmt1pmt6* null mutant is much more similar to the *pmt1* mutant, suggesting Pmt6p has a different protein target(s) than Pmt1p with regard to O-linked mannosylation. A *pmt6* null mutant also has a reduced ability to adhere to cells in a monolayer, and the strains exhibit reduced virulence in a mouse model (122).

After addition of the first mannose, the second mannose is attached in the Golgi complex and the transfer reaction is catalyzed by the *C. albicans* homolog of *MNT1.* Buurman et al. identified this gene by Southern analysis using the *ScMNT1* sequence as a probe (9). They further demonstrated that *CaMNT1* encodes an α-1,2-mannosyl transferase. In addition, Thompson et al. have demonstrated that *CaMNT1* is specifically involved in O-glycosylation (120). A strain lacking *CaMNT1* shows a reduced ability to adhere to human buccal cells and also has reduced virulence in a mouse model (9). The *Camnt1* null mutant also has a low residual addition of second and third mannoses to O-linked residues, suggesting that there are other proteins capable of performing the same function, albeit at a much lower level than *CaMNT1.* In fact, analysis of the *C. albicans* genome has identified four other *MNT* genes that encode proteins showing significant homology to *CaMNT1*; however, the functions of these genes have yet to be examined (120).

CHITIN

Chitin constitutes a minor (0.5 to 3.0%) but important structural polymer that is essential for cell viability. Chitin is a linear polymer of repeating units of β-1,4-*N*-acetylglucosamine. These linear polysaccharides are hydrogen bonded between the adjacent sugar units in an antiparallel manner, resulting in the formation of microfibrils. In electron micrographs of chitin preparations, the microfibrils appear in a range of forms, such as short chains from yeast cells and long entangled chains in hyphal walls. These microfibrils aggregate with the glucan complexes (67) to form a crystalline complex that constitutes a structural scaffold on which the rest of the cell wall is built. Chitin can be detected by staining with Calcofluor white, a fluorescent brightener, and with fluorescein-labeled wheat germ agglutinin, a plant lectin, both of which have high affinity for chitin.

Organization in the Cell Wall

Although the basic cell wall architecture is conserved between *S. cerevisiae* and *C. albicans*, there are some subtle differences, i.e., in *C. albicans* there is less β-1,3 glucan linked to chitin as compared to β-1,6 glucan-chitin linkage (48). Under cell stress conditions in *Candida* sp. there is an increase in chitin synthesis and more chitin is linked to the β-1,6 glucan as compared to the β-1,3 glucan (48). The terminal residue of chitin is linked to the nonreducing end of a β-1,3 glucan chain by a β-1,4 linkage (67). Covalent linkage between chitin and β-1,6 glucan is through a glycosidic linkage at position 6 of *N*-acetylglucosamine and position 1 of the glucose in the glucan. Kollar et al. (68) demonstrated that the reducing terminus of the chitin chain is linked in β-1,4 or β-1,6 linkage to the β-1,3 glucan, which in turn is linked to the β-1,6 glucan. The chitin found in the cell wall and some of the chitin found in the ring of dividing cells are linked to the β-1,6 glucan, whereas some portion of the ring chitin is directly linked to the β-1,3 glucan (68). In *S. cerevisiae* the Chs3p is responsible for the synthesis of chitin, which is linked to glucans (67). In *S. cerevisiae* this chitin is found in the cell wall and in the base of the rings of an emerging bud (67). It is speculated that both the chitin and the glucans (23) are synthesized at the plasma membrane and secreted into the periplasmic space where the final linkages take place (68). As far as the timing is concerned, cell wall chitin is synthesized by Chs3p only after the primary septum formation occurs, which is late in the cell cycle after cytokinesis. During the final phase of the bud maturation late in the cell cycle, linkages with glucans are formed (67, 102).

As in *S. cerevisiae, C. albicans* has three chitin synthases, which are encoded by *CaCHS1, CaCHS2,* and *CaCHS3*. These three genes correspond to the *S. cerevisiae CHS1, CHS2,* and CHS3.

CaCHS1 was cloned by functional complementation of the *S. cerevisiae chs1* null mutant (1). At the amino acid level, CaChs1p was 37% identical to the ScChs1p. CaChs1p is required for the primary septum formation, cell viability, cell shape, and integrity (84). Conditional null mutants of *CaCHS1* were reconstituted with *CaCHS1* under the control of a glucose repressible promoter. Under repressing conditions, yeast cells grew but failed to separate as daughter cells. These conditional mutants also failed to form septa in hyphae, which after several generations, led to the hyphal swelling that in turn resulted in lysis either at the hyphal apex or at other locations not associated with septum formation. Therefore, CaChs1p not only is responsible for primary septum formation but also is responsible for the integrity of the lateral cell wall. The conditional mutant was also avirulent in a mouse model of systemic candidiasis (84).

The *CaCHS2* of *C. albicans* encodes a chitin synthase, which is active in the hyphal phase. The *cachs2* null mutants were viable and exhibited normal morphology although germ tubes exhibited a 40% reduction in their chitin content (33). The *cachs2* mutants did not show any loss of virulence in a mouse model of systemic candidiasis. In *S. cerevisiae* the *chs2* mutant exhibits abnormal morphology showing a normal or an increase in chitin content and a lack of the chitinous primary septum. These results indicate that the *CaCHS2* may not be a functional homolog of the *CHS1* and *CHS2* of the *S. cerevisiae* (33).

CaChs3 was cloned from *C. albicans* using the *S. cerevisiae CAL1* gene as a probe. The *C. albicans chs3* null mutant shows about an 80% reduction in the amount of chitin in the cell wall in the yeast phase, and these mutants show attenuated virulence in a mouse model of systemic candidiasis. The CaChs3p is required for the synthesis of chitin rings but is not needed for septa formation (7).

In the presence of RO-09-3143, which is a novel inhibitor specific for *CaCHS1, C. albicans* failed to form septa, displayed aberrant morphology, and arrested cell growth. RO-09-3143 is lethal to the *cachs2* mutant but not so with the *cachs3* mutant; double mutants of *cachs2* and *cachs3* are viable (79). In *S. cerevisiae* a double disruption of *CHS1* and *CHS2* is still viable, and only the simultaneous inactivation of *CHS2* and *CHS3* is lethal whereas in *C. albicans* the simultaneous inactivation of *CaCHS1* and *CaCHS2* is lethal (113).

A gene corresponding to the *S. cerevisiae CHS4* gene has also been identified in *C. albicans* (112). *CHS4* in *S. cerevisiae* is a posttranslational regulator of the Chs3p complex (87). In *S. cerevisiae* it has been shown that the Chs3p and Chs4p physically interact. Chs5p and Chs6p are also involved in regulating the activity of Chs3p in *S. cerevisiae* (112).

Chitinase

Chitinases are important for remodeling the chitin in the cell wall of fungi and play an important role in the formation of hyphae, probably by regulating the plasticity of the expanding areas of the cell wall during branching and apical hyphal growth (96). Three genes, *CHT1*, *CHT2*, and *CHT3*, have been isolated from *C. albicans* that encode chitinases (77). Transcripts of *CHT2* and *CHT3* are highly expressed in the yeast as compared to the hyphae, whereas expression of the *CHT1* was not detected (77). Subsequently, it was found that the *CHT1* encodes a truncated form of a chitinase that lacks the conserved Ser/Thr-rich region, which might explain its lack of expression (76). Null mutants of *CHT2* form cell aggregates, indicating the role of this chitinase in cell separation (77).

GLYCOLIPIDS

Glycolipids account for only 1 to 7% by dry weight of the cell wall of *Candida* species (10) but have important functions. Their carbohydrate moieties protrude from the exterior surface of the cell membrane, just as do glycoproteins, and frequently function as receptors or antigens in cells. But this is only our traditional understanding of glycolipids. More and more data, derived from eukaryotic organisms other than *C. albicans,* have hinted broadly that glycolipids also play an important role in signal transduction, cell wall synthesis, and antigen processing of macrophages or T cells.

With respect to the immunoreactivity of pathogenic *C. albicans,* another important glycolipid, phospholipidomannan (PLM), must be mentioned. PLM corresponds to a family of glycolipids in *C. albicans,* consisting of a single inositol and glycophosphalipids (Fig. 5). The linear chains of β-1,2-oligomannose are the major PLM component. This unusual type of linkage is also found in the immunogenic component of the cell wall, phosphopeptidomannan, of *C. albicans* via a phosphodiester bridge (105). The specific humoral response, anti-β-1,2-oligomannoside antibodies, has been shown to protect mice from candidiasis under laboratory conditions (34). Therefore, it is not surprising that PLM with these same sugar residues has been investigated for its role in virulence and immunomodulation in *C. albicans* (124) with the results described below.

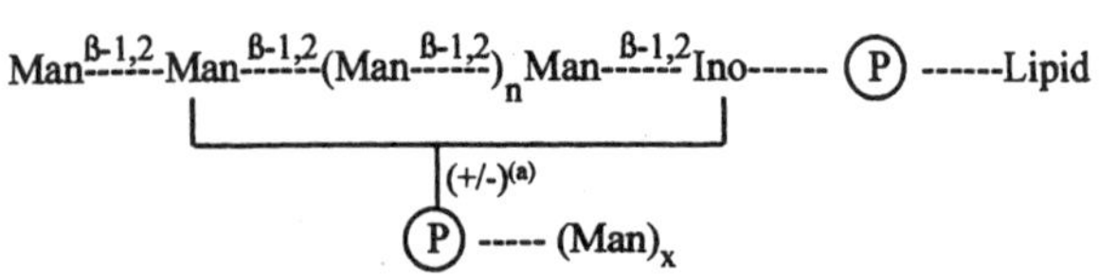

Figure 5. The proposed structure of the glycolipid PLM of *C. albicans*. Reprinted from reference 124 with permission.

PLM has been shown to be released from the cell wall of *C. albicans,* binding to the macrophage membrane mannose receptor through β-1,2-oligomannosides (44) and triggering cytokine synthesis, such as tumor necrosis factor-α through a phosphotyrosine kinase-dependent signaling pathway. Experimental evidence indicates that β-1,2-oligomannosides are involved in virulence and immunomodulation and that they elicit protective antibody responses in candidiasis. Therefore, current data have shown that PLM should be considered in any analysis of host-*C. albicans* relationships.

Compared with α-mannosides, β-1,2-oligomannosides have a less favorable stereochemical structure and are expressed only in *C. albicans* and *C. tropicalis,* which are the most pathogenic *Candida* species. They can act as epitopes for a large number of anti-*C. albicans* phosphopeptidomannan monoclonal antibodies (24), suggesting that β-1,2-oligomannosides are strong immunogens. Although very little is known about β-1,2-mannosyltransferases of *C. albicans,* either their activation or substrate specificity, PLM can be synthesized by *C. albicans* even under growth conditions that prevent attachment of β-1,2-oligomannosides to phosphopeptidomannan. Whether this property is significant remains to be investigated.

Glycosphingolipids, which are amphipathic compounds of sugar and ceramide moieties, have been investigated in a variety of eukaryotic cells including yeast. Previously, it was thought that the only role for phospholipids and sphingolipids was as structural components of the cell wall that establish a barrier for cell permeability or formed a matrix for the attachment of proteins to the cell wall. However, the new results show that sphingosine lipids seem to be an inhibitor of protein kinase C, which led us to explore the role of sphingolipid and their intermediates in signal transduction and cell cycle regulation.

Lipid-dependent signaling transduction is currently a rapidly expanding area of interest. Observations from *S. cerevisiae* are that the sphingoid and ceremides are directly involved in various aspects of stress responses, such as heat shock (21, 22, 42) and endocytosis (126). Although the precise processes still remain to be discovered, the ceramides have been put forward as possibly the key compounds in the metabolism of sphingolipids and also as a possible second message, playing an important role in various cellular processes including signal transduction, cell regulation, transportation of secretory vesicles from the endoplasmic reticulum to the Golgi apparatus (2), and even in the immune response by intracellular interaction with cytokines or through carbohydrate antigen processing (95).

Structurally, ceramides consist of a long chain

amino alcohol (sphingosine or sphinganine) covalently linked to a fatty acyl chain via some type of amide linkage (17). The fatty acid chain can vary in length or undergo unsaturation or hydroxylation in different ceramide molecules. However, the study of ceramide metabolism is impeded at present because of its very low levels in cells, as well as its apolar nature and the enormous diversity of molecules. Several means have been used in the identification and quantitation of cellular ceramide levels, such as high-performance liquid chromatography and mass spectrometry. The glucosylceramides and galactosylceramides could be synthesized by a transmembrane protein, ceramide glucosyltransferase, which transfers glucose or galactose to the ceramide. However, glucosylceramides appear not to be essential for vegetative growth of *C. albicans,* based on a preliminary study of the ceramide glucosyltransferase-knockout strain of *C. albicans* (70).

GPI, a complex glycolipid that acts as a membrane anchor for many CWPs in eukaryotic organisms, accounts for roughly 88% of all covalently linked CWPs in *C. albicans* (48). Studies on the assembly of the yeast cell wall have recently shown that some of the GPI-anchored proteins have an important enzymatic function in *Candida* cell wall synthesis and in the modification of cross-linking polymers. A series of GPI-anchored proteins, β-1,3 glucanosyltransferase, has been cloned and characterized in several varieties of yeast and in *A. fumigatus,* respectively. These proteins are thought to be responsible for the elongation of 1,3-β glucan side chains and are also thought to be necessary for correct morphogenesis in yeast when the antibiotic aculeacin A (inhibiting 1,3-β glucan synthesis) is present. The utility of these glycolipids as a biochemical tool remains to be investigated (82, 88, 94). Few functional studies of the GPI moiety in CWP modifications have been done in *Candida* spp., but studies in *S. cerevisiae* have revealed that the proteins that are supposedly covalently linked to β-1,6 glucan are initially anchored by GPI and then are incorporated into the cell wall by means of a transglycosidation reaction between the glucan part of GPI and β-1,6 glucan. It is very likely that *C. albicans* follows the same basic rules as *S. cerevisiae* in constructing the cell wall, so that GPI-anchored CWPs are attached to 1,3-β glucan or chitin or both through 1,6-β glucan (45).

Biosynthesis of GPI is initiated by the transfer of *N*-acetylglucosamine to phosphatidylinositol to form GlcNAc-PI. At least 10 enzymatic reactions are required before linkage to a protein in the endoplasmic reticulum occurs (55). GPI can exist on the cell surface itself, or it can be covalently bound to the carboxyl terminus of a protein that has a GPI-attachment signal peptide, with this GPI-anchored protein finally being transported to the cell surface through the secretory pathway.

The majority of the enzymes required for biosynthesis of GPI have been cloned and characterized in *S. cerevisiae.* These include *MCD4* (ethanolaminephosphate transferase) and *GPI7* (exact function not determined), which are also involved in mannose modification by ethanolaminephosphate in the biosynthesis of GPI. The mutants derived from these two genes have a cell wall fragility and a reduction in GPI anchoring (3, 26). The difference in GPI biosynthesis between mammalian cells and yeast (26, 37) may offer a clue to the development of new antifungal agents by inhibiting some fungal-specific enzyme in GPI synthesis.

A great deal of progress has been made in our understanding of *C. albicans* glycolipid function. However, a complete elucidation of the structures of the various *C. albicans* glycolipids, particularly their biosynthetic pathways and metabolism, will still be necessary to provide a structural basis for understanding their immunochemical and signal transduction properties, their protein sorting mechanisms, and their role in the pathogenesis of *C. albicans* infections.

REFERENCES

1. **Au-Young, J., and P. W. Robbins.** 1990. Isolation of a chitin synthase gene (CHS1) from *Candida albicans* by expression in *Saccharomyces cerevisiae. Mol. Microbiol.* **4:**197–207.
2. **Bagnat, M., S. Keränen, A. Shevchenko, A. Shevchenko, and K. Simons.** 2000. Lipid rafts function in biosynthetic delivery of proteins to the cell surface in yeast. *Proc. Natl. Acad. Sci. USA* **97:**3254–3259.
3. **Benachour, A., G. Sipos, I. Flury, F. Reggiori, E. Canivenc-Gansel, C. Vionnet, A. Conzelmann, and M. Benghezal.** 1999. Deletion of GPI7, a yeast gene required for addition of a side chain to the glycosylphosphatidylinositol (GPI) core structure, affects GPI protein transport, remodeling, and cell wall integrity. *J Biol Chem.* **274:**15251–15261.
4. **Boone, C., A. Sdicu, M. Laroche, and H. Bussey.** 1991. Isolation from *Candida albicans* of a functional homolog of the *Saccharomyces cerevisiae* KRE1 gene, which is involved in cell wall beta-glucan synthesis. *J. Bacteriol.* **173:**6859–6864.
5. **Braun, P. C., and R. A. Calderone.** 1978. Chitin synthesis in *Candida albicans:* comparison of yeast and hyphal forms. *J. Bacteriol.* **133:**1472–1477.
6. **Brawner, D. L., J. E. Cutler, and W. L. Beatty.** 1990. Caveats in the investigation of form-specific molecules of *Candida albicans. Infect. Immun.* **58:**378–383.
7. **Bulawa, C. E., D. W. Miller, L. K. Henry, and J. M. Becker.** 1995. Attenuated virulence of chitin-deficient mutants of *Candida albicans. Proc. Natl. Acad. Sci. USA* **92:** 10570–10574.
8. **Burda, P., and M. Aebi.** 1999. The dolichol pathway of N-linked glycosylation. *Biochim. Biophys. Acta* **1426:**239–257.
9. **Buurman, E. T., C. Westwater, B. Hube, A. J. Brown, F. C. Odds, and N. A. Gow.** 1998. Molecular analysis of CaMnt1p, a mannosyl transferase important for adhesion

and virulence of *Candida albicans. Proc. Natl. Acad. Sci. USA* **95**:7670–7675.

10. **Calderone, R. A., and P. C. Braun.** 1991. Adherence and receptor relationships of *Candida albicans. Microbiol. Rev.* **55**:1–20.
11. **Chaffin, W. L., J. L. Lopez-Ribot, M. Casanova, D. Gozalbo, and J. P. Martinez.** 1998. Cell wall and secreted proteins of *Candida albicans:* identification, function, and expression. *Microbiol. Mol. Biol. Rev.* **62**:130–180.
12. **Chambers, R. S., M. J. Broughton, R. D. Cannon, A. Carne, G. W. Emerson, and P. A. Sullivan.** 1993. An exo-beta-(1,3)-glucanase of *Candida albicans:* purification of the enzyme and molecular cloning of the gene. *J. Gen. Microbiol.* **139**: 325–334.
13. **Chattaway, F. W., M. R. Holmes, and A. J. Barlow.** 1968. Cell wall composition of the mycelial and blastospore forms of *Candida albicans. J. Gen. Microbiol.* **51**:367–376.
14. **Cid, V. J., A. Duran, F. del Rey, M. P. Snyder, C. Nombela, and M. Sanchez.** 1995. Molecular basis of cell integrity and morphogenesis in *Saccharomyces cerevisiae. Microbiol. Rev.* **59**:345–386.
15. **Coen, M. L., C. G. Lerner, J. O. Capobianco, and R. C. Goldman.** 1994. Synthesis of yeast cell wall glucan and evidence for glucan metabolism in a *Saccharomyces cerevisiae* whole cell system. *Microbiology* **140**:2229–2237.
16. **Cohen, R. E., L. Ballou, and C. E. Ballou.** 1980. *Saccharomyces cerevisiae* mannoprotein mutants. Isolation of the mnn5 mutant and comparison with the mnn3 strain. *J. Biol. Chem.* **255**:7700–7707.
17. **Cremesti, A. E., and A. S. Fischl.** 2000. Current methods for the identification and quantitation of ceramides: an overview. *Lipids* **35**:937–945.
18. **Cutfield, S., G. Brooke, P. Sullivan, and J. Cutfield.** 1992. Crystallization of the exo(1,3)-beta-glucanase from *Candida albicans. J. Mol. Biol.* **225**:217–218.
19. **Cutfield, S. M., G. J. Davies, G. Murshudov, B. F. Anderson, P. C. Moody, P. A. Sullivan, and J. F. Cutfield.** 1999. The structure of the exo-beta-(1,3)-glucanase from *Candida albicans* in native and bound forms: relationship between a pocket and groove in family 5 glycosyl hydrolases. *J. Mol. Biol.* **294**:771–783.
20. **Dean, N.** 1999. Asparagine-linked glycosylation in the yeast Golgi. *Biochim. Biophys. Acta* **1426**:309–322.
21. **Dickson, R. C.** 1998. Sphingolipid functions in *Saccharomyces cerevisiae:* comparison to mammals. *Annu. Rev. Biochem.* **67**:27–48.
22. **Dickson, R. C., E. E. Nagiec, M. Skrzypek, P. Tillman, G. B. Wells, and R. L. Lester.** 1997. Sphingolipids are potential heat stress signals in *Saccharomyces. J. Biol. Chem.* **272**: 30196–30200.
23. **Drgonova, J., T. Drgon, K. Tanaka, R. Kollar, G. C. Chen, R. A. Ford, C. S. Chan, Y. Takai, and E. Cabib.** 1996. Rho1p, a yeast protein at the interface between cell polarization and morphogenesis. *Science* **272**:277–279.
24. **Faille, C., J. C. Michalski, G. Strecker, D. W. Mackenzie, D. Camus, and D. Poulain.** 1990. Immunoreactivity of neoglycolipids constructed from oligomannosidic residues of the *Candida albicans* cell wall. *Infect. Immun.* **58**:3537–3544.
25. **Fonzi, W. A.** 1999. PHR1 and PHR2 of *Candida albicans* encode putative glycosidases required for proper cross-linking of beta-1,3- and beta-1,6-glucans. *J. Bacteriol.* **181**: 7070–7079.
26. **Gaynor, E. C., G. Mondesert, S. J. Grimme, S. I. Reed, P. Orlean, and S. D. Emr.** 1999. MCD4 encodes a conserved endoplasmic reticulum membrane protein essential for glycosylphosphatidylinositol anchor synthesis in yeast. *Mol. Biol. Cell.* **10**:627–648.
27. **Gentzsch, M., T. Immervoll, and W. Tanner.** 1995. Protein O-glycosylation in *Saccharomyces cerevisiae:* the protein O-mannosyltransferases Pmt1p and Pmt2p function as heterodimer. *FEBS Lett.* **377**:128–130.
28. **Gentzsch, M., S. Strahl-Bolsinger, and W. Tanner.** 1995. A new Dol-P-Man:protein O-D-mannosyltransferase activity from *Saccharomyces cerevisiae. Glycobiology* **5**:77–82.
29. **Gentzsch, M., and W. Tanner.** 1996. The PMT gene family: protein O-glycosylation in *Saccharomyces cerevisiae* is vital. *EMBO J.* **15**:5752–5759.
30. **Gentzsch, M., and W. Tanner.** 1997. Protein-O-glycosylation in yeast: protein-specific mannosyltransferases. *Glycobiology* **7**:481–486.
31. **Goldman, R. C., P. A. Sullivan, D. Zakula, and J. O. Capobianco.** 1995. Kinetics of beta-1,3 glucan interaction at the donor and acceptor sites of the fungal glucosyltransferase encoded by the BGL2 gene. *Eur. J. Biochem.* **227**:372–378.
32. **Gonzalez, M. M., R. Diez-Orejas, G. Molero, A. M. Alvarez, J. Pla, C. Nombela, and M. Sanchez-Perez.** 1997. Phenotypic characterization of a *Candida albicans* strain deficient in its major exoglucanase. *Microbiology* **143**:3023–3032.
33. **Gow, N. A., P. W. Robbins, J. W. Lester, A. J. Brown, W. A. Fonzi, T. Chapman, and O. S. Kinsman.** 1994. A hyphal-specific chitin synthase gene (CHS2) is not essential for growth, dimorphism, or virulence of *Candida albicans. Proc. Natl. Acad. Sci. USA* **91**:6216–6220.
34. **Han, Y., and J. E. Cutler.** 1995. Antibody response that protects against disseminated candidiasis. *Infect. Immun.* **63**: 2714–2719.
35. **Hartland, R. P., C. A. Vermeulen, F. M. Klis, J. H. Sietsma, and J. G. Wessels.** 1994. The linkage of (1-3)-beta-glucan to chitin during cell wall assembly in *Saccharomyces cerevisiae. Yeast* **10**:1591–1599.
36. **Hayette, M. P., G. Strecker, C. Faille, D. Dive, D. Camus, D. W. Mackenzie, and D. Poulain.** 1992. Presence of human antibodies reacting with *Candida albicans* O-linked oligomannosides revealed by using an enzyme-linked immunosorbent assay and neoglycolipids. *J. Clin. Microbiol.* **30**: 411–417.
37. **Hong, Y., Y. Maeda, R. Watanabe, K. Ohishi, M. Mishkind, H. Riezman, and T. Kinoshita.** 1999. Pig-n, a mammalian homologue of yeast Mcd4p, is involved in transferring phosphoethanolamine to the first mannose of the glycosylphosphatidylinositol. *J. Biol. Chem.* **274**:35099–35106.
38. **Ikuta, K., N. Shibata, H. Kanehiko, H. Kobayashi, S. Suzuki, and Y. Okawa.** 1997. NMR assignment of the galactomannan of *Candida lipolytica. FEBS Lett.* **414**:338–342.
39. **Immervoll, T., M. Gentzsch, and W. Tanner.** 1995. PMT3 and PMT4, two new members of the protein-O-mannosyltransferase gene family of *Saccharomyces cerevisiae. Yeast* **11**:1345–1351.
40. **Inoue, S. B., N. Takewaki, T. Takasuka, T. Mio, M. Adachi, Y. Fujii, C. Miyamoto, M. Arisawa, Y. Furuichi, and T. Watanabe.** 1995. Characterization and gene cloning of 1,3-beta-D-glucan synthase from *Saccharomyces cerevisiae. Eur. J. Biochem.* **231**:845–854.
41. **Jars, M. U., S. Osborn, J. Forstrom, and V. L. MacKay.** 1995. N- and O-glycosylation and phosphorylation of the bar secretion leader derived from the barrier protease of *Saccharomyces cerevisiae. J. Biol. Chem.* **270**:24810–24817.
42. **Jenkins, G. M., A. Richards, T. Wahl, C. Mao, L. Obeid, and Y. Hannun.** 1997. Involvement of yeast sphingolipids in the heat stress response of *Saccharomyces cerevisiae. J. Biol. Chem.* **272**:32566–32572.

43. **Jigami, Y., and T. Odani.** 1999. Mannosylphosphate transfer to yeast mannan. *Biochim. Biophys. Acta* **1426:**335–345.
44. **Jouault, T., C. Fradin, P. A. Trinel, A. Bernigaud, and D. Poulain.** 1998. Early signal transduction induced by *Candida albicans* in macrophages through shedding of a glycolipid. *J. Infect. Dis.* **178:**792–802.
45. **Jouault, T., C. Fradin, P. A. Trinel, and D. Poulain.** 2000. *Candida albicans*-derived beta-1,2-linked mannooligosaccharides induce desensitization of macrophages. *Infect. Immun.* **68:**965–968.
46. **Kandasamy, R., G. Vediyappan, and W. L. Chaffin.** 2000. Evidence for the presence of pir-like proteins in *Candida albicans. FEMS Microbiol. Lett.* **186:**239–243.
47. **Kapteyn, J. C., G. J. Dijkgraaf, R. C. Montijn, and F. M. Klis.** 1995. Glucosylation of cell wall proteins in regenerating spheroplasts of *Candida albicans. FEMS Microbiol. Lett.* **128:**271–277.
48. **Kapteyn, J. C., L. L. Hoyer, J. E. Hecht, W. H. Muller, A. Andel, A. J. Verkleij, M. Makarow, H. Van Den Ende, and F. M. Klis.** 2000. The cell wall architecture of *Candida albicans* wild-type cells and cell wall-defective mutants. *Mol. Microbiol.* **35:**601–611.
49. **Kapteyn, J. C., R. C. Montijn, G. J. Dijkgraaf, and F. M. Klis.** 1994. Identification of beta-1,6-glucosylated cell wall proteins in yeast and hyphal forms of *Candida albicans. Eur. J. Cell Biol.* **65:**402–407.
50. **Kapteyn, J. C., R. C. Montijn, G. J. Dijkgraaf, H. Van den Ende, and F. M. Klis.** 1995. Covalent association of beta-1,3-glucan with beta-1,6-glucosylated mannoproteins in cell walls of *Candida albicans. J. Bacteriol.* **177:**3788–3792.
51. **Kapteyn, J. C., R. C. Montijn, E. Vink, J. de la Cruz, A. Llobell, J. E. Douwes, H. Shimoi, P. N. Lipke, and F. M. Klis.** 1996. Retention of *Saccharomyces cerevisiae* cell wall proteins through a phosphodiester-linked beta-1,3-/beta-1,6-glucan heteropolymer. *Glycobiology* **6:**337–345.
52. **Kapteyn, J. C., A. F. Ram, E. M. Groos, R. Kollar, R. C. Montijn, H. Van Den Ende, A. Llobell, E. Cabib, and F. M. Klis.** 1997. Altered extent of cross-linking of beta1,6-glucosylated mannoproteins to chitin in *Saccharomyces cerevisiae* mutants with reduced cell wall beta1,3-glucan content. *J. Bacteriol.* **179:**6279–6284.
53. **Kapteyn, J. C., H. Van Den Ende, and F. M. Klis.** 1999. The contribution of cell wall proteins to the organization of the yeast cell wall. *Biochim. Biophys. Acta* **1426:**373–383.
54. **Kapteyn, J. C., P. Van Egmond, E. Sievi, H. Van Den Ende, M. Makarow, and F. M. Klis.** 1999. The contribution of the O-glycosylated protein Pir2p/Hsp150 to the construction of the yeast cell wall in wild-type cells and beta 1,6-glucan-deficient mutants. *Mol. Microbiol.* **31:**1835–1844.
55. **Kinoshita, T., and N. Inoue.** 2000. Dissecting and manipulating the pathway for glycosylphosphatidylinositol-anchor biosynthesis. *Curr. Opin. Chem. Biol.* **4:**632–638.
56. **Kobayashi, H., M. Komido, M. Watanabe, K. Matsuda, M. Suzuki, T. Ikeda, H. Oyamada, N. Shibata, and S. Suzuki.** 1994. Structure of cell wall mannan of *Candida kefyr* IFO 0586. *Infect. Immun.* **62:**4425–4431.
57. **Kobayashi, H., K. Matsuda, T. Ikeda, M. Suzuki, S. Takahashi, A. Suzuki, N. Shibata, and S. Suzuki.** 1994. Structures of cell wall mannans of pathogenic *Candida tropicalis* IFO 0199 and IFO 1647 yeast strains. *Infect. Immun.* **62:** 615–622.
58. **Kobayashi, H., H. Mitobe, K. Takahashi, T. Yamamoto, N. Shibata, and S. Suzuki.** 1992. Structural study of a cell wall mannan-protein complex of the pathogenic yeast *Candida glabrata* IFO 0622 strain. *Arch. Biochem. Biophys.* **294:** 662–669.
59. **Kobayashi, H., N. Shibata, M. Nakada, S. Chaki, K. Mizugami, Y. Ohkubo, and S. Suzuki.** 1990. Structural study of cell wall phosphomannan of *Candida albicans* NIH B-792 (serotype B) strain, with special reference to 1H and 13C NMR analyses of acid-labile oligomannosyl residues. *Arch. Biochem. Biophys.* **278:**195–204.
60. **Kobayashi, H., N. Shibata, T. Osaka, Y. Miyagawa, Y. Ohkubo, and S. Suzuki.** 1992. Structural study of cell wall mannan of a *Candida albicans* (serotype A) strain. *Phytochemistry* **31:**1147–1153.
61. **Kobayashi, H., N. Shibata, A. Suzuki, S. Takahashi, M. Suzuki, K. Matsuda, K. Hisamichi, and S. Suzuki.** 1994. Expression of alpha-1,3 linkage-containing oligomannosyl residues in a cell-wall mannan of *Candida tropicalis* grown in yeast extract-Sabouraud liquid medium under acidic conditions. *FEBS Lett* **342:**19–22.
62. **Kobayashi, H., J. Suzuki, S. Tanaka, Y. Kiuchi, H. Oyamada, N. Iwadate, H. Suzuki, N. Shibata, S. Suzuki, and Y. Okawa.** 1997. Structure of a cell wall mannan from the pathogenic yeast, *Candida catenulata:* assignment of 1H nuclear magnetic resonance chemical shifts of the inner alpha-1,6-linked mannose residues substituted by a side chain. *Arch. Biochem. Biophys.* **341:**70–74.
63. **Kobayashi, H., S. Takahashi, N. Shibata, M. Miyauchi, M. Ishida, J. Sato, K. Maeda, and S. Suzuki.** 1994. Structural modification of cell wall mannans of *Candida albicans* serotype A strains grown in yeast extract-Sabouraud liquid medium under acidic conditions. *Infect. Immun.* **62:**968–973.
64. **Kobayashi, H., M. Takaku, Y. Nishidate, S. Takahashi, M. Takikawa, N. Shibata, and S. Suzuki.** 1992. Structure of the D-mannan of the pathogenic yeast, *Candida stellatoidea* ATCC 20408 (type II) strain, in comparison with that of *C. stellatoidea* ATCC 36232 (type I) strain. *Carbohydr. Res.* **231:**105–116.
65. **Kobayashi, H., S. Tanaka, J. Suzuki, Y. Kiuchi, N. Shibata, S. Suzuki, and Y. Okawa.** 1997. Amended structure of side chains in a cell wall mannan from *Candida albicans* serotype A strain grown in yeast extract-Sabouraud liquid medium under acidic conditions: detection of the branched side chains corresponding to antigenic factor 4. *FEMS Microbiol Lett.* **152:**235–242.
66. **Kogan, G., V. Pavliak, J. Sandula, and L. Masler.** 1988. Novel structure of the cellular mannan of the pathogenic yeast *Candida krusei. Carbohydr. Res.* **184:**171–182.
67. **Kollar, R., E. Petrakova, G. Ashwell, P. W. Robbins, and E. Cabib.** 1995. Architecture of the yeast cell wall. The linkage between chitin and beta(1—>3)-glucan. *J. Biol. Chem.* **270:** 1170–1178.
68. **Kollar, R., B. B. Reinhold, E. Petrakova, H. J. Yeh, G. Ashwell, J. Drgonova, J. C. Kapteyn, F. M. Klis, and E. Cabib.** 1997. Architecture of the yeast cell wall. Beta(1—>6)-glucan interconnects mannoprotein, beta(1—>)3-glucan, and chitin. *J. Biol. Chem.* **272:**17762–17775.
69. **Kondoh, O., Y. Tachibana, Y. Ohya, M. Arisawa, and T. Watanabe.** 1997. Cloning of the RHO1 gene from *Candida albicans* and its regulation of beta-1,3-glucan synthesis. *J. Bacteriol.* **179:**7734–7741.
70. **Leipelt, M., D. C. Warnecke, B. Hube, U. Zahringer, and E. Heinz.** 2000. Characterization of UDP-glucose:ceramide glucosyltransferases from different organisms. *Biochem. Soc. Trans.* **28:**751–752.
71. **Lipke, P. N., and R. Ovalle.** 1998. Cell wall architecture in yeast: new structure and new challenges. *J. Bacteriol.* **180:** 3735–3740.
72. **Lu, C. F., R. C. Montijn, J. L. Brown, F. Klis, J. Kurjan, H. Bussey, and P. N. Lipke.** 1995. Glycosyl phosphatidylinosi-

tol-dependent cross-linking of alpha-agglutinin and beta 1,6-glucan in the *Saccharomyces cerevisiae* cell wall. *J. Cell Biol.* **128:**333–340.

73. **Lussier, M., M. Gentzsch, A. M. Sdicu, H. Bussey, and W. Tanner.** 1995. Protein O-glycosylation in yeast. The PMT2 gene specifies a second protein O-mannosyltransferase that functions in addition to the PMT1-encoded activity. *J. Biol. Chem.* **270:**2770–2775.
74. **Lussier, M., A. M. Sdicu, F. Bussereau, M. Jacquet, and H. Bussey.** 1997. The Ktr1p, Ktr3p, and Kre2p/Mnt1p mannosyltransferases participate in the elaboration of yeast O- and N-linked carbohydrate chains. *J. Biol. Chem.* **272:** 15527–15531.
75. **Lussier, M., A. M. Sdicu, S. Shahinian, and H. Bussey.** 1998. The *Candida albicans* KRE9 gene is required for cell wall beta-1,6-glucan synthesis and is essential for growth on glucose. *Proc. Natl. Acad. Sci. USA* **95:**9825–9830.
76. **McCreath, K. J., C. A. Specht, Y. Liu, and P. W. Robbins.** 1996. Molecular cloning of a third chitinase gene (CHT1) from *Candida albicans. Yeast* **12:**501–504.
77. **McCreath, K. J., C. A. Specht, and P. W. Robbins.** 1995. Molecular cloning and characterization of chitinase genes from *Candida albicans. Proc. Natl. Acad. Sci. USA* **92:** 2544–2548.
78. **Mio, T., M. Adachi-Shimizu, Y. Tachibana, H. Tabuchi, S. B. Inoue, T. Yabe, T. Yamada-Okabe, M. Arisawa, T. Watanabe, and H. Yamada-Okabe.** 1997. Cloning of the *Candida albicans* homolog of *Saccharomyces cerevisiae* GSC1/FKS1 and its involvement in beta-1,3-glucan synthesis. *J. Bacteriol.* **179:**4096–4105.
79. **Mio, T., T. Yabe, M. Sudoh, Y. Satoh, T. Nakajima, M. Arisawa, and H. Yamada-Okabe.** 1996. Role of three chitin synthase genes in the growth of *Candida albicans. J. Bacteriol.* **178:**2416–2419.
80. **Mio, T., T. Yamada-Okabe, T. Yabe, T. Nakajima, M. Arisawa, and H. Yamada-Okabe.** 1997. Isolation of the *Candida albicans* homologs of *Saccharomyces cerevisiae* KRE6 and SKN1: expression and physiological function. *J. Bacteriol.* **179:**2363–2372.
81. **Montijn, R. C., E. Vink, W. H. Muller, A. J. Verkleij, H. Van Den Ende, B. Henrissat, and F. M. Klis.** 1999. Localization of synthesis of beta 1,6-glucan in *Saccharomyces cerevisiae. J. Bacteriol.* **181:**7414–7420.
82. **Mouyna, I., T. Fontaine, M. Vai, M. Monod, W. A. Fonzi, M. Diaquin, L. Popolo, R. P. Hartland, and J. P. Latge.** 2000. Glycosylphosphatidylinositol-anchored glucanosyltransferases play an active role in the biosynthesis of the fungal cell wall. *J. Biol. Chem.* **275:**14882–14889.
83. **Mouyna, I., M. Monod, T. Fontaine, B. Henrissat, B. Lechenne, and J. P. Latge.** 2000. Identification of the catalytic residues of the first family of beta(1–3)glucanosyltransferases identified in fungi. *Biochem. J.* **347**(Pt. 3)**:**741–747.
84. **Munro, C. A., K. Winter, A. Buchan, K. Henry, J. M. Becker, A. J. Brown, C. E. Bulawa, and N. A. Gow.** 2001. Chs1 of *Candida albicans* is an essential chitin synthase required for synthesis of the septum and for cell integrity. *Mol. Microbiol.* **39:**1414–1426.
85. **Nakajima, T., and C. E. Ballou.** 1974. Characterization of the carbohydrate fragments obtained from *Saccharomyces cerevisiae* mannan by alkaline degradation. *J. Biol. Chem.* **249:**7679–7684.
86. **Okubo, Y., N. Shibata, T. Ichikawa, S. Chaki, and S. Suzuki.** 1981. Immunochemical study on bakers' yeast mannan prepared by fractional precipitation with cetyltrimethylammonium bromide. *Arch. Biochem. Biophys.* **212:**204–215.
87. **Ono, N., T. Yabe, M. Sudoh, T. Nakajima, T. Yamada-Okabe, M. Arisawa, and H. Yamada-Okabe.** 2000. The yeast Chs4 protein stimulates the trypsin-sensitive activity of chitin synthase 3 through an apparent protein-protein interaction. *Microbiology* **146:**385–391.
88. **Osumi, M.** 1998. The ultrastructure of yeast: cell wall structure and formation. *Micron* **29:**207–233.
89. **Peat, S., W. J. Whelan, and T. E. Edwards.** 1961. Polysaccharides of bakers yeast. IV. *Mannan* **1:**29–34.
90. **Phaff, H. J.** 1963. Cell wall of yeasts. *Annu. Rev. Microbiol.* **17:**15–30.
91. **Podzorski, R. P., G. R. Gray, and R. D. Nelson.** 1990. Different effects of native *Candida albicans* mannan and mannan-derived oligosaccharides on antigen-stimulated lymphoproliferation in vitro. *J. Immunol.* **144:**707–716.
92. **Popolo, L., D. Gilardelli, P. Bonfante, and M. Vai.** 1997. Increase in chitin as an essential response to defects in assembly of cell wall polymers in the ggp1delta mutant of *Saccharomyces cerevisiae. J. Bacteriol.* **179:**463–469.
93. **Popolo, L., and M. Vai.** 1998. Defects in assembly of the extracellular matrix are responsible for altered morphogenesis of a *Candida albicans* phr1 mutant. *J. Bacteriol.* **180:** 163–166.
94. **Popolo, L., and M. Vai.** 1999. The Gas1 glycoprotein, a putative wall polymer cross-linker. *Biochim. Biophys. Acta* **1426:** 385–400.
95. **Prigozy, T. I., O. Naidenko, P. Qasba, D. Elewaut, L. Brossay, A. Khurana, T. Natori, Y. Koezuka, A. Kulkarni, and M. Kronenberg.** 2001. Glycolipid antigen processing for presentation by CD1d molecules. *Sciences* **291:**664–667.
96. **Rast, D. M., M. Horsch, R. Furter, and G. W. Gooday.** 1991. A complex chitinolytic system in exponentially growing mycelium of *Mucor rouxii:* properties and function. *J. Gen. Microbiol.* **137:**2797–2810.
97. **Reiss, E.** 1986. *Candida albicans,* p. 191–239. *In Molecular Immunology of Mycotic and Actinomycotic Infections.* Elsevier, New York, N.Y.
98. **Sanjuan, R., J. Zueco, J. Perez, C. Penarroja, and R. Sentandreu.** 1996. A comparative study of the incorporation of a 1,6-beta-glucan and an O-glycosylated protein epitope into the cell wall of *Candida albicans. Microbiology* **142:** 2255–2262.
99. **Sanjuan, R., J. Zueco, R. Stock, J. Font de Mora, and R. Sentandreu.** 1995. Identification of glucan-mannoprotein complexes in the cell wall of *Candida albicans* using a monoclonal antibody that reacts with a (1,6)-beta-glucan epitope. *Microbiology* **141:**1545–1551.
100. **Sarthy, A. V., T. McGonigal, M. Coen, D. J. Frost, J. A. Meulbroek, and R. C. Goldman.** 1997. Phenotype in *Candida albicans* of a disruption of the BGL2 gene encoding a 1,3-beta-glucosyltransferase. *Microbiology* **143:**367–376.
101. **Shahinian, S., and H. Bussey.** 2000. Beta-1,6-glucan synthesis in *Saccharomyces cerevisiae. Mol. Microbiol.* **35:**477–489.
102. **Shaw, J. A., P. C. Mol, B. Bowers, S. J. Silverman, M. H. Valdivieso, A. Duran, and E. Cabib.** 1991. The function of chitin synthases 2 and 3 in the *Saccharomyces cerevisiae* cell cycle. *J. Cell Biol.* **114:**111–123.
103. **Shepherd, M. G.** 1987. Cell envelope of *Candida albicans. Crit. Rev. Microbiol.* **15:**7–25.
104. **Shibata, N., M. Arai, E. Haga, T. Kikuchi, M. Najima, T. Satoh, H. Kobayashi, and S. Suzuki.** 1992. Structural identification of an epitope of antigenic factor 5 in mannans of *Candida albicans* NIH B-792 (serotype B) and J-1012 (serotype A) as beta-1,2-linked oligomannosyl residues. *Infect. Immun.* **60:**4100–4110.
105. **Shibata, N., T. Ichikawa, M. Tojo, M. Takahashi, N. Ito, Y. Okubo, and S. Suzuki.** 1985. Immunochemical study on

the mannans of *Candida albicans* NIH A-207, NIH B-792, and J-1012 strains prepared by fractional precipitation with cetyltrimethylammonium bromide. *Arch. Biochem. Biophys.* **243:**338–348.

106. **Shibata, N., K. Ikuta, T. Imai, Y. Satoh, R. Satoh, A. Suzuki, C. Kojima, H. Kobayashi, K. Hisamichi, and S. Suzuki.** 1995. Existence of branched side chains in the cell wall mannan of pathogenic yeast, *Candida albicans*. Structure-antigenicity relationship between the cell wall mannans of *Candida albicans* and *Candida parapsilosis*. *J. Biol. Chem.* **270:** 1113–1122.
107. **Shibata, N., M. Onozawa, N. Tadano, Y. Hinosawa, A. Suzuki, K. Ikuta, H. Kobayashi, S. Suzuki, and Y. Okawa.** 1996. Structure and antigenicity of the mannans of *Candida famata* and *Candida saitoana:* comparative study with the mannan of *Candida guilliermondii*. *Arch. Biochem. Biophys.* **336:** 49–58.
108. **Smits, G. J., J. C. Kapteyn, H. van den Ende, and F. M. Klis.** 1999. Cell wall dynamics in yeast. *Curr. Opin. Microbiol.* **2:** 348–352.
109. **Southard, S. B., C. A. Specht, C. Mishra, J. Chen-Weiner, and P. W. Robbins.** 1999. Molecular analysis of the *Candida albicans* homolog of *Saccharomyces cerevisiae* MNN9, required for glycosylation of cell wall mannoproteins. *J. Bacteriol.* **181:**7439–7448.
110. **Strahl-Bolsinger, S., M. Gentzsch, and W. Tanner.** 1999. Protein O-mannosylation. *Biochim. Biophys. Acta* **1426:** 297–307.
111. **Stubbs, H. J., D. J. Brasch, G. W. Emerson, and P. A. Sullivan.** 1999. Hydrolase and transferase activities of the beta-1,3-exoglucanase of *Candida albicans*. *Eur. J. Biochem.* **263:** 889–895.
112. **Sudoh, M., K. Tatsuno, N. Ono, A. Ohta, H. Chibana, H. Yamada-Okabe, and M. Arisawa.** 1999. The *Candida albicans* CHS4 gene complements a *Saccharomyces cerevisiae* skt5/chs4 mutation and is involved in chitin biosynthesis. *Microbiology* **145:**1613–1622.
113. **Sudoh, M., T. Yamazaki, K. Masubuchi, M. Taniguchi, N. Shimma, M. Arisawa, and H. Yamada-Okabe.** 2000. Identification of a novel inhibitor specific to the fungal chitin synthase. Inhibition of chitin synthase 1 arrests the cell growth, but inhibition of chitin synthase 1 and 2 is lethal in the pathogenic fungus *Candida albicans*. *J. Biol. Chem.* **275:** 32901–32905.
114. **Sullivan, P. A., C. Y. Yin, C. Molloy, M. D. Templeton, and M. G. Shepherd.** 1983. An analysis of the metabolism and cell wall composition of *Candida albicans* during germ-tube formation. *Can. J. Microbiol.* **29:**1514–1525.
115. **Surarit, R., P. K. Gopal, and M. G. Shepherd.** 1988. Evidence for a glycosidic linkage between chitin and glucan in the cell wall of *Candida albicans*. *J. Gen. Microbiol.* **134:** 1723–1730.
116. **Suzuki, A., N. Shibata, M. Suzuki, F. Saitoh, H. Oyamada, H. Kobayashi, S. Suzuki, and Y. Okawa.** 1997. Characterization of beta-1,2-mannosyltransferase in *Candida guilliermondii* and its utilization in the synthesis of novel oligosaccharides. *J. Biol. Chem.* **272:**16822–16828.
117. **Suzuki, A., N. Shibata, M. Suzuki, F. Saitoh, Y. Takata, A. Oshie, H. Oyamada, H. Kobayashi, S. Suzuki, and Y. Okawa.** 1996. Characterization of alpha-1,6-mannosyltransferase responsible for the synthesis of branched side chains in *Candida albicans* mannan. *Eur. J. Biochem.* **240:**37–44.
118. **Suzuki, A., Y. Takata, A. Oshie, A. Tezuka, N. Shibata, H. Kobayashi, Y. Okawa, and S. Suzuki.** 1995. Detection of beta-1,2-mannosyltransferase in *Candida albicans* cells. *FEBS Lett.* **373:**275–279.
119. **Symons, M.** 1996. Rho family GTPases: the cytoskeleton and beyond. *Trends Biochem. Sci.* **21:**178–181.
120. **Thomson, L. M., S. Bates, S. Yamazaki, M. Arisawa, Y. Aoki, and N. A. Gow.** 2000. Functional characterization of the *Candida albicans* MNT1 mannosyltransferase expressed heterologously in *Pichia pastoris*. *J. Biol. Chem.* **275:** 18933–18938.
121. **Timpel, C., S. Strahl-Bolsinger, K. Ziegelbauer, and J. F. Ernst.** 1998. Multiple functions of Pmt1p-mediated protein O-mannosylation in the fungal pathogen *Candida albicans*. *J. Biol. Chem.* **273:**20837–20846.
122. **Timpel, C., S. Zink, S. Strahl-Bolsinger, K. Schroppel, and J. Ernst.** 2000. Morphogenesis, adhesive properties, and antifungal resistance depend on the Pmt6 protein mannosyltransferase in the fungal pathogen *Candida albicans*. *J. Bacteriol.* **182:**3063–3071.
123. **Trinel, P. A., G. Lepage, T. Jouault, G. Strecker, and D. Poulain.** 1997. Definitive chemical evidence for the constitutive ability of *Candida albicans* serotype A strains to synthesize beta-1,2 linked oligomannosides containing up to 14 mannose residues. *FEBS Lett.* **416:**203–206.
124. **Trinel, P. A., Y. Plancke, P. Gerold, T. Jouault, F. Delplace, R. T. Schwarz, G. Strecker, and D. Poulain.** 1999. The *Candida albicans* phospholipomannan is a family of glycolipids presenting phosphoinositolmannosides with long linear chains of beta-1,2-linked mannose residues. *J. Biol. Chem.* **274:** 30520–30526.
125. **Yu, L., K. K. Lee, K. Ens, P. C. Doig, M. R. Carpenter, W. Staddon, R. S. Hodges, W. Paranchych, and R. T. Irvin.** 1994. Partial characterization of a *Candida albicans* fimbrial adhesin. *Infect. Immun.* **62:**2834–2842.
126. **Zanolari, B., S. Friant, K. Funato, C. Sutterlin, B. J. Stevenson, and H. Riezman.** 2000. Sphingoid base synthesis requirement for endocytosis in *Saccharomyces cerevisiae*. *EMBO J.* **19:**2824–2833.

IV. IMMUNITY

Candida and Candidiasis
Edited by Richard A. Calderone

Chapter 13

Host Defense against Oral, Esophageal, and Gastrointestinal Candidiasis

HERBERT L. MATHEWS AND LINDA WITEK-JANUSEK

Although *Candida* spp. are frequently isolated from various mucosal sites within the oral cavity, esophagus, and gastrointestinal (GI) tract, few healthy carriers develop clinical signs of disease. Rather, it is a change in the environment of the host that ultimately determines whether the fungus simply remains as a commensal or proliferates, invades tissues, and produces candidiasis. The commensal relationship is dependent on the maintenance of host tissue integrity with normal microbial flora as well as on an intact immune system. As long as these host conditions are maintained, mucosal candidiasis is not observed clinically. However, a breakdown in anatomic integrity or a change in the resident microbial flora can lead to environmental conditions that are favorable for the growth of *Candida* spp. with the potential for host invasion by the fungus. Such environmental conditions in conjunction with an imbalance of host cytokine response can lead to increased tissue colonization and fungal burden resulting in mucosal candidiasis. These conditions most likely contribute to oropharyngeal candidiasis, thrush, and enhanced localization of the fungus within the lower intestinal tract. Endogenously disseminated candidiasis is also a consequence of local environmental and immunological factors, as well as systemic changes in host immune function (primarily neutropenia). This combination of local and systemic conditions leads to dissemination of the fungus from mucosal sites within the GI tract. A breakdown in mucosal barrier defense and decreased polymorphonuclear leukocyte (PMN) function permit endogenous mucosal colonization to initiate localized mucosal disease and fungal dissemination systemically. Mucosal candidiasis of the oropharyngeal cavity in human immunodeficiency virus (HIV)-infected individuals is the prime example of mucosal candidiasis of the mouth and esophagus. Neutropenic patients, immunosuppressed critical care patients, and neonates are individuals at greatest risk for disseminated infection by the fungus. This chapter will focus on *Candida* infections of the oral cavity, esophagus, and GI tract of humans and will include descriptions of existent experimental models employed to understand the infectious process and in particular the immune response to the fungus.

CANDIDA ASSOCIATION WITH THE NORMAL HUMAN GI TRACT

In humans, the GI microbial flora establishes itself a few days after birth. Once established, the resident microbial flora is maintained in a relatively stable state. Approximately 10^{14} microorganisms live in the entire GI tract, with the oral cavity and the colon being the most densely colonized regions. Of the bacteria, obligate anaerobe bacteria extensively outnumber the aerobes. Fungi are important contributors to the microbial flora of the GI tract. Of the fungi present, yeasts predominate and *Candida* is the major genus. *Candida* spp. can be found in the oral cavity, stomach, duodenal secretions, and feces. Although a variety of *Candida* species have been found to occupy the GI tract, most are present transiently. *Candida albicans* often inhabits the GI tract for prolonged periods and is considered part of the resident microbial flora (99). *Candida* colonization begins early in the postnatal period, and on the basis of mother-infant pair studies, infants are typically colonized by strains of *C. albicans* that are derived from the infant's mother (7, 59, 123).

Up to 60% of healthy individuals harbor *C. albi-*

Herbert L. Mathews • Department of Microbiology and Immunology, Stritch School of Medicine, Loyola University of Chicago, 2160 South First Avenue, Maywood, IL 60153-3304. **Linda Witek-Janusek** • Department of Maternal Child Health Nursing, Niehoff School of Nursing, Loyola University of Chicago, 2160 South First Avenue, Maywood, IL 60153-3304.

cans as a commensal in their oral cavity (56). In particular, yeasts colonize the surfaces of the tongue, where oral thrush is the most common and severe. *Candida* spp. are also found on other surfaces of the oral cavity. A survey of healthy dental patients found *Candida* spp. to be most frequently isolated from the tongue (58.5%), followed by the palate (35%), upper jaw (27%), and lower jaw (19.5%). *C. albicans* was the predominant species found in these patients and was most frequent in those individuals 60 years of age and older. Colonization was mild in 46% of these patients, moderate in 12%, and heavy in 9% (15).

In the stomach, *Candida* colonization is, in part, pH dependent. In healthy volunteers, with a gastric juice pH of less than 3, *Candida* spp. colonization was 47%. When gastric pH was greater than 3, colonization increased to 70%. The main species found in the stomach were *C. albicans, C. krusei,* and *C. tropicalis.* Both *C. albicans* and *C. krusei* were present independent of the degree of acidity. *C. tropicalis* was more common in nonacidic gastric juice. When gastric pH was greater than 3, *C. glabrata* was found (15). The effect of gastric pH on *Candida* colonization is most dramatic in critically ill patients treated with hydrogen ion blockers to decrease gastric acidity. These patients are at a much greater risk for the development of candidemia (108). *Candida* spp. also populate the small intestine. In duodenal juice, *Candida* spp. were found in 23% of healthy volunteers with less than 10^3 CFU/ml. In patients with GI disease, 26% were colonized (at less than 10^3 CFU/ml) whereas 6% of the patients had counts greater than 10^3 CFU/ml. The major species found in duodenal juice were *C. albicans* (61%), *C. tropicalis* (18%), and *C. glabrata* (10%) (15).

The balance of the fungal ecosystem within the large intestine is dependent on the presence of the indigenous bacterial flora. In vitro experiments have shown that *Escherichia coli, Salmonella* sp., *Shigella* spp., *Proteus* spp., *Pseudomonas aeruginosa,* and *Lactobacillus acidophilus* inhibit the growth of *C. albicans* (51, 65, 88). Within the large intestine *Candida* spp. are found typically at no more than 3.3 log CFU/g of fecal material (15). In a continuous flow culture system, when fecal flora was added subsequent to the establishment of *Candida* in monoculture, *Candida* germ tube number counts and mycelial formation decreased (15). Using the same system, lactulose, which increased growth of bifidobacteria, also resulted in a decrease in *Candida* numbers. Similar increases in *Candida* colonization and fungal numbers have been observed in animals in which the microbial flora was altered with antibiotics (72, 73) and in humans treated with broad-spectrum antibiotics (110). Further, the resident bacteria inhibit *Candida* adhesion to mucosal cells (73). Thus, with reduced numbers of these bacteria, *Candida* is thought to colonize, bind to the mucosa, and potentially translocate out of the bowel if there is a breach in the mucosal barrier. Fungal overgrowth within the intestinal tract and the development of candidiasis are often a consequence of the liberal use of broad-spectrum antibiotics in modern medical practice that disrupts the balance of the intestinal microbial flora (40). This is often the case in neutropenic patients and critically ill patients who are hospitalized in intensive-care units (ICU).

ORAL, ESOPHAGEAL, AND GI *CANDIDA* INFECTIONS OF PATIENTS

Candidiasis from Endogenous GI Sources

Cancer patients receiving antineoplastic therapy and organ transplant patients are often immunosuppressed, have impaired nutrition, and can be debilitated due to their underlying disease. Oral thrush and localized candidal esophagitis are common in cancer (especially leukemia) and transplant patients. When neutropenic, these patients are at high risk for more serious disseminated *Candida* infections (24). In addition to neutropenia, these patients have a variety of risk factors that compound their susceptibility to *Candida* infections and include the presence of central venous catheters, mucositis (often severe), total parenteral nutrition, and long-term administration of broad-spectrum antibiotics (20). It is well recognized that neutropenia in cancer and transplant patients places them at high risk for colonization by *Candida* spp. (4, 100). Although PMNs serve as a primary defense against tissue invasion and dissemination of *Candida* spp., other factors interact to place the neutropenic patient at risk for disseminated *Candida* infections. Most important to this discussion is that these patients have disruptions of mucosal barriers that can provide sites for local infection and hematogenous dissemination (20). Many of these patients have mucositis and ulcerations of the oropharynx and GI tract. Antineoplastic agents destroy the proliferating epithelial cells of the GI tract, further disrupting the integrity of the gut mucosal barrier (4). This, together with unchecked fungal colonization of GI mucosal surfaces subsequent to antibiotic therapy, leads to excess fungal burden that is hypothesized to spread hematogenously and to cause acute and/or chronic disseminated candidiasis (4, 100, 109). In neutropenic patients with disseminated *Candida* infections the GI tract is involved in 100% of cases, the spleen in 94%, and the liver in 75%, implying that the GI tract is the site of origin from which *Candida* spp. invade (20, 86). Surveillance cultures of bone marrow transplant patients revealed that of 65% with high-level colonization, 82% had *C. albicans* and 18% had non-*C. albicans Candida* sp. colonization (44). In a study of neutropenic patients the *Candida* spp. that were most frequently isolated from the oropharynx and the GI tract were, in decreasing order, *C. albicans, C. glabrata, C. tropicalis, C. krusei,* and *C. parapsilosis*. The majority (74%) of the *C. albicans* isolated were of the smooth phenotype (122). A case-control study of patients with acute lymphocytic leukemia with candidemia found that significant risk factors included previous bacteremia, prolonged neutropenia, prolonged fever, prolonged administration of antimicrobial agents, treatment with multiple antimicrobial agents, and a relatively high concentration of *Candida* in the stool. Others have also demonstrated that broad-spectrum antibiotics given to cancer patients produce an increase in the concentration of yeasts in stool specimens (110). Fecal *Candida* CFU were found to be increased in patients with acute myeloid leukemia and Hodgkin's lymphoma only if the patient had received antibiotic prophylaxis (4, 16). In patients with acute lymphocytic leukemia, antibiotic administration (vancomycin or imipenem in this case) proved to be an independent risk factor for candidemia. Moreover, vancomycin was associated with a greater than 3-log increase in the numbers of *Candida* in stool and was predictive of subsequent candidemia (100). Autopsy studies of cancer patients with fungal infections indicate that 20% of these patients exhibited lesions in the small or large intestine (48).

Alterations of the oral mucosal environment have also been associated with the development of candidiasis in cancer patients. Irradiated head and neck cancer patients with xerostomia were found to have a significantly increased carriage of *Candida* spp., predominantly *C. albicans*. It is hypothesized that *Candida* spp. undergo genetic and phenotypic adaptation that supports their survival in the oral cavity of those individuals with impaired salivary defenses (79). Overall, evidence in cancer patients supports the contention that in susceptible hosts the GI tract can serve as a reservoir for fungi that are able to breach the mucosal barrier and evade the compromised immune system of debilitated cancer and organ transplant patients.

The incidence of disseminated *Candida* infections in critical care patients, including burn, trauma, and surgical patients, has surged in recent years to become the fourth most common cause of nosocomial bloodstream infections (13). The pathogenesis of systemic candidiasis in these patients remains unresolved. However, invasion from a colonized GI tract is believed to be an important portal of entry for *Candida* spp. in patients in ICUs (40). Although animal models support the GI tract as a site of fungal dissemination, in humans, other alternative sources of invasive *Candida* infection include intravascular catheters, long-term parenteral nutrition, surgery (especially surgery that transects the gut wall), and breaches of skin integrity as a result of injury or burns (55). Despite the lack of conclusive proof, there is a growing body of clinical evidence that candidemia can develop as a result of endogenous colonization of the GI tract with fungi that are subsequently translocated across the GI mucosal barrier. Although never proven, evidence from animal models as well as clinical evidence has accumulated that supports the idea that microorganisms can escape the GI tract and cause disseminated disease (41). A demonstration of the invasive potential of *Candida* from the GI tract was documented when Krause et al. recovered *Candida* spp. in both the urine and the blood after ingestion of the organism by an individual with a normally functioning intestine (75). This same group also described a case report in which the onset of symptoms suggestive of septicemia occurred 2 h following ingestion of a suspension of 10^{12} cells of *Candida*. In 1974, *Candida* was shown to migrate across an intact healthy GI lumen by the mechanism then termed persorption (or paracellular or intracellular passage of particles through an intact epithelium), which is now termed translocation (118). The concept of fungal translocation is further supported by the findings that *Candida* can adhere to and invade epithelial surfaces by activation of phospholipases and proteinases (25, 54). On the other hand, Rantala et al. performed multiple blood cultures on patients during reoperations with intestinal manipulation and found no evidence for immediate perioperative fungemia (98). Nevertheless, there is evidence, although not conclusive, to suggest that *Candida* in appreciable quantities in the GI tract may migrate across a normal intestinal mucosal barrier. More importantly, the translocation of *Candida* across the GI barrier is more apt to occur in those with impaired gut barrier function and deficient host defense. This contention is supported by the escalation of disseminated *Candida* infections in critical care and surgical patients (13, 55). Three critical promoting factors are believed to promote translocation: (i) disruption of the ecological balance of the host's intestinal microbial flora, (ii) impaired host immune defenses, and (iii) physical disruption or injury of the gut mucosal barrier (41).

Numerous clinical and experimental studies suggest that critical illness, trauma, and burns are accompanied by diminished mucosal barrier integrity. The defects in mucosa barrier function result from direct effects of surgery, low perfusion to the bowel, and lack of enteral nutrition. These defects place the patient at greater risk for fungal invasion via the GI tract (40). In addition, critical care patients are often immunosuppressed due to underlying disease and this, together with an increase in GI fungal burden, interacts to result in candidiasis and/or candidemia. These patients have often experienced altered intestinal function subsequent to intestinal ischemia or manipulation during surgery, blood loss, or a major hypotensive state; are immunocompromised and/or malnourished; and have received pharmacologic agents that alter the GI microbial flora (e.g., broad-spectrum antibiotics, antacids, or histamine-2 blockers) (55, 64, 98, 128). Case studies of nosocomial bloodstream infections caused by *Candida* spp. all implicate GI manipulation or disease, with colonization subsequent to prior antibiotic usage (128).

In trauma patients, as in other critically ill patients, total parental nutrition (TPN) increases the risk of *Candida* infection and has been found to be an independent risk factor for infection (21, 53). TPN is a highly concentrated mixture of electrolytes, trace metals, protein, and fats and is often provided as the sole means of nutrition in patients with gut dysfunction (21, 40, 53). These nutritional solutions are excellent media in which microorganisms can grow, and in vitro *Candida* spp. have selective advantage over bacteria in replicative capacity and growth (114). However, hematogenous spread of *Candida* subsequent to TPN administration may not be the only likely mechanism for the development of candidiasis in patients nutritionally managed with TPN. TPN administration has been linked to reduced *Candida* phagocytosis in animal models (115) and to increased microbial translocation from the GI tract (3, 115). Further, the use of TPN in lieu of enteral feedings leads to atrophy of the intestinal mucosa, perhaps secondary to a deficiency of glutamine (2). Conversely, enteral nutrition, which supports gut barrier function, reduces infection rates in surgical patients (76, 84). It is likely that yeast traverses the GI barrier more easily in patients in whom the gut barrier is disrupted by surgery, trauma, hyperperfusion, or diffuse atrophy associated with TPN. Impaired immune defenses would then permit the translocated microorganisms to disseminate and produce systemic infection (40).

Critical to the dissemination of *Candida* spp. from endogenous GI sources is an impairment of immune function. An important relationship exists between the state of intestinal barrier function and Kupffer cell activity, such that impaired Kupffer cell function potentiates the systemic spread of GI-derived fungi (41). Individuals with orthotopic liver transplantation are prone to fungal infection, especially from *Candida* spp., due to apparent derangement of the hepatic macrophage-monocyte system (28). Tertiary peritonitis syndrome is also postulated to result from the inability of the exhausted peritoneal macrophage to halt translocated *Candida* spp. after repeated abdominal surgery that involved perforations (55). Focal hepatosplenic candidiasis (a syndrome of disseminated fungal infection involving the liver and spleen of leukemic patients receiving intensive chemotherapy) is also thought to arise from dissemination of the fungus to the portal circulation from the GI tract after fungal colonization and mucosal ulceration of the gut (46, 71).

It has been increasingly recognized that infants hospitalized in neonatal intensive-care units (NICU) are at risk for developing late-onset sepsis from *Candida* spp. (117). In addition to access via hematogenous sources (i.e., indwelling vascular lines) and breaches in skin integrity, fungal colonization of the GI tract has also been implicated in neonatal candidiasis (12, 92, 108). Infants swallow *Candida* spp. at birth, and other risk factors (e.g., lack of enteral feedings and prolific use of antibiotics) promote GI fungal overgrowth and fungal burden (7, 22, 59). In a prospective study of infants in an NICU, almost two-thirds were colonized by the first week of life (7). The perirectal area is most commonly colonized, and colonization occurs more often in low-birth-weight infants (7, 59, 63). In the infant, *Candida* spp. are not limited to mucosal disease but readily disseminate and are associated with a mortality ranging from 25 to 50% (112, 126). Especially in low-birth-weight infants, *C. albicans* can cause severe and even fatal disseminated infection, with involvement of almost all tissues of the body including kidneys, liver, spleen, lung, heart, blood vessels, brain, bones, and joints (22, 126). The propensity for *Candida* spp. theoretically to disseminate from the GI tract is likely related to compounding risk factors, including bouts of intestinal ischemia, deficient mucosal immunity (sIgA), and an underdeveloped GI mucosal barrier. Similar to what is hypothesized in adult critical care patients, excessive GI fungal burden, together with a breach of the mucosal barrier, is proposed to lead to translocation of *Candida* spp. across the intestinal wall (22, 92). Recently published results from the National Epidemiology of Mycosis Survey (NEMS) support the role of GI tract colonization in the pathogenesis of candidemia in the neonate. The NEMS was a prospective multicenter study that assessed risk factors for candidemia in the NICU. Multivariate logistic regression analysis, which adjusted for birth weight and abdominal surgery, revealed a number of risk factors for neonatal candidemia, including gestational age, Apgar score, shock, antibiotic usage, parenteral nutrition, central catheters, H_2 blockers, length of stay, and intubation. Additionally, GI tract colonization was identified as a univariate risk factor for candidemia. Most important, GI tract colonization preceded candidemia in a significant number of cases compared to non-case patients (45.5 versus 21.9%). Molecular typing confirmed the importance of GI colonization in the development of candidemia in that a greater number of patients had preceding fungal colonization with the identical clone that produced the candidemia (108). Others have also linked GI tract colonization in the infant with the development of candidemia. In a study by Pappu-Katikanenni et al., half of very-low-birth-weight infants colonized with $>8 \times 10^6$ *Candida* spp. in the GI tract developed feeding intolerance or bloody stools and 28.5% of these infants developed candidemia (92). Excess fungal burden in an infant with inadequate antifungal host defense mechanisms, including GI mucosal barrier function, likely intensifies the risk for fungal dissemination (113, 116). Although a precise understanding of infant antifungal defense is sorely lacking, Shareef et al. demonstrated that direct lymphocyte-mediated antifungal defense is impaired in infants. This impairment was most marked in infants under 32 weeks gestational age (113) and with severity of illness scores (Score for Neonatal Acute Physiology; SNAP) greater than 10 (129). Similarly, the NEMS epidemiological study found that a gestational age of <32 weeks was a significant predictor of risk for candidemia, and SNAP scores greater than 10 were an important risk factor in the univariate analysis (108). These authors speculate that low-birth-weight and/or gestational age are surrogate markers for immune function. This highlights the need for future studies directed at understanding the precise defects in the infants' immune response to *Candida* spp. to develop better preventive strategies for infant candidiasis of which the GI tract is a contributing source of *Candida* spp.

Candida Infections in Individuals with HIV

Mucosal candidiasis is prevalent in HIV infection and occurs in almost all patients at some time during the course of their disease. The widespread use of highly active antiretroviral therapy has significantly reduced the incidence of opportunistic fungal infections of the GI tract in patients with HIV disease (91). However, oropharyngeal candidiasis (OPC) and esophageal candidiasis still occur and remain common opportunistic infections in those infected with HIV. *C. albicans* is the primary fungal pathogen of both OPC and esophageal candidiasis. However, other non-*C. albicans* species, including *C. krusei, C. tropicalis, C. parapsilosis,* and *C. glabrata,* cause the same disease (39, 60, 74, 89). Isolates of *C. albicans* obtained from HIV-infected patients have been shown to adhere to buccal epithelial cells in greater numbers than control isolates (93). OPC is most often characterized by white plaques, which may be focal or become confluent to involve almost the entire oropharynx. Yet OPC may occasionally present as diffuse erythema without plaques or angular cheilitis (127). Clinical experience shows that as many as 90% of the cases of OPC in HIV-positive individuals (with systemic $CD4^+$ lymphocytes >400) are atrophic and limited to the tongue and soft and hard palates. As the $CD4^+$ lymphocyte numbers drop to <200, symptomatic disease is 90% pseudomembranous. Under these conditions, lesions appear on the buccal mucosa, floor of the mouth, soft palate, retromolar pad, alveolar ridges, and tongue. The majority of cases of OPC are defined as primary and/or sporadic, i.e., without prior bouts of OPC or with only sporadic episodes (<1 to 2 per annum). In addition, there is a select group of HIV-positive individuals who are diagnosed with recurrent OPC. These individuals respond adequately to antifungal therapy but have intractable recurrences within 1 month of cessation of therapy. OPC produces oral pain and dysphasia and leads to poor nutrition and debilitation and, therefore, impacts negatively on the quality of life (50). Although the efficacy of antifungal medications such as fluconazole is good, an increasing number of resistant strains have been identified (52, 111). Infections by non-*C. albicans* species have also become increasingly prevalent in HIV-positive individuals, especially those on fluconazole prophylactic therapy (43, 89). OPC is often the first clinical sign of immunosuppression (62, 94). Moreover, esophageal candidiasis is considered an AIDS-defining illness (80). *Candida* spp. do not appear to disseminate into adult tissues beyond the mucosal epithelium, in that candidemia is only rarely associated with HIV infections (90). However, it is clear that OPC is an important complication of HIV infection that critically diminishes the quality of life in an already vulnerable patient population.

Since the primary site of *Candida* infection is the mucosal surface, it is logical to presume that host susceptibility or resistance is dependent on the mucosal immune system. On the basis of early life exposure to *C. albicans,* most healthy individuals have anti-*Candida* immunity demonstrable by delayed-type hypersensitivity and in vitro peripheral blood lymphocyte proliferation in response to *Candida* antigens (33). These forms of cell-mediated immunity (CMI) seem to play an important role in host defense against *C. albicans* at mucosal surfaces (33, 78). In addition, significantly increased circulating antibodies to *Candida* have been demonstrated in patients with esophageal candidiasis (17). However, the location of the infection and the fact that most forms of candidiasis are limited to the epithelial surface suggest that secretory immunity may play a role in disease modulation (33). Considerable attention has been paid to the relationship between IgA and HIV infection. There is a well-documented IgA hyperglobulinemia in patient sera during the course of HIV infection, which increases very early during the course of HIV infection and relates to HIV disease progression (97). There is an inverse relationship between serum and salivary IgA levels (85, 119). This is true for both IgA subclasses and in either whole or parotid saliva. IgA antibody titers to *C. albicans* are increased in whole and parotid saliva from HIV patients but reduced in AIDS patients. The avidity of salivary IgA antibodies for *Candida* spp. is unimpaired in HIV patients but reduced in AIDS patients. Further, antibody levels have been significantly correlated with the numbers of *Candida* organisms isolated from saliva of HIV-positive individuals, indicative of a response to antigenic challenge by the infecting *Candida* spp. (33, 34, 97).

Analysis of CMI in OPC is limited, but salivary cytokine profiles have been assessed in HIV-positive individuals and compared with healthy HIV-negative immunocompetent adults (78). In the saliva, the HIV-positive individuals have a Th2 type of cytokine profile composed primarily of interleukin (IL)-4 and IL-10, whereas the HIV-negative individuals had a constitutive ThO profile with little cytokine production. Moreover, HIV-positive patients with OPC showed evidence for a more profound Th2 cytokine profile, consistent with susceptibility to OPC. The origin, systemic versus local production, of these salivary cytokines remains to be determined (78). At the systemic level, reductions in delayed cutaneous skin test reactivity to *Candida* antigens have been observed in HIV-positive individuals with <200 $CD4^+$ T lymphocytes per μl of blood, irrespective of mucosal infection. However, limited in vitro differences in *Candida*-specific lymphoproliferation and Th1/Th2 cytokine production suggest that deficiencies in *Candida*-specific CMI do not solely account for the susceptibility to OPC of HIV-infected individuals (77). The authors postulate that a threshold number of $CD4^+$ T lymphocytes are required to protect the oral mucosa against infection, below which the occurrence of OPC depends exclusively on the status of local immune mechanisms. At a cellular level, ultrastructural and immunohistochemical analyses of OPC have revealed a dense mononuclear cell infiltrate at sites of infection with *Candida* spp. The lamina propria and basal epithelial layer of the oral mucosa of HIV-infected patients were infiltrated by dendritic macrophages and $CD8^+$ T lymphocytes. This cellular infiltration was most marked at sites of erythema and pseudomembranous candidiasis and was remarkable for its absence of $CD4^+$ T lymphocytes (102). Epithelial candidiasis was associated with submucosal accumulations of lymphocytes and macrophages and not only was there an alteration in the number of cells present but also in the surface expression of markers associated with lymphocyte activation. These alterations in the mucosal immune response were more pronounced with the pseudomembranous form of the disease and less pronounced with the erythematous form.

In summary, *Candida* colonization of the GI tract does not present any risk to the healthy host. It is only in those individuals who are immunosuppressed that the GI fungal flora can be viewed as an infectious reservoir. Those susceptible hosts include individuals debilitated by cancer (especially leukemic patients), transplant patients receiving immunosuppressive therapy, those infected with HIV, the elderly, the low-birth-weight and premature infant, and critically ill patients who occupy ICUs. Oral, esophageal, and GI candidiasis may also develop in individuals receiving steroid therapy, pregnant women, and those with endocrinopathies such as diabetes mellitus and hypoparathyroidism (56). In the bowel, *Candida* spp. are not major components of the microbial flora. However, destruction of the normal GI microbial flora leads to multiplication of *Candida* spp. and in immunocompromised and/or debilitated hosts, GI overgrowth of *Candida* spp. is often the origin of candidiasis that frequently complicates clinical management of these patients.

EXPERIMENTAL MODELS OF *CANDIDA* INFECTION

Murine

Three main models of oral and/or GI candidiasis have been developed to evaluate the infectious process by and the immune response to the fungus. *C. albicans* is not a component of the indigenous microbial flora of the rodent gut, and *Candida* colonization of normal adult mice is difficult to accomplish due to innate host defense mechanisms, the mucosal barriers of the gut, and the resident microbial flora (38). However, it is possible to establish GI candidiasis in immunocompetent neonatal mice challenged by the oral-intragastric route. Typically, 2×10^8 yeast cells are delivered in saline into 6-day-old mice that have not been fed 3 to 4 h before the inoculation (38). Initial defenses are minimal in these immunocompetent animals, and the mucin barrier of the GI tract appears to be breached by the fungus within 1 h after oral-intragastric inoculation. Over a period of 2 to 4 days the fungus colonizes the keratinized epithelium, which extends from the esophagus to the cardiac-atrial fold. The fungus penetrates the keratinized surface and reaches the epithelial layer (35). A portion of the oral-intragastric inoculum passes through the stomach of the neonate and associates with the mucosal surfaces of the jejunum and ileum. Yeast cells are visible with the mucin layer and are also associated with the columnar epithelial surfaces of the microvillous layer of the gut. One hundred percent of these animals can be observed to be colonized 5 weeks after inoculation, with some animals retaining the fungus as long as 16 weeks. The duration of colonization is dependent on both the mouse and *Candida* strains employed (58).

In these infected animals, the most remarkable colonization by yeast and hyphae is detected in the region of the cardiac-atrial fold. (In the mouse this portion of the stomach is at the junction of the keratinized and glandular epithelium. In humans the keratinized layer of the upper alimentary tract extends only to the cardiac sphincter.) Multiple intraepithelial abscesses can be found in association with fungal colonization and consist of a thickened keratinized outer layer that partly envelops a dense aggregate of PMNs. Surrounding the PMNs is a layer of keratin, keratinocytes, and remnants of epithelial cells. In addition, a large number of mononuclear cells, including T lymphocytes and macrophages, are localized in the lamina propria as well as submucosal layers and regions of the stomach (38). This immune response, most likely in conjunction with the innate host defenses of the GI tract, appears to be sufficient to protect the mature adult in that, with time, colonization by the fungus decreases in these oral-intragastrically challenged animals.

In addition to GI candidiasis, this model has been demonstrated to be useful for the analysis of hematogenously disseminated candidiasis. Administration of cyclophosphamide and cortisone acetate approximately 2 weeks post oral-intragastric challenge results in the spread of the fungus from the GI tract to the liver, lungs, spleen, and kidneys (30, 35). Treatment with these drugs results in alterations of the normal integrity of the epithelium of the gut and produces a severe neutropenia, permitting the translocation and spread of the fungus. These and similar drugs lead to disseminated candidiasis in humans as well, and as such, this model is an excellent mimic of the human disease.

An alternative model has been developed that uses germ-free mice that are mono-associated with *C. albicans*. Gnotobiotic neonatal mice are introduced into cages that house mice colonized with pure cultures of *C. albicans*. These neonatal animals become colonized intestinally with the fungus within 1 day and remain chronically and stably colonized (10^7 to 10^8 CFU/g of cecal material) for the life of the animal (8, 69). Before the introduction of the fungus to these germ-free animals, the mice exhibit no detectable response to the fungus. However, upon introduction, an immune response to the fungus is produced. Since infection of the gnotobiotic model does not require the use of immunosuppressive agents or cytotoxic drugs (that may simultaneously suppress phagocytic cell function, CMI, and T- and B-lymphocyte function) (19, 23, 107), a direct analysis of individual components of the immune response to the fungus can be accomplished.

Other Models

Other animal models of oral, esophageal, and GI candidiasis have been developed. These models in the rabbit, rat, pig, and hamster have been used either to evaluate chemotherapeutic treatment of these forms of candidiasis (125) or to determine fungal pathogenic factors that may contribute to disease development (5, 42, 130). With few exceptions (32, 47) the immune response to the fungus has been most fully described in the murine models described above.

EXPERIMENTAL INFECTIONS AND IMMUNE RESPONSE TO *CANDIDA* SPP.

The murine models of oral, GI, and systemic candidiasis simulate the conditions found in humans (35–38). In these murine models, defects in both T-lymphocyte and phagocytic cell function are necessary for murine susceptibility to disseminated candidiasis of endogenous origin. In contrast, defects solely in T-lymphocyte function increase susceptibility of the animals to mucosal candidiasis (9, 25, 27). SCID mice (deficient in T and B lymphocytes) and SCID-beige mice (congenital T and B lymphocyte and phagocytic cell deficient) when given an intragastric or oral inoculation of *C. albicans* develop a persistent GI infection. Conversely, mice that solely lack phagocytic cells are capable of clearing this type of infection efficiently (25).

The specific mucosal immune mechanisms that control *Candida* spp. as commensals within the GI tract are not fully defined, and it is clear that *C. albicans* readily colonizes the GI tract of both immunodeficient and immunocompetent mice (8, 66, 69). Oral colonization of immunocompetent and some immunodeficient mice evokes immunity to mucosal candidiasis. Adoptive transfer of lymphocytes from immune mice can transfer resistance to candidiasis in susceptible SCID and SCID-beige mice (8, 9, 57). To date, no role has been demonstrated for antibody in protection from GI candidiasis, although other forms of mucosal infection (e.g., vaginal) have been shown to be responsive to specific antibody (47, 68). Athymic mice depleted of T-cell receptor (TCR) $\gamma\delta+$ T lymphocytes manifest exacerbated gastric candidiasis but do not develop systemic disease (69). Immunocompetent euthymic mice, depleted of TCR $\gamma\delta+$ T lymphocytes do not manifest as dramatic an increase in susceptibility to orogastric candidiasis as that observed in the TCR $\gamma\delta+$ T lymphocyte-depleted athymic mice. These data suggest that both TCR $\gamma\delta+$ T lymphocyte and thymic-derived T lymphocytes work in conjunction to protect the host. The precise means by which these lymphocytes protect the host is unknown, but the production of gamma interferon (IFN)-γ and the activation of macrophages are likely to be a significant candidacidal mechanism. Since nitric oxide has not been found to be cytocidal for *C. albicans*, peroxynitrite has been proposed as the macrophage-derived fungicidal molecule. Such a mechanism is less likely to contribute to host protection in humans (121).

Gnotobiotic, *Candida*-colonized mice, deficient in $CD8^+$ T lymphocytes (β_2-microglobulin knockout) have been shown to be susceptible to gastric and disseminated candidiasis of endogenous origin (10, 69, 70). Analysis of TCR $\alpha\beta+$ T lymphocyte-deficient mice (α chain knockout) has shown these mice to succumb to lethal infection after natural colonization of infant mice by contact with *Candida* colonized mothers. Hyphae and budding yeast cells were present on mucosal surfaces of TCR $\alpha\beta+$ T lymphocyte-deficient mice as well as upon mucosal surface of TCR $\gamma\delta+$ T lymphocyte-deficient mice (δ chain knockout), suggesting that both TCR $\alpha\beta+$ and TCR $\gamma\delta+$ T lymphocytes participate in host resistance to mucosal candidiasis. No disseminated candidiasis was detected in either of these TCR-deficient mice, regardless of the grade of mucosal infection. This is a surprising observation in that *Candida* colonization of $CD8^+$ lymphocyte-deficient mice (β_2-microglobulin knockout) leads to dissemination from the mucosal surface to internal organs (10). These results suggest that distinct differences exist in these two separate types of gene-disrupted animals and that alternative functions may exist for $CD8^+$ T lymphocytes that are independent of TCR and that may control dissemination of the fungus from mucosal sites. Since $CD8^+$ T lymphocytes can directly interact with *C. albicans* and inhibit growth of the fungus, it is possible that these antifungal $CD8^+$ T lymphocytes may function to prevent oroesophageal candidiasis and disseminated candidiasis of endogenous origin (14). Further, in HIV-positive individuals who have had prior episodes of OPC, such antifungal lymphocytes are readily demonstrable in the peripheral circulation (81). The numbers and antifungal capacity of these lymphocytes directly correlated with prior episodes of OPC and inversely correlated with the number of $CD4^+$ T lymphocytes per μl of blood.

In summary, orogastric and disseminated candidiasis in immunosuppressed patients likely results from several immune defects that are caused by either the patient's disease or the use of immunosuppressive and/or cytotoxic chemotherapeutic drugs (23, 61, 107). Data from these murine models are in agreement with these clinical observations and demonstrate that defects in one arm of immunity (e.g., $CD4^+$ and/or $CD8^+$ T lymphocytes) can predispose to oroesophageal candidiasis. However, defects in at least two arms of immunity (T cell-mediated functions and PMN function) appear to be necessary for *Candida* spp. to cause mucosal infections and disseminate out of the GI tract and invade systemic tissues (69, 121).

MUCOSAL IMMUNIZATION AND RESPONSE TO *CANDIDA* SPP.

Mucosal immunization with *C. albicans* confers protection against subsequent systemic challenge (45, 124). T lymphocytes are important determinants of this anamnestic response, and mucosal immunization with *C. albicans* leads to an expansion of effector and memory phenotypes that are coincident with the acquisition of fungal host defense (26, 30). The acquisition of host resistance is accompanied by an expansion of both $CD4^+$, TCR $\alpha\beta+$ and $CD8^+$, TCR $\alpha\beta+$ T lymphocytes within the spleen (26, 67, 124). In the GI tract of the mouse, colonization with *C. albicans* leads to the expansion of $CD8^-$, $CD4^-$, TCR $\gamma\delta+$ T lymphocytes in the stomach as well as an infiltration of TCR $\gamma\delta+$ T lymphocytes into the oral cavity (32, 69). In the gastric mucosa, both $CD4^+$ and $CD8^+$, TCR $\alpha\beta+$ T lymphocytes numbers are increased (18, 69, 85). Oral colonization alone induces major changes within the $CD8^+$, TCR $\alpha\beta+$, and TCR $\gamma\delta+$ T lymphocyte (47) subsets of interstitial epithelial lymphocytes, but such an infection has no apparent effect on intraepithelial $CD4^+$ T lymphocytes (68).

Although $CD4^+$ T cells may not contribute to the intraepithelial response to *C. albicans,* they certainly do contribute to the systemic immune response to the fungus (68). Striking increases have been observed in $CD4^+$ and $CD8^+$ T lymphocyte responses in the spleen of animals orally challenged with *Candida* sp. Although $CD4^+$ T lymphocyte depletion or deficiencies do not appear to enhance the susceptibility of mice to candidiasis of endogenous origin (38, 87), the role of CD4+ T cells in resistance and susceptibility to experimental systemic candidiasis has been clearly demonstrated in immunocompetent mice (105, 106). Experimental infections of animals genetically resistant to *Candida* spp. exhibit a Th1 lymphocyte response with the production of IL-2, IFN-γ, and IL-12 (6, 95), whereas mice genetically susceptible to candidiasis exhibit a Th2 response with the production of IL-4 and IL-10. These experimental results appear to mirror the immunological response to *Candida* spp. in humans in that normal healthy humans produce IL-2, IFN-γ, and granulocyte-macrophage colony-stimulating factor (GM-CSF) in response to *Candida* spp. (6). In murine candidiasis both resistance to mucosal infection and subsequent systemic reinfection are dependent on the activation of Th1 responses. IFN-γ unresponsive mice (α-chain receptor deficient) are highly susceptible to mucosal infection and are unable to develop resistance to subsequent reinfection with the fungus (29). Susceptibility to mucosal infection correlates with a decreased frequency of intragastric T lymphocytes producing IFN-γ, IL-4, and IL-5. Decreased production of IL-2 was also observed in the draining lymph nodes of these animals, indicating the failure of IFN-γ deficient mice to mount effective *Candida* Th1 responses at the mucosal level. It would appear that IFN-γ is a major component of the Th1 response to the fungus; however, the role of the cytokine in host defense is disputed. IFN-γ-deficient knockout mice, with a normal GI microbial flora, have been reported to be no more susceptible to gastric or systemic candidiasis of endogenous origin than immunocompetent control animals (96). However, germ-free IFN-γ-deficient mice (IFN-γ knockout), chronically colonized and mono-infected with a large viable population of *C. albicans,* were more susceptible to gastric and anorectal candidiasis than immunocompetent littermate control animals. These germ-free IFN-γ-deficient mice (IFN-γ knockout) were resistant to candidiasis at many other oral and GI mucosal sites (palate, tongue, esophagus, small and large intestine, and cecum) and did not show any enhanced susceptibility to systemic candidiasis of endogenous origin. A number of experimental differences exist between these two reports (11), but chief among these was the large viable population of *C. albicans* resident in the mono-infected, germ-free mice. The resident bacterial flora in the non-germ-free animals may have protected those animals from mucosal candidiasis. It is well known that oral antibiotic therapy increases *Candida* sp. numbers in mammals and that such therapies predispose to candidiasis. Hence, the resident microbial flora may have been disadvantageous to the necessary development of *Candida* fungal burden.

In a consistent fashion, tumor necrosis factor alpha (TNF-α)-deficient mice (TNF-α knockout) are also highly susceptible to GI candidiasis, and this lack of host protection correlated with impaired development of a protective Th1 immune response (82). In GI infections, stomach section from TNF-α-deficient mice revealed the presence of numerous intraepithelial abscesses consisting of a thickened, keratinized outer layer that enveloped a dense aggregate of hyphae and a few infiltrating PMNs. Large numbers of mononuclear cells were also detected in the histological sections of the submucosal region of the stomach, with conspicuous signs of acanthosis and hyperkeratosis. Abscesses and mucosal infiltration were observed in regions other than the cardiac-atrial fold. In wild-type mice only a few yeast cells were present in the keratinized layer with a limited inflammatory reaction at the mucosal level, mainly observed in the cardiac-atrial fold. In the TNF-α deficient mice, numerous abscesses containing hyphal and infiltrating cells were also observed in the esophagus with extensive mononuclear cell responses in the submucosal region. In these GI infections, a significant reduction in fecal content of IFN-γ, IL-6, and IgA was observed in the TNF-α deficient mice.

IFN-γ and TNF-α are capable of mobilizing and activating antifungal effector phagocytes, and the production of these cytokines is typically a result of an IL-12-dependent Th1 CMI response. Production of IFN-γ is greatly impaired in IL-12-deficient mice upon reinfection with *Candida* spp. (83). In those animals, host susceptibility correlated with a failure to activate CD4+ Th1 lymphocytes producing IFN-γ and IL-2. Hence, it appears that a Th1 immune response is protective and that a Th2 immune response may inhibit the development of protective antifungal responses. IL-10 suppresses the antifungal effector functions of phagocytes and reduces the expression of costimulatory molecules and cytokines necessary for the development of effective antifungal immunity. IL-10-deficient mice (IL-10 knockout) in response to *Candida* spp. produce larger amounts of IL-1-α, TNF-α, and IL-6 than do wild-type mice, and these molecules appear to contribute to host protection from GI *C. albicans* infections (30, 31).

A role for Th2 cytokines in host protection has been proposed as well (104). It has been suggested that the down-regulation of a strong potentially immunopathologic Th1 immune response could be beneficial to the host (1, 101). Th2 cytokines may limit the GI damage caused by *Candida* colonization and subsequent inflammatory stimuli (30, 103). It is possible that commensal yeast may have evolved mechanisms to down-regulate effector Th1 immune responses. The immune response in such a mucosal environment would be typically a mixture of both a Th1 and a Th2 immune response in the mouse (26, 30) and presumably in humans as well (6). Phagocyte-dependent and nondependent resistance to *Candida* spp. would then be an outcome of two sets of opposing cytokine responses. In models of oral and gastric candidiasis, a combined Th1 immune response in conjunction with the production of IL-4 results in optimal host protection (30, 47, 83). IL-4 appears to promote the development of a protective Th1 response. Essentially all humans have encountered *Candida* spp. early as a neonate, then in adult life *Candida* diseases would develop in the presence of underlying immune reactivity (6, 49). *Candida* infectivity is typically associated with immunosuppressive or antibacterial therapy, neutropenia, or the breakdown of anatomic defenses as well as alterations in cytokine balance, coinfection, or immunomodulatory therapy, which may lead to changes in fungal burden and/or localization of infection. These changes would affect *Candida* carriage/infection and related pathology. Treatment of self-limiting GI candidiasis with IL-4 and/or IL-10 greatly exacerbates the course of primary disease and renders resistant mice susceptible to infection (120). However, neither cytokine separately nor in combination renders mice susceptible to systemic candidemia when a predominate Th1 reactivity was initially established in the animals. Thus, overproduction of Th2 cytokines may exacerbate disseminated candidiasis only in the absence of a strong established protective immune response. These results may explain the relative rarity of disseminated candidiasis in AIDS patients, in spite of the high frequency of mucosal disease. If HIV induces a moderate bias toward a Th0 or a Th2 immune response, the result might be an increase in fungal burden or mucosal colonization as a consequence of a reduced Th1 response. Under these conditions *Candida* may no longer remain a commensal, and increased fungal burden could result in infection. This change in mucosal status would not be apparent systemically unless a marked drop in CD4$^+$ T lymphocytes occurred, resulting in mucosal candidiasis. The host would continue to oppose candidemia and the onset of systemic disease. The absence of CD4$^+$ T lymphocytes has been found to be highly detrimental in most experimental models of mucosal infection (18, 45). Once an environmental change has occurred, then the immune effector mechanisms described above are mobilized to protect the host. Such immune responsiveness is summarized in Fig. 1. Within the GI tract, the predominant effector cell populations that encounter the invading fungus are PMNs, CD4$^+$ and CD8$^+$ T lymphocytes, and NK cells. Each of these cells has the capacity to produce a number of cytokines that can activate and/or mobilize other cell populations to heightened antifungal capacity. PMNs and CD8$^+$ T lymphocytes are also capable of direct contact-mediated effects against the fungus. A defect in any of these mechanisms can lead to increased localized fungal burden and the requirement for other components of the immune effector response to compensate to achieve host defense.

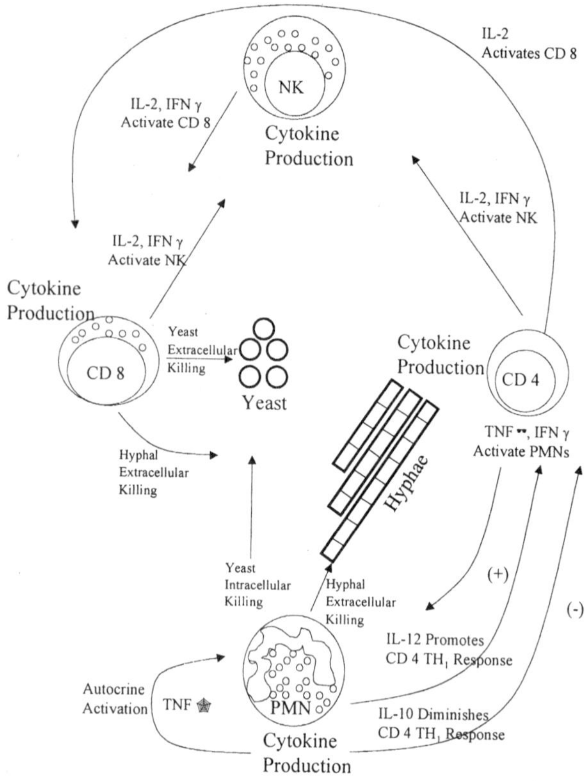

Figure 1. Effector mechanisms of host defense against oral, esophageal, and GI candidiasis. Host defense against *Candida* can be mediated by a number of effector cell populations of the immune system. These include PMN, NK cells, and CD8$^+$ and CD4$^+$ lymphocytes. PMNs have the capacity to phagocytose the yeast form of the fungus, whereas the hyphal and yeast forms of the fungus can be affected by antifungal extracellular mechanisms of both PMNs and CD8$^+$ lymphocytes. When PMNs, CD8$^+$, and NK cells encounter *Candida* spp., they are induced to produce a subset of cytokines that can affect antifungal effector cell populations in either an autocrine or paracrine fashion. Further, CD4$^+$ lymphocytes, when presented with *Candida* antigen, produce a large number of diverse cytokines that regulate overall antifungal immunity. Th1 responses are associated with resistance to infection, whereas Th2 responses are associated with susceptibility to infection, especially when Th1 responses are diminished.

SUMMARY AND FUTURE DIRECTIONS

This chapter has focused on infections of the oral cavity, esophagus, and GI tract caused by *Candida* spp. These infections are most prevalent in individuals who are receiving cytotoxic chemotherapy for neoplastic disease, undergoing solid-organ and bone marrow transplantation, beset with acquired or primary immunodeficiencies, very young or very old, or critically ill. In these immunocompromised individuals *Candida* spp. are a major cause of morbidity and mortality. Significant advances have been made in the development of strategies to treat fungal infection in these individuals, yet *Candida* spp. remain a common clinical problem. Current antifungal therapies are inadequate, and clinical data demonstrate increased incidence of *Candida* infection and of *Candida* resistance to antifungal drugs. These observations underscore the need for the development of innovative therapeutic approaches to treat oral, esophageal, and GI tract *Candida* infections and to enhance host resistance to *Candida* spp. Such approaches should include the development of immunologically based procedures that limit disease development. To facilitate such approaches, a clear understanding of host defense against the fungus is required, not just in the existent experimental models but also in infected humans. Of necessity, the role in host protection of phagocytic and nonphagocytic cell populations, T and B lymphocytes, NK cells, associated cytokines and chemokines, and specific antibody will need to be understood at the cellular and molecular level. The immune response to such a commensal opportunistic fungus is complex and a number of host factors contribute to not only infection but also to its resolution. Much is known about the host factors that contribute to the infectious process. Less is known about the immunological factors necessary to resolve infections in experimental animals, and even less is known about the human immune response to *Candida* spp. It is essential to understand the immune response to the human forms of the disease, so that it will be possible to develop strategies that contain *Candida* spp. as a commensal and improve the quality of life of individuals at risk for infection with this opportunistic pathogen.

Acknowledgments. This work was supported in part by AI-31127, NR-00085, and the Cancer Federation.

REFERENCES

1. **Adorini, L., J. Magram, and S. Trembeau.** 1995. The role of endogenous IL-12 in the induction of Th-1cell-mediated autoimmune diseases. *Res. Immunol.* **146**:645–651.
2. **Alverdy, J., E. Aoy, P. Weiss-Carrington, and D. A. Burk.** 1992. The effect of glutamine-enriched TPN on gut immune cellularity. *J. Surg. Res.* **52**:34–39.
3. **Alverdy, J. C., S. Aoy, and G. S. Moss.** 1988. Total parenteral nutrition promotes bacterial translocation from the gut. *Surgery* **104**:185–190.
4. **Anaissie, E., and G. P. Bodey.** 1990. Fungal infection in patients with cancer. *Pharmacology* **10**(Suppl.):1645–1695.
5. **Andrutis, K. A., P. J. Riggle, C. A. Kumamoto, and S. Tzipori.** 2000. Intestinal lesions associated with disseminated candidiasis in an experimental animal model. *J. Clin. Microbiol.* **38**: 2317–2323.
6. **Ausiello, C. M., F. Urbani, S. Gessani, G. C. Spagnoli, M. Gomez, and A. Cassone.** 1993. Cytokine gene expression in human peripheral blood mononuclear cells stimulated by mannoprotein constituents from *Candida albicans. Infect. Immun.* **61**:4105–4111.
7. **Baley, J. E., R. M. Kliegman, B. Boxerbaum, and A. A. Fanaroff.** 1986. Fungal colonization in the very low birth weight infant. *Pediatrics* **78**:225–232.
8. **Balish, E., and H. Filutowicz.** 1991. Serum antibody response of gnotobiotic athymic and euthymic mice following alimentary tract colonization and infection with *Candida albicans. Can. J. Microbiol.* **37**:204–210.
9. **Balish, E., H. Filutowicz, and T. D. Oberlev.** 1990. Correlates of cell-mediated immunity in *Candida albicans*-colonized gnotobiotic mice. *Infect. Immun.* **58**:107–113.
10. **Balish, E., F. A. Vasquez-Torres, J. Jones-Carson, R. D. Wagner, and T. Warner.** 1996. Importance of β_2 microglobulin in murine resistance to mucosal and systemic candidiasis. *Infect. Immun.* **64**:5092–5097.
11. **Balish, E., R. D. Wagner, A. Vasquez-Torres, C. Pierson, and T. Warner.** 1998. Candidiasis in interferon-γ knockout (IFN-$\gamma^{-/-}$) mice. *J. Infect. Dis.* **178**:478–487.
12. **Beck-Sague, C. M., P. Azimi, S. N. Fonseca, R. S. Baltimore, D. A. Powell, Bland, M. J. Arduino, S. K. McAllister, R. S. Huberman, R. L. Sinkowitz, R. A. Ehrenkranz, and W. R. Jarvis.** 1994. Bloodstream infection in neonatal intensive care unit patients: results of a multicenter study. *Pediatr. Infect. Dis.* **13**:1110–1116.
13. **Beck-Sague, C. M., W. R. Jarvis, and the National Nosocomial Infections Surveillance System.** 1993. Secular trends in the epidemiology of nosocomial fungal infections in the United States, 1980–1990. *J. Infect. Dis.* **167**:1247–1251.
14. **Beno, D. W. A., A. G. Stöver, and H. L. Mathews.** 1995. Growth inhibition of *Candida albicans* hyphae by CD8+ lymphocytes. *J. Immunol.* **154**:5273–5281.
15. **Bernhardt, H., and M. Knoke.** 1997. Mycological aspects of gastrointestinal microflora. *Scand. J. Gastroenterol.* **222**: 102–106.
16. **Bernhardt, H., M. Schwenke, M. Knoke, T. Bootz, and R. Mollmann.** 1989. Veranderungen der fakalflora bei Patienten mit hamatologischen erkankungen. *Zeitschr. Antimikrob. Antineoplast. Chemotherapie* **7**:49–57.
17. **Bernhardt, J.** 1999. Orointestinal candidiasis with special emphasis on esophageal candidiasis. *Mycoses* **42**(Suppl. 1): 68–72.
18. **Bistoni, F., E. Cenci, A. Mencacci, E. Schiafella, P. Mosci, P. Puccetti, and L. Romani.** 1993. Mucosal and systemic T helper cell function after intragastric colonization of adult mice with *Candida albicans. J. Infect. Dis.* **168**:1449–1457.
19. **Bodey, G. P.** 1984. Candidiasis in cancer patients. *Am. J. Med.* 77(Suppl. 4D):13–19.
20. **Bodey, G. P.** 1997. Disseminated candidiasis in neutropenic patients. *Int. J. Infect. Dis.* **1**(Suppl. 1):S2–S6.
21. **Borzotta, A. P., and K. Beardsley.** 1999. *Candida* infections in critically ill trauma patients: a retrospective case-control study. *Arch. Surg.* **134**:657–665.
22. **Butler, K. M., and C. J. Baker.** 1988. *Candida:* an increasingly important pathogen in the nursery. *Pediatr. Clin. N. Am.* **35**: 543–563.
23. **Butler, W. T., and R. D. Rosen.** 1973. Effects of corticoste-

roids in immunity in man. 1. Decreased serum IG concentrations caused by 3 or 5 days of high dose methyl prednisolone. *J. Clin. Invest.* **52**:2629–2633.

24. **Calderone, R. A.** 1989. Host parasite relationships in candidiasis. *Mycoses* **32**(Suppl. 2):12–17.
25. **Cantorna, M., and E. Balish.** 1990. Mucosal and systemic candidiasis in congenitally immunodeficient mice. *Infect. Immun.* **58**:1093–1100.
26. **Cantorna, M. T., and E. Balish.** 1991. Role of CD4$^+$ lymphocytes in resistance to mucosal candidiasis. *Infect. Immun.* **29**: 2447–2455.
27. **Cantorna, M. T., and E. Balish.** 1991. Acquired immunity to systemic candidiasis in immunodeficient mice. *J. Infect. Dis.* **164**:936–943.
28. **Castaldo, P., R. J. Stratta, R. P. Wood, R. S. Markin, K. D. Patil, M. S. Shaefer, A. N. Langas, E. C. Reed, S. Li, T. J. Pillen, and B. W. Shaw, Jr.** 1991. Clinical spectrum of fungal infections after orthotopic liver transplantation. *Arch. Surg.* **126**:149–156.
29. **Cenci, E., A. Mencacci, G. Del Sero, C. Fe' d'Ostiani, P. Mosci, A. Bacci, C. Montagnoli, M. Kopf, and L. Romani.** 1998. IFN-γ is required for IL-12 responsiveness in mice with *Candida albicans* infection. *J. Immunol.* **161**:3543–3550.
30. **Cenci, E., A. Mencacci, R. Spaccapelo, L. Tonnetti, P. Mosci, K. H. Enssle, P. Puccetti, L. Romani, and F. Bistoni.** 1995. T helper cell type 1 (Th1)- and Th2-like responses are present in mice with gastric candidiasis but protective immunity is associated with Th1 development. *J. Infect. Dis.* **171**: 1279–1288.
31. **Cenci, E., L. Romani, A. Mencacci, R. Spaccapelo, E. Schiafella, P. Puccetti, and F. Bistoni.** 1993. Interleukin-4 and interleukin-10 inhibit nitric oxide-dependent macrophage killing of *Candida albicans. Eur. J. Immunol.* **23**:1034–1038.
32. **Chakir, J., L. Côte, L. Coulombe, and N. Deslauriers.** 1994. Differential pattern of infection and immune response during experimental oral candidiasis in BALB/c and DBA/2(H-2^d) mice. *Oral Microbiol. Immunol.* **9**:88–94.
33. **Challacombe, S. J.** 1990. Immunology of oral candidosis, p. 104–123. *In* L. P. Samaranayake and T. W. MacFarlane (ed.), *Oral Candidosis.* Wright, London, United Kingdom.
34. **Challacombe, S. J., and S. P. Sweet.** 1997. Salivary and mucosal immune responses to HIV and its co-pathogens. *Oral Dis.* **3**(Suppl. 1):S79–S84.
35. **Cole, G. T., A. A. Halawa, and E. J. Anaissie.** 1996. The role of the gastrointestinal tract in hematogenous candidiasis: from the laboratory to the bedside. *Clin. Infect. Dis.* **22**(Suppl 2):S73–S88.
36. **Cole, G. T., K. T. Lynn, K. R. Seshan, and M. Franco.** 1993. Gastrointestinal candidiasis: histopathology of *Candida*-host interactions in a murine model. *Mycol. Res.* **97**:385–408.
37. **Cole, G. T., K. T. Lynn, K. R. Seshan, and L. M. Pope.** 1989. Gastrointestinal and systemic candidiasis in immunocompromised mice. *J. Med. Vet. Mycol.* **27**:363–380.
38. **Cole, G. T., K. R. Seshan, K. T. Lynn, and M. Franco.** 1993. Gastrointestinal candidiasis: histopathology of *Candida*-host interactions in a murine model. *Mycol. Res.* **97**:385–408.
39. **Coleman, D. C., D. E. Bennett, D. J. Sullivan, P. J. Gallagher, M. C. Henman, D. B. Shanley, and R. J. Russell.** 1993. Oral *Candida* in HIV infection and AIDS: new perspectives/new approaches. *Crit. Rev. Microbiol.* **19**:61–82.
40. **Dean, D. A., and K. W. Burchard.** 1996. Fungal infections in surgical patients. *Am. J. Surg.* **171**:374–382.
41. **Deitch, E. A.** 1990. The role of intestinal barrier failure and bacterial translocation in the development of systemic infection and multiple organ failure. *Arch. Surg.* **125**:403–404.
42. **de Repentigny, L., F. Aumont, K. Bernard, and P. Belhumeur.** 2000. Characterization of binding of *Candida albicans* to small intestinal mucin and its role in adherence to mucosal epithelial cells. *Infect. Immun.* **68**:3172–3179.
43. **Dick, J., W. Merz, and R. Saral.** 1980. Incidence of polyene-resistant yeast recovered from clinical specimens. *Antimicrob. Agents Chemother.* **18**:158–163.
44. **Dictar, M., M. T. Veron, S. Arduino, C. Foncuberta, M. Zylberman, and G. Kusminsky.** 1997. Prevention of candidiasis in bone marrow transplantation patients: a comparison of different approaches. *Int. J. Infect. Dis.* **1**(Suppl. 1):S56–S59.
45. **Domer, J. E.** 1988. Intragastric colonization or infant mice with *Candida albicans* induces systemic immunity demonstrable challenge as adults. *J. Infect. Dis.* **157**:950–958.
46. **Edwards, J. E.** 1991. Invasive *Candida* infections: evolution of a fungal pathogen. *N. Engl. J. Med.* **324**:1060–1062.
47. **Elahi, S., G. Pang, R. Clancy, and R. B. Ashman.** 2000. Cellular and cytokine correlates of mucosal protection in murine model of oral candidiasis. *Infect. Immun.* **68**:5771–5777.
48. **Eras, P., M. J. Goldstein, and P. Sherlock.** 1972. *Candida* infection of the gastrointestinal tract. *Medicine* **51**:367–379.
49. **Fischer, A., J. J. Ballet, and C. Griscelli.** 1978. Specific inhibition of in vitro *Candida*-induced lymphocyte proliferation by polysaccharide antigens present in serum of patients with chronic mucocutaneous candidiasis. *J. Clin. Invest.* **62**: 1005–1013.
50. **Fisher-Hoch, S. P., and L. Hutwagner.** 1995. Opportunistic candidiasis: an epidemic of the 1980s. *Clin. Infect. Dis.* **21**: 897–904.
51. **Fitzsimmons, N., and D. R. Berry.** 1994. Inhibition of *C. albicans* by *Lacidobacillus acidophilus:* evidence for the involvement of a peroxidase system. *Microbios* **88**:125–133.
52. **Fox, R., K. R. Neal, C. L. S. Leen, M. E. Ellis, and B. K. Mandal.** 1991. Fluconazole resistant *Candida* in AIDS. *J. Infect.* **22**:201–204.
53. **Fraser, V. J., M. Jones, J. Dunkel, S. Storfer, G. Medoff, and W. C. Dunagan.** 1992. Candidemia in a tertiary care hospital: epidemiology, risk factors, and predictors of mortality. *Clin. Infect. Dis.* **15**:414–421.
54. **Ghannoum, M. A., and K. H. Abu-Elteen.** 1990. Pathogenicity determinants of *Candida. Mycoses* **6**:265–282.
55. **Giamarellou, H., and A. Antoniadou.** 1996. Epidemiology, diagnosis, and therapy of fungal infections in surgery. *Infect. Control Hosp. Epidemiol.* **17**:558–564.
56. **Glick, M., and M. A. Siegel.** 1999. Viral and fungal infections of the oral cavity in immunocompetent patients. *Infect. Dis. Clin. N. Am.* **13**:817–831.
57. **Greenfield, R. A.** 1992. Host defense system interactions with *Candida. J. Med. Vet. Mycol.* **30**:89–104.
58. **Guentzel, M. N., G. T. Cole, and L. M. Pope.** 1985. Animal models for candidiasis. *Curr. Top. Med. Mycol.* **1**:57–116.
59. **Hageman, H. R., J. Stenske, H. Keuler, and E. Randall.** 1985. *Candida* colonization and infection in very low birth weight infants. *J. Perinatol.* **6**:251–254.
60. **Hauman, C. H., I. O. Thompson, F. Theunissen, and P. Wolfaart.** 1993. Oral carriage of *Candida* in healthy and HIV-seropositive persons. *Oral. Surg. Med. Oral. Pathol.* **76**: 570–572.
61. **Hess, A. D., P. M. Colombani, and A. H. Esa.** 1986. Cyclosporine and the immune response aspects. *Crit. Rev. Immunol.* **6**:123–149.
62. **Holmberg, K., and R. D. Meyer.** 1986. Fungal infections in patients with AIDS and AIDS-related complex. *Scand. J. Infect. Dis.* **18**:179–185.
63. **Huang, Y., C. Li, T. Lin, R. Lien, Y. Chou, J. Wu, and C. Hsueh.** 1998. Association of fungal colonization and invasive

disease in very low birth weight infants. *Pediatr. Infect. Dis.* 17:819–822.

64. **Inone, S., J. A. Wirman, J. W. Alexander, O. Trocki, and R. R. Cardel.** *Candida albicans* translocation across the gut mucosa following burn injury. *J. Surg. Res.* **44**:479–492.
65. **Jack, M., B. J. B. Wood, and D. R. Berry.** 1990. Evidence for the involvement of thiocyanate in the inhibition of *Candida albicans* by *Lactobacillus acidophilus*. *Microbios* **62**:37–46.
66. **Jensen, J., T. Warner, and E. Balish.** 1993. Resistance of SCID mice to *Candida albicans* administered intravenously or colonizing the gut: role of polymorphonuclear leukocytes and macrophages. *J. Infect. Dis.* **167**:912–919.
67. **Jensen, J., T. Warner, C. Johnson, and E. Balish.** 1996. Oral immunization of mice against candidiasis. *J. Infect. Dis.* **174**: 133–140.
68. **Jones-Carson, J., F. A. Vasquez-Torres, and E. Balish.** 1997. B cell-independent selection of memory T cells after mucosal immunization with *Candida albicans*. *J. Immunol.* **158**: 4328–4335.
69. **Jones-Carson, J., A. Vasquez-Torres, H. C. van der Heyde, T. Warner, R. D. Wagner, and E. Balish.** 1995. γδ T cell-induced nitric oxide production enhances resistance to mucosal candidiasis. *Nature Med.* **1**:552–557.
70. **Jones-Carson, J., A. Vasquez-Torres, T. Warner, and E. Balish.** 2000. Disparate requirement for T cells in resistance to mucosal and acute systemic candidiasis. *Infect. Immun.* **68**: 2363–2365.
71. **Kapur, A., R. Vasudeva, and C. W. Howden.** 1997. Candida splenic abscess in the absence of obvious immunodeficiency. *Am. J. Gastroenterol.* **92**:509–512.
72. **Kennedy, M. J., A. L. Rogers, and R. J. Yancey, Jr.** 1988. An anaerobic continuous-flow culture model of interactions between intestinal microflora and *Candida albicans*. *Mycopathology* **103**:125–134.
73. **Kennedy, M. J., and P. A. Volz.** 1985. Ecology of *Candida albicans* gut colonization: inhibition of *Candida* adhesion, colonization, and dissemination from the gastrointestinal tract by bacterial antagonism. *Infect. Immun.* **49**(3): 654–663.
74. **Klein, R. S., C. A. Harris, C. B. Small, B. Moll, M. Lesser, and G. H. Friedland.** 1984. Oral candidiasis in high-risk patients as the initial manifestation of the acquired immunologic deficiency syndrome. *N. Engl. J. Med.* **311**:354–358.
75. **Krause, W., H. Matheis, and K. Wulf.** 1969. Fungaemia and funguria after oral administration of *Candida albicans*. *Lancet* **i**:598–599.
76. **Kudsk, K. A., M. A. Croce, and T. C. Fabian.** 1991. Enteral versus parenteral feeding. *Ann. Surg.* **215**:503–513.
77. **Leigh, J. E., M. Barousse, R. K. Swoboda, T. Myers, S. Hager, N. A. Wolf, J. L. Cutright, J. Thompson, and P. L. Fidel.** 2001. *Candida*-specific systemic cell-mediated immune reactivities in HIV-positive persons with mucosal candidiasis. *J. Infect. Dis.* **183**:277–285.
78. **Leigh, J. E., C. Steele, F. L. Wormley, W. Luo, R. A. Clark, W. Gallaher, and P. L. Fidel.** 1998. Th1/Th2 cytokine expression in saliva of HIV-positive and HIV-negative individuals: a pilot study in HIV-positive individuals with oropharyngeal candidiasis. *J. Acquir. Immune Defic. Syndr. Hum. Retrovirol.* **19**:373–380.
79. **Leung, W. K., R. S. Dassanayake, J. Y. Y. Yau, L. J. Jin, W. C. Yam, and L. P. Samaranayake.** 2000. Oral colonization, phenotypic, and genotypic profiles of *Candida* species in irradiated, dentate, xerostomic nasopharyngeal carcinoma survivors. *J. Clin. Microbiol.* **38**:2219–2226.
80. **Macher, A. M.** 1988. The pathology of AIDS. *Public Health Rep.* **103**:246–250.
81. **Mathews, H. L., and L. Witek-Janusek.** Antifungal capacity of peripheral blood lymphocytes derived from HIV+ individuals. Unpublished observations.
82. **Mencacci, A., E. Cenci, G. Del Sero, C. Fe' d'Ostiani, P. Mosci, C. Montagnoli, A. Bacci, F. Bistoni, V. F. J. Quesniaux, B. Ryffel, and L. Romani.** 1998. Defective co-stimulation and impaired Th1 development in tumor necrosis factor/lymphotoxin-α double deficient mice infected with *Candida albicans*. *Int. Immun.* **10**:37–48.
83. **Mencacci, A., E. Cenci, G. Del Sero, C. Fe' d'Ostiani, P. Mosci, G. Trinchieri, L. Adorini, and L. Romani.** 1998. IL-10 is required for development of protective Th1 responses in IL-12 deficient mice upon *Candida albicans* infection. *J. Immunol.* **161**:6228–6237.
84. **Moore, F. A., D. V. Feliciano, and R. J. Andrassy.** 1992. Early enteral feeding, compared with parenteral, reduces postoperative septic complications: the results of a metanalysis. *Ann. Surg.* **216**:172–183.
85. **Muller, F., S. S. Froland, M. Hvatum, J. Radl, and P. Brandtzaeg.** 1991. Both IgA subclasses are reduced in parotid saliva from patients with AIDS. *Clin. Exp. Immun.* **83**(2): 203–209.
86. **Myerwitz, R. L., G. J. Pazin, and C. M. Allen.** 1977. Disseminated candidiasis. Changes in incidence, underlying diseases and pathology. *Am. J. Clin. Pathol.* **68**:29–38.
87. **Narayanan, R., W. A. Joyce, and R. A. Greenfield.** 1991. Gastrointestinal candidiasis in a murine model of severe combined immunodeficiency syndrome. *Infect. Immun.* **59**: 2116–2119.
88. **Odds, F. C.** 1988. *Candida and Candidosis*, 2nd ed. Bailliere Tindall, London, United Kingdom.
89. **Odds, F. C.** 1994. *Candida* species and virulence. *ASM News* **60**:313–318.
90. **Palacios, R., J. Santos, C. Romero, V. Garcia, A. Rivero, and M. Marquez.** 1999. Fungemia by *Candida* non *albicans* in patients with HIV infection. *Enferm. Infec. Microbiol. Clin.* **17**:279–282.
91. **Palella, F. J., Jr., K. M. Melaney, A. C. Moorman, M. O. Loveless, and J. Fuhrer.** 1998. Declining morbidity and mortality among patients with advanced human immunodeficiency virus infection. HIV Outpatient Study Investigators. *N. Engl. J. Med.* **338**:853–860.
92. **Pappu-Katikaneni, L. D., K. P. P. Roa, and E. Banister.** 1990. Gastrointestinal colonization with yeast species and *Candida* septicemia in very low birth weight infants. *Mycoses* **33**: 20–23.
93. **Pereiro, M., Jr., A. Losada, and J. Toribio.** 1997. Adherence of *Candida albicans* strains isolated from AIDS patients. Comparison with pathogenic yeasts isolated from patients without HIV infection. *Br. J. Dermatol.* **137**:76–80.
94. **Phelan, J. A., B. R. Salzman, G. H. Friendland, and R. S. Klein.** 1987. Oral findings in patients with acquired immune deficiency syndrome. *Oral Surg.* **64**:50–56.
95. **Puccetti, P., A. Mencacci, E. Cenci, R. Spaccapelo, P. Mosci, K. H. Enssle, L. Romani, and F. Bistoni.** 1994. Cure of murine candidiasis by recombinant soluble interleukin-4. *J. Infect. Dis.* **169**:1325–1331.
96. **Qian, Q., and J. E. Cutler.** 1997. Gamma interferon is not essential in host defense against disseminated candidiasis in mice. *Infect. Immun.* **65**:1748–1753.
97. **Quesnel, A., P. Moja, F. Lucht, J. L. Touraine, B. Pozzetto, and C. Genin.** 1994. Is there IgA of gut mucosal origin in the serum of HIV1 infected patients? *Gut* **35**(6):803–808.
98. **Rantala, A., J. Niinnikoski, and O. P. Lehtonen.** 1990. Pathogenesis of postoperative candidiasis: no detectable fungemia

during reoperations after abdominal surgery. *Mycoses* **34:** 47–52.

99. **Reagan, D. R., M. A. Pfaller, R. J. Hollis, and R. P. Wensel.** 1995. Evidence of nosocomial spread of *Candida albicans* causing blood stream infection in a neonatal intensive care unit. *Diagn. Microbiol. Infect. Dis.* **21:**191–194.
100. **Richet, H. M., A. Andremont, C. Tancrede, J. L. Pico, and W. R. Jarvis.** Risk factors for candidemia in patients with acute lymphocytic leukemia. *Rev. Infect. Dis.* **13:**211–215.
101. **Romagnani, S.** 1994. Regulation of the development of type-2 T-helper cells in allergy. *Curr. Opin. Immunol.* **6:**838–846.
102. **Romagnoli, P., N. Pimpinelli, M. Mori, P. A. Reichart, L. R. Eversole, and G. Ficarra.** 1997. Immunocompetent cells in oral candidiasis of HIV-infected patients: an immunohistological and electron microscopical study. *Oral Dis.* 3(2): 99–105.
103. **Romani, L., F. Bistoni, A. Mencacci, E. Cenci, R. Spaccapelo, and P. Puccetti.** 1995. IL-12 in *Candida albicans* infections. *Res. Immunol.* **146:**532–538.
104. **Romani, L., F. Bistoni, and P. Puccetti.** 1997. Initiation of T-helper cell immunity to *Candida albicans* by IL-12: the role of the neutrophils. *Chem. Immun.* **68:**110–135.
105. **Romani, L., A. Mencacci, U. Grohmann, S. Mocci, P. Mosci, P. Puccetti, and F. Bistoni.** 1992. Neutralizing antibody to interleukin 4 induces systemic protection and T helper type 1-associated immunity in murine candidiasis. *J. Exp. Med.* **176**(Suppl. 1):19–25.
106. **Romani, L., S. Mocci, C. Bietta, L. Lanfaloni, P. Puccetti, and F. Bistoni.** 1991. Th1 and Th2 cytokine secretion patterns in murine candidiasis: association of Th1 responses with acquired resistance. *Infect. Immun.* **59**(12):4647–4654.
107. **Roy, M. J., and T. J. Walsh.** 1992. Histopathologic and immunohistochemical changes in gut-associated lymphoid tissues after treatment of rabbits with dexamethasone. *Lab. Invest.* **64:**437–443.
108. **Saiman, L., E. Ludington, M. Pfaller, S. Rangel-Frausto, R. T. Wiblin, J. Dawson, H. M. Blumberg, J. E. Patterson, M. Rinaldi, J. E. Edwards, R. P. Wenzel, W. Jarvis, and the National Epidemiology of Mycosis Survey Study Group.** 2000. Risk factors for candidemia in neonatal intensive care unit patients. *Pediatr. Infect. Dis. J.* **19:**319–324.
109. **Samonis, G., and D. Bafaloukos.** 1992. Fungal infections in cancer patients: an escalating problem. *In Vivo* **6:**183–194.
110. **Samonis, G., A. Gikas, P. Toloudis, S. Maraki, G. Vrentzos, Y. Tselentis, N. Tsaparas, and G. Bodey.** 1994. Prospective study of the impact of broad-spectrum antibiotics on the yeast flora of the human gut. *Eur. J. Clin. Microbiol. Infect. Dis.* **13:**665–667.
111. **Sangeorzan, J. A., S. F. Bradley, X. He, L. T. Zarins, G. L. Ridenour, R. N. Tiballi, and C. A. Kauffman.** 1994. Epidemiology of oral candidiasis in HIV-infected patients: colonization, infection, treatment, and emergence of fluconazole resistance. *Am. J. Med.* 97(4):339–346.
112. **Saxen, H., M. Virtanen, P. Carlson, K. Hoppu, M. Pohjavuori, M. Vaara, J. Vuopio-Varkila, and H. Peltola.** 1995. Neonatal *Candida parapsilosis* outbreak with a high case fatality rate. *Pediatr. Infect. Dis. J.* **14:**776–781.
113. **Shareef, M. J., T. F. Myers, H. L. Mathews, and L. Witek-Janusek.** 1999. Reduced capacity of neonatal lymphocytes to inhibit the growth of *Candida albicans. Biol. Neonate* **75:** 31–39.
114. **Sherertz, R. J., K. S. Gledhill, and K. D. Hamptom.** 1992. Outbreak of *Candida* bloodstream infections associated with retrograde medication administration in a neonatal ICU. *J. Pediatr.* **120:**455–461.
115. **Shou, J., J. Lappin, E. A. Minnard, and J. M. Daly.** 1994. Total parenteral nutrition, bacterial translocation, and host immune function. *Am. J. Surg.* **167:**145–150.
116. **Spencer, J., and T. T. MacDonald.** 1990. Ontogeny of human mucosal immunity, p. 230–250. *In* T. T. MacDonald (ed.), *Ontogeny of the Immune System of the Gut.* CRC Press, Boca Raton, Fla.
117. **Stoll, B. J., T. Gordon, S. B. Korones, S. Shankaran, J. E. Tyson, C. R. Bauer, A. A. Fanaroff, J. A. Lemons, E. F. Donovan, W. Oh, D. K. Stevenson, R. A. Ehrenkranz, L. Papile, J. Verter, and L. L. Wright.** 1996. Late-onset sepsis in very low birth weight neonates: a report from the National Institute of Child Health and Human Development Neonatal Research Network. *J. Pediatr.* **129:**63–71.
118. **Stone, H. H., L. D. Kolb, C. A. Currie, C. E. Geheger, and J. Z. Cuzzell.** 1974. *Candida* sepsis: pathogenesis and principles of treatment. *Ann. Surg.* **179:**697–710.
119. **Sweet, S. P., D. Rahman, and S. J. Challacombe.** 1995. Serum and saliva immunoglobulin-a concentrations show an inverse relationship in HIV-infection and AIDS. *AIDS* **9**(11): 1288–1289.
120. **Tonnetti, L., R. Spaccapelo, E. Cenci, A. Mencacci, P. Puccetti, R. L. Coffman, F. Bistoni, and L. Romani.** 1995. Interleukin-4 and -10 exacerbate candidiasis in mice. *Eur. J. Immunol.* **25:**1559–1565.
121. **Vasquez-Torres, A., J. Jones-Carson, and E. Balish.** 1995. Nitric oxide production does not directly increase macrophage candidacidal activity. *Infect. Immun.* **63:**1142–1144.
122. **Velegraki, A., D. Papalambrou, S. Soremi, and N. J. Legakis.** 1996. Variable antifungal susceptibility of wild-type *Candida albicans* phenotypes from neutropenic hosts. *Eur. J. Clin. Microbiol. Infect. Dis.* **15:**854–860.
123. **Waggoner-Fountain, L., M. Walker, R. J. Hollis, M. A. Pfaller, J. E. Ferguson, R. P. Wenzel, and L. G. Donowitz.** 1996. Vertical and horizontal transmission of unique *Candida* species to premature newborns. *Clin. Infect. Dis.* **22:** 803–808.
124. **Wagner, R., A. Vazquez-Torres, J. Jones-Carson, T. Warner, and E. Balish.** 1994. B cell "knockout" mice are resistant to mucosal and systemic candidiasis. *J. Infect. Dis.* **174:** 589–593.
125. **Walsh, T. J., C. E. Gonzalez, S. Piscitelli, J. D. Bacher, J. Peter, R. Torres, D. Shetti, V. Katsov, K. Kligys, and C. A. Lyman.** 2000. Correlation between in vitro and in vivo antifungal activities in experimental fluconazole-resistant oropharyngeal and esophageal candidiasis. *J. Clin. Microbiol.* 38:2369–2373.
126. **Weese-Mayer, D. E., D. W. Fondriest, R. T. Brouillett, and S. T. Shulman.** 1987. Risk factors associated with candidemia in the neonatal intensive care unit: a case-control study. *Pediatr. Infect. Dis. J.* **6:**190–196.
127. **Weinert, M., R. M. Grimes, and D. P. Lynch.** 1996. Oral manifestations of HIV infection. *Ann. Intern. Med.* **125:** 485–496.
128. **Wenzel, R. P.** 1995. Nosocomial candidemia: risk factors and attributable mortality. *Clin. Infect. Dis.* **20:**1531–1534.
129. **Witek-Janusek, L., and H. L. Mathews.** Infant susceptibility to *Candida albicans:* reduced lymphocyte mediated antifungal capacity. Unpublished observations.
130. **Zhao, X., G. E. McElhaney-Feser, W. H. Bowen, M. F. Cole, S. E. Broedel, Jr., and R. L. Cihlar.** 1996. Requirement for *Candida albicans FAS2* gene for infection in a rat model of oropharyngeal candidiasis. *Microbiology* **142:**2509–2514.

Candida and Candidiasis
Edited by Richard A. Calderone
© 2002 ASM Press, Washington, D.C.

Chapter 14

Host Defense against Vaginal Candidiasis

PAUL L. FIDEL, JR., AND JACK D. SOBEL

Vulvovaginal candidiasis (VVC) is a common mucosal infection caused by *Candida* species that affects a significant number of women predominantly in their reproductive years (51, 93, 94). In fact, up to 75% of all women will experience at least one lifetime episode of acute VVC (93, 94). *Candida albicans* is the causative agent in approximately 85 to 90% of VVC cases, followed by *C. glabrata* and *C. tropicalis* as a distant third. A host of other *Candida* species cause VVC even less frequently (93, 94).

Acute VVC has several known predisposing factors, including antibiotic and oral contraceptive usage, hormone replacement therapy, pregnancy, uncontrolled diabetes mellitus, immunosuppressive therapy, and possibly human immunodeficiency virus (HIV) infection (51, 93, 94). Recurrent VVC (RVVC) occurs in a small subset of women (5 to 10%) and, although multifactorial in etiology, is usually defined as idiopathic, with no known predisposing factors in the majority of those affected (93, 94). In women with RVVC, antifungal therapy is highly effective for individual symptomatic attacks but does not prevent subsequent recurrence. There is little evidence that antifungal resistance plays a role in the pathogenesis of RVVC (61). Instead, susceptibility to RVVC is postulated to be immune-based and that these women experience repeated symptomatic episodes as a result of some immunological dysfunction or deficiency. However, host defense mechanisms functioning at the vaginal mucosa are poorly understood, not to mention those specifically acting against *C. albicans*. Accordingly, animal models of experimental vaginal candidiasis have been employed to investigate vaginal host defense mechanisms against *C. albicans*. To date, much of these data have come from both a mouse and a rat model, although recently a nonhuman primate model has also been explored.

Protective immunity against pathogenic organisms may occur in the form of adaptive/acquired immunity. The protection can be long-lived from as little as one exposure to antigen or short-lived, requiring repeated antigen exposures, depending on the strength of the memory response, and can be induced by vaccination or in response to the live organism. Protective immunity may also only be partial, allowing the organism to colonize mucosal surfaces but not invade or cause disease. This graded protection can be in the form of innate or adaptive immunity. Innate responses must be activated at each exposure since memory does not exist. The adaptive response must be tightly controlled by positive immunity and tolerance or immunoregulation to allow for asymptomatic colonization. If either of these immune mechanisms (which may not be mutually exclusive) is overwhelmed or even dysfunctional, symptomatic infection will ensue. Protection against *C. albicans* mucosal infection falls into this latter category. However, the actual protective mechanisms are poorly understood. This chapter will review the most current data on human and animal host defense mechanisms acting at the vaginal mucosa against *C. albicans*, including both systemic and local mechanisms; discuss the limited information known regarding vaginal host defense against *C. glabrata;* and lastly, provide hypotheses regarding the mechanisms of local host protection against vaginitis.

EXPERIMENTAL MODELS OF VAGINITIS

C. albicans Vaginitis

The majority of experimental studies to date have employed rodent models of experimental vaginitis. These models require that the animals be in a state of pseudoestrus at the time of intravaginal inoculation to obtain a persistent infection that can be studied for

Paul L. Fidel, Jr., and Jack D. Sobel • Department of Microbiology, Immunology, and Parasitology, Louisiana State University Medical Center, New Orleans, LA 70112.

immunological or therapeutic purposes (26, 88, 104). Additionally, rats must be oophorectomized to obtain a state of pseudoestrus. Moreover, the pseudoestrus condition must be maintained throughout the infection period with weekly injections of estradiol. Estrogen converts vaginal columnar epithelium to thick stratified squamous epithelium and increases glycogen content and growth substrates, all of which increase the avidity of the yeast for the tissue and enhances growth of the yeast (52). Animals are usually treated subcutaneously with estradiol (0.2 to 0.5 mg/rodent) 48 to 72 h prior to vaginal inoculation although a similar infection can be achieved if estrogen is administered several days postinoculation (19). The inoculum consists of a stationary-phase *C. albicans* culture given intravaginally in a small volume of phosphate-buffered saline. The vaginal infection resulting under this pseudoestrus state is usually persistent in mice ($>10^4$ CFU) lasting for weeks as long as the hormonal condition is maintained (19). In rats, however, the infection spontaneously resolves ($<10^3$ CFU) in 3 to 4 weeks despite the maintenance of pseudoestrus (14). In the absence of pseudoestrus in mice or rats, a similar short-lived (1 to 2 week) infection ensues, with fungal titers in most animals declining to undetectable levels by the second week (19, 27). Progesterone, on the other hand, plays no role in the development of the infection in rodents and cannot reverse the effects that estrogen has on promoting or maintaining the infection (19). The actual dose of estradiol administered to mice can be used to control the persistence of the infection. Under lower concentrations of estradiol (0.1 mg/mouse), the infection resolves more rapidly (19). Since reproductive hormones are known to inhibit immune responses (55, 62, 64), the enhanced reduction of vaginal fungal burden under reduced estradiol conditions may be reflective of a more significant immune response and/or less favorable local growth conditions for *C. albicans*.

The experimental infection is usually monitored by quantitative vaginal lavage culture or micropipet culture (9, 26). The vaginal fungal burden in CFU is then used as a measure of the level of infectivity. Animals can be sampled independently over time or longitudinally. It should be noted, however, that repeated lavages may influence the vaginal fungal titers leading to skewed results/interpretations. Additionally, a wet mount slide preparation of the fluid is usually used as a qualitative measure of infectivity evidenced by the presence of hyphae either free or associated with sheets of epithelial cells. One interesting caveat of the rodents is their general resistance to yeast colonization and subsequent lack of *C. albicans*-derived immune sensitization (delayed-type hypersensitivity, lymphocyte responses) to *C. albicans* antigen in the naive state. This is in contrast to humans, in whom *C. albicans* is often detected colonizing mucosal surfaces in the absence of symptoms, as well as immune sensitization to *C. albicans* that is demonstrable in normal healthy adults by the presence of *Candida*-specific immunoglobulin, and peripheral blood lymphocyte responses and cutaneous delayed skin test reactivity in response to *Candida* antigens (25, 73). Additionally, the vaginal pH of rodents is significantly higher (7 to 9) compared to that of the human vagina (4 to 4.5). It is unclear what the implications of these differences may be. Certainly, the lack of asymptomatic colonization or of recognizable symptomatic infection in rodents makes it difficult to make direct comparisons with the human disease. On the other hand, experimental infection in rodents remarkably parallels the human condition (i.e., fungal titers, persistent infection) and has been highly predictive of efficacy of antifungal drugs. Moreover, the murine models have been invaluable in identifying and studying host defense mechanisms against vaginal *C. albicans* infection.

Because of the apparent limitations of the rodent model, nonhuman primates have been considered as an alternative model to study pathogenesis of human *C. albicans* vaginal infection. As in humans, both rhesus and pigtailed macaques were found to have detectable yeast colonization at mucosal sites and evidence of positive immune sensitization at both the local mucosal and systemic levels (*Candida*-specific peripheral blood lymphocyte responses, *Candida*-specific vaginal antibody expression, and vaginal-associated cytokine expression) (101). However, only the rhesus macaques were susceptible to an experimental *C. albicans* vaginal infection, either untreated, after antibiotic-mediated reduction of normal vaginal flora, or following the induction of a state of estrus. In each case, although the experimental vaginal infection resolved spontaneously in some animals, most had to be treated with topical antifungal agents. Figure 1 shows a typical progression of an experimental *C. albicans* vaginal infection in mice, rats, and primates.

C. glabrata Vaginitis

In general, models of *C. glabrata* mucosal infections had been difficult to establish. To this end, while standard immunocompetent mice used for *C. albicans* vaginitis were not susceptible to a vaginal *C. glabrata* infection, non-obese diabetic (NOD/Lt) mice were susceptible to *C. glabrata* vaginal infection (20) (Fig. 2). In comparison to *C. albicans* infections, although a higher inoculum of *C. glabrata* is routinely used (1×10^7 blastoconidia) compared to *C. albicans* (5×10^5 blastoconidia), inocula as low as 5×10^5 CFU are capable of establishing *C. glabrata* infections. The

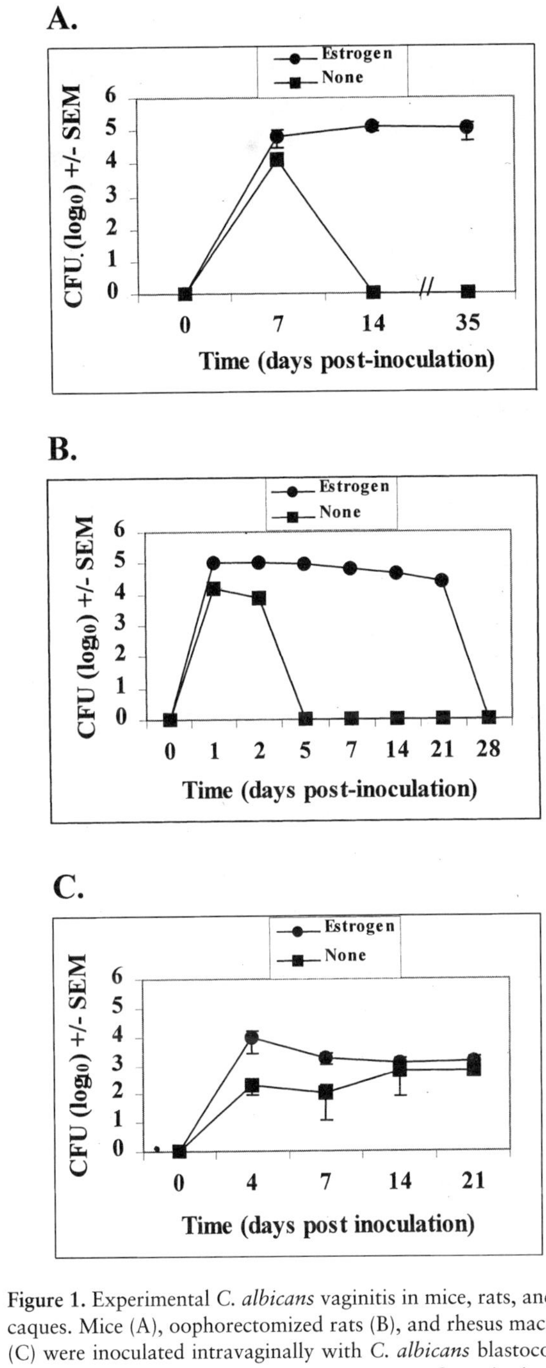

Figure 1. Experimental *C. albicans* vaginitis in mice, rats, and macaques. Mice (A), oophorectomized rats (B), and rhesus macaques (C) were inoculated intravaginally with *C. albicans* blastoconidia with or without exogenous estrogen treatment. Quantitative vaginal lavages were used to quantify the vaginal fungal burden over time. Rats and primates were tested longitudinally, whereas separate mice were tested at each time interval. Data for rats were kindly provided by F. DeBernardis, Rome, Italy.

infection is usually sustained for 14 days at high titers and resolves in most animals by 21 days. Another interesting feature of the *C. glabrata* vaginal infection in NOD mice is the relative lack of a requirement for pseudoestrus. Although rates of infection are generally greater in pseudoestrus-treated mice, the vaginal fungal burden is comparable in pseudoestrus-treated or untreated mice. This observation is in keeping with the clinical observation that *C. glabrata* is frequent in postmenopausal women developing *Candida* vaginitis (95).

The use of NOD mice as a means of studying diabetes has an interesting caveat in this model. The model was originally conceived based on the high susceptibility that women with diabetes mellitus have to *C. glabrata* and *C. albicans* vaginitis (34, 83, 93, 96). However, the NOD mice that were susceptible to the vaginal *C. glabrata* infection were not yet hyperglycemic. In fact, the NOD mice used at 7 to 10 weeks of age in the named study did not become hyperglycemic until 22 weeks of age. These results suggested that NOD mice may be susceptible to *C. glabrata* vaginal infection, not by virtue of a state of hyperglycemia, but by their genetic susceptibility to diabetes mellitus. This experimental model of *C. glabrata* vaginitis provides an opportunity to study the pathogenesis of *C. glabrata* vaginal infections, as well as to dissect the genetic issues related to susceptibility to infection.

PROTECTIVE HOST DEFENSE MECHANISMS AGAINST *C. ALBICANS* VAGINITIS

Innate, humoral, and cell-mediated immunity (CMI) is involved in protection against *C. albicans* infections. Although each may contribute to some extent at any tissue site, innate immunity by polymorphonuclear leukocytes (PMNL) and macrophages dominates protection against systemic candidiasis, whereas CMI is predominant at mucosal surfaces. The role of humoral immunity is controversial, especially clinically, but has been shown to act at both systemic and mucosal sites. Because immune mechanisms against *Candida* spp. at various sites and settings are covered in other chapters, the discussion of host defense in this chapter will be restricted to only those involved against vaginitis.

Role of Systemic CMI

Until recently, little was known regarding host defense mechanisms important at the vaginal mucosa against any vaginal pathogen, including *C. albicans.* On the basis of data suggesting that T cells and CMI were the predominant host defense mechanisms against mucosal candidiasis, clinical and animal studies were designed and conducted to evaluate the role of CMI against vaginal candidiasis. In our laboratory, recognizing that a systemic Th1-type response was generated as a result of a vaginal *C. albicans* infection

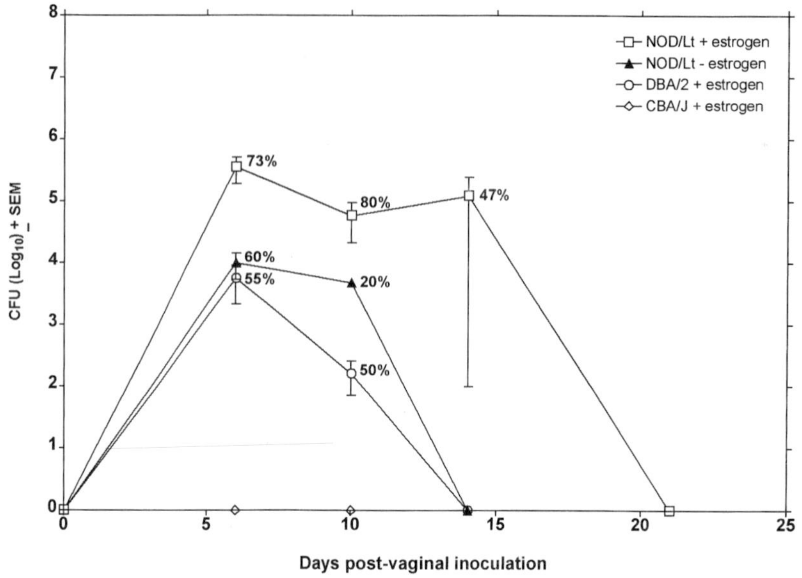

Figure 2. Experimental *C. glabrata* infections in nonobese diabetic (NOD/Lt) mice, DBA/2 mice, and CBA/J mice. Data points represent mean CFU ± standard errors of the mean (SEM) of animals with positive cultures only. Percentage of animals with positive cultures at each time point is shown.

and that this response had also been reported to be associated with protection against systemic and mucosal *C. albicans* infection (10, 86, 87), preinduced *Candida*-specific systemic CMI was evaluated with regard to impact on vaginal *Candida* burden during experimental *Candida* vaginitis. Results showed, however, that in this model system, neither CD4$^+$ Th1-type CMI nor the presence of *Candida*-specific suppressor T cells that suppressed the infection-induced delayed-type hypersensitivity (DTH) reactivity had any effect on vaginal fungal titers (28). These results were the first evidence that systemic CMI expressed in the peripheral circulation may not represent a dominant host defense mechanism at the vaginal mucosa. Partial protection against vaginitis was, however, achieved in animals given a second inoculation of *C. albicans* following the spontaneous resolution of a primary infection in the absence of estrogen (24) (Fig. 3). Interestingly, although anamnestic DTH occurred during the secondary infection, suppression of this systemic Th1-type reactivity, either by *Candida*-specific suppressor T cells or depletion of all systemic CD4$^+$ cells, had no effect on the protection against vaginitis (24), providing additional evidence that systemic CMI had a limited role in protection against vaginal candidiasis. Also in support of this, we showed that mice either resistant or susceptible to systemic *C. albicans* infection (39) were equally susceptible to vaginitis and could equally be partially protected against a second vaginal infection (18). This was supported further by another study that employed six different strains of mice representing four haplotypes (2). We concluded from these studies that some form of locally acquired mucosal immunity, T

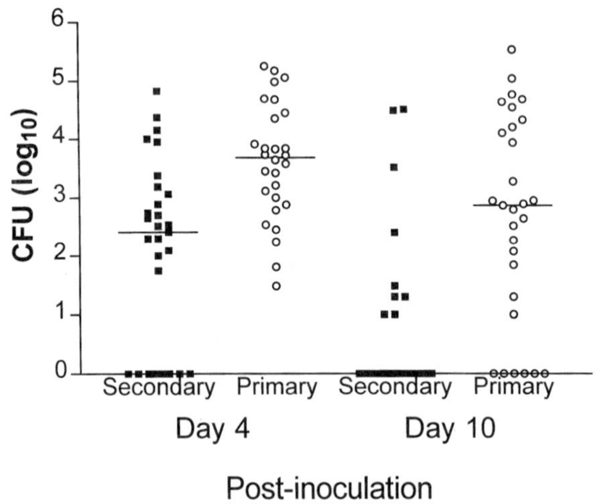

Figure 3. Partial protection from vaginal candidiasis following primary vaginal immunization in nonestrogenized mice. Four weeks after mice were given a primary (1°) vaginal inoculation of *C. albicans* and the infection had resolved, the mice were reinoculated in the presence of exogenous estrogen (squares). Control mice received a primary vaginal inoculation in the presence of estrogen (circles). Vaginal fungal burden was monitored on days 4 and 10 postsecondary inoculation. Fungal burden in secondary-infected mice was significantly reduced compared to that in primary-infected mice ($P <$ 0.001).

cell- and/or antibody-mediated, was responsible for protecting mice against vaginal *C. albicans* infection and that the vaginal mucosa had some level of immunological independence or immune compartmentalization. In support of the concept of immune compartmentalization, complement-fixing antibodies specific for T cells given intravenously to mice depleted T cells in the periphery, but not in the vagina, whereas intravaginal administration of the same antibodies depleted T cells in both the vagina and the periphery (22). Additionally, adoptive transfer of *Candida*-sensitized T cells into T-cell deficient (nude) mice had no effect on vaginitis (4). Despite this overwhelming evidence for a lack of effects of systemic responses against a vaginal *C. albicans* infection, a group has recently described T cell-mediated protection against vaginitis by systemic immunization in a particular strain of mice (69, 70). Although it is unclear what type of immunity was generated (Th1/Th2), this suggests that under some circumstances (i.e., genetic background, antigen) systemic responses may have some effect at the vaginal mucosa. These studies, however, reflect a minority view of the protective role of systemic CMI.

Overall, these animal data correlated well with clinical studies conducted in women with RVVC although such studies have not been without controversy. In a comprehensive study from our laboratory, we showed that although some RVVC patients may experience a loss in *Candida*-specific cutaneous delayed skin test reactivity, the majority of RVVC patients, both during symptomatic infections and infection-free periods of remission, had normal levels of *Candida*-specific systemic CMI detected by both peripheral blood lymphocyte proliferation and cytokine expression (25). Interestingly, not only was the systemic CMI response present in RVVC patients, the cytokine expression was identified as the $CD4^+$ Th1-type (interleukin [IL]-2, gamma interferon [IFN-γ], and IL-12) known to be associated with resistance to candidiasis (10, 86, 87). We concluded from these results that the immune dysfunction or deficiency, if present in RVVC patients, was at the local rather than systemic level and that the loss of *Candida*-specific skin test reactivity was the result rather than a cause of infection (25). This is supported further by the fact that women with idiopathic RVVC rarely experience oral, esophageal, or cutaneous candidiasis (86). However, studies previous to this that examined solely delayed cutaneous skin test responses and/or peripheral blood lymphocyte (PBL) proliferative responses showed that women with RVVC had some form of impairment of systemic CMI (32, 42, 107, 108) either at the T-cell or macrophage level or had no detectable defect (32, 66, 102). The controversy continues into the present with a limited number of additional studies that examined *Candida*-specific CMI (lymphocyte proliferation, cytokine production). One described a dysfunction in proliferation and IFN-γ and tumor necrosis factor alpha (TNF-α) production during acute episodes of RVVC that was restored in remission (72). A second reported reduced responsiveness in RVVC patients during the follicular phase of the menstrual cycle (least influence of hormones) (12). Although it is unclear what significance the latter carries since most women with RVVC do not show a pattern of episodic recurrences during the follicular stage of the menstrual cycle, it does emphasize that stage of the menstrual cycle should be taken into account when examining local or systemic immune reactivity to *C. albicans*. These data also confirm the systemic cytokine profile in response to *Candida* antigen in all studies to date showing that control women and RVVC patients have some level of Th1-type responses in the virtual absence of Th2-type responses (12, 21, 25). Our results specifically showing that most episodes of RVVC occur in the presence of normal levels of *Candida*-specific Th1-type CMI correlate with two relevant clinical observations: women with RVVC are generally not susceptible to oral, esophageal, or other forms of cutaneous candidiasis (93), and women with chronic mucocutaneous candidiasis are rarely susceptible to RVVC (73). On the basis of this information, we have postulated, similar to the animal studies, that the proposed immune deficiency in RVVC patients is primarily localized to the vaginal mucosa and does not involve systemic CMI.

The lack of effects of systemic CMI at the vaginal mucosa appears to extend as well to the HIV patient although again the studies are not without controversy. Some reports have suggested both that vaginitis is more common in the HIV patient and the incidence of infection increases as the CD4 cell counts decrease (5, 16, 98). In contrast, other reports have suggested that vaginitis is not more common in the HIV-positive or AIDS patients than in HIV-negative women (11, 58, 92, 106), or at least does not correlate with decreased CD4 cell counts if present (44, 85). There are several possible explanations for these controversial findings. A serious problem with these studies is the lack of appropriate control groups. For example, comparing parameters between HIV-positive and HIV-negative individuals requires several matched groups, including age and associated behavioral risk factors. However, the design of too many studies failed to include an unmatched control group that can be used to identify true baseline levels. Additionally, the lack of knowledge of host defense mechanisms important for protection against vaginal candidiasis has hampered the ability to interpret adequately data from the clinical studies. Nevertheless, the controversy itself indicates that the effects of HIV and systemic immunocompromising conditions on the vaginal mucosa are different from those observed at the oral mucosa where it is clear that reduced blood CD4 cell counts correlate with increased incidence of oropharyngeal and esophageal candidiasis and a high prevalence of infection (44, 54, 56, 91). A recent study conducted in our laboratory that examined *Candida*-specific systemic CMI in HIV-positive women with or without VVC showed that although delayed cutaneous skin test reactivity to *Candida* antigen was reduced in HIV-positive women with less than 200 CD4 cells/μl, there was no correlation of reduced skin test reactivity to VVC. Furthermore, PBL proliferation and Th1/Th2 cytokine production in response to *Candida* antigens were relatively similar in HIV-positive women with or without symptomatic VVC although one cytokine, IFN-γ, was reduced in HIV- and VVC-positive women compared to HIV-negative women (58). This provides yet another example for the virtual lack of any role for *Candida*-specific systemic CMI against vaginal *C. albicans* infections. The differences in incidence of oral and vaginal candidiasis relative to the prevalence of candidiasis under immunocompromised conditions are intriguing. In the past, because few formal studies were conducted in women, the vaginal mucosa was grouped with other mucosal sites in discussions of mucosal candidiasis during immunosuppression. However, with the increased attention women's health has received in the recent past, these mucosal distinctions have become more fully recognized and need to be studied independently.

Role of Local CMI

In light of little evidence suggesting a role for systemic CMI against *C. albicans* vaginal infection, recent work has focused on the presence of T-cell subpopulations at the vaginal mucosa and the role of local CMI against vaginal *C. albicans* infection. The murine vaginal mucosa, although not containing organized lymphoid areas as that in the gastrointestinal tract (i.e., Peyer's patches, tonsils), nevertheless has all the necessary components for competent adaptive immune responses. This includes immunoglobulin expression, T cells, and major histocompatibility complex (MHC) class II-positive cells (i.e., Langerhan's cells, macrophages) to serve as antigen-presenting cells (74, 75). Of critical importance, several investigators have reported that vaginal lymphocytes in mice are phenotypically distinct from those in the periphery (30, 43, 46, 71). Similar observations have been made in humans (41, 45, 47). In mice, flow cytometric data suggest that although $CD4^+$, α/β T-cell receptor (TCR)-positive cells predominate the T-cell repertoire at the vaginal mucosa in a manner similar to lymph node cells or PBLs, there is a 5- to 40-fold higher percentage of γ/δ TCR-positive cells (15 to 50%) (30, 43, 46, 71) and very few if any $CD8^+$ cells (normally 20% in blood) (30). In humans, the ratios of α/β and γ/δ T cells are similar to those in mice (41, 45), but there are abundant $CD8^+$ T cells (41) that have cytotoxic T lymphocyte function (105). Similar findings have been reported in nonhuman primates (60, 67). These observations further support the concept of immunological independence or compartmentalization of vaginal T cells.

Through several independent studies (i.e., flow cytometry, immunohistochemistry, and reverse transcriptase [RT] PCR), our laboratory has evidence suggesting that murine vaginal $CD4^+$ T cells atypically express the CD4 protein compared to their systemic counterparts in peripheral blood or lymph nodes. This was first observed by the differential recognition by epitope-distinct anti-CD4 antibodies under nondenatured conditions (30). Specifically, flow cytometry experiments showed that in contrast to lymph node cells that stained positively with anti-CD4 antibodies specific for both the N terminus and C terminus of the CD4 protein, vaginal lymphocytes stained positively with antibodies only directed against the C terminus (30). A similar atypical expression of the CD4 protein on the vaginal cells was observed in situ using the intravaginal administration of complement-fixing antibodies (30). Evidence for the masking of the N-terminal epitope of the CD4 protein rather the absence of the epitope came from positive and negative immunohistochemical staining of collagense-treated vaginal cells under denatured and nondenatured conditions, respectively, using anti-CD4 antibodies directed to the N terminus (112).

The uniqueness of the murine vaginal CD4 protein was also found to extend to the level of transcription (112). RT-PCR analyses using several murine systemic T-cell-specific primer sets showed that despite the consistent positive amplification of mRNA specific for CD3, TCRβ, and TCRδ chain constant regions, but not CD8, in vaginal tissue (consistent with flow cytometry), amplification of CD4 mRNA in vaginal tissue was only rarely observed. This was true for multiple strains of mice using a panel of systemic cell-derived CD4 primer sets spanning the length of the cDNA that all consistently amplified lymph node mRNA. The inability to amplify CD4 mRNA from a purified population of the unique $CD4^+$ vaginal lymphocytes confirmed the absence of CD4 mRNA in the cells. Possibilities for the presence of the atypical CD4 protein on vaginal $CD4^+$ T cells include differential splicing or a passive acquisition from a source or soluble CD4 in the tissue.

Regardless of the means by which the altered CD4 protein is acquired, an atypical expression of the vaginal CD4 protein may have significant implications in host defense. Since the CD4 protein interacts with major histocompatibility complex class II during T-cell activation and certain signals are initiated through CD4, an altered conformation may significantly affect TCR-mediated vaginal $CD4^+$ T-cell activation. Furthermore, if it is passively acquired, there may be little to no functional cytoplasmic signal potential.

The ultimate question is whether this unique CD4 protein is specific to the vagina as opposed to other mucosal tissues, and whether a similar unique CD4 protein is present in human vaginal tissue. Recent evidence, however, suggests that this expression is unique to the murine vagina and possibly to mice alone as a similar expression of CD4 has not been observed on human $CD4^+$ T cells isolated from nondiseased vaginal cuff tissue obtained from hysterectomy surgery (31).

Some interesting observations have also recently been made regarding vaginal γ/δ T cells. It appears that in contrast to γ/δ T cells at other mucosal sites, the γ/δ T cells in the vaginal mucosa of mice express a homogenous Vγ4/Vδ1 TCR lacking N-region junctional diversity (71, 81). Although all γ/δ T cells share a limited repertoire of antigenic recognition, the site-specific phenotype of the vaginal γ/δ T cells implies compartmentalization and the potential for a unique function(s). Furthermore, the murine vaginal γ/δ T cells lack both CD2 and CD28, two potent costimulatory signals, but show an effector phenotype with the expression of CD44, CD45RB, and LFA-1 (81, 82). These cells too can be expanded by the intravenous injection of pan anti-γδ TCR antibodies (82). Taken together, it appears that both types of T cells in the murine vaginal mucosa are phenotypically and potentially functionally distinct from their peripheral and other mucosal tissue counterparts.

Studies have now been conducted to evaluate potential changes in vaginal T cells during a *C. albicans* experimental infection. The predominance of $CD4^+$ α/β TCR-positive cells in the vaginal mucosa provides the cells that are critical for host defense against candidal infections at other mucosal sites in close proximity to the site of infection. Previously, the only studies that examined the role of local T cells during vaginitis were conducted by Balish and coworkers. In those studies, immunodeficient mice were used to study the natural history of *Candida* vaginal infections (7). The nude strain of mice deficient in T cells (*nu*/*nu*) showed no increase in susceptibility to vaginitis compared to the immunocompetent controls. However, since the animals were not maintained in a state of pseudoestrus and vaginal T cells were not evaluated, it is difficult to interpret these findings. Recently, however, these studies were repeated under pseudoestrus conditions with similar findings (4). With regard to the role of γ/δ T cells, a study showed that mice depleted of γ/δ T cells had an increased susceptibility to vaginitis, suggesting a potential role for these cells as a first-line defense mechanism (48). In stark contrast to this, however, vaginitis in δ-chain TCR knockout mice has been found to be less severe, suggestive of a tolerance role for vaginal γ/δ T cells (113). Clearly more investigation is required to fully understand the role of these vaginal T cells against *Candida* spp.

Studies to examine changes in vaginal T cells using flow cytometry, immunohistochemistry, and RT-PCR all show little evidence for modulation of α/β or γ/δ vaginal T cells during either primary or secondary experimental vaginal *C. albicans* infections and no evidence for systemic T-cell infiltration during a vaginal *Candida* infection (23). These results are consistent with those from the immunodeficient or knockout mice (4, 7) as well as the systemic immune studies in immunocompetent mice (18, 24, 28, 29). This lack of responsiveness to *Candida* infection is in direct contrast to comprehensive studies conducted in a murine model of a genital *Chlamydia trachomatis* infection in which it was determined that lymphocytes in the genital tract were increased in infected mice and responded to *Chlamydia* antigens by proliferation (6). However, the responding cells were found to have been derived from the periphery, namely, the draining lymph nodes (50). In other recent studies, it was determined that vaginal infection with herpes simplex virus-2 (HSV-2) stimulates a similar infiltration of $CD4^+$ cells from the periphery (77, 78). In both infections, Th1-type $CD4^+$ T cells were found to predominate in the infiltrate. These distinct differences between the immune responses to *Candida* and *Chlamydia* or HSV-2 genital tract infections, together with the fact that *Chlamydia* sp. and HSV-2, as opposed to *C. albicans*, are not recognized vaginal commensal organisms, emphasize further the uniqueness of the host vaginal response(s) against *C. albicans*. Interestingly, a recent study examining a dual infection with a *Candida* sp. and a *Chlamydia* sp. showed a complete independence of "responsiveness" in the upper genital tract (*Chlamydia* sp.) and "lack of responsiveness" in the lower tract (*Candida* sp.) (49), showing further the complexity of genital tract immunity.

Experimental studies with *Candida* spp. have since focused on local cytokines and chemokines during infection to better understand the lack of vaginal responsiveness to *C. albicans*. Examination of chemokines showed that MCP-1 (chemotactic for macrophages and T cells) was increased in the vaginal mucosa during infection and MIP-2 (chemotactic for PMNL) was constitutively expressed at high levels in the vagina (89). Furthermore, in vivo neutralization of MCP-1 with anti-MCP-1 antibodies resulted in increased vaginal fungal burden, suggesting some role for the chemokine in the host response. However, elevated levels of MCP-1 did not result in any demonstrable increases in T cells or macrophages in vaginal lavage fluid (previously shown as well in vaginal tissue [23]). Thus, either MCP-1 is playing a role independent of chemotaxis or it is regulated such that a stronger function is prohibited. When local Th1/Th2 cytokines were evaluated, high constitutive levels of transforming growth factor-beta (TGF-β) were found whereas other Th1/Th2 cytokines (i.e., IL-2, IFN-γ, IL-12, IL-4, IL-10) were low or undetectable (103). During pseudoestrus and/or infection, TGF-β, but not the other cytokines, was transiently increased (Fig. 4). Furthermore, TGF-β was significantly higher in the lower genital tract than in the upper genital tract. These results suggest a possible Th3-type condition whereby TGF-β contributes to immunoregulation or tolerance in the tissue. This may explain the lack of responsiveness in the vagina during a *Candida* infection and demonstrable responses in the upper tract during a *Chlamydia* infection. Furthermore, TGF-β has been shown to inhibit chemokine receptors (90), which may explain the lack of stronger effects by MCP-1 during infection (89). Current analyses are focused on the effects of TGF-β neutralization and manifestations of such immunoregulation through the activation status of vaginal T cells as well as adhesion molecule expression in the vaginal mucosa during *C. albicans* vaginal infections. Interestingly, although not yet identified in vaginal secretions, a T-cell derived antigen-binding molecule has been identified in serum of RVVC patients, and to a lesser extent in control women, that can become associated with TGF-β and

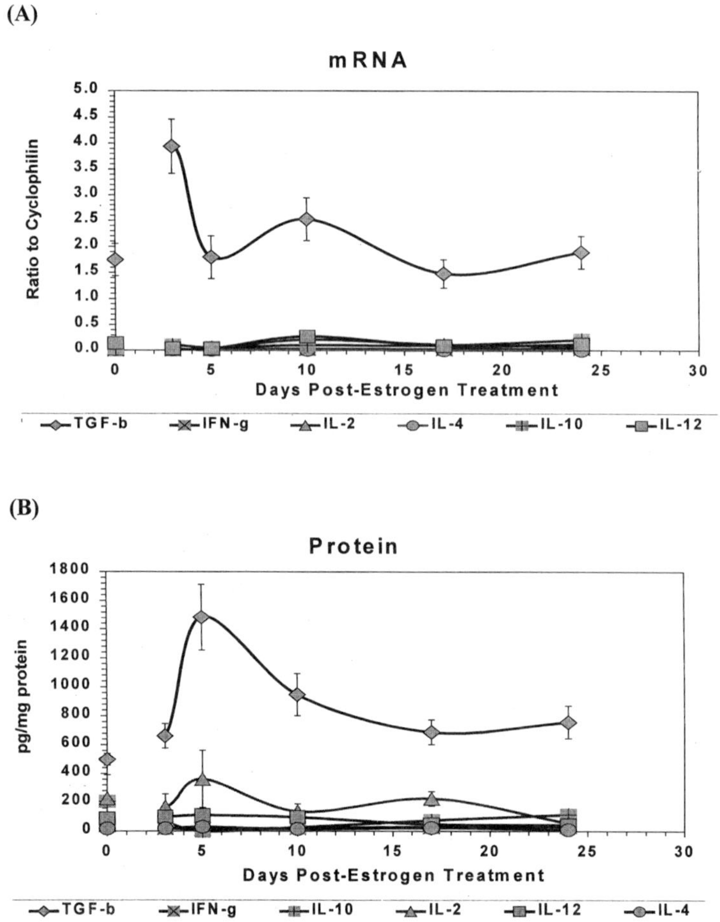

Figure 4. Vaginal presence of Th1/Th2 cytokines in estrogen-treated infected mice, revealing the predominance of TGF-β. (A) mRNA expression. (B) Protein. Unconnected points on the left represent the levels in naive mice.

inhibit *Candida*-specific PBL proliferation and cytokine production (59).

In contrast to these results in mice, a recent study in the rat model revealed quite different findings. Although the rat model has been used predominantly to study the role of humoral immunity against vaginal *C. albicans* infection, the same model was most recently used to examine the role of T cells during an infection (14). As mentioned earlier, an important difference between the rat and mouse model is the fact that under a state of pseudoestrus, the infection in rats resolves spontaneously over a 2- to 3-week period (14), whereas the infection in mice remains persistent for several weeks (26, 27) (Fig. 1). With this fact in mind, although the relative percentages of vaginal-associated T cells were similar in rats and mice (infected or uninfected), significant numbers of $CD8^+$ T cells were identified in the rat vagina similar to that in humans (41). During successive infections, the protection was enhanced, indicative of a secondary response (Fig. 5), together with a change in the ratio of CD4 : CD8 cells, with increases in $CD4^+$ α/β T cells expressing CD25. Additionally, Th1-type cytokines (IL-12, IL-2, and IFN-γ) in vaginal lavage fluid increased as well during the infections. Finally, vaginal lymphocytes, but not draining lymph nodes, from infected rats proliferated in vitro to *Candida* antigen, indicating an extremely restricted local response compared to the predominant systemic responsiveness with little evidence for

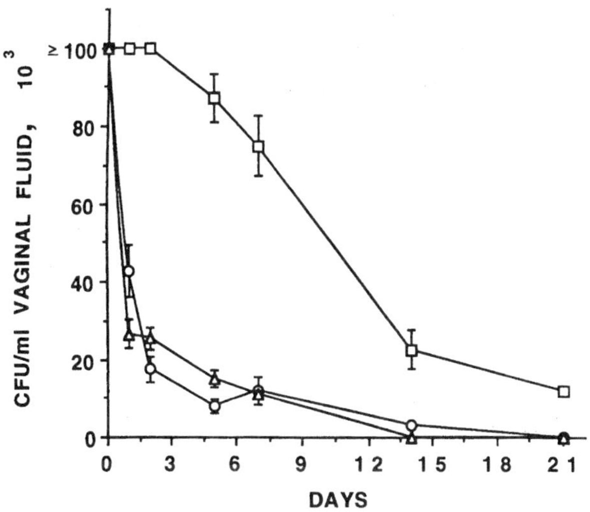

Figure 5. Natural protection against *C. albicans* vaginitis in rats. Oophorectomized rats were inoculated under pseudoestrus conditions (squares) while other rats were reinoculated with the identical numbers of organisms once (circles) or twice (triangles) following spontaneous resolution of the preceding infection. (Reproduced from reference 9 with the permission of Antonio Cassone, Rome, Italy, and *Infection and Immunity*.)

a local CMI response in mice (23, 89, 103). These results are consistent with the relative outcomes for each. Furthermore, on the basis of these results, it would not appear that the immunoregulation or tolerance predicted in mice and humans is operative in the rat.

In uninfected nonhuman primates, a Th2-type cytokine profile was observed in vaginal secretions (cervicovaginal lavage fluid) predominated by IL-4 and IL-10 (101). Under estrogen and infected conditions (rhesus) the vaginal-associated cytokines declined, suggesting a potential protective role of Th2-type cytokines. However, a similar profile was observed in pigtailed macaques that were resistant to infection (101). Clearly, these models are distinct with respect to local immunity during an infection. Although disparate, each may serve in its own right to elucidate aspects of the host response(s) to vaginal *C. albicans* infection.

Although much can be learned from animal models, how does one learn about local CMI in humans and control for the effects of reproductive hormones? To begin to evaluate CMI at the vaginal mucosa, useful information can be obtained by evaluating the presence of cytokines and chemokines in vaginal secretions. Accordingly, one experimental design is to perform vaginal lavages in a cross-sectional analysis (i.e., women with symptomatic infection compared with healthy controls) and to correlate the vaginal cytokine and chemokine expression with prevalence of infection and hormonal status.

Taking into account the general view that $CD4^+$ Th1- and Th2-type cellular reactivity is associated with resistance and susceptibility, respectively, to *Candida* infection at other mucosal sites (i.e., oral, gastrointestinal) (10, 86, 87), we recently evaluated Th1 (IL-2, IL-12, IFN-γ)- and Th2 (IL-4, IL-5, IL-10)-type cytokines in vaginal lavage fluid from women with RVVC (21). Interestingly, we found a constitutive presence of Th1-type, but not Th2-type, cytokines in cervicovaginal lavage fluid of normal healthy control women that might reflect a natural immune homeostasis, possibly in response to normal flora, including *C. albicans*. Constitutive levels of *Candida*-specific immunoglobulins (IgG, IgA, and IgE) were also observed. With respect to patients in the study, although some differences in cytokine expression were detected between fluids collected from control women and RVVC patients with or without a symptomatic infection (namely, reduction in IL-12 and IL-5 in those with RVVC), we did not detect any characteristic pattern of cytokine changes that would reflect a major deviation or shift from the profile in control women. We recognized, however, that reductions in IL-12 may reflect a lack of innate resistance that may follow with some form of reduced Th1-type reactivity. There is some recent evidence for the presence of heat shock proteins in vaginal secretions and/or sera of women with RVVC that are postulated to down-regulate local Th1-type CMI, creating susceptibility to RVVC (35, 36). However, there is little evidence, based on data in the above study, that vaginal cytokines are vastly affected in RVVC if such proteins are present. In these same local immunological studies, similar to previous studies (63, 84, 109, 110), local levels of *Candida*-specific IgG and IgA were similar between controls and RVVC patients, whereas *Candida*-specific IgE antibodies were significantly elevated in some RVVC patients.

Although a cross-sectional analysis conducted in real time is preferred, there are several unavoidable limitations in the experimental design that affect confidence in the interpretations of these data. These include (i) dynamics of local immune reactivity in subjects sampled at various times postinitiation of infection, (ii) lack of known influence of *Candida* spp. on the local cytokines measured, and (iii) lack of control for hormonal influences. Thus, the largely negative results of the cross-sectional study may have been of limited significance. To circumvent this, we designed an alternative strategy involving intravaginal antigenic challenge with *C. albicans* antigen (i.e., killed organisms or soluble antigen). In essence, we would perform a type of skin test analysis in the vaginal mucosa and detect a putative response (i.e., cytokine production) in vaginal lavage fluid. Because most humans are sensitized to *C. albicans* (25, 53, 63, 73), most healthy women would be expected to respond and the administration of a soluble antigen or killed organism posed no risk of contracting a vaginal yeast infection. A small pilot study without controlling for time of the menstrual cycle showed a small but significant elevation in Th1-type cytokines (IL-2, IL-12, and IFN-γ) in lavage fluid 16 to 18 h after intravaginal *Candida* antigen administration. In contrast, neither Th2-type cytokines (IL-4, IL-5, IL-10) nor total or *Candida*-specific IgA, IgG, and IgE were elevated in response to antigen administration (21). With respect to noncytokine immunomodulators, we found a significant elevation in histamine (21), but not prostaglandin E_2 (PGE_2) (17). The increase in histamine provided support for the presence of IgE antibodies in the lavage fluid of some women. The induced Th1-type response observed following intravaginal challenge is consistent with the constitutive vaginal cytokine expression observed in normal healthy women, and is that which is associated with protection against mucosal *C. albicans* infection (10, 86, 87). Although these results were preliminary, the intravaginal antigenic challenge represents a novel approach for studying *Candida*-specific vaginal CMI and its regulation. This approach is currently being used in large numbers of normal healthy women during different stages of the menstrual cycle to gain a better understanding of the role of reproductive hormones in vaginal immunity to *Candida* antigens. These studies may also provide information relative to putative local immunoregulatory mechanisms in humans. Ultimately, the design could be applied to other commensal organisms or to those organisms in which some form of immune sensitization is detectable, including pathogens of sexually transmitted diseases.

Role of Antibodies

In addition to resident T cells and cytokines, immunoglobulins may represent another protective mechanism functioning against *C. albicans* vaginal infections. Immunoglobulins are clearly present in vaginal secretions, including *Candida*-specific antibodies (IgG and IgA) (84, 109, 110). Interestingly though, B cells are a minor constituent of the mouse, rat, or human vaginal mucosa (76), and in contrast to other mucosal sites, IgG antibodies predominate over IgA antibodies, at least on the basis of total immunoglobulin (21, 57). Irrespective, clinical studies show that serum IgG and vaginal IgG and IgA are similar in women with RVVC (symptomatic or in remission) and healthy control women with no history of RVVC (21, 53, 63). Similar results were observed in infected and uninfected rhesus macaques, including the predominance of vaginal IgG over IgA immunoglobulins (101). Despite these experimental and clinical observations that largely fail to support a role for antibody against candidiasis, there are studies in rodents that indicate a protective role for humoral immunity in experimental vaginal candidiasis. Pollonelli and coworkers showed that rats given an intravaginal immunization using antibodies that neutralize the anti-*Candida* activity of a yeast killer toxin were protected against a vaginal infection (79). The protection was found to be associated with rising vaginal titers of anti-idiotypic IgA antibodies that could passively transfer protection to nonimmunized rats. Interestingly, similar killer toxin anti-idiotypic-like antibodies were also detected in women with symptomatic vaginitis (80). Similarly, Cassone and colleagues have shown that a primary *C. albicans* vaginal infection in estrogen-treated rats induces anti-mannan and anti-aspartyl IgA antibodies in vaginal secretions that protected those same rats against a secondary vaginal infection or recipient rats treated intravaginally with vaginal fluids from primary-infected rats (9, 13) (Fig.

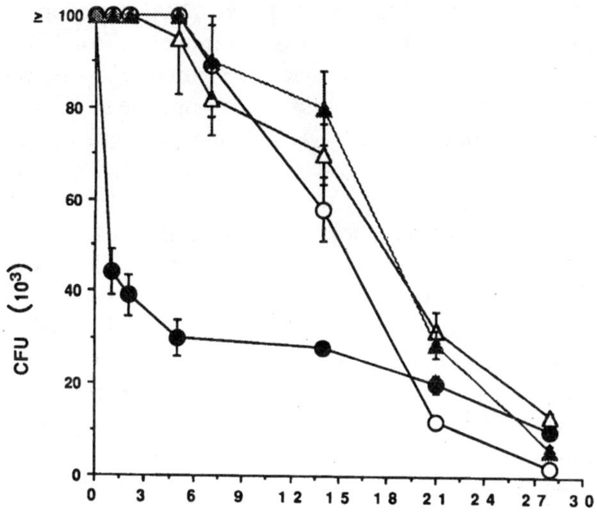

Figure 6. Protection against experimental vaginitis by vaginal fluids from primary infected rats. Oophorectomized, estradiol-treated *C. albicans*-infected rats treated with vaginal fluids from rats inoculated with germinative virulent *C. albicans* (closed circles), agerminative avirulent *C. albicans* (closed triangles), or *C. parapsilosis* (open triangles). Vaginal fungal burden was compared to that of rats given a primary inoculation of virulent *C. albicans* (open circles). The vaginal fluids from animals inoculated with germinative *C. albicans* protected rats against vaginitis. (Reproduced from reference 9 with the permission of Antonio Cassone, Rome, Italy, and *Infection and Immunity*.)

6). Moreover, vaginal lymphocyte analysis during primary or secondary vaginal *C. albicans* infections revealed an increase in B cells in the tissue (14). Successful protection against vaginitis in the presence of these IgA antibodies possibly may reflect "protective" antibodies based on the Casadevall concept of nonprotective, protective, and indifferent *Candida*-specific antibodies (8). In support of this, Cutler and coworkers have shown that two different "protective" antibodies specific for mannan (IgM and IgG3) protect mice against *Candida* vaginitis when given either locally or systemically (37, 38). Taking this into account, one might speculate that where antibodies are detected clinically, but do not appear to have a demonstrable effect, a predominance of indifferent or nonprotective antibodies may be in the highest concentration or dominate the antibody pool. If, indeed, there is some precedent for this, it appears to be the norm rather than the exception.

In contrast to complement-fixing antibodies, IgE antibodies represent another form of humoral immunity that may play a role in pathogenesis of, rather than host defense against, vaginitis. We and others have shown that small numbers of women with RVVC have elevated concentrations of *Candida*-specific IgE antibodies (21, 84, 109). It has, therefore, been postulated that in some women, an IgE-mediated immediate hypersensitivity may promote some of the characteristic histamine-associated symptoms observed in *Candida* vaginitis (i.e., itching, burning, edema). It should be noted that the presence of elevated antibodies, including IgE, during an infection is indicative of a local Th2-type response reported to be associated with susceptibility to systemic and mucosal *Candida* infections or at least a lack of protection (10, 86, 87). One mechanism for the immunopathogenesis of RVVC via allergy is that histamine plus *Candida* antigen induces the release of PGE_2 from macrophages that inhibits Th1-type cytokines (68). Although this was supported by studies showing PGE_2 production by PBL from control women and RVVC patients in response *Candida* antigen and histamine (111), the lack of locally produced PGE_2 (17) in response to intravaginal challenge with *Candida* antigen that induced significant histamine (21) challenges a putative role for PGE_2 in the immunopathogenesis of RVVC through allergic responses.

Role of Innate Resistance

Innate immunity may also play a significant role in protection against vaginitis. This was initially predicted based on a leukocytic infiltrate of predominantly PMNL that is sometimes observed in vaginal lavage fluid of infected animals. These leukocytic cells are usually associated with or attached to the hyphae and/or sheets of epithelial cells. On the other hand, when this infiltrate is present during infection, it does not correlate with lower vaginal fungal titers (23, 89). Additionally, this leukocytic infiltrate is generally not observed in clinical cases of *Candida* vaginitis. Although PMNL and macrophages (two types of leukocytes with considerable effector function against *C. albicans* [73]) are potential candidates for anti-*Candida* innate resistance and are present at or near the vaginal mucosa, Balish and coworkers showed that animals with the beige mutation and immunodeficient in phagocytic cells (*bg*/*bg*) were not more susceptible to a natural *C. albicans* infection under nonestrogenized conditions (7). More recently a study addressed the specific role of PMNL during experimental vaginitis. The results showed that depletion of PMNL under pseudoestrus conditions had no effect on vaginal fungal burden, although microabscesses within the tissue were significantly reduced (3). Although no differences in fungal titers were observed, the authors nevertheless speculated that PMNL may in fact play a significant role against *C. albicans* in the vagina, but they cannot consistently be deployed in high enough numbers during pseudoestrus to be effective. We recently tested this hypothesis by examining the effects of PMNL depletion both in estrogen- and nonestrogen-treated mice. Results similarly showed that depletion of PMNL had no effect on vaginal fungal burden under either hormonal condition (23), suggesting that PMNL do not in fact appear to play a significant role against *C. albicans* in the vagina despite their presence in the vaginal lumen during some experimental infections. Perhaps this reflects their inability to function against *C. albicans* in the vaginal microenvironment compared to blood or tissue culture as a result of putative immunoregulatory mechanisms. Alternatively, the presence of PMNL during an infection might not represent a response to the yeast, but simply reflect their normal presence during the diestrus stage of the menstrual cycle (every 2 days in mice) when they are deployed to phagocytize the apoptotic squamous epithelial cells from the estrus (2-day cycle) stage. This is supported by the variable and erratic presence of the PMNL infiltrate and the observation that a similar PMNL infiltrate occurs in pseudoestrus-treated mice not infected with *C. albicans*. This suggests that PMNL deployment into the vagina during diestrus is not under the same hormonal regulation that controls the stage of the menstrual cycle. In support of this, a recent study described a role for the chemokine, MIP-2, in the recruitment of PMNL during diestrus (97). The constitutive presence of MIP-2 in vaginal tissue (89) is consistent with this concept.

Natural killer (NK) cells may represent another potential innate resistance mechanism against *C. albicans* at the vaginal mucosa. However, most studies have shown little or no role for NK cells against *C. albicans* (1, 15). Furthermore, NK cells do not appear to be resident cells in the vaginal mucosa (76). Thus, although NK cells may have the potential to be recruited into the vaginal mucosa in response to *C. albicans*, it is unlikely that NK cells play a major role in innate resistance against *C. albicans* at the vaginal mucosa.

In light of the uncertainties regarding the role of conventional innate resistance against *C. albicans* at the vaginal mucosa, some attention has shifted to somewhat unconventional immune cells (i.e., epithelial and endothelial cells) in the vaginal mucosa as potential anti-*Candida* effector cells. Epithelial cells have recently been shown to produce several cytokines and chemokines (40), and endothelial cells have been shown to be phagocytic for *Candida* spp. (33). Epithelial cells are particularly intriguing as innate effectors as they represent the cell type most often associated with *Candida* spp. in the vagina. Recognizing this, we recently examined whether vaginal cells had any anti-*Candida* activity. Results demonstrated that indeed an epithelial-enriched fraction of vaginal cells extracted from the naive mice, or collected from human and nonhuman primate vaginal lavages, inhibited the growth of *C. albicans* blastoconidia and/or hyphae in vitro (100, 101) (Fig. 7). Interestingly, this putative epithelioid cell-mediated anti-*Candida* activity appears to be hormonally regulated, with less inhibitory activity in cells from estrogen-treated mice and macaques (19, 101). We found as well that soluble factors from the epithelial cell/*Candida* sp. coculture cannot replace the cellular requirement for the

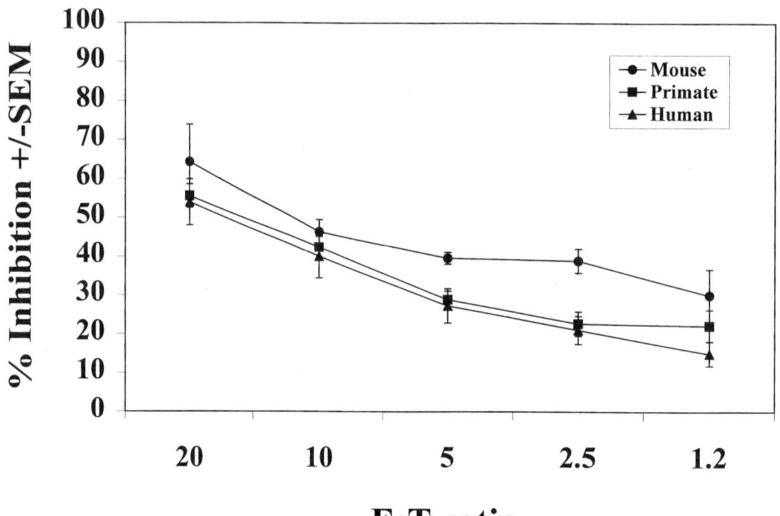

Figure 7. Epithelioid cell-mediated anti-*Candida* activity. Epithelioid-enriched cells from collagenase-treated naive mouse vaginae, and nonhuman primate and human vaginal lavages, were tested at various effector to target (E:T) ratios for growth inhibition of *C. albicans* in vitro using a 9-h ^{3}H-glucose-uptake assay.

anti-*Candida* activity. Interestingly, human oral epithelial cells have recently been shown to have a similar activity through an apparent same mechanism (cellular contact with viable effectors cells and without any role for soluble factors) (99). Thus, although more studies need to be performed to identify the mechanism of action, epithelial cells may represent important innate resistance effector cells against *C. albicans* at the vaginal mucosa.

Host Defense against *C. glabrata* Vaginitis

There is extremely limited information on host defense against *C. glabrata* vaginitis despite the prevalence of these infections, and most information that has been collected is very preliminary. As a commensal organism similar to *C. albicans,* there are likely to be normal host mechanisms that effectively control *C. glabrata,* holding its presence "in check" at mucosal sites, thereby preventing infection. However, the relative low pathogenicity of *C. glabrata* in animal models compared to *C. albicans* suggests that control of *C. glabrata* may not require mechanisms that are as stringent as that required to hold *C. albicans* in check. Nevertheless, the increased prevalence of *C. glabrata* infections in immunocompromised individuals indicates that some level of host defense does indeed exist.

There has been only one formal study that examined humoral and innate cellular defenses in patients with *C. glabrata* infections (65). Measured in each woman were secretory IgA (sIgA), IgA, and numbers of granulocytes and macrophages in vaginal secretions, and IgA in blood. The only difference detected in women with *C. glabrata* vaginitis was a small but significantly lower level of sIgA in vaginal secretions (65). Although no clear pattern of local or systemic innate or humoral immune deficiency was observed in women with *C. glabrata* vaginitis, and although local or systemic T-cell function in response to *C. glabrata* was not evaluated, it appears that identifying immunological deficiencies or dysfunctions in *C. glabrata*-infected women may be as difficult as it has been for those with *C. albicans* vaginitis (21, 25, 32, 65).

Our laboratory has performed a limited number of experiments involving immune reactivity to *C. glabrata.* In a limited number of tests performed with human PBLs, we recently found that human PBLs respond in vitro to heat-killed *C. glabrata* in a manner similar to that observed for *C. albicans* (PBLs from approximately 80 to 85% of normal healthy persons positively responded) (17). Thus, normal healthy adults appear to be sensitized to *C. glabrata* with demonstrable cell-mediated responsiveness, although we recognize that such responses may be the result of cross-reactive antigens with *C. albicans*-specific cells. Also, oral epithelial cells have been shown to inhibit the growth of *C. glabrata* in vitro similar to that of *C. albicans* (99). We predict a similar action by vaginal epithelial cells, although this has not been confirmed. In an animal model, we found that NOD mice infected vaginally with *C. glabrata* did not respond by DTH to *C. albicans* culture filtrate antigen (CaCF) (17), whereas mice used in the experimental *C. albicans* vaginitis model (CBA/J) readily respond to CaCF by DTH following vaginal infection (26). This suggests that a vaginal *C. glabrata* infection does not induce a systemic cell-mediated immune response that is cross-reactive or responsive to *C. albicans* antigen. Understanding the important host defenses against *C. glabrata* vaginitis will require controlled studies conducted in animal models.

CONCLUSIONS

From experimental studies using the animal model of vaginal candidiasis as well as clinical studies and observations, it is clear that the local immune response is more relevant than the systemic response in protecting the vaginal mucosa against *C. albicans* infection. In addition, the mechanisms responsible for protection against *Candida* vaginitis are different from those that protect against candidal infections at other mucosal surfaces. What is still unclear is whether the innate or adaptive immune response is more critical following exposure, and which adaptive response (humoral or CMI) is the dominant protective mechanism. With all the available information, is it possible to predict or speculate what the dominant protective mechanisms might be? In mice and humans the protection is certainly not complete, but partial at best. Clinical experience shows that some women are highly resistant to *Candida* vaginitis, never acquiring a symptomatic episode, whereas others acquire infections frequently following exposure to known exogenous predisposing factors. Still others are highly susceptible to intractable recurrent vaginitis with no known predisposing factors. In humans, too, it is important not to lose sight of the fact that *C. albicans* is also a vaginal commensal organism, and as a result, the protective host response must be sensitively programmed and controlled by positive reactivity and potential tolerizing mechanisms as is predicted from studies in mice. To this end, it appears that the vaginal immune response has evolved to keep the organism in check without promoting a vigorous inflammatory response. This appears a reasonable task for the local tissue, with its lack of organized lymphoid areas but seemingly compartmentalized property. Furthermore, recent data suggest that *C. albicans* may not be a strict vaginal opportunistic pathogen as defined by the characteristic increased incidence of infection during periods of reduced systemic immunity, although it remains unclear if it is an opportunist relative to local immunity. In actuality, the protective immune mechanisms at the vaginal mucosa probably involve several entities functioning at different levels in any one individual. Our view based on data in humans and mice is as follows. The local compartmentalized response(s) could involve innate as well as adaptive immune responses by the phenotypically distinct resident cells (i.e., $CD4^+$ α/β T cells, γ/δ T cells). The interaction of *C. albicans* with epithelial cells may be involved to control the numbers of *Candida* organisms following entry into the vagina and to produce some early cytokines, some of which may be responsible for inhibiting the systemic T-cell infiltration to avoid chronic inflammation in response to the colonizing yeast. With the lack of large numbers of resident vaginal T cells, little change in them during a *C. albicans* infection, and a strong down-regulatory cytokine response, a seemingly weak T-cell response, *Candida*-specific IgA antibodies, or action by epithelial cells, alone or in combination, could serve to maintain the immune homeostasis as well as small numbers of *Candida* organisms. However, in the absence of a systemic response, a large organism pool or inoculum brought on by any one of a number of factors (i.e., antibiotic usage, hormones, immune deficiency, behavioral factors) can easily overwhelm the existing defenses, resulting in a persistent vaginal infection that usually requires some form of antifungal therapy. Additionally, a change in antigen concentration or modulation of antigenic determinants in a genetically predisposed host, away from that recognized as commensal, may shift a weak protective response to one that promotes susceptibility to infection (i.e., Th1/Th2). Another hypothesis is that nonprotective *Candida*-specific antibodies may be produced in high titers at the expense of protective antibodies. Under these circumstances, one might speculate that the host could benefit from a systemic anti-*Candida* response to aid the relatively weak or dysfunctional local response. Thus, a key to effective absolute immune protection may be to provide the necessary immunomodulators (cytokines/chemokines) to up-regulate adhesion molecules and initiate the systemic infiltration of CMI and the associated inflammation at a time when it is needed the most. Clearly the rat appears to have these factors, based on the fairly vigorous response observed during a vaginal infection. Therefore, the rat model appears more valuable to understand what a protective response against the vaginal infection should be, whereas the value of the mouse model lies in the ability to better understand the apparent vaginal immunoregulation or tolerance predicted in humans. Together, the results from both models may lead to immunotherapies that can be used together with antifungal agents to prevent or treat *Candida* vaginitis. The nonhuman primate model, too, with more characteristics similar to the human conditions, might also be useful for future immunotherapeutic or immunopathogenic studies relative to *Candida* vaginal infections. Is vaccination an option? The preexisting *Candida*-specific adaptive immunity precludes the use of a strict vaccination strategy. Rather, an immunotherapeutic approach directing or redirecting the existing immune response is probably more appropriate. The continued use of animal models and clinical studies will be critical to achieving these goals.

Acknowledgments. We thank Floyd L. Wormley, Jr., Chad Steele, Brad Taylor, Michael Saavedra, Mace Scott, Wei Luo, Vitali Lounev, and Marc Baker of Louisiana State University Health Sciences, New Orleans, and Norbert Wolf and Jessica Cutright of Wayne State University School of Medicine, Detroit, for their scientific contributions in the mouse and nonhuman primate models of experimental vaginitis as well as clinical studies described in the manuscript. We also thank Antonio Cassone and Flavia De Bernardis of Rome, Italy, for their scientific contributions in the rat model of *Candida* vaginitis. Finally, we acknowledge the National Institute of Allergy and Infectious Diseases for supporting a considerable portion of the work summarized in this chapter (AI-32556; AI-41693).

REFERENCES

1. **Arancia, G., A. Molinari, P. Crateri, A. Stringaro, C. Ramoni, M. L. Dupuis, M. J. Gomez, A. Torosantucci, and A. Cassone.** 1995. Noninhibitory binding of human interleukin-2-activated natural killer cells to the germ tube forms of *Candida albicans*. *Infect. Immun.* **63:**280–288.
2. **Black, C. A., F. M. Eyers, M. L. Dunkley, R. L. Clancy, and K. W. Beagley.** 1999. Major histocompatibility haplotype does not impact the course of experimentally induced murine vaginal candidiasis. *Lab Anim. Sci.* **49:**668–672.
3. **Black, C. A., F. M. Eyers, A. Russell, M. L. Dunkley, R. L. Clancy, and K. W. Beagley.** 1998. Acute neutropenia decreases inflammation associated with murine vaginal candidiasis but has no effect on the course of infection. *Infect. Immun.* **66:**1273–1275.
4. **Black, C. A., F. M. Eyers, A. Russell, M. L. Dunkley, R. L. Clancy, and K. W. Beagley.** 1999. Increased severity of *Candida* vaginitis in BALB/c *nu/nu* mice versus the parent strain is not abrogated by adoptive transfer of T cell enriched lymphocytes. *J. Reprod. Immunol.* **45:**1–18.
5. **Burns, D. N., R. Tuomala, B. H. Chang, R. Hershow, H. Minkoff, E. Rodriquez, C. Zorrilla, H. Hammill, and J. Regan.** 1997. Vaginal colonization or infection with *Candida albicans* in human immunodeficiency virus-infected women during pregnancy and during postpartum period. *Clin. Infect. Dis.* **24:**201–210.
6. **Cain, T. K., and R. G. Rank.** 1995. Local Th1-like responses are induced by intravaginal infection of mice with the mouse

pneumonitis biovar of *Chlamydia trachomatis*. *Infect. Immun.* **63**:1784–1789.

7. **Cantorna, M. T., D. Mook, and E. Balish.** 1990. Resistance of congenitally immunodeficient gnotobiotic mice to vaginal candidasis. *Infect. Immun.* **58**:3813–3815.
8. **Casadevall, A.** 1995. Antibody immunity and invasive fungal infections. *Infect. Immun.* **63**:4211–4218.
9. **Cassone, A., M. Boccanera, D. A. Adriani, G. Santoni, and F. De Bernardis.** 1995. Rats clearing a vaginal infection by *Candida albicans* acquire specific, antibody-mediated resistance to vaginal infection. *Infect. Immun.* **63**:2619–2624.
10. **Cenci, E., A. Mencacci, R. Spaccapelo, L. Tonnetti, P. Mosci, K. H. Enssle, P. Puccetti, L. Romani, and F. Bistoni.** 1995. T helper cell type 1 (Th1)- and Th2-like responses are present in mice with gastric candidiasis but protective immunity is associated with Th1 development. *J. Infect. Dis.* **171**: 1279–1288.
11. **Clark, R. A., S. A. Blakley, J. Rice, and W. Brandon.** 1995. Predictors of HIV progression in women. *J. Acquir. Immune. Defic. Syndr. Hum. Retrovirol.* **9**:43–50.
12. **Corrigan, E. M., R. L. Clancy, M. L. Dunkley, F. M. Eyers, and K. W. Beagley.** 1998. Cellular immunity in recurrent vulvovaginal candidiasis. *Clin. Exp. Immunol.* **111**:574–578.
13. **De Bernardis, F., M. Boccanera, D. Adriana, E. Spreghini, G. Santoni, and A. Cassone.** 1997. Protective role of antimannan and anti-aspartyl proteinase antibodies in an experimental model of *Candida albicans* vaginitis in rats. *Infect. Immun.* **65**:3399–3405.
14. **De Bernardis, F., G. Santoni, M. Boccanera, E. Spreghini, D. Adriana, L. Morelli, and A. Cassone.** 2000. Local anticandidal immune responses in a rat model of vaginal infection by and protection against *Candida albicans*. *Infect. Immun.* **68**: 3297–3304.
15. **Djeu, J. Y., and D. K. Blanchard.** 1987. Regulation of human polymorphonuclear neutrophil (PMN) activity against *Candida albicans* by large granular lymphocytes via release of a PMN-activating factor. *J. Immunol.* **139**:2761–2767.
16. **Duerr, A., M. F. Sierra, J. Feldman, L. M. Clarke, I. Ehlich, and J. Dehovitz.** 1997. Immune compromise and prevalence of Candida vulvovaginitis in human immunodeficiency virus-infected women. *Obstet. Gynecol.* **90**:252–256.
17. **Fidel, P. L. Jr.** Unpublished observations.
18. **Fidel, P. L., Jr., J. L. Cutright, and J. D. Sobel.** 1995. Effects of systemic cell-mediated immunity on vaginal candidiasis in mice resistant and susceptible to *Candida albicans* infections. *Infect. Immun.* **63**:4191–4194.
19. **Fidel, P. L., Jr., J. L. Cutright, and C. Steele.** 2000. Effects of reproductive hormones on experimental vaginal candidiasis. *Infect. Immun.* **68**:651–657.
20. **Fidel, P. L., Jr., J. L. Cutright, L. Tait, and J. D. Sobel.** 1996. A murine model of *Candida glabrata* vaginitis. *J. Infect. Dis.* **173**:425–431.
21. **Fidel, P. L., Jr., K. A. Ginsburg, J. L. Cutright, N. A. Wolf, D. Leaman, K. Dunlap, and J. D. Sobel.** 1997. Vaginal-associated immunity in women with recurrent vulvovaginal candidiasis: evidence for vaginal Th1-type responses following intravaginal challenge with *Candida* antigen. *J. Infect. Dis.* **176**: 728–739.
22. **Fidel, P. L., Jr., W. Luo, J. Chabain, N. A. Wolf, and E. Van Buren.** 1997. Use of cellular depletion analysis to examine circulation of immune effector function between the vagina and the periphery. *Infect. Immun.* **65**:3939–3943.
23. **Fidel, P. L., Jr., W. Luo, C. Steele, J. Chabain, M. Baker, and F. L. Wormley.** 1999. Analysis of vaginal cell populations during experimental vaginal candidiasis. *Infect. Immun.* **67**: 3135–3140.
24. **Fidel, P. L., Jr., M. E. Lynch, D. H. Conaway, L. Tait, and J. D. Sobel.** 1995. Mice immunized by primary vaginal *C. albicans* infection develop acquired vaginal mucosal immunity. *Infect. Immun.* **63**:547–553.
25. **Fidel, P. L., Jr., M. E. Lynch, V. Redondo-Lopez, J. D. Sobel, and R. Robinson.** 1993. Systemic cell-mediated immune reactivity in women with recurrent vulvovaginal candidiasis (RVVC). *J. Infect. Dis.* **168**:1458–1465.
26. **Fidel, P. L., Jr., M. E. Lynch, and J. D. Sobel.** 1993. *Candida*-specific cell-mediated immunity is demonstrable in mice with experimental vaginal candidiasis. *Infect. Immun.* **61**: 1990–1995.
27. **Fidel, P. L., Jr., M. E. Lynch, and J. D. Sobel.** 1993. *Candida*-specific Th1-type responsiveness in mice with experimental vaginal candidiasis. *Infect. Immun.* **61**:4202–4207.
28. **Fidel, P. L., Jr., M. E. Lynch, and J. D. Sobel.** 1994. Effects of preinduced *Candida*-specific systemic cell-mediated immunity on experimental vaginal candidiasis. *Infect. Immun.* **62**: 1032–1038.
29. **Fidel, P. L., Jr., M. E. Lynch, and J. D. Sobel.** 1995. Circulating CD4 and CD8 T cells have little impact on host defense against experimental vaginal candidiasis. *Infect. Immun.* **63**: 2403–2408.
30. **Fidel, P. L., Jr., N. A. Wolf, and M. A. KuKuruga.** 1996. T lymphocytes in the murine vaginal mucosa are phenotypically distinct from those in the periphery. *Infect. Immun.* **64**: 3793–3799.
31. **Fidel, P. L., Jr., F. L. Wormley, Jr., and V. Lounev.** 2001. Analysis of the CD4 protein on human vaginal $CD4^+$ T cells. *Am. J. Reprod. Immunol.* **45**:200–204.
32. **Fong, I. W., P. McCleary, and S. Read.** 1992. Cellular immunity of patients with recurrent or refractory vulvovaginal moniliasis. *Am. J. Obstet. Gynecol.* **166**:887–890.
33. **Fratti, R. A., M. A. Ghannoum, J. E. Edwards, Jr., and S. G. Filler.** 1996. Gamma interferon protects endothelial cells from damage by *Candida albicans* by inhibiting endothelial cell phagocytosis. *Infect. Immun.* **64**:4714–4718.
34. **Geiger, A. M., B. Foxman, and J. D. Sobel.** 1995. Chronic vulvovaginal candidiasis: characteristics of women with *Candida albicans, Candida glabrata,* and no *Candida*. *Genitourin. Med.* **71**:304–307.
35. **Giraldo, P., A. Neuer, I. L. Korneeva, A. Ribeiro-Filho, J. A. Simoes, and S. S. Witkin.** 1999. Vaginal heat shock protein expression in symptom-free women with a history of recurrent vulvovaginitis. *Am. J. Obstet. Gynecol.* **180**:524–529.
36. **Giraldo, P. C., A. D. Ribeiro-Filho, J. A. Simoes, A. Neuer, S. B. Feitosa, and S. S. Witkin.** 1999. Circulating heat shock proteins in women with a history of recurrent vulvovaginitis. *Infect. Dis. Obstet. Gynecol.* **7**:128–132.
37. **Han, Y., R. P. Morrison, and J. E. Cutler.** 1998. A vaccine and monoclonal antibodies that enhance mouse resistance to *Candida albicans* vaginal infection. *Infect. Immun.* **66**: 5771–5776.
38. **Han, Y., M. H. Riesselman, and J. E. Cutler.** 2000. Protection against candidiasis by an immunoglobulin G3 (IgG3) monoclonal antibody specific for the same mannotriose as an IgM protective antibody. *Infect. Immun.* **68**:1649–1654.
39. **Hector, R. F., J. E. Domer, and E. W. Carrow.** 1982. Immune responses to *Candida albicans* in genetically distinct mice. *Infect. Immun.* **38**:1020–1028.
40. **Hedges, S. R., W. W. Agace, and C. Svanborg.** 1995. Epithelial cytokine responses and mucosal cytokine networks. *Trends Microbiol.* **3**:266–270.
41. **Hladik, F., G. Lentz, E. Delpit, A. McElroy, and M. J. McElrath.** 1999. Coexpression of CCR5 and IL-2 in human genital

but not blood cells: implications for the ontogeny of the CCR5+ Th1 phenotype. *J. Immunol.* **163**:2306–2313.

42. **Hobbs, J. R., D. Briden, F. Davidson, M. Kahan, and J. K. Oates.** 1977. Immunological aspects of candidal vaginitis. *Proc. R. Soc. Med.* **70**:11–14.
43. **Ibraghimov, A. R., R. E. Sacco, M. Sandor, Z. Iakoubov, and R. G. Lynch.** 1995. Resident CD4^{+} $\alpha\beta$ T cells of the murine female genital tract: a phenotypically distinct T cell lineage that rapidly proliferates in response to systemic T cell activation stimuli. *Int. Immunol.* **7**:1763–1769.
44. **Imam, N., C. C. J. Carpenter, K. H. Mayer, A. Fisher, M. Stein, and S. B. Danforth.** 1990. Hierarchical pattern of mucosal *Candida* infections in HIV-seropositive women. *Am. J. Med.* **89**:142–146.
45. **Inghirami, G., B. Y. Zhu, L. Chess, and D. M. Knowles.** 1990. Flow cytometric and immunohistochemical characterization of the gamma/delta T-lymphocyte population in normal human lymphoid tissue and peripheral blood. *Am. J. Pathol.* **136**:357–367.
46. **Itohara, S., A. G. Farr, J. J. Lafaille, M. Bonneville, Y. Takagaki, W. Haas, and S. Tonegawa.** 1990. Homing of a gamma/delta thymocyte subset with homogenous T-cell receptors to mucosal epithelia. *Nature* **343**:754–757.
47. **Johansson, E.-L., A. Rudin, L. Wassen, and J. Holmgren.** 2000. Distribution of lymphocytes and adhesion molecules in human cervix and vagina. *Immunology* **96**:272–277.
48. **Jones-Carson, J., A. Vazquez-Torres, H. C. van der Heyde, T. Warner, R. D. Wagner, and E. Balish.** 1995. γ/δ T cell-induced nitric oxide production enhances resistance to mucosal candidiasis. *Nat. Med.* **6**:552–557.
49. **Kelly, K. A., H. L. Gray, J. C. Walker, R. G. Rank, F. L. Wormley, Jr., and P. L. Fidel, Jr.** 2001. *Chlamydia trachomatis* infection does not enhance local cellular immunity against concurrent *Candida albicans* vaginal infection. *Infect. Immun.* **69**:3451–3454.
50. **Kelly, K. A., and R. G. Rank.** 1997. Identification of homing receptors that mediate the recruitment of CD4 T cells to the genital tract following intravaginal infection with *Chlamydia trachomatis. Infect. Immun.* **65**:5198–5208.
51. **Kent, H. L.** 1991. Epidemiology of vaginitis. *Am. J. Obstet. Gynecol.* **165**:1168–1175.
52. **Kinsman, O. S., and A. E. Collard.** 1986. Hormonal factors in vaginal candidiasis in rats. *Infect. Immun.* **53**:498–504.
53. **Kirkpatrick, C. H., R. R. Rich, and J. E. Bennett.** 1971. Chronic mucocutaneous candidiasis: model building in cellular immunity. *Ann. Intern. Med.* **75**:955–978.
54. **Klein, R. S., C. A. Harris, C. B. Small, B. Moll, M. Lesser, and G. H. Friedland.** 1984. Oral candidiasis in high-risk patients as the initial manifestation of the acquired immunodeficiency syndrome. *N. Engl. J. Med.* **311**:354–357.
55. **Klink, M., B. Rozalaska, and W. Rudnicka.** 1993. Weakness of cellular response to Listeria antigens in pregnant mice. *Medycyna Doswiadczalna i Mikrobiologia* **45**:51–54. (In Polish.)
56. **Knight, L., and J. Fletcher.** 1971. Growth of *Candida albicans* in saliva: stimulation by glucose associated with antibiotics, corticosteroids and diabetes mellitus. *J. Infect. Dis.* **123**: 371–377.
57. **Kutteh, W. H., Z. Moldoveanu, and J. Mestecky.** 1998. Mucosal immunity in the female reproductive tract: correlation of immunoglobulins, cytokines, and reproductive hormones in human cervical mucus around the time of ovulation. *AIDS Res. Hum. Retrovir.* **14**:51–55.
58. **Leigh, J. E., M. Barousse, R. K. Swoboda, T. Myers, S. Hager, N. A. Wolf, J. L. Cutright, J. Thompson, J. D. Sobel, and P. L. Fidel, Jr.** 2001. *Candida*-specific systemic cell-mediated immune reactivities in HIV-infected persons with and without mucosal candidiasis. *J. Infect. Dis.* **183**:277–285.
59. **Little, C. H., G. M. Georgiou, A. Marceglia, H. Ogedgebe, R. E. Cone, and D. Mazza.** 2000. Measurement of T-cell-derived antigen binding molecules and immunoglobulin G specific to *Candida albicans* mannan in sera of patients with recurrent vulvovaginal candidiasis. *Infect. Immun.* **68**: 3840–3847.
60. **Lohman, B., C. J. Miller, and M. B. McChesney.** 1995. Antiviral cytotoxic T lymphocytes in vaginal mucosa of simian immunodeficiency virus-infected rhesus macaques. *J. Immunol.* **155**:5855–5860.
61. **Lynch, M. E., J. D. Sobel, and P. L. Fidel, Jr.** 1996. Role of antifungal drug resistance in the pathogenesis of recurrent vulvovaginal candidasis. *J. Med. Vet. Mycol.* **34**:337–339.
62. **Mathur, S., R. S. Mathur, J. M. Goust, H. O. Williamson, and H. H. Fundenberg.** 1979. Cyclic variations in white cell subpopulations in the human menstrual cycle: correlations with progesterone and estradiol. *Clin. Immunol Immunopathol.* **13**:246–253.
63. **Mathur, S., G. Virella, J. Koistinen, E. O. Horger, T. A. Mahvi, and H. H. Fudenberg.** 1977. Humoral immunity in vaginal candidiasis. *Infect. Immun.* **15**:287–294.
64. **Mazumder, D. N., N. Ghose, J. Mirta, G. Dutta, and A. Santra.** 1990. Immunological status of women with prolonged oral contraceptives and occurrence of giardiasis. *J. Indian Med. Assoc.* **88**:129–131.
65. **Mendling, W., and U. Koldovsky.** 1996. Immunological investigations in vaginal mycoses. *Mycoses* **39**:177–183.
66. **Mendling, W., and U. Koldovsky.** 1996. Investigations by cell-mediated immunologic tests and therapeutic trials with thymopentin in vaginal mycoses. *Infect. Dis. Obstet. Gynecol.* **4**:225–231.
67. **Miller, C. J., M. McChesney, and P. F. Moore.** 1992. Langerhans cells, macrophages, and lymphocyte subsets in the cervix and vagina of rhesus macaques. *Lab. Invest.* **67**: 628–634.
68. **Mossman, T. R., and R. L. Coffman.** 1989. Th1 and Th2 cells: different patterns of lymphokine secretion lead to different functional properties. *Ann. Rev. Immunol.* **7**:145–173.
69. **Mulero-Marchese, R. D., K. J. Blank, and T. G. Sieck.** 1998. Genetic basis for protection against experimental vaginal candidiasis by peripheral immunization. *J. Infect. Dis.* **178**: 227–234.
70. **Mulero-Marchese, R. D., K. J. Blank, and T. G. Sieck.** 1999. Strain-dependent migration of lymphocytes to the vaginal mucosa after peripheral immunization. *Immunogenetics* **49**: 973–980.
71. **Nandi, D., and J. P. Allison.** 1991. Phenotypic analysis and gamma/delta-T cell receptor repertoire of murine T cells associated with the vaginal epithelium. *J. Immunol.* **147**: 1773–1778.
72. **Nawrot, U., K. Grzybek-Hryncewicz, U. Zielska, A. Czarny, and J. Podwinska.** 2000. The study of cell-mediated immune response in recurrent vulvovaginal candidiasis. *FEMS Immunol. Med. Microbiol.* **29**:89–94.
73. **Odds, F. C.** 1988. Chronic mucocutaneous candidiosis, p. 104–110. *In Candida and Candidosis.* University Park Press, Baltimore, Md.
74. **Parr, M. B., L. Kepple, and E. L. Parr.** 1991. Antigen recognition in the female reproductive tract. II. Endocytosis of horseradish peroxidase by Langerhans cells in murine vaginal epithelium. *Biol. Reprod.* **45**:261–265.
75. **Parr, M. B., and E. L. Parr.** 1990. Antigen recognition in the female reproductive tract: I. Uptake of intraluminal protein

tracers in the mouse vagina. *J. Reprod. Immunol.* **17:** 101–114.
76. **Parr, M. B., and E. L. Parr.** 1991. Langerhans cells and T lymphocyte subsets in the murine vagina and cervix. *Biol. Reprod.* **44:**491–498.
77. **Parr, M. B., and E. L. Parr.** 1997. Protective immunity against HSV-2 in the mouse vagina. *J. Reprod. Immunol.* **36:**77–92.
78. **Parr, M. B., and E. L. Parr.** 1998. Mucosal immunity to herpes simplex virus type 2 infection in the mouse vagina is impaired by in vivo-depletion of T lymphocytes. *J. Virol.* **72:** 2677–2685.
79. **Polonelli, L., F. De Bernardis, S. Conti, M. Boccanera, M. Gerloni, G. Morace, W. Magliani, C. Chezzi, and A. Cassone.** 1994. Idiotypic intravaginal vaccination to protect against candidal vaginitis by secretory, yeast killer toxin-like anti-idiotypic antibodies. *J. Immunol.* **152:**3175–3182.
80. **Polonelli, L., F. De Bernardis, S. Conti, M. Boccanera, W. Magliani, M. Gerloni, C. Cantella, and A. Cassone.** 1996. Human natural yeast killer toxin-like candidicidal antibodies. *J. Immunol.* **156:**1880–1885.
81. **Rakasz, E., M. Hagen, M. Sandor, and R. G. Lynch.** 1997. $\gamma\delta$ T cells of the murine vagina: T cell response in vivo in the absence of the expression of CD2 and CD28 molecules. *Int. Immunol.* **9:**161–167.
82. **Rakasz, E., M. Sandor, M. Hagen, and R. G. Lynch.** 1996. Activation features of intraepithelial $\gamma\delta$ T-cells of the murine vagina. *Immunol. Lett.* **54:**129–134.
83. **Redondo-Lopez, V., M. Lynch, C. Schmitt, R. Cook, and J. D. Sobel.** 1990. *Torulopsis glabrata* vaginitis: clinical aspects and susceptibility to antifungal agents. *Obstet. Gynecol.* **76:** 651–655.
84. **Regulez, P., J. F. Garcia Fernandez, M. D. Moragues, J. Schneider, G. Quindos, and J. Ponton.** 1994. Detection of anti-*Candida albicans* IgE antibodies in vaginal washes from patients with acute vulvovaginal candidiasis. *Gynecol. Obstet. Invest.* **37:**110–114.
85. **Rhoads, J. L., D. C. Wright, R. R. Redfield, and D. S. Burke.** 1987. Chronic vaginal candidiasis in women with human immunodeficiency virus infection. *JAMA* **257:**3105–3107.
86. **Romani, L., A. Mencacci, E. Cenci, R. Spaccapelo, P. Mosci, P. Puccetti, and F. Bistoni.** 1993. CD+ subset expression in murine candidiasis. *J. Immunol.* **150:**925–931.
87. **Romani, L., S. Mocci, C. Bietta, L. Lanfaloni, P. Puccetti, and F. Bistoni.** 1991. Th1 and Th2 cytokine secretion patterns in murine candidiasis: association of Th1 responses with acquired resistance. *Infect. Immun.* **59:**4647–4654.
88. **Ryley, J. F., and S. McGregor.** 1986. Quantitation of vaginal *Candida albicans* infections in rodents. *J. Med. Vet. Mycol.* **24:**455–460.
89. **Saavedra, M., B. Taylor, N. W. Lukacs, and P. L. Fidel, Jr.** 1999. Local production of chemokines during experimental vaginal candidiasis. *Infect. Immun.* **67:**5820–5829.
90. **Sallusto, F., A. Lanzavecchia, and C. R. Mackay.** 1998. Chemokines and chemokine receptors in T-cell priming and Th1/Th2-mediated responses. *Immunol. Today* **19:**568–574.
91. **Samaranayake, L. P.** 1992. Oral mycoses in HIV infection. *Oral Surg. Oral Med. Oral Pathol.* **73:**171–180.
92. **Schuman, P., J. D. Sobel, S. Ohmit, K. H. Mayer, A. Rompalo, A. Duerr, D. K. Smith, D. Warren, and R. S. Klein.** 1998. Mucosal candidal colonization and candidiasis in women with or at risk for human immunodeficiency virus infection. *Clin. Infect. Dis.* **27:**1161–1167.
93. **Sobel, J. D.** 1988. Pathogenesis and epidemiology of vulvovaginal candidiasis. *Ann. N. Y. Acad. Sci.* **544:**547–557.
94. **Sobel, J. D.** 1992. Pathogenesis and treatment of recurrent vulvovaginal candidiasis. *Clin. Infect. Dis.* **14:**S148–S153.
95. **Sobel, J. D.** Unpublished observations.
96. **Sobel, J. D., and W. Chaim.** 1997. Treatment of *Torulopsis glabrata* vaginitis: retrospective review of boric acid therapy. *Clin. Infect. Dis.* **24:**649–652.
97. **Sonoda, Y., N. Mukaida, J. Wang, M. Shimada-Hiratsuka, M. Naito, T. Kasahara, A. Harada, M. Inoue, and K. Matsushima.** 1998. Physiologic regulation of postovulatory neutrophil migration into vagina in mice by a C-X-C chemokine. *J. Immunol.* **160:**6159–6165.
98. **Spinillo, A., G. Michelone, C. Cavanna, L. Colonna, E. Capuzzo, and S. Nicola.** 1994. Clinical and microbiological characteristics of symptomatic vulvovaginal candidiasis in HIV-seropositive women. *Genitourin. Med.* **70:**268–272.
99. **Steele, C., J. E. Leigh, R. K. Swoboda, and P. L. Fidel, Jr.** 2000. Growth inhibition of *Candida* by human oral epithelial cells. *J. Infect. Dis.* **182:**1479–1485.
100. **Steele, C., H. Ozenci, W. Luo, M. Scott, and P. L. Fidel, Jr.** 1999. Growth inhibition of *Candida albicans* by vaginal cells from naive mice. *J. Med. Mycol.* **37:**251–260.
101. **Steele, C., M. Ratterree, and P. L. Fidel, Jr.** 1999. Differential susceptibility to experimental vaginal candidiasis in macaques. *J. Infect. Dis.* **180:**802–810.
102. **Syverson, R. A., H. Buckley, J. Gibian, and J. J. M. Ryan.** 1979. Cellular and humoral immune status in women with chronic *Candida* vaginitis. *Am. J. Obstet. Gynecol.* **134:** 624–627.
103. **Taylor, B. N., M. Saavedra, and P. L. Fidel, Jr.** 2000. Local Th1/Th2 cytokine production during experimental vaginal candidiasis. *J. Med. Mycol.* **38:**419–431.
104. **Valentin, A., C. Bernard, M. Mallie, M. Huerre, and J. M. Bastide.** 1993. Control of *Candida albicans* vaginitis in mice by short-duration butoconazole treatment in situ. *Mycoses* **36:**379–384.
105. **White, H. D., K. M. Crassi, A. L. Givan, J. E. Stern, J. L. Gonzalez, V. A. Memoli, W. R. Green, and C. R. Wira.** 1997. CD3+ CD8+ CTL activity within the human female reproductive tract: influence of stage of the menstrual cycle and menopause. *J. Immunol.* **158:**3017–3027.
106. **White, M. H.** 1996. Is vulvovaginal candidiasis an AIDS-related illness. *Clin. Infect. Dis.* **22**(Suppl. 2):S124–S127.
107. **Witkin, S. S.** 1986. Inhibition of *Candida*-induced lymphocyte proliferation by antibody to *Candida albicans. Obstet. Gynecol.* **68:**696–699.
108. **Witkin, S. S., J. Hirsch, and W. J. Ledger.** 1986. A macrophage defect in women with recurrent *Candida* vaginitis and its reversal in vitro by prostaglandin inhibitors. *Am. J. Obstet. Gynecol.* **155:**790–795.
109. **Witkin, S. S., J. Jeremias, and W. J. Ledger.** 1988. A localized vaginal allergic response in women with recurrent vaginitis. *J. Allergy Clin. Immunol.* **81:**412–416.
110. **Witkin, S. S., J. Jeremias, and W. J. Ledger.** 1989. Vaginal eosinophils and IgE antibodies to *Candida albicans* in women with recurrent vaginitis. *J. Med. Vet. Mycol.* **27:**57–58.
111. **Witkin, S. S., A. Kalo-Klein, L. Galland, M. Teich, and W. J. Ledger.** 1991. Effect of *Candida albicans* plus histamine on prostaglandin E2 production by peripheral blood mononuclear cells from healthy women and women with recurrent candidal vaginitis. *J. Infect. Dis.* **164:**396–399.
112. **Wormley, F. L., Jr., M. Scott, W. Luo, M. Baker, J. Chaiban, and P. L. Fidel, Jr.** 2000. Evidence for a unique expression of CD4 on murine vaginal $CD4^+$ cells. *Immunology* **100:** 300–308.
113. **Wormley, F. L., Jr., C. Steele, K. Wozniak, K. Fujihashi, J. R. McGhee, and P. L. Fidel, Jr.** Resistance of TCR δ-chain-deficient mice to experimental *Candida* vaginitis. *Infect. Immun.*, in press.

Candida and Candidiasis
Edited by Richard A. Calderone

Chapter 15

Immunology of Cutaneous Candidiasis

Peter G. Sohnle, Maqsood Bhatti, and David K. Wagner

This chapter will review the major mechanisms involved in the defense against cutaneous candidiasis. In this condition the epidermis of the skin is infected by *Candida albicans* and occasionally certain non-*C. albicans* species, with chronic mucocutaneous candidiasis representing a subgroup of syndromes with particularly chronic and recalcitrant superficial *Candida* infections. Local and systemic defenses against *Candida* spp. and cutaneous candidiasis will be reviewed with an emphasis on the immunological predispositions that have been described in chronic mucocutaneous candidiasis. In particular, this discussion will cover the elements of the cutaneous immune system, the mechanisms of immunologic deficits in chronic mucocutaneous candidiasis, and the role of cytokines in the defense against cutaneous *Candida* infections. Implications for possible reversal of the immunologic abnormalities as an adjunct to the use of antifungal drugs for the treatment of chronic mucocutaneous candidiasis will also be addressed.

CHARACTERISTICS OF CUTANEOUS CANDIDIASIS

Cutaneous candidiasis is an infection of the skin that is generally caused by the fungus *C. albicans* and that can be either acute or chronic in nature. Cases are sometimes seen of cutaneous candidiasis caused by other *Candida* species, including *C. parapsilosis* or *C. tropicalis,* but these are rare. Recently, *C. glabrata* has developed increased importance as a cause of human disease and currently ranks second or third as the agent of superficial (cutaneous or mucosal) or deep candidiasis (34). *C. albicans* is part of the normal flora of the gastrointestinal tract rather than that of the skin, although it can be found on the skin on occasion. This organism can grow as either yeast cells or filamentous forms, with mixtures of the two phases often seen in the cutaneous infections. As discussed elsewhere, the virulence of *C. albicans* has been attributed variously to its ability to grow at particular temperatures, its ability to produce filamentous forms, its adherence capabilities, and the activity of its different enzymes.

Acute cutaneous candidiasis may present as intertrigo, with production of intense erythema, edema, creamy exudate, and satellite pustules within folds of the skin. Other infections may be more chronic, as in the feet where there can be a thick white layer of infected stratum corneum overlaying the epidermis of the interdigital spaces. *Candida* paronychia is marked by infections of the periungual skin and the nail itself, resulting in the typical swelling and redness of this type of *Candida* infection.

In some cases superficial *C. albicans* infections may be particularly severe and recalcitrant to treatment, producing the uncommon disorder known as chronic mucocutaneous candidiasis. This condition consists of persistent and recurrent infections of the mucous membranes, skin, and nails, along with a variety of other manifestations. The superficial infections last for years in the affected patients unless they are properly treated; however, deep *Candida* infections are very rare in this situation (46). Oral thrush and *Candida* vaginitis are fairly common in patients with chronic mucocutaneous candidiasis. There is often infection of the esophagus, although further extension into the viscera is unusual. The typical skin lesions are generally red, raised, and hyperkeratotic, but usually are not painful. Epidermal neutrophilic microabscesses, which are common in acute cutaneous candidiasis, are rare in the lesions of chronic mucocutaneous candidiasis. Nail involvement can be severe

Peter G. Sohnle, Maqsood Bhatti, and David K. Wagner • Division of Infectious Diseases, Department of Medicine, Medical College of Wisconsin, Milwaukee, WI 53226, and Infectious Diseases Section, Consultant Care Division, VA Medical Center, Milwaukee, WI 53295.

in this condition, producing marked thickening, distortion, and fragmentation of the nails, with chronic swelling of the distal phalanx. The oral thrush and vaginitis in chronic mucocutaneous candidiasis closely resemble the acute mucous membrane infections in other patients, except that they are more chronic in nature. The oral lesions are generally tender and painful.

There are a number of other disorders that are associated with the syndrome of chronic mucocutaneous candidiasis (35, 49). Especially prominent are certain types of endocrine dysfunction, such as hypoadrenalism, hypoparathyroidism, hypothyroidism, ovarian insufficiency, pernicious anemia, and diabetes mellitus. The combination of chronic superficial candidiasis and endocrine hypofunction has been termed the "*Candida* endocrinopathy" syndrome. More recently the term autoimmune polyendocrinopathy-candidiasis-ectodermal dystrophy (APECED) has been used to describe this syndrome (11). A particular gene, AIRE (for autoimmune regulator), appears to be responsible for this syndrome in both humans and mice (57, 75). The product of the AIRE gene is predicted as a proline-rich polypeptide with two zinc-finger motifs and a putative nuclear targeting signal, suggesting involvement in the regulation of transcription; this protein is expressed in the thymus, as well as the pancreas and adrenal cortex, and may be involved in the molecular pathogenesis of APECED and other types of autoimmunity (10).

Sometimes found in patients with chronic mucocutaneous candidiasis are alopecia totalis, vitiligo, malabsorption, chronic hepatitis, dysplasia of the dental enamel, congenital thymic dysplasia, thymomas, and other infections. Among the latter, chronic dermatophytosis, recurrent bacterial infections, and occasional opportunistic infections such as cryptococcosis, histoplasmosis, and *Pneumocystis carinii* pneumonia are the most common (31, 35, 47). In these patients dermatophytosis may cause extensive skin lesions that may be misidentified as cutaneous candidiasis and then perhaps not be treated optimally (18). Chronic mucocutaneous candidiasis no doubt represents a group of syndromes, in addition to APECED, with a variety of predisposing or secondary abnormalities in host defense function. Therefore, it may be difficult to describe an immunologic pattern that includes all patients. The most common deficiency appears to be one of cell-mediated immune responses against *Candida* antigens, as discussed below, although abnormalities in chemotaxis or phagocytic cell function have also been reported; other host defense mechanisms, such as humoral immunity and the complement system, have generally been found to be normal in these patients.

Although the superficial infections of chronic mucocutaneous candidiasis are generally not life threatening, they can be very disfiguring. Before the azole antifungal agents became available, the treatment of this condition was quite difficult. Whereas amphotericin B produced prompt clearance of the cutaneous lesions, relapses usually occurred, presumably because of the underlying immunodeficiency state. At the present, long-term treatment with azole antifungal drugs can produce good results in chronic mucocutaneous candidiasis, although occasional failures have occurred due to the development of resistant strains of *C. albicans*. Also, endocrine dysfunction, including life-threatening adrenal crises, can develop after presentation of the candidiasis, so these patients need to be followed for this possibility. Patients who present with chronic mucocutaneous candidiasis should also be evaluated for the presence of infection with the human immunodeficiency virus (HIV), and if presenting as adults, for the possibility of thymoma.

CUTANEOUS DEFENSES

Predisposing Factors to Cutaneous Candidiasis

A variety of local and systemic factors predispose to superficial fungal infections. Cutaneous candidiasis most frequently occurs when there are warm, moist conditions such as in skin folds, under the diapers of newborns, and also in tropical climates or during the summer months. Otherwise, treatments with corticosteroids, cytotoxic agents, broad-spectrum antibiotics, and oral contraceptives all predispose to various forms of candidiasis. Diabetes mellitus and infection with HIV are both strongly associated with superficial candidiasis, although disseminated candidiasis is unusual in these conditions. In diabetes mellitus a variety of disturbances in immune and phagocytic cell functions may be involved in the increased susceptibility to infection, and particularly with *C. albicans,* there may be increased adherence to diabetic cells (40). Deficiency of the neutrophil enzyme myeloperoxidase may be associated with cutaneous candidiasis, presumably because of diminished ability to produce fungicidal oxidants (65). In fact, addition of recombinant human myeloperoxidase enhances the ability of activated macrophages to kill *C. albicans* in vitro (55). Genetic predisposition may be important in chronic mucocutaneous candidiasis in that approximately 25% of these patients have relatives with this disease (43). The hyper-immunoglobulin E (IgE) syndrome is another condition in which cutaneous candidiasis as well as recurrent staphylococcal abscesses are common; this syndrome has complicated effects on the host defense system, possibly mediated in part by IgE antibodies against *Candida* or staphylococcal antigens (18, 24).

Nonimmunologic Cutaneous Defenses

Structure of the skin

The physical and chemical structure of the skin represents a form of defense against fungal pathogens. In keratinized epithelia the stratum corneum has a structure of protein-enriched corneocytes embedded in a continuous, lipid-enriched, intercellular matrix in the "bricks and mortar" model (29, 79). This makeup lends tensile strength to the skin and also may protect it from invasion by microorganisms. In addition, the skin surface is relatively inhospitable to fungal growth because of exposure to ultraviolet light, low moisture conditions, and competition from the normal bacterial flora of this site. Therefore, this surface acts as a barrier to the entry of fungi. The stratum corneum is made up of keratin, which most microorganisms cannot use for nutrition. However, *C. albicans* produces proteases (keratinases) that hydrolyze this substance and facilitate the growth of these organisms in the stratum corneum itself (63). These enzymes are secreted aspartyl proteases and in one study of *C. parapsilosis* were found in higher concentrations in skin versus blood isolates (23). The very superficial site of infection in the stratum corneum may protect the infecting organisms from direct contact with at least some of the effector cells of the immune system. Although neutrophils and small numbers of lymphocytes may enter the epidermis, the major infiltrates of cell-mediated immune responses are generally confined to the dermis.

Keratinization and epidermal proliferation

The process by which the stratum corneum is continually renewed through keratinization of the epidermal cells may also present a form of defense against organisms infecting this site. The anatomy of the normal skin is shown in Fig. 1. Basal epidermal cells produce continued growth of the epidermis as they undergo repeated cell divisions that move the resulting daughter cells (keratinocytes) outward, toward the surface. As they mature, these cells lose their nuclei and become flattened to form the keratinized cells. This process results in shedding of the stratum corneum, which also may remove infecting fungal microorganisms residing there. Keratinocytes in the periphery of a similar kind of superficial fungal infection, annular dermatophytosis, have been found to divide at an increased rate (7). Inflammation, including that produced by cell-mediated immune reactions, appears to enhance epidermal proliferation so that rates of transit of epidermal cells toward the stratum corneum are increased (53). Epidermal proliferation in experimental cutaneous candidiasis appears to be enhanced by cell-mediated immune responses to fungal antigens in the infected skin and may play a role in the defense against cutaneous candidiasis (85).

Antifungal substances

Lipids of adult hair contain saturated fatty acids that are fungistatic against *Microsporum audouini*, formerly a common cause of hair and scalp infections (76). In particular, various types of sphingosines have recently been found to be active against certain dermatophytes and *C. albicans* (8). Whereas the sebum of adults may not be significantly more fungistatic than that from children on a weight-per-weight basis, older individuals appear to produce quantitatively more of this material than do children (51). In addition, fungicidal proteins have been isolated from normal epidermis and could play some role in the defense against cutaneous fungal infections (45). *C. albicans* and the dermatophytes seem to be capable of infecting

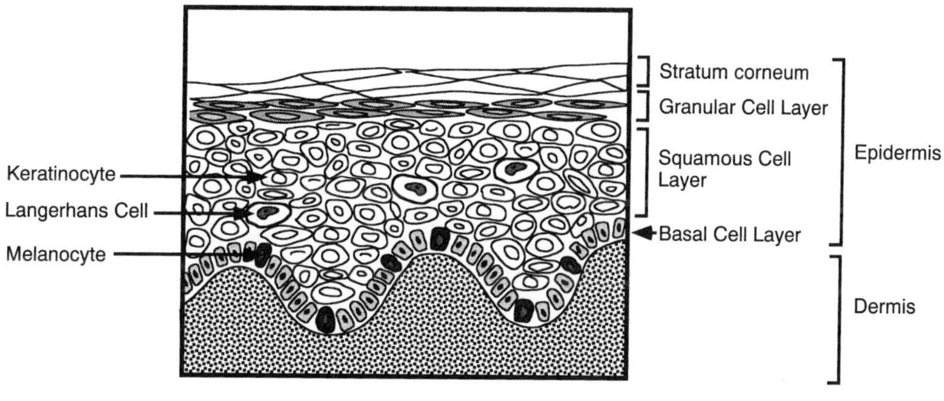

Figure 1. Anatomy of the normal skin.

the keratinized layers of the skin, and in some cases seem to be inhibited from deeper invasion. This phenomenon has been related to the presence in the dermis of unsaturated transferrin, which may prevent growth of the organisms in the deeper layers of the skin by competition for iron (32).

The Inflammatory Response

Chemotactic mechanisms

Although cutaneous candidiasis is generally limited to the most superficial layers of the skin, these infections can be highly inflammatory even in patients with evidence for various kinds of immune dysfunction. One can observe in the infected skin a variety of gross changes including scaling, pustules, and erythema. Evidence of epidermal proliferation may also be seen in the chronic infections as hyperkeratosis and parakeratosis. Microscopically, the lesions are characterized by an accumulation of neutrophils in the infected skin of acute infections, or a mononuclear cell infiltrate in the dermis of the more chronic ones. The acute inflammatory responses may be manifested as epidermal microabscesses in which the *Candida* yeast cells or filamentous forms can be seen by using appropriate special stains.

A variety of mechanisms have been described by which inflammatory cells are attracted into the sites of cutaneous fungal infections, including cutaneous candidiasis. *C. albicans* has been shown to activate complement through the alternative pathway (68). Similarly, a collagenous serum lectin, called mannose-binding lectin, has been shown to bind strongly to a variety of microorganisms including *Candida* species and promote C4 deposition in a concentration-dependent manner (64); this mechanism may be of importance in innate immunity and may represent a type of first-line defense against these organisms. *C. albicans* also produces low-molecular-weight chemotactic factors analogous to the ones made by growing bacteria (22). These factors may be of two different types, including one that seems to act through the formyl peptide receptor of neutrophils, and another that is not inhibited by an antagonist to this receptor and appears to attract macrophages through a different mechanism (28). Finally, as discussed more fully below, keratinocytes can generate chemotactic cytokines that could also be responsible for some of the inflammation in the lesions of cutaneous fungal infections. Other elements of the cutaneous immune system may also be involved in generating an inflammatory response in the infected skin of cutaneous candidiasis.

Antifungal mechanisms of phagocytic cells

Neutrophils and monocytes/macrophages appear to be important in the defense against fungi, including those involved in the cutaneous mycoses. Neutrophils can directly attack pathogens using a variety of microbicidal processes (reviewed in reference 62). Some of these processes depend on microbicidal oxidants, including superoxide, hydrogen peroxide, hypochlorous acid, and monochloramine (42, 92). Alternatively, the neutrophil killing mechanisms may involve nonoxidative granule microbicidal substances, such as the defensins (38), bactericidal/permeability-increasing protein (97), lactoferrin (2), lysozyme (21), azuricidin (15) and cathelicidin (99). Most of these substances have been studied primarily for their ability to kill the organisms, although lactoferrin may have both microbistatic and microbicidal effects (3). In studies of neutrophil-mediated damage to *C. albicans* hyphae, confocal microscopy and quantification of cell wall glycoprotein release reveal that both oxidative and nonoxidative mechanisms are required for maximal effects on the target fungal cells (20). Macrophages have an additional antimicrobial mechanism whereby they can use production of nitric oxide to inhibit growth of ingested fungal pathogens, such as *Cryptococcus neoformans* (1). This mechanism might potentially be active against the organisms causing superficial fungal infections also.

Neutrophils also appear to have significant growth-inhibitory activity in addition to their microbicidal processes. These cells contain large amounts of a calcium and zinc binding protein, called calprotectin or MRP 8/14, that has potent microbistatic activity against *C. albicans* and other fungi (82, 86). This protein is released into inflammatory exudates as neutrophils die at sites of infection (82) and could supplement other host defenses in the infected skin by controlling growth of *C. albicans* or other fungi there.

The Cutaneous Immune System

Potential role in cutaneous candidiasis

Because cutaneous fungal infections are more frequent and more severe in patients with immunologic defects, immune responses to fungal antigens would seem to play an important role in the host defense against these infections. Immunologic host defense mechanisms in normal hosts seem to be effective even when the infections are limited to superficial locations such as the stratum corneum. A number of studies suggest that the epidermis of the skin acts as a unique immunologic organ in addition to its role as a passive barrier against entry of infecting organisms. In 1983, a hypothesis regarding the skin-associated lymphoid tissue (SALT) concept was advanced wherein the skin acted as an immune surveillance unit (90). A variety of cell types are believed to have involvement in this cutaneous immune system and will be reviewed below. The mechanisms employed are complex, involving a network of fixed or mobile cells interacting either by trafficking of the cells themselves from one site to another or by the production of cytokines that influence the function of other cells. Such skin-initiated immune responses act against a broad spectrum of foreign antigens and it is likely that they are also active against *C. albicans* when it is involved in infections of the stratum corneum. Therefore, this system is probably responsible for initiating immune responses that eliminate the infecting organisms in the immune host. In addition, such responses may also produce some of the inflammation that results in much of the symptomatology of these infections. The cutaneous immune system has been reviewed in detail recently (69, 89) and will be summarized briefly here.

Cells with immunologic potential in the skin

Epidermal Langerhans cells. Langerhans cells develop as dendritic cells from bone marrow stem cells and home in to selected tissues. At least five distinct subsets of dendritic cells have been recognized, including Langerhans cells in epithelial tissues, dendritic cells in peripheral blood or lymph, interdigitating dendritic cells in T-cell dependent areas of lymphoid tissues, follicular dendritic cells in B-cell dependent areas, and dermal dendritic cells (6). Epidermal Langerhans cells make up approximately 2 to 5% of the total epidermal cell population and vary in density depending on anatomic location. These cells express a variety of antigenic markers on their surface (88) and function to present antigens in an immunologically relevant fashion to both naive and sensitized T lymphocytes.

Dermal dendritic cells. The dermis contains a population of antigen-presenting cells that constitute one of the five subsets described above. These cells have dendritic processes, are motile, and express a variety of markers, including high levels of class II major histocompatibility complex (MHC) antigen as well as certain proteins involved in adherence of one cell type to another. These cells also act as antigen-presenting cells and probably are important in the initiation of immunologic responses in the skin, particularly those involving antigens in the dermis.

Epidermal T lymphocytes. Although the lymphoid infiltrates characteristic of cutaneous cell-mediated immune responses are generally confined to the dermis of the skin, there are small numbers of T lymphocytes that are present within the epidermis (12). T lymphocyte antigen receptors are of two types, with most being of the $\alpha\beta$ heterodimer phenotype and a small population expressing the $\gamma\delta$ heterodimer. In the papillary dermis up to 80% of T lymphocytes are $\alpha\beta$ positive and approximately 7% are $\gamma\delta$ positive. In contrast, only 60% of the T lymphocytes in the epidermis are $\alpha\beta$ positive, with 18 to 29% being $\gamma\delta$ positive. Sensitized T lymphocytes can be found in the epidermis, either through antigenic stimulation of resting T lymphocytes at this site or attraction of already sensitized T lymphocytes by chemotactic cytokines, possibly including members of the interleukin (IL)-8 family produced by keratinocytes.

Keratinocytes. Keratinocytes not only have an important structural role in forming a physical barrier to foreign antigens and microorganisms, but are also important functionally in mediating cutaneous immune reactions. These cells are by far the most numerous in the epidermis, although other cell types including melanocytes and Langerhans cells are also found there (see Fig. 1). The interfollicular epidermis is divided into a series of proliferating units, known as epidermal proliferative units (67). Within an epidermal proliferative unit there are slow and fast cycling basal keratinocytes, which are distinct populations that could possibly have different functions. Other neighboring cells, Langerhans cells, and cells in the dermis appear to have a regulatory effect on keratinocytes and may lead to cellular diversity within the basal layer. Keratinocytes secrete a number of soluble factors that are capable of up-regulating and down-regulating immune responses. The IL-7 that they produce has been shown to serve as a growth factor for epidermal T lymphocytes in mice (56).

Microvascular endothelial cells. Microvascular endothelial cells are located near the microenvironment where the important cutaneous immunologic reactions occur. Endothelial cells are known to be active participants in a variety of functions, including wound healing, angiogenesis, production of clotting factors, and maintenance of vascular tone. Their role in epidermal immunologic events is not entirely clear, although there is increasing evidence for their participation in this area. Like the keratinocytes, microvascular endothelial cells secrete a number of soluble factors capable of inducing inflammation and recruiting leukocytes, and express a variety of adhesion molecules.

Initiation and expression of cutaneous immune responses

According to the SALT concept, the skin contains an immune surveillance system consisting of antigen-presenting Langerhans cells, cytokine-producing keratinocytes, epidermotropic T lymphocytes, and draining peripheral lymph nodes. Much work has been done to confirm and expand this concept. In the working hypothesis proposed for mechanisms and pathways involved in these cutaneous immune responses (69, 88), foreign antigens entering the epidermis are first ingested and processed by Langerhans cells so that the antigenic fragment is complexed to MHC-encoded antigens. Concomitantly, there is antigen-induced enhancement of cytokine production by keratinocytes, leading to activation of the Langerhans cells. Within a short time, the antigen-processing Langerhans cells leave the epidermis, enter the dermal lymphatics, and migrate as veiled cells to the draining lymph nodes. Here they present the antigen-MHC complex on their surface to the proper receptors on resting T lymphocytes and elicit an antigen-specific response in these cells. Through a second signal (IL-1) produced by the Langerhans cells, there is T-lymphocyte stimulation and subsequent clonal expansion. The resulting T-lymphocyte blasts then migrate back to the dermis and epidermis by homing to cytokine-activated microvascular endothelial cells in this area. Once in this location, the T lymphocytes can be further stimulated by other antigen-presenting cells to undergo continued clonal expansion and generation of effector cells that can help eliminate the pathogenic microorganisms. Other aspects of this immune surveillance mechanism are continuing to be elucidated and include possible other functions for the dermal dendritic cells, keratinocytes, and epidermal T lymphocytes. Each of these cell types may have other less well-defined roles in the above-described immune pathway, or they may play a more or less prominent role against a particular type of infection or other antigenic insult to the skin. The exact role of each cell type in producing immune responses against the organisms causing cutaneous mycoses has not yet been defined, although it is very likely that the immune surveillance mechanism described above is heavily involved in the defense against cutaneous candidiasis.

IMMUNOLOGY OF CUTANEOUS CANDIDIASIS

Immune Responses to *Candida* Antigens

Inoculation into the skin of viable *C. albicans* yeast cells in mice has been shown to elicit cell-mediated immune responses to various antigens of this organism (60). Experimental cutaneous candidiasis also sensitizes the infected animals so that a second infection is cleared more rapidly than is the initial one in both guinea pigs (83) and mice (98). Clearance of the organisms in these experimental infections appears to be mediated at least in part by a vigorous epidermal proliferative response associated with cell-mediated immune responses to the antigens of the organisms (83, 85). On the other hand, a certain degree of epidermal proliferation occurs in the infected skin of immunosuppressed mice, suggesting that other factors are also involved (84).

Depending on environmental conditions, *C. albicans* can grow in either yeast or filamentous forms. Therefore, it is possible that phase-specific immune responses could develop to antigens that are different between the two phases. Indeed, specific antigens have been found on the surface of cultured hyphal forms that are not present on yeast cells (91). In addition, it has been shown that antibodies in sera from some patients with candidiasis react only with germinating *C. albicans,* whereas those from normal individuals react preferentially with yeast cells (44).

Antibody against *C. albicans* is often found in high titers in human patients with chronic mucocutaneous candidiasis (4, 47, 58). Whereas an occasional patient with this condition lacks anti-*Candida* antibodies in either serum (19, 43) or saliva (52), most seem to have intact humoral immunity to *C. albicans.* Also, the patients who have been reported to have abnormal antibody production appear to be indistinguishable from other patients with chronic mucocutaneous candidiasis, so the significance of these abnormalities is uncertain. More specific tests of B-cell function may show abnormalities in patients with this condition in that Schick tests have been reported to be abnormal in some patients (14) and in vitro antibody production to *Candida* mannan by cells from patients with active *Candida* infection was found to be deficient in another study (27). Patients with the hyper-IgE syndrome often have chronic superficial *C. albicans* infections along with elevated levels of IgE antibodies to this organism (5, 78).

Most noninfected humans have evidence of cell-mediated immunity to *C. albicans,* as demonstrated by skin testing (33, 80), in vitro lymphocyte stimulation (9, 41), and lymphokine production (9, 81). On the other hand, patients with chronic mucocutaneous candidiasis often demonstrate significant immunologic defects in cell-mediated immune responses to *C. albicans* antigens, as discussed below. Even so, the pattern of immunologic abnormalities does not correlate very well with other manifestations of chronic mucocutaneous candidiasis. Also, since some uninfected relatives of patients with this condition also have diminished responsiveness to *Candida* antigens (77), this abnormality cannot entirely explain why the patients are susceptible to the fungal infections.

Mechanisms of Immunologic Defects in Cutaneous Candidiasis

Deficient cell-mediated immunity to *Candida* antigens

In patients with chronic mucocutaneous candidiasis, the most common immunologic abnormalities found are defects in cell-mediated immunity (35, 43, 47, 49). Although most of the patients have normal numbers of T lymphocytes, they often do not manifest delayed hypersensitivity responses to *Candida* extracts when skin tested. Obviously lack of exposure to the antigens cannot explain the negative skin tests since the patients are chronically infected with the organism. In vitro correlates of delayed hypersensitivity responses, including lymphocyte transformation and lymphokine production, are also abnormal in many of these patients. These deficient responses fall into the general patterns of anergy to all antigens tested, unresponsiveness to *Candida* antigens only, and normal responses to all antigens, including those from *Candida*. For example, in one study, 10 of 26 patients appeared to have normal cell-mediated immunity to *Candida* antigens (94). However, other patients appear to have significant abnormalities in lymphocyte function, with some having complete anergy to a battery of recall antigens and negative in vitro lymphocyte proliferation responses to mitogens and all antigens (49).

The abnormalities in either cutaneous delayed hypersensitivity responses or in vitro lymphocyte function do not appear to relate directly to the clinical manifestations of the mucocutaneous *Candida* infections (35). For example, subgroups of chronic mucocutaneous candidiasis patients, such as those with APECED or thymoma, do not all have the same patterns of reactivity in skin testing or in vitro lymphocyte assays, and some in each group may have apparently normal responses to *Candida* antigens in all the standard assays. Normal persons, without evidence of chronic superficial *Candida* infections, do not all react to *Candida* antigens in these assays, either; however, in this case it is possible that lack of exposure may account for negative tests in some people. In any event, it seems likely that the predisposition to chronic *Candida* infections in some patients with chronic mucocutaneous candidiasis and normal immunologic responsiveness may be due to factors other than deficient cell-mediated immunity; on the other hand, it may be that our immunologic assays are too crude to pick up subtle defects in cell-mediated immunity that do predispose the patients to these infections. In other cases it is possible that some nonimmunologic factor like antibiotic usage could initiate superficial *Candida* infections that suppress cell-mediated immunity secondarily and lead to more chronic infections; possible mechanisms involved in this type of suppression are discussed below.

Serum inhibitors

Serum inhibitors appear to account for some of the immunologic defects in patients with chronic mucocutaneous candidiasis (13, 50, 93, 94), and sometimes these defects disappear after antifungal therapy (26, 48, 93). Parenteral administration of viable *C. albicans* yeast cells or extracts of this organism to experimental animals can result in suppression of cell-mediated immunity (16, 70, 72). Carbohydrate antigens from *C. albicans,* primarily mannans, have been shown to persist in the serum of patients with chronic mucocutaneous candidiasis and suppress lymphocyte proliferation responses of cells from control subjects (36). Defective handling of mannan by monocytes from patients with chronic mucocutaneous candidiasis has been postulated as the reason why this substance accumulates in the serum of these patients (37). Mannan-derived oligosaccharides from *C. albicans* can inhibit in vitro lymphocyte proliferation induced by *Candida* antigens (66). Therefore, catabolism of mannan in vivo may generate immunoinhibitory oligosaccharides that cause the defects in cell-mediated immunity in some patients with chronic mucocutaneous candidiasis. However, other patients with this syndrome probably have immunologic abnormalities due to other mechanisms, and still others have no demonstrable immunologic abnormalities at all and may be susceptible to chronic superficial *C. albicans* infections for other reasons.

Imbalance of Th1 versus Th2 responses

T-lymphocyte subpopulations include the CD4 helper cells that secrete cytokines and the CD8 cells that are mainly cytotoxic killer cells. There are two major types of CD4 cells, including type 1 (Th1) helper cells that secrete IL-2 and gamma interferon (IFN-γ) and type 2 (Th2) cells that secrete IL-4, -5, -6, and -10, but not IL-2 or IFN-γ (25). Cytokine production influences the type of immune response needed to protect against particular types of infectious agents and may also normally reduce allergic or autoimmune responses. In particular, the production of cytokines by Th1 cells facilitates cell-mediated immunity, including the activation of macrophages and T-cell-mediated cytotoxicity; alternatively, Th2 cells help the B lymphocytes to produce antibodies. Th1 and Th2 cells may inhibit each other; for example, secretion of IFN-γ by Th1 cells inhibits Th2 cells, and secretion of IL-10 by Th2 cells reciprocally inhibits Th1 cells (61). Since the activity of Th1 cells promotes protective cell-mediated immune responses, overactivity by Th2 cells might work to inhibit these responses and predispose the host to certain types of infection.

Studies in mice have demonstrated that resistance to *C. albicans* infections results from the development of Th1 cell responses that generate cytokines that activate macrophages and neutrophils and increase their candidacidal abilities (74). Alternatively, IL-4, a Th2 cytokine, has been shown to inhibit uptake and killing of *C. albicans* cells by human mononuclear phagocytes (73). Therefore, coordination of Th1 and Th2 responses is required for efficient host defense against this organism. Lymphocytes from patients with chronic mucocutaneous candidiasis have been found to show impaired in vitro secretion of IL-2 (a Th1 cytokine), but increased secretion of IL-6 (a Th2 cytokine) in response to stimulation by *Candida* antigens; therefore, these antigens appear to trigger predominantly a Th2 response in these patients, perhaps leading to their increased susceptibility to this type of infection (54).

Role of cytokines in cutaneous candidiasis

Cytokines appear to enhance the ability of phagocytic cells to damage or kill *C. albicans* cells. Three types of colony-stimulating factors, including granulocyte colony-stimulating factor (G-CSF), macrophage colony-stimulating factor (M-CSF), and granulocyte macrophage colony-stimulating factor (GM-CSF), as well as IL-2, IFN-γ, and tumor necrosis factor alpha (TNF-α), have been shown in vitro to enhance the fungicidal activity of phagocytic cells against *Candida* species (reviewed in reference 71). GM-CSF also appears to work in concert with neutrophil myeloperoxidase to augment killing of *C. albicans* by macrophages (55). Neutrophils from human volunteers given G-CSF were found in one study to more effectively damage the pseudohyphae of *C. albicans* (39). Other cytokines, including IL-12 and IL-15, may also act to enhance neutrophil killing of *Candida* spp. (71, 96). Alternatively, IL-4 and IL-10 characterize the Th2 response and appear to decrease the antifungal activity of macrophages against *C. albicans* (17). Since neutrophils can enter the stratum corneum and contact the infecting organisms in cutaneous candidiasis, it is likely that modulation of the fungicidal mechanisms of these cells by various cytokines, in either a positive or negative manner, could significantly affect the ability of the host to clear this type of infection.

THERAPEUTIC IMPLICATIONS

Standard therapy of chronic mucocutaneous candidiasis involves long treatment courses (6 to 9 months) with oral azole antifungal agents such as ketoconazole or fluconazole. For other forms of cutaneous candidiasis, therapy can be attempted with topical preparations of azoles, amphotericin B or nystatin, or cyclopirox. These therapies are generally effective, although relapses can occur, particularly in chronic mucocutaneous candidiasis when the treatment is stopped or if a resistant organism is encountered. Therefore, in chronic mucocutaneous candidiasis, maintenance therapy is usually required after the initial antifungal treatment has cleared the cutaneous and mucosal lesions. In some patients, the defects in cell-mediated immunity may resolve after antifungal therapy; this improvement may be due to the disappearance of circulating inhibitory serum factors related to mannan products from the organism itself, as discussed above.

Early attempts at immunological treatment used transplants of whole thymic tissue, lymphocytes, or bone marrow, or leukocyte-derived factors such as transfer factor or thymosin (35, 48). In some cases immunologic reconstitution was achieved, but generally these therapies were difficult and only marginally effective. The development and approval of various cytokines for use in humans have provided a possible new therapy for difficult mucocutaneous *Candida* infections. To date, there are only limited data on the use of cytokines as adjuvant therapy for fungal infections in general. However, in experimental animals, in vivo synergy between antifungal drugs and various cytokines has been convincingly demonstrated (reviewed in reference 87). Formal clinical trials will be required to determine if administration of cytokines can significantly enhance the treatment of fungal infections, perhaps including relapsing forms of chronic mucocutaneous candidiasis.

SUMMARY

Cutaneous candidiasis represents infections of the epidermis, primarily the stratum corneum of the skin, with *C. albicans* and occasionally certain non-*C. albicans* species. The condition known as chronic mucocutaneous candidiasis consists of a variety of syndromes with varying degrees of immune dysfunction and resulting chronic infections of the skin and mucous membranes with *Candida* organisms. The various forms of cutaneous candidiasis have a number of predispositions, such as warmth, moisture, and occlusion at the local site; various kinds of natural or iatrogenic immunosuppression; and perhaps some degree of inherited susceptibility. The immune system, particularly cell-mediated immunity, appears to be important in the defense against this type of infection. In the skin the mechanisms involved in generating immunologic reactions are particularly complex, with epidermal Langerhans cells, other dendritic cells, lymphocytes, microvascular endothelial cells, and the keratinocytes themselves all playing important roles. Studies of cutaneous candidiasis have elucidated a number of immunologic defects, which in some cases may be preexistent and in others may be secondary to the infection itself. Different mechanisms may cause immunologic dysfunction in individual patients and lead to the development of chronic infections. Although an inability to develop protective immune responses appears to be involved in the chronicity of certain cutaneous *Candida* infections, treatment at the present time depends primarily on antifungal medications; therapeutic modalities aimed at reversing the underlying immunologic defects remain experimental.

REFERENCES

1. **Alspaugh, J. A., and D. L. Granger.** 1991. Inhibition of *Cryptococcus neoformans* replication by nitrogen oxides supports the role of these molecules as effectors of macrophage-mediated cytostasis. *Infect. Immun.* **59:**2291–2296.
2. **Arnold, R. R., M. Brewer, and J. J. Gauthier.** 1980. Bactericidal activity of human lactoferrin: sensitivity of a variety of microorganisms. *Infect. Immun.* **23:**893–898.
3. **Arnold, R. R., J. E. Russell, W. J. Champion, and J. J. Gauthier.** 1981. Bactericidal activity of human lactoferrin: influence of physical conditions and metabolic state of the target microorganism. *Infect. Immun.* **32:**655–660.
4. **Axelsen, N. H., C. H. Kirkpatrick, and R. H. Buckley.** 1974. Precipitins to *Candida albicans* in chronic mucocutaneous candidiasis studied by crossed immunoelectrophoresis with intermediate gels. *Clin. Exp. Immunol.* **17:**385–394.
5. **Berger, M., C. H. Kirkpatrick, P. K. Goldsmith, and J. I. Gallin.** 1980. IgE antibodies to *Staphylococcus aureus* and *Candida albicans* in patients with the syndrome of hyperimmunoglobulin E and recurrent infections. *J. Immunol.* **125:**2437–2443.
6. **Bergstresser, P. R., P. D. Cruz, Jr., J. Y. Niederkorn, and A. Takashima.** 1992. Third International Workshop on Langerhans cells: discussion overview. *J. Invest. Dermatol.* **99:** 1S–4S.
7. **Berk, S. H., N. S. Penneys, and G. D. Weinstein.** 1976. Epidermal activity in annular dermatophytosis. *Arch. Dermatol.* **112:** 485–488.
8. **Bibel, D. J., R. Aly, S. Shah, and H. R. Shinefield.** 1993. Sphingosines: antimicrobial barriers of the skin. *Acta Derm. Venereol.* (Stockholm) **73:**407–411.
9. **Bice, D. E., M. Lopez, H. Rothschild, and J. Salvaggio.** 1974. Comparison of *Candida* delayed hypersensitivity skin test size with lymphocyte transformation, migration inhibitory factor production and antibody titer. *Int. Arch. Allergy Appl. Immunol.* **47:**54–62.
10. **Bjorses, P., J. Aaltonen, N. Horelli-Kuitunen, M. L. Yaspo, and L. Peltonen.** 1998. Gene defect behind APECED: a new clue to autoimmunity. *Hum. Mol. Genet.* **7:**1547–1553.
11. **Bjorses, P., M. Halonen, J. J. Palvimo, M. Kolmer, J. Aaltonen, P. Ellonen, J. Perheentupa, I. Ulmanen, and L. Peltonen.** 2000. Mutations in the AIRE gene: effects on subcellular location and transactivation function of the autoimmune polyendocrinopathy-candidiasis-ectodermal dystrophy protein. *Am. J. Hum. Genet.* **66:**378–392.
12. **Bos, J. D., M. B. M. Teunissen, I. Cairo, S. R. Krieg, M. L. Kapsenberg, P. K. Das, and J. Borst.** 1990. T-cell receptor $\gamma\delta$ bearing cells in normal human skin. *J. Invest. Dermatol.* **94:** 37–42.
13. **Burford-Mason, A. P., R. C. Matthews, and J. R. B. Williams.** 1987. Transient abrogation of immunosuppression in a patient with chronic mucocutaneous candidiasis following vaccination with *Candida albicans. J. Infect.* **14:**147–157.
14. **Cahill, L. T., E. Ainbender, and P. R. Glade.** 1974. Chronic mucocutaneous candidiasis: T cell deficiency associated with B cell dysfunction in man. *Cell. Immunol.* **14:**215–225.
15. **Campanelli, D., P. A. Detmers, C. F. Nathan, and J. E. Gabay.** 1990. Azuricidin and a homologous serine protease from neutrophils. Differential antimicrobial and proteolytic properties. *J. Clin. Invest.* **85:**904–915.
16. **Carrow, E. W., and J. E. Domer.** 1985. Immunoregulation in experimental murine candidiasis: specific suppression induced by *Candida albicans* cell wall glycoprotein. *Infect. Immun.* **49:** 172–181.
17. **Cenci, E., L. Romani, A. Mencacci, R. Spaccapelo, E. Schiaffella, P. Pucetti, and F. Bistoni.** 1993. Interleukin-4 and IL-10 inhibit nitric oxide-dependent macrophage killing of *Candida albicans. Eur. J. Immunol.* **23:**1034–1038.
18. **Chappler, R. R., H. I. Maibach, M. K. A. Conant, and R. Aly.** 1978. Mucocutaneous candidiasis or mucocutaneous microbiosis. *JAMA.* **239:**428–429.
19. **Chipps, B. E., F. T. Saulsbury, S. H. Hsu, W. T. Hughes, and J. A. Winkelstein.** 1979. Non-candidal infections in children with chronic mucocutaneous candidiasis. *Johns Hopkins Med. J.* **144:**175–179.
20. **Christin, L., D. R. Wysong, T. Meshulam, S. Wang, and R. D. Diamond.** 1997. Mechanisms and target sites of damage in killing of *Candida albicans* hyphae by human polymorphonuclear neutrophils. *J. Infect. Dis.* **176:**1567–1578.
21. **Collins, M. S., and D. Pappagianis.** 1974. Inhibition by lysozyme of growth of the spherule phase of *Coccioides immitis* in vitro. *Infect. Immun.* **10:**616–623.
22. **Cutler, J. E.** 1977. Chemotactic factor produced by *Candida albicans. Infect. Immun.* **18:**568–573.
23. **De Bernardis, F., F. Mondello, R. San Millan, J. Ponton, and A. Cassone.** 1999. Biotyping and virulence properties of skin isolates of *Candida parapsilosis. J. Clin. Microbiol.* **37:** 3481–3486.
24. **de la Torre Morin, F., J. C. Garcia Robaina, C. Bonnet Moreno, and G. L. Fonta.** 1997. Hyper IgE syndrome. Presentation of three cases. *Allerg. Immunopathol.* **25:**30–35.
25. **Delves, P. J., and I. M. Riott.** 2000. The immune system. *N. Engl. J. Med.* **343:**108–117.
26. **Drouhet, E., and B. Dupont.** 1980. Chronic mucocutaneous candidiasis and other superficial and systemic mycoses successfully treated with ketoconazole. *Rev. Infect. Dis.* **2:**606–619.
27. **Durandy, A., A. Fischer, F. Le Deist, E. Drouhet, and C. Gris-**

celli. 1987. Mannan-specific and mannan-induced T-cell suppressive activity in patients with chronic mucocutaneous candidiasis. *J. Clin. Immunol.* **7:**400–409.

28. **Edens, H. A., C. A. Parkos, T. W. Liang, A. J. Jesaitis, J. E. Cutler, and H. M. Miettinen.** 1999. Non-serum-dependent chemotactic factors produced by *Candida albicans* stimulate chemotaxis by binding to the formyl peptide receptor on neutrophils and to an unknown receptor on macrophages. *Infect. Immun.* **67:**1063–1071.
29. **Elias, P. M.** 1983. Epidermal lipids, barrier function, and desquamation. *J. Invest. Dermatol.* **80:**44s–49s.
30. **Elias, P. M., and K. R. Feingold.** 1999. Skin as an organ of protection, p. 164–174. *In* I. M. Freedberg, A. Z. Eisen, K. Wolff, K. F. Austen, L. A. Goldsmith, S. I. Katz, and T. B. Fitzpatrick (ed.), *Dermatology in General Medicine.* McGraw-Hill, New York, N.Y.
31. **Eppinger, T. M., J. E. Aronson, L. S. Fonacier, and C. Cunningham-Rundles.** 1999. *Pneumocystis carinii* pneumonia in a 15 year old with chronic mucocutaneous candidiasis. *Scand. J. Infect. Dis.* **31:**203–206.
32. **Esterly, N. B., S. R. Brammer, and R. G. Crounse.** 1967. The relationship of transferrin and iron to serum inhibition of *Candida albicans. J. Invest. Dermatol.* **49:**437–442.
33. **Ferguson, A. C., H. E. Kershnar, W. K. Collin, and E. R. Stiehm.** 1977. Correlation of cutaneous hypersensitivity with lymphocyte response to *Candida albicans. Am. J. Clin. Pathol.* **68:**499–504.
34. **Fidel, P. L., Jr., J. A. Vazquez, and J. D. Sobel.** 1999. *Candida glabrata:* review of epidemiology, pathogenesis, and clinical disease with comparison to *C. albicans. Clin. Microbiol. Rev.* **12:**80–96.
35. **Filler, S. G., and J. E. Edwards, Jr.** 1993. Chronic mucocutaneous candidiasis, p. 117–133. *In* J. W. Murphy, H. Friedman, and M. Bendinelli (ed.), *Fungal Infections and Immune Responses.* Plenum Press, New York, N.Y.
36. **Fischer, A. J., J. J. Ballet, and C. Griscelli.** 1987. Specific inhibition of the in vitro *Candida* induced lymphocyte proliferation by polysaccharide antigens present in the serum of patients with chronic mucocutaneous candidiasis. *J. Clin. Invest.* **62:**1005–1013.
37. **Fischer, A. J., L. Pichat, M. Audinot, and C. Griscelli.** 1982. Defective handling of mannan by monocytes in patients with chronic mucocutaneous candidiasis resulting in a specific cellular unresponsiveness. *Clin. Exp. Immunol.* **47:**653–660.
38. **Ganz, T., M. E. Selsted, D. Szklarek, S. S. L. Harwig, K. Dahler, D. F. Bainton, and R. I. Lehrer.** 1985. Defensins: natural peptide antibiotics of human neutrophils. *J. Clin. Invest.* **76:**1427–1435.
39. **Gavira, J. M., J. A. van Burik, D. C. Dale, R. K. Root, and W. C. Liles.** 1999. Modulation of neutrophil-mediated activity against the pseudohyphal form of *Candida albicans* by granulocyte colony-stimulating factor (G-CSF) administered in vivo. *J. Infect. Dis.* **179:**1301–1304.
40. **Geerlings, S. E., and A. I. Hoepelman.** 1999. Immune dysfunction in patients with diabetes mellitus. *FEMS Immunol. Med. Microbiol.* **26:**259–265.
41. **Gettner, S. M. M., and D. W. R. Mackenzie.** 1981. Responses of human peripheral lymphocytes to soluble and insoluble antigens of *Candida albicans. J. Med. Microbiol.* **14:**333–340.
42. **Grisham, M. B., M. M. Jefferson, D. F. Melton, and E. L. Thomas.** 1983. Chlorination of exogenous amines by isolated neutrophils. Ammonia dependent bactericidal, cytotoxic, and cytolytic activities of the chloramines. *J. Biol. Chem.* **258:**10404–10413.
43. **Herrod, H. G.** 1990. Chronic mucocutaneous candidiasis in childhood and complications of non-*Candida* infection: a report of the pediatric immunodeficiency study group. *J. Pediatr.* **116:**377–382.
44. **Ho, Y., M. Ng, and C. T. Huang.** 1979. Antibodies to germinating and yeast cells of *Candida albicans* in human and rabbit sera. *J. Clin. Pathol.* **32:**399–405.
45. **Kashima, M., H. Takahashi, M. Shimozuma, W. L. Epstein, and K. Fukuyama.** 1989. Candidacidal activities of proteins partially purified from rat epidermis. *Infect. Immun.* **57:**186–190.
46. **Kauffman, C. A., M. J. Shea, and P. T. Frame.** 1981. Invasive fungal infections in patients with chronic mucocutaneous candidiasis. *Arch. Intern. Med.* **141:**1076–1078.
47. **Kirkpatrick, C. H., R. R. Rich, and J. E. Bennett.** 1971. Chronic mucocutaneous: model building in cellular immunity. *Ann. Intern. Med.* **74:**955–978.
48. **Kirkpatrick, C. H., and T. K. Smith.** 1974. Chronic mucocutaneous candidiasis: immunologic and antibiotic therapy. *Ann. Intern. Med.* **80:**310–320.
49. **Kirkpatrick, C. H., and P. G. Sohnle.** 1981. Chronic mucocutaneous candidiasis, p. 495–514. *In* B. Safai and R. A. Good (ed.), *Immunodermatology.* Plenum Press, New York, N.Y.
50. **Kirkpatrick, C. H., and D. B. Windhorst.** 1979. Mucocutaneous candidiasis and thymoma. *Am. J. Med.* **66:**939–945.
51. **Kligman, A. M., and D. Ginsberg.** 1950. Immunity of the adult scalp to infection with *Microsporum audouini. J. Invest. Dermatol.* **14:**345–356.
52. **Lehner, T. J., M. A. Wilton, and L. Ivanyi.** 1972. Immunodeficiencies in chronic mucocutaneous candidiasis. *Immunology* **22:**775–787.
53. **Lepper, A. W. D., and H. S. Anger.** 1976. Experimental bovine *Trichophyton verrucosum* infection. Comparison of the rate of epidermal cell proliferation and keratinization in non-infected and reinoculated cattle. *Res. Vet. Sci.* **20:**117–121.
54. **Lilic, D., A. J. Cant, M. Abinum, J. E. Calvert, and G. P. Spickett.** 1996. Chronic mucocutaneous candidiasis. I. Altered antigen-stimulated IL-2, IL-4, IL-6 and interferon-gamma (IFN-gamma) production. *Clin. Exp. Immunol.* **105:**205–212.
55. **Marodi, L., C. Tournay, R. Kaposzta, R. B. Johnston, Jr., and N. Moguilevsky.** 1998. Augmentation of human macrophage candidacidal capacity by recombinant human myeloperoxidase and granulocyte-macrophage colony-stimulating factor. *Infect. Immun.* **66:**2750–2754.
56. **Matsue, H., P. R. Bergstresser, and A. Takashima.** 1993. Keratinocyte-derived IL-7 serves as a growth factor for dendritic epidermal T cells in mice. *J. Immunol.* **151:**6012–6019.
57. **Mittaz, L., C. Rossier, M. Heino, P. Peterson, K. J. Krohn, A. Gos, M. A. Morris, J. Judoh, N. Shimizu, S. E. Antonarakis, and H. S. Scott.** 1999. Isolation and characterization of the mouse Aire gene. *Biochem. Biophys. Res. Comm.* **255:**483–490.
58. **Mobacken, H., L. Lindholm, and S. Olling.** 1977. Deficient neutrophil function in a patient with chronic mucocutaneous candidiasis, thymoma and myasthenia gravis. *Acta Derm. Venereol.* **57:**335–339.
59. **Montes, L. F.** 1992. Candidiasis, p. 913–923. *In* S. L. Moschella and H. J. Hurley (ed.), *Dermatology,* 3rd ed. W. B. Saunders, Philadelphia, Pa.
60. **Moser, S. A., J. E. Domer, and F. J. Mather.** 1980. Experimental murine candidiasis: cell-mediated immunity after cutaneous challenge. *Infect. Immun.* **27:**140–149.
61. **Mosmann, T. R., and S. Sad.** 1996. The expanding universe of T cell subsets: Th1, Th2 and more. *Immunol. Today* **17:**138–146.
62. **Nauseef, W. M., and R. A. Clark.** 2000. Granulocytic phagocytes, p. 89–112. *In* G. L. Mandel, J. E. Bennett, and R. Dolin

(ed), *Principles and Practice of Infectious Diseases.* Churchill Livingstone, Philadelphia, Pa.

63. **Negi, M., R. Tsuboi, T. Matsui, and H. Ogawa.** 1984. Isolation and characterization of proteinase from *Candida albicans:* substrate specificity. *J. Invest. Dermatol.* **83:**32–36.
64. **Neth, O., D. L. Jack, A. W. Dodds, H. Holzel, N. J. Klein, and M. W. Turner.** 2000. Mannose-binding lectin binds to a range of clinically relevant microorganisms and promotes complement deposition. *Infect. Immun.* **68:**688–693.
65. **Nguyen, C., and H. P. Katner.** 1997. Myeloperoxidase deficiency manifesting as pustular candidal dermatitis. *Clin. Infect. Dis.* **24:**258–260.
66. **Podzorski, R. P., G. R. Gray, and R. D. Nelson.** 1990. Different effects of native *Candida albicans* mannan and mannan-derived oligosaccharides on antigen-stimulated lymphoproliferation in vitro. *J. Immunol.* **144:**707–716.
67. **Potten, C. S.** 1974. The epidermal proliferative unit: the possible role of the central basal cell. *Cell Tissue Kinet.* **7:**77–88.
68. **Ray, T. L., and K. D. Wuepper.** 1976. Activation of the alternative (properdin) pathway of complement by *Candida albicans* and related species. *J. Invest. Dermatol.* **67:**700–703.
69. **Ring, J., and M. Thewes.** 1999. The clinical expression of allergy in the skin. *Allergy* **54:**192–197.
70. **Rivas, V., and T. J. Rogers.** 1983. Studies on the cellular nature of *Candida albicans*-induced suppression. *J. Immunol.* **130:** 376–379.
71. **Rodriguez-Adrian, L. J., M. L. Grazziutti, J. H. Rex, and E. J. Anaissie.** 1998. The potential role of cytokine therapy for fungal infections in patients with cancer: is recovery from neutropenia all that is needed? *Clin. Infect. Dis.* **26:**1270–1278.
72. **Rogers, T. J., and E. Balish.** 1978. Suppression of lymphocyte blastogenesis by *Candida albicans. Clin. Immunol. Immunopathol.* **10:**298–305.
73. **Roilides, E., I. Kadiltsoglou, A. Dimitriadou, M. Hatzistilianou, A. Manitsa, J. Karpouzas, P. A. Pizzo, and T. J. Walsh.** 1997. Interleukin 4 suppresses antifungal activity of human mononuclear phagocytes against *Candida albicans* in association with decreased uptake of blastoconidia. *FEMS Immunol. Med. Microbiol.* **19:**169–180.
74. **Romani, L.** 1999. Immunity to *Candida albicans:* Th1, Th2 cells and beyond. *Curr. Opin. Microbiol.* **2:**363–367.
75. **Rosatelli, M. C., A. Meloni, A. Meloni, M. Devoto, A. Cao, H. S. Scott, P. Peterson, M. Heino, K. J. Krohn, K. Nagamine, J. Kodoh, N. Shimizu, and S. E. Antonarakis.** 1998. A common mutation in Sardinian autoimmune polyendocrinopathy-candidiasis-ectodermal dystrophy patients. *Hum. Genet.* **103:** 428–434.
76. **Rothman, S., A. Smiljanic, A. L. Shapiro, and A. W. Weitkamp.** 1947. The spontaneous cure of tinea capitis in puberty. *J. Invest. Dermatol.* **8:**81–98.
77. **Rothschild, H., M. Wilson, M. Lopez, J. Salvaggio, and D. Bice.** 1976. An immunological investigation of a family with chronic mucocutaneous candidiasis. *Int. Arch. Allergy Appl. Immunol.* **52:**291–296.
78. **Schmitt, C., and J. J. Ballet.** 1983. Serum IgE and IgG antibodies to tetanus toxoid and candidin in immunodeficient children with the hyper-IgE syndrome. *J. Clin. Immunol.* **3:**178–183.
79. **Schurer, N. Y., and P. M. Elias.** 1991. The biochemistry and function of stratum corneum lipids. *Adv. Lipid Res.* **24:**27–56.
80. **Shannon, D. C., G. Johnson, F. S. Rosen, and K. F. Austen.** 1966. Cellular reactivity to *Candida albicans* antigen. *N. Engl. J. Med.* **275:**690–693.
81. **Sohnle, P. G., C. Collins-Lech, and K. E. Huhta.** 1983. Kinetics of lymphokine production by lymphocytes from elderly humans. *Gerontology* **29:**169–175.
82. **Sohnle, P. G., C. Collins-Lech, and J. H. Wiessner.** 1991. The zinc-reversible antimicrobial activity of neutrophil lysates and abscess fluid supernatants. *J. Infect. Dis.* **164:**137–142.
83. **Sohnle, P. G., M. M. Frank, and C. H. Kirkpatrick.** 1976. Mechanisms involved in elimination of organisms from experimental cutaneous *Candida albicans* infection in guinea pigs. *J. Immunol.* **117:**523–530.
84. **Sohnle, P. G., and B. L. Hahn.** 1989. Epidermal proliferation and the neutrophilic infiltrates of experimental cutaneous candidiasis in mice. *Arch. Dermatol. Res.* **281:**279–283.
85. **Sohnle, P. G., and C. H. Kirkpatrick.** 1978. Epidermal proliferation in the defense against cutaneous candidiasis. *J. Invest. Derm.* **70:**130–133.
86. **Steinbakk, M., C. F. Naess-Andresen, E. Lingass, I. Dale, P. Brandtzaeg, and M. K. Fagerhol.** 1990. Antimicrobial actions of calcium binding leucocyte L1 protein, calprotectin. *Lancet* **336:**763–765.
87. **Stevens, D. A.** 1998. Combination immunotherapy and antifungal chemotherapy. *Clin. Infect. Dis.* **26:**1266–1269.
88. **Stingl, G.** 1993. This skin: initiation and target site of immune responses. *Recent Results Cancer Res.* **128:**45–57.
89. **Stingl, G., D. Maurer, C. Hauser, and K. Wolff.** 1999. The epidermis: an immunologic microenvironment, p. 343–370. *In* I. M. Freedberg, A. Z. Eisen, K. Wolff, K. F. Austen, L. A. Goldsmith, S. I. Katz, and T. B. Fitzpatrick (ed.), *Dermatology in General Medicine.* McGraw-Hill, New York, N.Y.
90. **Streilein, J. W.** 1983. Skin-associated lymphoid tissues (SALT): origins and functions. *J. Invest. Dermatol.* **80:**12S–16S.
91. **Sundstrom, P. M., and G. E. Kenny.** 1984. Characterization of antigens specific to the surface of germ tubes of *Candida albicans* by immunofluorescence. *Infect. Immun.* **43:**850–855.
92. **Test, S. T., M. B. Lampert, P. J. Ossanna, J. G. Thoene, and S. J. Weiss.** 1984. Generation of nitrogen-chlorine oxidants by human phagocytes. *J. Clin. Invest.* **74:**1341–1349.
93. **Twomey, J. T., C. C. Waddel, S. Krantz, R. O'Reilly, P. L'Esperance, and R. A. Good.** 1975. Chronic mucocutaneous candidiasis with macrophage dysfunction, a plasma inhibitor and coexistent aplastic anemia. *J. Lab. Clin. Med.* **85:** 968–977.
94. **Valdimarsson, H., J. M. Higgs, R. S. Wells, M. Yamamura, J. R. Hobbs, and P. J. L. Holt.** 1973. Immune abnormalities associated with chronic mucocutaneous. *Cell Immunol.* **6:** 348–361.
95. **Van der Meer, J. W. M., P. C. J. Leijh, M. Van den Barselaar, and R. Van Furth.** 1978. Functions of phagocytic cells in chronic mucocutaneous candidiasis. *Br. Med. J.* **1:**147–148.
96. **Vazquez, N., T. J. Walsh, D. Friedman, S. J. Chanock, and C. A. Lyman.** 1998. Interleukin-15 augments superoxide production and microbicidal activity of human monocytes against *Candida albicans. Infect. Immun.* **66:**145–150.
97. **Weiss, J., P. Elsbach, I. Olsson, and H. Odeberg.** 1978. Purification and characterization of a potent bactericidal and membrane active protein from the granules of human polymorphonuclear leukocytes. *J. Biol. Chem.* **253:**2664–2672.
98. **Wilson, B. D., and P. G. Sohnle.** 1986. Participation of neutrophils and cell-mediated immunity in the defense against experimental cutaneous candidiasis in mice. *Am. J. Pathol.* **123:** 241–249.
99. **Zanetti, M., R. Gennaro, and D. Romeo.** 1996. Cathelicidins: a novel protein family with a common proregion and a variable C-terminal antimicrobial domain. *FEBS Lett.* **374:**1–5.

Candida and Candidiasis
Edited by Richard A. Calderone
© 2002 ASM Press, Washington, D.C.

Chapter 16

Immunology of Invasive Candidiasis

Luigina Romani

Candida albicans is a unique parasite capable of colonizing mucosal tissues, infecting the same tissues as well as organs, persisting on mucosal surfaces, and stimulating mucosal immune responses. As a pathogen, it is associated with a wide spectrum of diseases in humans, including systemic forms of infection, that may arise as localized primary diseases of deep organs or as hematogenously disseminated infection (83). *Candida* spp. now rank fourth among microbes most frequently isolated from blood cultures (48), and mortality rates from systemic candidiasis can be as high as 50%. Not only are bloodstream infections with *C. albicans* and non-*C. albicans* species occurring more frequently, but the relative proportion due to non-*C. albicans* species is increasing, including species such as *C. glabrata, C. tropicalis, C. parapsilosis, C. krusei*, and *C. lusitaniae*. Common risk factors for bloodstream candidiasis include extremes of age (low-birth-weight infants and the elderly), immunosuppression, malignancy with leukopenia, major abdominal surgery, or trauma, as well as exposure to multiple antibacterial agents, central venous catheterization, prolonged length of stay in intensive care units, and parenteral nutrition (48).

Because early diagnosis of invasive infection is difficult, strategies to prevent it seem to be attractive. The beneficial effect of immunomodulators in clinical and preclinical models of the infection (56, 85, 118) suggests that maneuvers aimed at restoring the host defective antifungal immune responsiveness can be exploited in adjunctive antifungal therapies (43, 56, 92).

An essential point to be considered is the acknowledgment of the redundancy of the anticandidal immune responses with respect to protection. In the context of the antagonistic relationships that characterize the host-pathogen interactions, the strategies used by the host to limit fungal infectivity are necessarily disparate (102 and references therein) and, in retaliation, the fungus has developed its own elaborate tactics to evade or overcome these defenses (19, 47). This may have resulted in an expanded repertoire of cross-regulatory and overlapping antifungal host responses that makes it extremely difficult to define the relative contribution of individual components of the immune system in the antifungal defense.

Within the limitations imposed by the above considerations, this chapter will analyze the role of the innate and adaptive immune systems, and their reciprocal regulation in resistance to nonmucosal *C. albicans* infection. Much of the information has been obtained from experimental models of disseminated candidiasis, in which the infection can be established under controlled, reproducible conditions. For example, the intravenous injection of a suitable fungal inoculum into mice of different strains is sufficient to establish an acute disseminated visceral infection with multiple deep organs involved, clearly mimicking the disseminated infection in humans (83, 100). Data from such experimental and clinical studies will be comparatively analyzed, with the intent to put forward a unitary view for cell-mediated immunity in anticandidal resistance that may operate from commensalism to the different forms of infection.

IMMUNITY TO *C. ALBICANS*: AN INTEGRATED VIEW

Innate immunity and acquired cell-mediated immunity have been acknowledged as the primary mediators of host resistance to *C. albicans* (7, 101, 102). With the recognition of the reciprocal influences between the innate and the adaptive T helper (Th) immunity (35), it appears that an integrated immune response determines the lifelong commensalism of the

Luigina Romani • Microbiology Section, Department of Experimental Medicine and Biochemical Sciences, University of Perugia, Via del Giochetto, 06122 Perugia, Italy.

fungus at the mucosal level, as well as the transition from mucosal saprophyte to pathogen (97, 98).

For many years, innate immunity has been considered as a separate entity from the adaptive immune response to pathogens and has been regarded to be of secondary importance in the hierarchy of immune functions. However, evidence is now accumulating for an essential role of the innate immunity in orchestrating the subsequent adaptive immunity to pathogens (35, 69). In the vertebrate host, the innate and adaptive immune responses are integrated as a single immune system, with the innate response preceding, and being necessary for, the adaptive immune response. Through the involvement of a set of germline-encoded receptors (referred to as pattern recognition receptors, PRRs) (1, 68, 69), cells of the innate immune system not only discriminate between different forms of fungi, but also contribute to discrimination between self and pathogens at the level of the adaptive Th immunity (36, 100) (Fig. 1). As the different Th cell subsets are endowed with the ability to release a distinct panel of cytokines, capable of activating and deactivating signals to effector phagocytes, the activation of an appropriate Th subset may be instrumental in the generation of a successful or unsuccessful immune response to fungal pathogens in general or *C. albicans* specifically (39, 88, 96, 97, 107) (Fig. 2). In its basic conception, the paradigm calls for (i) an association between Th1 responses and the onset and maintenance of phagocyte-dependent immunity, critical for opposing infectivity of the commensals or clearing pathogenic fungi from infected tissue; (ii) the

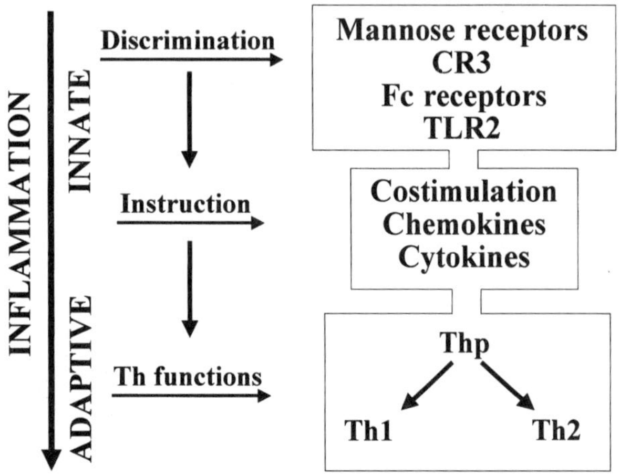

Figure 1. An integrated view of the innate and adaptive immune responses to *C. albicans*. The innate immune system discriminates between different forms of the fungus and produces sets of cytokines and costimulatory molecules that signal the adaptive T helper (Th) immunity. CR3, complement receptor 3; TLR2, Toll-like receptor 2; Thp, T-helper precursor.

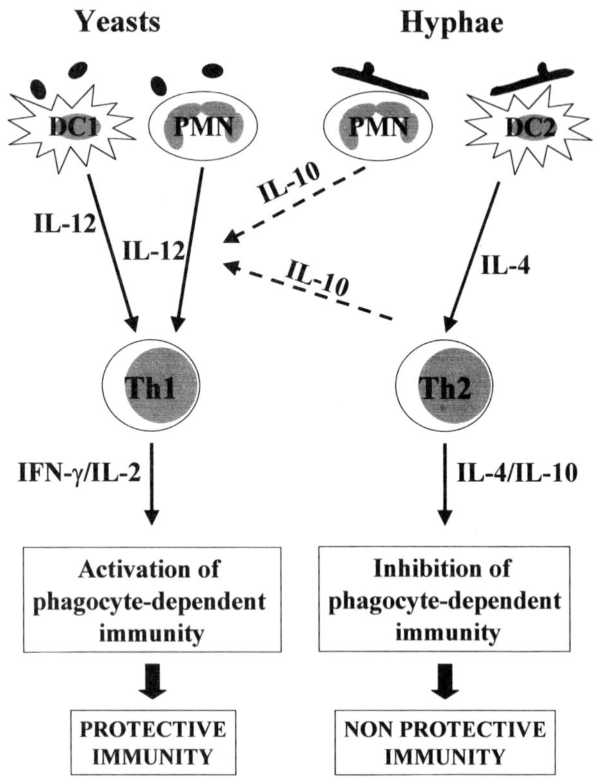

Figure 2. A simplified view of pathways of induction of T helper responses to *C. albicans*. Upon recognition of *Candida* yeasts, dendritic cells 1 (DC1) and polymorphonuclear neutrophils (PMN) produce IL-12, which is absolutely required for the activation of Th1 cells producing IFN-γ and IL-2 that both stimulate effector phagocytes to a fungicidal state. In contrast, upon interaction with *Candida* hyphae, DC2 produce IL-4, which is absolutely required for activation of Th2 cells producing IL-4 and IL-10, both deactivating effector phagocytes. Meanwhile, production of IL-10 by PMN further contributes to the inhibition of Th1 development. Solid and dotted lines refer to positive and negative regulatory pathways, respectively.

occurrence of Th2 responses in fungal infections and fungal diseases; (iii) the reciprocal regulation of Th1 and Th2 cells, occurring either directly or through regulatory T cells, resulting in a dynamic balance between these two types of reactivity, that may operate from commensalism to infection, and may contribute to the induction and maintenance of protective, memory antifungal responses with minimum immunopathology.

All of these aspects will be dealt with in the following sections.

Innate Immunity

The observation that invasive candidiasis occurs concomitantly with defects in neutrophil number and functions (16), together with the detection of cells and mediators of the innate immune system with antifungal effector activities (7), has led to the central dogma of resistance to candidiasis, i.e., that resistance to invasive candidiasis is mediated by the innate immune system, which includes circulating polymorphonuclear neutrophils (PMNs) and monocytes, tissue macrophages, natural killer (NK) cells, and soluble molecules, including opsonins (specific antibodies and components of classical and alternative complement pathways), mannose-binding proteins, collectins, and defensins (7, 99, 102). Evidence suggests that platelets and endothelial and epithelial cells may also serve as nonconventional antifungal effectors (99) and that the serum level of iron (73) or lipoproteins (80) may determine the susceptibility and outcome of invasive candidiasis.

Although the effectiveness of this effector system is undoubtedly acknowledged, it is important to emphasize the new emerging concepts in the field: first, that optimal antifungal immune resistance is achieved through the combined and interdependent efforts of innate and adaptive immune mechanisms and, second, that the innate immune system functions as both a guide and instructor of the subsequent adaptive immunity.

Antifungal effector function of the innate immune system

Figure 3 illustrates cells, factors, and functions that contribute to innate resistance against *C. albicans*.

Phagocytes. Fungal cells possess a variety of cell surface analogs of the integrin family and complement receptors (CRs) and adhesins, which may facilitate attachment (opsonization) and phagocytosis by phagocytic cells (reviewed in reference 99). These include macrophages, continuously maturing from circulat-

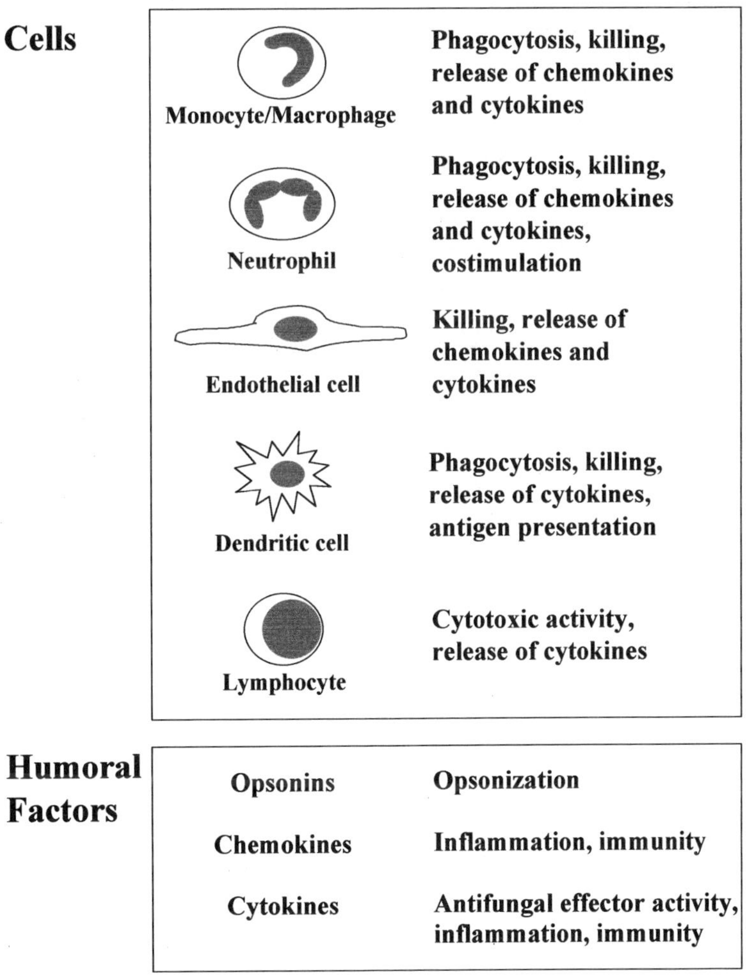

Figure 3. The innate immune resistance to *C. albicans:* cells, humoral factors, and functions.

ing monocytes, and circulating neutrophils that engulf opsonized and unopsonized fungal cells through various receptors, among which are the mannose receptors (MRs), CRs, and Fc receptors (FcRs).

The MRs belong to a family of lectins that mediate nonopsonic phagocytosis of the fungus, through recognition of α-linked oligomannoses with branched structures (68 and references therein). MR ligation results in the release of some proinflammatory cytokines and chemokines (see below), and can be linked to induction of effector functions, but the link is dependent on activation.

CR3 is a heterodimeric molecule (CD11b/CD18) that belongs to the β2-integrin family of cell adhesion molecules (68 and references therein). A remarkable characteristic of CR3 is its broad capacity for recognition of diverse ligands, such as iC3b, β-glucan, and zymosan. Thus, the multiplicity of binding sites of CR3 creates both opsonic and nonopsonic recognition. CR3 and CR1 mediate binding of the fungus and, when appropriately activated, they also mediate phagocytosis. However, they are incapable of initiating other cellular activities that ensue upon FcR ligation, such as the generation of oxidative burst.

The FcRs comprise a family of molecules that bind to the Fc portion of immunoglobulin molecules, each member of the family recognizing immunoglobulin of one or a few closely related isotypes (68 and references therein). Cross-linking of FcRs by antibody-coated fungi activates phagocytosis with enhanced antigen presentation, increases the production of fungicidal oxidants, and promotes cytokine and chemokine release.

PMNs, more than monocytes/macrophages, represent the first line of defense in the control of *C. albicans* infections (7, 112). Accumulating experimental evidence indicates that defects in PMN number or function increase the susceptibility to disseminated *C. albicans* infection (10, 31, 49, 103, 104, 106, 125). Depression in *Candida* phagocytosis and/or killing by PMNs and monocytes has been noted in several naturally occurring disorders in human patients, for example, myeloperoxidase deficiency and chronic granulomatous disease, lymphomas, chronic leukemias and acute leukemias in relapse, premature neonates, insulin-dependent diabetes, and patients receiving intensive cancer chemotherapy (83). Phagocytosis of *C. albicans* yeasts by PMNs may occur in the absence of serum opsonins, but opsonins are required for optimal intracellular killing of the fungus. Although phagocytosis and killing of blastoconidia by PMNs are superior to that of germ tubes and longer hyphae, only a fraction of engulfed *Candida* yeasts are digested. Other studies have shown that phagocytosis of unopsonized fungi by PMNs stimulates only a limited oxidative burst when occurring through a mannose-inhibitable mechanism (30). Thus, it appears that phagocytosis of yeasts by PMNs through a mannose-inhibitable receptor may not be coupled with the activation of the metabolic burst. In contrast to ingestible yeasts, extracellular hyphal elements are more susceptible to attack by PMNs.

As binding of the fungus to macrophages occurs in vivo, macrophages clearly play a role in the host response to *Candida* (20, 128). Most of the evidence suggests that PMNs are frequently more important than macrophages in host resistance to *Candida* challenge (83). Equivocal and disparate effects were recorded in studies on the role of macrophages in infection. It has been suggested that macrophages play a major role in the pathology of disseminated candidiasis (128). Macrophages are recruited in tissues, and yeast and filamentous forms of *Candida* can be detected both within cells and extracellularly. Interestingly, the phagocytic and microbicidal activities of macrophages are enhanced by myeloperoxidase that is released by neutrophils, a finding suggesting a possible cell cooperativity in the activation of macrophages as sites of infection (reference 100 and references therein).

The killing of yeast and hyphal forms of *C. albicans* by activated macrophages and neutrophils involves both oxidative and nonoxidative burst and production of nitric oxide (NO) (reference 100 and references therein). Initiation of the oxidative metabolic burst and hydrogen peroxide production by neutrophils in response to opsonized or unopsonized forms of the fungus occurs through different modalities and involves different intracellular events (references 99 and 100 and references therein). This means that if different events mediate phagocyte activation by opsonized and unopsonized fungal elements, candidacidal activity in vivo may vary under the divergent conditions that exist at specific localized sites of infection. As gamma interferon (IFN-γ) and tumor necrosis factor alpha (TNF-α) have disparate effects on the fungicidal activity of neutrophils, the candidacidal activity in vivo also reflects the local cytokine microenvironment (99, 100 and references therein).

Although freshly isolated phagocytic cells clearly express intrinsic anti-*Candida* activity, numerous studies have demonstrated that expression of the full candidacidal function of both neutrophils and monocytes/macrophages requires activation by colony-stimulating factors (CSFs) (7, 56, 57). However, optimal expression of the antifungal effector activity of cells of the innate immune system is attained in association with antigen-driven immune responses (6, 90, 97). This may occur through the release of cytokines with activating (IFN-γ/TNF-α) or deactivating (interleukin [IL]-4/IL-10) signals to effector phagocytes (33).

As already emphasized, the engagement of each receptor on phagocytic cells may result in profoundly different downstream intracellular events that have important consequences in the expression of the overall antifungal immune defense.

CR3 binds iC3b-opsonized fungal particles, a finding indicating that fungal cells have receptors for cleavage fragments of C3 (19, 47). Stimulation of CR3-dependent phagocytosis or degranulation requires the simultaneous ligation of two distinct sites within CR3, one specific for iC3b and a second site specific for the fungal cell wall β-glucan (40). Although binding and internalization of fungal cells by PMNs may occur through MRs (30), CR3 (40), and FcRs (114), effective phagocytosis and killing of *C. albicans* occur via targeting FcγRI (CD64) and FCαRI (CD89) receptors (126), a finding supporting the notion that opsonization is required for effective killing of the fungus after phagocytosis. It is important to realize that phagocytosis of antibody-opsonized yeasts also induces TNF-α release (12), although β2 integrins have a major role in the regulation of cytokine gene expression in neutrophils (131). However, a degree of cooperatively between FcR- and CR-dependent processes appears to exist (123).

Phagocytosis of *Candida* cells by macrophages is mediated by a combination of lectin-like receptor and FcR- and CR3-dependent processes and is influenced by many factors, including C3, soluble mannose-binding proteins, and vibronectin (100 and references therein). As with PMNs, internalization via constitutively competent MRs does not represent an effective way of clearing yeasts by macrophages. Unopsonized *C. albicans* yeasts can be internalized through the macrophage MR; however, the highest killing activity is observed against opsonized yeasts (62–64, 111). Actually, the enhancement of phagocytosis and killing of *C. albicans* by macrophages correlated with a decreased number of mannose receptors (64). The most efficient uptake is dependent on CR3-mediated phagocytosis of both serum opsonized and unopsonized yeasts, a process inhibitable by cell wall components of the fungus (121). However, interaction with macrophage CR3 leads to suppression of the immune response to the microorganism (121). Thus, macrophages use different receptors to phagocytose opsonized and unopsonized *Candida* cells. This has important consequences, as the candidacidal activity and secretory function of macrophages largely depend on the anatomical site, cell source, and the mode of internalization: uptake of opsonized yeasts results in higher killing activity with increased activation of respiratory burst, compared with unopsonized yeasts (100). Accordingly, the mannose receptor-mediated uptake of unopsonized *Candida* yeasts may lead to phagocyte abuse if not accompanied by the coordinate activation of the cell cytotoxic machinery (64). Increased expression of the receptor with no induced cytotoxicity is induced upon exposure of macrophages to IL-4 (93, 117). In contrast, IFN-γ down-regulates the expression of macrophage mannose receptors and, nevertheless, results in effective killing, presumably via increased coupling of the receptor to cytotoxic functions (64). Interestingly, production of some cytokines, such as IL-1α, IL-6, and granulocyte-macrophage CSF are mediated by the mannose receptor, while some chemokine responses may be mediated by other receptors (133).

Recent studies have shed new light on the different mechanisms, and consequences, through which phagocytes interact with the different forms of *Candida* spp. The two forms of the fungus differ not only in the way they enter and are killed by macrophages but also elicit functionally different secretory responses (100). Whereas PMNs appear to be able to phagocytose the fungal yeasts, the filamentous form of *Candida* sp. is not phagocytosed by a murine macrophage cell line (13) but can penetrate intact macrophages even when phagocytosis is blocked (52). Hyphae, however, are capable of inducing production of inflammatory cytokines to a higher extent than phagocytosed yeasts (52). In contrast, uptake of *Candida* yeasts and germ tubes by macrophages has the characteristics of phagocytosis, requires intact actin filaments, depends on the activity of protein kinase C, and occurs through a nonmannose receptor (52). Once inside the cells, *Candida* phagosomes rapidly fuse with late endosome and lysosomes. However, the yeasts may develop germ tubes within phagolysosomes, escaping from them and destroying the macrophages (52).

Recent studies indicate that dendritic cells (DCs) also behave as potent antifungal effector cells in *C. albicans* infection (36). These cells may be of particular importance in candidiasis, considering that the fungus behaves as a commensal as well as a true pathogen of skin and mucosal surfaces (83), known to be highly enriched with DCs. DCs phagocytose both yeast and hyphal forms of the fungus. Apparently, DCs phagocytose more yeasts than do neutrophils. Interestingly, the yeasts and hyphae of *C. albicans* are internalized through different receptors and phagocytic mechanisms (Fig. 4). Engulfment of yeasts occurs via coiling, overlapping phagocytosis, eventually leading to phagolysosome formation, in which different stages of progressive yeast degradation are seen. In contrast, internalization of hyphae appears to occur through a more conventional zipper-type phagocyto-

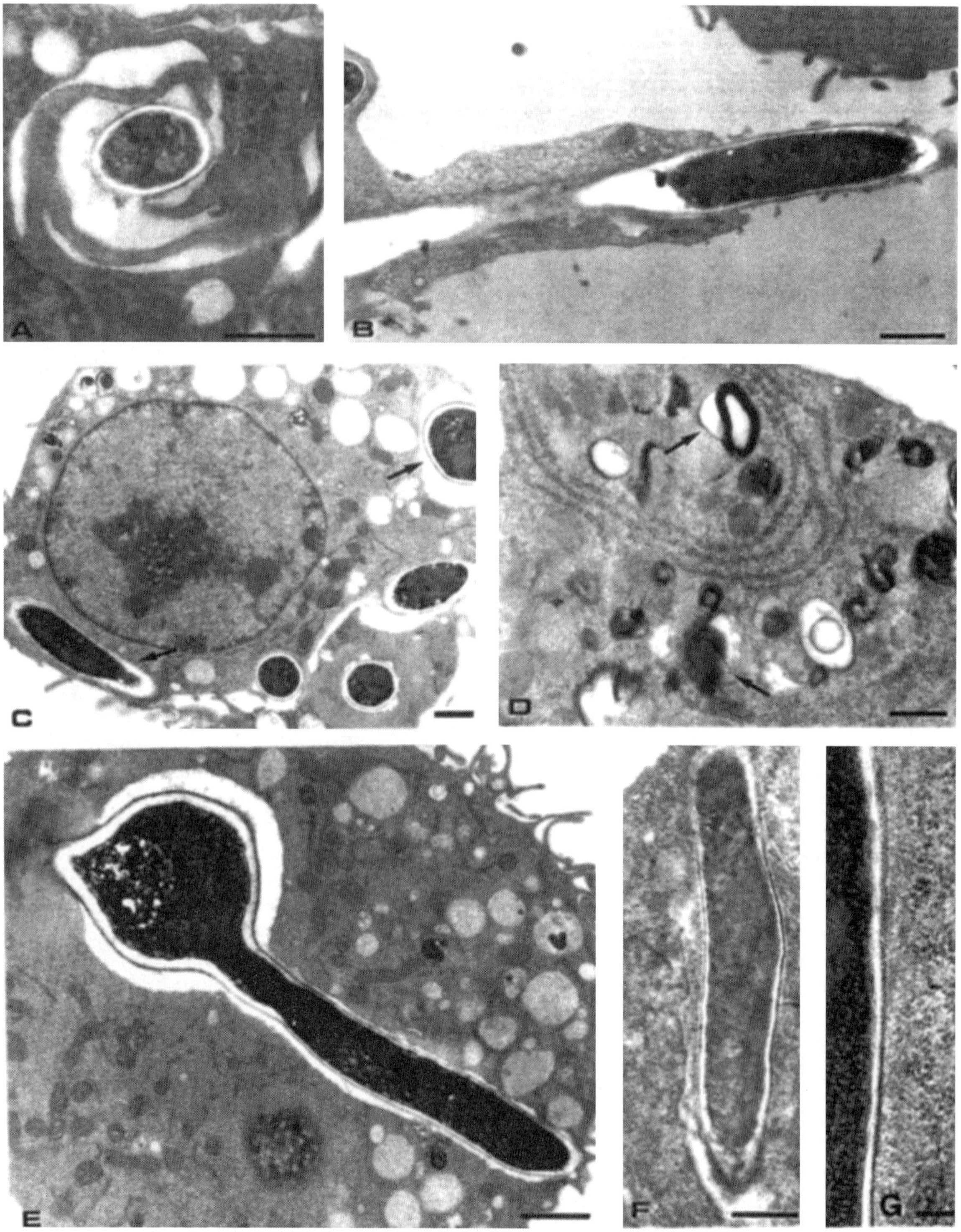

Figure 4. Transmission electron microscopy of phagocytosis of *C. albicans* by a dendritic cell. (A) Yeast engulfment through coiling phagocytosis; (B) hypha uptake through zipper-type phagocytosis at 15 min; (C) fungal elements inside phagolysosomes at 2 h; (D) partially degraded at 4 h; (E) hyphae escaping the phagolysosomes at 2 h; and (F and G) lying free in the cytoplasm. Reproduced from the *Journal of Experimental Medicine* (36) by copyright permission of The Rockefeller University Press.

sis. Internalization of either form is inhibitable, although to a different extent, by soluble mannan. Once inside the cells, hyphae appear to promote rupture of the phagosomal membrane and escape into the cytoplasm. Thus, not only are yeasts and hyphae ingested through different forms of phagocytosis, but, once inside the cells, they reside in distinct cellular compartments. After phagocytosis of yeasts or hyphae, the downstream cellular events are clearly different. Ingestion of yeasts, but not hyphae, activates dendritic cells for candidacidal activity, including nitric oxide production. Thus, these results indicate that DCs may fulfill the requirement of a cell uniquely capable of sensing the different forms of fungi in terms of antifungal effector functions and type of Th immune responses elicited (further discussed below).

In regard to the antifungal activity of NK cells, both human and murine NK cells do not have direct killing activity toward *C. albicans,* although the fungus may interact with NK cells and affect NK cell function. This interaction, however, may initiate the release of cytokines affecting the activity of phagocytic effector cells (reference 100 and references therein).

Opsonins. In vivo studies have provided convincing evidence that the complement system is an important component of innate resistance to fungi through opsonization and induction of an inflammatory response (55). Mice with congenital deficiencies in C5 production show decreased resistance to disseminated candidiasis, likely due to a failure to mount an adequate inflammatory response (reference 100 and references therein). *C. albicans* yeasts activate the complement cascade through both the classical and alternative pathways of initiation, eventually leading to deposition of C3 on the cell surface (55). Indeed, C3 deposition is greatly accelerated through activation of the classical pathway by naturally occurring antimannan IgG antibody. This finding, while suggesting that the different pathways normally operate together, also points to the important role of antibodies directed against the cell surface to serve as an amplification of C3b deposition and opsonization once either the classical or lectin pathway has been activated (55).

The expression of complement receptors on *C. albicans* yeasts and hyphae is influenced by growth conditions and by morphology, being greatest on hyphae than blastoconidia. The presence of complement receptors on most pathogenic *Candida* spp. suggests a role in pathogenesis (55). Indeed, complement receptors that act as fungal adhesins may play a role in iron acquisition by the fungus, and C3b deposition on fungal surfaces signals the ultimate destruction of the pathogen by phagocytic cells. This occurs by the specific recognition of bound complement components by CRs on phagocytes (reference 99 and references therein). By targeting specific CRs on phagocytic cells, the complement system not only fulfills the requirement of a first-line defense against the fungus, but also contributes to the innate control of the subsequent adaptive immunity.

For many years the role of antibodies in candidiasis has been neglected, mainly due to the observation that B-cell deficiency does not increase the susceptibility to infection, and because experiments with polyclonal sera have produced evidence for and against an important role of antibody in host defense (21). However, specific antibody plays a role in the initiation and regulation of complement activation by the fungus (55) as well as augmenting host immune defenses.

The existence of protective and nonprotective monoclonal antibodies to *C. albicans* (22, 23) has greatly helped clarify the controversial issue on the role of antibodies in the infection. It is now clear that differences in the composition and proportion of protective and nonprotective antibodies produced in infection may underlie the variable results obtained with polyclonal sera in experimental infections as well as the lack of correlation of the presence of specific antibody with protection against infection (21). However, the presence of antibodies to a 47-kDa breakdown product of heat shock protein 90 is associated with recovery from *C. albicans* infections and protection against disseminated disease in patients with AIDS (66, 67). Sera from patients who have recovered from disseminated candidiasis confer protection upon passive transfer into infected mice. Additional evidence points to the existence of protective antibody. First, both polyclonal sera and IgM monoclonal antibodies to a mannan adhesin fraction are able to passively transfer protection against disseminated and vaginal candidiasis in mice (44–46). A crude extract of the phosphomannan complex encapsulated into a liposome and given to intact or immunocompromised mice elicits protection, clearly attributable to agglutinating antibodies. The sharing of the same isotype, specificity, and agglutinating function is not sufficient to confer protective value to other monoclonal antibodies. Second, antibodies specific for the idiotype of antibodies reactive with yeast killer toxin (anti-idiotypic antibodies) are lethal to strains of *C. albicans* expressing the receptor for toxin (24, 61). Naturally occurring antibodies with killer toxin-like activity are present in the vaginal fluid and serum of patients with vaginal candidiasis. Anti-idiotypic antibodies as well as single chain variable antibodies confer protection upon passive transfer in a rat model of vaginal candidiasis. Thus, antibody-dependent protection is certainly operative in mucosal defense. Finally, indirect evidence for the protective role of antibodies comes from the observation that *C. albicans* has evolved strategies to evade antibody immunity, such as the production of proteases that may degrade immunoglobulins and antigenic variation (21). Altogether, these results indicate that humoral immunity, either independently or through augmentation of complement activity or protective cell-mediated immunity, may contribute to host resistance to *C. albicans.*

Cytokines. Upon contact with *C. albicans,* cells of the innate immune system release a battery of chemokines and cytokines that have profound effects on the functional activity of the innate response and on subsequent events of adaptive immune. The local release of these effector molecules serves to regulate cell trafficking of various types of leukocytes, thus initiating the inflammatory response, and to activate phagocytic cells to a microbicidal state. TNF-α, IL-1β, and IL-6 are proinflammatory cytokines readily produced upon interaction of phagocytes with fungal cells and are detected in *Candida* sepsis (87). TNF-α is essential in the innate control of disseminated infection caused by *C. albicans* (72, 82, 102). It is produced by PMNs in an opsonic-dependent manner (12) and by macrophages in response to beta-1,2 linked mannooligosaccharides (51) and in a Fas-FasL-dependent interaction (81). TNF-α is also produced by endothelial cells in response to the fungus and mediates the secretion of IL-8 by these cells (84). The cytokine regulates the recruitment of inflammatory cells, triggers the respiratory burst, and induces expression of costimulatory molecules. Although IL-1 shares many properties with TNF-α, both IL-1β and IL-6, which mainly act through recruitment of PMNs, do not seem to be as essential as TNF-α in the innate antifungal response. Administration of IL-1β has been beneficial in mice with candidiasis; nevertheless, IL-1 deficiency does not increase the susceptibility of mice to the infection as does IL-6 deficiency (72).

IFN-γ is a key cytokine in the innate control of an infection (78, 119). It stimulates migration, adherence, phagocytosis, and oxidative killing of PMNs and activates macrophages and endothelial cells for fungicidal activity. Studies in mice and humans have clearly shown the importance of IFN-γ as one major determinant of innate resistant to candidiasis (78, 119). However, other studies have revealed the dispensability of IFN-γ as an effector molecule (27, 89), thus revealing the complex role of IFN-γ in the interactions between the innate and the Adaptive immunity to the fungus (further discussed below).

IL-12 is recognized as essential for the induction of protective Th1 responses to the fungus (108). Upon phagocytosis of the fungus, IL-12 is produced by different cells, including PMNs (108), monocytes (29), and DCs (36) (see further below). Both IL-12 and IL-18 are produced during infection and induce IFN-γ (70, 108).

One of the most important cytokines produced during infection is IL-10. It is readily produced by PMNs (109) and macrophages (32) upon phagocytosis of the fungus and plays a crucial role in determining susceptibility to the infection (72, 124). High levels of IL-10 are seen in patients with chronic disseminated candidiasis (95). IL-10 acts by impairing the antifungal effector functions of phagocytes, including secretion of inflammatory cytokines and IL-12, and by inhibiting the development of protective cell-mediated immunity (72, 91, 94). It also acts as a major cytokine that discriminates between virulent and less virulent forms of the fungus (109, 132). Similar to IL-10, transforming growth factor beta (TGF-β) is produced by macrophages and appears to discriminate between virulent and less virulent forms of the fungus in mice with candidiasis (72).

In addition to IL-10, IL-4 may act as a major discriminating factor in the susceptibility and resistance of disseminated candidiasis (72). Ablation of IL-4 renders susceptible mice resistant to candidiasis. Although IL-4 may inhibit the fungicidal activity of phagocytes (33, 93), it also activates phagocytes (90, 117). Thus, one likely mechanism of the inhibitory activity of IL-4 in infection relies on its ability to promote Th2 reactivity, thus dampening protective Th1 responses. One major unresolved issue concerns the cell source of IL-4 in infection. Only recently has decisive evidence been obtained in this regard. It has been found that DCs produce IL-4 upon phagocytosis of hyphae but not yeasts of *C. albicans* (36), thus sensing the different forms of the fungus in terms of cytokine production (see below).

Instructive role of the innate immune system

Evidence is accumulating suggesting that cells of the innate immune system sense the different forms of the fungus through the different PRRs. How the innate immune system, through the use of different PRRs, discriminates between yeasts and hyphae of the fungus, produces qualitatively different responses to them, and promotes different Th responses will be the subject of the following sections and is illustrated in Fig. 1.

Discrimination. The innate responses to pathogens involve recognition mechanisms that are based on germ-line encoded PRRs that recognize invariant molecular structures shared by large groups of pathogens (also known as PAMPs, pathogen-associated molecular patterns). The Toll-like receptors (TLRs) can be considered as PRRs that subserve this recognition. Toll was originally defined as a *Drosophila* gene important for ontogenesis and antimicrobial resistance (1). TLRs are type I transmembrane proteins that activate specialized antifungal genes through the activation of NF-κB family members. Distinct PRRs and TRLs now appear to be involved in the recognition of PAMPs on different classes of pathogens: lipopolysaccharide (LPS) of gram-negative bacteria, lipoteichoic acid and peptoglycan of gram-positive bacteria, mannan and glucan of fungi, and phosphoglycan of parasites. TLR4, identified as an essential component of the LPS receptor signaling complex, is expressed on cells of the immune system, and its overexpression causes the release of cytokines (IL-1 and IL-6) and the expression of costimulatory molecules that are essential for activation of the adaptive immunity. TRL2, in contrast, mediates responses to gram-positive bacteria and yeasts (1).

PRRs are expressed by PMNs, macrophages, DC and NK cells, and probably also epithelial and endothelial cells in the lung, kidney, skin, and gastrointestinal tract. Mammalian PRRs include MRs, TLRs, scavenger receptors, integrins, collectins, and other clusters of differentiation antigens (68 and references therein). MRs, CR3, β-glucan receptors, and CD14 are known receptors on neutrophils, macrophages, and DCs that may work as PRRs recognizing PAMPs of fungi (99). The early observation that phagocytes from different anatomical sites exhibit a heterogeneous secretory response in response to the different forms of *C. albicans* (14) may have to be revisited in terms of activation of different PRRs by distinct PAMPs.

Although few studies have addressed, as yet, the issue of the involvement of PRRs in response to fungi, several considerations can be drawn. Experimental evidence indicates that production of IL-12 during *C. albicans* infection occurs normally in C3H/HeJ mice, known to have a functional TLR4 deficiency (95a). However, these mice show a moderate resistance to the invasive infection with the fungus (100), a finding suggesting that IL-12 production, more than Th1 induction, occurs independently of TLR4 signaling. In contrast, both IL-12 production and yeast but not hyphal phagocytosis by DCs (36) occur through a mannose-inhibitable receptor, a finding suggesting that MRs are involved in the production of IL-12 in response to *C. albicans*. Thus, not only are different PRRs involved in the recognition of the different forms of the fungus, but also the engagement of different PRRs results in different cellular responses. From this scenario, it follows that if the entry of fungal cells occurs through a phagocyte receptor other than the MRs, this may result in failure to activate IL-12-dependent protective Th1 responses. Alternatively, the use of different PRRs by different forms of fungi may represent one important strategy of immune evasion and parasitism by the fungus. This seems to be the case. CR3 engagement is one of the most efficient receptors for uptake of opsonized yeasts (121). However, as already stated, for effective killing and cytokine release to occur, the concomitant engagement of the FcγRI or FCαRI receptors is required (126). Thus, signaling through CR3 may not lead to phagocyte activation. It has recently been shown that signaling via CR3 down-regulates IL-12 production in response to *Histoplasma capsulatum* (65). In the case of *C. albicans,* the interaction with macrophage CR3 led to suppression of the immune response to the fungus (121). Interestingly, CR3 has more binding sites for *Candida* hyphae than yeasts (40) and therefore may represent one of the most important binding sites for the hyphal form. This situation may result in the failure to induce IL-12 and protective Th1 immunity in response to *Candida* hyphae. Chiani et al. have recently reported that human monocytes fail to induce IL-12 in response to the hyphal form of the fungus (29).

One further important observation is that the functioning of PRRs is sensitive to cytokines. The mannose receptor-mediated uptake of unopsonized *Candida* yeasts may lead to phagocyte abuse if not accompanied by the coordinate activation of the cell cytotoxic machinery (64). Increased expression of the receptor with no induced cytotoxicity occurs upon exposure of macrophages to IL-4 (117). In contrast, IFN-γ down-regulates the expression of macrophage mannose receptors and, nevertheless, results in effective killing, presumably via increased coupling of the receptor to cytotoxic functions (64). Thus, Th1 and Th2 cytokines may cooperate to stimulate mannose-receptor-mediated phagocytosis (90).

Altogether, these observations suggest that the use of the different PRRs, either alone or simultaneously, may result in the coupling or uncoupling of phagocytosis from inflammatory and immunological responses. Hence, the innate immune system appears to have the ability to autonomously decide whether to implicate the adaptive immune system. In addition, should different PRRs be used by opsonized and unopsonized fungi, this implies that the activation of phagocytes in vivo may vary according to the divergent conditions at specific, localized sites of infection.

Instruction. The instructive role of the innate immune system in the adaptive immune responses to *C.*

albicans occurs at different levels (72, 98). Qualitative or quantitative defects of antifungal effector and immunoregulatory functions of phagocytic cells result in the development of anticandidal Th2, rather than Th1, cell responses (72, 109). As $CD4^+$ Th cell differentiation in vivo was found to be critically affected by the tissue fungal load (72), an important role of phagocytic cells relies on their ability to control the fungal growth through their antifungal effector mechanisms. In addition to this, however, the instructive role of the innate immune system in the adaptive immune response to the fungus is operative at the levels of cytokine release and expression of costimulatory molecules (72, 98).

An important instructive role has recently been attributed to neutrophils and DCs by virtue of their ability to produce opposing cytokines upon recognition of different forms of the fungus. Neutrophils, more than macrophages, are endowed with the ability to produce directive cytokines, such as IL-10 and IL-12. Most important, IL-12 appears to be released in response to a *Candida* strain that initiates Th1 development in vivo, but IL-10 is released in response to a virulent strain (109). By producing IL-10 and IL-12, neutrophils may influence antifungal Th cell development, as evidenced by the inability of neutropenic mice to mount protective anticandidal Th1 responses. However, Th1-mediated resistance is increased upon IL-12 administration in neutropenic mice or IL-10 neutralization in nonneutropenic mice. Thus, neutrophils, through the differential production of directive cytokines, may directly contribute to discriminative Th responses to virulent or nonvirulent forms of the fungus. Human neutrophils also produce bioactive IL-12 in response to a mannoprotein fraction of *C. albicans* and are capable of inducing Th1 cytokine expression in peripheral blood mononuclear cells (108). Production of IL-12 by neutrophils occurs independently of TNF-α and IFN-γ, is impaired upon iron overload, but increases upon in vitro priming with IL-4, through up-regulation of IL-4 receptor expression (75). Because of the large number of neutrophils present in the blood or inflammatory tissues during infection (109), it is likely that neutrophil production of cytokines may influence the development and/or maintenance of the Th repertoire to *C. albicans*. Interestingly, it has recently been reported that neutrophils quickly release *Candida* antigens upon phagocytosis (3). Thus, it is likely that the immunoregulatory role of neutrophils in candidiasis may go beyond their cytokine production, to include signaling through antigen presentation and costimulation.

It has been found that expression of costimulatory molecules by cells of the innate immune system, including PMNs, is affected in invasive candidiasis (72). Both TNF-α and IL-10 are important cytokines regulating costimulatory antigen expression during infection (72). Interestingly, the expression of these molecules on PMNs is differentially regulated upon exposure to *Candida* yeasts or hyphae and correlates with the ability of PMNs to release IL-10 and to affect T-cell activation (69a). Human studies confirmed the multiple and complex role neutrophils may have in candidiasis. First, risk factors for invasive fungal infections are not the same in all neutropenic patients (130). Second, chronic systemic candidiasis initiated by neutropenia may persist in spite of normal neutrophil counts and adequate antifungal therapy (15). Third, some patients, particularly transplant recipients who have adequate or even normal neutrophil counts, may be at high risk for invasive mycoses (110). Figure 5 depicts the central role of PMNs in anticandidal immunity.

Among the important virulence factors of *C. albicans* is its ability to reversibly switch from a unicellular yeast form into various filamentous forms, all of which can be found in tissues (54, 76). Recent studies have clearly shown that the ability to switch from yeast to filamentous form is required for virulence (41, 60). It is likely that a host cell exists that finely discriminates between the two forms of the fungus in terms of class of immune response elicited. Accumulating evidence points to a unique role of the DCs in infections, as they are regarded as both sentinel for innate recognition and initiator of of Th cell differentiation and functional commitment (11). In candidiasis, DCs were found to be uniquely able to phagocytose both yeasts or hyphae of the fungus. However, the downstream cellular events after internalization of either form of the fungus are clearly different. In vitro, ingestion of yeasts activates dendritic cells for IL-12 and NO production and priming of Th1 cells, whereas ingestion of hyphae inhibits IL-12, NO, and Th1 priming. In vivo, generation of antifungal protective immunity is observed upon injection of DCs ex vivo pulsed with *C. albicans* yeasts but not hyphae. The immunization capacity of yeast-pulsed DCs is lost in the absence of IL-12, whereas that of hypha-pulsed DCs is gained in the absence of IL-4 (36). These results indicate that DCs fulfill the requirement of a cell uniquely capable of sensing the different forms of the fungus in terms of the type of immune responses elicited. Considering that the morphogenesis of *C. albicans* is activated in vivo by a wide range of signals (18) and that human DCs also phagocytose *C. albicans* (28) and activate T-cell responses to the fungus, DCs appear to meet the challenge of Th priming and education in *C. albicans* saprophytism and infections.

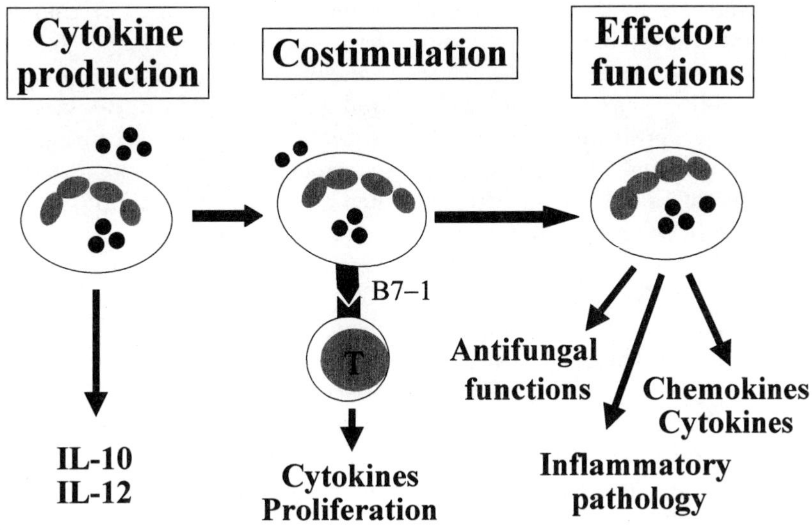

Figure 5. The central role of PMNs in anticandidal immunity. Besides their antifungal effector activity, the PMNs participate in the initial host defense by the discriminative production of cytokines, such as IL-10 and IL-12, and expression of costimulatory molecules, such as B7–1. Both activities have an impact on the subsequent development of adaptive T helper immunity and place neutrophils squarely in a regulatory role.

Adaptive Immunity: the Th Paradigm

The clinical circumstances in which recurrent *Candida* infections occur definitely suggest an association with impaired cell-mediated immunity, yet only in the last decade has direct evidence of this relationship been obtained in experimental models of mucosal or invasive candidiasis (7, 39, 88, 96, 97, 107).

In conditions in which the animals are overwhelmed by a high dose of virulent cells given intravenously, mice of different inbred strains die within a few days. Therefore, any contribution of T-cell-mediated immunity could hardly be assessed in this setting and, thus, resistance of naive mice to the acute infection mostly reflects the activity of natural immune mechanisms. This may help explain the controversial results earlier obtained in mice rendered functionally T-cell deficient by different means (7 and references therein). However, upon intravenous challenge with sublethal fungal doses or with low-virulence yeast cells, or after gastrointestinal infection, an infection is sustained long enough so that it is possible to evaluate the contribution of both nonspecific and specific effector immune mechanisms in the control of the infection and its pathology (88, 96, 97, 107). A combination of defects in both phagocytic cell function and T-cell-mediated immune responses predisposes mice to disseminated candidiasis of endogenous origin (49), thus emphasizing the interdependency between the innate and adaptive immune systems in infection. Corroborative evidence was provided by the transfer of a *Candida*-specific T-cell line into sublethally irradiated mice (113); the T-cell line confers resistance against primary intravenous challenge. Further evidence indicated that both $CD4^+$ and $CD8^+$ cells contribute to the host response against the infection (88, 96, 107). Interestingly, *C. albicans* was able to induce selective expansion of T lymphocytes bearing a particular T-cell receptor Vβ specificity, raising the possibility that molecules with superantigen activity may be displayed by the fungus (97).

The general thrust of the results described above indicates that the major function of the T lymphocytes in *Candida* infections is the production of cytokines with activating and deactivating signals to fungicidal effector phagocytes. Therefore, host resistance to the fungus appears to be dependent on the induction of cellular immunity, mediated by T lymphocytes and nonspecific effector phagocytes (7, 97). Not surprisingly, delayed-type hypersensitivity (DTH) to *Candida* antigens is a standard in vivo assay for T-cell-mediated immunity in humans. DTH reactivity is usually detectable in more than 80% of the normal adult population (83). The expression of this cutaneous reactivity is often defective in neonates, in immunocompromised individuals, and in patients with recurrent or persistent infection with the fungus, or immunopathology associated with it (39, 88, 96, 107).

The discovery that subsets of $CD4^+$ Th cells could be distinguished according to their ability to produce discrete patterns of cytokines (77) offered the conceptual framework of adaptive immunity in *C. albicans*

(39, 88, 96, 101, 107). Th1 cells, by their production of IFN-γ and TNF-α, are responsible for directing cell-mediated immune responses to the fungus. Th2 cells by producing IL-4 and IL-10 have been strongly implicated in dampening the protective antifungal Th1 immunity and mediating fungal allergy. The relative importance of the different Th cells and of effector phagocytes to the outcome of the infection depends on numerous factors, including localization and virulence of the primary infection, early cytokine response of the host to the fungus, and the predominant type of Th cells activated by challenge. The qualitative pattern of cytokines secreted by T cells will ultimately determine the efficacy of the effector response mediated by phagocytes. Accordingly, in evaluating the relative contributions of various Th-dependent effector mechanisms in murine candidiasis, it is important to distinguish between those that are responsible for recovery from the primary infection and those that mediate protection upon reinfection.

Primary resistance

In studying the immune response to *C. albicans* in genetically distinct mice, circumstantial evidence was reported that active suppression of protective immunity might occur in inbred strains of mice that are classified as genetically susceptible to candidiasis and are characterized by high antibody levels and poor DTH responses (5). More recent studies indicate that susceptibility and resistance to primary disseminated infection with low-virulence *C. albicans* vary among inbred strains of mice of different MHC haplotypes (100 and references therein). This genetically determined resistance to the primary infection correlates with the balance occurring between protective Th1 and nonprotective Th2 $CD4^+$ cells. Induction of Th1 response requires IFN-γ, IL-12, and $CD4^+$ cells in the afferent induction, and $CD8^+$ cells in the effector phase. Nonspecifically activated macrophages and granulocytes with microbicidal properties act as the final effector cells of this response. The induction of $CD4^+$ Th1 cells requires the presence of an activated innate immune system, such as the ability of phagocytic cells to inhibit fungal growth and to release cytokines. In contrast, in mice not surviving the primary infection, high-level production of Th2 cytokines, such as IL-4 and IL-10, is observed early in the infection and until the animal's death. In this case, $CD4^+$ cells from these mice release Th2 cytokines in vitro in response to specific antigen (105). Neutralization of IL-4 or IL-10 early in infection allows the activation of $CD4^+$ Th1 cells and renders mice resistant to primary and secondary infections (72). The general conclusion from these studies is that resistance to disseminated *C. albicans* infection is determined by nonspecific phagocytic mechanisms, the activity of which is augmented or reinforced by Th1 cytokines and impaired by Th2 cytokines. Of interest, systemic activation of host-protective $CD4^+$ Th1 cells is detected in mice with mucosal yeast colonization of limited grade and duration (39, 88, 96, 107). This condition, which simulates saprophytic yeast carriage by healthy humans with peripheral Th1-type reactivity (8, 9), is associated with increased resistance to systemic reinfection. Therefore, the expression of Th1-mediated resistance at both mucosal and nonmucosal effector sites may involve common mechanisms in humans who develop systemic immunity as a consequence of their mucosal colonization. This could explain why the absence of $CD4^+$ cells is consistently detrimental in mucosal colonization with the fungus (where a strong Th1 response typically develops).

Recent studies on the genetic control of the host susceptibility and/or resistance invasive *C. albicans* infection have shed new and important light on the role of antifungal cell-mediated immunity. Two Mendelian-type resistance genes control the host response to infection in mice (4). These genes appear to affect distinct parameters of infection, such as tissue destruction and kidney colonization.

Acquired resistance

In models of sustained protective anticandidal responses, such as the mucosal exposure to the fungus or the vaccine-induced resistance, $CD4^+$ T but not B lymphocytes and IFN-γ are required for the expression of acquired resistance to the fungus (7, 50, 101). Th1 reactivity is associated with acquired resistance to either disseminated or vaginal infection. That acquired immunity to *C. albicans* correlates with the expression of local or peripheral Th1 reactivity has also been confirmed by studies in adult healthy humans (38, 59). Underlying acquired immunity to the fungus, such as the expression of a positive DTH, is demonstrable in adult immunocompetent individuals and is presumed to prevent mucosal colonization from progression to symptomatic infection (39, 88, 96, 107). Human lymphocytes show strong proliferative responses after stimulation with *Candida* antigens (8) and produce a number of different cytokines (9). Due to their action on circulating leukocytes, the cytokines produced by *Candida*-specific T cells may be instrumental in mobilizing and activating anticandidal effectors (97, 117), thus providing prompt and effective control of infectivity once *Candida* sp. has established itself in mucosal tissues or spread to internal organs. In atopic subjects, in women with recurrent vaginal candidiasis, and in patients with chronic

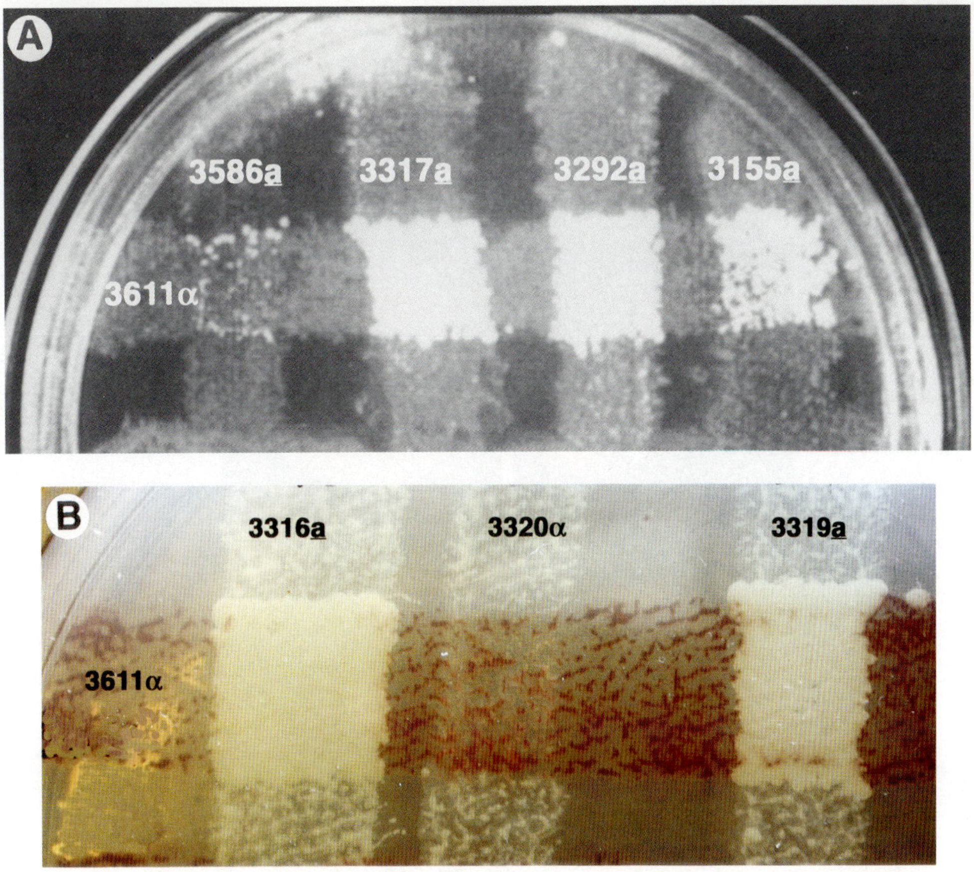

Color plate 1. Matings of the strains listed below were plated on YEPD then replicated after 7 days to minimal medium. (A) 3586 (*ade2 ura3 MTL***a**), 3317 (*trp1 lys2 MTL***a**), 3292 (*ura3MTL***a**), 3155 (*ade2 ura3 MTL***a**/*Δa*), 3611 (*ade1 MTL***a**). The *ura3* strains are derivatives of CAI4. Strain 3155 is derived from a deletion of the "**a**" region of chromosome 5 (22). The other strains were made homozygous for mating type by growth on sorbose. Strain 3611 is derived from B792-P1. (B) 3316 (*trp1 lys2 MTL***a**), 3320 (Arg^- Ilv^- *MTL***a**), 3319 (Arg^- Ilv^- *MTL***a**), 3611 (*adel MTL***a**), Strains 3316, 3319, and 3320 are derived from FC18. Strains 3319 and 3320 are sorbose derivatives of the same parent (A658).

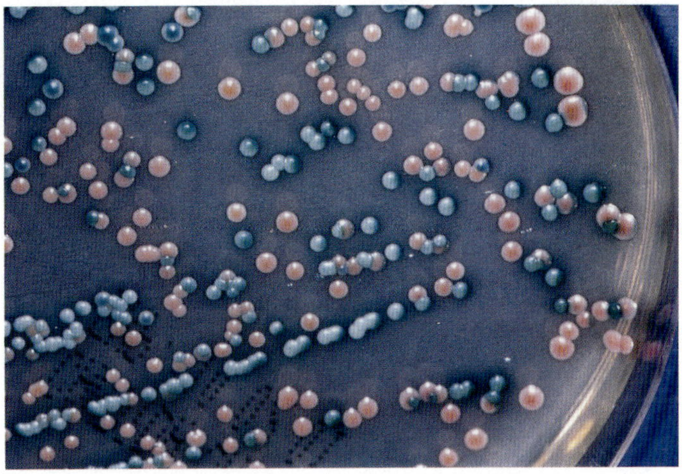

Color plate 2. Colonies of *Candida albicans* (green colonies) and *Candida glabrata* (pink colonies) following 48 h of growth at 37°C on CHROMagar Candida medium.

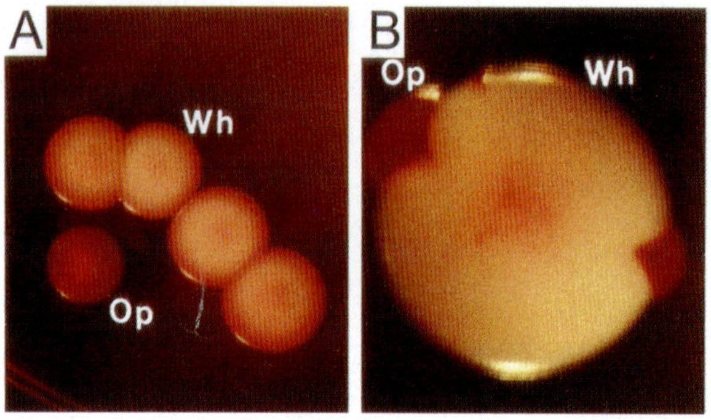

Color plate 3. "White opaque transition" in *C. albicans* WO-1. (A) A switch from white (Wh) to opaque (Op). (B) Opaque sectors (Op) in a white (Wh) colony.

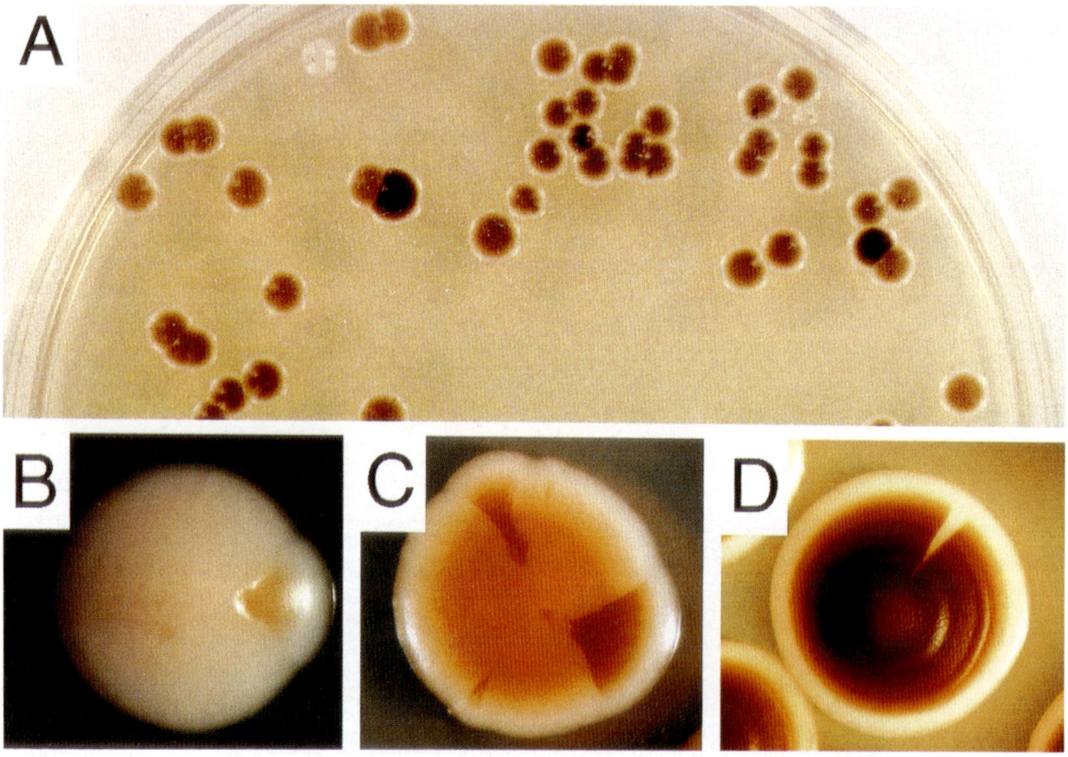

Color plate 4. Switching between the white, light brown, and dark brown phenotypes in *Candida glabrata*. (A) Field of colonies generated from cells of a single light brown colony that includes white, light brown, and dark brown colonies. (B) White colony with a light brown sector. (C) Light brown colony with dark brown sectors. (D) Dark brown colony with a white sector. (Reprinted from Lachke, S., T. Srikantha, L. Tsai, K. Daniels, and D. R. Soll, *Infect. Immun.* **68**:884–895, 2000.)

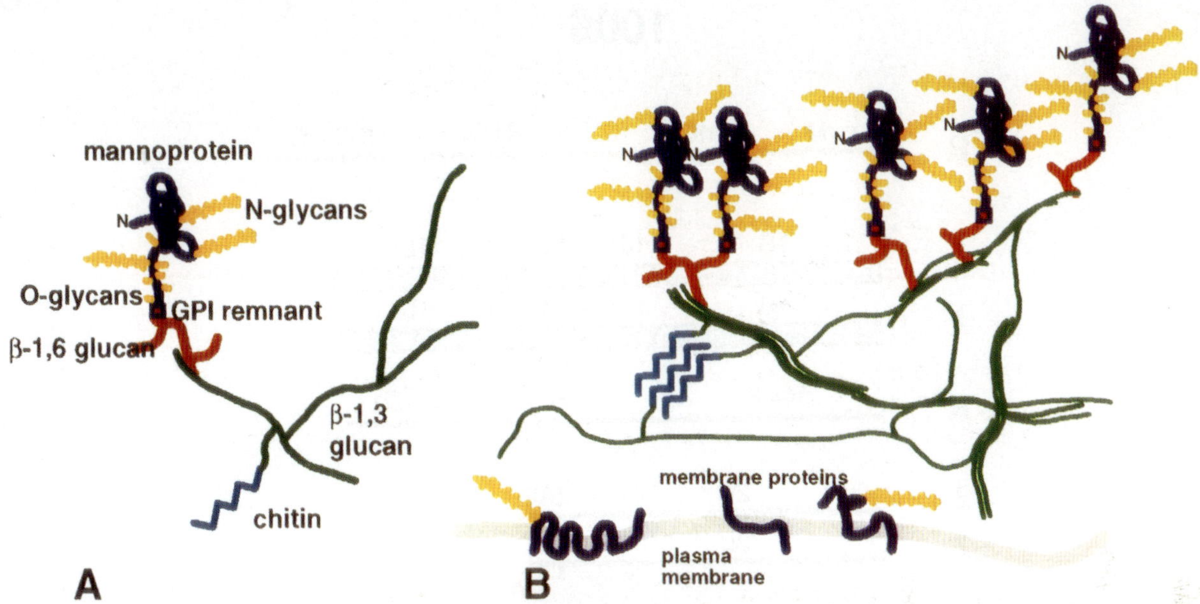

Color plate 5. (A) The prototypical module of the *Saccharomyces cerevisiae* cell wall. Individual components are color-coded: blue, mannoprotein polypeptide; yellow, oligosaccharides. Components are labeled as N or O linked. Chitin and the β-glucans are indicated, but not all branch points are indicated. (B) Representation of modules in a cell wall lattice. The β-glucans are interassociated in a triple helice, while chitin is represented as a crystalline domain. (Reprinted with permission from Lipke, P. N., and R. Ovalle, *J. Bacteriol.* **180**:3735–3740, 1998.)

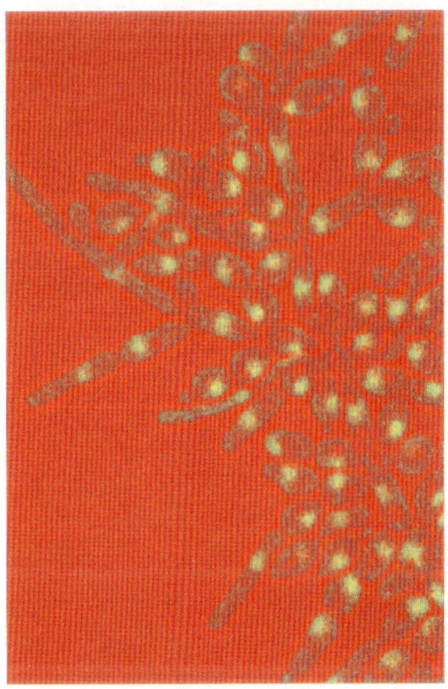

Color plate 6. Localization of a Efg1p-yEGFP fusion protein in *Candida albicans*. A *EFG1-yEGFP* fusion was overexpressed in *C. albicans* CAI4 by the *PCK1* promoter, which led to extensive pseudohyphae. The photo shows an overlay of the GFP fluorescence (green) and a differential interference contrast image (red), taken with a confocal laser microscope. The fusion protein is visible in nuclei of pseudohyphal cells by its green fluorescence.

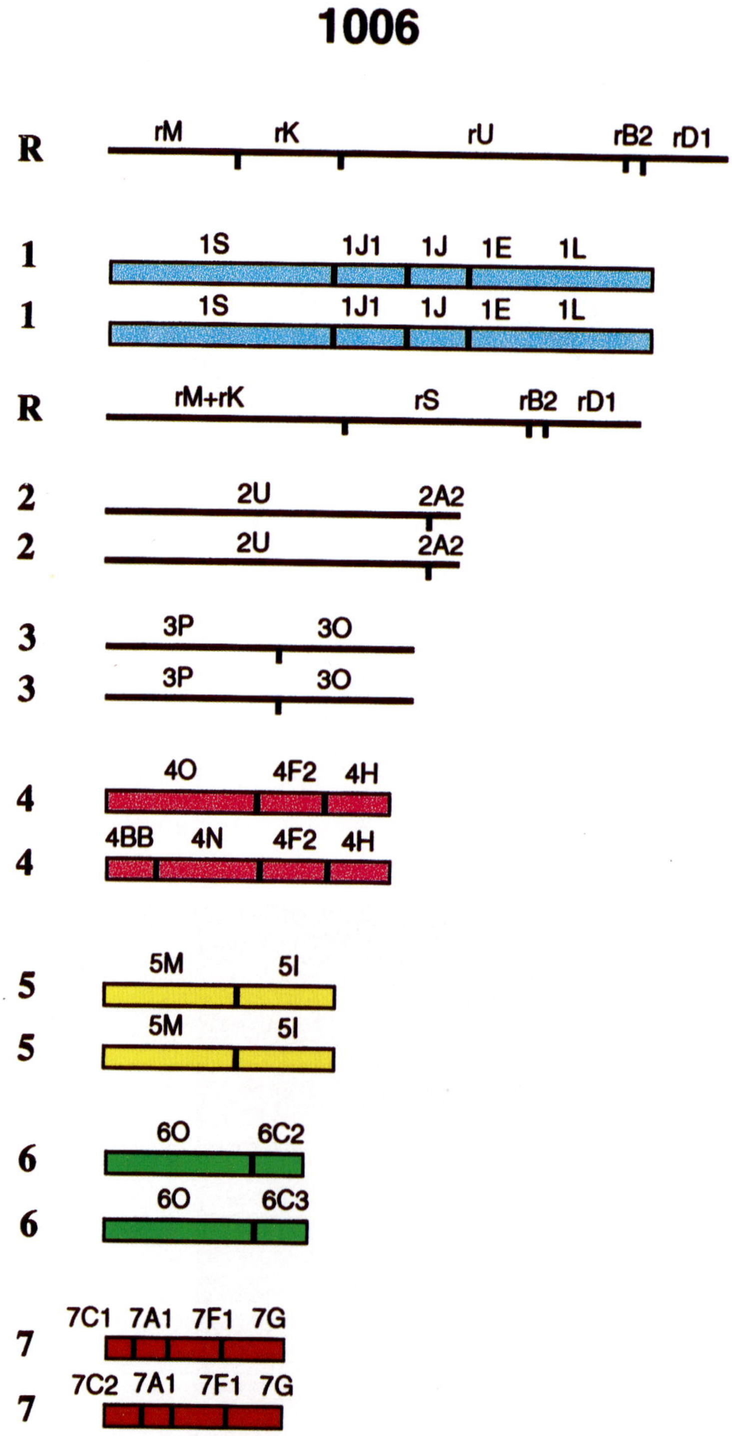

Color plate 7. Diagrams of the *Sfi*I restriction maps of the chromosomes of *Candida albicans* strains 1006 and WO-1. The breaks in the chromosomes indicate the *Sfi*I sites. The *Sfi*I fragments are colored according to their origin on the homologous chromosomes of strain 1006.

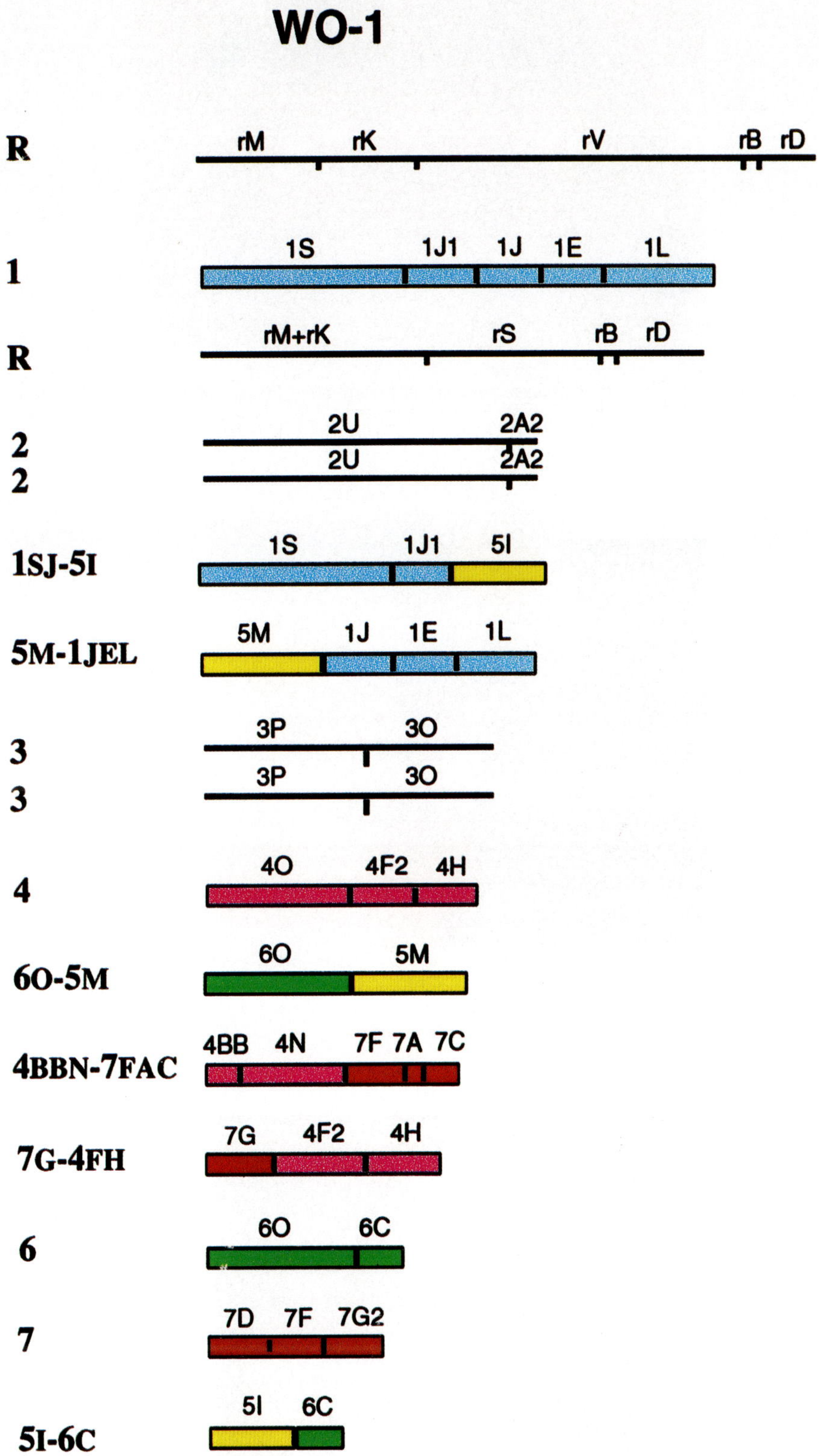

Color plate 7. *Continued.*

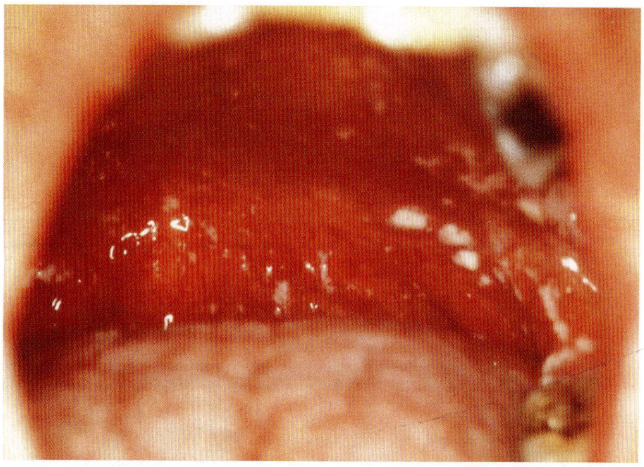

Color plate 8. Acute pseudomembranous candidiasis (oral thrush) with white plaques and diffuse erythematous areas in the oral cavity of a patient with AIDS.

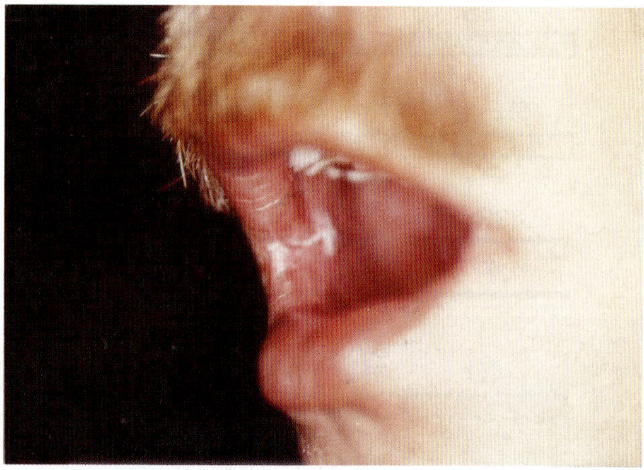

Color plate 9. Angular cheilitis with plaque-like candidiasis of the buccal mucosa in a patient with AIDS.

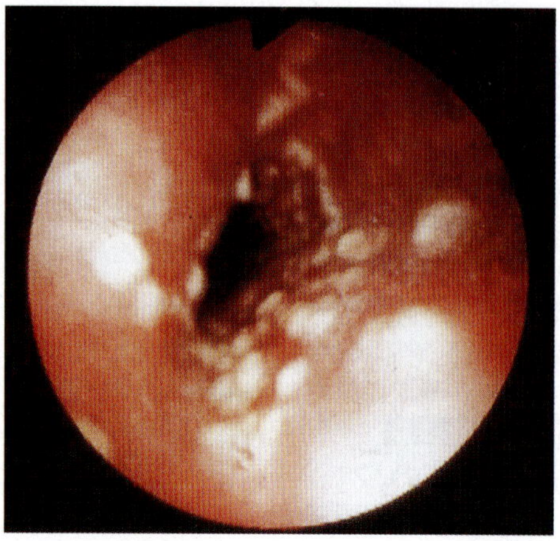

Color plate 10. *Candida* esophagitis, grade III, with confluent plaques combined with ulceration in a patient with AIDS.

mucocutaneous candidiasis, the suppressed delayed skin responses to the fungus show an inverse relationship with elevated levels of *Candida*-specific immunoglobulins IgE, IgA, and IgG (39, 88, 96, 107). These data argue for the reciprocal regulation of humoral and cell-mediated immunity to the fungus and suggest that the yeast/host relationship in saprophytism and disease presents features compatible with the Th1/Th2 paradigm of acquired immunity. A Th1-type reactivity may characterize the saprophytic yeast carriage of healthy subjects, whereas Th2-type responses would be mostly associated with susceptibility to recurrent or persistent infection (122) and allergy (96). For example, in patients with defective IL-12/IFN-γ pathway, such as those with hyperimmunoglobulinemia E syndrome, both an impaired IL-12 response to the fungus (17) and visceral candidiasis (134) are observed. Of interest, suppression of cell-mediated immunity may be a consequence of *C. albicans* infection, as demonstrated by much experimental and clinical evidence. Polysaccharide antigens of the fungus generate a complex series of interactions resulting in the suppression of both T- and B-cell responses to the homologous antigen. These effects are mediated by antigen-nonspecific inhibitory factors that are able to block the synthesis of cytokines by human monocytes and T cells (reviewed in reference 107).

It is important to note that experimental and clinical evidence indicates that differences may exist in cell and cytokine requirements for antifungal resistance at mucosal or peripheral levels (37, 88, 107), a notion exemplified by the long-recognized association between disseminated candidiasis and qualitative and quantitative defects of neutrophils and between chronic mucosal infections and T-cell abnormalities (83). The concept of a reciprocal regulation between the phagocyte system and the T-cell compartment may provide a unifying thread between the systemic immune responses and events occurring at the mucosal surface. This notion emphasizes that the anticandidal responses that have been characterized in invasive and mucosal infections are not unique to either condition. The expression of acquired resistance at both mucosal and nonmucosal effector sites may involve common mechanisms in humans who develop systemic immunity as a consequence of their mucosal colonization. These mechanisms likely operate through the action of Th1 lymphocytes, the cytokines they release, and nonspecifically activated effector cells. The unitary role for cell-mediated immunity in anticandidal resistance would predict that, for example, eradication of an established infection, whether superficial or deep seated, could be accelerated by recruitment of antigen-specific cells that would provide the locally high cytokine concentrations needed for optimal activation of the anticandidal effector phagocytes.

IMMUNOREGULATION: THE CYTOKINE PARADOXES

Th1 and Th2 $CD4^+$ T cells develop from a common naive $CD4^+$ T cell precursor, and several parameters have been reported to influence the pathway of differentiation of $CD4^+$ T-cell precursors (107). Among these, cytokines appear to play a major role, acting not only as modulators of antifungal effector functions but also as key regulators in the development of the different Th subsets from precursor Th cells. Development of protective anticandidal Th1 responses against invasive infection requires the concerted actions of several cytokines such as IFN-γ, TGF-β, IL-6, TNF-α, and IL-12 in the relative absence of inhibitory Th2 cytokines, such as IL-4 and IL-10, which inhibit the induction of Th1 responses (101, 107). Early in infection, neutralization of Th1 cytokines (IFN-γ and IL-12) leads to the onset of Th2 rather than Th1 responses, while neutralization of Th2 cytokines (IL-4 and IL-10) allows for the development of Th1 rather than Th2 cell responses (101, 107). However, further studies have clearly revealed that individual cytokines can produce opposing effects depending on dose and timing of their participation in the immune response and that some cytokines exert their effects on both the innate and adaptive immunity. For instance, both qualitative and quantitative changes in antifungal effector functions of phagocytic cells, particularly neutrophils, and the activation of nonprotective Th2 responses are observed in the absence of TNF-α or IL-6 (72). One likely mechanism of Th2 development in mice with candidiasis is the increased fungal burden in organs, as the production of IL-4, and hence Th2 activation, is strictly dependent on the fungal dose (101). Therefore, the defective antifungal effector functions of phagocytes and consequently the unopposed fungal growth may account for the failure to mount a protective Th1 response in the absence of TNF-α or IL-6. However, TNF-α was also found to be required for optimal expression of costimulatory molecules on phagocytic cells and for IL-12 responsiveness in $CD4^+$ Th1 cells, whereas decreased production of IL-12 and increased production of IL-10 occurred in the absence of IL-6 (72).

IFN-γ is not necessary for induction and expression of anticandidal Th2 responses (27, 89). Instead, the absence of IFN-γ correlated with the failure to mount protective anticandidal Th1 responses due to an impaired IL-12 responsiveness rather than IL-12 production (27). The activities of IL-12 are mediated through a high-affinity receptor composed of two subunits, designated β1 and β2. Of these two subunits, β2 is more restricted in its distribution, and regulation of its expression is likely a central mechanism by which IL-12 responsiveness is controlled (42). Indeed, the IL-12Rβ2 subunit expression on activated $CD4^+$ Th1 cells is known to correspond to loss of IL-12 responsiveness and represents an early step in the commitment of T cells to the Th2 pathway (120). Because IFN-γ is necessary to override the IL-4-induced inhibition of IL-12β2 receptor expression in Th1 cells (120), it is likely that in murine candidiasis the Th1-promoting activity of IFN-γ may rely on its ability to maintain IL-12 responsiveness on $CD4^+$ cells, through sustaining the IL-12Rβ2 expression.

Although IL-4 induces anticandidal Th2 development and exogenous IL-4 exacerbates candidiasis in mice, IL-4 also primes neutrophils for IL-12 synthesis (72). This may account for the requirement for IL-4 in the generation of memory anticandidal Th1 response. Paradoxically, the induction and maintenance of memory Th1 resistance also require IL-10 and TGF-β (97). Thus, cytokines with inhibitory activity in developing Th1 cell responses are indeed required for sustained Th1 reactivity to the fungus. The possible regulatory cells and mechanisms underlying the expression of immunological memory to *C. albicans* are not yet understood. However, it is intriguing that different Th cells and cytokines are produced in response to different fungal antigens (25). It is possible that the temporally distinct expressions of different antigens during fungal growth in vivo have a role in the expression of immunological memory responses to *C. albicans,* through the induction of regulatory T cells.

Altogether, the data indicate that (i) the cytokine requirement for the expression of innate antifungal defense may be different from that required for the expression of Th1-mediated protection; (ii) a single cytokine may participate in both the innate and the adaptive phase of the response to the fungus, sometimes exhibiting opposite effects; and (iii) a hierarchic pattern exists of cytokine-mediated regulation of antifungal Th cell development and effector function. Early in infection, production of some proinflammatory cytokines (TNF-α and IL-6) appears to be essential for the successful control of infection and the resulting protective Th1-dependent immunity. Both IL-12 production and IL-12 responsiveness are required for the development of Th1 cell responses that are maintained in the presence of physiological levels of IL-4, IL-10, TGF-β, and IL-18. Thus, a finely regulated balance of directive cytokines, rather than the relative absence of opposing cytokines, appears to be required for optimal development and maintenance of Th1 reactivity in mice with candidiasis. Table 1

Table 1. Major features of the most important cytokines in the innate and adaptive immunity to *C. albicans*

Cytokine	Immunity (reference)	
	Innate	Adaptive
TNF-α	Recruits and activates effector phagocytes (72, 82) Induces costimulatory molecules (72)	Required for Th1 induction (72)
IL-1	Recruits and activates effector phagocytes (58)	Unknown
IFN-γ	Activates oxidative burst (33) Enhances coupling of macrophage mannose receptors to candidacidal function (64)	Required for Th1 induction (27)
IL-2	Activates PMNs to a candidacidal state (34)	Not required for Th1 induction (115)
IL-4	Increases macrophage mannose receptors (90, 117) Suppresses phagocytosis and antifungal activity of effector phagocytes (93) Increases IL-12 production by PMNs (75)	Promotes Th2 responses (75) Required for memory responses (75)
IL-6	Recruits and activates effector phagocytes (72, 125)	Required for Th1 induction (72)
IL-8	Recruits inflammatory cells (10)	Unknown
IL-10	Suppresses phagocytosis and antifungal activity of effector phagocytes (94, 95) Regulates costimulatory molecule expression (72)	Down-regulates Th1 responses (72)
IL-12	Increases the IFN-γ-dependent production of NO (72)	Required for Th1 induction (72)
IL-15	Stimulates proinflammatory and antifungal activity of phagocytes (79, 129)	Unknown
IL-18	Increases the IFN-γ-dependent production of NO (70)	Required for memory responses (70)
TGF-β	Inhibits NO production by phagocytes (116)	Required for Th1 induction (116)

summarizes the most important cytokines and their functions in candidiasis.

CONCLUSIONS: PERSPECTIVES FOR THERAPY

As clinical resistance represents a significant component of the overall drug resistance of the antifungals (2), one major strategy to prevent antifungal drug resistance is to improve the immune functions of the immunocompromised host. A variety of cytokines, including chemokines (53) and growth factors (57, 127), proved to be beneficial in experimental fungal infections (78, 119). However, establishing the clinical utility of cytokines as therapy for fungal infections in patients has been difficult (118). The basic strategies pursued include the increase in number, function, and mobility of phagocytic effector cells, as cytokines, effector cells, and antifungal agents work synergistically to oppose fungal growth. The identification of PRRs as critical components of the innate recognition system is a fundamental breakthrough in immunology, but much remains to be learned. The discoveries of PRRs may have important clinical implications and improve our understanding of PRR functions and dysfunctions in candidal infections. Recently, the Th1/Th2 balance itself was found to be the target of immunotherapy (26, 71, 74, 86). The therapeutic efficacy of antifungal agents in experimental candidiasis is significantly increased by the concomitant inhibition of Th2 cytokines or the addition of Th1 cytokines, although host immune reactivity is critical (26, 71). Thus, the deliberate targeting of cells and pathways of cell-mediated immunity to the fungus may represent a useful strategy in the prophylaxis and treatment of invasive candidiasis in immunocompromised and nonimmunocompromised patients.

Acknowledgments. Many thanks are due to numerous collaborators over the years in different sections of the work described. This work was supported by grants from AIDS 50B.33 and ICS 120.5/RF 98/97 projects.

REFERENCES

1. **Aderem, A., and R. J. Ulevitch.** 2000. Toll-like receptors in the induction of the innate immune response. *Nature* **406:** 782–787.
2. **Alexander, B. D., and J. R. Perfect.** 1997. Antifungal resistance trends towards the year 2000. Implications for therapy and new approaches. *Drugs* **54:**657–678.
3. **Ashley, C., M. Morhart, R. Rennie, and B. Ziola.** 1997. Release of *Candida albicans* yeast antigens upon interaction with human neutrophils in vitro. *J. Med. Microbiol.* **46:** 747–755.
4. **Ashman, R. B.** 1998. *Candida albicans:* pathogenesis, immunity and host defence. *Res. Immunol.* **149:**281–288.
5. **Ashman, R. B.** 1990. Murine candidiasis: cell-mediated immune responses correlate directly with susceptibility and resistance to infection. *Immunol. Cell. Biol.* **68:**15–20.
6. **Ashman, R. B., and J. M. Papadimitriou.** 1990. What's new in the mechanisms of host resistance to *Candida albicans* infection? *Pathol. Res. Pract.* **186:**527–534.
7. **Ashman, R. B., and J. M. Papadimitriou.** 1995. Production and function of cytokines in natural and acquired immunity to *Candida albicans* infection. *Microbiol. Rev.* **59:**646–672.
8. **Ausiello, C. M., G. C. Spagnoli, M. Boccanera, I. Casalinuovo, F. Malavasi, C. U. Casciani, and A. Cassone.** 1986. Proliferation of human peripheral blood mononuclear cells induced by *Candida albicans* and its cell wall fractions. *J. Med. Microbiol.* **22:**195–202.
9. **Ausiello, C. M., F. Urbani, S. Gessani, G. C. Spagnoli, M. J. Gomez, and A. Cassone.** 1986. Cytokine gene expression in human peripheral blood mononuclear cells stimulated by mannoprotein constituents from *Candida albicans. Infect. Immun.* **61:**4105–4111.
10. **Balish, E., R. D. Wagner, A. Vasquez-Torres, J. Jones-Carson, C. Pierson, and T. Warner.** 1999. Mucosal and systemic candidiasis in IL-8R/h-/- BALB/c mice. *J. Leukoc. Biol.* **66:** 144–150.
11. **Banchereu, J., and R. M. Steinman.** 1998. Dendritic cells and the control of immunity. *Nature* **392:**245–252.
12. **Bazzoni, F., M. A. Cassatella, C. Laudanna, and F. Rossi.** 1991. Phagocytosis of opsonized yeast induces tumor necrosis factor-alpha mRNA accumulation and protein release by human polymorphonuclear leukocytes. *J. Leukoc. Biol.* **50:** 223–228.
13. **Blasi, E., L. Pitzurra, M. Puliti, L. Lanfrancone, and F. Bistoni.** 1992. Early differential molecular response of a macrophage cell line to yeast and hyphal forms of *Candida albicans. Infect. Immun.* **60:**832–837.
14. **Blasi, E., M. Puliti, L. Pitzurra, A. Bartoli, and F. Bistoni.** 1994. Heterogeneous secretory response of phagocytes from different anatomical districts to the dimorphic fungus *Candida albicans. Cell Immunol.* **153:**239–247.
15. **Bodey, G. P., and E. J. Anaissie.** 1989. Chronic systemic candidiasis. *Eur. J. Clin. Microbiol. Infect. Dis.* **8:**855–857.
16. **Bodey, G. P., M. Buckley, Y. S. Sathe, and E. J. Freireich.** 1986. Quantitative relationship between circulating leukocytes and infection in patients with acute leukemia. *Ann. Intern. Med.* **64:**328–340.
17. **Borges, W. G., N. H. Augustine, and H. R. Hill.** 2000. Defective interleukin-12/interferon-gamma pathway in patients with hyperimmunoglobulinemia E syndrome. *J. Pediatr.* **136:** 176–180.
18. **Brown, A. J. P., and N. A. R. Gow.** 1999. Regulatory networks controlling *Candida albicans* morphogenesis. *Trends Microbiol.* **7:**333–338.
19. **Calderone, R.** 1994. Molecular pathogenesis of fungal infections. *Trends Microbiol.* **2:**461–463.
20. **Calderone, R., and J. Sturtevant.** 1994. Macrophage interactions with *Candida. Immunol. Ser.* **60:**505–515.
21. **Casadevall, A.** 1995. Antibody immunity and invasive fungal infections. *Infect. Immun.* **63:**4211–4218.
22. **Casadevall, A.** 1998. Antibody-mediated protection against intracellular pathogens. *Trends Microbiol.* **6:**5–10.
23. **Casadevall, A., A. Cassone, F. Bistoni, J. E. Cutler, W. Magliani, J. W. Murphy, L. Polonelli, and L. Romani.** 1998. Antibody and/or cell-mediated immunity, protective mechanisms in fungal diseases: an ongoing dilemma or an unnecessary dispute? *Med. Mycol.* **36**(S1)**:**45–51.

24. **Cassone, A., S. Conti, F. De Bernardis, and L. Polonelli.** 1997. Antibodies, killer toxins and antifungal immunoprotection: a lesson from nature? *Immunol. Today* **18:**164–169.

25. **Cassone, A., F. De Bernardis, C. M. Ausiello, M. J. Gomez, M. Boccanera, R. La Valle, and A. Torosantucci.** 1998. Immunogenic and protective *Candida albicans* constituents. *Res. Immunol.* **149:**289–299.

26. **Cenci, E., A. Mencacci, G. Del Sero, F. Bistoni, and L. Romani.** 1997. Induction of protective ThI responses to *Candida albicans* by antifungal therapy alone or in combination with an interleukin-4 antagonist. *J. Infect. Dis.* **176:**217–226.

27. **Cenci, E., A. Mencacci, G. Del Sero, C. Fè d'Ostiani, P. Mosci, M. Kopf, and L. Romani.** 1998. IFN-γ is required for IL-12 responsiveness in mice with *Candida albicans* infection. *J. Immunol.* **161:**3543–3550.

28. **Chen, B.-G., Y. Shi, J. D. Smith, D. Choi, J. D. Geiger, and J. J. Mulè.** 1998. The role of tumor necrosis factor-α in modulating the quantity of peripheral blood-derived, cytokine-driven human dendritic cells and its role in enhancing the quality of dendritic cell function in presenting soluble antigens to $CD4^+$ T cells in vitro. *Blood* **91:**4652–4661.

29. **Chiani, P., C. Bromuro, and A. Torosantucci.** 2000. Defective induction of interleukin-12 in human monocytes by germ-tube forms of *Candida albicans. Infect. Immun.* **68:** 5628–5634.

30. **Danley, D. L., and A. E. Hilger.** 1981. Stimulation of oxidative metabolism in murine polymorphonuclear leukocytes by unopsonized fungal cells: evidence for a mannose-specific mechanisms. *J. Immunol.* **127:**551–556.

31. **Davis, S. L., E. P. Hawkins, E. O. Mason, Jr., C. W. Smith, and S. L. Kaplan.** 1996. Host defenses against disseminated candidiasis are impaired in intercellular adhesion molecule 1-deficient mice. *J. Infect. Dis.* **174:**435–439.

32. **Del Sero, G., A. Mencacci, E. Cenci, C. Fè d'Ostiani, C. Montagnoli, A. Bacci, P. Mosci, and L. Romani.** 1999. Antifungal type 1 responses are upregulated in IL-10-deficient mice. *Microbes Infect.* **1:**1169–1180.

33. **Djeu, J. Y.** 1993. Modulators of immune response to fungi, p. 521–532. *In* J. W. Murphy, H. Friedman, and M. Bendinelli (ed.), *Fungal Infections and Immune Responses.* Plenum Press, New York, N.Y.

34. **Djeu, J. Y., J. H. Liu, S. Wei, H. Rui, C. A. Pearson, M. J. Leonard, and D. K. Blanckard.** 1993. Function associated with IL-2 receptor-beta on human neutrophils. Mechanism of activation of antifungal activity against *Candida albicans* by IL-2. *J. Immunol.* **150:**960–970.

35. **Fearon, J. D., and R. M. Locksley.** 1996. The instructive role of innate immunity in the acquired immune response. *Science* **272:**50–54.

36. **Fè d'Ostiani, C., G. Del Sero, A. Bacci, C. Montagnoli, A. Spreca, A. Mencacci, P. Ricciardi-Castagnoli, and L. Romani.** 2000. Dendritic cells discriminate between yeasts and hyphae of the fungus *Candida albicans:* implications for initiation of Th immunity in vitro and in vivo. *J. Exp. Med.* **191:** 1661–1674.

37. **Fidel, P. L., Jr.** 1999. Host defense against oropharyngeal and vaginal candidiasis: site-specific differences. *Rev. Iberoam. Mycol.* **16:**8–15.

38. **Fidel, P. L., K. A. Ginsburg, J. L. Cutright, N. A. Wolf, D. Leaman, K. Dunlap, and J. D. Sobel.** 1997. Vaginal-associated immunity in women with recurrent vulvovaginal candidiasis: evidence for vaginal Th1-type responses following intravaginal challenge with *Candida* antigen. *J. Infect. Dis.* **176:** 728–739.

39. **Fidel, P. L., Jr., and J. D. Sobel.** 1994. The role of cell-mediated immunity in candidiasis. *Trends Microbiol.* **6:** 202–206.

40. **Forsyth, C. B., E. F. Plow, and L. Zang.** 1998. Interaction of the fungal pathogen *Candida albicans* with integrin CD11b/CD18: recognition by the I domain is modulated by the lectin-like domain and the CD18 subunit. *J. Immunol.* **161:** 6198–6205.

41. **Gale, C. A., C. M. Bendel, M. McClellan, M. Hauser, J. M. Becker, J. Berman, and M. K. Hostetter.** 1998. Linkage of adhesion, filamentous growth, and virulence in *Candida albicans* to a single gene, INT1. *Science* **279:**1355–1358.

42. **Gately, M. K., L. M. Renzetti, J. Magram, A. S. Stern, L. Adorini, U. Gubler, and D. H. Presky.** 1998. The interleukin-12/interleukin-12-receptor system: role in normal and pathologic immune responses. *Annu. Rev. Immunol.* **16:**495–521.

43. **Georgopapadakou, N. H., and T. J. Walsh.** 1996. Antifungal agents: chemotherapeutic targets and immunologic strategies. *Antimicrob. Agents Chemother.* **40:**279–291.

44. **Han, Y., and J. E. Cutler.** 1995. Antibody response that protects against disseminated candidiasis. *Infect. Immun.* **63:** 2714–2719.

45. **Han, Y., and J. E. Cutler.** 1997. Assessment of a mouse model of neutropenia and the effect of an anti-candidiasis monoclonal antibody in these animals. *J. Infect. Dis.* **175:** 1169–1175.

46. **Han, Y., M. A. Ulrich, and J. E. Cutler.** 1999. *Candida albicans* mannan extract-protein conjugates induce a protective immune response against experimental candidiasis. *J. Infect. Dis.* **179:**1477–1484.

47. **Hogan, L. H., B. S. Klein, and S. M. Levitz.** 1994. Virulence factors of medically important fungi. *Clin. Microbiol. Rev.* **9:**469–488.

48. **Jarvis, W. R.** 1995. Epidemiology of nosocomial fungal infections, with emphasis on *Candida* species. *Clin. Infect. Dis.* **20:**1526–1530.

49. **Jensen, J., T. Warner, and E. Balish.** 1993. Resistance of SCID mice to *Candida albicans* administered intravenously or colonizing the gut: role of polymorphonuclear leukocytes and macrphages. *J. Infect. Dis.* **167:**912–919.

50. **Jones-Carson, J., F. A. Vasquez-Torres, and E. Balish.** 1997. B cell-independent selection of memory T cells after mucosal immunization with *Candida albicans. J. Immunol.* **158:** 4328–4335.

51. **Jouault, T., C. Fradin, P. A. Trinel, A. Bernigaud, and D. Poulain.** 1998. Early signal transduction induced by *Candida albicans* in macrophages through shedding of a glycolipid. *J. Infect. Dis.* **178:**792–802.

52. **Kàpostza, R., L. Marodi, M. Hollinshead, S. Gordon, and R. P. da Silva.** 1999. Rapid recruitment of late endosomes and lysosomes in mouse macrophages ingesting *Candida albicans. J. Cell. Sci.* **112:**3237–3248.

53. **King, A. G., K. Johanson, C. L. Frey, P. L. deMarssh, J. R. White, P. McDevitt, D. McNulty, J. Balcarek, Z. L. Jonak, P. K. Bhatnagar, and L. M. Pelus.** 2000. Identification of unique truncated KC/GRO beta chemokines with potent hematopoietic and anti-infective activities. *J. Immunol.* **164:** 3774–3782.

54. **Kobayashi, S. D., and J. E. Cutler.** 1998. *Candida albicans* hyphal formation and virulence: is there a clearly defined role? *Trends Microbiol.* **6:**2–4.

55. **Kozel, T. R.** 1998. Complement activation by pathogenic fungi. *Res. Immunol.* **149:**309–320.

56. **Kullberg, B. J., and E. J. Anaissie.** 1998. Cytokines as therapy for opportunistic fungal infections. *Res. Immunol.* **149:** 478–488.

57. **Kullberg, B. J., M. G. Netea, J. H. Curfs, M. Keuter, J. F.**

Meis, and J. W. van der Meer. 1998. Recombinant murine granulocyte colony-stimulating factor protects against acute disseminated *Candida albicans* infection in nonneutropenic mice. *J. Infect. Dis.* **177:**175–181.

58. **Kullberg, B. J., M. G. Netea, A. G. Vonk, and J. W. van der Meer.** 1999. Modulation of neutrophil function in host defense against disseminated *Candida albicans* infection in mice. *FEMS Immunol. Med. Micobiol.* **26:**299–307.
59. **La Sala, A., F. Urbani, A. Torosantucci, A. Cassone, and C. Ausiello.** 1996. Mannoproteins from *Candida albicans* elicit a Th1-type-1 cytokine profile in human *Candida* specific long-term T cell cultures. *J. Biol. Regul. Homeost. Agents* **10:** 8–12.
60. **Lo, H.-J., J. R. Kohler, B. DiDomenico, D. Loebenberg, A. Cacciapuoti, and G. R. Fink.** 1997. Nonfilamentous *C. albicans* mutants are avirulent. *Cell* **90:**939–949.
61. **Magliani, W., S. Conti, F. De Bernardis, M. Gerloni, D. Bertolotti, P. Mozzoni, A. Cassone, and L. Polonelli.** 1997. Therapeutic potential of antiidiotypic chain antibodies with yeast killer toxin activity. *Nat. Biotechnol.* **15:**155–158.
62. **Marodi, L., J. R. Forehand, and R. B. Johnston, Jr.** 1991. Mechanisms of host defense against *Candida* species. II. Biochemical basis for the killing of *Candida* by mononuclear phagocytes. *J. Immunol.* **146:**2790–2794.
63. **Marodi, L., H. M. Korchak, and R. B. Johnston, Jr.** 1991. Mechanisms of host defense against *Candida* species. I. Phagocytosis by monocytes and monocyte-derived macrophages. *J. Immunol.* **146:**2783–2789.
64. **Marodi, L., S. Schreiber, D. C. Anderson, R. P. MacDermott, H. M. Korchak, and R. B. Johnston, Jr.** 1993. Enhancement of macrophage candidacidal activity by interferon-γ increased phagocytosis, killing and calcium signal mediated by a decreased number of mannose receptors. *J. Clin. Invest.* **91:** 2596–2601.
65. **Marth, T., and B. L. Kelsall.** 1997. Regulation of interleukin-12 by complement receptor 3 signaling. *J. Exp. Med.* **185:** 1987–1995.
66. **Matthews, R., and J. Burnie.** 1996. Antibodies against *Candida:* potential therapeutics? *Trends Microbiol.* **4:**354–358.
67. **Matthews, R., and J. Burnie.** 1998. The role of antibodies in protection against candidiasis. *Res. Immunol.* **149:**343–352.
68. **Mcknight, A., and S. Gordon.** 2000. Forum in immunology: innate recognition systems. *Microbes Infect.* **2:**239–336.
69. **Medzihitov, R., and C. A. Janeway, Jr.** 1997. Innate immunity: impact on the adaptive immune response. *Curr. Opin. Immunol.* **12:**13–19.

69a. **Mencacci, A.** Unpublished data.

70. **Mencacci, A., A. Bacci, E. Cenci, C. Montagnoli, S. Fiorucci, A. Casagrande, R. A. Flavell, F. Bistoni, and L. Romani.** 2000. Interleukin 18 restores defective Th1 immunity to *Candida albicans* in caspase 1-deficient mice. *Infect. Immun.* **68:** 5126–5131.
71. **Mencacci, A., E. Cenci, A. Bacci, F. Bistoni, and L. Romani.** 2000. Host immune reactivity determine the efficacy of combination immunotherapy and antifungal chemotherapy in candidiasis. *J. Infect. Dis.* **181:**686–694.
72. **Mencacci, A., E. Cenci, F. Bistoni, G. Del Sero, A. Bacci, C. Montagnoli, C. Fe' d'Ostiani, and L. Romani.** 1998. Specific and non-specific immunity to *Candida albicans:* a lesson from genetically modified animals. *Res. Immunol.* **149:**352–361.
73. **Mencacci, A., E. Cenci, J. R. Boelaert, P. Bucci, P. Mosci, C. Fè d'Ostiani, Bistoni F., and L. Romani.** 1997. Iron overload alters innate and T helper cell responses to *Candida albicans* in mice. *J. Infect. Dis.* **175:**1467–1476.
74. **Mencacci, A., E. Cenci, R. Spaccapelo, L. Tonnetti, L. Romani, P. Puccetti, and F. Bistoni.** 1995. Rationale for cytokine and anticytokine therapy of *Candida albicans* infection. *J. Med. Mycol.* **5:**25–30.
75. **Mencacci, A., G. Del Sero, E. Cenci, C. Fè d'Ostiani, A. Bacci, C. Montagnoli, M. Kopf, and L. Romani.** 1998. IL-4 is required for development of protective $CD4^+$ T helper type 1 cell responses to *Candida albicans. J. Exp. Med.* **187:** 307–317.
76. **Mitchell, A. P.** 1998. Dimorphism and virulence in *Candida albicans. Curr. Opin. Microbiol.* **1:**687–692.
77. **Mosmann, T. R., and R. L. Coffman.** 1989. TH1 and TH2 cells: different patterns of lymphokine secretion lead to different functional properties. *Annu. Rev. Immunol.* **7:**145–173.
78. **Murphy, J. W., F. Bistoni, G. S. Deepe, R. A. Blackstock, K. Buchanan, R. B. Ashman, L. Romani, A. Mencacci, E. Cenci, C. Fè d'Ostiani, G. Del Sero, V. L. Calich, and S. S. Kashino.** 1998. Type 1 and type 2 cytokines: from basic science to fungal infections. *Med. Mycol.* **36**(S1)**:**109–118.
79. **Musso, T., L. Calosso, M. Zucca, M. Millesimo, M. Puliti, S. Bulfone-Paus, C. Merlino, D. Savoia, R. Cavallo, A. N. Ponzi, and R. Badolato.** Interleukin-15 activates proinflammatory and antimicrobial functions in polymorphonuclear cells. *Infect. Immun.* **66:**2640–2607.
80. **Netea, M. G., P. N. Demacker, N. de Bont, O. G. Boerman, A. F. Stalenhoef, J. W. van der Meer, and B. J. Kullberg.** 1997. Hyperlipoproteinemia enhances susceptibility to acute disseminated *Candida albicans* infection in low-density-lipoprotein-receptor-deficient mice. *Infect. Immun.* **7:** 2663–2667.
81. **Netea, M. G., J. W. van Der Meer, J. F. Meis, and B. J. Kullberg.** 1999. Fas-FasL interactions modulate host defense against systemic *Candida albicans* infection. *J. Infect. Dis.* **180:**1648–1655.
82. **Netea, M. G., L. J. van Tits, J. H. Curfs, F. Amiot, J. F. Meis, J. W. van der Meer, and B. J. Kullberg.** 1999. Increased susceptibility of TNF-alpha lymphotoxin-alpha double knockout mice to systemic candidiasis through impaired recruitment of neutrophils and phagocytosis of *Candida albicans. J. Immunol.* **163:**1498–1505.
83. **Odds, F. C.** 1989. *Candida and Candidosis,* 2nd ed. Baillière-Tindall, London, United Kingdom.
84. **Orozco, A. S., X. Zhou, and S. G. Filler.** 2000. Mechanisms of the proinflammatory response of endothelial cells to *Candida albicans* infection. *Infect. Immun.* **68:**1134–1141.
85. **Polonelli, L., and A. Cassone.** 1999. Novel strategies for treating candidiasis. *Curr. Opin. Infect. Dis.* **12:**61–69.
86. **Poynton, C. H., R. A. Barnes, and J. Rees.** 1998. Interferon γ and granulocyte-macrophage colony-stimulating factor for the treatment of hepatosplenic candidosis in patients with acute leukemia. *Clin. Infect. Dis.* **26:**239–240.
87. **Presterl, E., A. Lassnigg, P. Mueller-Uri, I. El-Menyaw, and W. Graninger.** 1999. Cytokines in sepsis due to *Candida albicans* and in bacterial sepsis. *Eur. Cytokine Netw.* **10:** 423–430.
88. **Puccetti, P., L. Romani, and F. Bistoni.** 1995. A T_H1-T_H2-like switch in candidiasis: new perspectives for therapy. *Trends Microbiol.* **3:**237–240.
89. **Qian, Q., and J. E. Cutler.** 1997. Gamma interferon is not essential in host defense against disseminated candidiasis in mice. *Infect. Immun.* **65:**1748–1756.
90. **Raveh, D., B. A. Kruskal, J. Farland, and R. A. Ezekowitz.** 1998. Th1 and Th2 cytokines cooperate to stimulate mannose-receptor-mediated phagocytosis. *J. Leukoc. Biol.* **64:** 108–113.
91. **Roilides, E., A. Anastasiou-Katsiardani, A. Dimitriadou-Georgiadou, I. Kadiltsoglou, S. Tsaparidou, C. Panteliadis, and T. J. Wash.** 1998. Suppressive effects of interleukin-10

on human mononuclear phagocyte function against *Candida albicans* and *Staphylococcus aureus*. *J. Infect. Dis.* **178:** 1734–1742.

92. **Roilides E., M. C. Dignani, E. J. Anaissie, and J. H. Rex.** 1998. The role of immunoreconstitution in the management of refractory opportunistic fungal infections. *Med. Mycol.* **1:** 12–25.

93. **Roilides, E., I. Kadiltsoglou, A. Dimitriadou, M. Hatzistilianou, A. Manitsa, J. Karpouzas, P. A. Pizzo, and T. J. Wash.** 1997. Interleukin-4 suppresses antifungal activity of human mononuclear phagocytes against *Candida albicans* in association with decreased uptake of bastoconidia. *FEMS Immunol. Med. Microbiol.* **19:**169–180.

94. **Roilides, E., H. Katsifa, S. Tsaparidou, T. Stergiopoulos, C. Panteliadis, and T. J. Wash.** 2000. Interleukin-10 suppresses phagocytic and antihyphal activities of human neutrophils. *Cytokine* **12:**370–387.

95. **Roilides, E., T. Sein, R. Schaufele, S. J. Chanock, and T. J. Walsh.** 1998. Increased serum concentrations of interleukin-10 in patients with hepatosplenic candidiasis. *J. Infect. Dis.* **178:**589–592.

95a. **Romani , L.** Unpublished data.

96. **Romani, L.** 1997. The T cell response to fungi. *Curr. Opin. Immunol.* **9:**484–490.

97. **Romani, L.** 1999. Immunity to *Candida albicans:* Th1, Th2 cells and beyond. *Curr. Opin. Microbiol.* **2:**363–367.

98. **Romani, L.** 2000. Innate and adaptive immunity in *Candida albicans* infections and saprophytism. *J. Leukoc. Biol.* **68:** 175–179.

99. **Romani, L.** 2001. Innate immunity against fungal pathogens, p. 401–432. *In* R. Chilar and R. Calderone (ed.), *Fungal Pathogenesis: Principles and Clinical Applications.* Marcel Dekker, Inc., New York, N.Y.

100. **Romani, L., and F. Bistoni.** 2001. Systemic immunity in candidiasis, p. 483–514. *In* R. Chilar and R. Calderone (ed.), *Fungal Pathogenesis: Principles and Clinical Applications.* Marcel Dekker, Inc., New York, N.Y.

101. **Romani, L., and D. H. Howard.** 1995. Mechanisms of resistance to fungal infections. *Curr. Opin. Immunol.* **7:**517–523.

102. **Romani, L., and S. H. E. Kaufmann.** 1998. Immunity to fungi. *Res. Immunol.* **149:**277–281.

103. **Romani, L., A. Mencacci, E. Cenci, G. Del Sero, F. Bistoni, and P. Puccetti.** 1997. An immunoregulatory role for neutrophils in CD4+ T helper subset selection in mice with candidiasis. *J. Immunol.* **158:**2356–2362.

104. **Romani, L., A. Mencacci, E. Cenci, R. Spaccapelo, G. Del Sero, I. Nicoletti, G. Trinchieri, F. Bistoni, and P. Puccetti.** 1997. Neutrophils production of IL-12 and IL-10 in candidiasis and efficacy of IL-12 therapy in neutropenic mice. *J. Immunol.* **158:**5349–5356.

105. **Romani, L., A. Mencacci, E. Cenci, S. Spaccapelo, P. Mosci, P. Puccetti, and F. Bistoni.** 1993. $CD4^+$ subset expression in murine candidiasis. Th responses correlate directly with genetically determined susceptibility or vaccine-induced resistance. *J. Immunol.* **150:**925–931.

106. **Romani, L., A. Mencacci, E. Cenci, R. Spaccapelo, C. Toniatti, P. Puccetti, F. Bistoni, and V. Poli.** 1996. Impaired neutrophil response and $CD4^+$ T helper cell 1 development in interleukin-6-deficient mice infected with *Candida albicans.* *J. Exp. Med.* **183:**1–11.

107. **Romani, L., P. Puccetti, and F. Bistoni.** 1996. Biological role of helper T-cell subsets in candidiasis. *Chem. Immunol.* **63:** 113–137.

108. **Romani, L., P. Puccetti, and F. Bistoni.** 1997. Interleukin-12 in infectious diseases. *Clin. Microbiol. Rev.* **10:**611–636.

109. **Romani, L., P. Puccetti, and F. Bistoni.** 1997. Initiation of T-helper cell immunity to *Candida albicans* by IL-12: the role of neutrophils. *Chem. Immunol.* **68:**110–135.

110. **Sable, C. A., and G. R. Donowitz.** 1994. Infections in bone marrow transplant recipients. *Clin. Infect. Dis.* **18:**273–284.

111. **Sasada, M., and R. B. Johnston, Jr.** 1980. Macrophage microbicidal activity: correlation between phagocytosis associated oxidative metabolism and the killing of *Candida* by macrophages. *J. Exp. Med.* **152:**85–98.

112. **Schaffner, A., C. E. Davis, T. Schaffner, and M. Markert.** 1986. In vitro susceptibility of fungi to killing by neutrophil granulocytes discriminates between primary pathogenicity and opportunism. *J. Clin. Invest.* **78:**511–524.

113. **Sieck, T. G., M. A. Moors, H. R. Buckley, and K. J. Blank.** 1993. Protection against disseminated candidiasis mediated by a *Candida albicans*-specific T-cell line. *Infect. Immun.* **61:** 3540–3543.

114. **Solomkin, J. S., E. L. Mills, G. S. Gienbink, R. D. Nelson, R. L. Simmons, and P. G. Quie.** 1978. Phagocytosis of *Candida albicans* by human leukocytes: opsonic requirements. *J. Infect. Dis.* **137:**30–37.

115. **Spaccapelo, R., G. Del Sero, P. Mosci, F. Bistoni, and L. Romani.** 1997. Early T cell unresponsiveness in mice with candidiasis and reversal by IL-2. Effect on T helper cell development. *J. Immunol.* **158:**2294–2302.

116. **Spaccapelo, R., L. Romani, L. Tonnetti, E. Cenci, A. Mencacci, G. Del Sero, R. Tognellini, S. G. Reed, P. Puccetti, and F. Bistoni.** 1995. TGF-β is important in determining the in vivo patterns of susceptibility or resistance in mice infected with *Candida albicans.* *J. Immunol.* **155:**1349–1360.

117. **Stein, M., S. Keshav, N. Harris, and S. Gordon.** 1992. Interleukin 4 potently enhances murine macrophages mannose receptor activity: a marker of alternative immunologic macrophage activation. *J. Exp. Med.* **176:**287–292.

118. **Stevens, D. A.** 1998. Combination immunotherapy and antifungal chemotherapy. *Clin. Infect. Dis.* **26:**1266–1269.

119. **Stevens, D. A., T. J. Walsh, F. Bistoni, E. Cenci, K. V. Clemons, G. Del Sero, C. Fè d'Ostiani, B. J. Kullberg, A. Mencacci, E. Roilides, and L. Romani.** 1998. Cytokines and mycoses. *Med. Mycol.* **36**(S1)**:**171–182.

120. **Szabo, S. J., A. S. Dighe, U. Gubler, and K. M. Murphy.** 1997. Regulation of the interleukin (IL)-12Rβ2 subunit expression in developing T. helper 1(Th1) and Th2 cells. *J. Exp. Med.* **185:**817–824.

121. **Szabo, I., L. Guan, and T. J. Rogers.** 1995. Modulation of macrophage phagocytic activity by cell wall components of *Candida albicans.* *Cell. Immunol.* **164:**182–188.

122. **Talluri, G., V. K. Marella, D. Shirazian, and G. J. Wise.** 1999. Immune response in patients with persistent candiduria and occult candidemia. *J. Urol.* **162:**1361–1364.

123. **Tang, T., A. Rosenkranz, K. J. M. Assmann, M. J. Goodman, J. C. Gutierrez-Ramos, M. C. Carroll, R. S. Cotran, and T. N. Mayadas.** 1997. A role for Mac-1 (CD11b/CD18) in immune complex-stimulated neutrophil function in vivo: Mac-1 deficiency abrogates sustained Fcgamma receptor-dependent neutrophil adhesion and complement-dependent proteinuria in acute glomerulonephritis. *J. Exp. Med.* **186:**1853–1863.

124. **Tavares, D., P. Ferreira, and M. Arala-Chaves.** 2000. Increased resistance to systemic candidiasis in athymic or interleukin-10-depleted mice. *J. Infect. Dis.* **182:**266–273.

125. **Van Enckevort, F. H., M. G. Netea, A. R. Hermus, C. G. Sweep, J. F. Meis, J. W. Van Der Meer, and B. J. Kullberg.** 1999. Increased susceptibility to systemic candidiasis in interleukin-6 deficient mice. *Med. Mycol.* **37:**419–426.

126. **van Spriel, A. B., I. E. van den Herik-Oudijk, H. A. van Sorge, and J. G. van de Winkel.** 1999. Effective phagocytosis and killing of *Candida albicans* via targeting FCgammaRI (CD64)

or FCalphaRI (CD89) on neutrophils. *J. Infect. Dis.* **179:** 661–669.

127. **van Spriel, A. B., I. E. van den Herik-Oudijk, and J. D. van den Winkel.** 2000. A single injection of polyethylene-glycol granulocyte colony-stimulating factor strongly prolongs survival of mice with systemic candidiasis. *Cytokine* **12:** 666–670.
128. **Vasquez-Torres, A., and E. Balish.** 1997. Macrophages in resistance to candidiasis. *Microbiol. Mol. Rev.* **61:**170–192.
129. **Vazquez, N., T. J. Walsh, D. Friedman, S. J. Chanock, and C. A. Lyman.** 1998. Interleukin-15 augments superoxide production and microbicidal activity of human monocytes against *Candida albicans. Infect. Immun.* **66:**145–150.
130. **Walsh, T. J., J. Hiemenz, and P. A. Pizzo.** 1994. Evolving risk factors for invasive fungal infections: all neutropenic patients are not the same. *Clin. Infect. Dis.* **18:**793–798.
131. **Walzog, B., P. Weinmann, F. Jeblonski, K. Scharffetter-Kochanek, K. Bommert, and P. Gaehtgens.** 1999. A role for beta(2) integrins (CD11/CD18) in the regulation of cytokine gene expression of polymorphonuclear neutrophils during the inflammatory response. *FASEB J.* **13:**1855–1865.
132. **Xiong, J., K. Kang, L. Liu, Y. Yoshida, K. Cooper, and M. Ghannoum.** 2000. *Candida albicans* and *Candida krusei* differentially induce human blood mononuclear cell interleukin-12 and gamma interferon production. *Infect. Immun.* **68:** 2464–2469.
133. **Yamamoto, Y., T. W. Klein, and H. Friedman.** 1997. Involvement of mannose receptor in cytokine interleukin-1β (IL-1β), IL-6, and granulocyte-macrophage colony stimulating factor responses, but not chemokine macrophage inflammatory protein 1α (MIP-1α), MIP-2, and KC responses, caused by attachment of *Candida albicans* to macrophages. *Infect. Immun.* **65:**1877–1082.
134. **Yates, A. B., D. Mehrotra, and J. E. Moffitt.** 1997. *Candida* endocarditis in a child with hyperimmuneglobulinemia E syndrome. *J. Allergy Clin. Immunol.* **99:**770–702.

Candida and Candidiasis
Edited by Richard A. Calderone

Chapter 17

Immunoprotection against Candidiasis

Jim E. Cutler, Bruce L. Granger, and Yongmoon Han

The history of research on candidiasis has been interesting in that the name of the disease has undergone profound changes over the past 150 years or so, and even to this day there is disagreement as to whether it should be referred to as candidiasis or candidosis. Likewise, the genera and epithet names, and the taxonomic and phylogenetic positions of the etiologic agents responsible for the disease, have also changed during that time. During the 1970s, the importance of host neutrophils and cell-mediated immunity (CMI) in defense against candidiasis became the predominant theme, whereas over the past 10 years or so an impressive literature supporting the role of protective antibodies has amassed. These latter developments are the subject of this chapter.

Experimental data supporting the existence of protective antibodies against candidiasis imply that the human host, through development and use of an appropriate vaccine, could advantage this arm of the immune system. The incidence and prevalence of disease, paucity of antifungal drugs, and emergence of drug-resistant strains provide a rationale for pursuit of immunological approaches to prevention and therapy of candidiasis. Unlike many infectious disease agents, the most prevalent cause of candidiasis, *Candida albicans,* is a normal and common inhabitant of mucosal surfaces. Other *Candida* species of clinical importance also may be occasionally associated with the mucosa (94, 146). The presence of these fungi, along with likely subclinical and occasional clinically apparent bouts of candidiasis, leads to immunological sensitization manifested by the almost universal presence of serum antibodies and hypersensitivities specific to candidal antigens in humans.

A reasonable question regarding vaccine development is that if most people are naturally sensitized to *Candida,* what is the benefit of vaccination? Because of the antigenic complexity of the etiologic agents of candidiasis, there is no guarantee that natural exposure to these agents will result in production of antibodies of appropriate specificity, isotype, and titer for protection. Short-term protection via passive transfer of protective antibodies should be considered for those patients who will undergo medical procedures that could place them at high risk of developing hematogenously disseminated candidiasis. These procedures include abdominal surgeries (46, 91, 166, 167), transplantations (22, 27, 67, 109, 197), and other major surgical interventions (7, 37, 51, 146, 165, 192). Active immunization should be given to all women. The majority of women in the United States will experience at least one bout of *Candida* vaginitis; approximately 50% of these will have more than one episode, and many will develop chronic disease (53, 98). A safe, long-lasting immunity that prevents disease would certainly be preferable to treatment with antifungal drugs after disease onset. Risk factors such as the use of dentures (120, 199), late-onset diabetes (189), surgical interventions, placement of indwelling catheters (145, 169, 171), and long-term stays in intensive care units (152, 171, 193) are especially associated with the aged, suggesting that active immunization against candidiasis should be considered for everyone over the age of 65.

In this chapter, we will emphasize immunoprotection against candidiasis. The major focus will be the discussion of candidate vaccines that induce protective antibodies. Not all of the literature or immunoprotection will be presented; instead we selected observations that strongly suggest an efficacy that warrants phase I clinical trials. Other chapters in the text are more representative of specific types of immunity against pathogens (chapters 13–16).

Jim E. Cutler, Bruce L. Granger, and Yongmoon Han • Department of Microbiology, Montana State University, Bozeman, MT 59717-3520.

COMMON BELIEF THAT ANTIBODIES ARE NOT PROTECTIVE

An accumulation of clinical and experimental observations led to the conclusion that antibodies specific for *C. albicans* are not protective. As discussed above, the presence of *Candida*-reactive antibodies in the blood of people is common (43) but does not preclude development of candidiasis either as disseminated life-threatening disease or as superficial lesions at mucosal and dermal sites (5, 61, 108). In Kirkpatrick, Rich, and Bennett's now classic paper, which reported the results of clinical studies on 12 patients with chronic mucocutaneous candidiasis (108), the authors observed normal or elevated serum agglutinin and precipitin titers, and normal parotid fluid agglutinin levels in every subject. Because eight of the patients were severely depleted in cell-mediated immune functions, the authors concluded that this arm of the immune system is responsible for host defense against mucocutaneous candidiasis.

In controlled experiments, mice developed enhanced resistance to disseminated candidiasis following a mucosal sensitization to whole yeast cells, and the protection was associated with CMI (17). T-cell-mediated immunity was also implicated as the important acquired specific host defense against hematogenously disseminated candidiasis in studies involving immunodeficient mice (16). Bistoni, Romani, and coworkers have published an impressive amount of data showing that resistance against experimental candidiasis in mice is associated with Th1-type responses (9, 23, 24, 52, 164, 173–175), whereas others have obtained support for Th1 and Th2 responses (191). Some investigators have obtained data that antibodies may be detrimental to the host (14, 114, 195), whereas other studies indicated that antibodies were of no consequence to disease outcome (29).

HOW MIGHT ANTIBODIES BE PROTECTIVE AGAINST CANDIDIASIS?

Yeast cells have an enormous number of epitopes associated with their surface. We hypothesize that antibody to a small subset of these epitopes will show protection against candidiasis. People who are exposed to *C. albicans* will not necessarily respond by making "protective" antibodies in sufficient concentration to be of any benefit against development of candidiasis. If this hypothesis is correct, then merely finding antibodies in the sera of patients or experimental animals with candidiasis is not reason to reject a positive role for antibodies in host defense against various forms of candidiasis. The more important questions to consider are the specificities and titers of antibodies that are present in the serum of each patient. The ideal antibody-inducing vaccine formulation against candidiasis may consist of either a cocktail of a select number of purified antigens or an extract of the fungus that is highly enriched for so-called protective epitopes. The remainder of the formulation will consist of appropriate carriers or adjuvants to ensure responses of appropriate titer and isotype.

Our hypothesis may be best understood in the context of a consideration of *Candida*-host interactions. *C. albicans* is usually a noninvasive mucosal commensal that can express certain characteristics that allow for its survival at a host site co-occupied by competing microbes (33). These characteristics act as virulence traits in the immunocompromised patient in whom the fungus is able to invade tissues. Events that occur naturally, such as onset of diabetes or AIDS, or as a result of medical procedures, are risk factors for development of candidiasis (11, 37, 54, 57, 95, 100, 126, 170, 171, 194, 197, 200). The immunologic defense dysfunction may be innate, such as destruction of mucosal surfaces or decreased neutrophil activities, or acquired specific immunity as alluded to above. More than likely, the factors involved in protection are complex and include others, such as endocrine dysfunction (6, 44), hypercalcemia (106), thyroiditis (44), and malignancies (3, 128), or the fact that people without apparent immunodeficiency also may develop candidiasis (26, 44, 107).

In previous chapters, the discussion of immunity has included the hypothesis that a particular defect in immunity may not necessarily predispose that individual to all forms of candidiasis. Other immune systems that remain intact are sufficient to compensate for the defect and suppress these fungi of low virulence. The relative importance of a given defense mechanism also will be dependent on the specific site within the body to which the fungus has gained access. For example, neutropenia is clearly a high-risk factor for development of hematogenously disseminated candidiasis (2, 54, 121, 156, 196, 198), but nonneutropenic patients are also susceptible (13, 45, 47, 112, 147, 153, 179). This may indicate that susceptibility to disseminated candidiasis depends on both access of the fungus to the circulatory system and the inoculum dose. Severe reduction in circulating neutrophils renders the experimental animal more susceptible to fatal disseminated candidiasis, but in such experiments the animals usually receive the challenge dose of viable yeast cells directly into the bloodstream (10, 59, 74, 101, 131, 132, 181, 188), thus bypassing host defense systems on mucosal surfaces. The clinical parallel to this situation may be the neutropenic patient with an indwelling central venous line on which biofilms of *C. albicans* develop and serve as a continuous inoculum of fungi into the circulatory system (54, 156). On the other hand, AIDS patients rarely develop invasive disease since their neutrophil counts remain at near normal levels, especially in early AIDS.

Adding to the complexity of host-*Candida* interactions is the virulence state of the fungus, which is decidedly related to its growth conditions (147). While forming a biofilm on a catheter, *C. albicans* will likely grow as a mixture of hyphae, pseudohyphae, and yeast forms, and during such morphogenetic changes, each of these growth forms varies dramatically in regard to their cell surface properties. For example, the degree of cell surface hydrophobicity (CSH) changes as an inverse function of cell wall protein mannosylation, with high CSH associated with low mannosylation and low CSH (i.e., hydrophilicity) associated with high levels of protein mannosylation (88, 129). An interesting feature is that high CSH yeast forms of a given isolate of this species are more virulent than are their hydrophilic counterparts (4, 48, 68). The definitive reason for the increased virulence of hydrophobic yeast forms may relate to increased adherence properties of these fungal cells for tissues (48, 49, 84, 85, 130, 178). Likewise, a surface change from hydrophilicity to hydrophobicity precedes germination (83) and yeast forms with high CSH germinate more readily than hydrophilic yeast forms. This latter observation is consistent with recent work on gene knockout/complementation experiments that suggest (110) that the hyphal form is an essential component of virulence (1, 28, 30, 31, 60, 92, 115, 119, 141). In reality, probably all growth forms are required for pathogenesis.

On the basis of the complexity of *Candida*-host interactions, we propose that under the appropriate clinical or experimental conditions, virtually any host defense mechanism plays an important role. Antibodies are included as a possible defense, but an important point is that mere detection of polyclonal antibodies in the circulation of people with candidiasis does not preclude a possible beneficial role of antibodies against the disease. Indeed, predominant antibody responses to *C. albicans* may be against cytosolic proteins (149), which would not be expected to be of much benefit to the host during pathogenesis of candidiasis. Instead, the minimum criteria of antibody specificity, predominant immunoglobulin isotype, antibody titer, and availability of effector function components must be considered when assessing a functional role for antibodies. As an example regarding this last criterion, a patient deficient in complement component C3 will not be protected against candidiasis by opsonizing antibodies that work by causing rapid deposition of C3 onto the fungal surface.

These criteria are meant to illustrate the specificity of the requirements for a protective antibody. Clearly, cell-mediated immunity is also important, as are other host defense mechanisms. There is a multitude of innate and acquired host defenses that collectively form an effective barrier to development of clinically apparent candidiasis. The dysfunction or loss (i.e., AIDS) of one or more of these barriers can render the host susceptible to candidiasis, but a deficiency in one barrier may also be compensated by overcompensation of another. Indeed, specific antibodies, whether produced by the patient or given passively, should benefit the patient if the action of the antibodies results in sufficient decrease in tissue fungal burden, allowing existing defenses to eliminate any remaining viable fungal elements.

EARLY EVIDENCE THAT SUGGESTED A PROTECTIVE ROLE FOR ANTIBODIES

A report prior to the 1960s was of special interest because, contrary to the widely accepted belief that candidiasis patients have circulating antibodies against the fungus (146), some of the subjects were without detectable *Candida*-specific agglutinins (127). Furthermore, one of the patients recovered from candidiasis following administration of rabbit serum containing a high titer of *Candida*-specific antibodies.

The earliest convincing experimental results showing a positive effect due to specific antibodies were by Mourad and Friedman in the 1960s (142, 143). Mice given repeated doses of a vaccine composed of sonically disrupted *C. albicans* yeast cells developed enormous agglutinin titers and their sera transferred protection to naive mice against a lethal intravenous (i.v.) challenge with viable yeast form cells of the fungus. In these experiments, all of the control animals died by day 50 after challenge, but 33% of the test animals survived the 140-day observation period and the organs taken from the sacrificed survivors were culture negative for *C. albicans*. Comparisons with actively immunized mice were favorable; 50% of the animals survived the challenge (142).

Two other aspects of the Mourad-Friedman experiments deserve additional comment. First, the investigators achieved slide agglutinin titers up to 1,280 in mice, which is more than one order of magnitude greater than titers we have observed in immunization work spanning more than 30 years (our unpublished data). Considering the antigenic complexity of whole yeast cells, the titers obtained by these researchers may have been key to their success, as opposed to others who have done similar experiments but obtained negative results (97). Second, the investigators began passive transfer of antisera 1 day after the animals were challenged with viable *C. albicans,* which suggests that antibodies may have therapeutic potential in patients who develop hematogenously disseminated candidiasis.

A total of 10 years elapsed before conclusions reached by Mourad and Friedman were confirmed by investigations led by Pearsall et al. (153). These investigators developed a mouse-thigh lesion model for experimental candidiasis and noted first that lesions that were generated in response to a large inoculum of *C. albicans* yeast cells into the thigh muscle resolved by 6 weeks, yet there was little evidence of a granulomatous response (151). This result was surprising considering the already accepted doctrine that CMI was the prevalent mechanism of host defense against candidiasis. They found further that recovered animals were more resistant to a second challenge of viable yeast cells into their thigh muscle, which suggested that the animals had developed an acquired immunity against candidiasis. The most striking result, however, was that sera from immunized mice transferred protection to naive mice, but immune lymphocytes had little or no effect (150).

In 1978, Domer's group determined that in an experimental *C. albicans* cutaneous murine infection, antibodies specific for the fungus that made animals less susceptible to disseminated candidiasis than controls were induced (66). When these investigators depleted mice of B cells, by anti-μ therapy, the animals became more susceptible to disseminated disease than controls (113). Other investigators essentially confirmed these experiments (125). Although the early literature was scant, the evidence for antibodies in host defense against candidiasis was beginning to accumulate.

RECENT STUDIES ON PROTECTIVE ANTIBODIES

Anti-Heat Shock Protein 90

Beginning in the mid-1980s, Matthews, Burnie, and coworkers showed that the development of antibodies against *C. albicans* heat shock protein 90 (hsp90) is protective in both human and animal disease. These investigations have culminated in current pilot-scale production of genetically engineered human antibody against hsp90 with the prospect of its use in phase IIa clinical trials in patients with disseminated candidiasis (140). In accordance with nomenclature promoted by these investigators, we will refer to the key protein in question as hsp90, even though homology of the *C. albicans* protein to the cognate heat shock protein of *Saccharomyces cerevisiae* and work by others (12, 25, 89) indicate that it might best be referred to as hsp82.

In their initial observations, the Matthews group found that the sera from patients who had recovered from disseminated candidiasis tended to have a relatively high and protracted titer of antibody against a 47-kDa fungal antigen (138, 139), which is apparently a breakdown product of a larger and immunodominant antigen (136, 138, 139) of similar size to (136, 138) immunodominant antigens reported by others (56, 72). By use of immunoelectron microscopic analysis (136), the 47-kDa antigen was detected in the cytosol primarily near the plasmalemma and in discrete areas on the outer aspects of the cell wall; it also appeared to traverse the cell wall in a manner reminiscent of channels hypothesized by Poulain and coworkers (163). Results of cloning and sequencing (133) of part of the coding region for the 47-kDa antigen supported the breakdown product hypothesis (89, 133).

Through the use of epitope mapping strategies, a conserved epitope of hsp90 (LKVIRK) was identified (137) as responsible for induction of the most significant protective antibodies. LKVIRK is located at positions 317 to 322 from the carboxy terminus of the 47-kDa antigen and hsp90, and is also found in mouse and human hsp90 (137). In these same studies, the investigators obtained an important monoclonal antibody, CA-Str7-1, specific for LKVIRK, by use of hybridoma technology in which splenocytes were obtained from mice hyperimmunized with the peptide LKVIRKNIVKKMIE conjugated to keyhole limpet hemocyanin. Mice had increased resistance to a lethal challenge with *C. albicans* if before challenge they received either patient's serum containing anti-hsp90, an Ig fraction of patient's serum, or monoclonal antibody (MAb) CA-Str7-1.

Protection also occurred in mice pretreated with phage displaying a human antibody fragment specific for LKVIRK (135). The approaches used to demonstrate the protection were a bit unconventional, but the results were especially interesting for two reasons: (i) only a very small amount of anti-LKVIRK is apparently required for a protective effect and (ii) the antibody can be given after the initiation of disease, which, in addition to the Mourad-Friedman results, implies a possible therapeutic application of antibodies.

A hypothesis was formulated that the fungal hsp90 is a toxin that is released from the fungal cells during pathogenesis of disease much like an endotoxic reaction that may occur during sepsis caused by a gram-negative rod (134, 135). The toxin hypothesis seems consistent with similar studies completed by these investigators on *S. cerevisiae* (89). Overexpression of its hsp82, which is >78% identical to the *C. albicans* hsp90, led to increased virulence of the *S. cerevisiae* (89). Strains PMY1-3A and PMY1-82 were used, which are isogenic except that PMY1-82 contains multiple episomal copies of the homologous heat-inducible HSP82 gene (described previously [25]). Both strains were grown for 48 h at 30°C, and then each was heat shocked at 39°C for 75 min just prior to virulence testing in mice. Virulence comparisons of the two strains grown at 30°C were unfortunately not done, which precludes evaluation of possible non-HSP82 differences between the strains. However, high i.v. dosages of yeast (at least 10^8 cells) were required to produce a lethal infection in mice, but in all three experiments, significant differences were recorded between the two strains with respect to resultant tissue burden of *S. cerevisiae* (i.e., CFU) mortality (89). The authors believe that hsp90 is a virulence factor. Their conclusion that hsp90 is a toxin is also consistent with their results indicating that antibodies can be given after the infection has been established. As a possible limitation to the clinical implementation of the above approaches, because human hsp90 also contains the LKVIRK epitope, there may well be undesirable short- and long-term effects from administering an autoantibody to patients.

Anti-Mannan Responses

Cutler and coworkers initially began studies on the adherence properties of *C. albicans* in order to understand the pathogenesis of hematogenously disseminated candidiasis. Mannans were found as entirely responsible for the attachment of yeast cells to mouse splenic marginal zone macrophages (103, 104, 117), and antibodies specific for certain mannan epitopes enhanced resistance of mice against both hematogenously disseminated candidiasis and against vaginal infection (73, 75–77, 79–81).

By using an ex vivo assay, hydrophilic *C. albicans* yeast cells were found to adhere specifically to certain macrophage populations in mouse splenic marginal zones and to subcapsular and trabecular sinus areas of peripheral lymph nodes (34, 78, 82, 102, 105, 172). These results also occur in vivo, as attested by the pattern of yeast cell binding to tissues following an appropriate in vivo administration of the fungal cells (34, 187; Cutler, Riesselman, Tripp, unpublished data).

The nature of the host cell (i.e., macrophage) receptor for yeast cell attachment has not been definitively identified. Evidence, however, has been obtained that the receptor is not sialoadhesin (78), but may be a unique kind of mannose receptor (105) or galectin-3 (55).

Through the use of the ex vivo assay, we arrived at a chemical definition of the *Candida* adhesin responsible for adherence to splenic and lymph node macrophages. According to a model as proposed by Suzuki and coworkers (177), yeast cell wall phosphomannans are N-linked to cell wall protein, and the mannan-protein conjugates are collectively referred to as the phosphomannoprotein complex (PMC) (104). The PMC is composed of an acid-stable component consisting of a mannan backbone composed of α-1,6 glycosidic linkages, as well as α-linked mannose units of oligomannosyl side chains (primarily). Acid hydrolysis results in cleavage of the phosphate bond, which releases oligomannosyl residues composed of mannose units linked exclusively by β-1,2-glycosidic bonds (177) and are thus termed the acid-labile part of the PMC. A strong adhesin activity is associated with certain moieties within the acid-stable part of the PMC (102, 103). A β-1,2-mannotetraose, which is also one of the acid-labile components, is another adhesin site (102, 117) responsible for yeast adherence to the specific kinds of mouse macrophages. These results led to the rather obvious question as to the effects of PMC-specific antibodies on pathogenesis of candidiasis.

Encapsulation of the PMC into conventional-type liposomes provided a reliable immunogen for antibody responses by mice against mannan epitopes (73, 79). Immunized mice were more resistant to an i.v. challenge of a lethal dose of live *C. albicans* yeast cells than animals that received liposomes alone or buffer diluent prior to the challenge. The protection was due at least in part to antibody as strongly indicated by the transfer of protection to naive mice of whole sera and immunoglobulin fractions of the sera obtained from immune animals. The polyclonal antiserum protected mice against disseminated disease due to serotype A and B strains of *C. albicans* and against a strain of *C. tropicalis* (73). Furthermore, immune sera preabsorbed with *C. albicans* yeast cells did not transfer protection (73).

In more recent work, immunogenic preparations were obtained by conjugating the mannan extract to a protein carrier. Antisera obtained from mice immunized with mannan-bovine serum albumin (BSA) complexes had the same ability to transfer protection to naive animals as sera from mannan-liposome immunized mice (81). In addition to eliminating the need for liposomes, the mannan-BSA conjugate vaccine formulation is superior because the vaccine can be administered intraperitoneally instead of i.v. and enhanced resistance to candidiasis can be induced by a priming dose followed by a single booster.

By use of hybridoma technology, two MAbs, B6.1 and B6, were isolated. Although both antibodies are IgM and agglutinate whole yeast cells, only MAb B6.1 enhances resistance of mice to hematogenously disseminated candidiasis, and this antibody is markedly more effective in reducing vaginal colonization by *C. albicans* or *C. tropicalis* than MAb B6 (73, 77, 79). By use of various fractionation and chemical analytical approaches, the epitope recognized by MAb B6.1 was defined as an acid-labile β-1,2-mannotriose and the B6 epitope as an acid-stable moiety in the PMC (77). The B6.1 epitope is expressed in vivo and in vitro and is uniformly distributed along the cell surface of hydrophilic yeast cells. The B6 epitope tends to have a more patchy distribution (77).

Speculations on Mechanisms by Which Antibodies Protect against Candidiasis

While MAb B6.1 antibody is an IgM, this isotype is not a requisite for protection. When the polyclonal antiserum obtained from mice vaccinated against the mannan-liposomal preparation was fractionated, protective activities associated with both the IgM and IgG fractions were observed (73). For example, MAb C3.1 (an IgG3 monoclonal antibody), with an epitope specificity similar to that of MAb B6.1, demonstrated a protective activity like that of MAb B6.1 (80).

Complement activation is required for protection by antibodies. Mouse neutrophils (in the presence of MAb B6.1 plus complement) showed the highest ability to ingest and kill *C. albicans* yeast cells compared with that of either MAb B6.1 in the absence of complement or MAb B6 with or without complement (15).

The Cutler laboratory, in collaboration with Dr. Kozel's laboratory at the University of Nevada, is currently testing the hypothesis that protective antimannan antibodies induce very rapid deposition of complement onto the surface of yeast cells, which favors an interaction of the opsonized yeast cells with host phagocytic cells. In addition to an in vitro requirement of complement for enhanced neutrophil candidacidal activity by MAb B6.1, compelling evidence has been obtained that the protective activities of MAbs B6.1 and C3.1 require the presence of complement in vivo (78a).

Other Protective Antibodies that May Be Specific for Mannan and/or Protein

In studies on experimental vaginal infection in rats, Cassone and coworkers concluded that antibodies specific for a *Candida* mannan and antibodies specific for the protein portion of secreted aspartyl proteinase 2 (Sap 2) are protective (21, 39, 40). The putative antimannan was identified on the basis of its reactivity in an enzyme-linked immunosorbent assay, but since the capture antigen was a crude mannoprotein preparation (21, 186), the conclusion that only antimannan responses were measured remains uncertain. Regardless, following intravaginal infection the investigators detected IgM, IgG, and IgA antibodies specific for mannan and secreted proteinase in the vaginal contents (21), but how protection is achieved is unclear.

Since the secreted proteinases (SAPs) are virulence factors (33, 38, 63, 90, 96, 111, 123, 148, 168), then intuitively, anti-Sap antibodies may neutralize the proteinase activity (39, 40). The cell-wall-associated nature of the secreted proteinase (69) could, however, promote formation of agglutinates in the presence of antibody with resultant reduction of infectious units. The binding of antibody to cell-wall surface proteinases may also facilitate yeast-phagocyte interactions through antibody- and antibody-complement-mediated opsonic activity.

As alluded to earlier in this chapter, any defense mechanism that keeps the number of fungal viable units to a certain threshold number should enhance resistance. The mechanisms would be expected to vary depending on the predominant tissue location of the infection and immunologic status of the host. The mechanisms may include direct effects of antibodies on the ability of the fungus to germinate (19, 70), neutralization of toxins (64, 65, 134, 135), reduction of infectious units by agglutination (122), and inhibition of adherence to host tissue sites and opsonic activity (as discussed above). A few of these aspects have been studied and are considered in the following sections.

SOME ANTIBODIES MAY DIRECTLY INHIBIT *C. ALBICANS*

Inhibition of Morphogenesis

Two independent research teams reported that certain antibodies can prevent a yeast to hyphal transition in *C. albicans*. Assuming that ability to make hyphae is a virulence trait, there is obvious potential clinical application of such antibodies in the prevention and treatment of candidiasis. On the basis of observations by Grappel, Ferthiere, and Blank that antibodies against dermatophytes affect morphological development and may even inhibit growth of these fungi (71), Grappel and Calderone (70) also conducted similar experiments with *C. albicans*. One serotype A strain and two serotype B strains of *C. albicans* were grown in a chemically defined medium as yeast cells in shake culture at room temperature for 16 h to, presumably, late log phase. Under these conditions, the cells would be expected to have relatively thin cell walls. Washed and resuspended yeast cells in buffer were mixed twice with either pooled rabbit anti-*C. albicans* serum (agglutinin titers of at least 320), a gamma globulin fraction of the antiserum, normal rabbit serum, or buffer. All cultures were incubated at 37°C for 30 min, and the induction of germination was followed at 27 and 37°C while oxygen consumption was measured at 27°C. Normal rabbit serum-treated yeast cells of all isolates had increased oxygen consumption and cells germinated normally. However, yeast cells treated with either pooled antiserum or the gamma globulin fraction showed a dramatic decrease in respiratory function and an inability to undergo morphogenesis.

Casanova, Martinez, and Chaffin have reported that Fab fragments of MAb 4C12 inhibits germination of *C. albicans* (19). These investigators previously showed that MAb 4C12 is an IgG1 that has a specificity for the protein portion of a 260-kDa cell wall mannoprotein of *C. albicans* (18) that is apparently only expressed in hyphae. *C. albicans* (strain 3153A) was grown to stationary phase in the medium of Lee, Buckley, and Campbell (116). Cells (5×10^7 per ml of the same medium) were incubated for 2 h at 37°C, and then the appropriate antibody or control material was added. The presence of germ tubes was measured after an additional 3 h of incubation at 37°C. At a high yeast cell concentration, germination should be inhibited (86, 87) or only short germlings should be apparent after a 1.5- to 2.5-h incubation (50). Regardless, the data indicated that Fabs, but not intact IgG1, of MAb 4C12 inhibited germ tube formation. Irrelevant Fabs from human IgG used as a control did not inhibit germination, although the control Fabs were apparently a commercial preparation. A more ideal control would have been irrelevant Fabs prepared exactly as the test Fabs (yeast cell germination is readily inhibited by a multitude of environmental factors and contaminants [35, 87a]), since MAb 4C12 is directed against the surface of germ tubes, as shown by indirect fluorescence antibody (IFA) techniques, and IFA was not able to detect the 4C12 epitope in yeast cell extracts (18). While the distribution of the epitope reactive with MAb 4C12 appeared rather uniformly distributed over the hyphal cell surface, yeast inhibited from germinating showed a punctate appearance of the epitope (19), possibly representing the point of germ tube emergence. The authors believe that the Fabs of MAb 4C12 may alter the conformation of the 260-kDa protein, which would adversely affect the ability of the yeast cell to germinate (19).

These observations warrant further investigation, since the antibodies are specific for certain epitopes and may have direct inhibitory effects on *C. albicans*. Certainly these epitopes could be considered in the formulation of a vaccine against candidiasis. Further, antibodies such as MAb 4C12 may be useful in experiments designed to test the importance of morphogenesis in the candidal pathogenesis.

Antibody Specific for Killer Factor Receptor

Killer factors are proteins (8, 176, 201) secreted by one strain of yeast that are capable of killing other strains of yeast by various mechanisms; sensitive strains must possess a receptor specific for the killer factor. Such systems have been described in *Saccharomyces* sp. (8, 201), *Ustilago* sp., *Kluyveromyces* sp., *Pichia* sp., *Hansenula* sp., *Candida* sp. (157, 160), and even in prokaryotes (99, 160). Polonelli and coworkers have investigated the potential use of yeast killer factors in the treatment of fungal diseases; positive in vivo results were reported when killer factor 25F from *Pichia anomala* was directly applied topically for treatment of experimental dermatitis and otitis externa due to *Malassezia furfur* and *Malassezia pachydermatis* (159). Among the most intriguing observations of the Polonelli group, however, has been the finding that antibody raised against the combining site of antibody specific for a yeast killer factor (i.e., anti-idiotypic antibody) behaves as does the killer factor itself and is thus directly toxic to *C. albicans* cells expressing the killer factor receptor. Use of such an anti-idiotypic antibody might obviate the problems associated with purification and inherent instability of killer factors as therapeutic agents.

The Polonelli group has focused most recently on killer factor UCSF25 from *P. (Hansenula) anomala*. A monoclonal mouse IgG1 (MAbKT4) that precipitates and neutralizes this factor was tested as a vaccine in rabbits. Sera and affinity-purified antibody from these rabbits directly inhibited the growth of *C. albicans* (161) (see Fig. 4 in reference 161), presumably through the action of anti-idiotypic antibodies, although other antibodies against MAbKT4 must have also been present. It would thus be important to determine whether the antiserum has the same effect (mode of action) as the killer factor.

In follow-up experiments, MAbKT4 was used as an immunogen in BALB/c mice (i.e., syngeneic animals with respect to MAbKT4) and in rats for testing induction of enhanced resistance against disseminated and vaginal candidiasis, respectively. Immune sera showed some ability to inhibit growth of *C. albicans* in vitro, and this inhibition was blocked by MAbKT4. In another study, oophorectomized rats received an intravaginal bolus of MAbKT4 emulsified in Freund adjuvant on days 0, 7, 14, and 21, and the animals were infected intravaginally on day 30 and, in some cases, again on day 124 (158). The *C. albicans* infection boosted the anti-idiotypic antibody response in MAbKT4-immunized rats, and nonimmunized rats infected several times developed antikiller toxin antibodies in their vaginal tracts, consistent with the hypothesized antigenic similarity between the MAbKT4 idiotype and the *Candida* receptor, and between killer factor and the anti-idiotype.

In other work, a monoclonal anti-idiotypic antibody has been isolated and characterized (162); this rat IgM binds to *C. albicans* and inhibits its growth. Concomitant with the above rat infection studies, 9 of 13 human volunteers symptomatic for *Candida* vaginitis had evidence of the anti-idiotypic antibodies (designated as KTIdAb for antibodies that mimic the killer toxin) in their vaginal fluid. KTIdAb was not detectable in asymptomatic volunteers (158). Evidence was obtained that the human KTIdAb enhanced resistance of rats to vaginal candidiasis. These results imply that KTIdAb responses occur in humans during a natural infection with *C. albicans* and such antibodies may be of benefit to the host. Because anti-idiotypic antibodies may be difficult to raise reliably, it would be of interest to determine the usefulness of killer factor receptor as a vaccine candidate.

The authors also showed that anti-idiotypic single-chain Fv antibody constructs (ScFv) had a function similar to that of the native intact KTIdAb (124). Rather than using the rat monoclonal anti-idiotype mentioned above for these constructs, cDNAs from splenocytes that bound MAbKT4 (from mice immunized with MAbKT4) were used. Bacteria expressing ScFv with MAbKT4-binding activity were then identified, and the purified ScFv were found to inhibit growth of *C. albicans* in vitro, an inhibition that could be neutralized by prior incubation with MAbKT4. Complications due to possible endotoxin contamination and agglutinating potential of the ScFv were not assessed, however. When tested in vivo using the rat vaginitis model, the greatest reduction in recoverable *C. albicans* CFUs from vaginal material occurred when animals were treated with the recombinant anti-idiotypic preparation at the time of challenge. Negative controls had no effect compared with untreated infected controls. It would, of course, be interesting to learn whether these recombinant molecules protect against disseminated candidiasis.

Confounding the application of the antibody killer factor mimic approach in therapy is the fact that the specific etiologic agent of disease must express the killer factor receptor. As stated above, a useful vaccine for the generation of antibodies that directly kill *C. albicans,* then, might require a formulation that consists of several monoclonal antibodies with diversity sufficient to affect most isolates of *C. albicans.*

FUTURE PERSPECTIVES AND CONCLUSIONS

The literature supports the hypothesis that antibodies are protective against both disseminated and cutaneous forms of candidiasis and that a useful vaccine formulation should consist of a limited number of *Candida* antigens, rather than a whole cell preparation. The erratic success of the latter approach is likely due to the enormous antigenic complexity of whole *C. albicans* and the relatively few antigens that may lead to a protective antibody response. In this chapter, we reviewed several targets of putative protective antibodies; these targets may be useful in the formulation of vaccines. Several additional antigens that have been recently described merit closer examination as well.

Immunosuppressive and immunoenhancing activities of *C. albicans* antigens have been associated with whole cells, cell-wall fractions, proteins, and mannans (20, 32, 36, 41, 42, 118, 154, 155, 182, 183). Of these, the p43 antigen, which apparently nonspecifically stimulates B cells but suppresses the ability of experimental animals to respond to sheep erythrocytes and candidal antigens (182, 184), is the most defined. The activities of p43 in part appear similar to those of the "suppressor B cells" induced in mice by soluble extracts of *C. albicans,* as reported by Rogers and coworkers (32). Both factors suppress antibody responses, probably through the production of certain cytokines (182, 190). Since mice that were either immunized against p43 or received antisera from immune animals were protected against disseminated candidiasis (183), the molecular and functional characterization of the p43 antigen is needed in order to define it as a possible vaccine candidate.

Candidal adhesins that promote mucosal colonization or adherence to endothelial cells, and attachment to extracellular matrix proteins are likely to benefit the fungus. As described in chapter 6, *C. albicans* Hwp1, *ALS1,* and *ALA1* (62, 93, 180) may be potential vaccine candidates. Finally, antibodies against certain *C. albicans* hydrophobic cell-wall proteins inhibit attachment of the fungus to extracellular matrix proteins (130). A potentially useful vaccine may consist of a mixture of each of these surface proteins. Finally, the most ideal vaccine should be broad spectrum in its activity to include additional *Candida* species, such as *C. dubliniensis, C. glabrata, C. tropicalis, C. krusei, C. lusitaniae, C. parapsilosis,* and *C. guilliermondii.*

The pursuit of an antibody-inducing vaccine against candidiasis in humans is rational. The identification of potential vaccine candidates is already in place, so that a vaccine should be realized in the near future. The experimental and clinical evidence favors a role of antibodies, including the recent application of bovine anti-*C. albicans* polyclonal antisera to reduce oral carriage of *C. albicans* in bone marrow transplant recipients (185). Not curative by itself, antibody promotes the rapid resolution of candidiasis if applied along with standard antifungal therapies.

Acknowledgments. The topic of this chapter overlaps a more extensive chapter written by the authors for a book in press titled *Fungal Pathogenesis: Principles and Clinical Applications* (Marcel Dekker). The reader is referred to that text for a more thorough consideration of some of the topics covered in this chapter. The research reported from the Cutler laboratory was supported by grants from the National Institute of Allergy and Infectious Diseases (RO1 AI24912, RO1 AI41502, and PO1 AI37194).

REFERENCES

1. **Alonso-Monge, R., F. Navarro-Garcia, G. Molero, R. Diez-Orejas, M. Gustin, J. Pla, M. Sanchez, and C. Nombela.** 1999. Role of the mitogen-activated protein kinase Hog1p in morphogenesis and virulence of *Candida albicans. J. Bacteriol.* **181:**3058–3068.
2. **Anaissie, E.** 1992. Opportunistic mycoses in the immunocompromised host: experience at a cancer center and review. *Clin. Infect. Dis.* **14:**S43–S53.
3. **Anaissie, E. J., and G. P. Bodey.** 1990. Fungal infections in patients with cancer. *Pharmacotherapy* **10:**164–169.
4. **Antley, P. P., and K. C. Hazen.** 1988. Role of yeast cell growth temperature on *Candida albicans* virulence in mice. *Infect. Immun.* **56:**2884–2890.
5. **Aronson, I. K., and K. Soltani.** 1976. Chronic mucocutaneous candidosis: a review. *Mycopathologia* **60:**17–25.
6. **Arulanantham, K., J. M. Dwyer, and M. Genel.** 1979. Evidence for defective immunoregulation in the syndrome of familial candidiasis endocrinopathy. *N. Engl. J. Med.* **300:** 164–168.
7. **Berrouane, Y., H. Bisiau, F. Le Baron, C. Cattoen, P. Duthilleul, and E. Dei Cas.** 1998. *Candida albicans* blastoconidia in peripheral blood smears from non-neutropenic surgical patients. *J. Clin. Pathol.* **51:**337–338.
8. **Bevan, E. A., A. J. Herring, and D. J. Mitchell.** 1973. Preliminary characterization of two species of dsRNA in yeast and their relationship to the "killer" character. *Nature* **142:** 81–86.
9. **Bistoni, F., A. Vecchiarelli, E. Cenci, P. Puccetti, P. Marconi, and A. Cassone.** 1986. Evidence for macrophage-mediated protection against lethal *Candida albicans* infection. *Infect. Immun.* **51:**668–674.
10. **Bistoni, F., A. Vecchiarelli, E. Cenci, G. Sbaraglia, S. Perito, and A. Cassone.** 1984. A comparison of experimental pathogenicity of *Candida* species in cyclophosphamide-immunodpresses mice. *Sabouraudia J. Med. Vet. Mycol.* **22:**409–418.
11. **Bodey, G. P.** 1988. The emergence of fungi as major hospital pathogens. *J. Hosp. Infect.* **11:**411–426.
12. **Borkovich, K. A., F. W. Farrelly, D. B. Finkelstein, J. Taulien, and S. Lindquist.** 1989. HSP82 is an essential protein that is required in higher concentrations for growth of cells at higher temperatures. *Mol. Cell. Biol.* **9:**3919–3930.
13. **British Society for Antimicrobial Chemotherapy Working Party.** 1994. Management of deep *Candida* infection in surgical and intensive care unit patients. *Intensive Care Med.* **20:** 522–528.
14. **Bromuro, C., R. La Valle, S. Sandini, F. Urbani, C. M. Ausiello, L. Morelli, C. Fe d'Ostiani, L. Romani, and A. Cassone.** 1998. A 70-kilodalton recombinant heat shock protein of *Candida albicans* is highly immunogenic and enhances systemic murine candidiasis. *Infect. Immun.* **66:**2154–2162.
15. **Caesar-TonThat, T. C., and J. E. Cutler.** 1997. A monoclonal antibody to *Candida albicans* enhances mouse neutrophil candidacidal activity. *Infect. Immun.* **65:**5354–5357.
16. **Cantorna, M. T., and E. Balish.** 1991. Acquired immunity to systemic candidiasis in immunodeficient mice. *J. Infect. Dis.* **164:**936–943.
17. **Cardenas-Freytag, L., E. Cheng, P. Mayeux, J. E. Domer, and J. D. Clements.** 1999. Effectiveness of a vaccine composed of heat-killed *Candida albicans* and a novel mucosal adjuvant, LT(R192G), against systemic candidiasis. *Infect. Immun.* **67:** 826–833.
18. **Casanova, M., M. L. Gil, L. Cardenoso, J. P. Martinez, and R. Sentandreu.** 1989. Identification of wall-specific antigens synthesized during germ tube formation by *Candida albicans. Infect. Immun.* **57:**262–271.
19. **Casanova, M., J. P. Martinez, and W. L. Chaffin.** 1990. Fab fragments from a monoclonal antibody against a germ tube mannoprotein block the yeast-to-mycelium transition in *Candida albicans. Infect. Immun.* **58:**3810–3812.
20. **Cassone, A.** 1995. Immunogenic and immunomodulatory properties of mannoproteins from *Candida albicans. Can. J. Bot.* **73:**1192–1198.
21. **Cassone, A., M. Boccanera, D. Adriani, G. Santoni, and F. De Bernardis.** 1995. Rats clearing a vaginal infection by *Candida albicans* acquire specific, antibody-mediated resistance to vaginal reinfection. *Infect. Immun.* **63:**2619–2624.
22. **Castald, P., R. J. Stratta, R. P. Wood, R. S. Markin, K. D. Patil, M. S. Shaefer, A. N. Langnas, E. C. Reed, S. Li, T. J. Pillen, and B. W. Shaw.** 1991. Clinical spectrum of fungal infections after orthotopic liver transplantation. *Arch. Surg.* **126:**149–156.
23. **Cenci, E., A. Mencacci, G. Del Sero, F. Bistoni, and L. Romani.** 1997. Induction of protective Th1 responses to *Candida albicans* by antifungal therapy alone or in combination with an interleukin-4 antagonist. *J. Infect. Dis.* **176:**217–226.
24. **Cenci, E., A. Mencacci, R. Spaccapelo, L. Tonnetti, P. Mosci, K.-H. Enssle, P. Puccetti, L. Romani, and F. Bistoni.** 1995. T helper cell type 1 (Th1)- and Th2-like responses are present in mice with gastric candidiasis but protective immunity is associated with Th1 development. *J. Infect. Dis.* **171:** 1279–1288.
25. **Cheng, L., K. Hirst, and P. W. Piper.** 1992. Authentic temperature-regulation of a heat shock gene inserted into yeast on a high copy number vector. Influences of overexpression of HSP90 protein on high temperature growth and thermotolerance. *Biochim. Biophys. Acta* **1132:**26–34.
26. **Christensson, B., L. Ryd, L. Dahlberg, and S. Lohmander.** 1993. *Candida albicans* arthritis in a nonimmunocompromised patient. *Acta Orthop. Scand.* **64:**695–698.
27. **Collins, L. A., M. H. Samore, M. S. Roberts, R. Luzzati, R. L. Jenkins, W. D. Lewis, and A. W. Karchmer.** 1994. Risk factors for invasive fungal infections complicating orthotopic liver transplantation. *J. Infect. Dis.* **170:**644–652.

28. **Corner, B. E., and P. T. Magee.** 1997. *Candida* pathogenesis: unravelling the threads of infection. *Curr. Biol.* **7:** R691–R694.
29. **Costantino, P. J., N. F. Gare, and J. R. Warmington.** 1995. Humoral immune responses to systemic *Candida albicans* infection in inbred mouse strains. *Immunol. Cell Biol.* **73:** 125–133.
30. **Csank, C., C. Makris, S. Meloche, K. Schröppel, M. Röllinghoff, D. Dignard, D. Y. Thomas, and M. Whiteway.** 1997. Derepressed hyphal growth and reduced virulence in a VH1 family-related protein phosphatase mutant of the human pathogen *Candida albicans. Mol. Biol. Cell* **8:**2539–2551.
31. **Csank, C., K. Schroppel, E. Leberer, D. Harcus, O. Mohamed, S. Moleche, D. Y. Thomas, and M. Whiteway.** 1998. Roles of *Candida albicans* mitogen-activated protein kinase homolog, Cek1p, in hyphal development and systemic candidiasis. *Infect. Immun.* **66:**2713–2721.
32. **Cuff, C. F., B. J. Packer, and T. J. Rogers.** 1989. A further characterization of *Candida albicans*-induced suppressor B-cell activity. *Immunology* **68:**80–86.
33. **Cutler, J. E.** 1991. Putative virulence factors of *Candida albicans. Ann. Rev. Microbiol.* **45:**187–218.
34. **Cutler, J. E., D. L. Brawner, K. C. Hazen, and M. A. Jutila.** 1990. Characteristics of *Candida albicans* adherence to mouse tissue. *Infect. Immun.* **58:**1902–1908.
35. **Cutler, J. E., and K. C. Hazen.** 1983. Yeast/mold dimorphism, p. 267–306. *In* J. W. Bennett and A. Ciegler (ed.), *Secondary Metabolism and Differentiation in Fungi.* Marcel Dekker, Inc., New York, N.Y.
36. **Cutler, J. E., and R. K. Lloyd.** 1982. Enhanced antibody responses induced by *Candida albicans* in mice. *Infect. Immun.* **38:**1102–1108.
37. **Dean, D. A., and K. W. Burchard.** 1996. Fungal infection in surgical patients. *Am. J. Surg.* **171:**374–382.
38. **De Bernardis, F., S. Arancia, L. Morelli, B. Hube, D. Sanglard, W. Schäfer, and A. Cassone.** 1999. Evidence that members of the secretory aspartyl proteinase gene family, in particular *SAP2,* are virulence factors for *Candida* vaginitis. *J. Infect. Dis.* **179:**201–208.
39. **De Bernardis, F., M. Boccanera, D. A. Adriani, E. Spreghini, G. Santoni, and A. Cassone.** 1997. Protective role of antimannan and anti-aspartyl proteinase antibodies in an experimental model of *Candida albicans* vaginitis in rats. *Infect. Immun.* **65:**3399–3409.
40. **De Bernardis, F., G. Santoni, M. Boccanera, E. Spreghini, D. A. Adriani, L. Morelli, and A. Cassone.** 2000. Local anticandidal immune responses in a rat model of vaginal infection by and protection against *Candida albicans. Infect. Immun.* **68:**3297–3304.
41. **Domer, J. E.** 1989. *Candida* cell wall mannan: a polysaccharide with diverse immunologic properties. *Crit. Rev. Microbiol.* **17:**33–51.
42. **Domer, J. E., L. G. Human, G. B. Andersen, J. A. Rudbach, and G. L. Asherson.** 1993. Abrogation of suppression of delayed hypersensitivity induced by *Candida albicans*-derived mannan by treatment with monophosphoryl lipid A. *Infect. Immun.* **61:**2122–2130.
43. **Domer, J. E., and R. I. Lehrer.** 1993. Introduction to *Candida:* systemic candidiasis, p. 49–116. *In* J. W. Murphy, H. Friedman, and M. Bendinelli (ed.), *Infectious Agents and Pathogenesis: Fungal Infections and Immune Responses.* Plenum Press, New York, N.Y.
44. **Dwyer, J. M.** 1981. Chronic mucocutaneous candidiasis. *Annu. Rev. Med.* **32:**491–497.
45. **Edwards, J. E., and S. G. Filler.** 1992. Current strategies for treating invasive candidiasis: emphasis on infections in non-neutropenic patients. *Clin. Infect. Dis.* **14**(Suppl 1): S106–S113.
46. **Eggimann, P., P. Francioli, J. Bille, R. Schneider, M.-M. Wu, G. Chapuis, R. Chiolero, A. Pannatier, J. Schilling, S. Geroulanos, M. P. Glauser, and T. Calandra.** 1999. Fluconazole prophylaxis prevents intra-abdominal candidiasis in high-risk surgical patients. *Crit. Care Med.* **27:**1066–1072.
47. **El-Ebiary, M., A. Torres, N. Fàbregas, J. P. de la Bellacasa, J. González, J. Ramirez, D. del Baño, C. Hernández, and M. T. Jiménez de Anta.** 1997. Significance of the isolation of *Candida* species from respiratory samples in critically ill, non-neutropenic patients: an immediate postmortem histologic study. *Am. J. Respir. Crit. Care Med.* **156:**583–590.
48. **Ellepola, A. N. B., and L. P. Samaranayake.** 1998. The effect of limited exposure to antimycotics on the relative cell-surface hydrophobicity and the adhesion of oral *Candida albicans* to buccal epithelial cells. *Arch. Oral Biol.* **43:**879–887.
49. **Ener, B., and L. J. Douglas.** 1992. Correlation between cell-surface hydrophobicity of *Candida albicans* and adhesion to buccal epithelial cells. *FEMS Microbiol. Lett.* **99:**37–42.
50. **Evans, E. G. V., F. C. Odds, M. D. Richardson, and K. T. Holland.** 1974. The effect of growth medium on filament production in *Candida albicans. Sabouraudia* **12:**112–119.
51. **Fass, R. J., D. A. Goff, and S. J. Sierawski.** 1996. Candida infections in the surgical intensive care unit. *J. Antimicrob. Chemother.* **38:**915–916.
52. **Fidel, P. L., K. A. Ginsburg, J. L. Cutright, N. A. Wolf, D. Leaman, K. Dunlap, and J. D. Sobel.** 1997. Vaginal-associated immunity in women with recurrent vulvovaginal candidiasis: evidence for vaginal Th1-type responses following intravaginal challenge with *Candida* antigen. *J. Infect. Dis.* **176:** 728–739.
53. **Fidel, P. L., and J. D. Sobel.** 1996. Immunopathogenesis of recurrent vulvovaginal candidiasis. *Clin. Microbiol. Rev.* **9:** 335–348.
54. **Filler, S. G., and J. E. Edwards.** 1995. When and how to treat serious candidial infections: concepts and controversies. *Curr. Clin. Top. Infect. Dis.* **15:**1–18.
55. **Fradin, C., D. Poulain, and T. Jouault.** 2000. Beta-1,2-linked oligomannosides from *Candida albicans* bind to a 32-kilodalton macrophage membrane protein homologous to the mammalian lectin galectin-3. *Infect. Immun.* **68:**4391–4398.
56. **Franklyn, K. M., J. R. Warmington, A. K. Ott, and R. B. Ashman.** 1990. An immunodominant antigen of *Candida albicans* shows homology to the enzyme enolase. *Immunol. Cell Biol.* **68:**173–178.
57. **Fridkin, S. K., and W. R. Jarvis.** 1996. Epidemiology of nosocomial fungal infections. *Clin. Microbiol. Rev.* **9:**499–511.
58. **Fu, Y., G. Rieg, W. A. Fonzi, P. H. Belanger, J. E. Edwards, and S. G. Filler.** 1998. Expression of the *Candida albicans* gene ALS1 in *Saccharomyces cerevisiae* induces adherence to endothelial and epithelial cells. *Infect. Immun.* **66:** 1783–1786.
59. **Fulurija, A., R. B. Ashman, and J. M. Papadimitriou.** 1995. Neutrophil depletion increases susceptibility to systemic and vaginal candidiasis in mice, and reveals differences between brain and kidney in mechanisms of host resistance. *Microbiology* **142:**3487–3496.
60. **Gale, C. A., C. M. Bendel, M. McClellan, M. Hauser, J. M. Becker, J. Berman, and M. K. Hostetter.** 1998. Linkage of adhesion, filamentous growth, and virulence in *Candida albicans* to a single gene, INT1. *Science* **279:**1355–1358.
61. **García-Ruiz, J. C., M. Del Carmen Arilla, P. Regúlez, G. Quindos, A. Álvarez, and J. Pontón.** 1997. Detection of antibodies to *Candida albicans* germ tubes for diagnosis and therapeutic monitoring of invasive candidiasis in patients with

hematologic malignancies. *J. Clin. Microbiol.* **35:** 3284–3287.

62. **Gaur, N. K., S. A. Klotz, and R. L. Henderson.** 1999. Overexpression of the *Candida albicans ALA1* gene in *Saccharomyces cerevisiae* results in aggregation following attachment of yeast cells to extracellular mattrix proteins, adherence properties similar to those of *Candida albicans. Infect. Immun.* **67:**6040–6047.
63. **Ghannoum, M., and K. A. Elteen.** 1986. Correlative relationship between proteinase production, adherence and pathogenicity of various strains of *Candida albicans. J. Med. Vet. Mycol.* **24:**407–413.
64. **Ghannoum, M. A.** 2000. Potential role of phospholipases in virulence and fungal pathogenesis. *Clin. Microbiol. Rev.* **13:** 122–143.
65. **Ghannoum, M. A., and K. H. Abu-Elteen.** 1990. Pathogenicity determinants of *Candida. Mycoses* **33:**265–282.
66. **Giger, D. K., J. E. Domer, and J. T. McQuitty.** 1978. Experimental murine candidiasis: pathological and immune responses to cutaneous inoculation with *Candida albicans. Infect. Immun.* **19:**499–509.
67. **Gladdy, R. A., S. E. Richardson, H. D. Davies, and R. A. Superina.** 1999. *Candida* infection in pediatric liver transplant recipients. *Liver Transplant. Surg.* **5:**16–24.
68. **Glee, P. M., P. Sundstrom, and K. C. Hazen.** 1995. Expression of surface hydrophobic proteins by *Candida albicans* in vivo. *Infect. Immun.* **63:**1373–1379.
69. **Goldman, R. C., D. J. Frost, J. O. Capobianco, S. Kadam, R. R. Rasmussen, and C. Abad-Zapatero.** 1995. Antifungal drug tests: *Candida* secreted aspartyl protease and fungal wall β-glucan synthesis. *Infect. Agents Dis.* **4:**228–247.
70. **Grappel, S. F., and R. A. Calderone.** 1976. Effect of antibodies on the respiration and morphology of *Candida albicans. S. Afr. Med. J.* **14:**51–60.
71. **Grappel, S. F., A. Ferthiere, and F. Blank.** 1971. Effect of antibodies on growth and structure of *Trichophyton mentagrophytes. Sabouraudia* **9:**50–55.
72. **Greenfield, R. A., and J. M. Jones.** 1981. Purification and characterization of a major cytoplasmic antigen of *Candida albicans. Infect. Immun.* **32:**469–477.
73. **Han, Y., and J. E. Cutler.** 1995. Antibody response that protects against disseminated candidiasis. *Infect. Immun.* **63:** 2714–2719.
74. **Han, Y., and J. E. Cutler.** 1996. Monoclonal antibody B6.1 protects neutropenic mice and enhances the therapeutic potential of antifungal drugs against disseminated candidiasis, abstr. F87, p. 121. *Proc. Gen. Meet. Am. Soc. Microbiol.* American Society for Microbiology, Washington, D.C.
75. **Han, Y., and J. E. Cutler.** 1997. Assessment of a mouse model of neutropenia and the effect of an anti-candidiasis monoclonal antibody in these animals. *J. Infect. Dis.* **175:** 1169–1175.
76. Deleted in proof.
77. **Han, Y., T. Kanbe, R. Cherniak, and J. E. Cutler.** 1997. Biochemical characterization of *Candida albicans* epitopes that can elicit protective and nonprotective antibodies. *Infect. Immun.* **65:**4100–4107.
78. **Han, Y., S. Kelm, M. H. Riesselman, P. R. Crocker, and J. E. Cutler.** 1994. Mouse sialoadhesin is not responsible for *Candida albicans* yeast cell binding to splenic marginal zone macrophages. *Infect. Immun.* **62:**2115–2118.

78a. **Han, Y., T. R. Kozel, M. X. Xhang, R. S. MacGill, M. C. Carroll, and J. E. Cutler.** Complement is essential for protection by an IgM and an IgG monoclonal antibody against experimental hematogenously disseminated candidiasis. *J. Immunol.*, in press.

79. **Han, Y., R. P. Morrison, and J. E. Cutler.** 1998. A vaccine and monoclonal antibodies that enhance mouse resistance to *Candida albicans* vaginal infection. *Infect. Immun.* **66:** 5771–5776.
80. **Han, Y., M. H. Riesselman, and J. E. Cutler.** 2000. Protection against candidiasis by an immunoglobulin G3 (IgG3) monoclonal antibody specific for the same mannotriose as an IgM protective antibody. *Infect. Immun.* **68:**1649–1654.
81. **Han, Y., M. A. Ulrich, and J. E. Cutler.** 1999. *Candida albicans* mannan extract-protein conjugates induce a protective immune response against experimental candidiasis. *J. Infect. Dis.* **179:**1477–1484.
82. **Han, Y., N. van Rooijen, and J. E. Cutler.** 1993. Binding of *Candida albicans* yeast cells to mouse popliteal lymph node tissue is mediated by macrophages. *Infect. Immun.* **61:** 3244–3249.
83. **Hazen, B. W., and K. C. Hazen.** 1988. Dynamic expression of cell surface hydrophobicity during initial yeast cell growth and before germ tube formation of *Candida albicans. Infect. Immun.* **56:**2521–2525.
84. **Hazen, K. C.** 1989. Participation of yeast cell surface hydrophobicity in adherence of *Candida albicans* to human epithelial cells. *Infect. Immun.* **57:**1894–1900.
85. **Hazen, K. C., D. L. Brawner, M. H. Riesselman, M. A. Jutila, and J. E. Cutler.** 1991. Differential adherence between hydrophobic and hydrophilic yeast cells of *Candida albicans. Infect. Immun.* **59:**907–912.
86. **Hazen, K. C., and J. E. Cutler.** 1979. Autoregulation of germ tube formation by *Candida albicans. Infect. Immun.* **24:** 661–666.
87. **Hazen, K. C., and J. E. Cutler.** 1983. Isolation and purification of morphogenic autoregulatory substance produced by *Candida albicans. J. Biochem.* **94:**777–783.

87a. **Hazen, K. C., and J. E. Cutler.** Unpublished data.

88. **Hazen, K. C., and P. M. Glee.** 1995. Cell surface hydrophobicity and medically important fungi, p. 1–31. *In* M. Borgers, R. Hay, and M. G. Rinaldi (ed.), *Current Topics in Medical Mycology.* Prous Science, Barcelona, Spain.
89. **Hodgetts, S., R. Matthews, G. Morrissey, K. Mitsutake, P. Piper, and J. Burnie.** 1996. Over-expression of *Saccharomyces cerevisiae* hsp90 enhances the virulence of this yeast in mice. *FEMS Immunol. Med. Microbiol.* **16:**229–234.
90. **Hoegl, L., M. Ollert, and H. C. Korting.** 1996. The role of *Candida albicans* secreted aspartic proteinase in the development of candidoses. *J. Mol. Med.* **74:**135–142.
91. **Hoerauf, A., S. Hammer, B. Müller-Myhsok, and H. Ruprecht.** 1998. Intra-abdominal *Candida* infection during acute necrotizing pancreatitis has a high prevalence and is associated with increased mortality. *Crit. Care. Med.* **26:** 2010–2015.
92. **Hostetter, M. K.** 1998. Linkage of adhesion, morphogenesis, and virulence in *Candida albicans. J. Lab. Clin. Med.* **132:** 258–263.
93. **Hoyer, L. L., T. L. Payne, and J. E. Hecht.** 1998. Identification of *Candida albicans* ALS2 and ALS4 and localization of Als proteins to the fungal cell surface. *J. Bacteriol.* **180:** 5334–5343.
94. **Huang, Y.-C., T.-Y. Lin, H.-S. Leu, J.-L. Wu, and J.-H. Wu.** 1998. Yeast carriage on hands of hospital personnel working in intensive care units. *J. Hosp. Infect.* **39:**47–51.
95. **Hughes, W. T., D. Armstrong, G. P. Bodey, A. E. Brown, J. E. Edwards, R. Feld, P. Pizzo, K. V. I. Rolston, J. L. Shenep, and L. S. Young.** 1997. 1997 Guidelines for the use of antimicrobial agents in neutropenic patients with unexplained fever. *Clin. Infect. Dis.* **25:**551–573.
96. **Hunter, P. R., and C. A. M. Fraser.** 1989. Application of a

numerical index of discriminatory power to a comparison of four physiochemical typing methods for *Candida albicans. J. Clin. Microbiol.* **27**:2156–2160.

97. **Hurd, R. C., and C. H. Drake.** 1953. *Candida albicans* infections in actively and passively immunized animals. *Mycopathol. Mycologia Applic.* **6**:290–297.

98. **Irving, G., D. Miller, A. Robinson, S. Reynolds, and A. J. Copas.** 1998. Psychological factors associated with recurrent vaginal candidiasis: a preliminary study. *Sex. Transm. Infect.* **74**:334–338.

99. **Izgu, F., and D. Altinbay.** 1997. Killer toxins of certain yeast strains have potential growth inhibitory activity on gram-positive pathogenic bacteria. *Microbios.* **89**:15–22.

100. **Jarvis, W. R.** 1995. Epidemiology of nosocomial fungal infections, with emphasis on *Candida* species. *Clin. Infect. Dis.* **20**:1526–1530.

101. **Jensen, J., T. Warner, and E. Balish.** 1994. The role of phagocytic cells in resistance to disseminated candidiasis in granulocytopenic mice. *J. Infect. Dis.* **170**:900–905.

102. **Kanbe, T., and J. E. Cutler.** 1994. Evidence for adhesin activity in the acid-stable moiety of the phosphomannoprotein complex of *Candida albicans. Infect. Immun.* **62**:1662–1668.

103. **Kanbe, T., and J. E. Cutler.** 1998. Minimum chemical requirements for adhesin activity of the acid-stable part of *Candida albicans* cell wall phosphomannoprotein complex. *Infect. Immun.* **66**:5812–5818.

104. **Kanbe, T., Y. Han, B. Redgrave, M. H. Riesselman, and J. E. Cutler.** 1993. Evidence that mannans of *Candida albicans* are responsible for adherence of yeast forms to spleen and lymph node tissue. *Infect. Immun.* **61**:2578–2584.

105. **Kanbe, T., M. A. Jutila, and J. E. Cutler.** 1992. Evidence that *Candida albicans* binds via a unique adhesion system on phagocytic cells in the marginal zone of the mouse spleen. *Infect. Immun.* **60**:1972–1978.

106. **Kantarjian, H. M., M. F. Saad, E. H. Estey, R. V. Sellin, and N. A. Samaan.** 1983. Hypercalcemia in disseminated candidiasis. *Am. J. Med.* **74**:721–724.

107. **Kapur, A., R. Vasudeva, and C. W. Howden.** 1997. *Candida* splenic abscess in the absence of obvious immunodeficiency. *Am. J. Gastroenterol.* **92**:509–512.

108. **Kirkpatrick, C. H., R. R. Rich, and J. E. Bennett.** 1971. Chronic mucocutaneous candidiasis: model-building in cellular immunity. *Ann. Intern. Med.* **74**:955–978.

109. **Klingspor, L., G. Stintzing, A. Fasth, and J. Tollemar.** 1996. Deep *Candida* infection in children receiving allogeneic bone marrow transplants: incidences, risk factors and diagnosis. *Bone Marrow Transpl.* **17**:1043–1049.

110. **Kobayashi, S. D., and J. E. Cutler.** 1998. *Candida albicans* hyphal formation and virulence: is there a clearly defined role? *Trends Microbiol.* **6**:92–94.

111. **Kondoh, Y., K. Shimizu, and K. Tanaka.** 1987. Proteinase production and pathogenicity of *Candida albicans.* II. Virulence for mice of *C. albicans* strains of different proteinase activity. *Microbiol. Immunol.* **31**:1061–1069.

112. **Kullberg, B. J., M. G. Netea, J. H. A. J. Curfs, M. Keuter, J. F. G. M. Meis, and J. M. W. Van der Meer.** 1998. Recombinant murine granulocyte colony-stimulating factor protects against acute disseminated *Candida albicans* infection in non-neutropenic mice. *J. Infect. Dis.* **177**:175–181.

113. **Kuruganti, U., L. A. Henderson, R. E. Garner, R. Asofsky, P. J. Baker, and J. E. Domer.** 1988. Nonspecific and *Candida*-specific immune responses in mice suppressed by chronic administration of anti-μ. *J. Leukoc. Biol.* **44**:422–433.

114. **LaForce, F. M., D. M. Mills, K. Iverson, R. Cousins, and E. D. Everett.** 1975. Inhibition of leukocyte candidacidal activity by serum from patients with disseminated candidiasis. *J. Lab. Clin. Med.* **86**:657–666.

115. **Leberer, E., K. Ziegelbauer, A. Schmidt, D. Harcus, D. Dignard, J. Ash, L. Johnson, and D. Y. Thomas.** 1997. Virulence and hyphal formation of *Candida albicans* require the Ste20p-like protein kinase CaCla4p. *Curr. Biol.* **7**:539–546.

116. **Lee, K. L., H. R. Buckley, and C. C. Campbell.** 1975. An amino acid liquid synthetic medium for the development of mycelial and yeast forms of *Candida albicans. Sabouraudia* **13**:148–153.

117. **Li, R.-K., and J. E. Cutler.** 1993. Chemical definition of an epitope/adhesin molecule on *Candida albicans. J. Biol. Chem.* **268**:18293–18299.

118. **Li, S. P., S.-I. Lee, and J. E. Domer.** 1998. Alterations in frequency of interleukin-2 (IL-2)-, gamma interferon-, or IL-4-secreting splenocytes induced by *Candida albicans* mannan and/or monophosphoryl lipid A. *Infect. Immun.* **66**:1392–1399.

119. **Lo, H.-J., J. R. Köhler, B. DiDomenico, D. Loebenberg, A. Cacciapuoti, and G. R. Fink.** 1997. Nonfilamentous *C. albicans* mutants are avirulent. *Cell* **90**:939–949.

120. **Lockhart, S. R., S. Joly, K. Vargas, J. Swails-Wenger, L. Enger, and D. R. Soll.** 1999. Natural defenses against *Candida* colonization breakdown in the oral cavities of the elderly. *J. Dent. Res.* **78**:857–868.

121. **Lortholary, O., and B. Dupont.** 1997. Antifungal prophylaxis during neutropenia and immunodeficiency. *Clin. Microbiol. Rev.* **10**:477–504.

122. **Louria, D. B., J. K. Smith, R. G. Brayton, and M. Buse.** 1972. Anti-*Candida* factors in serum and their inhibitors. *J. Infect. Dis.* **125**:102–114.

123. **Macdonald, F.** 1984. Secretion of inducible proteinase by pathogenic *Candida* species. *Sabouraudia J. Med. Vet. Mycol.* **22**:79–82.

124. **Magliani, W., S. Conti, F. De Bernardis, M. Gerioni, D. Bertolotti, P. Mozzoni, A. Cassone, and L. Polonelli.** 1997. Therapeutic potentials of antiidiotypic single chain antibodies with yeast killer toxin activity. *Nat. Biotech.* **15**:155–158.

125. **Maiti, P. K., A. Kumar, R. Kumar, and L. N. Mohapatra.** 1985. Role of antibodies and effect of BCG vaccination in experimental candidiasis in mice. *Mycopathologia* **91**:79–85.

126. **Marodi, L.** 1997. Local and systemic host defense mechanisms against *Candida:* immunopathology of candidal infections. *Pediatr. Infect. Dis. J.* **16**:795–801.

127. **Martin, D. S.** 1941. The practical application of some immunologic principles to the diagnosis and treatment of certain fungus infections. *J. Invest. Dermatol.* **4**:471–481.

128. **Martino, R., R. Lopez, A. Sureda, S. Brunet, and A. Domingo-Albós.** 1997. Risk of reactivation of a recent invasive fungal infection in patients with hematological malignancies undergoing further intensive chemo-radiotherapy: a single-center experience and review of the literature. *Haematologica* **82**:297–304.

129. **Masuoka, J., and K. C. Hazen.** 1997. Cell wall protein mannosylation determines *Candida albicans* cell surface hydrophobicity. *Microbiology* **143**:3015–3021.

130. **Masuoka, J., G. Wu, P. M. Glee, and K. C. Hazen.** 1999. Inhibition of *Candida albicans* attachment to extracellular matrix by antibodies which recognize hydrophobic cell wall proteins. *FEMS Immunol. Med. Microbiol.* **24**:421–429.

131. **Matsumoto, M., S. Matsubara, T. Matsuno, M. Tamura, K. Hattori, H. Nomura, M. Ono, and T. Yokota.** 1987. Protective effect of human granulocyte colony-stimulating factor on microbial infection in neutropenic mice. *Infect. Immun.* **55**:2715–2720.

132. **Matsumoto, M., S. Matsubara, T. Matsuno, M. Tamura, K.**

Hattori, H. Nomura, M. Ono, and T. Yokota. 1993. Protective effect of human granulocyte colony-stimulating factor on microbial infection in neutropenic mice. *Infect. Immun.* 55: 2715–2720.

133. **Matthews, R., and J. Burnie.** 1989. Cloning of a DNA sequence encoding a major fragment of the 47 kilodalton stress protein homologue of *Candida albicans*. *FEMS Microbiol. Lett.* 60:25–30.
134. **Matthews, R., and J. Burnie.** 1992. The role of hsp90 in fungal infection. *Immunol. Today* 13:345–348.
135. **Matthews, R., S. Hodgetts, and J. Burnie.** 1995. Preliminary assessment of a human recombinant antibody fragment to hsp90 in murine invasive candidiasis. *J. Infect. Dis.* 171: 1668–1671.
136. **Matthews, R., C. Wells, and J. P. Burnie.** 1988. Characterisation and cellular localisation of the immunodominant 47-Kda antigen of *Candida albicans*. *J. Med. Microbiol.* 27:227–232.
137. **Matthews, R. C., J. P. Burnie, D. Howat, T. Rowland, and F. Walton.** 1991. Autoantibody to heat-shock protein 90 can mediate protection against systemic candidosis. *Immunology* 74:20–24.
138. **Matthews, R. C., J. P. Burnie, and S. Tabaqchali.** 1984. Immunoblot analysis of the serological response in systemic candidosis. *Lancet* ii:1415–1418.
139. **Matthews, R. C., J. P. Burnie, and S. Tabaqchali.** 1987. Isolation of immunodominant antigens from sera of patients with systemic candidiasis and characterization of serological response to *Candida albicans*. *J. Clin. Microbiol.* 25:230–237.
140. **Matthews, R. C., G. Rigg, S. Hodgetts, and J. Nelson.** 2000. Human recombinant antibody to hsp90 in the treatment of disseminated candidiasis, abstr. O63, p. 510. *Proc. Gen. Meet. Am. Soc. Microbiol.*, American Society for Microbiology, Washington, D.C.
141. **Mitchell, A. P.** 1998. Dimorphism and virulence in *Candida albicans*. *Curr. Opin. Microbiol.* 1:687–692.
142. **Mourad, S., and L. Friedman.** 1961. Active immunization of mice against *Candida albicans*. *Proc. Soc. Exp. Biol. Med.* 106:570–572.
143. **Mourad, S., and L. Friedman.** 1968. Passive immunization of mice against *Candida albicans*. *Sabouraudia* 6:103–105.
144. **Nolla-Salas, J., A. Sitges-Serra, C. León-Gil, J. Martínez-González, M. A. León-Regidor, P. Ibáñez-Lucía, and J. M. Torres-Rodriguez.** 1997. Candidemia in non-neutropenic critically ill patients: analysis of prognostic factors and assessment of systemic antifungal therapy. *Intensive Care Med.* 23:23–30.
145. **Nucci, M., A. L. Colombo, F. Silveira, R. Richtmann, R. Salomão, M. L. Branchini, and N. Spector.** 1998. Risk factors for death in patients with candidemia. *Infect. Control Hosp. Epidemiol.* 19:846–850.
146. **Odds, F. C.** 1988. *Candida and Candidosis*. Bailliere Tindall, London, United Kingdom.
147. **Odds, F. C., L. Van Nuffel, and N. A. Gow.** 2000. Survival in experimental *Candida albicans* infections depends on inoculum growth conditions as well as animal host. *Microbiology* 146:1881–1889.
148. **Ollert, M. W., C. Wende, M. Gorlich, C. G. McMullan-Vogel, M. Borg-Von Zepelin, C.-W. Vogel, and H. C. Korting.** 1995. Increased expression of *Candida albicans* secretory proteinase, a putative virulence factor, in isolates from human immunodeficiency virus-positive patients. *J. Clin. Microbiol.* 33:2543–2549.
149. **Pardo, M., M. Ward, A. Pitarch, M. Sanchez, C. Nombela, W. Blackstock, and C. Gil.** 2000. Cross-specific identification of novel *Candida albicans* immunogenic proteins by combination of two-dimensional polyacrylamide gel electrophoresis and mass spectroscopy. *Electrophoresis* 21:2651–2659.
150. **Pearsall, N. N., B. L. Adams, and R. Bunni.** 1978. Immunologic responses to *Candida albicans*. III. Effects of passive transfer of lymphoid cells or serum on murine candidiasis. *J. Immunol.* 120:1176–1180.
151. **Pearsall, N. N., and D. Lagunoff.** 1974. Immunological responses to *Candida albicans*. *Infect. Immun.* 9:999–1002.
152. **Pfaller, M. A., S. A. Messer, A. Houston, M. S. Rangel-Frausto, T. Wiblin, H. M. Blumberg, J. E. Edwards, W. Jarvis, M. A. Martin, H. C. Neu, L. Saiman, J. E. Patterson, J. C. Dibb, C. M. Roldan, M. G. Rinaldi, and R. P. Wenzel.** 1998. National epidemiology of mycoses survey: a multicenter study of strain variation and antifungal susceptibility among isolates of *Candida* species. *Diagn. Microbiol. Infect. Dis.* 31:289–296.
153. **Phillips, P., S. Shafran, G. Garber, C. Rotstein, F. Smaill, I. Fong, I. Salit, M. Miller, K. Williams, J. M. Conly, J. Singer, and S. Ioannou.** 1997. Multicenter randomized trial of fluconazole versus amphotericin B for treatment of candidemia in non-neutropenic patients. *Eur. J. Clin. Microbiol. Infect. Dis.* 16:337–345.
154. **Piccolella, E., G. Lombardi, and R. Morelli.** 1981. Generation of suppressor cells in the response of human lymphocytes to a polysaccharide from *Candida albicans*. *J. Immunol.* 126: 2151–2155.
155. **Piccolella, E., G. Lombardi, and R. Morelli.** 1981. Mitogenic response of human peripheral blood lymphocytes to a purified *C. albicans* polysaccharide fraction: lack of helper activities is responsible for the in vitro unresponsiveness to a second antigenic challenge. *J. Immunol.* 126:2156–2160.
156. **Pizzo, P. A., M. Rubin, A. Freifeld, and T. J. Walsh.** 1991. The child with cancer and infection. I. Empiric therapy for fever and neutropenia, and preventive strategies. *J. Pediatr.* 119:679–693.
157. **Polonelli, L., S. Conti, M. Gerloni, W. Magliani, C. Chezzi, and G. Morace.** 1991. Interfaces of the yeast killer phenomenon. *Crit. Rev. Microbiol.* 18:47–87.
158. **Polonelli, L., F. De Bernardis, S. Conti, M. Boccanera, W. Magliani, M. Gerloni, C. Cantelli, and A. Cassone.** 1996. Human natural yeast killer toxin-like candidacidal antibodies. *J. Immunol.* 156:1880–1885.
159. **Polonelli, L., R. Lorenzini, F. De Bernardis, and G. Morace.** 1986. Potential therapeutic effect of yeast killer toxin. *Mycopathologia* 96:103–107.
160. **Polonelli, L., and G. Morace.** 1986. Reevaluation of the yeast killer phenomenon. *J. Clin. Microbiol.* 24:866–869.
161. **Polonelli, L., and G. Morace.** 1988. Yeast killer toxin-like anti-idiotypic antibodies. *J. Clin. Microbiol.* 26:602–604.
162. **Polonelli, L., N. Seguy, S. Conti, M. Gerloni, Bertolotti, Cantelli, Magliani, and J. Cailliez.** 1997. Monoclonal yeast killer toxin-like candidacidal anti-idiotypic antibodies. *Clin. Diagn. Lab. Immunol.* 4:142–146.
163. **Poulain, D., J.-C. Cailliez, and J.-F. Dubremetz.** 1989. Secretion of glycoproteins through the cell wall of *Candida albicans*. *Eur. J. Cell Biol.* 50:94–99.
164. **Puccetti, P., L. Romani, and F. Bistoni.** 1995. A T_H1-T_H2-like switch in candidiasis: new perspectives for therapy. *Trends Microbiol.* 3:237–240.
165. **Rabinovici, R., D. Szewczyk, P. Ovadia, J. R. Greenspan, and J. J. Sivalingam.** 1997. *Candida* pericarditis: clinical profile and treatment. *Ann. Thorac. Surg.* 63:1200–1204.
166. **Rantala, A.** 1993. Postoperative candidiasis. *Ann. Chir. Gynaecol. Suppl.* 205:6–52.
167. **Rantala, A., J. Niinikoski, and O.-P. Lehtonen.** 1993. Early *Candida* isolations in febrile patients after abdominal surgery. *Scand. J. Infect. Dis.* 25:479–485.
168. **Ray, T. L., and C. D. Payne.** 1988. Scanning electron micros-

copy of epidermal adherence and cavitation in murine candidiasis: a role for *Candida* acid proteinase. *Infect. Immun.* **56:** 1942–1949.

169. **Rex, J. H.** 1996. Editorial response: catheters and candidemia. *Clin. Infect. Dis.* **22:**467–470.
170. **Rex, J. H., T. J. Walsh, and E. J. Anaissie.** 1998. Fungal infections in iatrogenically compromised hosts. *Adv. Int. Med.* **43:**321–371.
171. **Richards, M. J., J. R. Edwards, D. H. Culver, R. P. Gaynes, and National Nosocomial Infections Surveillance System.** 1998. Nosocomial infections in coronary care units in the United States. *Am. J. Cardiol.* **82:**789–793.
172. **Riesselman, M. H., T. Kanbe, and J. E. Cutler.** 1991. Improvements and important considerations of an ex vivo assay to study interactions of *Candida albicans* with splenic tissue. *J. Immunol. Methods* **1450:**153–160.
173. **Romani, L.** 1999. Immunity to *Candida albicans:* Th1, Th2 cells and beyond. *Curr. Opin. Microbiol.* **2:**363–367.
174. **Romani, L., A. Mencacci, U. Grohmann, S. Mocci, P. Mosci, P. Puccetti, and F. Bistoni.** 1992. Neutralizing antibody to interleukin 4 induces systemic protection and T helper type 1-associated immunity in murine candidiasis. *J. Exp. Med.* **176:**19–25.
175. **Romani, L., P. Puccetti, A. Mencacci, E. Cenci, R. Spaccapelo, L. Tonnetti, U. Grohmann, and F. Bistoni.** 1994. Neutralization of IL-10 up-regulates nitric oxide production and protects susceptible mice from challenge with *Candida albicans. J. Immunol.* **152:**3515–3521.
176. **Schmitt, M. J., P. Klavehn, J. Wang, I. Schonig, and D. J. Tipper.** 1996. Cell cycle studies on the mode of action of yeast K28 killer toxin. *Microbiology* **142:**2655–2662.
177. **Shibata, N., K. Ikuta, T. Imai, Y. Satoh, R. Satoh, A. Suzuki, C. Kojima, H. Kobayashi, K. Hisamichi, and S. Suzuki.** 1995. Existence of branched side chains in the cell wall mannan of pathogenic yeast, *Candida albicans. J. Biol. Chem.* **270:** 1113–1122.
178. **Silva, T. M. J., P. M. Glee, and K. C. Hazen.** 1995. Influence of cell surface hydrophobicity on attachment of *Candida albicans* to extracellular matrix proteins. *J. Med. Vet. Mycol.* **33:** 117–122.
179. **Solomkin, J. S.** 1993. Pathogenesis and management of *Candida* infection syndromes in non-neutropenic patients. *New Horizons* **1:**202–213.
180. **Staab, J. F., S. D. Bradway, P. L. Fidel, and P. Sundstrom.** 1999. Adhesive and mammalian transglutaminase substrate properties of *Candida albicans* Hwp 1. *Science* **283:** 1535–1538.
181. **Steinshamn, S., K. Bergh, and A. Waage.** 1993. Effects of stem cell factor and granulocyte colony-stimulating factor on granulocyte recovery and *Candida albicans* infection in granulocytopenic mice. *J. Infect. Dis.* **168:**1444–1448.
182. **Tavares, D., P. Ferreira, and M. Arala-Chaves.** 2000. Increased resistance to systemic candidiasis in athymic or interleukin-10-depleted mice. *J. Infect. Dis.* **182:**266–273.
183. **Tavares, D., P. Ferreira, M. Vilanova, A. Videira, and M. Arala-Chaves.** 1995. Immunoprotection against systemic candidiasis in mice. *Int. Immunol.* **7:**785–796.
184. **Tavares, D., A. Salvador, P. Ferreira, and M. Arala-Chaves.** 1993. Immunological activities of a *Candida albicans* protein which plays an important role in the survival of the microorganism in the host. *Infect. Immun.* **61:**1881–1888.
185. **Tollemar, J., N. Gross, N. Dolgiras, C. Jarstrand, O. Ringden, and L. Hammarstrom.** 1999. Fungal prophylaxis by reduction of fungal colonization by oral administration of bovine anti-*Candida* antibodies in bone marrow transplant recipients. *Bone Marrow Transpl.* **23:**283–290.
186. **Torosantucci, A., C. Palma, M. Boccanera, C. M. Ausiello, G. C. Spagnoli, and A. Cassone.** 1990. Lymphoproliferative and cytotoxic responses of human peripheral blood mononuclear cells to mannoprotein constituents of *Candida albicans. J. Gen. Microbiol.* **136:**2155–2163.
187. **Tripp, D., and J. E. Cutler.** 1994. Evidence for complement independent in vivo adherence of *Candida albicans* yeast cells to mouse splenic marginal zone, abstr. F31, p. 48. *Proc. Gen. Meet. Am. Soc. Microbiol.* American Society for Microbiology, Washington, D.C.
188. **Van't Wout, J. W., H. Mattie, and R. van Furth.** 1989. Comparison of the efficacies of amphotericin B, fluconazole, and itraconazole against a systemic *Candida albicans* infection in normal and neutropenic mice. *Antimicrob. Agents Chemother.* **33:**147–151.
189. **Vazquez, J. A., and J. D. Sobel.** 1995. Fungal infections in diatetes. *Infect. Dis. Clin. N. Am.* **9:**97–116.
190. **Vazquez, N., H. R. Buckley, and T. J. Rogers.** 1996. Production of IL-6 and TNF-α by the macrophage-like cell line RAW 264.7 after treatment with a cell wall extract of *Candida albicans. J. Interferon Cytokine Res.* **16:**465–470.
191. **Vazquez-Torres, A., J. Jones-Carson, R. D. Wagner, T. Wagner, and E. Balish.** 1999. Early resistance of interleukin-10 knockout mice to acute systemic candidiasis. *Infect. Immun.* **67:**670–674.
192. **Verghese, S., A. Mullasari, P. Padmaja, P. Sudha, M. C. Sapna, and K. M. Cherian.** 1998. Fungal endocarditis following cardiac surgery. *Indian Heart J.* **50:**418–422.
193. **Vincent, J.-L., E. Anaissie, H. Bruining, W. Demajo, M. El-Ebiary, J. Haber, Y. Hiramatsu, G. Nitenberg, D. Pittet, T. Rogers, P. Sandven, G. Sganga, M.-D. Schaller, J. Solomkin, and P.-O. Nyström.** 1998. Epidemiology, diagnosis and treatment of systemic *Candida* infection in surgical patients under intensive care. *Intensive Care Med.* **24:**206–216.
194. **Voss, A., J. L. M. L. le Noble, F. M. Verduyn Lunel, N. A. Foudraine, and J. F. G. M. Meis.** 1997. Candidemia in intensive care unit patients: risk factors for mortality. *Infection* **25:**8–10.
195. **Walker, S. M., and S. J. Urbaniak.** 1980. A serum-dependent defect of neutrophil function in chronic mucocutaneous candidiasis. *J. Clin. Pathol.* **33:**370–372.
196. **Walsh, T. J., and J. W. Lee.** 1993. Prevention of invasive fungal infections in patients with neoplastic diseases. *Clin. Infect. Dis.* **17**(Suppl. 2):S468–S480.
197. **Warnock, D. W.** 1995. Fungal complications of transplantation: diagnosis, treatment and prevention. *J. Antimicrob. Chemother.* **36:**73–90.
198. **Warren, R. E.** 1993. Chemoprophylaxis for candidosis and aspergillosis in neutropenia and transplantation: a review and recommendations. *J. Antimicrob. Chemother.* **32:**5–21.
199. **Webb, B. C., C. J. Thomas, M. D. P. Willcox, D. W. S. Harty, and K. W. Knox.** 1998. Candida-associated denture stomatitis. Aetiology and management: a review. *Aust. Dental J.* **43:** 45–50.
200. **Wenzel, R. P.** 1995. Nosocomial candidemia: risk factors and attributable mortality. *Clin. Infect. Dis.* **20:**1531–1534.
201. **Woods, D. R., and E. A. Bevan.** 1968. Studies on the nature of the killer factor produced by *Saccharomyces cerevisiae. J. Gen. Microbiol.* **51:**115–126.

V. GENOMICS

Candida and Candidiasis
Edited by Richard A. Calderone

Chapter 18

Gene Discovery and Comparative Genomics: Progress and Prospects

STEWART SCHERER

Since molecular genetics techniques were first applied to *Candida albicans,* many routes have been employed for gene discovery. Complementation of *Saccharomyces cerevisiae* mutants was one of the earliest methods used (6). It was rapidly determined that a number of genes could be cloned in this fashion (22). The method was not limited to complementation of auxotrophs but also worked for diverse functions such as genes involved in control of the cell cycle (26). Of interest for the development of the DNA transformation system (see chapter 19) was the cloning of genes corresponding to the known *C. albicans* auxotrophs.

In some cases, especially with more highly conserved genes, hybridization-based methods relying on sequence homology were used. This approach was of particular importance because it was used to isolate a number of genes known to contain introns in other species. In the case of β-tubulin, the location and structure of the introns were conserved when compared with those of other fungi (27). The size and frequency of introns had important implications for the decisions to embark on large-scale DNA sequencing to find genes.

Both of the above methods rely on similarities of *Candida* genes to those in other species. Of great interest in the examination of *Candida* pathogenesis is the set of genes unique to *C. albicans* or only present in its closest relatives. Although it is possible to clone *Candida* genes through complementation of *Candida* mutants (8), this approach has not been widely employed. The intrinsic difficulties with the *Candida* genetic system, including the lack of a complete sexual cycle for laboratory manipulations and its diploid nature, have limited the number of available mutants. Additional complications are presented by the DNA transformation system.

In some cases, investigators have used the more versatile *Saccharomyces* system to isolate *Candida* genes on the basis of their ability to confer a new function in *S. cerevisiae.* Areas investigated in this way include drug resistance (5) and pheromone arrest of the cell cycle (30). In both cases, the novel genes encoded proteins with enough similarity to proteins known in other species to give indications about their function. The CUG codon, translated as serine rather than the standard leucine (see chapter 20), does not appear to have significantly affected efforts of this type because of its relatively infrequent use in *C. albicans,* particularly in more abundantly expressed genes.

Although DNA transformation of *C. albicans* has not been used extensively to isolate genes by complementation of mutants, the relatively effective methods for reverse genetics (see chapter 19) have, in many ways, driven the needs for more extensive collections of *C. albicans* genes involved in various processes in the cell. One route to expanding the set of cloned genes has been the use of differential screening methods. Examples of areas investigated in this manner include the yeast-to-hyphal transition (3), the white-opaque switching system (28), and the response to pH changes (24). One advantage of this approach is that it does not rely on conservation of sequence or function across species to identify genes, giving it the potential to identify genes of types not known in other species.

With increases in DNA sequencing capabilities, it became clear that genome sequencing would provide the most efficient route to discover all of the genes of *C. albicans.* After initial pilot studies using both genome shotgun and clone-based methods, a large-scale whole-genome shotgun sequencing project was initiated. The goal was not only to determine a complete haploid genome sequence as has been done with

Stewart Scherer • 3938 Paseo Grande, Moraga, CA 94556.

S. cerevisiae but to obtain sufficient sequence to explore allelic variation as well. Toward this end, mean coverage was taken to 10.4× (29), which is considerably higher than that used to sequence other species. Unfinished sequences from the project have been made available to the community to facilitate more directed efforts on specific areas of *Candida* biology (7, 25, 29). Although the genome sequence is not yet complete (in terms of closing gaps and aligning it with the physical map), the large collection of genes cloned from directed studies, combined with indications from the pilot projects, has provided considerable information about the genome and the initial tools for comparisons with other species.

GENERAL ASPECTS OF COMPARATIVE GENOMICS

Many of the principal questions in the basic biology and pathogenesis of *C. albicans* can be addressed by asking if it contains genes corresponding to those involved in similar processes in other species. However, there are some general caveats to be considered in such an analysis.

First, even with the complete *Candida* genome sequence being available, the absence of a particular gene does not mean that *C. albicans* does not perform such a function. An example is provided with the *URA1* gene. Searches with the corresponding *S. cerevisiae* gene would not reveal any gene in *C. albicans* with strong sequence similarity. While *Candida* appears to do de novo pyrimidine biosynthesis via the same intermediates as *Saccharomyces*, an entirely different enzyme is used for the dihydro-orotate dehydrogenase step. A soluble enzyme that reduces fumarate in the cytoplasm is found in *Saccharomyces* and several other organisms. In contrast, *Candida*, like *Escherichia coli*, *Schizosaccharomyces pombe*, and humans, produces a mitochondrial or membrane-bound enzyme that is coupled to the electron transport chain (Table 1).

Second, many proteins found within a species are in families with closely related members. When two such species are compared, it can be extremely difficult to determine, by sequence analysis alone, which gene corresponds to which gene in the other. In other cases, a single gene in one species may be related to a family in the other. One route toward generating candidates for the cognate pairs is to start with a gene in one species, find the closest match in the other, and use that second gene to search against the starting genome. Such analyses are further complicated in *C. albicans* because of the existence of significantly diverged alleles. If the best match returns to the gene that was used to start the process, it is more likely that the cognate pair has been found. Such efforts are most successful when complete genome sequences are available. An example of how refinements in such results are made is seen with *C. albicans* genes for DNA ligase (1).

Finally, rRNA sequences have been a very effective tool in establishing or confirming the relationship of species. With proteins such as cytochrome *c*, these relationships are generally reproduced (14). However, in a number of cases, the trees derived from the examination of a gene present in a single copy may not recapitulate the rRNA tree. An example is seen with the *C. albicans PHO85* gene being more closely related to a gene in *Aspergillus fumigatus* than *S. cerevisiae PHO85* (19). Selective pressure, horizontal transmission, or genetic drift (especially with smaller proteins) can account for these observations. It will be possible to detect more examples of this type as

Table 1. Dihyroorotate dehydrogenase (*URA1*) proteins[a]

C. albicans		*S. cerevisiae*	
Species	E value	Species	E value
S. pombe	10^{-103}	*L. lactis*	10^{-129}
Homo sapiens	10^{-84}	*S. pneumoniae*	10^{-112}
Drosophila melanogaster	10^{-69}	*T. cruzi*	10^{-92}
E. coli	10^{-52}	*E. coli*	10^{-24}
Lactococcus lactis	10^{-16}	*S. pombe*	10^{-12}
Trypanosoma cruzi	10^{-13}	*D. melanogaster*	10^{-10}
S. cerevisiae	10^{-7}	*H. sapiens*	10^{-10}
Streptococcus pneumoniae	10^{-6}	*C. albicans*	10^{-7}

[a]Similarity between *Candida* and *Saccharomyces URA1* proteins was measured using blastp to search all proteins (449 aa query for *C. albicans* and 314 aa query for *S. cerevisiae*). The match between *Candida* and *Saccharomyces* is of borderline significance in a search of such a large database.

the collection of sequences from even more species becomes available.

IDENTIFICATION OF *C. ALBICANS* GENES FROM SEQUENCE DATA

All evidence to date points to *Candida* genes typically being organized like those in *Saccharomyces* and usually lacking introns. This is in contrast to the situation in *Cryptococcus neoformans* in which coding regions are more widely interrupted. In addition, genes are relatively densely packed compared with mammalian genomes. These features make gene identification much more like the problem in bacteria where it is reduced to finding open reading frames of sufficient size to make their occurrence by chance alone unlikely. Typically, 100 amino acids are used as a cutoff in this type of analysis, but genomes do contain some smaller proteins. Even when genome sequencing projects are completed, the gene discovery process continues.

In genes where they occur, *C. albicans* introns are similar in their structure and conserved elements to those in *S. cerevisiae* (12, 19, 27). As a result, one would expect that gene-finding programs designed to assemble gene from exons, using a model developed using *S. cerevisiae* gene sets, would be relatively effective with *Candida* DNA in cases where the coding exons are of sufficient size.

No matter how sequences are first identified from genes of interest, conservation across species is generally the very first tool employed to obtain additional functional information. Most *C. albicans* genes show some degree of relatedness to ones found in *S. cerevisiae,* but the degree of conservation varies widely (10). Not surprisingly, structural proteins such as actin and tubulin are among the most conserved. Most enzymes in metabolism fall into a broad peak of 45 to 75% identity at the protein level. Some small proteins such as those encoded by *TRP1* and *DFR1* show reduced identity at the protein level, but this may merely reflect the statistical drift less likely to be seen with larger genes. Of greater interest are larger proteins that fall with limited sequence similarity, such as *TRL1* and *PDE1*. Here the greater divergence may indicate as yet undetermined functional differences.

Confounding almost all studies of newly identified *C. albicans* genes is the question of whether a second band seen on a Southern blot or a variant sequence obtained in clones derived from the same strain is simply allelic variation or whether one has discovered that the function is encoded by a second gene at a different chromosomal location. In some cases, the differences are readily explained by variation in simple sequence repeats in coding regions, such as runs of glutamines (16). Genes containing trinucleotide repeats are a rich source of polymorphisms for genetic and epidemiologic studies (see chapters 5 and 28). Although one can generally expect that the extent of single nucleotide changes between alleles will be very low, the existence of extreme examples, such as the mating-type and adjacent genes, limits the reliability of such an approach (12). Assignment of genes to the *Sfi*I fragments of the chromosomes or fosmids being used to build the physical map can help resolve some issues (see chapter 21). Closely linked gene family members can be detected by studies of individual fosmids and eventually will be identified as the complete genome sequence is assembled.

In a number of cases, allelic variation of single-copy genes has been studied in detail. Initially, nearby restriction site polymorphisms were valuable for the interpretation of gene disruption experiments, but those variations were assumed to be neutral from the perspective of function. Variation in genes in the ergosterol pathway has been of particular interest to explore mechanisms of resistance to azole antifungal agents. Whereas *Candida* loss of function mutants generally are expected to have arisen initially on one chromosome and subsequently become homozygous by mitotic recombination, the *ERG3* locus of the Darlington strain was found to have one allele with a nonsense mutation and the other with multiple missense mutations (20). Variation of about 1% between alleles of *PHR1* demonstrates the practical implications of low-level polymorphism for gene disruption studies. Strong bias for integration into the homolog containing the allele identical to that being used for DNA transformation has been observed (31).

One of the striking results with regard to gene discovery in *C. albicans* is that after a gene is identified as being involved in a process suspected to be important for pathogenesis, further investigation reveals it to be part of a large gene family (see also chapter 9). This has been reported to date for the secreted aspartyl proteinases, lipases, and the ALS genes. Such observations were initially made using Southern blots or while screening libraries to isolate additional (or larger) clones for the prototypical family member. Now the genome sequence data can be used to search for family members more quickly and with much greater sensitivity. Much effort has gone into determining the precise size of these gene families (9, 11, 21). Recent entries in the public sequence databases report 10 aspartyl proteinases, 10 lipases, and 9 ALS genes. Large gene families of this type are not a major feature of the *S. cerevisiae* genome.

Allelic variation, combined with relatively close

chromosomal locations for some family members, makes the task of counting gene family members difficult in the absence of the completed genome sequence combined with a high-resolution physical map. It is not yet clear how widely the gene family sizes obtained with one strain of *C. albicans* will translate to others. One significant effort that has been made was to determine if the aspartyl proteinase family extends to *C. tropicalis*. To date, four members of the family have been identified in that species (32). Such studies are likely to be of great assistance in determining the roles for each member of these gene families in *Candida* pathogenesis.

GENES SPECIFIC TO *C. ALBICANS*

The first *C. albicans* species-specific sequences were identified in the search for DNA probes for molecular epidemiology (see chapter 28). Species specificity and high-copy-number sequences were sought, and several families of sequences were identified. The development of the physical map demonstrated that these sequences were dispersed across the genome. The most widely used of these sequences, a part of the Ca3/27A family, although absent in *C. tropicalis*, is present to some degree in *C. dubliniensis*.

More recent studies have focused on the retroviral-related elements in the *C. albicans* genome. The genome sequence already available has enabled investigators to catalog these elements relatively thoroughly and establish their relationship to other families previously described (7). *C. albicans* has a much greater number of retrotransposon families than *S. cerevisiae*. Only 3 of these 34 families appear to have a functional copy in the genome. Some defective elements may remain mobile through the protein products of others acting in *trans*. Subtelomeric regions are a particularly rich source of retrotransposon sequences.

Although most *C. albicans* low-copy-number genes identified to date are related to genes in other species, a significant number lack clear counterparts in other species. Whereas this number depends in large degree on the precise level of similarity judged to be relevant in searches of the sequence databases, the few cosmids sequenced in their entirety (25) suggested this will be considerable. Such results have been observed with all microbial genome sequencing projects where essentially every organism has a significant fraction of species-specific genes.

Beyond this set of *C. albicans*-specific genes, one finds many genes with quite limited similarity to proteins known in other species, but some reasonable guess as to function can be made, often relying on the presence of sequence motifs rather than overall similarity. Thus, many genes identified only as zinc-finger transcription factors or dehydrogenases by this approach may prove to have specialized functions for *Candida* not known in other organisms.

GENOME EVOLUTION

Molecular approaches have largely confirmed the relationships among the *Candida* spp. established by other methods (see chapter 28). Whereas *C. stellatoidea* and *C. clausenii* are distinguished from *C. albicans* by clear phenotypic differences, molecular data suggest that they are within the range of sequence variation observed among *C. albicans* strains (18). *C. dubliniensis*, however, is clearly more distant than the other *Candida* spp. mentioned above. Although only a few genes have been cloned and sequenced from *C. dubliniensis*, there are generally more substitutions at the DNA and protein levels than one would expect for *C. albicans* allele or strain variants. The sequence of the actin gene reveals considerable divergence in its intron (84% identity) in contrast to the 98% identity of nucleotides in the exons (4). The *URA3* coding sequences are 93% identical at the nucleotide level (97% at the protein level) (see Table 2).

In the taxonomic branch of the yeasts that contains the species with CUG encoding serine, *C. tropicalis* and *C. maltosa* are roughly equidistant from *C. albicans*, with *C. parapsilosis* more distant. Relatively few genes have been sequenced from the other species. Currently the only protein sequence available from all is from *URA3*. A comparison of these sequences is shown in Table 2. Sequences for other genes in which the set is not yet complete support these relationships.

In contrast, some *Candida* spp., such as *C. glabrata*, have been found to be well within the *Saccharomyces* branch of the phylogenetic tree (2) using the

Table 2. Comparison of *URA3* protein sequences[a]

Species	E value
C. albicans	1.0×10^{-142}
C. dubliniensis	9.3×10^{-140}
C. maltosa	4.2×10^{-121}
C. tropicalis	8.7×10^{-121}
C. parapsilosis	3.0×10^{-111}
S. cerevisiae	3.8×10^{-104}

[a]Comparison of the *C. albicans URA3* protein to those in other species. The E values were obtained in a blastp search against all known proteins. The self-comparison provides a reference point as the scores depend on the length and composition of the query protein.

conventional nuclear code for genes. This higher degree of relatedness to *S. cerevisiae* facilitates many efforts with *C. glabrata* but limits the ability to use results obtained with it for interpretation of the *C. albicans* genome.

Although most early DNA sequences obtained from *C. albicans* focused on individual genes, a number did extend far enough to indicate that the neighboring genes in *Candida* were generally not the same neighbors found in *S. cerevisiae.* From this work and pilot efforts from the sequencing project, some cases were identified in which gene order, but not necessarily orientation, was conserved. One of the first examples of this type involved *LYS2* and *RAD16*.

By using sequence data from several complete cosmids and preliminary data from the genome project, it was possible to extend these analyses to show that small regions of the *Candida* genome often contain several genes from the same neighborhood of a *Saccharomyces* chromosome, with precise order and orientation not being conserved (25). To explain these observations, it has been estimated that approximately 1,100 small inversions occurred in the chromosomes as the two species followed their separate histories. As more extensive sequence data become available for other yeasts, it should be possible to discern when some of these events are likely to have occurred. It is important to note that such studies are complicated by *C. albicans* having half the chromosome number of *S. cerevisiae,* with a genome duplication believed to have occurred in the evolution of *Saccharomyces* after the species diverged. Extensive chromosomal additions and deletions must have subsequently occurred as most *S. cerevisiae* genes are not obviously duplicated and with *C. albicans* having a slightly larger haploid genome (see also chapter 21). Part of the increase in the genome size for *C. albicans* may be explained by the additional transposon families mentioned above.

Some adjacent gene pairs such as *GAL1* and *GAL10* share a regulatory region in *Saccharomyces,* making conservation of order and orientation more likely. As is the case with *Saccharomyces,* it is relatively rare in *Candida* for genes of related function to be clustered together. One other notable example is the genes for *N*-acetylglucosamine utilization where one sees a hexokinase adjacent to the coding regions for two enzymes in that pathway (15).

CONSERVATION OF GENE FUNCTION AND *C. ALBICANS* BIOLOGY

A number of questions about the basic biology of *C. albicans* have already been addressed through gene discovery and comparative genomics. The most important of these have been the efforts to determine the nature of the *C. albicans* sexual cycle (see chapter 2). The first work in this regard was the observation that a G protein α subunit gene from *C. albicans* would complement the mating defect as well as the lethality of corresponding *S. cerevisiae* mutants. Complementation of the mating defect suggested that it would interact with the *S. cerevisiae* pheromone receptors. Surprisingly, the gene also was regulated in *Saccharomyces* by mating type as is the corresponding *S. cerevisiae* gene (23). Many *Candida* genes corresponding to important components of the *Saccharomyces* mating system have subsequently been cloned or identified in the genome sequence (29). Although there is as yet no experimental evidence for pheromones in *C. albicans* mating, homologs of the *Saccharomyces* pheromone receptor, components of the downstream MAK kinase signaling pathway, and several pheromone processing enzymes were found in the *Candida* genome.

The genome sequence provided a route to the identification of the mating loci themselves (12). Although the structure of the mating-type loci is different from that seen in *Saccharomyces,* the overall function appears to be similar. The same regulatory proteins are present and strains heterozygous for the mating alleles do not mate. The negative regulators **a**1 and α2 are more readily identified from the complete sequence; the counterpart of the *Saccharomyces* positive regulator α1 would not be so convincingly established solely by searching the entire *Candida* genome sequence data. In addition, there are genes at the mating-type loci not obviously related to the mating process as understood from work with *Saccharomyces.* These include a polyA-polymerase, a PI-kinase, and an oxysterol binding protein (12).

In the case of the *Candida* mating-type locus, one also observes more variation between the two alleles than is seen in *S. cerevisiae.* The local chromosomal rearrangements in the mating-type locus alleles are not fundamentally different from the large number of small inversions described above in the more global genome comparison with *Saccharomyces.* It is not known if similar rearrangements leading to different structures on generally homologous chromosomes are found in other locations in the genome.

On the basis of expected behavior of allele combinations from work in *Saccharomyces,* construction of mutations of the mating-type loci or creation of strains homozygous for that chromosome led to the demonstration of mating in *C. albicans* (13, 17). Although many other genes have been found in *Candida,* indicating that mating portions of the sexual cycle are likely similar between *Candida* and *Sacchar-*

omyces, some genes important for meiosis in *Saccharomyces* have not yet been found (29). This class includes a key regulator of meiosis, *IME1,* and several genes involved in initiation of recombination and formation of synaptonemal complexes. It remains to be determined if genes unrelated at the sequence level are present to do similar functions, akin to the situation described above for the *URA1* gene. The *Candida* genome also contains genes implicated in the sexual cycles of other species but absent in *Saccharomyces,* but their role in *Candida* is not known.

CONCLUSIONS

The complete genome sequence of *Candida* will provide the starting material for a large number of new methods of investigation with this species. The sequence can be used to design microarrays for expression studies and the constructs needed for systematic gene disruption efforts. Further efforts to use sequence comparison to study *Candida* biology or pathogenesis will soon become limited not by our knowledge of *C. albicans* but instead by the available information on other species.

To date, genome projects have emphasized the study of diverse species ranging from bacteria to humans. Even as the other principal fungal pathogens are sequenced, there will be limits to their utility in understanding *C. albicans. C. glabrata* is evolutionarily as distant from *C. albicans* as *S. cerevisiae* is from *C. albicans.* Genera such as the aspergilli and cryptococci are far more distant.

Unless a surprising degree of convergent evolution is detected, the most powerful sequence-based approach to understanding *C. albicans* will come from comparisons with its closest relatives or other strains within the species with distinct phenotypic characteristics. In this way, one can attempt to correlate the presence of specific genes with particular aspects of pathogenesis. Although one can use DNA hybridization to ask if related species contain similar genes, the overall divergence of the genome sequences and the presence of gene families limit this approach. Whereas sequencing another closely related species is a significant undertaking, the numbers of differences with *C. albicans* will be much smaller, making it much easier to understand which genes may be responsible for the success of *C. albicans* as a pathogen. Computational approaches are far more sensitive than hybridization methods for more diverged sequences and also can be more effective with gene families.

When one examines other strains within the species, such an effort effectively becomes a "resequencing" project that can be accomplished with much greater economy. Although the strain being used for the genome sequencing, Sc5314, has been widely used in laboratory studies (frequently through mutants derived from it such as CAI-4 [see chapter 19]) and has a typical karyotype, it may be missing some genes frequently found in other isolates. When phenotypic characteristics are used for species identification, some are known to be variable within *C. albicans.* The genes controlling these characteristics, as well as significant allelic variation at other loci, will likely be determined through sequencing from other *C. albicans* isolates. One can expect that a combination of expression studies, disruption experiments, and additional sequence comparisons will soon give us a much deeper understanding of the function of the genes of *C. albicans.*

Acknowledgment. The complete *C. albicans URA1* sequence was kindly provided by Ted Jones, Stanford Genome Technology Center. See www-sequence.stanford.edu/group/candida.

REFERENCES

1. **Andaluz, E., A. Ciudad, J. Rubio Coque, R. Calderone, and G. Larriba.** 1999. Cell cycle regulation of a DNA ligase-encoding gene (CaLIG4) from *Candida albicans. Yeast* **15:** 1199–1210.
2. **Barns, S. M., D. J. Lane, M. L. Sogin, C. Bibeau, and W. G. Weisburg.** 1991. Evolutionary relationships among pathogenic *Candida* species and relatives. *J. Bacteriol.* **173:**2250–2255.
3. **Braun, B. R., W. S. Head, M. X. Wang, and A. D. Johnson.** 2000. Identification and characterization of TUP1-regulated genes in *Candida albicans. Genetics* **156:**31–44.
4. **Donnelly, S. M., D. J. Sullivan, D. B. Shanley, and D. C. Coleman.** 1999. Phylogenetic analysis and rapid identification of *Candida dubliniensis* based on analysis of *ACT1* intron and exon sequences. *Microbiology* **145:**1871–1882.
5. **Fling, M. E., J. Kopf, A. Tamarkin, J. A. Gorman, H. A. Smith, and Y. Koltin.** 1991. Analysis of a *Candida albicans* gene that encodes a novel mechanism for resistance to benomyl and methotrexate. *Mol. Gen. Genet.* **227:**318–329.
6. **Gillum, A. M., E. Y. Tsay, and D. R. Kirsch.** 1984. Isolation of the *Candida albicans* gene for orotidine-5′-phosphate decarboxylase by complementation of *S. cerevisiae ura3* and *E. coli pyrF* mutations. *Mol. Gen. Genet.* **198:**179–182.
7. **Goodwin, T. J., and R. T. Poulter.** 2000. Multiple LTR-retrotransposon families in the asexual yeast *Candida albicans. Genome Res.* **10:**174–191.
8. **Goshorn, A. K., S. M. Grindle, and S. Scherer.** 1992. Gene isolation by complementation in *Candida albicans* and applications to physical and genetic mapping. *Infect. Immun.* **60:** 876–884.
9. **Hoyer, L. L., and J. E. Hecht.** 2000. The *ALS6* and *ALS7* genes of *Candida albicans. Yeast* **16:**847–855.
10. **Hoyer, L. L., B. B. Magee, E. H. Rikkerink, and S. Scherer.** 1994. The *ARG4* gene of *Candida albicans. Gene* **142:** 213–218.
11. **Hube, B., F. Stehr, M. Bossenz, A. Mazur, M. Kretschmar, and W. Schafer.** 2000. Secreted lipases of *Candida albicans:* cloning, characterisation and expression analysis of a new gene family with at least ten members. *Arch. Microbiol.* **174:** 362–374.

12. **Hull, C. M., and A. D. Johnson.** 1999. Identification of a mating type-like locus in the asexual pathogenic yeast *Candida albicans. Science* **285:**1271–1275.
13. **Hull, C. M., R. M. Raisner, and A. D. Johnson.** 2000. Evidence for mating of the "asexual" yeast *Candida albicans* in a mammalian host. *Science* **289:**307–310.
14. **Janbon, G., E. P. Rustchenko, S. Klug, S. Scherer, and F. Sherman.** 1997. Phylogenetic relationships of fungal cytochromes c. *Yeast* **13:**985–990.
15. **Kumar, M. J., M. S. Jamaluddin, K. Natarajan, D. Kaur, and A. Datta.** 2000. The inducible *N*-acetylglucosamine catabolic pathway gene cluster in *Candida albicans:* Discrete *N*-acetylglucosamine-inducible factors interact at the promoter of *NAG1. Proc. Natl. Acad. Sci. USA* **97:**14218–14223.
16. **Lunel, F. V., L. Licciardello, S. Stefani, H. A. Verbrugh, W. J. Melchers, J. F. Meis, S. Scherer, and A. van Belkum.** 1998. Lack of consistent short sequence repeat polymorphisms in genetically homologous colonizing and invasive *Candida albicans* strains. *J. Bacteriol.* **180:**3771–3778.
17. **Magee, B. B., and P. T. Magee.** 2000. Induction of mating in *Candida albicans* by construction of MTLa and MTLα strains. *Science* **289:**310–313.
18. **Mahrous, M., A. D. Sawant, W. R. Pruitt, T. Lott, S. A. Meyer, and D. G. Ahearn.** 1992. DNA relatedness, karyotyping and gene probing of *Candida tropicalis, Candida albicans* and its synonyms *Candida stellatoidea* and *Candida claussenii. Eur. J. Epidemiol.* **8:**444–451.
19. **Miyakawa, Y.** 2000. Identification of a *Candida albicans* homologue of the *PHO85* gene, a negative regulator of the PHO system in *Saccharomyces cerevisiae. Yeast* **16:**1045–1051.
20. **Miyazaki, Y., A. Geber, H. Miyazaki, D. Falconer, T. Parkinson, C. Hitchcock, B. Grimberg, B. Nyswaner, and J. E. Bennett.** 2000. Cloning, sequencing, expression and allelic sequence diversity of *ERG3* (C-5 sterol desaturase gene) in *Candida albicans. Gene* **236:**43–51.
21. **Monod, M., B. Hube, D. Hess, and D. Sanglard.** 1998. Differential regulation of *SAP8* and *SAP9,* which encode two new members of the secreted aspartic proteinase family in *Candida albicans. Microbiology* **144:**2731–2737.
22. **Rosenbluh, A., M. Mevarech, Y. Koltin, and J. A. Gorman.** 1985. Isolation of genes from *Candida albicans* by complementation in *Saccharomyces cerevisiae. Mol. Gen. Genet.* **200:**500–502.
23. **Sadhu, C., D. Hoekstra, M. J. McEachern, S. I. Reed, and J. B. Hicks.** 1992. A G-protein α subunit from asexual *Candida albicans* functions in the mating signal transduction pathway of *Saccharomyces cerevisiae* and is regulated by the a1-α2 repressor. *Mol. Cell. Biol.* **12:**1977–1985.
24. **Saporito-Irwin, S. M., C. E. Birse, P. S. Sypherd, and W. A. Fonzi.** 1995. *PHR1,* a pH-regulated gene of *Candida albicans,* is required for morphogenesis. *Mol. Cell. Biol.* **15:**601–613.
25. **Seoighe, C., N. Federspiel, T. Jones, N. Hansen, V. Bivolarovic, R. Surzycki, R. Tamse, C. Komp, L. Huizar, R. W. Davis, S. Scherer, E. Tait, D. J. Shaw, D. Harris, L. Murphy, K. Oliver, K. Taylor, M. A. Rajandream, B. G. Barrell, and K. H. Wolfe.** 2000. Prevalence of small inversions in yeast gene order evolution. *Proc. Natl. Acad. Sci. USA* **97:**14433–14437.
26. **Sherlock, G., A. M. Bahman, A. Mahal, J. C. Shieh, M. Ferreira, and J. Rosamond.** 1994. Molecular cloning and analysis of *CDC28* and cyclin homologues from the human fungal pathogen *Candida albicans. Mol. Gen. Genet.* **245:**716–723.
27. **Smith, H. A., H. S. Allaudeen, M. H. Whitman, Y. Koltin, and J. A. Gorman.** 1988. Isolation and characterization of a β-tubulin gene from *Candida albicans. Gene* **63:**53–63.
28. **Srikantha, T., and D. R. Soll.** 1993. A white-specific gene in the white-opaque switching system of *Candida albicans. Gene* **131:**53–60.
29. **Tzung, K.-W., R. M. Williams, S. Scherer, N. Federspiel, T. Jones, N. Hansen, V. Bivolarevic, L. Huizar, C. Komp, R. Surzycki, R. Tamse, R. W. Davis, and N. Agabian.** Genomic evidence for a complete sexual cycle in *Candida albicans. Proc. Natl. Acad. Sci. USA,* in press.
30. **Whiteway, M., D. Dignard, D. Y. Thomas.** 1992. Dominant negative selection of heterologous genes: isolation of *Candida albicans* genes that interfere with *Saccharomyces cerevisiae* mating factor-induced cell cycle arrest. *Proc. Natl. Acad. Sci. USA* **89:**9410–9414.
31. **Yesland, K., and W. A. Fonzi.** 2000. Allele-specific gene targeting in *Candida albicans* results from heterology between alleles. *Microbiology* **146:**2097–2104.
32. **Zaugg, C., M. Borg-Von Zepelin, U. Reichard, D. Sanglard, and M. Monod.** 2001. Secreted aspartic proteinase family of *Candida tropicalis. Infect. Immun.* **69:**405–412.

Candida and Candidiasis
Edited by Richard A. Calderone
© 2002 ASM Press, Washington, D.C.

Chapter 19

Gene Expression and Genetic Techniques

JOACHIM F. ERNST AND DIRK P. BOCKMÜHL

CLASSICAL GENETICS

Candida albicans

Because *C. albicans* is diploid, it has been difficult to isolate homozygous mutants carrying recessive mutations. Depending on the strain background, mild mutagenesis generated only specific auxotrophs, which very likely was due to heterozygosity of the gene locus involved (39, 94). A combination of mild mutagenesis by a chemical mutagen and UV expanded the range of mutations that could be obtained, presumably because a transient heterozygous state was resolved by UV-induced mitotic recombination (39). Auxotrophs could be enriched using inositol starvation and treatments by amphotericin B or folate pathway inhibitors (14, 32, 67); morphological mutants were enriched by filtration (5). The mutants thus obtained were expected to contain multiple unwanted and independent genomic alterations and thus could not be considered as genetically defined mutants.

As was expected from the difficulty of isolating specific mutants, *C. albicans* spontaneously produces high frequencies of a wide range of chromosomal aberrations (74). Such rearrangements occur especially at lowered temperatures (<25°C), and it has been suggested that they are the means to generate genetic variability in an organism that lacks a sexual cycle. Chromosomal rearrangements were shown to be associated with changes in cellular and colony morphology, as well as fluconazole resistance (63, 74). Monosomy of a specific chromosome (chromosome 5) allowed *C. albicans* to grow on L-sorbose, presumably because of reduced expression of a gene encoding a negative factor regulating expression of the *SOU1* gene, which is required for sorbose utilization (38). Monosomy of chromosome 4 also contributed to the development of fluconazole resistance (63). Experimentally, chromosome loss can be easily induced by temperature shock or by treatment with the microtubule inhibitor benzimidazole (2, 34).

Spheroplasts of *C. albicans* can be fused in the presence of polyethylene glycol and "fusants" can be regenerated on selective media (68). Fusion of two auxotrophic strains produced heterozygous prototrophic fusants with a cell volume twice that of the original strains (68). Heat shock treatment and mitotic recombination led to random chromosome loss in the fusants, and linkage groups could be defined by mutations, which cosegregated in the derivative strains (34, 39). Spheroplast fusion initially produces heterokaryons, which may undergo nuclear fusion to become tetraploids and may reduce their chromosome number, or they can transfer individual chromosomes from one nucleus to another (78). The formation of tetraploids by spheroplast fusion followed by chromosome loss can generate a complete parasexual cycle. Spheroplast fusion is applicable for linkage analysis of mutated alleles in *C. albicans* (22); even fusants of *C. tropicalis* and *C. albicans* spheroplasts can be obtained (14).

It has been described that *C. albicans* contains a locus on chromosome 5 with homology to the mating type locus of *Saccharomyces cerevisiae (MTL),* which encodes components similar to the Mata1, Matα1, and Matα2 transcriptional regulators and which is heterozygous in many *C. albicans* strains (36). Such a strain was rendered homozygous by gene disruption or by selecting growth on sorbose, in which one or the other chromosome 5-homolog was lost (37, 55). Homozygous *MAT***a**-like strains were shown to mate specifically to *MAT*α-like strains and to produce tetraploids, which appeared to lose chromosomes with time. Thus, this discovery opens a new route for genetic analysis and manipulation of *C. albicans,* in addition to parasexual genetics. The importance of mating in *C. albicans* population genetics is unclear,

Joachim F. Ernst and Dirk P. Bockmühl • Institut für Mikrobiologie, Heinrich-Heine-Universität, Universitätsstr. 1/26.12, D-40225 Düsseldorf, Germany.

because natural populations reproduce mainly clonally, although a minor contribution of recombination has been observed (27).

Other *Candida* Species

Like *C. albicans, C. tropicalis* is diploid and lacks a sexual cycle. Auxotrophic mutants of *C. tropicalis* have been isolated following heavy mutagenesis (14, 28); mutants can be enriched by nystatin treatment or inositol starvation (28, 64). *C. glabrata* is asexual but haploid, which facilitates the generation and detection of mutants (13).

TRANSFORMATION

Reliable transformation systems have been developed for *Candida* species, consisting of marked host strains and matching transformation vectors. Existing methods generate transformed strains containing plasmids either in an integrated or in an episomal state.

Host Strains and Selection Markers

Auxotrophic strains have been used as hosts for transformation experiments in *C. albicans*. Mutations complemented by the respective wild-type genes on transformation vectors or fragments include *ura3, ade2, leu2, his1, arg4,* and *arg5,6* mutations (Table 1). The current strains in use are mainly derivatives of strain SC5314, e.g., strain CAI4 (21), or, for the analysis of white-opaque phenotypic switching, derivatives of strain WO-1 (80); because these strains were constructed by gene disruption, they are genetically defined and the mutations are not revertible. The level of complementation of these mutations, e.g., by wild-type genes on transformation vectors, may be important for virulence studies, because the expression status of any of these genes may have an effect on virulence (48). Auxotrophic mutations significantly lower virulence characteristics of *C. albicans* (10, 42). A heterologous dominant resistance marker suitable for routine transformation of *C. albicans* wild-type strains has not yet been developed. However, a method has been described, which relies on overexpression of the *C. albicans IMH3* gene conferring resistance to mycophenolic acid (45); recently, a variant *IMH3* gene able to confer mycophenolic acid-resistance by single-copy integration was used for gene disruption in a clinical isolate (3).

Auxotrophic host strains, which can be transformed, have also been established in *C. glabrata* and *C. tropicalis* (Table 1); a method based on resistance to mycophenolic acid has been described for *C. dubliniensis* (89). Recently it has been reported that a mutated *hph* gene encoding hygromycin B phosphotransferase, in which nine CTG codons were exchanged according to the unusual codon usage of *C. tropicalis,* was functional as a dominant resistance marker in *C. tropicalis,* and it could be used to directly select

Table 1. *Candida* host strains

Species	Name	Auxotrophic marker(s)	Reference
C. albicans	SGY 243	*ura3*	41
	CAI4	*ura3*	21
	hOG300	*ade2*	69
	SGY129	*ade2*	41
	CNC44	*arg5,6*	61
	SGY 484	*ura3, leu2*	41
	CAI8	*ura3, ade2*	21
	RM1000	*ura3, his1*	61
	CNC43	*ura3, his1, arg5,6*	61
	BWP17	*ura3, his1, arg4*	96
C. glabrata	Q	*ura3*	99
	BG14	*ura3*	12
	BG87b, 88b	*ura3, his3*	12
	BG98, 99	*his3*	12
	CGA2-21-2	*ura3, ade2*	30
	2001TU	*ura3, trp1*	44
	2001HT	*trp1, his3*	44
	2001HTU	*ura3, trp1, his3*	44
C. tropicalis	SU2	*ura3*	28
	Ha900	*ade2*	76

transformants on media containing hygromycin B (31).

Transformation Vectors

Homologous recombination occurs frequently between a plasmid-resident *C. albicans* gene or a gene fragment with its chromosomal counterpart. Although circular plasmids integrate spontaneously at the site of homology, integration frequency is improved drastically by cutting the plasmid within the region of homology, which generates recombinogenic ends. Integration frequencies are highest into highly expressed genes (85), which may explain the different rates of integration into genes. Specific integration vectors allowing a high-frequency transformation into neutral chromosomal sites have been described (91). Chromosomal integration ensures that the plasmid is inserted as a single copy and is stably inherited, thus preventing changes in copy number. On the other hand, expression levels of some genes to be tested, e.g., reporter gene fusions present on integrated plasmids, may be too low to allow their convenient detection.

Episomal plasmids do not require a homologous recombination event for transformation and, therefore, they are transformed into host strains at high frequencies (Table 2). While autonomously replicating sequences (*ARS*) derived from *S. cerevisiae* are functional in *C. glabrata* (30), they are inactive in *C. albicans*. Three *ARS*-elements from *C. albicans* have been described. *CARS1* (46), which is also functional in *C. tropicalis* (76), frequently forms multimers in transformants. Transformation with a *CARS1*-containing plasmid led to two types of transformants identifiable by their colony sizes (41, 46). Most transformant colonies were small and typically contained free oligomeric plasmids consisting of tandemly arranged plasmid repeats (average copy number of 5 to 10), which were mitotically unstable; few large transformant colonies contained tandem plasmid repeats integrated into the genome. Vectors containing *CARS2*, which is situated next to sequences encoding 5S RNA, were described by Cannon and coworkers (6). While the majority of transformants containing the *ARS2*-carrying plasmid pRC2312 carried two to three free plasmids in a monomeric form, few large transformant colonies also contained tandemly arranged plasmids integrated into the genome. A third replicator of *C. albicans, CARS3,* which is derived from an unknown genomic location presumably after a rearrangement, is also functional in *S. cerevisiae* and *C. albicans; C. albicans* transformants with *CARS3*-containing vectors contain episomal and integrated plasmid copies (33). Plasmids containing both *CARS2* and *CARS3* show increased copy numbers and stabilities (66). Although a *C. glabrata* centromere was already described in 1996 (43), until today no centromere-containing plasmids have been described for *C. albicans,* which would allow their stable inheritance in transformants at a copy number of about one to two plasmids per cell.

Table 2. *C. albicans* cloning vectors

Name	Marker gene(s)	*CARS*	Reference
pMK22	*URA3*	1	46
pCARS1	*URA3*	1	41
pRM10	*URA3*	2, 3	66
pMK16	*ADE2*	1	46
pBT4	*ADE2*	2	82
pEM7	*TCM1*	3	33
pRC2312	*URA3, LEU2*	2	6
pRM1	*URA3, LEU2*	2, 3	66

Transformation Methods

Transformation methods for *Candida* species are similar to methods used in *S. cerevisiae,* including the use of spheroplasts (35), a salt (lithium acetate) method, and electroporation. In the classical method spheroplasts prepared by treatment of whole cells with zymolyase or glusulase are incubated and coprecipitated with the transforming DNA, followed by wall regeneration on osmotically stabilized medium. This method may fail, e.g., for disruptions of genes affecting wall regeneration. On the other hand, spheroplasts can be stored for several weeks, which makes this transformation system versatile. The use of electroporation for transformation purposes has been described for many *Candida* species including *C. tropicalis* (73) and *C. albicans* (4). Although transformation frequencies were low initially, they were recently improved (16). Following electroporation there is no need for cell wall regeneration and cells can be plated on regular media, which are not osmotically stabilized. This is also true for the lithium acetate transformation method, which has been described for *Candida* species (30, 77). Although simple and fast, the transformation efficiencies are low with this method.

GENE DISRUPTION

The possibility of generating specific genomic deletions has been crucial for the analysis of *Candida* species. Gene disruptions have generated auxotrophic mutants, which can be complemented by transformation plasmids, and have provided essential information on the function of genes. Methods to obtain deletions all rely on integrative transformation via homologous recombination, which occurs frequently in *Candida* species. The construction of null mutants for a given gene is relatively easy in haploid fungi such as *S. cerevisiae* or *C. glabrata,* whereas in diploid species including *C. albicans* and *C. tropicalis* both gene copies have to be mutated in succession.

C. albicans

Specific genomic deletions are constructed in *C. albicans* by the use of a disruption fragment, in which a marker sequence replaces the deleted sequences and whose flanking regions allow genomic integration by homologous recombination. In initial approaches the marker sequence on the disruption fragment could not be selected and rare disrupted strains had to be uncovered by PCR screening (21); alternatively, co-transformation of the disruption with a replicative, selectable plasmid (which subsequently was evicted) was used to enrich for cells, in which the disruption had taken place (41). Since *C. albicans* is diploid, mutant alleles thus introduced were rendered homozygous to generate a complete null mutant for the respective gene and to uncover recessive phenotypes. Homozygosity was induced by a mild UV treatment, which stimulates mitotic recombination and specifically induces recombination between the disrupted gene and the centromere, which by segregation form homozygous mutants (41, 75). In the method described by Sadhu et al. (75), which is based on the *ADE2* gene as the selectable marker, homozygous disrupted cells could be detected in red/white-sectoring colonies, because red sectors are indicative of homozygous *ade2* mutants arising during reciprocal recombination. A method to directly select for mitotic recombination leading to homozygosity was described recently, in which the selectable marker is composite, allowing either *ARG4* or *URA3* expression following homologous recombination between flanking repeats (18). Selection for both markers is indicative of homozygously disrupted cells. Although mitotic recombination is a convenient method to generate homozygosity, it suffers the major drawback that distal to the induced recombination event an undefined number of gene loci are rendered homozygous; thus, heterozygote parent and homozygote progeny cells cannot be considered as isogenic strains.

Another approach leading to homozygosity of a disrupted allele involved the use of a selectable marker flanked by direct repeats, whose presence and absence could be selected. In a first approach the *GAL1* gene flanked by bacterial *cat* sequences was used as the marker gene, whose presence could be selected in a *gal1* host background by growth on galactose and whose absence was selectable on media containing 2-deoxy-D-galactose (25). Modification and extension of this work led to the "*URA*-blaster" method, which at present is the most frequently used method to disrupt genes in *C. albicans* (21). In this method the *URA3* marker, which is selectable in a *ura3* genetic background by growth in the absence of uridine, is flanked by direct repeats of bacterial *hisG* sequences (Fig. 1A). Following positive selection for the presence of the disruption cassette in the first allele, the heterozygous disruptant cells are plated on media containing 5′-fluoroorotic acid (FOA), which only allows growth of Ura-negative cells lacking *URA3* sequences, because FOA is converted by the *URA3* gene product into a toxic agent. Ura-negative cells arise spontaneously, most likely because of homologous recombination between the *hisG* repeats. These cells can be used for a second round of transformation and of FOA selection to delete the second allele and to remove *URA3* sequences; the resulting null mutant is then commonly transformed with an empty plasmid or a plasmid containing the deleted gene to construct a pair of prototrophic strains only differing in the presence of the gene to be tested. Although this method has been used successfully many times for gene disruptions, there are several important drawbacks. First, repeated use of the Ura-blaster cassette leaves *hisG* sequences in the disrupted strains, thus providing a site of homology at which unwanted integration events can occur. This is especially important in the case of gene families, but it was also reported as a problem during the deletion of the second allele of the *RAS1* gene (20). A solution may be the use of a different disruption cassette for disruption of the second allele, e.g., a *URA3* gene flanked by *hph* sequences (20), by *cat* sequences (70), or by repeated *URA3* sequences (95). A second problem may arise once a null mutant containing one *hisG*- and one Ura-blaster-disrupted allele has been constructed, because FOA selection may generate a Ura-negative strain not only by recombination between *hisG* sequences in the second disrupted allele, but also by mitotic recombination between the centromere and the gene locus, which leads to homozygosity of all distal loci. This problem has not yet been reported as a major problem in practice, but any such cases of unwanted mitotic recombination could be at least identified, if disruptions of both alleles are carried out by different disruption cassettes, e.g., containing different flanking repeats. A third problem may arise if the sequences flanking the desired deletion are different in both chromosomal alleles. In such a case, the use of a single disruption cassette will greatly favor integration of the Ura-blaster only to the one allele, whose sequences

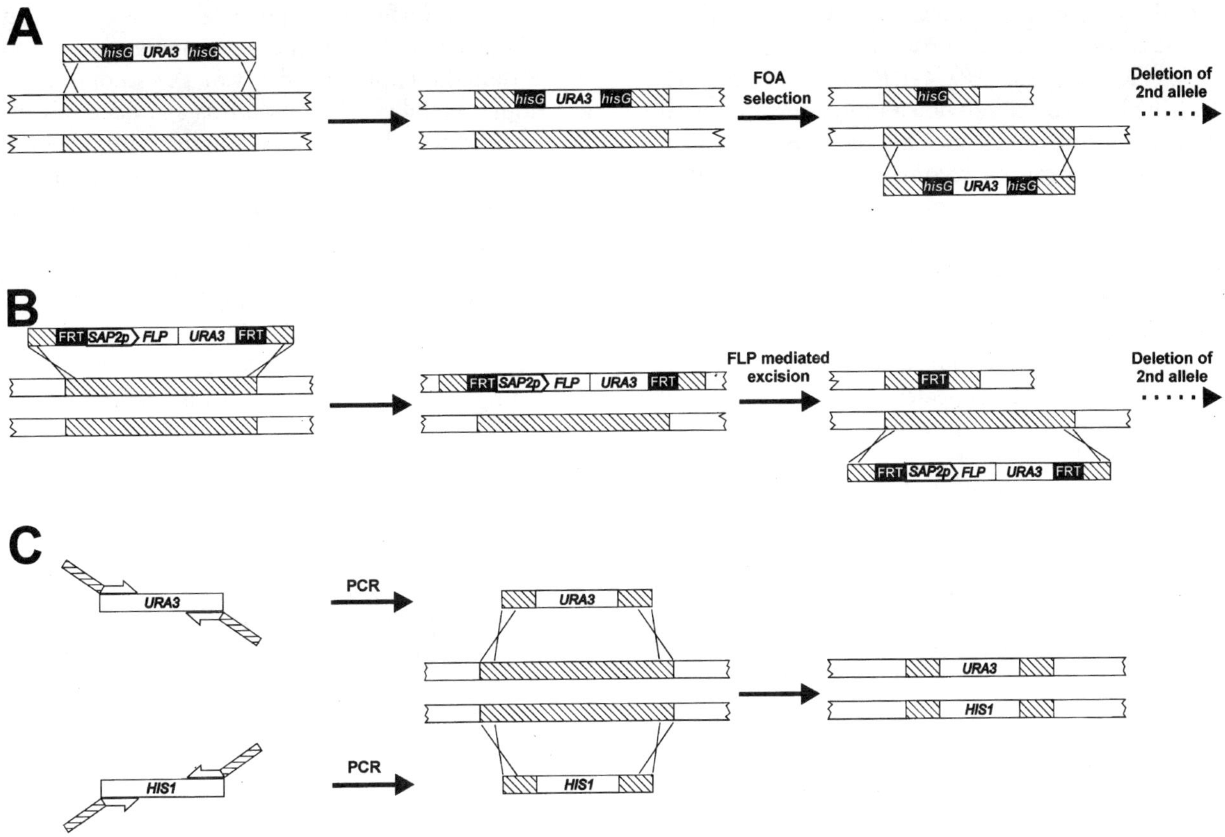

Figure 1. Methods for gene disruptions in *C. albicans*. The procedures for (A) the Ura-blaster method (20), (B) the Ura-flipper method (57), and (C) the PCR approach (93) are shown. The target gene to be disrupted is shown as hatched box. Primers used to generate the disruption fragments in (C) by PCR are shown as open arrows (not drawn to scale).

are present on the disruption fragment (79, 98). Spontaneous loss of the *URA3* marker is a rare event, occurring at a frequency of 10^{-5} to 10^{-6} (21). To remove the selectable marker effectively in a disruption cassette, the Flp recombinase of *S. cerevisiae* has been used (58). In this method the *URA3* marker is flanked by direct repeats of the minimal Flp recognition target (FRT) and, in addition, the "Ura3 flipper cassette" contains the gene encoding the Flp recombinase under control of the inducible promoter of the *SAP2* gene (Fig. 1B). After disruption of the first allele, the *SAP2* promoter is induced and the Flp recombinase efficiently removes *URA3* and *FLP* sequences, leaving behind a disrupted allele with the FRT sequences.

The most straightforward approach to generate a *C. albicans* null mutant is to use different selectable markers for the disruption of both alleles. Selection for both markers can be performed even simultaneously in doubly marked auxotroph (47, 61). An efficient variant of this procedure has been presented recently, in which PCR-generated disruption fragments carrying different selectable markers were used for transformation of a doubly auxotrophic strain (96). The genes encoding selectable markers were amplified using oligonucleotide primers containing about 60 bp of homology to the target region and were then transformed. An analysis of the transformants revealed that about 5 to 10% of all transformants contained the correctly disrupted alleles. A disadvantage of this method is the inability to disrupt more than one gene (two alleles). To circumvent this problem and because the size of the original Ura-blaster cassette did not allow efficient PCR amplification, a "mini-blaster" consisting of a partially duplicated *URA3* sequence was constructed and used (95). Alternatively, the Ura-blaster was amplified in two overlapping parts as a split-marker cassette (19) from each end; cotransformation of both PCR-generated parts, by in vivo recombination, led to the desired gene disruption (16).

The collective experience on gene disruptions in *C. albicans* obtained in several laboratories suggests several caveats and pitfalls. First, it is obviously impossible to disrupt both alleles of an essential gene. The hypothesis, that this is indeed the case, is based initially on negative evidence, but should be proven by the use of regulated promoters (see below). The use of the composite *ARG4-URA3* selectable marker described above will provide a rapid indication of the essentiality of a gene, since all viable Arg^+ Ura^+ isolates arising by mitotic recombination will be triploid (18). Second, the choice of the host strain is important, because some *C. albicans* strains, e.g., strain SGY243, are at least partially triploid (26) and even isolates of the commonly used strain CAI4 have been described to be triploid in some loci (56, 71). Third, intergenic regions in *C. albicans* are small (9) and the possibility should be considered that by deleting the coding region of a gene the expression of a neighboring gene could be affected as well. An extreme case has been reported, in which the coding regions of two essential genes in *C. albicans* were shown to overlap (23), but in more subtle cases it is conceivable that transcript levels could be affected by neighboring deletions, e.g., in the case of divergently transcribed genes. Finally, the null mutant strains should not only be analyzed by PCR, but also by Southern blotting experiments, because null strains may contain additional copies of the disruption cassette in undefined locations.

Other *Candida* Species

Disruption of *C. glabrata* genes is facilitated by its haploid genome and the possibility of using *S. cerevisiae* marker genes (44). On the other hand, disruption methods for the diploid species *C. tropicalis* have to cope with the same problems as discussed for *C. albicans*. A laborious method for sequential gene disruption in *C. tropicalis* has been described, in which *URA3* within the disruption cassette was destroyed by mutation following disruption of the first allele (64). This method was improved recently by a Ura-blaster method (40).

ADJUSTING GENE EXPRESSION LEVELS

Phenotypes arising during a lowered and/or an elevated state of gene expression provide important clues on the functions of a gene to be characterized. Several regulated and constitutive *Candida* promoters have been developed, which have been used to experimentally modify gene expression levels.

Lowering Gene Expression

It has become standard procedure to lower gene expression in *C. albicans* by complete disruptions of both alleles of the gene in question. Typically, deletion of the second allele is not possible in the case of an essential gene, and a regulatable promoter is used to prove that the expression level of the second allele determines viability or growth. It is an added advantage of conditional gene expression that initial phenotypes closely related to gene function can be monitored in a depletion experiment, whereas a complete gene disruption only reveals an "endpoint" phenotype, which may be caused by a series of secondary events; furthermore, reconstitution of the mutant by addition of the wild-type allele is not necessary in this case. The promoter of the *PCK1* gene is strongly repressed by glucose and its levels of induction depend on medium components (51). A selectable *URA3-PCK1* promoter cassette was used to replace the promoter of the *EFG1* gene, which is a central regulator of *C. albicans* morphogenesis (90). Growth in glucose-containing medium prevented the induction of hyphae by serum and led to an elongated abnormal yeast phenotype, indicating that Efg1p plays a dual role as an activator of hypha formation and a repressor of normal yeast growth. The *MAL2* promoter is inducible by maltose and repressed in media containing other carbon sources such as glucose or glycerol (4). Replacement of the promoter of the *DPB2* gene in the second remaining allele led to transformants able to grow on maltose, but not on glucose, indicating that it is essential for growth (1). In a depletion experiment a shift of maltose-growing cells to glucose media led to filament formation, suggesting a role of Dpb2p in cell division. The *MET3* promoter is another highly regulated promoter in *C. albicans* that is repressed by methionine or cysteine (7). The *GAL1* promoter has also been described to allow regulatable gene expression (25). Experiments with the essential *SEC20* gene revealed advantages and disadvantages in the types of promoters used for conditional gene expression (93). Replacement of the *SEC20* by the *MET3* promoter caused transformants to stop growing in the presence of a combination of methionine and cysteine, thereby proving the essentiality of *SEC20*. Interestingly, single additions of either methionine or cysteine did not prevent growth of transformants, indicating leakiness of the *MET3* promoter in this condition. Transformants, in which the *SEC20* promoter was replaced by the *PCK1* promoter, were tested as well and still grew in high-glucose media, which repress the *PCK1* promoter. However, even though the *PCK1-SEC20* transformants grew, they showed new phenotypes including sensitivities to aminoglycoside antibiotics and agents affecting cell-wall integrity. These experiments suggested that although the *MET3* and *PCK1* promoters are highly regulated, the *MET3* promoter is relatively weak, which may be advantageous in maximally lowering expression levels; nevertheless, the experiments with the *PCK1* promoter also indicate that moderate reductions in expression may reveal phenotypes related to low expression that escape detection with the *MET3* promoter. On the other hand, in the case of the *EFG1* gene, the *PCK1* promoter fusion lowered *EFG1* expression below a threshold level, creating a similar phenotype as in a strain containing a complete *EFG1* disruption (90). Nakayama et al. (60) adopted the tetracycline-regulatable expression system for use in *C. albicans* by using a recombinant TetR-HAP4AD transactivator, whose gene was codon-adapted to *C. albicans* on one plasmid, in conjunction with a "readout" plasmid containing a composite promoter encompassing the *tetO* binding site for the transactivator. In transformants containing both plasmids, the presence of doxycycline to transformants was able to repress promoter activity up to 1,000-fold, depending on the nature of the promoter containing *tetO*. This system was validated by placing essential genes under control of the *tetO*-containing promoter, which prevented growth of transformants in the presence of doxycycline in vitro and even in vivo, in a mouse model of systemic infection.

Clearly, various factors other than promoter strength, including transcript stability and translation efficiency, may be altered by replacing promoters of test genes by any of the promoters mentioned. Thus, the usefulness of any of the mentioned promoters highly depends on the nature of the respective gene and has to be tested empirically. In a recent report, an antisense approach was used to downregulate gene expression and to identify essential genes (15a); however, the factors required to reliably obtain antisense regulation remain to be established.

Gene Overexpression

Overexpression of a gene may generate a phenotype that reflects an increased activity of the main functions of the encoded protein, although nonphysiological phenotypes due to amplifications of secondary functions may arise as well. Overexpression of *EFG1* by full derepression of the *PCK1* promoter-*EFG1* fusion in some media resulted in *C. albicans* cells growing in the form of extremely elongated pseudohyphae carrying constrictions at cellular junctions and terminal buds (Color plate 6) (90). This phenotype, which did not arise if the *PCK1p-EFG1* fusion was expressed moderately, appears nonphysiological, because it did not occur in any environmental condition in wild-type cells. Gene overexpression has been extremely useful in epistasis analyses to obtain genetic evidence for the sequence of cellular reactions. Components in the signaling pathway activating the Cek1 MAP kinase and the Cph1 transcription factor were established by overexpression of genes encoding downstream components in mutants defective in upstream components (15, 49), e.g., the *cek1* morphogenesis-defective phenotype was suppressed by overexpression of *CPH1,* but not *HST7* (15). Similarly, *EFG1* overexpression reconstituted the phenotype of a *tpk2* mutant, suggesting that protein kinase A functions upstream of Efg1p (81). Such suppression results are only possible if the downstream component has some basal activity, which is independent of activation by the upstream component. Promoters that have been used for gene overexpression include promoters of the *ACT1* (54), *ADH1* (15, 49), and *PCK1* (51) genes. Elevated gene expression has been achieved also by placing complete *C. albicans* genes on episomal vectors, which increase the gene copy number (15, 49, 81).

REPORTERS OF GENE EXPRESSION

Reporter genes encoding easily assayable products have been used as convenient tools to analyze gene expression in *Candida* species. Such genes are fused (i) to the promoter, (ii) to promoter and coding regions, or (iii) solely to the coding regions of genes to be characterized. In general, promoter fusions may not reflect transcript stabilities and intracellular localization, which in principle can be determined using approaches ii and iii, but may be obscured by high production levels of the reporter fusions.

C. albicans

Because CUG codons determine serine instead of leucine residues in *C. albicans* (62), standard reporter genes containing CUG codons, e.g., *lacZ,* were not functional. Heterologous expression of a heterologous CUG-decoding *S. cerevisiae* $tRNA^{Leu}$ was found to be toxic and thus did not remedy this problem (52). The *LAC4* gene of the milk yeast *Kluyveromyces lactis,* which encodes β-galactosidase, was the first functional heterologous reporter gene for *C. albicans* (50). The *LAC4* transcript contains two CUG codons, which do not prevent β-galactosidase activity. The Lac4 protein can be easily assayed in cell-free assays and with whole cells using enzymatic substrates used for the determination of LacZ β-galactosidase activity, and its activity is apparent in colonies growing on agar by the use of the X-Gal substrate. The moderate sensitivities of colorimetric substrates were dramatically increased using a bioluminescent substrate for Lac4p (51). Using the latter method, a greater than 100-fold regulation of the *PCK1* promoter in a

PCK1p-LAC4 fusion was determined. Another β-galactosidase-encoding gene, *lacZ* of *Streptococcus thermophilus,* has been established recently as an efficient reporter of gene expression (91a).

The luciferase of the sea pansy *Renilla reniformis* does not contain residues encoded by CUG codons and its functional expression in *C. albicans* proved successful (84). The level of the RrLuc protein has been assayed in a cell-free system or with whole cells using a bioluminescent substrate over a 20,000-fold range. Fusions of *RrLUC* downstream of different promoters revealed the sensitivities of the assays using this reporter gene (53, 84, 86). This bioluminescent system is about 60-fold less efficient using intact cells compared with cell extracts.

Initial attempts to functionally express the green fluorescent protein (GFP) of *Aequoria victoria* in *C. albicans* failed, but replacement of the single CUG codon in the *GFP* gene sufficed to detect GFP fluorescence in cells containing a fusion of the *ACT1* promoter to *GFP* (57). In another successful approach, the entire *GFP* gene was optimized according to the codon usage of highly expressed *C. albicans* genes and by replacement of two residues to enhance fluorescence (11). The yEGFP (yeast enhanced GFP) was detected in immunoblots of cellular extracts and by fluorescence of whole cells. An example for the use of yEGFP is shown in Color plate 6; an Efg1p-yEGFP fusion protein is detected in the nucleus of cells overproducing this fusion. Further derivatives of the *yEGFP* gene encoding replacements of residues known to change excitation and emission wavelengths were constructed and shown to result in yellow, cyan, and red fluorescence (24). In the future, combinations of yEGFP will be certainly useful to detect simultaneously levels and localizations of fusion proteins. Although there are no comparative studies on the sensitivities and other advantages of reporter genes, it appears that the sensitivity of the *GFP* reporter gene is severalfold lower compared to the *LAC4* and *LUC* reporters. Furthermore, GFP is known as a very stable protein; therefore, promoter down-regulation cannot be reliably monitored (83) unless GFP stability is lowered by its fusion to a destabilizing protein (29).

A codon-optimized version of the *FLP* gene encoding the Flp recombinase of *S. cerevisiae* has been used in another approach as a reporter gene to monitor expression of regulated promoters in *C. albicans* (87). Production of Flp causes recombination between repeated Flp target sequences, FRT, flanking another reporter gene system, the *C. albicans IMH3* gene under transcriptional control of the strong *ACT1* promoter, which causes mycophenolic acid (MPA) resistance. Flp-mediated recombination leads to loss of the *ACT1-IMH3* fusion gene and thereby to MPA sensitivity. Thus, the final readouts in this system are MPA-sensitive or -resistant *C. albicans* cells, which on a solid medium containing limiting MPA amounts form small and large colonies, respectively. By this method the activation of a *C. albicans* promoter can be monitored during infection, as in in vivo expression technologies used in other species. This has been demonstrated for the *SAP2* promoter, which was found to be active during disseminated infections, but not esophageal infections of mice (87). The exchange of four residues in the Flp recombinase led to a protein with enhanced recombinase activity that could be used to monitor the differential activities of promoters of the *SAP1* through *6* genes during different stages of mice infections (88). One drawback of the method is that any promoter down-regulation occurring in vivo cannot be determined.

Besides *IMH3,* other homologous genes of *C. albicans* have been used as reporters of gene expression. The *URA3* gene encoding orotidine monophosphate carboxylase has served as a sensitive reporter, allowing the detection of weakly expressed single-copy genes but requires the preparation of cell extracts and of *ura3* auxotrophic strains to lower background activities (59). The *XOG1* gene encoding the major glucanase of *C. albicans* has been used as another homologous reporter gene (8). The *XOG1* gene product is detected on solid and in liquid media, allowing the use of flow cytometry, but this method requires the use of specific strains deleted for *XOG1.* A glycosylphosphatidylinositol anchoring domain to the C-terminal end of Xog1p anchors its activity to the cellular surface, which improves quantification in flow cytometry (cited in reference 65). Recently, it was reported that a homozygous *met15* mutant strain develops a brown colony color, which is complemented by the wild-type *MET15* gene (92).

Other *Candida* Species

C. dubliniensis in recent years has been identified as a species that is closely related to *C. albicans.* A modified *GFP* gene, in which the single CUG codon was exchanged and which had been functionally expressed in *C. albicans,* was shown to function in *C. dubliniensis* (89). The *K. lactis LAC4* gene encoding β-galactosidase was functional in *C. tropicalis* as well as in *C. albicans* (50). In addition, unlike *C. albicans* transformants, *C. tropicalis* transformants expressing *LAC4* at high levels were able to grow with lactose as the sole carbon source, indicating that a lactose transporter exists in this species. A dominant resistance marker for *C. tropicalis* was constructed by exchanging the nine CUG codons of the *Escherichia coli hph* gene; expression of the modified *hph* gene led to hygromycin B resistance (31).

Genes of *C. glabrata* are translated according to the standard codon usage. Therefore, it was not surprising that the *E. coli lacZ* gene could be used as a reporter gene in this species (17). β-Galactosidase activities directed by *lacZ* were detected by an indirect filter assay and quantitatively from permeabilized cells. Recently, it has been communicated that expression of the bacterial *hph* and *nat* genes in *C. glabrata* leads to resistance to hygromycin B and to nourseothricin, respectively (24a).

FUTURE DIRECTIONS

Knowledge of the *C. albicans* genome will certainly be used within the next years to significantly increase the knowledge of *C. albicans* biology and virulence. As for *S. cerevisiae,* DNA array technology will be employed to monitor changes in gene expression of all open reading frames, which is of particular interest for *C. albicans* because of its dimorphism, its contact with various host cells and molecules, and its resistance mechanisms to antifungal agents. DNA arrays of intergenic regions will allow a genomewide screening for the binding sites of transcription factors (72), and protein arrays will be a convenient method to obtain a genomewide overview of protein function and specificities, as in *S. cerevisiae* (100).

Besides array technologies, future approaches will be centered to systematically elucidate protein profiles (proteome), especially in different conditions relevant to infection, an approach that will reveal actual protein concentrations and posttranslational modifications. The patterns of intracellular metabolites specific, for example, for certain host environments, will be determined and will result in metabolic profiling of *C. albicans*. Furthermore, it will be of great interest to determine the interactions of *C. albicans* proteins, e.g., by two-hybrid analysis or by biochemical methods; this applies not only to interactions between fungal proteins, but also between fungal and host proteins, which may be relevant for virulence. In addition, it will be highly desirable to systematically disrupt all open reading frames in *C. albicans,* preferably marking the deletions by specific sequence tags, which will allow the identification of specific deletants within pools of mutants (97), e.g., those mutants that are affected in specific conditions such as contact with host cells. This approach will reveal genes involved in host interaction and thereby in fungal virulence. The feasibility of this approach has already been shown for *C. glabrata* by using a limited set of random mutants (13).

REFERENCES

1. **Backen, A. C., I. D. Broadbent, R. W. Fetherston, J. D. C. Rosamond, N. F. Schnell, and M. J. R. Stark.** 2000. Evaluation of the *CaMAL2* promoter for regulated expression of genes in *Candida albicans. Yeast* **16:**1121–1129.
2. **Barton, R. C., and K. Gull.** 1992. Isolation, characterization, and genetic analysis of monosomic, aneuploid mutants of *Candida albicans. Mol. Microbiol.* **6:**171–177.
3. **Beckerman, J., H. Chibana, J. Turner, and P. T. Magee.** 2001. Single-copy *IMH3* allele is sufficient to confer resistance to mycophenolic acid in *Candida albicans* and to mediate transformation of clinical *Candida* species. *Infect. Immun.* **69:**108–114.
4. **Brown, D. H., Jr., I. V. Slobodkin, and C. A. Kumamoto.** 1996. Stable transformation and regulated expression of an inducible reporter construct in *Candida albicans* using restriction enzyme-mediated inegration. *Mol. Gen. Genet.* **251:**75–80.
5. **Cannon, R. D.** 1986. Isolation of a mycelial mutant of *Candida albicans. J. Gen. Microbiol.* **132:**2405–2407.
6. **Cannon, R. D., H. F. Jenkinson, and M. G. Sheperd.** 1992. Isolation and nucleotide sequence of an autonomously replicating sequence (ARS) element functional in *Candida albicans* and *Saccharomyces cerevisiae. Mol. Gen. Genet* **221:**210–218.
7. **Care, R. S., J. Trevethick, K. M. Binley, and P. E. Sudbery.** 1999. The *MET3* promoter: a new tool for *Candida albicans* molecular genetics. *Mol. Microbiol.* **34:**792–798.
8. **Chambers, R. S., M. J. Broughton, R. D. Cannon, A. Carne, G. W. Emerson, and P. A. Sullivan.** 1993. An exo-beta-(1,3)-glucanase of *Candida albicans:* purification of the enzyme and molecular cloning of the gene. *J. Gen. Microbiol.* **139:**325–334.
9. **Chibana, H., B. B. Magee, S. Grindle, Y. Ran, S. Scherer, and P. T. Magee.** 1998. A physical map of chromosome 7 of *Candida albicans. Genetics* **149:**1739–1752.
10. **Cole, M. F., W. H. Bowen, X. J. Zhao, and R. L. Cihlar.** 1995. A virulence of *Candida albicans* auxotrophic mutants in a rat model of oropharyngeal candidiasis. *FEMS Microbiol. Lett.* **126:**177–180.
11. **Cormack, B. P., G. Bertram, M. Egerton, N. A. Gow, S. Falkow, and A. J. P. Brown.** 1997. Yeast-enhanced green fluorescent protein (YEGFP) a reporter of gene expression in *Candida albicans* and *C. tropicalis. Microbiology* **143:**303–311.
12. **Cormack, B. P., and S. Falkow.** 1999. Efficient homologous and illegitimate recombination in the opportunistic yeast pathogen *Candida glabrata. Genetics* **151:**979–987.
13. **Cormack, B. P., N. Ghori, and S. Falkow.** 1999. An adhesin of the yeast pathogen *Candida glabrata* mediating adherence to human epithelial cells. *Science* **285:**578–582.
14. **Corner, B. E., and R. T. M. Poulter.** 1989. Interspecific complementation analysis by protoplast fusion of *Candida tropicalis* and *Candida albicans* adenine auxotrophs. *J. Bacteriol.* **171:**3586–3589.
15. **Csank, C., K. Schröppel, E. Leberer, D. Harcus, O. Mohamed, S. Meloche, D. Y. Thomas, and M. Whiteway.** 1998. Roles of the *Candida albicans* mitogen-activated protein kinase homolog, Cek1p, in hyphal development and systemic candidiasis. *Infect. Immun.* **66:**2713–2721.

15a. **De Backer, M., B. Nelissen, M. Logghe, J. Viaene, I. Loonen, S. Vandoninck, R. de Hoogt, S. Dewaele, F. A. Simons, P. Verhasselt, G. Vanhoof, R. Contreras, and W. H. M. L. Luyten.** 2001. An antisense-based functional genomics approach for identification of genes critical for growth of *Candida albicans. Nat. Biotechnol.* **19:**235–241.

16. **De Hoogt, R., W. H. Luyten, R. Contreras, and M. D. De Backer.** 2000. PCR- and ligation-mediated synthesis of split-marker cassettes with long flanking homology regions for gene disruption in *Candida albicans*. *Biotechniques* **28:** 1112–1116.
17. **El Barkani, A., K. Haynes, H.-U. Mösch, M. Frosch, and F. A. Mühlschlegel.** 2000. *Candida glabrata* shuttle vectors suitable for translational fusions to *lacZ* and use of β-galactosidase as a reporter of gene expression. *Gene* **246:**151–155.
18. **Enloe, B., A. Diamond, and A. P. Mitchell.** 2000. A single-transformation gene function test in diploid *Candida albicans*. *J. Bacteriol.* **182:**5730–5736.
19. **Fairhead, C., B. Llorente, F. Denis, M. Soler, and B. Dujon.** 1996. New vectors for combinatorial deletions in yeast chromosomes and for gap-repair using 'split-marker' recombination. *Yeast* **12:**1439–1457.
20. **Feng, Q., E. Summers, B. Guo, and G. Fink.** 1999. Ras signaling is required for serum-induced hyphal differentiation in *Candida albicans*. *J. Bacteriol.* **181:**6339–6346.
21. **Fonzi, W. A., and M. Y. Irwin.** 1993. Isogenic strain construction and gene mapping in *Candida albicans*. *Genetics* **134:** 717–728.
22. **Fournier, P., A. Provost, C. Bourguignon, and H. Heslot.** 1977. Recombination after protoplast fusion in the yeast *Candida albicans*. *Arch. Microbiol.* **115:**143–149.
23. **Gerads, M., and J. F. Ernst.** 1998. Overlapping coding regions and transcriptional units of two essential chromosomal genes (*CCT8, TRP1*) in the fungal pathogen *Candida albicans*. *Nucleic Acids Res.* **26:**5061–5066.
24. **Gerami-Nejad, M., J. Berman, and C. Gale.** 2001. Cassettes for PCR-mediated construction of green, yellow and cyan fluorescent protein fusions in *Candida albicans*. *Yeast* **18:** 859–864.
24a. **Goldstein, A.** Unpublished results.
25. **Gorman, J. A., W. Chan, and J. W. Gorman.** 1991. Repeated use of *GAL1* for gene disruption in *Candida albicans*. *Genetics* **129:**19–24.
26. **Gow, N. A., P. W. Robbins, J. W. Lester, A. J. Brown, W. A. Fonzi, T. Chapman, and O. S. Kinsman.** 1994. A hyphal-specific chitin synthase gene (CHS2) is not essential for growth, dimorphism, or virulence of Candida albicans. *Proc. Natl. Acad. Sci. USA* **91:**6216–6220.
27. **Gräser, Y., M. Volovsek, J. Arrington, G. Schönian, W. Presber, T. G. Mitchell, and R. Vilgalys.** 1996. Molecular markers reveal that population structure of the human pathogen *Candida albicans* exhibits both clonality and recombination. *Proc. Natl. Acad. Sci. USA* **93:**12473–12477.
28. **Haas, L. O., J. M. Cregg, and M. A. Gleeson.** 1990. Development of an integrative transformation system for the yeast *Candida tropicalis*. *J. Bacteriol.* **172:**4571–4577.
29. **Hampton, Y. R., A. Koning, R. Wright, and J. Rine.** 1996. In vivo examination of membrane protein localization and degradation with green fluorescent protein. *Proc. Natl. Acad. Sci. USA* **93:**828–833.
30. **Hanic-Joyce, P. J., and P. B. M. Joyce.** 1998. A high-copy-number *ADE2*-bearing plasmid for transformation of *Candida glabrata*. *Gene* **211:**395–400.
31. **Hara, A., M. Ueda, S. Misawa, T. Matsui, K. Furuhashi, and A. Tanaka.** 2000. A mutated hygromycin resistance gene is functional in the n-alkane-assimilating yeast *Candida tropicalis*. *Arch. Microbiol.* **173:**187–192.
32. **Henson, O. E., and D. O. McClary.** 1979. Growth inhibition of *Candida albicans* by folate pathway inhibitors. Their potential in the selection of auxotrophs. *Antonie Van Leeuwenhoek* **45:**211–223.
33. **Herreros, E., M. I. Garcia-Sáez, C. Nombela, and M. Sánchez.** 1992. A reorganized *Candida albicans* DNA sequence promoting homologous non-integrative genetic transformation. *Mol. Microbiol.* **6:**3567–3574.
34. **Hilton, C., D. Markie, B. Corner, E. Rikkerink, and R. Poulter.** 1985. Heat shock induces chromosome loss in the yeast *Candida albicans*. *Mol. Gen. Genet.* **200:**162–168.
35. **Hinnen, A., J. B. Hicks, and G. R. Fink.** 1978. Transformation of yeast. *Proc. Natl. Acad. Sci. USA* **75:**1929–1933.
36. **Hull, C. M., and A. D. Johnson.** 1999. Identification of a mating type-like locus in the asexual pathogenic yeast *Candida albicans*. *Science* **285:**1271–1275.
37. **Hull, C. M., R. M. Raisner, and A. D. Johnson.** 2000. Evidence for mating of the "asexual" yeast *Candida albicans* in a mammalian host. *Science* **289:**307–310.
38. **Janbon, G., F. Sherman, and E. Rustchenko.** 1998. Monosomy of a specific chromosome determines L-sorbose utilization: a novel regulatory mechanism in *Candida albicans*. *Proc. Natl. Acad. Sci. USA* **95:**5150–5155.
39. **Kakar, S. N., R. M. Partridge, and P. T. Magee.** 1983. A genetic analysis of *Candida albicans:* isolation of a wide variety of auxotrophs and demonstration of linkage and complementation. *Genetics* **104:**241–255.
40. **Kanayama, N., U. Mitsuyoshi, A. Haruyuki, and A. Tanaka.** 1998. Genetic evaluation of physiological functions of thiolase isozymes in the n-alkane-assimilating yeast *Candida tropicalis*. *J. Bacteriol.* **180:**690–698.
41. **Kelly, R., S. M. Miller, and M. B. Kurtz.** 1987. One-step gene disruption by cotransformation to isolate double auxotrophs in *Candida albicans*. *Mol. Gen. Genet.* **214:**24–31.
42. **Kirsch, D. R., and R. R. Whitney.** 1991. Pathogenicity of *Candida albicans* auxotrophic mutants in experimental infections. *Infect. Immun.* **59:**3297–3300.
43. **Kitada, K., E. Yamaguchi, and M. Arisawa.** 1996. Isolation of a *Candida glabrata* centromere and its use in construction of plasmid vectors. *Gene* **175:**105–108.
44. **Kitada, K. E., E. Yamaguchi, and M. Arisawa.** 1995. Cloning of the *Candida glabrata TRP1* and *HIS3* genes, and construction of their disruptant strains by sequential integrative transformation. *Gene* **165:**203–206.
45. **Köhler, G. A., T. C. White, and N. Agabian.** 1997. Overexpression of a cloned IMP dehydrogenase gene of *Candida albicans* confers resistance to the specific inhibitor mycophenolic acid. *J. Bacteriol.* **179:**2331–2338.
46. **Kurtz, M. B., M. W. Cortelyou, S. M. Miller, M. Lai, and D. R. Kirsch.** 1987. Development of autonomously replicating plasmids for *Candida albicans*. *Mol. Cell. Biol.* **7:**209–217.
47. **Kurtz, M. B., and J. Marrinan.** 1989. Isolation of *hem3* mutants from *Candida albicans* by sequential gene disruption. *Mol. Gen. Genet.* **217:**47–52.
48. **Lay, J., L. K. Henry, J. Clifford, Y. Koltin, C. E. Bulawa, and J. M. Becker.** 1998. Altered expression of selectable marker *URA3* in gene-disrupted *Candida albicans* strains complicates interpretation of virulence studies. *Infect. Immun.* **66:** 5301–5306.
49. **Leberer, E., D. Harcus, I. D. Broadbent, K. L. Clark, D. Dignard, K. Ziegelbauer, A. Schmidt, N. A. R. Gow, A. J. P. Brown, and D. Y. Thomas.** 1996. Signal transduction through homologs of the Ste20p and Ste7p protein kinases can trigger hyphal formation in the pathogenic fungus *Candida albicans*. *Proc. Natl. Acad. Sci. USA* **93:**13217–13222.
50. **Leuker, C. E., A. M. Hahn, and J. F. Ernst.** 1992. β-Galactosidase of *Kluyveromyces lactis* (Lac4p) as reporter of gene expression in *Candida albicans* and *C. tropicalis*. *Mol. Gen. Genet.* **235:**235–241.
51. **Leuker, C. E., A. Sonneborn, S. Delbrück, and J. F. Ernst.** 1997. Sequence and regulation of the *PCK1* gene encoding

phosphoenolpyruvate carboxykinase of the fungal pathogen *Candida albicans*. *Gene* **192**:235–240.

52. **Leuker, C. E., and J. F. Ernst.** 1994. Toxicity of a heterologous leucyl-tRNA (anticodon CAG) in the pathogen *Candida albicans:* in vivo evidence for non-standard decoding of CUG codons. *Mol. Gen. Genet.* **245**:212–217.
53. **Lockhart, S. R., M. Nguyen, T. Srikantha, and D. R. Soll.** 1998. A MADS box protein consensus binding site is necessary and sufficient for activation of the opaque-phase-specific gene *OP4* of *Candida albicans. J. Bacteriol.* **180**:6607–6616.
54. **Losberger, C., and J. F. Ernst.** 1989. Sequence of the *Candida albicans* gene encoding actin. *Nucleic Acids Res.* **17**:9488.
55. **Magee, B. B., and P. T. Magee.** 2000. Induction of mating in *Candida albicans* by construction of *MTLα* and *MTLα* strains. *Science* **298**:310–313.
56. **Mio, T., M. Adachi-Shimizu, Y. Tachibana, H. Tabuchi, S. B. Inoue, T. Yabe, T. Yamada-Okabe, M. Arisawa, T. Watanabe, and H. Yamada-Okabe.** 1997. Cloning of the *Candida albicans* homolog of *Saccharomyces cerevisiae GSC1/FKS1* and its involvement in beta-1,3-glucan synthesis. *J. Bacteriol.* **179**:4096–4105.
57. **Morschhäuser, J., S. Michel, and J. Hacker.** 1998. Expression of a chromosomally integrated, single-copy GFP gene in *Candida albicans,* and its use as a reporter of gene regulation. *Mol. Gen. Genet.* **257**:412–420.
58. **Morschhäuser, J., S. Michel, and P. Staib.** 1999. Sequential gene disruption in *Candida albicans* by FLP-mediated site-specific recombination. *Mol. Microbiol.* **32**:547–556.
59. **Myers, K. K., P. S. Sypherd, and W. A. Fonzi.** 1995. Use of *URA3* as a reporter of gene expression in *C. albicans. Curr. Genet.* **27**:243–248.
60. **Nakayama, H., T. Mio, S. Nagahashi, M. Kokado, M. Arisawa, and Y. Aoki.** 2000. Tetracycline-regulatable system to tightly control gene expression in the pathogenic fungus *Candida albicans. Infect. Immun.* **68**:6712–6719.
61. **Negredo, A., L. Monteoliva, C. Gil, J. Pla, and C. Nombela.** 1997. Cloning, analysis and one-step disruption of the ARG5,6 gene of *Candida albicans. Microbiology* **143**: 297–302.
62. **Ohama, T., T. Suzuki, M. Mori, S. Osawa, T. Ueda, K. Watanabe, and T. Nakase.** 1993. Non-universal decoding of the leucine codon CUG in several *Candida* species. *Nucleic Acids Res.* **21**:4039–4045.
63. **Perepnikhatka, V., F. J. Fischer, M. Niimi, R. A. Baker, R. D. Cannon, Y.-K. Wang, F. Sherman, and E. Rustchenko.** 1999. Specific chromosome alterations in fluconazole-resistant mutants of *Candida albicans. J. Bacteriol.* **181**: 4041–4049.
64. **Picataggio, S., K. Deanda, and J. Mielenz.** 1991. Determination of *Candida tropicalis* acyl coenzyme A oxidase isozyme function by sequential gene disruption. *Mol. Cell. Biol.* **11**: 4333–4339.
65. **Pla, J., C. Gil, L. Monteoliva, F. Navarro-Garcia, M. Sánchez, and C. Nombela.** 1996. Understanding *Candida albicans* at the molecular level. *Yeast* **12**:1677–1702.
66. **Pla, J., R. M. Pérez-Díaz, F. Navarro-Garcia, M. Sánchez, and C. Nombela.** 1995. Cloning of *Candida albicans HIS1* gene by direct homologous complementation of a histidine auxotroph using an improved double-ARS shuttle vector. *Gene* **165**:115–120.
67. **Poulter, R., V. Hanrahan, K. Jeffery, D. Markie, M. G. Shepherd, and P. A. Sullivan.** 1982. Recombination analysis of naturally diploid *Candida albicans. J. Bacteriol.* **152**: 969–975.
68. **Poulter, R., K. Jeffery, M. J. Hubbard, M. G. Shepherd, and P. A. Sullivan.** 1981. Parasexual genetic analysis of *Candida albicans* by spheroplast fusion. *J. Bacteriol.* **146**:833–840.
69. **Poulter, R. T., and E. H. Rikkerink.** 1983. Genetic analysis of red, adenine requiring mutants of *Candida albicans. J. Bacteriol.* **156**:1066–1077.
70. **Rademacher, F., V. Kehren, V. R. Stoldt, and J. F. Ernst.** 1998. Chaperonins as specific dominant-negative suppressors of fungal morphogenesis and *RAS* signal transduction pathways. *Microbiology* **114**:2951–2960.
71. **Ramanan, N., and Y. Wang.** 2000. A high-affinity iron permease essential for *Candida albicans* virulence. *Science* **288**: 1062–1064.
72. **Ren, B., F. Robert, J. J. Wyrick, O. Aparicio, E. G. Jennings, I. Simon, J. Zeitlinger, J. Schreiber, N. Hannett, E. Kanin, T. L. Volkert, C. J. Wilson, S. P. Bell, and R. A. Young.** 2000. Genome-wide location and function of DNA binding proteins. *Science* **290**:2306–2309.
73. **Rohrer, T. L., and S. K. Picataggio.** 1991. Targeted integrative transformation of *Candida tropicalis* by electroporation. *Appl. Microbiol. Biotechnol.* **36**:650–654.
74. **Rutstchenko-Bulgac, E. P., F. Sherman, and J. Hicks.** 1990. Chromosomal rearrangements associated with morphological mutants provide a means for genetic variation of *Candida albicans. J. Bacteriol.* **172**:1276–1283.
75. **Sadhu, C., D. Hoekstra, M. J. McEachern, S. I. Reed, and J. B. Hicks.** 1992. A G-protein alpha subunit from asexual *Candida albicans* functions in the mating signal transduction pathway of *Saccharomyces cerevisiae* and is regulated by the a1-alpha2 repressor. *Mol. Cell. Biol.* **12**:1977–1985.
76. **Sanglard, D., and A. Fiechter.** 1992. DNA transformations of *Candida tropicalis* with replicating and integrative vectors. *Yeast* **8**:1065–1075.
77. **Sanglard, D., F. Ischer, M. Monod, and J. Bille.** 1996. Susceptibilities of *Candida albicans* multidrug transporter mutants to various antifungal agents and other metabolic inhibitors. *Antimicrobiol. Agents Chemother.* **40**:2300–2305.
78. **Sarachek, A., and D. A. Weber.** 1984. Temperature-dependent internuclear transfer of genetic material in heterokaryosis of *Candida albicans. Curr. Genet.* **8**:181–187.
79. **Sentandreu, M., M. V. Elorza, R. Sentandreu, and W. A. Fonzi.** 1998. Cloning and characterization of *PRA1,* a gene encoding a novel pH-regulated gene of *Candida albicans. J. Bacteriol.* **180**:282–289.
80. **Soll, D. R.** 1997. Gene regulation during high-frequency switching in *Candida albicans. Microbiology* **143**:279–288.
81. **Sonneborn, A., D. P. Bockmühl, M. Gerads, K. Kurpanek, D. Sanglard, and J. F. Ernst.** 2000. Protein kinase A encoded by *TPK2* regulates dimorphism of the human pathogen *Candida albicans. Mol. Microbiol.* **35**:386–396.
82. **Sonneborn, A., B. Tebarth, and J. F. Ernst.** 1999. Control of white-opaque phenotypic switching in *Candida albicans* by the Efg1p morphogenetic regulator. *Infect. Immun.* **67**: 4655–4660.
83. **Spellig, T., A. Bottin, and R. Kahmann.** 1996. Green fluorescent protein (GFP) as a new vital marker in the phytopathogenic fungus *Ustilago maydis. Mol. Gen. Genet.* **252**: 503–509.
84. **Srikantha, T., A. Klapach, W. W. Lorenz, L. K. Tsai, A. Laughlin, J. A. Gorman, and D. R. Soll.** 1996. The sea pansy *Renilla reniformis* luciferase serves as a sensitive bioluminescent reporter for differential gene expression in *Candida albicans. J. Bacteriol.* **178**:121–129.
85. **Srikantha, T., B. Morrow, K. Schröppel, and D. R. Soll.** 1995. The frequency of integrative transformation at phase-specific genes of *Candida albicans* correlates with their transcriptional state. *Mol. Gen. Genet.* **246**:342–352.

86. **Srikantha, T., L. K. Tsai, and D. R. Soll.** 1997. The *WH11* gene of *Candida albicans* is regulated in two distinct developmental programs through the same transcription activation sequences. *J. Bacteriol.* **179:**3837–3844.
87. **Staib, P., M. Kretschmar, T. Nichterlein, G. Köhler, S. Michel, H. Hof, J. Hacker, and J. Morschhäuser.** 1999. Host-induced, stage-specific virulence gene activation in *Candida albicans* during infection. *Mol. Microbiol.* **32:**533–546.
88. **Staib, P., M. Kretschmar, T. Nichterlein, H. Hof, and J. Morschhäuser.** 1999. Differential activation of a *Candida albicans* virulence gene family during infection. *Proc. Natl. Acad. Sci. USA* **97:**6102–6107.
89. **Staib, P., S. Michel, G. Köhler, and J. Morschhäuser.** 2000. A molecular genetic system for the pathogenic yeast *Candida dubliniensis. Gene* **242:**393–398.
90. **Stoldt, V. R., A. Sonneborn, C. Leuker, and J. F. Ernst.** 1997. Efg1, an essential regulator of morphogenesis of the human pathogen *Candida albicans,* is a member of a conserved class of bHLH proteins regulating morphogenetic processes in fungi. *EMBO J.* **16:**1982–1991.
91. **Swoboda, R. K., I. D. Broadbent, G. Bertram, S. Budge, G. Gooday, N. A. R. Gow, and A. J. P. Brown.** 1995. Structure and regulation of a *Candida albicans RP10* gene which encodes an immunogenic protein homologous to *Saccharomyces cerevisiae* ribosomal protein 10. *J. Bacteriol.* **177:** 1239–1246.
91a. **Uhl, M. A., and A. D. Johnson.** 2001. Development of *Streptococcus thermophilus lacZ* as a reporter gene for *Candida albicans. Microbiology* **147:**1189–1195.
92. **Viane, J., P. Tiels, M. Logghe, S. Dewaele, W. Martinet, and R. Contreras.** 2000. *MET15* as a visual selection marker for *Candida albicans. Yeast* **16:**1205–1215.
93. **Weber, Y., U. J. Santore, J. F. Ernst, and R. K. Swoboda.** 2000. Divergence of eukaryotic secretory components: the *Candida albicans* homolog to the *Saccharomyces cerevisiae* Sec20 protein is N-terminally truncated and its levels determine antifungal resistance and viability. *J. Bacteriol.* **183:** 46–54.
94. **Whelan, W. L., R. M. Partridge, and P. T. Magee.** 1980. Heterozygosity and segregation in *Candida albicans. Mol. Gen. Genet.* **180:**107–113.
95. **Wilson, R. B., D. Davis, B. M. Enloe, and A. P. Mitchell.** 2000. A recyclable *Candida albicans URA3* cassette for PCR product-directed gene disruptions. *Yeast* **16:**65–70.
96. **Wilson, R. B., D. Davis, and A. P. Mitchell.** 1999. Rapid hypothesis testing with *Candida albicans* through gene disruption with short homology regions. *J. Bacteriol.* **181:** 1868–1874.
97. **Winzeler, E. A., D. D. Shoemaker, A. Astromoff, H. Liang, K. Anderson, B. Andre, R. Bangham, R. Bonito, J. D. Boeke, H. Bussey, A. M. Chu, C. Connelly, K. Davis, F. Dietrich, S. Whelen Dow, M. El Bakkoury, F. Foury, S. H. Friend, E. Gentalen, G. Giaever, J. H. Hegemann, T. Jones, M. Laub, H. Liao, N. Liebundguth, D. J. Lockhart, A. Lucau-Danila, M. Lussier, N. M'Rabet, P. Menard, M. Mittman, C. Pai, C. Rebischung, J. L. Revuelta, L. Riles, C. J. Roberts, P. Ross-MacDonald, B. Scherens, M. Snyder, S. Sookhai-Mahadeo, R. K. Storms, S. Véronneau, M. Voet, G. Volckaert, T. R. Ward, R. Wysocki, G. S. Yen, K. Yu, K. Zimmerman, P. Philippsen, M. Johnston, and R. W. Davis.** 1999. Functional characterization of the *S. cerevisiae* genome by gene deletion and parallel analysis. *Science* **285:**901–906.
98. **Yesland, K., and W. A. Fonzi.** 2000. Allele-specific targeting in *Candida albicans* results from heterology between alleles. *Microbiology* **146:**2097–2104.
99. **Zhou, P., M. S. Szczypka, R. Young, and D. J. Thiele.** 1994. A system for gene cloning and manipulation in the yeast *Candida glabrata. Gene* **142:**135–140.
100. **Zhu, H., J. F. Klemic, S. Chang, P. Bertone, A. Casamayor, K. G. Klemic, D. Smith, M. Gerstein, M. A. Reed, and M. Snyder.** 2000. Analysis of yeast protein kinases using protein chips. *Nat. Genet.* **26:**283–289.

Candida and Candidiasis
Edited by Richard A. Calderone

Chapter 20

Standard and Nonstandard mRNA Decoding in *Candida*

JUSTIN M. O'SULLIVAN, MANUEL A. S. SANTOS, AND MICK F. TUITE

Transcription, the first step in the transfer of genetic information from DNA sequence to protein sequence, produces an mRNA template that in eukaryotes is transported to the cytoplasm via nuclear pores. In the cytoplasm, the fully processed mRNA is captured by ribosomes, which, together with tRNAs, proceeds to decode the open reading frame. Translation of the eukaryotic mRNA usually starts from the most 5′ AUG codon with the ribosome catalyzing the transfer of amino acids from the aminoacyl-tRNAs (aa-tRNA), present in the ribosomal A-site, to the nascent polypeptide chain bound to the P-site tRNA. Despite the obvious increases in complexity from unicellular to multicellular organisms, the underlying mechanisms of transcription and translation are highly conserved from yeast to humans.

There are several key stages within the processes of transcription and translation that ensure the maintenance of highly accurate decoding of the genetic code. These include codon:anticodon proofreading associated with the binding of the aa-tRNA at the ribosomal A-site, and the aminoacylation of the tRNA by its cognate aminoacyl-tRNA synthetase (aaRS). These two proofreading steps are important for ensuring that codons are accurately read and the correct amino acids are inserted into the growing polypeptide chain. However, given the nature of the genetic code and the means by which it is decoded, errors do occur. For example, the rate of codon mistranslation in *Escherichia coli* has been estimated to be of the order of one per 1,000 to 10,000 codons read (41) whereas our recent studies with the yeast *Saccharomyces cerevisiae* suggest a significantly greater level of decoding accuracy during mRNA decoding (57). It is, therefore, highly likely that the genetic code in all organisms has evolved to minimize decoding errors during translation since the failure to control such errors could be potentially devastating.

In the 1960s a combination of in vitro and in vivo experiments indicated that, despite a high degree of codon redundancy (i.e., the use of more than one codon for a given amino acid within the genetic code), codon meanings appeared to be universal (9, 11). Consequently Crick proposed the "frozen accident theory" in which he stated that "the (genetic) code is universal because at the present time any change would be lethal, or at least very strongly selected against" (11). This remained the accepted dogma until a number of unexpected deviations in prokaryotic, eukaryotic, and organellar genetic codes began to emerge at the beginning of the 1980s through comparative gene and protein sequencing studies of both mitochondrial and nuclear genes and their gene products (Table 1). These findings presented a clear challenge to acceptance of the universality of genetic code assignments.

The genetic code and its decoding present its nonuniversal nature in a number of different ways, with variation occurring in codon assignment and codon usage in different species, and even within different classes of genes or tissues in the same organism. Perhaps most dramatically, there exist a number of examples of wholesale reassignment of nonsense codons to sense meanings and vice versa (Table 1). However, sense-to-sense codon reassignments are much rarer, with only one well-established example in a nuclear genome, namely the reassignment of the CUG codon from leucine to serine in a large number of *Candida* species.

At the present time the *Candida* genus is unique in containing a large number of species that have undergone a wholesale codon reassignment within their nuclear genetic codes. In this chapter, we outline the current understanding of the genetic code within the *Candida* genus, both its composition gleaned from genome analysis and current thinking on how such a

Justin M. O'Sullivan and Mick F. Tuite • Department of Biosciences, University of Kent, Canterbury, Kent CT2 7NJ, United Kingdom. **Manuel A. S. Santos** • Department of Biology, University of Aveiro, 3810 Aveiro, Portugal.

Table 1. Known deviations from the "universal" genetic code in prokaryotes and eukaryotes[a]

Codon	Amino acid inserted		Organism in which described
	P	F	
Sense to sense			
CUG	Leu	Ser	*Candida* spp.
Sense to nonsense			
CGG	Arg	Stop	*Mycoplasma* spp.
AGA	Arg	Stop	*Micrococcus* spp.
AUA	Ile	Stop	*Micrococcus* spp.
Nonsense to sense			
UAR	Stop	Gln	*Tetrahymena* spp., *Paramecium* spp., *Stylonicia* sp., *Oxyticha* spp., *Acetabularia* spp.
UGA	Stop	Trp	*Mycoplasma* spp., *Spiroplasma* sp.
UGA	Stop	Cys	*Euplotes* sp.

[a]The standard three-letter code is used to designate amino acids. P, predicted by the universal genetic code; F, experimentally proven assignment of the codon; R, A or G.

potentially catastrophic reassignment could have evolved.

CODON USAGE IN *CANDIDA* SPECIES

Reassignment of the CUG Codon

Genomewide codon reassignments have been documented in a number of nuclear and mitochondrial systems (reviewed in 36, 38) (Table 1). Kawaguchi et al. (24) described the first example of a nuclear sense-to-sense codon reassignment within a eukaryotic organism, namely in *Candida cylindracea,* where the standard leucine CUG codon was found to code for a serine, not the predicted leucine residue. Earlier studies, using in vitro translation assays, had demonstrated that one (or more) aa-tRNAs from *Candida albicans* were able to mediate a nonstandard mRNA decoding event (62). This was subsequently confirmed to be due to CUG codons being decoded by a Ser-tRNA rather than a Leu-tRNA (45). Cytoplasmic Ser-tRNAs, with a 5′ CAG 3′ anticodon, from a number of *Candida* species were then isolated and shown to decode the CUG leucine codon as serine both in vitro and in vivo (24, 35, 46, 58, 59, 64). To date, in addition to *C. albicans,* a further 75 members of the *Candida* genus (Fig. 1) (58) have now been confirmed as decoding the CUG codon as serine in contravention of the universal genetic code. This finding raises three important questions: Why the CUG codon? Why *Candida* species? Are other aspects of mRNA decoding in *Candida* nonstandard?

Codon Sets and Bias within the *Candida* Genus

The standard and nonstandard genetic codes are degenerate (Table 2). This means, for example, that some members of the *Candida* genus, including *C. albicans,* have seven different codons available to code for serine. It can be argued that codons encoding one amino acid would be used equally throughout the coding sequences of an organism (52). However, the reality differs from this in that preferred and optimal codon sets have been identified in a wide variety of unicellular organisms and vertebrates (3, 5, 15, 20, 22, 23).

Up-to-date information on codon usage within the different members of the *Candida* genus can be obtained from the Codon Usage Database (32) (http://www.kazusa.or.jp/codon/). These data are compiled using the nucleotide sequences obtained from the latest major release of the GenBank sequence database (31). The most comprehensive data set on codon utilization within the *Candida* genus is for *C. albicans* coding sequences although significant data sets are also available for *C. maltosa, C. glabrata,* and *C. tropicalis.*

The codon usage data do not define the "optimal" codon set for a given organism, but rather they indicate the most frequently used or preferred codons within the coding sequences for the organism under study. That is, these data do not take into account the relative distribution of codons between genes that are expressed efficiently (and thus have a significant bias in the codons used) and poorly expressed genes where codon bias is usually much less obvious (29).

Brown et al. (7) were the first to assemble a codon usage table for *C. albicans* in which the preferred codons for this species were calculated from the fractional usage of synonymous codons within a very small number of verified coding sequences: *CaACT1, CaARF1, CaCMD1, CaCYP1, CaERG1, CaPRA1, CaTEF1, CaTEF2, CaTSA1, CaTUB2, CaURA3.*

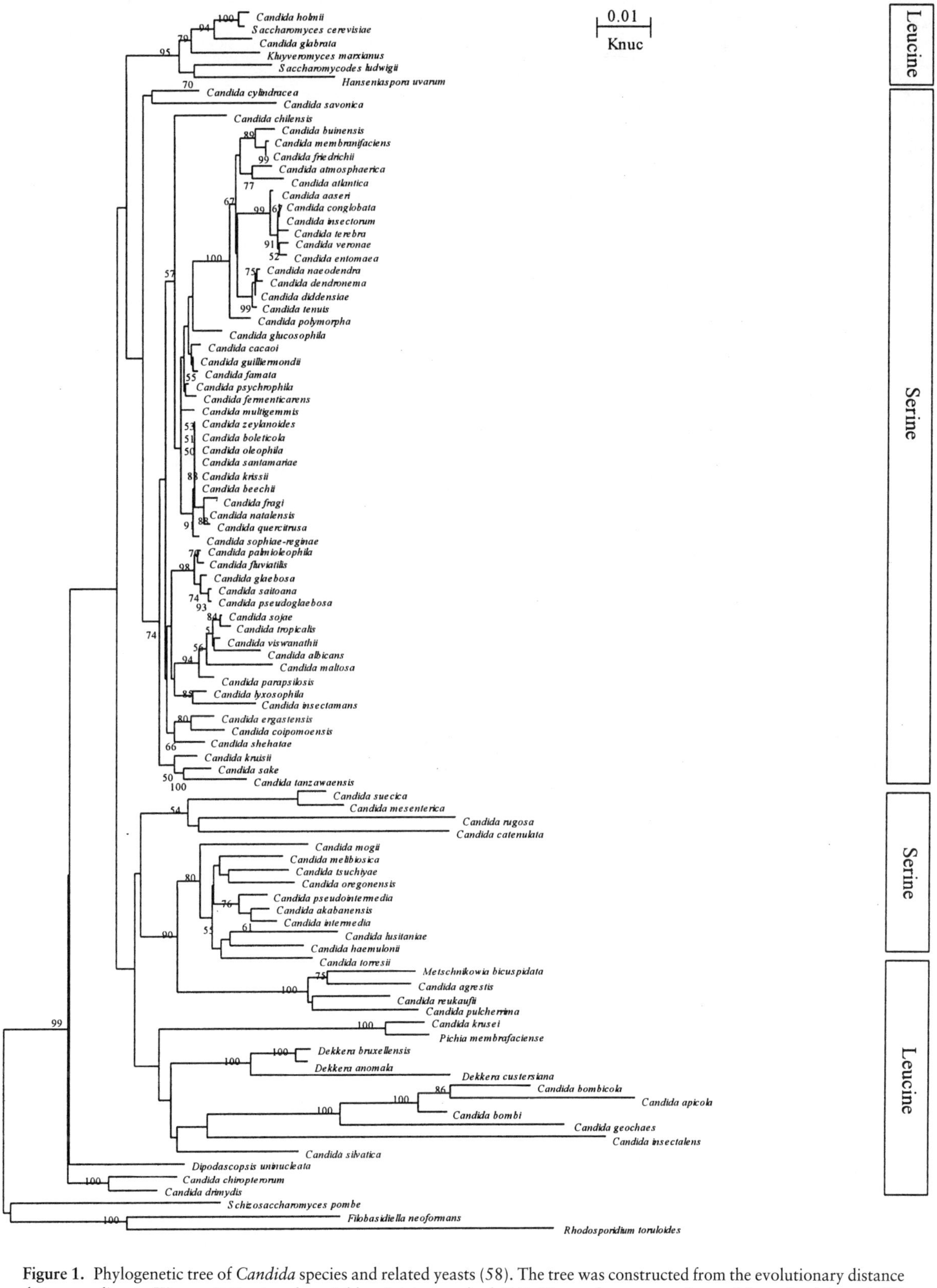

Figure 1. Phylogenetic tree of *Candida* species and related yeasts (58). The tree was constructed from the evolutionary distance data according to Kimura (25) using the neighbor-joining method (44). Numerals represent the confidence level from 1,000 replicate bootstrap samplings. Values for frequencies of less than 50% are not given. This figure was reprinted from Sugita and Nakase (58) with permission. The amino acid designations indicate the assignment of the CUG codon within species on the phylogenetic tree that fall within the confines of the box.

Table 2. The optimal codon set of *C. albicans*

Amino acid	Codon	Amino acid	Codon	Amino acid	Codon	Amino acid	Codon
Phe	UUU[a,b]	Ser	UCU[a–c]	Tyr	UAU[a,b]	Cys	UGU[a–d]
	UUC[a,c]		UCC[c]		UAC[a,c]		UGC
Leu	UUA[a]		UCA[b]	Ter	UAA	Ter	UGA
	UUG[a–c]		UCG	Ter	UAG	Trp[e]	UGG
Leu	CUU	Pro	CUU	His	CAU[a,b]	Arg	CGU
	CUC		CCC		CAC[c]		CGC
	CUA		CCA[a–c]	Gln	CAA[a–c]		CGA
Leu/Ser	CUG		CCG		CAG		CGG
Ile	AUU[a–c]	Thr	ACU[a–c]	Asn	AAU[a,b]	Ser	AGU
	AUC[c]		ACC[c]		AAC[a,c]		AGC
	AUA		ACA	Lys	AAA[a,b]	Arg	AGA[a–c]
Met[e]	AUG		ACG		AAG[c]		AGG
Val	GUU[a–c]	Ala	GCU[a–c]	Asp	GAU[a,b]	Gly	GGU[a–c]
	GUC[c]		GCC		GAC[c]		GGC
	GUA		GCA	Glu	GAA[a–c]		GGA
	GUG		GCG		GAG		GGG

[a]Preferred codons (7).
[b]Most frequently used codons in 510 coding sequences (CUTG Codon Usage Database) (32).
[c]Optimal codons (29).
[d]Apparently optimal, but does not show a significant difference between highly and lowly expressed gene sets (29).
[e]Amino acids, which only have one codon and must therefore be, by definition, optimal.

They compared the preferred codons from *C. albicans, Schizosaccharomyces pombe,* and *S. cerevisiae* and found that, although they overlapped, there were significant differences between the codon sets of these organisms. They attributed this to differences in the percentage of A+T within the respective genomes of these different yeast species, although analysis of the coding sequences of these three species gives % A+T values of 63.2, 60.2, and 60.3%, respectively (32) (Table 3).

Subsequently, Lloyd and Sharp (29) performed a more comprehensive survey of codon usage in *C. albicans* and, furthermore, attempted to define the optimal codons for this organism (Table 2). Codons were identified as optimal by using statistical comparisons of the frequency of the occurrence of the different codons in data extracted from *C. albicans* coding sequences, divided according to the predicted level of expression of the genes (29). This study identified a bias toward codons in which the third base was either an A or T, within the 28 *C. albicans* coding sequences examined. A detailed analysis of the G+C distribution within the coding sequences of *C. albicans,* compared to *S. cerevisiae* and *S. pombe,* is shown in Table 3. This confirms that *C. albicans* does indeed show a strong bias against G+C at the third base (wobble) position of the codons used. This is also seen for *S. pombe,* while there is much less bias in *S. cerevisiae.* A+T seems to be biased against at the first base position for all three species.

The optimal codon set defined by Lloyd and Sharp (29) differed from the preferred codons of Brown et al. (7) due to the definition of optimal codons as being those that occur "significantly" more frequently within highly expressed coding sequences when compared to lowly expressed coding sequences,

Table 3. %G+C within codons of *C. albicans* compared to two other yeast species, *S. cerevisiae* and *S. pombe*[a]

Species	%G+C			
	Total coding sequence	First base	Second base	Third base
C. albicans	36.8	43.9	37.7	28.9
S. cerevisiae	39.7	44.6	36.6	38.0
S. pombe	39.8	48.2	38.2	33.2

[a]These data were obtained from the 2000 release of the Codon Usage Database (32).

and not merely the most commonly used codon. Indeed, two codons (AAG and GAC) defined by Lloyd and Sharp (29) as being optimal are not the most frequently used, in either the high or low expression data sets (divided according to the Codon Adaptation Indices [CAI] of the genes [52]). However, the significant change in use between highly and lowly expressed genes indicates a preference for these two codons in translation (29). The failure to distinguish between highly and lowly expressed genes when defining optimal codons is a deficiency in the codon usage data tabulated from "all coding sequences" submitted to GenBank by Nakamura et al. (32). Despite this deficiency, these data do provide a general indication of the overall codon usage within the genome of *C. albicans* (Table 2).

It has been widely observed that closely related species often share identical or similar optimal codon sets (53), despite interspecies genetic variation (21, 53). Indeed, this is the situation for *S. cerevisiae* and *C. albicans* (29), which use essentially the same optimal codon sets. Yet these two species decode one codon—the CUG codon—with an entirely different meaning, which suggests that the evolutionary pressures that establish codon bias are distinct from those underlying the evolution of codon reassignment (see "The Evolutionary Significance of Codon Reassignment in *Candida* spp.," below). Comparison of the relative use of members of the leucine and serine codon families in four different *Candida* species, for which a significant amount of sequence data exist, is shown in Table 4. Interestingly, in these three *Candida* species in which the CUG codon is decoded as serine, the CUG codon is only used between 1 and 3 per 1,000 codons, whereas in *C. glabrata, S. cerevisiae,* and *S. pombe,* where the CUG codon is decoded as leucine, it is used between 6 and 12 per 1,000 codons read. However, in both classes of yeasts, the CUN codon family is used much less frequently in coding sequences than the UUA/UUG leucine codon pair. Therefore, the CUG codon is not part of the optimal codon set in either group of yeasts, although it does appear to be an optimal codon in at least one *Candida* species, namely *C. cylindracea,* where only preliminary sequence data are available (32).

CUG Codon Ambiguity in *Candida* Species

Rather than being a completed evolutionary event leading to a fixed codon reassignment, there is increasing evidence that the nuclear genetic code is continuing to evolve within the *Candida* genus. There is no single unifying genetic code for the *Candida* genus, but rather subtle variations, or steps in the evolution, of a nonstandard code where the CUG codon is variously translated in a given species as either serine or leucine (Fig. 1, Table 4). However, the situation is more complicated than simply some species decoding the CUG codon as a serine and others decoding it as leucine. This complication arises from the fact that, in some *Candida* species, the CUG codon is "polysemous" in nature, that is, the tRNA species that decodes the CUG codon can be aminoacylated either with leucine or serine. Thus, in a number of *Candida* species, the CUG codon appears to have two distinct assignments with serine insertion predominating (61).

Table 4. Leu/Ser codon usage in *Candida* species, *S. cerevisiae*, and *S. pombe*[a]

Codon	Amino acid	Frequency per 1,000 codons					
		S. cerevisiae	*S. pombe*	*C. albicans*	*C. glabrata*	*C. maltosa*	*C. tropicalis*
UUA	L	26.3	26.3	33.6	16.7	34.3	18.0
UUG	L	27.1	24.1	36.3	33.9	46.2	57.8
CUU	L	12.2	25.4	9.8	9.1	7.9	6.6
CUC	L	5.4	7.3	2.5	2.8	1.9	3.0
CUA	L	13.4	8.7	4.0	13.9	1.1	1.3
CUG	L/S	<u>10.4</u> (L)	<u>6.4</u> (L)	<u>3.1</u> (S)	<u>12.0</u> (L)	<u>1.2</u> (S)	<u>1.6</u> (S)
UCU	S	23.6	30.3	23.4	22.3	22.3	20.9
UCC	S	14.2	12.1	10.3	18.0	13.4	20.7
UCA	S	18.8	18.0	24.6	15.7	9.0	10.9
UCG	S	8.6	8.1	6.5	5.1	2.7	3.6
AGU	S	14.2	14.7	16.2	10.4	11.1	8.0
AGC	S	9.7	9.2	4.6	6.3	2.1	4.6
No. of coding sequences		11,651	5,717	542	39	41	61

[a]The data are taken from the Codon Usage Database (32). The frequency of CUG codon usage is underlined in all species and the identity of the predominant amino acid inserted at the CUG codon for a given species is given in parentheses.

This codon ambiguity is thought to arise from the CUG-decoding Ser-tRNA$_{CAG}$ possessing a mixed identity with respect to its recognition by the corresponding aaRSs, namely the LeuRS and SerRS. It does not appear to be the result of either the LeuRS or the SerRS activating two amino acids (39, 61).

The polysemous nature of the CUG codon is best exemplified by *C. zeylanoides* where 3% of the Ser-tRNA$_{CAG}$ is leucylated, with the remainder being serylated in vivo (61) and subsequently incorporated into polypeptides in this relative proportion. The CUG codon is also polysemous in *C. maltosa* while in vitro experiments, using the *C. zeylanoides* LeuRS, have indicated that the CUG codon is also likely to be polysemous in *C. albicans, C. lusitaniae,* and *C. tropicalis* (61). At present there is no conclusive proof whether this is also true in vivo for these species. Certainly at the level of sensitivity of modern protein sequencing and mass spectrometry technology, no significant levels of leucine appear to be incorporated at CUG codons in *C. albicans* in vivo (46, 66). In contrast, *C. cylindracea* appears to decode the CUG codon "exclusively" as serine (61) while *C. glabrata, C. krusei,* and other *Candida* species decode the CUG codon exclusively as leucine (Fig. 1) (58).

The finding that *Candida* species can variously decode the CUG codon as either leucine, serine, or both has obvious implications with regard to the accuracy of in silico translations of *Candida*-derived DNA sequences in predicting the encoded polypeptide sequence (40). The simple solution is that the identity of each of the 64 codons should be confirmed by comparative gene and protein sequencing. There are also implications for the use of heterologous reporter genes in *Candida* species although here the solution is relatively trivial; either use a reporter gene, that does not naturally contain a CUG codon (e.g., the *Renilla reniformis* luciferase gene [56]) or replace the CUG codons with the leucine codons UUA/UUG as was done, for example, in the construction of a green fluorescent protein (yeGFP) reporter gene for *C. albicans* (8).

tRNAs AND THEIR GENES IN *C. ALBICANS*

The tRNA Repertoire of *C. albicans*

The bias observed in the relative usage of codons in mRNA correlates well with the relative abundance of the corresponding isoacceptor tRNAs that decode those codons (16, 21–23). The availability of genome sequence data, coupled with software that aids in the identification of tRNA genes (e.g., tRNA scan-SE [27]), allows us to identify the complete set of tRNA genes for a given organism and thereby to provide an insight into the flexibility that is allowed during codon : anticodon pairing at the so-called wobble base position, the third base of the codon. It was first proposed by Crick (10) that nonstandard base-pair interactions were allowable between the third (3′) base of the codon and the first (5′) base of the anticodon. These so-called "wobble rules" were subsequently revised as a consequence of the discovery that modification of bases in or close to the anticodon can further influence the nature of the wobble pair during mRNA decoding (68). The cataloguing of tRNA gene sets from genome sequences has allowed the ubiquity of the wobble rules to be further explored (e.g., 16, 42).

Complete eukaryotic tRNA sets have been determined for *S. cerevisiae* (42) and *Caenorhabditis elegans* (16). The *S. cerevisiae* tRNA genes have 42 distinct anticodons and require four deviations (one A:I and three G:U pairings) from the wobble rules to decode all the codons present within its coding sequences (42). Interestingly, there is no Ser- or Leu-tRNA with a CAG anticodon in *S. cerevisiae* (42). *C. elegans* contains tRNAs with 46 distinct anticodons, including a Leu-tRNA$_{CAG}$ that has six copies of the corresponding gene in the genome (16).

The near-complete genome sequence for *C. albicans* has allowed us to catalogue this species tRNA gene set (Table 5), which we find to be almost identical to the *S. cerevisiae* set, except that *C. albicans* apparently lacks tRNAs with the CGU anticodon (which should decode the ACG codons) and the ACG anticodon (which should decode the CGU, CGC, and CGA codons). Although the set is not complete (being derived from the 7× coverage *C. albicans* genomic DNA sequence release, June 2000), the data set provides an interesting insight into codon recognition in *C. albicans*. However, we believe that the tRNAs with 5′ CGU 3′ and 5′ ACG 3′ anticodons are present in *C. albicans* as the codons they decode are present in *Candida* coding sequences, albeit a very low frequency; in fact, stop codons apart, the CGC codon is the least used codon of all 61 sense codons in *C. albicans* mRNAs (32).

tRNA Gene Organization

The genes encoding tRNAs are transcribed by RNA polymerase III, which recognizes the conserved short sequences known as the A and B boxes within the transcribed region downstream of the transcription initiation site (55). The predicted *C. albicans* tRNA genes show similar organization to other eukaryotic tRNA genes and range in size from 71 nucleotides (Gly-tRNA$_{CCG}$, Gly-tRNA$_{GCC}$, and Gly-tRNA$_{UCC}$) to a maximum of 121 nucleotides (Leu-

Table 5. *C. albicans* tRNA set[a]

tDNA anticodon (3′–5′)	No. of tRNA genes[b]	Anticodon[c]	Codon(s) recognized	Amino acid
TGC	2	UGC	GCA, GCG	Ala
AGC	3	IGC	GCU, GCC	Ala
TCT	5	UCU	**AGA**	Arg
CCG	1	CCG	CGG	Arg
CCT	1	CCU	AGG	Arg
GTT	1	GUU	AAU, **AAC**	Asn
GTC	3	GUC	GAU, **GAC**	Asp
GCA	4	GCA	UGU, UGC	Cys
TTG	4	UUG	**CAA**	Gln
CTG	1	CUG	CAG	Gln
CTC	1	CUC	GAG	Glu
TTC	6	UUC	**GAA**	Glu
CCC	1	CCC	GGG	Gly
GCC	5	GCC	**GGU**, GGC	Gly
TCC	2	UCC	GGA	Gly
GTG	4	GUG	CAU, **CAC**	His
AAT	3	IAU	**AUU**, AUC	Ile
TAT	1	UAU	AUA	Ile
CAA	3	CAA	**UUG**	Leu
AAG	1	IAG	CUC, CUU, CUA	Leu
TAA	3	UAA	UUA	Leu
TTT	6	UUU	AAA	Lys
CTT	1	CUU	**AAG**	Lys
CAT	3	CAU	AUG	Met
GAA	4	GAA	**UUU**, UUC	Phe
AGG	1	IGG	CCU, CCC	Pro
TGG	2	UGG	**CCA**, CCG	Pro
TGA	3	UGA	UCA	Ser
AGA	4	IGA	**UCU**, **UCC**	Ser
CGA	1	CGA	UCG	Ser
CAG	1	CAG	CUG	Ser
GCT	3	GCU	AGU, AGC	Ser
AGT	4	IGU	**ACU**, **ACC**	Thr
TGT	2	UGU	ACA	Thr
GTA	2	GUA	**UAU**, UAC	Tyr
CCA	1	CCA	UGG	Trp
TAC	1	UAC	GUA	Val
CAC	1	CAC	GUG	Val
AAC	4	IAC	**GUU**, GUC	Val

[a]A screen of the 7× coverage *C. albicans* genome sequence data release (http://www-sequence.stanford.edu/group/candida/) using BlastN (1) at the NCBI, tRNAScan-E (27), and the *S. cerevisiae* tRNA gene sequences (42) was performed to identify the set of tRNA genes within *C. albicans*. Optimal codons are denoted in bold. The most frequently used codons, within the total gene coding sets (7, 32), are underlined. NOTE: The *C. albicans* tRNA set illustrated in this table is available from http://wwwbio.ukc.ac.uk/tuite/.

[b]The number of tRNA genes present within the *C. albicans* genome is an estimate based on the occurrence within the 7× coverage release.

[c]tRNA anticodons were derived from the anticodons predicted by the tRNA sequence gene, identified by tRNAScan-E (http://www.genetics.wustl.edu/eddy/tRNAscan-SE/) (27). Anticodon base modifications are not shown except for adenosine to inosine conversion at the first position of the anticodon, which is a general occurrence in eukaryotic nuclear tRNAs (26).

$tRNA_{AAG}$). Following splicing, the predicted tRNAs range in size from 71 to 85 nucleotides (Leu-$tRNA_{UAA}$ being the largest), excluding the CCA trinucleotide that is added to the 3′ end of the tRNA posttranscriptionally by the enzyme tRNA nucleotidyl-transferase (encoded in *C. albicans* by the *CCA1* gene). In *S. cerevisiae* some 21% of the identified tRNA genes contain small introns immediately 3′ to the anticodon sequence (18) while over half of the predicted *C. albicans* tRNA genes, currently identified (Table 5), also contain introns. The *C. albicans* tRNA gene introns vary between 10 (Gln-$tRNA_{UUG}$) and 43 (Tyr-$tRNA_{GUA}$) nucleotides in length, and all are predicted to occur in the standard position within the tRNA precursors, that is one base 3′ to the anticodon (65). There are several examples of *C. albicans* tRNA fami-

```
                                                          — intron —
2657KTTT GCCTAGCTAGCTCAATCGGCTTAGAGCGTGAGACTTTTAttacaagagtgATCTCAAGGT
2669KTTT GCCTAGCTAGCTCAATCGGCTTAGAGCGTGAGACTTTTA-----------ATCTCAAGGT
         ***************************************          **********

2657KTTT TGCGGGTTCGAGTCCCGCGTTGGGCT
2669KTTT TGCGGGTTCGAGTCCCGCGTTGGGCT
         **************************
```

Figure 2. Alignment of two Lys-tRNA$_{UUU}$-encoding genes illustrating the absence of an intron in one copy of the gene. Sequences were obtained from the 7× coverage *C. albicans* genomic DNA sequence release. The intron sequence is given in lowercase bold.

lies containing isoacceptors, some members of which contain introns and other members that do not (e.g., serine, leucine, glutamate, glutamine, and arginine). This allows the possibility that defective splicing may have had a role in the evolution of the Ser-tRNA$_{CAG}$, as suggested by Yokogawa et al. (67). Interestingly, one copy of the Lys-tRNA$_{UUU}$ gene contains an intron while another, which is otherwise 100% identical (Fig. 2) lacks the intron, suggesting that these two tRNAs may be in the process of diverging, with the intron-lacking tRNA possibly being derived by reverse transcription. Interestingly, Suzuki et al. (60) discovered that all five genes encoding the Ser-tRNA$_{CAG}$ of *C. cylindracea* lacked introns, but encoded the 3′ CCA sequence consistent with the amplification of these tRNA genes occurring via a reverse transcription-driven mechanism. There is currently no evidence that any of the *C. albicans* tRNA genes, including the Lys-tRNA$_{UUU}$ (Fig. 2), encode the 3′ CCA sequence.

THE CUG-DECODING Ser-tRNA$_{CAG}$

The Ser-tRNA$_{CAG}$ that decodes the CUG codon in various *Candida* species, while showing the characteristic cloverleaf secondary structure, does have a number of unusual structural features that may provide a molecular insight into the mechanism by which an organism can undergo a wholesale codon reassignment without eventual extinction. Perhaps the most striking feature is the presence of a guanosine at position 33 within the tRNA's anticodon loop (Fig. 3). This position, which is immediately adjacent to the 5′ base of the anticodon 5′ CAG 3′, is almost invariably occupied by a U in all cytoplasmic and organellar tRNAs so far described in prokaryotes and eukaryotes, although there are a few examples of tRNAs with a C33 (reviewed in reference 13). However, the only characterized tRNAs with G33 are the CUG-decoding Ser-tRNA$_{CAG}$ from *Candida* species. The presence of G at this position results in a significant long-range distortion at the top of the anticodon stem of the tRNA resulting in the top of the anticodon stem (43) (Fig. 3) being less susceptible to V1 ribonuclease, which specifically targets helical or stacked structures in a tRNA molecule (28). A U residue at position 33 does not cause such a distortion, but rather ensures that there is a correct turn of the phosphate backbone at that point, thereby stacking the anticodon bases in the correct orientation for the codon : anticodon interaction (4, 19).

The ambiguity of CUG decoding in certain *Candida* species, caused by the misacylation of the CUG-decoding tRNA, raises the question of whether the Ser-tRNA$_{CAG}$ contains the "identity determinants" recognized by both the LeuRS and the SerRS of these species. In studies carried out in *S. cerevisiae,* the regions of the cognate tRNA molecule recognized by the LeuRS and the SerRS, respectively, are quite different.

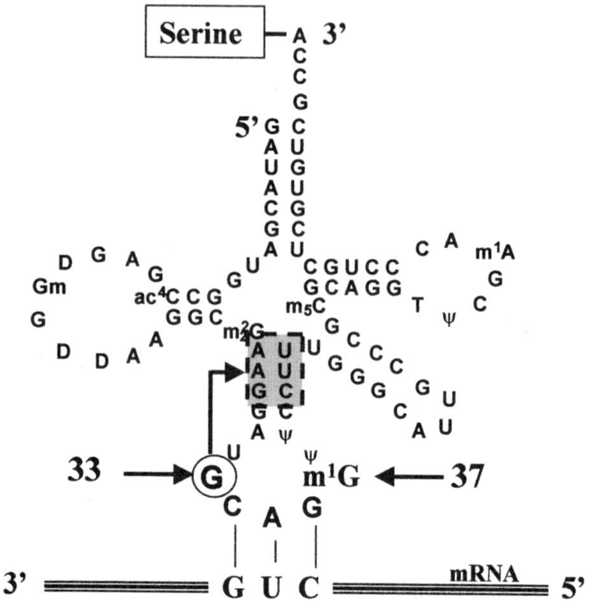

Figure 3. The ser-tRNA$_{CAG}$ that decodes the CUG codon in *C. albicans.* The positions of the G33 and m^{1}G37 nucleosides are indicated. The region of the anticodon stem, whose structure is influenced by G33, is indicated by the boxed and shaded region.

The *S. cerevisiae* LeuRS recognizes the D-loop and the anticodon stem (12) whereas the SerRS predominantly recognizes the variable arm and, to a lesser extent, the anticodon stem (14). Enzymatic and chemical probing of the *C. albicans* Ser-$tRNA_{CAG}$ has clearly shown that the key SerRS identity determinant of *S. cerevisiae* Ser-tRNA is structurally similar to the same region in the *C. albicans* Ser-$tRNA_{CAG}$ (43). This led to the conclusion that the *C. albicans* ser-$tRNA_{CAG}$ should be recognized by a normal cellular SerRS as opposed to a modified LeuRS recognizing a specialized tRNA. The fact that the *C. albicans* SerRS and LeuRS genes (*CaSES1* and *CaCDC60*, respectively) can functionally complement lethal knockouts of the corresponding genes in *S. cerevisiae* without detriment to the host (39, 40a) argues that neither can be considered as a specialized aaRS in *C. albicans*.

Comparison of the nucleotide sequence of the *C. albicans* ser-$tRNA_{CAG}$ genes (excluding introns) with the sequence of other Leu- and Ser-tRNA genes from *C. albicans* using ClustalW is consistent with it being more closely related to Ser-tRNAs. The *C. albicans* Ser-$tRNA_{CAG}$ shows 63 to 76% nucleotide identity with Ser-tRNAs, but only 52 to 63% identity with the Leu-tRNAs of the same species. The CUG-decoding Ser-$tRNA_{CAG}$ is most closely related in sequence terms to the UCG-decoding Ser-$tRNA_{CGA}$, suggesting that it may have evolved following a gene duplication event involving a Ser-$tRNA_{CGA}$ gene.

The sequences of Ser-$tRNA_{CAG}$ from a number of *Candida* species have now been deduced from cloned gene sequences and show between 74 and 98% nucleotide identity to the *C. albicans* tRNA (48 and references therein). All show the diagnostic G33 in the anticodon loop with the exception of *C. tropicalis*, which has C33 (64). The CUG-decoding tRNAs do, however, show a significant degree of variability at the top of the anticodon stem consistent with this region not being structurally constrained through evolution, presumably due to the distortion induced by the G33 (or C33), which disrupts intramolecular base pairing in this region (Fig. 3).

Significantly, all but one of the sequenced Ser-$tRNA_{CAG}$ contain the modified base methyl-1-guanosine (m^1G) at position 37, 3′ to the anticodon sequence (Fig. 3). m^1G37 is a key LeuRS determinant and Suzuki et al. (61) showed that this residue is critical for the leucylation of the Ser-$tRNA_{CAG}$. The presence of this base raises the issue of whether, in fact, this tRNA actually evolved from a Leu-tRNA (63). The absence of m^1G37 from the *C. cylindracea* Ser-$tRNA_{CAG}$ is consistent with that particular tRNA not being leucylated in vivo (61).

THE EVOLUTIONARY SIGNIFICANCE OF CODON REASSIGNMENT IN *CANDIDA* SPP.

Theories Proposed To Account for Codon Reassignment

The discovery, in the 1980s, of nonstandard genetic codes in mammalian mitochondria and later in bacteria, ciliates, and fungi has prompted much speculation about their origin and evolutionary significance (reviewed by in reference 38). However, the wide acceptance of the universality and immutability of the genetic code immortalized by the frozen accident theory (11) was a major obstacle to the development of new theories to explain how organisms and organelles evolved genetic codes that are different from the universal genetic code. The idea that alternative genetic codes were reminiscent versions of an ancient nonuniversal genetic code was rapidly rejected by molecular phylogenetic studies.

Until recently, the existence of alternative genetic codes was viewed as an aberration of nature and was believed to be of no true physiological or evolutionary significance. This conclusion arises from early work carried out on the effect of genomic G+C content fluctuations on codon usage that showed that rarely used codons can disappear from a genome under extreme G+C or A+T pressures (reviewed in reference 36). For example, in *Mycoplasma capricolum*, which has a very high genomic A+T content (75%), NNU/NNA codons predominate over NNC/NNG codons in this species mRNA, whereas the arginine CGG codon has yet to be detected (33). Interestingly, neither the tRNA with the anticodon 5′ CCG 3′ (decoding the codon CGG) nor its gene has been detected in this species (2, 30). Conversely, in *Micrococcus luteus*, which has a G+C-rich genome (75%), codons ending with G or C represent>95% of all codons and the AUA-Ile and AGA-Arg codons are apparently not used in the coding sequences of this microorganism (34). The apparent lack of the CGG, AUA, and AGA codons in both *M. capricolum* and *M. luteus* suggests that they were converted to synonymous codons and became unassigned in these organisms.

These observations prompted Jukes and Osawa to propose the "codon capture theory" to explain how codon reassignments can evolve. This theory postulates that codons that become unassigned can later be reassigned to other amino acids, through the mutation of other codons, provided mutant or natural tRNAs are available to decode them (37). The elegance of this theory is that it introduces evolutionary meaning to the genetic code and is not incompatible with a broad interpretation of the frozen accident theory (11). Furthermore, it introduces the concept that genetic code reassignments are a consequence of changes in genome G+C content that arise from alterations in the replication machinery. The existence of microorganisms containing unassigned codons can be taken to validate this theory.

A different view of the evolution of codon reassignment has been put forward by Schultz and Yarus (50). Their work on tRNA decoding, together with the recent work on CUG reassignment in *Candida* species, suggests that codon reassignment can occur without the need for codons to disappear from the genome (47, 51). This idea is based on the observations that tRNAs which reassign codons, in particular stop codons, are ambiguous decoders and furthermore codon ambiguity is not lethal if maintained under strict control (47). These observations are incorporated into the "ambiguous intermediate theory," which postulates that codon reassignment evolves in a stepwise manner through a mechanism requiring codon ambiguity (50).

The ambiguous intermediate theory is nonneutral and implies that aa-tRNA, aaRS, and release factor structural change, rather than alterations in genomic G+C content, are key factors in the evolution of genetic code changes (50, 51). That is, the translational machinery, rather than the transcriptional machinery, is the driving force of genetic code changes. It is not possible to exclude the complementarity of both theories in certain reassignments (Fig. 4); however, the two models are mechanistically distinct and have rather different evolutionary implications. The codon capture theory, being neutral, has no implication for the evolution of the coding sequences in the genome, since it does not increase the number of pseudogenes nor does it create new protein functionalities. Conversely, genetic code ambiguity introduces "mutations" during mRNA translation that have the potential to create new noninherited functionalities that are advantageous to the organism. Intriguingly, it is this apparent contradiction between decrease in fitness and increase in the potential to create functional diversity that might drive evolution of genetic code alterations. If so, it could be postulated that CUG reassignment in *Candida* species may have evolved to counteract the decrease in genetic diversity caused by the lack of a sexual cycle.

How CUG Codon Decoding Has Altered during the Evolutionary Divergence of *C. albicans* and *S. cerevisiae*

The reassignment of the CUG codon in *Candida* species is a paradigm for the evolution of codon reassignment through an ambiguous intermediate state (Fig. 4). The genetic code change is mediated by a novel Ser-$tRNA_{CAG}$, which has evolved a lower decoding efficiency to minimize the deleterious effects of serine-CUG decoding (45, 47, 61). That is, the novel Ser-$tRNA_{CAG}$ structure is in line with what would be predicted by the ambiguous intermediate theory, which postulates that tRNAs with unusual (i.e., ambiguous) decoding properties set the stage for codon reassignment (50, 51).

As described in "The CUG-Decoding Ser-$tRNA_{CAG}$" above, the novel CUG-decoding Ser-$tRNA_{CAG}$ has two main features: a guanosine at position 33 (G33) in place of the conserved pyrimidine 33 and both serine and leucine identity determinants (45, 47, 48, 62). Interestingly, these two features are apparently functionally contradictory in that G33 lowers the decoding efficiency of the Ser-$tRNA_{CAG}$ and is simultaneously a leucine identity antideterminant, that is, prevents leucylation of the tRNA at a high level (61). It is not yet clear why this is so, although it is likely that leucylation of the tRNA was acquired as a consequence of the introduction of a leucine anticodon-loop into a Ser-tRNA, hence incorporating two key leucine identity elements into the latter, i.e., A35 and m^1G37 (61). This is further confirmed by the fact that the Ser-$tRNA_{CAG}$ ancestor being a serine tRNA would have had an A37 (A37 or its modified derivatives are semiconserved in Ser-tRNA isoacceptors) and not m^1G37, which is characteristic of leucine tRNAs. That mutation of G37 to A37 in the *C. zeylanoides* Ser-$tRNA_{CAG}$, which is highly homologous to the *C. albicans* Ser-$tRNA_{CAG}$, abolishes leucine mischarging and the fact that the *C. cylindracea* Ser-$tRNA_{CAG}$, which also has A_{37}, is not leucylated confirms this hypothesis (61). That is, the important leucine identity element m^1G37 should have been a late acquisition in the evolution of the Ser-$tRNA_{CAG}$. Indeed, the requirement for m^1G37 might be structural because Leu-tRNAs containing G37 instead of m^1G37 lose decoding accuracy and frameshift (6, 17). If so, the decrease in decoding efficiency resulting from G33 is the key functional element of CUG reassignment because it allows for low-level Ser-CUG decoding, which is critical for maintaining serine substitution rates and hence toxicity to within tolerable limits.

Physiological Significance of CUG Reassignment

One of the most intriguing questions regarding the evolution of alternative genetic codes through decoding ambiguity is: "What selective advantages do they bring about to allow for their selection?" This is more intriguing if one considers that organisms have evolved highly accurate mechanisms to decode and

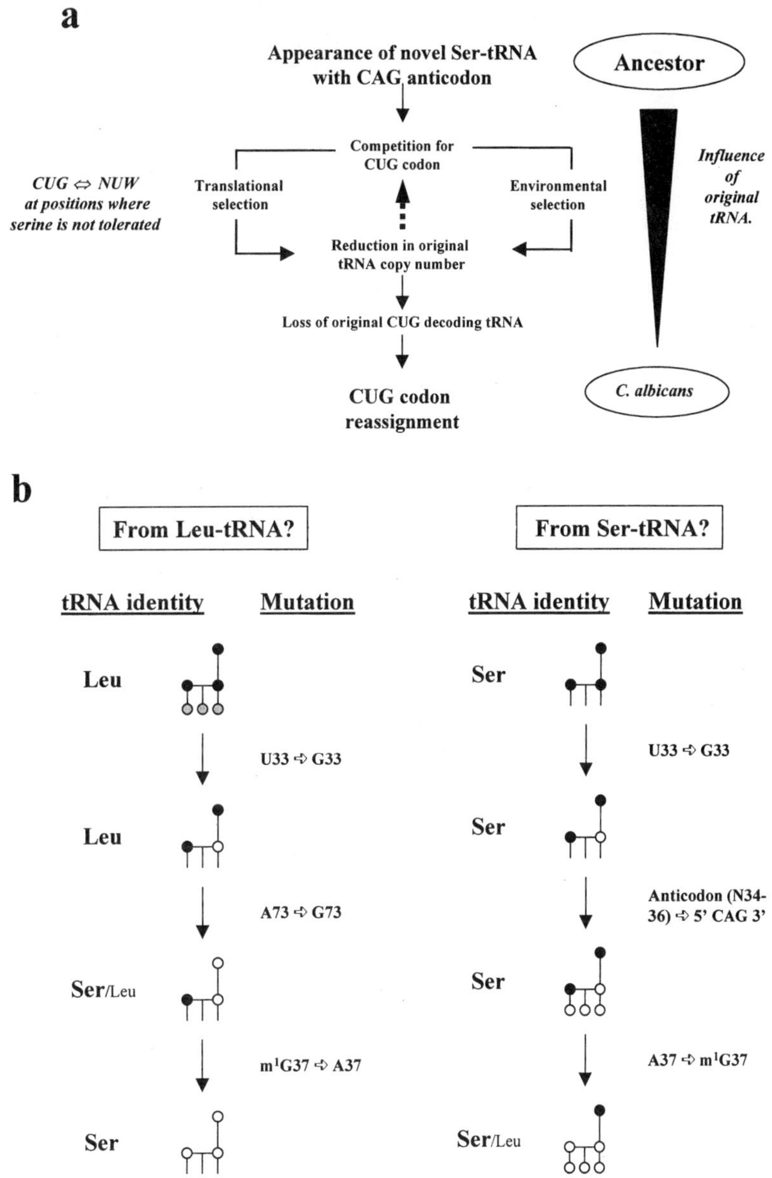

Figure 4. Pathway of CUG codon reassignment in *Candida* species. (A) Model for the evolution of codon reassignment. The model allows for the gradual reassignment in *Candida* spp. through a combination of the ambiguous intermediate theory and biased A + T pressure on genome composition. However, it does not explain the appearance of the novel CUG-decoding tRNA, which is explained in (B). The biased A + T pressure on genome composition is incorporated within the translational selection, in our model, which reduces the occurrence of the CUG codon within the coding sequences. The broken arrow indicates cycling until the eventual loss of the original CUG-decoding tRNA from the genome. N, any nucleotide (A, U, C, or G); W, A or U. (B) Model for the molecular evolution of the CUG-decoding tRNA. This model presents two possible progenitors for the CUG-decoding tRNA, either a Leu- or Ser-tRNA. Species designations next to tRNAs indicate the current situation in those species (see text). ○, position of important identity determinants and nucleotides within the tRNA. Alterations at positions other than those shown may have also been required to alter aminoacylation activity. Although not explicitly covered in this model, these substitutions can be accounted for by the insertion of more steps and have been excluded only for the sake of simplicity. ●, the ancestral base; ○, base substitution at that position; ◍, indicates that the ancestral Leu-tRNA may have contained an alternative anticodon and acquired a 5′ CAG 3′ anticodon through a nonlethal substitution, producing an isoaccepting tRNA, early in the evolution of the Ser-tRNA$_{CAG}$, prior to the acquisition of serine determinants.

transmit their genetic information and devote a significant part of their genomes and energy to ensure the high fidelity of DNA replication, transcription, and mRNA translation.

The first glimpse of a selective advantage produced by genetic code ambiguity was obtained from studies aimed at reconstructing the evolutionary pathway of CUG reassignment in *S. cerevisiae* (49). The data clearly show that CUG ambiguity, induced by expression of the *C. albicans* Ser-$tRNA_{CAG}$ in *S. cerevisiae,* triggers the general stress response, creating a heightened adaptation condition that allows the microorganism to tolerate lethal doses of stress agents, namely oxidants, heavy metals, and drugs (49). In a sense, this physiological condition mimics the increase in stress tolerance observed by preincubating a yeast culture for short periods in nonlethal doses of stress agents and then exposing it to lethal doses. Under these growth conditions, cells preadapt and are able to tolerate what would normally be lethal doses of that agent (reviewed by Siderius and Mager [54]).

Studies carried out by us clearly show that despite the dramatic decrease in growth rate, *S. cerevisiae* cells expressing CUG ambiguity are able to grow in the presence of doses of arsenite and cadmium that are lethal to wild-type cells (49). That is, the defect in growth rate is not an impediment to competition under these growth conditions and, therefore, these microorganisms have the potential for exploiting new ecological niches. The relevance of this to CUG reassignment in *C. albicans* needs to be determined; however, it indicates that genetic code ambiguity can create important selective advantages that could drive codon reassignment (49). It remains to be established whether the evolution of codon reassignment in *Candida* species contributed to the evolution of their pathogenicity.

Acknowledgments. Sequence data for *C. albicans* were obtained from the Stanford DNA Sequencing and Technology Center website at http://www-sequence.stanford.edu/group/candida. Sequencing of *C. albicans* was accomplished with the support of the NIDR and the Burroughs Wellcome Fund. Research on mRNA decoding in *Candida* species in the authors' laboratories was supported by research funds from the BBSRC (MFT), the Wellcome Trust (MFT/MAS), and the Portuguese Foundation for Science and Technology (MAS).

REFERENCES

1. **Altschul, S. F., T. L. Madden, A. A. Schäffer, J. Zhang, Z. Zhang, W. Miller, and D. J. Lipman.** 1997. Gapped BLAST and PSI-BLAST: a new generation of protein database search programs. *Nucleic Acids Res.* **25:**3389–3402.
2. **Andachi, Y., F. Yamao, M. Iwami, A. Muto, and S. Osawa.** 1989. Codon recognition patterns as deduced from sequences of the complete set of transfer RNA species in *Mycoplasma capricolum:* resemblance to mitochondria. *J. Mol. Biol.* **209:**37–54.
3. **Andersson, S. G. E., and C. G. Kurland.** 1990. Codon preferences in free living microorganisms. *Microbiol. Rev.* **54:**198–210.
4. **Ashraf, S. S., G. Ansari, R. Guenther, E. Sochacka, A. Malkiewicz, and P. Agris.** 1999. The uridine in "U-turn": contributions to tRNA-ribosomal binding. *RNA* **5:**503–511.
5. **Berg, O. G., and C. G. Kurland.** 1997. Growth rate-optimised tRNA abundance and codon usage. *J. Mol. Biol.* **270:**544–550.
6. **Björk, G. R., P. M. Wikstrom, and A. S. Byström.** 1989. Prevention of translational frameshifting by the modified nucleoside 1-methylguanosine. *Science* **244:**986–989.
7. **Brown, A. J. P., G. Bertram, J. F. Feldmann, M. W. Peggie, and R. K. Swoboda.** 1991. Codon utilisation in the pathogenic yeast, *Candida albicans. Nucleic Acids Res.* **19:**4298.
8. **Cormack, B. P., G. Bertram, M. Egerton, N. A. R. Gow, S. Falkow, and A. J. P. Brown.** 1997. Yeast-enhanced green fluorescent protein (yeGFP): a reporter of gene expression in *Candida albicans. Microbiology* **143:**303–311.
9. **Crick, F. H.** 1963. The recent excitement in the coding problem. *Prog. Nucleic Acid Res.* **1:**163–217.
10. **Crick, F. H.** 1966. Codon-anticodon pairing: the wobble hypothesis. *J. Mol. Biol.* **19:**548–555.
11. **Crick, F. H.** 1968. The origin of the genetic code. *J. Mol. Biol.* **38:**367–379.
12. **Dietrich, A., P. Romby, L. Marechal-Drouard, P. Guillemaut, and R. Giege.** 1990. Solution conformation of several free $tRNA^{Leu}$ species from bean, yeast and *Escherichia coli* and interaction of these tRNAs with bean cytoplasmic leucyl-tRNA synthetase. A phosphate alkylation study with ethylnitrosourea. *Nucleic Acids Res.* **18:**2589–2597.
13. **Dirheimer, G., G. Keith, P. Dumas, and E. Westhof.** 1995. Primary, secondary, and tertiary structures of tRNAs, p. 207–224. *In* D. Söll and U. L. Rajbhandary (ed.), *tRNA: Structure, Biosynthesis, and Function.* ASM Press, Washington, D.C.
14. **Dock-Bregeon, A. C., E. Westhof, R. Giege, and D. Moras.** 1989. Solution structure of a tRNA with a large variable region: yeast $tRNA^{Ser}$. *J. Mol. Biol.* **206:**707–722.
15. **Dong, H., L. Nilsson, and C. G. Kurland.** 1996. Co-variation of tRNA abundance and codon usage in *Escherichia coli* at different growth rates. *J. Mol. Biol.* **260:**649–663.
16. **Duret, L.** 2000. tRNA gene number and codon usage in the *C. elegans* genome are co-adapted for optimal translation of highly expressed genes. *Trends Genet.* **16:**287–289.
17. **Hagervall, T. G., T. M. Tohy, J. F. Atkins, and G. R. Björk.** 1993. Deficiency of 1-methylguanosine in tRNA from *Salmonella typhimurium* induces frameshifting by quadruplet translocation. *J. Mol. Biol.* **232:**5794–5801.
18. **Hani, J., and H. Feldman.** 1998. tRNA genes and retroelements in the yeast genome. *Nucleic Acids Res.* **26:**689–696.
19. **Hermann, T., and D. J. Patel.** 1999. Stitching together RNA tertiary architectures. *J. Mol. Biol.* **294:**829–849.
20. **Ikemura, T.** 1981. Correlation between the abundance of *Escherichia coli* transfer RNAs and the occurrence of the respective codons in its protein genes. *J. Mol. Biol.* **146:**1–21.
21. **Ikemura, T.** 1985. Codon usage and tRNA content in unicellular and multicellular organisms. *Mol. Biol. Evol.* **2:**13–34.
22. **Ikemura, T., and H. Ozeki.** 1982. Codon usage and transfer RNA contents: organism-specific codon-choice patterns in reference to the isoacceptor contents. *Symp. Quant. Biol.* **XLVII:**1087–1097.
23. **Kanaya, S., Y. Yamada, Y. Kudo, and T. Ikemura.** 1999. Studies of codon usage and tRNA genes of 18 unicellular organisms

and quantification of *Bacillus subtilis* tRNAs: gene expression level and species-specific diversity of codon usage based on multivariate analysis. *Gene* **238:**143–155.

24. **Kawaguchi, Y., H. Honda, J. Taniguchi-Morimura, and S. Iwasaki.** 1989. The codon CUG is read as serine in an asporogenic yeast *Candida cylindracea*. *Nature* **341:**164–166.
25. **Kimura, M.** 1980. A simple method for estimation of evolutionary rate of base substitutions through comparative studies of nucleotide sequences. *J. Mol. Evol.* **16:**111–120.
26. **Lim, V. I.** 1995. Analysis of action of the wobble adenine on codon reading within the ribosome. *J. Mol. Biol.* **252:** 277–282.
27. **Lowe, T., and S. R. Eddy.** 1997. tRNAscan-SE: a program for improved detection of transfer RNA genes in genomic sequence. *Nucleic Acids Res.* **25:**955–964.
28. **Lowman, H. B., and D. E. Draper.** 1986. On the recognition of helical RNA by cobra venom V_1 nuclease. *J. Biol. Chem.* **261:**5396–5403.
29. **Lloyd, A. T., and P. M. Sharp.** 1992. Evolution of codon usage patterns: the extent and nature of divergence between *Candida albicans* and *Saccharomyces cerevisiae*. *Nucleic Acids Res.* **20:** 5289–5295.
30. **Muto, A., Y. Andachi, H. Yuzawa, F. Yamao, and S. Osawa.** 1990. The organization and evolution of transfer RNA genes of *Mycoplasma capricolum*. *Nucleic Acids Res.* **18:** 5037–5043.
31. **Nakamura, Y., T. Gojobori, and T. Ikemura.** 1999. Codon usage tabulated from the international DNA sequence databases; its status 1999. *Nucleic Acids Res.* **27:**292.
32. **Nakamura, Y., T. Gojobori, and T. Ikemura.** 2000. Codon usage tabulated from the international DNA sequence databases: status for the year 2000. *Nucleic Acids Res.* **28:**292.
33. **Oba, T., Y. Andachi, A. Muto, and S. Osawa.** 1991. CGG, unassigned or nonsense codon: occurrence in *Mycoplasma capricolum*. *Proc. Natl. Acad. Sci. USA* **88:**921–925.
34. **Ohama, T., A. Muto, and S. Osawa.** 1990. Role of GC-biased mutation pressure on synonymous codon choice in *Micrococcus luteus*, a bacterium with a high genomic GC-content. *Nucleic Acids. Res.* **18:**1565–1569.
35. **Ohama, T., T. Suzuki, M. Mori, S. Osawa, T. Ueda, K. Watanabe, and T. Nakase.** 1993. Non-universal decoding of the leucine codon CUG in several *Candida* species. *Nucleic Acids Res.* **21:**4039–4045.
36. **Osawa, S.** 1995. *Evolution of the Genetic Code.* Oxford University Press, Oxford, United Kingdom.
37. **Osawa, S., and T. H. Jukes.** 1989. Codon reassignment (codon capture) in evolution. *J. Mol. Evol.* **28:**271–278.
38. **Osawa, S., T. H. Jukes, K. Watanabe, and A. Muto.** 1992. Recent evidence for evolution of the genetic code. *Microbiol. Rev.* **5:**229–264.
39. **O'Sullivan, J. M., M. J. Mihr, M. A. S. Santos, and M. F. Tuite.** 2001. An alteration in the structure and function of the seryl-tRNA synthetase is not responsible for the evolution of CUG codon reassignment in *Candida albicans*. *Yeast* **18:** 313–322.
40. **O'Sullivan, J. M., J. B. Davenport, and M. F. Tuite.** 2001. Codon reassignment and the evolving genetic code: problems and pitfalls in the sequencing era. *Trends Genet.* **17:**20–22.

40a. **O'Sullivan, J. M., M. J. Mihr, M. A. S. Santos, and M. F. Tuite.** The *Candida albicans* gene encoding the cytoplasmic leucyl-tRNA synthetase: implications for the evolution of CUG codon reassignment. *Gene,* in press.

41. **Parker, J.** 1989. Errors and alternatives in reading the universal genetic code. *Microbiol. Rev.* **53:**273–298.
42. **Percudani, R., A. Pavesi, and S. Ottonello.** 1997. Transfer RNA gene redundancy and translational selection in *Saccharomyces cerevisiae*. *J. Mol. Biol.* **268:**322–330.
43. **Perreau, V. M., G. Keith, W. M. Holmes, A. Przykorska, M. A. S. Santos, and M. F. Tuite.** 1999. The *Candida albicans* CUG-decoding ser-tRNA has an atypical anticodon stem-loop structure. *J. Mol. Biol.* **293:**1039–1053.
44. **Saito, N., and M. Nei.** 1987. The neighbour-joining method: a new method for reconstructing phylogenetic trees. *Mol. Biol. Evol.* **4:**406–425.
45. **Santos, M. A. S., G. Keith, and M. F. Tuite.** 1993. Non-standard translational events in *Candida albicans* mediated by a unusual $tRNA^{Ser}$ with a 5′-CAG-3′ (leucine) anticodon. *EMBO J.* **12:**607–616.
46. **Santos, M. A. S., and M. F. Tuite.** 1995. The CUG codon is decoded in vivo as serine and not leucine in *Candida albicans*. *Nucleic Acids Res.* **23:**1481–1486.
47. **Santos, M. A. S., M. V. Perreau, and M. F. Tuite.** 1996. Transfer RNA structural change is a key element in the reassignment of the CUG codon in *Candida albicans*. *EMBO J.* **15:** 5060–5068.
48. **Santos, M. A. S., T. Ueda, K. Watanabe, and M. F. Tuite.** 1997. The non-standard genetic code of *Candida* spp.: an evolving genetic code or a novel mechanism for adaptation? *Mol. Microbiol.* **26:**423–431.
49. **Santos, M. A. S., C. Cheesman, V. Costa, P. Moradas-Ferreira, and M. F. Tuite.** 1999. Selective advantages created by codon ambiguity allowed for evolution of an alternative genetic code in *Candida* spp. *Mol. Microbiol.* **31:**937–947.
50. **Schultz, D. W., and M. Yarus.** 1994. Transfer RNA mutation and the malleability of the genetic code. *J. Mol. Biol.* **235:** 1377–1380.
51. **Schultz, D. W., and M. Yarus.** 1996. On the malleability in the genetic-code. *J. Mol. Evol.* **42:**597–601.
52. **Sharp, P. M., and W.-H. Li.** 1986. An evolutionary perspective on synonymous codon usage in unicellular organisms. *J. Mol. Evol.* **24:**28–38.
53. **Sharp, P. M., E. Cowe, D. G. Higgins, D. C. Shields, K. H. Wolfe, and F. Wright.** 1988. Codon usage patterns in *Escherichia coli, Bacillus subtilis, Saccharomyces cerevisiae, Schizosaccharomyces pombe, Drosophila melanogaster* and *Homo sapiens:* a review of the considerable within-species diversity. *Nucleic Acids Res.* **16:**8207–8211.
54. **Siderius, M., and W. H. Mager.** 1997. General stress response: in search of a common denominator, p. 213–224. *In* S. Hohmann and W. H. Mager (ed.), *Yeast Stress Responses.* Chapman and Hall, New York, N.Y.
55. **Sprague, K. U.** 1995. Transcription of eukaryotic tRNA genes, p. 31–50. *In* D. Söll and U. L. Rajbhandary (ed.), *tRNA: Structure, Biosynthesis, and Function.* ASM Press, Washington, D.C.
56. **Srikantha, T., A. Klapach, W. W. Lorenz, L. K. Tsai, L. A. Laughlin, J. A. Gorman, and D. R. Soll.** 1996. The sea pansy *Renilla reniformis* luciferase serves as a sensitive bioluminescent reporter for differential gene expression in *Candida albicans*. *J. Bacteriol.* **178:**121–129.
57. **Stansfield, I., K. M. Jones, P. Herbert, A. Lewendon, W. V. Shaw, and M. F. Tuite.** 1998. Missense translation errors in *Saccharomyces cerevisiae*. *J. Mol. Biol.* **282:**13–24.
58. **Sugita, T., and T. Nakase.** 1999. Non-universal usage of the leucine CUG codon and the molecular phylogeny of the genus *Candida*. *System. Appl. Microbiol.* **22:**79–86.
59. **Sugiyama, H., M. Ohkuma, Y. Masuda, S. M. Park, A. Ohta, and M. Takagi.** 1995. In vivo evidence for non-universal usage of the codon CUG in *Candida maltosa*. *Yeast* **11:**43–52.
60. **Suzuki, T., T. Ueda, T. Yokogawa, K. Nishikawa, and K. Watanabe.** 1994. Characterisation of serine and leucine

tRNAs in an asporogenic yeast *Candida cyclindracea* and evolutionary implications of genes for $tRNA^{Ser}{}_{CAG}$ responsible for translation of a non-universal genetic code. *Nucleic Acids Res.* **22:**115–123.

61. **Suzuki, T., T. Ueda, and K. Watanabe.** 1997. Polysemous codon: a codon with multiple amino acid assignment caused by dual specificity of tRNA identity. *EMBO J.* **16:**1122–1134.
62. **Tuite, M. F., P. A. Bower, and C. S. McLaughlin.** 1986. A novel suppressor tRNA from the dimorphic fungus *Candida albicans. Biochim. Biophys. Acta* **866:**26–31.
63. **Tuite, M. F., and M. A. S. Santos.** 1996. Codon reassignment in *Candida* species: an evolutionary conundrum. *Biochimie* **78:** 993–999.
64. **Ueda, T., T. Suzuki, T. Yokogawa, K. Nishikawa, and K. Watanabe.** 1994. Unique structure of new serine tRNAs responsible for decoding leucine codon CUG in various *Candida* species and their putative ancestral tRNA genes. *Biochimie* **76:** 1217–1222.
65. **Westaway, S. K., and J. Abelson.** 1995. Splicing of tRNA precursors, p. 79–82. *In* D. Söll and U. L. Rajbhandary (ed.), *tRNA: Structure, Biosynthesis, and Function.* ASM Press, Washington, D.C.
66. **White, T. C., L. E. Andrews, D. Maltby, and N. Agabian.** 1995. The 'universal' leucine codon CTG in the secreted aspartyl proteinase 1 (*SAP1*) gene of *Candida albicans* encodes a serine in vivo. *J. Bacteriol* **177:**2953–2955.
67. **Yokogawa, T., T. Suzuki, T. Ueda, M. Mori, T. Ohama, Y. Kuchino, S. Yoshinari, I. Motoki, K. Nishikawa, S. Osawa, and K. Watanabe.** 1992. Serine tRNA complementary to the non-universal serine codon CUG in *Candida cylindracea:* evolutionary implications. *Proc. Natl. Acad. Sci. USA* **89:** 7408–7411.
68. **Yokoyama, S., and S. Nishimura.** 1995. Modified nucleosides and codon recognition, p. 207–224. *In* D. Söll and U. L. Rajbhandary (ed.), *tRNA: Structure, Biosynthesis, and Function.* ASM Press, Washington, D.C.

Candida and Candidiasis
Edited by Richard A. Calderone

Chapter 21

The Genomes of *Candida albicans* and Other *Candida* Species

P. T. Magee and Hiroji Chibana

For many years, the only way to analyze fungal genomes was via genetics, and genomic landmarks such as chromosome size and number and locations of centromeres were inferred from genetic data. However, the advent of pulse-field gel electrophoresis has allowed the direct observation of the DNA molecules that make up the chromosomes of fungi (as well as many other organisms), and analysis of the genome of *Candida albicans* is quite well advanced. We now know the number and physical size of the chromosomes, the locations of many of the genes, the location and structure of the telomeres and some of the centromeres, and the surprising variability of the chromosomal structure. In addition, the entire DNA sequence of the genome is known (see chapter 18). In this chapter we will discuss the physical features of the genome of *C. albicans* and will compare these results with the information available about other members of the genus.

GENOME SIZE OF *CANDIDA* SPECIES

C. albicans is diploid and has about 32 Mbp of nuclear DNA per cell; hence, the haploid genome size is 16 Mbp. That the organism is diploid was first suggested by Olaiya and Sogin, based on the fact that its sensitivity to UV light is similar to that of diploid *Saccharomyces cerevisiae* (54). However, since radiation sensitivity is a function of repair capacity as well as gene number, the ploidy could not be definitively determined in this way. Whelan and Magee demonstrated that natural isolates were heterozygous for several genes and suggested that the most likely explanation for this was that the organism is diploid (83, 84). Riggsby et al. used DNA-DNA hybridization to show that the amount of unique DNA per cell (15 to 20 pg) is about half the cellular DNA content (37 pg), providing physical confirmation of the genetic results (61). The estimate of repeated nuclear DNA was about 3% (61, 88). Whelan later showed genetically that *Candida parapsilosis* and *Candida krusei* are also diploid (81, 82). *Candida (Torulopsis) glabrata,* on the other hand, is haploid. Since this organism is more closely related to *S. cerevisiae* than to *C. albicans,* it is perhaps not so surprising that it differs from other *Candida* strains (33). Exhaustive analysis of the information content of species other than *C. albicans* has not been carried out.

BASIC STUDIES OF GENOMIC VARIABILITY

Early efforts at separation of the *C. albicans* chromosomes by use of pulse-field electrophoresis revealed that the electrophoretic karyotype of this organism is highly variable from isolate to isolate (34, 42, 47, 74, 75). The variability in the genome reflects a variety of genomic alterations. These include translocation, deletion, amplification, and loss of particular chromosomes (13, 23, 53, 64, 66–68, 79), aneuploidy and ploidy change (25, 44, 55, 76, 77), and chromosome length polymorphisms (CLP) (6).

The sequence of *C. albicans* strain SC5314 has been determined (see chapter 18); this strain was chosen because it is the progenitor of CAI4, which has become the major strain used for molecular genetics. In the end, the sequence data and the physical mapping data will provide mutual verification, and ambiguities from one approach will likely be resolved using data from the other. Mapping is also required because sequence data alone are not useful for the examination and elucidation of karyotypic alterations. This is particularly true since CAI4 was constructed from strain SC5314 partly because the latter has a "standard" karyotype; hence, the canonical sequence will

P. T. Magee • Department of Genetics, Cell Biology, and Genetics, University of Minnesota, St. Paul, MN 55105. Hiroji Chibana • Research Center for Pathogenic Fungi and Microbial Toxicoses, Chiba University, 1-8-1, Inohana, Chuo-Ku, Chiba 260-8673, Japan.

be that of the most frequent chromosomal configuration. All of the karyotypic variations are found in specific strains; sequencing of all the nonstandard strains is not feasible. In addition, many of the karyotypic changes are translocations, which take place around a repeated element of intermediate frequency. This element, called the major repeat sequence (MRS), will be described in detail below. Its size, which is much greater than the average sequencing run, means that the sequence assembly programs assemble unique DNA up to the edge of the MRS but cannot cross it; thus, these elements mark the end of unique DNA contigs in the assembled sequence.

Mapping is also required for the analysis of aneuploidy, since heterogeneity (heterozygosity) in the DNA sequence of a particular region indicates diploidy (or higher ploidy), but homozygosity does not necessarily indicate whether a chromosome is present in one or more than one copy. Mapping and sequence data together are useful for analyzing CLP, which may be due to a number of events, including deletion, addition, or expansion and contraction in the number of internal repeats.

Karyotype variability thus requires a physical map as well as the DNA sequence for elucidation, even though advanced computing power and sequencing methods make a map superfluous for organizing projects to sequence even very large genomes. For *C. albicans,* a sequence-tagged site map is being constructed using a 10× genomic library in a fosmid vector. The fosmid was constructed for cloning human DNA, which has a high number of repeats; hence, the tandemly repeated nature of the MRS is stably maintained in a fosmid library. The complete map of chromosome 7 has been determined using this library (8), and much of what was learned (for example, the nature of the telomeric sub-repeats) has been helpful in mapping the rest of the genome.

The standard karyotype of *C. albicans* is defined as that in which chromosomes containing largely homologous genetic information migrate together on a pulse-field gel. In this karyotype, the number of chromosomal bands is 8; hence, the diploid chromosome number of *C. albicans* is 16. The chromosomes are numbered from 1 (largest) to 7 (smallest). The largest chromosome is not numbered; it is denoted chromosome R because it contains the ribosomal DNA (rDNA) cistrons. The rDNA cistrons are found in tandem arrays on the two homologs of this chromosome, but the number of copies of the repeat usually differs between the two homologs. Furthermore, the number on a given homolog can change upon cultivation due to sister-chromatid exchange, which changes the number of tandem repeats on the chromosome. Chromosome R was not given a number, since the positions

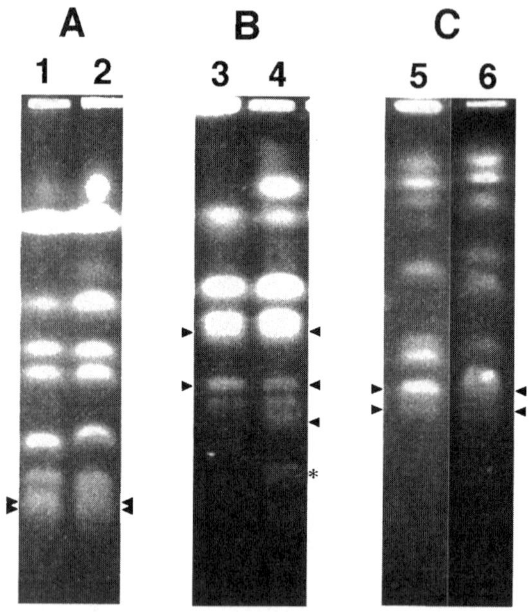

Figure 1. Contour-clamped homogeneous electric field pulse-field separations of *C. albicans* chromosomes. The procedures for DNA preparation and chromosome separation are described in reference 44. (A) Lane 1, strain 1006; lane 2, strain CAI4. (B) Lane 3, strain WO-2; lane 4, strain WO-1. (C) Lane 5, strain NUM114; lane 6, strain 1796. The arrows show chromosome 7 and its translocation products; in lanes 3 and 4, the upper two arrows show the chromosome 4,7 and 7,4 translocation products. The asterisk in lane 4 shows the 5,6 translocation in WO-1, which is lost in WO-2; the intact homolog of chromosome 7 in WO-1, indicated by the lowest arrowhead, is also lost in WO-2.

of its homologs on a pulse-field gel are variable because of the variation in distribution of the rDNA cistrons between them. Variation in the size of these homologs during serial culture has been demonstrated (21, 63). The estimated sizes of the various chromosomes in the karyotype of strain 1006 are discussed below. The most precisely measured is chromosome 7, where the physical map was calibrated by means of random breakage mapping in strain 1006 (8). The assembly of the complete sequence at the Stanford Genome Center has confirmed the physical map, including the order of markers and their relationship to the MRSs (http://www-sequence.stanford.edu/group/candida/).

The standard karyotype (Fig. 1A) is found in approximately 60 to 70% of clinical isolates of *C. albicans* (46). This karyotype has been well characterized and is the basis for the sequence assembly and for the map. There is a standard assignment of genes to the chromosomes; this assignment is given on the *C. albicans* web page (http://alces.med.umn.edu/candida.html). Slightly fewer than half of clinical isolates show variation in several parameters, including the size of chromosomes (often the two homologs are resolvable on pulse-field gels), the presence of extra bands, and/or the absence of particular bands. An example of a karyotype with both extra bands and absent bands is shown in Fig. 1B. This karyotype was made from strain WO-2, an aneuploid strain that arose from the clinical isolate WO-1 spontaneously in the laboratory (44). Note the new band between chromosomes 4 and 5 as well as the absence of chromosome 7 in this karyotype. Figure 1C shows a strain in which the two homologs of chromosome 7 are separable.

Diagrams of the karyotypes of *C. albicans* strains 1006 and WO-1 are shown in Color plate 7. The sizes of the chromosomes in the plate are not proportional; the breaks in the chromosomes correspond to sites for the 8-bp-specific restriction enzyme *Sfi*I. The fragments generated by *Sfi*I digestion are named according to their chromosomal origin and their size (4BB [45 kb] is the smallest and rV [2,500 kb] is the largest). The relationship of these sites to chromosome structure is described below.

Length polymorphism in *C. albicans* chromosomes is common, and the situation illustrated in Fig. 1C, homologs of unequal size, is often seen. However, before concluding that two closely adjacent bands are truly homologs of the same chromosome, one must verify their identity with probes whose chromosomal location is known (40, 85). Analysis of chromosome 7 in several strains with different-sized homologs suggests that much, if not all, of the length polymorphism is due to differences in the size of the MRS on different homologs (6). Other CLPs may be due to variation in the size of the telomeres or to small translocations, which add or subtract only a few tens of kilobases in size to the chromosome affected.

ROLE OF THE MRS IN GENOME VARIABILITY

It now seems clear that a great deal of the karyotypic variability found in *C. albicans* is associated with the intermediate repeat element called MRS. This element has been extensively studied by Tanaka and coworkers. It consists of three elements: HOK, about 5,200 bp; RPS, varying in size from 2 to 2.9 kb; and RB2, about 4 kb (7, 12, 20). The numbers are approximate because it is likely that copies on different chromosomes differ in size. The MRS is found on all chromosomes except chromosome 3; an analogous but largely nonhomologous sequence (26) is found in *C. dubliniensis* (44a). There is sequence variation in the separate copies of the MRS; for example, the different HOK sequences cloned from strain FC18 vary in homology from 82 to 97%. The arrangement of the MRS is shown in Color plate 7. We have adopted the convention of indicating its orientation by putting an arrowhead at the HOK side. The HOK sequence has a 35% GC content and has three small open reading frames, with one having homology to portions of the isocitrate dehydrogenase from *S. cerevisiae,* but this seems to be a pseudogene, since it contains many stop codons (12).

The RPS is usually tandemly repeated in the MRS, with the number of repeats of the whole unit varying from a few to as many as 50 (20, 35a). Within the RPS there are smaller tandem repeats called alts; these are about 172 bp in size. The alts are composed of 143 bp, which can vary in sequence between the different kinds of alt, followed by a sequence that is very highly conserved, COM29. This sequence contains a site for the 8-bp specific restriction enzyme, *Sfi*I. There are at least four different alts. The size of the RPS depends on the number of alt repeating units within it. The repeating alt region is flanked by DNA with high homology among the different RPS units. Homology of the RPS region is much higher than that of HOK, with the major difference coming from the number and kind of internal alt repeats (Fig. 2) (7, 20). Because of the *Sfi*I sites in the RPS, most of the *Sfi*I fragments generated from a digestion of the genome are generated by digestion in these repeats; however, there are several *Sfi*I sites that are in unique DNA.

The variability of composition of the MRS is the basis of a great deal of the genomic variability of *C. albicans.* Chibana et al. have shown that CLP is usually the result of variation in the sizes of the MRS on the specific chromosomes. In an intensive investigation of chromosome 7 they showed that size differences in the MRS accounted for almost all of the differences in length of the homologs both within and between strains (6). It seems likely, although it is of course not known at this time that this will be true throughout the genome.

Evidence that variation can occur in the MRS region within a strain lineage comes from the work of Soll and collaborators. This group showed that the differences in the restriction patterns are functions of the variation in the MRS. Since these can occur during culture, it seems clear that the structure of the MRS is dynamic both in vitro and in vivo (60).

What is the basis of the variation revealed by Ca3, 27A, and RPS? Ca3 (69), 27A (71), and RPS (20) have all been used as tools for the epidemiological analysis of *C. albicans.* Using Ca3 in particular, Soll and collaborators have published an extensive series of papers using molecular fingerprinting to examine both epidemiology and genomic changes during the course of infection and also during cultivation in the

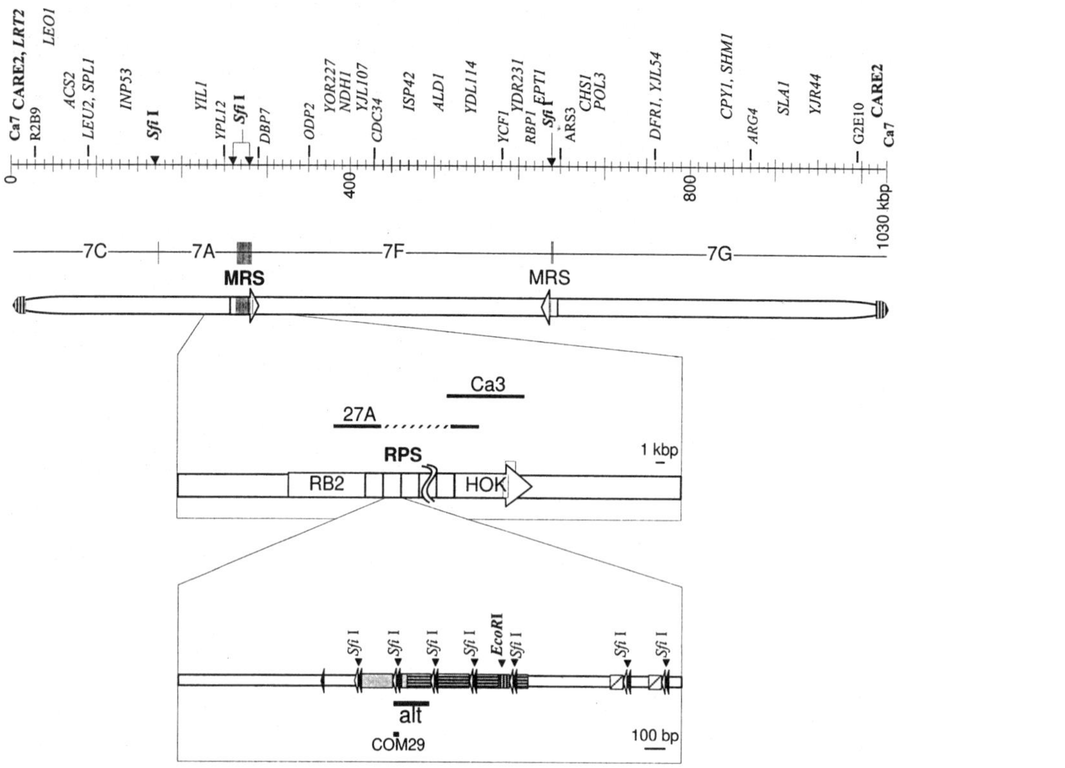

Figure 2. A map of chromosome 7 showing the orientation and fine structure of the MRS.

laboratory. Their technique involves digestion of genomic DNA with a restriction enzyme, usually *Eco*RI, followed by separation of the fragments and probing of the digest with a sequence that contains HOK and part of the RPS (1, 37, 38, 69, 72, 73). Each of the three probes, Ca3, 27A, and RPS, exhibits restriction fragment length polymorphisms (RFLPs) when used as probe on genomic Southern blots of various strains. Ca3 and 27A are included in the MRS, and a part of each overlaps with RPS (Fig. 2).

The first reason for the RFLPs is that each strain possesses a specific pattern with several different sizes of RPS, ranging from 1.7 to 3.5 kbp (7). The second reason is heterogeneity in the sites for *Eco*RI in the MRS, the sequence from which these probes come. The third reason is that, since the number of RPSs varies among different strains, the restriction fragments that include the RPS cluster exhibit RFLPs (6). The number of RPSs is alterable during culture in vitro and also in vivo, so fragments that include the RPS cluster display RFLP within a strain lineage (60).

The MRS also seems very important in the frequent chromosomal translocations that are found among *C. albicans* isolates (79). In WO-1, the strain whose translocations have been most completely characterized, all seem to have occurred at MRS sites. This inference is based on the fact that the *Sfi*I fragments in this strain are virtually identical to those in strain 1006, a strain with the "standard karyotype." The translocation products seem to be composed of the unique regions of two nonhomologous chromosomes that have undergone a crossover at the MRS (Color plate 7). Such products are found in strain 1001, another isolate whose genome has been characterized (53). Strains containing translocations can be analyzed by identifying the new locations of genes whose chromosomal location in the standard karyotype is known. In all cases so far examined in detail, the two reciprocal products of the translocation are present, although an aneuploid strain derived from WO-1, WO-2, has lost one of its translocation products as well as one intact copy of chromosome 7. McEachern et al. first showed that WO-1 can lose one of the translocation products and still survive (50).

Translocations at one of the repeated MRS sequences do not affect the organization of genes in the unique DNA between the repeats. Since RPS has several sites for the 8-bp-specific restriction enzyme *Sfi*I, the *Sfi*I fragment patterns of most *C. albicans* strains are similar. Chibana et al. demonstrated that translocations involving chromosome 7 in several clinical strains also occurred at the MRS and suggested that in *C. albicans,* synteny should be defined not as the association of genes on a chromosome but as association on an *Sfi*I fragment, since these fragments seem to be the conserved units of the *C. albicans* genome (6).

The frequency with which translocations are found in clinical isolates suggests that genomic rearrangement is either a cause or a result of the transition of *C. albicans* strains from commensal to pathogen. At the moment, there is no evidence in either direction. If translocations alter the patterns of gene expression, it is most likely to be via changes in chromatin structure, since the DNA sequences in the unique regions seem not to be altered.

TELOMERES AND SUBTELOMERIC REPEATS

A sequence corresponding to the *C. albicans* telomeric repeat was isolated in 1991 by Sadhu et al. (69). They cloned it by chance in a study of repeated genomic fragments. The *C. albicans* telomere is more complicated than that of most fungi: it consists of a 23-bp repeat (51). However, this repeat shares a conserved sequence motif with many budding yeasts (49). The size of the telomere in strain WO-1 is dependent on temperature; the number of repeats is greater at higher temperatures. Determination of the complete map of chromosome 7 (8) revealed that one of the intermediate repeated sequences previously isolated in two laboratories, CARE2 (Rel-1) (35, 80), constitutes a subtelomeric repeat in *C. albicans.* The absence of this repeated sequence was shown to be a differential diagnostic characteristic between *C. albicans* and *C. dubliniensis* (36, 52). The subtelomeric region contains sequences homologous to the reverse transcriptase of LINE-type retrotransposons (8).

C. ALBICANS CENTROMERES

Centromeres were identified in *S. cerevisiae* by segregation during meiosis. Since a complete sexual cycle has not been defined for *C. albicans,* this approach is not possible. The first attempts at genetic analysis of *C. albicans* after it was shown to be diploid were parasexual approaches using spheroplast fusion (27, 28, 59, 70). Attempts were made to identify the relationship of genes to the centromere on what was probably chromosome R, based on the linkage of Ade and Arg mutations (58), since *ADE1* and *ARG1* are both on this chromosome. The *S. cerevisiae* and *Schizosaccharomyces pombe* centromeres were isolated by taking advantage of the extensive genetic maps in those yeasts. Although the *S. pombe* centromere, ranging in size from 40 to 100 kb (10), is too large to use in most vectors, the *S. cerevisiae* functional unit is much smaller, about 120 bp (5). Hence, this centromere can be cloned into plasmids, and it confers stability on normally unstable vectors. Using such a test for centromere function, several laboratories tried to isolate the centromere of *C. albicans* without success. The complete and functional centromere has not yet been identified molecularly, although a sequence from chromosome 7, which confers stability on linear vectors of 40 kb, has been identified (9).

C. ALBICANS CHROMOSOMES

Chromosome R

Chromosome R is the largest of the chromosomes, comprising more than 4,000 kbp. It carries the rDNA cistrons. The size of the homologs varies in different strains because the partition of these cistrons is usually unequal. In Color plate 7, for example, rDNA is located on fragment rV on one homolog and fragment rS on the other; this repeated DNA accounts for the difference in size between these fragments. Chromosome R contains at least one copy of the MRS, but the exact number has not yet been determined. There are four *Sfi*I sites on one homolog and three on the other in strain 1006. No translocations involving chromosome R have been reported in *C. albicans.*

Chromosome 1 (3,400 kb)

Chromosome 1 has four to five *Sfi*I sites on each homolog. There is at least one MRS site located. Since in WO-1, one homolog of chromosome 1 is involved in a translocation with chromosome 5, and this translocation seems to occur between fragments 1J and $1J_1$, it seems likely, although not proven, that the MRS is located between these fragments.

Chromosome 2 (2,600 kb)

Chromosome 2 has an MRS sequence located close to one end, so that it contains one very large *Sfi*I fragment, 2U, and a very small one, 2A. Fragment 2A has been shown to be involved in translocations in several strains (53).

Chromosome 3 (1,800 kb)

Chromosome 3 is the only one of the eight *C. albicans* chromosomes that does not contain at least one copy of the MRS. It does have one of the repeated flanking sequences, RB2 (12), but it lacks HOK and RPS. No translocations involving this chromosome have been found.

Chromosome 4 (1,700 kb)

Chromosome 4, like chromosome 7, has two copies of the MRS sequence. The two are arranged as inverted repeats, flanking fragment 4N. In addition, there is one other *Sfi*I site on one homolog. Chromosome 4-chromosome 7 translocations have been identified in several strains (6, 13).

Chromosome 5 (1,200 kb)

Chromosome 5 contains one copy of the MRS (11). This copy can contain as many as 50 repeats of the RPS (35a). Perhaps because of this large MRS, chromosome 5 seems to be very frequently involved in translocations. Chromosome 5 is the site of the *MTL* loci (19, 43); hence, the two homologs contain a stretch of about 8.8 kb of nonhomologous DNA. Loss of one homolog of chromosome 5 leads to expression of the gene *SOU1,* which allows cells to metabolize L-sorbose (24, 25).

Chromosome 6 (1,100 kb)

Chromosome 6 contains one copy of the MRS. It is involved in a translocation with chromosome 5 in WO-1.

Chromosome 7 (1,000 kb)

Chromosome 7 is the most completely characterized of the *C. albicans* chromosomes, since a complete sequence-tagged site map has been published. This map, which included 79 markers assigned to 149 fosmids, verified that two of the *Sfi*I sites were associated with MRS sequences whereas the third (between fragments 7C and 7A) was located in unique DNA. The MRS sequences are arranged in an inverted repeat configuration although they are separated by 540 kb of unique DNA. An interesting question that has not been resolved is whether this arrangement ever leads to an inversion of *Sfi*I fragment 7F. The map also allowed the identification of the CARE-2 (Rel-2) element as a major subtelomeric repeat. Because it was the first chromosome for which the complete physical map was constructed, chromosome 7 polymorphism has been analyzed in several strains. This analysis has shown that both translocations and variations in the size of the MRS can lead to this polymorphism (6).

CHROMOSOME LOSS OR GAIN

A relatively common occurrence in *C. albicans* is chromosome loss. Chromosome loss can be induced in tetraploid spheroplast fusion products by heat shock (18). An aneuploid derivative of strain WO-1 was described by Magee and Magee (44). This strain WO-2, has lost two of the parental chromosome (the 6C,5M translocation product [Color plate 7]) and the intact homolog of chromosome 7), so it is aneuploid for about 10% of its genome. In contrast to the induced aneuploids described below, it is stable, although it grows slowly. The best explanation for its stability lies in its rearranged karyotype. Because the hemizygous information is present only in translocation products, there is no nondisjunction event that would return WO-2 to the euploid state. Apparently there is no karyotypic arrangement that can be arrived at by nondisjunction that confers a growth advantage sufficient for selection over the parental strain. McEachern et al. isolated derivatives of strain WO-1, which had lost the 6C,5M translocation and derivatives that had two copies of this product. The former were deficient in the phenotypic transition from white to opaque colony types characteristic of strain WO-1 and in germ-tube formation, whereas strains with an extra copy of this product showed an increased ability to form germ tubes (50). In contrast to these findings, strain WO-2 switches with a normal frequency from white to opaque and forms germ tubes and hyphae at a rate similar to that of the parent (44).

Barton and Gull showed that when diploid *C. albicans* is grown on methyl benzimidazole carbamate, strains that have undergone nondisjunction and lack one chromosome will arise at a frequency about 10-fold higher than that in the absence of the drug. These were identified by the appearance of pink colonies when a strain heterozygotic for the *ade2* mutation on chromosome 3 was used. These aneuploid cells gave rise to small colonies, which were unstable as shown by the appearance of larger colonies after growth overnight. The large colonies grew at the wild-type rate, suggesting that they had undergone a second nondisjunction event, resulting in the doubling of the remaining homolog and reconstitution of the euploid (diploid) state. Bands on pulse-field gels suggested that chromosome 3, the location of the *ADE2* gene, was about half as intense in the putative monosome as it was in the parent strain (3).

Subsequently Janbon et al. reported that strains plated on sorbose (a sugar normally considered nonutilizable by *C. albicans*) would give rise to a few colonies after about a week. The cells in these colonies all grow on sorbose, lack one homolog of chromosome 5 as indicated by pulse-field gels, and grow slowly on glucose medium; overnight culture in rich medium yields strains that have regained the diploid state and are no longer able to grow on sorbose. The structural gene for the enzyme that allows cells to metabolize sorbose (*SOU1*) is located on chromosome 4; Janbon et al. propose that chromosome 5 contains a gene for a repressor that is dose dependent, and the concentration of the regulator molecule in a hemizygous strain is insufficient to repress the *SOU1* gene (25). A study of the formation of the Sor$^+$ variants showed that they arose on the plates and that their rate of formation increased from about 10^{-6} to 10^{-1} during 8 days of incubation (24).

Perepnikhatka et al. examined fluconazole-resistant mutants and found that 7 days' exposure to the drug sometimes resulted in loss of one copy of chromosome 4, whereas long-term exposure could lead to trisomy for chromosome 3 (55). In another study of evolution to drug resistance, using a fresh clinical isolate, karyotypic changes leading to fluconazole resistance were not found, although there were random chromosomal alterations (14). It seems likely that the genetic heterogeneity of *C. albicans* isolates may determine whether chromosome loss gives rise to a particular phenotype.

MULTIPLE KARYOTYPE VARIATIONS

Although most laboratory strains of *C. albicans* show relatively stable karyotypes in vitro (except for chromosome R, as described above) (21, 63), several studies have demonstrated that karyotypic variation can be associated with phenotypic variation. The first to do so were Suzuki and coworkers, who demonstrated that the reversible transition in a clinical isolate from a smooth to a semirough colony morphology was accompanied by correlated changes in the electrophoretic karyotype (77). The semirough variant was avirulent in the mouse-tail-vein model. Their original isolate was approximately triploid, and the variants had an even greater DNA content. The karyotypes of the variants contained extra chromosomal bands but retained the five bands of the parent strain (all that were resolvable at that time). In a second paper, Suzuki and coworkers showed that colony morphology variants in *Candida tropicalis* were also associated with changes in the electrophoretic karyotype (78). However, in neither case was a causal relationship demonstrated.

In one case translocation was shown to occur at a frequency high enough so that it can be selected for by growth conditions. This first clear demonstration of a specific chromosome rearrangement related to a specific phenotypic change was the observation by Wickes et al. that when *Candida stellatoidea,* a subspecies of *C. albicans* that is normally unable to grow on sucrose, is plated on medium containing the sugar as sole carbon and energy source, spontaneous Suc$^+$ strains arise. These sucrose-metabolizing variants all contained four particular chromosome rearrangements (86). The mechanism by which these translocations render the cells able to grow on sucrose is not known, nor is the precise nature of the rearrangements, such as whether they occur at the MRS. Although the rearranged strains were selected for growth on sucrose, they had acquired several new phenotypes as well, including the ability to grow on glycerol, an increased growth rate, and heightened virulence.

Later, Barton and Scherer, using 1161, a stable strain, selected a mutant strain that showed a wrinkled colony phenotype and switched. It also had several new bands in its karyotype. They showed that chromosome breakage and rearrangement could be induced by transformation with a selectable marker, *URA3,* inserted into a piece of the MRS. Ten transformants of a total of 40 contained fragmented chromosomes when the unstable strain was transformed, whereas only 1 out of 37 transformants of stable strains had an altered karyotype. None of these strains had an obvious colony phenotype different from the parental strain. Interestingly, all of the translocations analyzed involved chromosomes 6 or 7 (4).

Rustchenko et al. found that karyotypic rearrangements were associated with colony morphology phenotypes in strain 3153A. However, there was no specific correlation of variant karyotype with colony phenotype (66–68). These authors suggested that karyotype variation is a means of achieving genetic variability in *C. albicans.* Many of the variations involved chromosome R (chromosome VIII in their numbering system); these variations seem to occur without affecting the phenotype in many strains (66).

The acquisition by *C. albicans* of the ability to assimilate L-sorbose or D-arabinose was shown to be accompanied by specific changes in the karyotype (64). In addition to the change in the copy number of chromosome 5, which they later characterized in detail, these workers observed an apparent deletion of part of chromosome 2 in cells that had acquired the ability to metabolize arabinose. The molecular basis of this rearrangement has not been determined. A later study demonstrated pleiotrophic phenotypic changes in strains selected for growth on arabinose or sorbose (65).

Taken together, these studies suggest that nondisjunction and probably translocation are relatively frequent events among *C. albicans* isolates and that the rate of karyotypic rearrangements is increased by conditions of stress, such as incubation on a nonutilizable carbon source. Further evidence for this conclusion was presented by Enloe et al., who designed a transformation cassette that allows for deletion of both alleles of a gene in one transformation step (16). This procedure relies on mitotic crossing over to make the strain homozygous for the original transformation product. If an essential gene is targeted, the result is a trisomic strain with the gene deleted on two of the chromosomes but intact on the third. This technique is described in more detail in chapter 19 of this volume. Since there is no step designed to induce either crossing over or nondisjunction in this procedure, one can infer that both processes normally occur at a fairly high rate.

It seems likely that the relatively frequent karyotypic rearrangements found in clinical isolates may arise from stress associated with host immune response or adaptation to an unaccustomed niche in the host. An open and important question is whether rearrangements generate a subpopulation that is more fit and therefore selected in vivo.

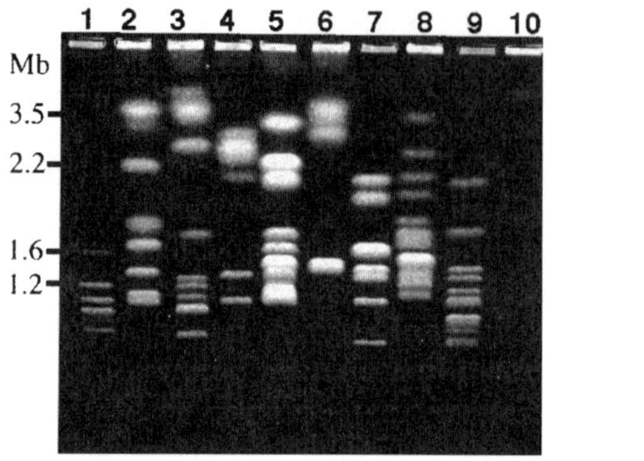

Figure 3. A contour-clamped homogeneous electric field separation of the chromosomes of eight different *Candida* species. Lane 1, *S. cerevisiae*; lane 2, *C. albicans* strain FC18; lane 3, *C. stellatoidea* strain IFO 1397; lane 4, *C. tropicalis* strain NUM37; lane 5, *C. parapsilosus* strain NUM303; lane 6, *C. krusei* strain IFO13; lane 7, *C. guilliermondii* strain NUM4; lane 8, *C. kefyr* strain IFO 586; lane 9, *C. glabrata* strain TIMM1063; lane 10, *S. pombe*. Reprinted from reference 22 with permission.

GENOMES OF OTHER *CANDIDA* SPECIES

Much less work has been expended on genomic analysis of *Candida* strains other than *C. albicans*. In part this is due to the importance of *C. albicans* in disease and in part to the paucity of genetic approaches to the other yeasts. *C. stellatoidea*, which is generally regarded as a subspecies of *C. albicans*, has a karyotype marked by numerous translocations (45, 62), but no careful characterization has been undertaken with any isolate. However, there is a reasonable amount of information on *C. glabrata, C. dubliniensis, C. krusei, C. parapsilosis,* and *C. tropicalis*. Among these species, too, the karyotypes of clinical isolates are highly variable. In the absence of a genome project for the particular species, the description of the genotype can only be provisional. Figure 3 (from reference 22) shows a typical electrophoretic separation of the most common clinical strains. It can be referred to in the following discussion, although the details of the karyotypes in different papers will, as discussed, vary.

C. glabrata

C. glabrata has been shown to be haploid, based on several studies of gene disruption (30, 89). There is one estimate of genome size, 14 Mb, based on an analysis of the electrophoretic karyotypes (15). The telomere sequence has been determined, and it is intermediate in complexity between the telomeres of other *Candida* species and the simple repeat of *S. cerevisiae*. Its sequence is CTGGGTGCTGTGGGGGT (49). A centromere has been cloned from *C. glabrata* and shown to be similar to that of *S. cerevisiae* (5). It contains orthologs of the three elements CDEI (8 bp), CDEII (79 bp and AT-rich), and CDEIII (26 bp). Centromere activity can be conferred by a 153-bp fragment. The *C. glabrata* centromere functions like the *S. cerevisiae* one; it confers mitotic stability and low copy number to plasmids containing it (31). However, despite the structural similarity, the *C. glabrata* centromere is not active in *S. cerevisiae* (32).

Several laboratories have examined the karyotypes of clinical isolates (2, 17, 42). Although these vary in detail, the general outline of the electrophoretic karyotype is relatively consistent. Usually 11 to 14 bands are resolved, ranging in size from 500 kbp to 2.5 Mbp. The sizes of the individual bands and their distribution vary from paper to paper and from isolate to isolate. The size of the genome determined from these analyses is between 11.9 and 14 Mbp.

C. tropicalis

Kamiryo et al. argued that *C. tropicalis* was diploid, based on the fact that several genes hybridized to two bands on the electrophoretic karyotype (29), while others showed that the acyl coenzyme A oxidase was present in two copies (56). Doi et al. found that *C. tropicalis* has a diploid DNA complement of about 30 Mb and 12 chromosome homologs (6 pairs). They analyzed three strains, two of which had seven bands, three of which hybridized with the tubulin, rDNA, and *PEP4* gene probes, respectively. In a third strain, the homologs carrying the rDNA were separable. They postulate that the number of homologous chromosome equivalents is 12 (6 pairs of homologs), based on a fluorimetric analysis of the intensity of the bands in their gels. Their karyotypes show seven bands except when the rDNA-containing homolog is resolved, giving eight. They point out that there are possible errors in the fluorimetric approach. In another study, seven bands were also seen (48). Without probes specific for every chromosome, it is impossible to determine the exact karyotype, but the estimated genome size is close to that for other *Candida* species. With this, as well as with other diploid yeasts, we will use the term "homologous chromosome equivalents," since the various bands seen on a gel may be due to reciprocal translocations, as is the case with *C. albicans* and *C. dubliniensis* (6, 13, 41), leaving no intact homologs of some chromosomes but preserving the diploid content of the genome.

C. parapsilosis

Whelan and Kwon-Chung presented evidence that *C. parapsilosis* and *C. krusei* were diploid or aneuploid, based on demonstrated heterozygosities in clinical isolates (82). *C. parapsilosis* was estimated to have a diploid genome of 25 Mb and 14 homologous chromosome equivalents (15); this determination is based on the appearance of 10 bands on the electrophoretic karyotype with separable homologs carrying the *PEP4* and tubulin gene (together) and another set of homologs carrying the rDNA cistrons. Other studies have given from 6 to 10 bands; from the gels shown by Pontieri et al. (57), one can estimate a diploid genome content of 28 to 30 Mb. Lott et al. have suggested that the maximum variation occurs in the smaller chromosomes (39); this would be in accord with the findings in *C. albicans* (21, 63), since the rDNA is located on the smaller bands of the pulse-field gel (15).

C. dubliniensis

C. dubliniensis is closely related to *C. albicans* as judged by the similarity in the rDNA cistrons. The genome size is similar to that of *C. albicans*. Isolates of this species have highly variable karyotypes; in fact, no "standard karyotype" has emerged from studies on this yeast and one cannot talk about the number of chromosomes, since this varies from isolate to isolate. However, like *C. albicans, C. dubliniensis* has a repeated sequence that may be analogous to the MRS; this sequence is found on every chromosome in some isolates (26). In addition, *C. dubliniensis* has an *Sfi*I digestion pattern that remains relatively constant from isolate to isolate, and the gene assignment to *Sfi*I fragments is similar to that of *C. albicans*. The chromosome map of each *C. dubliniensis* isolate seems to be derived from that of *C. albicans* by numerous different translocations, even involving the equivalent of chromosome 3, for which no translocation has been found in *C. albicans*.

C. krusei

Essayag et al. examined 43 *C. krusei* strains and found that the number of resolvable bands varied from three to six. The karyotype was highly variable, but all had one band around 3 Mb and one between 2.8 and 2.6 Mb (with one exception); the smaller chromosomes were highly variable. Wickes et al. postulated that *C. krusei* had five chromosomes (87). At this time, the exact karyotype cannot be determined.

CONCLUSION

A remarkable property of the genus *Candida* is the variability of karyotypes in many of its members. The implications of this variability are important. A large fraction of the isolates of *C. albicans,* the best-studied member of the genus, have pairs of homologous chromosomes of roughly the same size and containing allelic information, albeit with a high degree of heterozygosity. The remaining isolates have significantly diverse karyotypes, and the majority of these karyotypes have been shown to result from chromosomal rearrangements at the MRS. The recently discovered mating reaction in *C. albicans* suggests that meiosis may occur, albeit infrequently, in this species. If it does, the strains with rearrangements would necessarily be infertile, since meiosis would lead to aneuploid spores. However, the rearrangements may reflect a different way of generating genetic diversity.

The structural elements of the chromosomes of *Candida* species show high diversity, as might be expected from this genus, which is phylogenetically diverse. The telomeres and centromeres of the species that have been examined, *C. albicans* and *C. glabrata,* differ significantly. However, the most striking feature of the genome of *C. albicans* is the presence of the MRS, which seems to serve as a site for translocation. An analogous sequence seems to exist in *C. dubliniensis* and may occur in other members as well. Whether this sequence has any other important biological functions remains to be determined. The study of the mechanisms and phenotypic consequences of karyotype rearrangements will be an important part of *Candida* genomics in the next few years. It seems clear that analysis of the structure of *Candida* chromosomes and the dynamics of genomic variation will yield important clues to the biology of these yeasts.

Acknowledgments. We are grateful to Bebe Magee for a careful reading of the manuscript and to her, Paul Lephart, and Professor S. I. Iwaguchi for sharing unpublished results with us. The work from our laboratory was supported by USPHS grants R01AI16567, R01AI35109, R01AI46350, and contract N01AI05406.

REFERENCES

1. **Anderson, J., T. Srikantha, B. Morrow, S. H. Miyasaki, T. C. White, N. Agabian, J. Schmid, and D. R. Soll.** 1993. Characterization and partial nucleotide sequence of the DNA fingerprinting probe Ca3 of Candida albicans. *J. Clin. Microbiol.* **31:** 1472–1480.
2. **Asakura, K., S. Iwaguchi, M. Homma, T. Sukai, K. Higashide, and K. Tanaka.** 1991. Electrophoretic karyotypes of clinically isolated yeasts of *Candida albicans* and *C. glabrata*. *Gen. Microbiol.* **137:**2531–2538.
3. **Barton, R. C., and K. Gull.** 1992. Isolation, characterization, and genetic analysis of monosomic, aneuploid mutants of *Candida albicans*. *Mol. Microbiol.* **6:**171–177.
4. **Barton, R. C., and S. Scherer.** 1994. Induced chromosome rearrangements and morphologic variation in *Candida albicans*. *J. Bacteriol.* **176:**756–763.
5. **Carbon, J.** 1984. Yeast centromeres: structure and function. *Cell* **37:**351–353.
6. **Chibana, H., J. L. Beckerman, and P. T. Magee.** 2000. Fine-resolution physical mapping of genomic diversity in *Candida albicans*. *Genome Res.* **10:**1865–1877.
7. **Chibana, H., S. Iwaguchi, M. Homma, A. Chindamporn, Y. Nakagawa, and K. Tanaka.** 1994. Diversity of tandemly repetitive sequences due to short periodic repetitions in the chromosomes of *Candida albicans*. *J. Bacteriol.* **176:**3851–3858.
8. **Chibana, H., B. B. Magee, S. Grindle, Y. Ran, S. Scherer, and P. T. Magee.** 1998. A physical map of chromosome 7 of *Candida albicans*. *Genetics* **149:**1739–1752.
9. **Chibana, H., and P. T. Magee.** 1999. Cloning the centromere from *Candida albicans* using chromosome engineering techniques, p. B33. *In Am. Soc. Microbiol. Conf. Candida and Candidiasis*. American Society for Microbiology, Washington, D.C.
10. **Chikashige, Y., N. Kinoshita, Y. Nakaseko, T. Matsumoto, S. Murakami, O. Niwa, and M. Yanagida.** 1989. Composite motifs and repeat symmetry in *S. pombe* centromeres: direct analysis by integration of NotI restriction sites. *Cell* **57:** 739–751.
11. **Chindamporn, A., Y. Nakagawa, M. Homma, H. Chibana, M. Doi, and K. Tanaka.** 1995. Analysis of the chromosomal localization of the repetitive sequences (RPSs) in *Candida albicans*. *Microbiology* **141:**469–476.
12. **Chindamporn, A., Y. Nakagawa, I. Mizuguchi, H. Chibana, M. Doi, and K. Tanaka.** 1998. Repetitive sequences (RPSs) in the chromosomes of *Candida albicans* are sandwiched between two novel stretches, HOK and RB2, common to each chromosome. *Microbiology* **144:**849–857.
13. **Chu, W. S., B. B. Magee, and P. T. Magee.** 1993. Construction of an SfiI macrorestriction map of the *Candida albicans* genome. *J. Bacteriol.* **175:**6637–6651.
14. **Cowen, L. E., D. Sanglard, D. Calabrese, C. Sirjusingh, J. B. Anderson, and L. M. Kohn.** 2000. Evolution of drug resistance in experimental populations of *Candida albicans*. *J. Bacteriol.* **182:**1515–1522.
15. **Doi, M., M. Homma, A. Chindamporn, and K. Tanaka.** 1992. Estimation of chromosome number and size by pulsed-field gel electrophoresis (PFGE) in medically important *Candida species*. *J. Gen. Microbiol.* **138:**2243–2251.
16. **Enloe, B., A. Diamond, and A. P. Mitchell.** 2000. A single-transformation gene function test in diploid *Candida albicans*. *J. Bacteriol.* **182:**5730–5736.
17. **Espinel-Ingroff, A., J. L. Rodriguez-Tudela, and J. V. Martinez-Suarez.** 1995. Comparison of two alternative microdilution procedures with the National Committee for Clinical Laboratory Standards reference macrodilution method M27-P for in vitro testing of fluconazole-resistant and -susceptible isolates of *Candida albicans*. *J. Clin. Microbiol.* **33:**3154–3158.

17a. **Essayag, S. M., G. G. Baily, D. W. Denning, and J. P. Burnie.** 1996. Karyotyping of fluconazole-resistant yeasts with phenotype reported as *Candida krusei* or *Candida inconspicua*. *Int. J. Syst. Bacteriol.* **46:**35–40.

18. **Hilton, C., D. Markie, B. Corner, E. Rikkerink, and R. Poulter.** 1985. Heat shock induces chromosome loss in the yeast *Candida albicans*. *Mol. Gen. Genet.* **200:**162–168.
19. **Hull, C. M., and A. D. Johnson.** 1999. Identification of a mating type-like locus in the asexual pathogenic yeast *Candida albicans*. *Science* **285:**1271–1275.
20. **Iwaguchi, S., M. Homma, H. Chibana, and K. Tanaka.** 1992. Isolation and characterization of a repeated sequence (RPS1) of *Candida albicans*. *J. Gen. Microbiol.* **138:**1893–1900.
21. **Iwaguchi, S., M. Homma, and K. Tanaka.** 1992. Clonal variation of chromosome size derived from the rDNA cluster region in *Candida albicans*. *J. Gen. Microbiol.* **138:**1177–1184.
22. **Iwaguchi, S., M. Homma, and K. Tanaka.** 1990. Variation in the electrophoretic karyotype analysed by the assignment of DNA probes in *Candida albicans*. *J. Gen. Microbiol.* **136:** 2433–2442.
23. **Iwaguchi, S. I., T. Kanbe, T. Tohne, P. T. Magee, and T. Suzuki.** 2000. High-frequency occurrence of chromosome translocation in a mutant strain of *Candida albicans* by a suppressor mutation of ploidy shift. *Yeast* **16:**411–422.
24. **Janbon, G., F. Sherman, and E. Rustchenko.** 1999. Appearance and properties of L-sorbose-utilizing mutants of *Candida albicans* obtained on a selective plate. *Genetics* **153:**653–664.
25. **Janbon, G., F. Sherman, and E. Rustchenko.** 1998. Monosomy of a specific chromosome determines L-sorbose utilization: a novel regulatory mechanism in *Candida albicans*. *Proc. Natl. Acad. Sci. USA* **95:**5150–5155.
26. **Joly, S., C. Pujol, M. Rysz, K. Vargas, and D. R. Soll.** 1999. Development and characterization of complex DNA fingerprinting probes for the infectious yeast *Candida dubliniensis*. *J. Clin. Microbiol.* **37:**1035–1044.
27. **Kakar, S. N., and P. T. Magee.** 1982. Genetic analysis of *Candida albicans:* identification of different isoleucine-valine, methionine, and arginine alleles by complementation. *J. Bacteriol.* **151:**1247–1252.
28. **Kakar, S. N., R. M. Partridge, and P. T. Magee.** 1983. A genetic analysis of *Candida albicans:* isolation of a wide variety of auxotrophs and demonstration of linkage and complementation. *Genetics* **104:**241–255.
29. **Kamiryo, T., N. Mito, T. Niki, and T. Suzuki.** 1991. Assignment of most genes encoding major peroxisomal polypeptides to chromosomal band V of the asporogenic yeast *Candida tropicalis*. *Yeast* **7:**503–511.
30. **Kitada, K., E. Yamaguchi, and M. Arisawa.** 1995. Cloning of the *Candida glabrata* TRP1 and HIS3 genes, and construction of their disruptant strains by sequential integrative transformation. *Gene* **165:**203–206.
31. **Kitada, K., E. Yamaguchi, and M. Arisawa.** 1996. Isolation

of a *Candida glabrata* centromere and its use in construction of plasmid vectors. *Gene* **175**:105–108.

32. **Kitada, K., E. Yamaguchi, K. Hamada, and M. Arisawa.** 1997. Structural analysis of a *Candida glabrata* centromere and its functional homology to the *Saccharomyces cerevisiae* centromere. *Curr. Genet.* **31**:122–127.
33. **Kurtzman, C. P., and C. J. Robnett.** 1998. Identification and phylogeny of ascomycetous yeasts from analysis of nuclear large subunit (26S) ribosomal DNA partial sequences. *Antonie Van Leeuwenhoek* **73**:331–371.
34. **Lasker, B. A., G. F. Carle, G. S. Kobayashi, and G. Medoff.** 1989. Comparison of the separation of *Candida albicans* chromosome-sized DNA by pulsed-field gel electrophoresis techniques. *Nucleic Acids Res.* **17**:3783–3793.
35. **Lasker, B. A., L. S. Page, T. J. Lott, and G. S. Kobayashi.** 1992. Isolation, characterization, and sequencing of *Candida albicans* repetitive element 2. *Gene* **116**:51–57.

35a. **Lephart, P.** Unpublished data.

36. **Lischewski, A., D. Harmsen, K. Wilms, G. Baier, U. Gunzer, H. Klinker, M. Wilhelm, A. Schwinn, and J. Hacker.** 1999. Molecular epidemiology of *Candida albicans* isolates from AIDS and cancer patients using a novel standardized CARE-2 DNA fingerprinting technique. *Mycoses* **42**:371–383.
37. **Lockhart, S. R., J. J. Fritch, A. S. Meier, K. Schroppel, T. Srikantha, R. Galask, and D. R. Soll.** 1995. Colonizing populations of *Candida albicans* are clonal in origin but undergo microevolution through C1 fragment reorganization as demonstrated by DNA fingerprinting and C1 sequencing. *J. Clin. Microbiol.* **33**:1501–1509.
38. **Lockhart, S. R., B. D. Reed, C. L. Pierson, and D. R. Soll.** 1996. Most frequent scenario for recurrent *Candida vaginitis* is strain maintenance with "substrain shuffling": demonstration by sequential DNA fingerprinting with probes Ca3, C1, and CARE2. *J. Clin. Microbiol.* **34**:767–777.
39. **Lott, T. J., R. J. Kuykendall, S. F. Welbel, A. Pramanik, and B. A. Lasker.** 1993. Genomic heterogeneity in the yeast *Candida parapsilosis. Curr. Genet.* **23**:463–467.
40. **Magee, B. B., Y. Koltin, J. A. Gorman, and P. T. Magee.** 1988. Assignment of cloned genes to the seven electrophoretically separated *Candida albicans* chromosomes. *Mol. Cell. Biol.* **8**: 4721–4726.
41. **Magee, B. B., M. Sanchez, and P. T. Magee.** 1999. Karyotypic analysis of the recently identified oral pathogen, *Candida dubliniensis,* p. C52. *In Am. Soc. Microbiol. Conf. Candida and Candidiasis.* American Society for Microbiology, Washington, D.C.
42. **Magee, B. B., and P. T. Magee.** 1987. Electrophoretic karyotypes and chromosome numbers in *Candida* species. *J. Gen. Microbiol.* **133**:425–430.
43. **Magee, B. B., and P. T. Magee.** 2000. Induction of mating in *Candida albicans* by construction of *MTL* a and *MTL* alpha strains. *Science* **289**:310–313.
44. **Magee, B. B., and P. T. Magee.** 1997. WO-2, a stable aneuploid derivative of *Candida albicans* strain WO-1, can switch from white to opaque and form hyphae. *Microbiology* **143**: 289–295.

44a. **Magee, B. B., M. Sanchez, H. Chibana, and P. T. Magee.** Unpublished data.

45. **Magee, P. T.** 1993. Variations in chromosome size and organization in *Candida albicans* and *Candida stellatoidea. Trends Microbiol.* **1**:338–342.
46. **Magee, P. T., L. Bowdin, and J. Staudinger.** 1992. Comparison of molecular typing methods for *Candida albicans. J. Clin. Microbiol.* **30**:2674–2679.
47. **Magee, P. T., E. H. Rikkerink, and B. B. Magee.** 1988. Methods for the genetics and molecular biology of *Candida albicans. Anal. Biochem.* **175**:361–372.
48. **Mahrous, M., A. D. Sawant, W. R. Pruitt, T. Lott, S. A. Meyer, and D. G. Ahearn.** 1992. DNA relatedness, karyotyping and gene probing of *Candida tropicalis, Candida albicans* and its synonyms *Candida stellatoidea* and *Candida claussenii. Eur. J. Epidemiol.* **8**:444–451.
49. **McEachern, M. J., and E. H. Blackburn.** 1994. A conserved sequence motif within the exceptionally diverse telomeric sequences of budding yeasts. *Proc. Natl. Acad. Sci. USA* **91**: 3453–3457.
50. **McEachern, M. J., and J. B. Hicks.** 1991. Dosage of the smallest chromosome affects both the yeast-hyphal transition and the white-opaque transition of *Candida albicans* WO-1. *J. Bacteriol.* **173**:7436–7442.
51. **McEachern, M. J., and J. B. Hicks.** 1993. Unusually large telomeric repeats in the yeast *Candida albicans. Mol. Cell. Biol.* **13**:551–560.
52. **Morschhauser, J., M. Ruhnke, S. Michel, and J. Hacker.** 1999. Identification of CARE-2-negative *Candida albicans* isolates as *Candida dubliniensis. Mycoses* **42**:29–32.
53. **Navarro-Garcia, F., R. M. Perez-Diaz, B. B. Magee, J. Pla, C. Nombela, and P. Magee.** 1995. Chromosome reorganization in *Candida albicans* 1001 strain. *J. Med. Vet. Mycol.* **33**: 361–366.
54. **Olaiya, A. F., and S. J. Sogin.** 1979. Ploidy determination of *Candida albicans. J. Bacteriol.* **140**:1043–1049.
55. **Perepnikhatka, V., F. J. Fischer, M. Niimi, R. A. Baker, R. D. Cannon, Y. K. Wang, F. Sherman, and E. Rustchenko.** 1999. Specific chromosome alterations in fluconazole-resistant mutants of candida albicans. *J. Bacteriol.* **181**:4041–4049.
56. **Picataggio, S., K. Deanda, and J. Mielenz.** 1991. Determination of *Candida tropicalis* acyl coenzyme A oxidase isozyme function by sequential gene disruption. *Mol. Cell. Biol.* **11**: 4333–4339.
57. **Pontieri, E., L. Gregori, M. Gennarelli, T. Ceddia, G. Novelli, B. Dallapiccola, F. De Bernardis, and G. Carruba.** 1996. Correlation of SfiI macrorestriction endonuclease fingerprint analysis of *Candida parapsilosis* isolates with source of isolation. *J. Med. Microbiol.* **45**:173–178.
58. **Poulter, R., and V. Hanrahan.** 1983. Conservation of genetic linkage in nonisogenic isolates of *Candida albicans. J. Bacteriol.* **156**:498–506.
59. **Poulter, R., K. Jeffery, M. J. Hubbard, M. G. Shepherd, and P. A. Sullivan.** 1981. Parasexual genetic analysis of *Candida albicans* by spheroplast fusion. *J. Bacteriol.* **146**:833–840.
60. **Pujol, C., S. Joly, B. Nolan, T. Srikantha, and D. R. Soll.** 1999. Microevolutionary changes in *Candida albicans* identified by the complex Ca3 fingerprinting probe involve insertions and deletions of the full-length repetitive sequence RPS at specific genomic sites. *Microbiology* **145**:2635–2646.
61. **Riggsby, W. S., L. J. Torres-Bauza, J. W. Wills, and T. M. Townes.** 1982. DNA content, kinetic complexity, and the ploidy question in *Candida albicans. Mol. Cell. Biol.* **2**: 853–862.
62. **Rikkerink, E. H., B. B. Magee, and P. T. Magee.** 1990. Genomic structure of *Candida stellatoidea:* extra chromosomes and gene duplication. *Infect. Immun.* **58**:949–954.
63. **Rustchenko, E. P., T. M. Curran, and F. Sherman.** 1993. Variations in the number of ribosomal DNA units in morphological mutants and normal strains of *Candida albicans* and in normal strains of *Saccharomyces cerevisiae. J. Bacteriol.* **175**: 7189–7199.
64. **Rustchenko, E. P., D. H. Howard, and F. Sherman.** 1994. Chromosomal alterations of *Candida albicans* are associated

with the gain and loss of assimilating functions. *J. Bacteriol.* **176**:3231–3241.

65. **Rustchenko, E. P., D. H. Howard, and F. Sherman.** 1997. Variation in assimilating functions occurs in spontaneous *Candida albicans* mutants having chromosomal alterations. *Microbiology* **143**:1765–1778.
66. **Rustchenko-Bulgac, E. P.** 1991. Variations of *Candida albicans* electrophoretic karyotypes. *J. Bacteriol.* **173**:6586–6596.
67. **Rustchenko-Bulgac, E. P., and D. H. Howard.** 1993. Multiple chromosomal and phenotypic changes in spontaneous mutants of *Candida albicans. J. Gen. Microbiol.* **139**:1195–1207.
68. **Rustchenko-Bulgac, E. P., F. Sherman, and J. B. Hicks.** 1990. Chromosomal rearrangements associated with morphological mutants provide a means for genetic variation of *Candida albicans. J. Bacteriol.* **172**:1276–1283.
69. **Sadhu, C., M. J. McEachern, E. P. Rustchenko-Bulgac, J. Schmid, D. R. Soll, and J. B. Hicks.** 1991. Telomeric and dispersed repeat sequences in *Candida* yeasts and their use in strain identification. *J. Bacteriol.* **173**:842–850.
70. **Sarachek, A., D. D. Rhoads, and R. H. Schwarzhoff.** 1981. Hybridization of *Candida albicans* through fusion of protoplasts. *Arch. Microbiol.* **129**:1–8.
71. **Scherer, S., and D. A. Stevens.** 1988. A *Candida albicans* dispersed, repeated gene family and its epidemiologic applications. *Proc. Natl. Acad. Sci. USA* **85**:1452–1456.
72. **Schmid, J., E. Voss, and D. R. Soll.** 1990. Computer-assisted methods for assessing strain relatedness in *Candida albicans* by fingerprinting with the moderately repetitive sequence Ca3. *J. Clin. Microbiol.* **28**:1236–1243.
73. **Schroppel, K., T. Srikantha, D. Wessels, M. DeCock, S. R. Lockhart, and D. R. Soll.** 1996. Cytoplasmic localization of the white phase-specific WH11 gene product of *Candida albicans. Microbiology* **142**:2245–2254.
74. **Snell, R. G., I. F. Hermans, R. J. Wilkins, and B. E. Corner.** 1987. Chromosomal variations in *Candida albicans. Nucleic Acids Res.* **15**:3625.
75. **Snell, R. G., and R. J. Wilkins.** 1986. Separation of chromosomal DNA molecules from *C. albicans* by pulsed field gel electrophoresis. *Nucleic Acids Res.* **14**:4401–4406.
76. **Suzuki, T., A. Hitomi, P. T. Magee, and S. Sakaguchi.** 1994. Correlation between polyploidy and auxotrophic segregation in the imperfect yeast *Candida albicans. J. Bacteriol.* **176**: 3345–3353.
77. **Suzuki, T., I. Kobayashi, T. Kanbe, and K. Tanaka.** 1989. High frequency variation of colony morphology and chromosome reorganization in the pathogenic yeast *Candida albicans. J. Gen. Microbiol.* **135**:425–434.
78. **Suzuki, T., Y. Miyamae, and I. Ishida.** 1991. Variation of colony morphology and chromosomal rearrangement in *Candida tropicalis* pK233. *J. Gen. Microbiol.* **137**:161–167.
79. **Thrash-Bingham, C., and J. A. Gorman.** 1992. DNA translocations contribute to chromosome length polymorphisms in *Candida albicans. Curr. Genet.* **22**:93–100.
80. **Thrash-Bingham, C., and J. A. Gorman.** 1993. Identification, characterization and sequence of *Candida albicans* repetitive DNAs Rel-1 and Rel-2. *Curr. Genet.* **23**:455–462.
81. **Whelan, W. L.** 1987. The genetics of medically important fungi. *Crit. Rev. Microbiol.* **14**:99–170.
82. **Whelan, W. L., and K. J. Kwon-Chung.** 1988. Auxotrophic heterozygosities and the ploidy of *Candida parapsilosis* and *Candida krusei. J. Med. Vet. Mycol.* **26**:163–171.
83. **Whelan, W. L., and P. T. Magee.** 1981. Natural heterozygosity in *Candida albicans. J. Bacteriol.* **145**:896–903.
84. **Whelan, W. L., R. M. Partridge, and P. T. Magee.** 1980. Heterozygosity and segregation in *Candida albicans. Mol. Gen. Genet.* **180**:107–113.
85. **Wickes, B., J. Staudinger, B. B. Magee, K. J. Kwon-Chung, P. T. Magee, and S. Scherer.** 1991. Physical and genetic mapping of *Candida albicans:* several genes previously assigned to chromosome 1 map to chromosome R, the rDNA-containing linkage group. *Infect. Immun.* **59**:2480–2484.
86. **Wickes, B. L., J. E. Golin, and K. J. Kwon-Chung.** 1991. Chromosomal rearrangement in *Candida stellatoidea* results in a positive effect on phenotype. *Infect. Immun.* **59**:1762–1771.
87. **Wickes, B. L., J. B. Hicks, W. G. Merz, and K. J. Kwon-Chung.** 1992. The molecular analysis of synonymy among medically important yeasts within the genus *Candida. J. Gen. Microbiol.* **138**:901–907.
88. **Wills, J. W., B. A. Lasker, K. Sirotkin, and W. S. Riggsby.** 1984. Repetitive DNA of *Candida albicans:* nuclear and mitochondrial components. *J. Bacteriol.* **157**:918–924.
89. **Zhou, P., M. S. Szczypka, R. Young, and D. J. Thiele.** 1994. A system for gene cloning and manipulation in the yeast *Candida glabrata. Gene* **142**:135–140.

VI. DISEASES CAUSED BY *CANDIDA* SPP.

Candida and Candidiasis
Edited by Richard A. Calderone

Chapter 22

Skin and Mucous Membrane Infections

Markus Ruhnke

ORAL CANDIDIASIS

Candida albicans is a normal part of the gastrointestinal flora, and as an opportunistic pathogen, *Candida* species may establish an infection when immunologic and mechanical host defenses are immunocompromised. The clinical entity of oral thrush has probably been known for several centuries since it was described by Hippocrates in 400 B.C. as oral ulcers (1). It may be assumed that various pathological conditions in the oral cavity were categorized as this condition. More clearly, in 1839 Langenbeck was the first to describe the detection of fungi in the oral cavity (115). Finally, in 1846 Berg demonstrated that oral thrush is caused by fungi when he infected healthy newborns with material from "apthous lesions" that produced the thrush in those children (16). Today, this approach is certainly no longer feasible because of ethical, legal, and other reasons. However, infecting healthy "volunteers" with an infectious agent to understand the pathogenicity of a disease was common practice until the middle of the 20th century when Krause caused candidemia after drinking a *Candida* suspension (108).

Infections of the skin and the mucous membranes due to *Candida* spp. may occur either in immunocompromised or in nonimmunocompromised patients. This is in contrast to systemic candidiasis (e.g., candidemia), which is only seen in severely immunocompromised patients. It may be assumed that infections of the skin and the mucous membranes due to *Candida* spp. are growing in incidence because of the increasing numbers of immunocompromised patients. Essentially, the beginning of the AIDS epidemic has focused almost all studies and research on oral *Candida* infections in human immunodeficiency virus (HIV)-infected individuals. Therefore, two groups of patients may be characterized as at risk of developing oropharyngeal candidiasis (OPC), the HIV-infected and non-HIV-infected patients.

Epidemiology

Oral carriage of *Candida* spp. in "healthy" persons and in various patient groups has been described in numerous reports (see reference 152 for further references). As demonstrated by Russell and Lay, the frequency of carriage at birth is 5.7%, 14.2% by the time infants are discharged from the hospital, which then increases after 1 month at home and decreases again at 1 year of age (182). Wilkieson et al. found that 88% of elderly individuals hospitalized in a long-term-care facility carried *Candida* spp. in the oral cavity, and wearing a denture may contribute considerably to these findings (185, 220). The prevalence of oral colonization with *Candida* species was studied by Haumann et al. in 28 HIV-seropositive and 28 healthy persons. *Candida* was cultured from 75 and 68% of HIV-positive and control persons, respectively, with a significantly higher density carriage in the HIV-seropositive group (75). Summarizing the data of several papers published between 1960 and 1985, the published carriage frequencies of yeasts in healthy persons range from 2 to 71% (median, 34%) and in patients from 13 to 76% (median, 55%). As can be seen above, recoveries vary substantially between surveys, mostly because sample collections were done with different methods such as oral/pharyngeal swabs, saliva/mouthwashes, or imprint cultures. Imprint cultures or cultures of saliva or mouthwash generally yield higher colony counts than the swab method, but oral swabs are more easily done to collect samples in larger studies. Furthermore, oral hygiene may contribute considerably to the rate of oral yeast carriage. The majority of reports are descriptive in nature and consider *C. albicans* as the most prevalent yeast. However, considering the appli-

Marcus Ruhnke • Charité Campus Mitte der Humboldt-Universität Berlin, Department of Medicine, Division of Hematology/Oncology, Schumannstr. 20/21, 10117 Berlin, Germany.

cability of modern molecular typing techniques, it remains open as to how frequently misidentification of clinical isolates occurs. At least for the new species, the misidentification of *Candida dubliniensis* as *C. albicans* has been estimated to be as high as 17% (41). DNA fingerprinting studies detected not only "new" species, but revealed that the frequency, intensity, species, and strains of oral yeasts may vary as a function of host age (103).

Data about the "true" incidence of oral *Candida* colonization or infection in different patient groups other than HIV-infected individuals are rare. From the more than 150 *Candida* spp. that are known, only a few are considered to be pathogenic for humans. *C. albicans* is the most commonly isolated species (>70%) from samples taken from mucous membranes such as oral cavity and digestive and vaginal tracts. Less often (<7%), other *Candida* spp. (so-called non-*C. albicans Candida* spp.), including *C. tropicalis, C. glabrata, C. parapsilosis, C. krusei, C. kefyr, C. guilliermondii, Saccharomyces cerevisiae,* rarely *C. sake,* and the relatively new species *C. dubliniensis,* are isolated from nonsterile superficial sites (41, 82, 152). Non-*C. albicans* species are more likely to occur in patients who receive or have received antifungal therapy with azoles. The vast majority of data on OPC published in the last 10 years emphasizes the HIV-infected patient who frequently receives long-term or intermittent therapy with fluconazole and other agents (44). Almost all cases of OPC are caused by *C. albicans,* but rarely it has been claimed (in HIV-positive patients) that *C. glabrata, C. parapsilosis, C. tropicalis, C. krusei,* or *C. dubliniensis* by itself may cause OPC or even esophagitis (83, 94, 203, 206). However, in three reports, this has been observed in HIV-positive patients after therapy with either ketoconazole or fluconazole only. Interestingly, the presentations in these reports were either as erythematous candidiasis or as ulcers, suggesting that the "typical" pseudomembranous candidiasis may be caused by *C. albicans* only. In a small study by Dronda et al., the clinical significance of mixed oropharyngeal *Candida* infections (*C. albicans* cultivated together with non-*C. albicans* strains such as *C. krusei* or *C. glabrata*) was examined in 12 HIV-infected patients. It was concluded that non-*C. albicans* strains of *Candida,* less sensitive to azole drugs than their *C. albicans* counterparts, are not clinically relevant in episodes of mixed oropharyngeal candidiasis in HIV-1-infected patients (55).

C. dubliniensis has drawn much attention since it was described in 1995 to be a species distinct from other *Candida* species (203). *C. dubliniensis* may colonize the oral cavity as well as the vagina in HIV-infected and noninfected patients. In a study from Ireland, *C. dubliniensis* was recovered from the oral cavities of 27% (34 of 126) of HIV-infected individuals and 32% (24 of 76) of AIDS patients with clinical symptoms of OPC and from 19% (29 of 152) of HIV-infected individuals and 25% (7 of 28) of AIDS patients without clinical symptoms of OPC (41). The vast majority of HIV-infected and HIV-negative individuals who were found to harbor *C. dubliniensis* also harbored other *Candida* species in the oral cavity. However, the definite role of non-*C. albicans* yeasts as a causative pathogenic agent of OPC has not been clearly established. Several predisposing factors have been claimed to cause OPC. These may be divided into either systemic or local factors (Table 1), as suggested by Budtz-Jorgensen (24).

Table 1. Predisposing factors for oral candidiasis[a]

Systemic factors	Local factors
Physiological (elderly, infancy, pregnancy)	Dentures (changes in environmental conditions, trauma, denture usage, cleanliness)
Endocrine disorders (diabetes mellitus, hypothyroidism)	Endogenous epithelial changes (atrophy, hyperplasia, dysplasia)
Nutritional deficiencies (iron, folate, vitamin B_{12})	Saliva—quantitative changes (xerostomia, Sjögren's syndrome, radiotherapy, drug therapy)
Malignancies (acute leukemia, agranulocytosis)	Saliva—qualitative changes (pH, glucose concentration)
Immune defects, immunosuppression (AIDS, thymic, aplasia, corticosteroids, anticancer drugs)	Commensal flora
	High-carbohydrate diet
	Smoking (?)

[a] Adapted from reference 24.

Pathogenesis

Adhesion of yeasts to the mucosa of the oral cavity and dentures is an important initial step in the pathogenesis of oral yeast infections. Furthermore, a direct relationship between the adhesion capacity of various *Candida* species and their ability to cause infection has been observed (28, 97–99, 137). Adherence mechanisms known to be used by *C. albicans* are hydrophobicity, protein-protein binding via integrin-like surface proteins, and lectin-like proteins (27, 90). Local defense mechanisms play a central role in preventing yeast colonization of the oral cavity. These mechanisms include the physical local barrier of the epithelia, antimicrobial peptides, secretory immunoglobulin A, and salivary factors such as saliva flow rate and salivary molecules (e.g., lysozyme, histatins, and lactoferrin) (107). Observations in the late 1960s have shown that persistent *Candida* infection is common in patients with cell-mediated immunodeficiencies (79). Consequently, it was suggested in subsequent studies in chronic mucocutaneous candidiasis (CMC) that impaired cell-mediated immune response leads to this chronic infection (118, 119). In the pre-AIDS era the scant published data proposed a relationship between immunological parameters and response to therapy in oral candidiasis other than CMC (126). Experimental evidence supporting a role for T lymphocytes in resistance to mucosal candidiasis has come from studies with germ-free athymic mice (30). Further experimental studies supported the clinical observation in HIV-infected individuals that $CD4^+$ lymphocytes play a critical role in resistance to mucosal candidiasis (31, 66). Recently, Jones-Carson et al. provided evidence that, although highly susceptible to orogastric candidiasis, T-cell receptor delta- and alpha-chain knockout mice, deficient in gamma-delta and alpha-beta T cells, respectively, were found to be resistant to disseminated candidiasis of endogenous origin and to acute systemic candidiasis (93). The most important predisposing factor for OPC other than T-cell immunodeficiency is the wearing of removable dentures (20, 193). Other conditions that may contribute to OPC are radiation therapy for head and neck cancer, reduced salivary flow rates, diabetes mellitus, and gastrointestinal disorders (29, 59, 173, 209).

Clinical Presentation

Various presentations of OPC have been described, from which the pseudomembranous candidiasis (oral thrush) represents the most prevalent form (Color plate 8). Pseudomembranous candidiasis is characterized by removable white plaques that may be scraped away to reveal a bleeding surface. Symptoms of OPC usually include an alteration of taste ("furry" taste), inflammation in the mouth with oral pain and burning of mouth, and xerostomia. Occasionally patients complain that their breath smells like a brewery. In most cases, patients are able to maintain their oral nutritional intake, despite discomfort, and do not lose weight. Laboratory tests may confirm the diagnosis of candidiasis by microscopy with a 10 to 20% potassium hydroxide preparation of lesions for detection of pseudohyphae and yeast forms or by fungal culture on specialized media (e.g., 2% Sabouraud's glucose agar). More recently, the use of chromogenic media (e.g., CHROMagar, Albicans ID, and others) allows the detection of yeasts in mixed cultures by differences in colony color (123, 153, 189). According to the classification of the EEC-Clearinghouse on oral problems related to HIV infection, four subtypes were defined in HIV-infected individuals: erythematous, hyperplastic, pseudomembranous candidiasis and angular cheilitis (57). In addition to patients with HIV infection, the occurrence of pseudomembranous candidiasis has been described in neonates, the elderly, patients with malignancies and/or undergoing chemotherapy, and those with nutritional deficiency, deficiencies of cell-mediated immunity, or phagocyte dysfunction and after broad-spectrum antibiotics or steroids (29). The erythematous OPC has been reported primarily in patients with HIV infection, and it has been suggested that this form is more difficult to recognize and hence is underdiagnosed (53). In a study by Dodd et al., of 169 HIV-positive patients with OPC, 92 had pseudomembranous candidiasis, 37 had erythematous candidiasis, and 40 patients had both types of lesions (53). Data from Samaranayake et al. suggested that almost equal numbers of cases present with either the erythematous or pseudomembranous form, but Dodd et al. found a threefold-higher incidence of the pseudomembranous form compared to the erythematous presentation, and the examination of 456 consecutive HIV-infected patients in a study by Palmer et al. revealed erythematous candidiasis in 24%, pseudomembranous candidiasis in 14%, and angular cheilitis (Color plate 9) in 6% (53, 156, 184). These data may reflect the fact that the erythematous form is more difficult to diagnose and may be missed on oral examination. However, a clear definition of erythematous candidiasis (other than a red area without removable white spots or plaques) as seen in HIV-infected individuals is lacking (57). In non-HIV-infected individuals the presentation of erythematous candidiasis has been observed in patients with denture stomatitis, but definite epidemiologic data are rare (22). Furthermore, in non-HIV-positive patients other forms such as chronic atrophic candidiasis and acute atrophic candidiasis (antibiotic sore tongue) have been described and associated with denture wearing, habitual thumb-sucking, or use of corticosteroid aerosols or broad-spectrum antibiotics (29). Chronic hyperplastic candidiasis (*Candida* leukoplakia) and angular cheilitis (perlèche) have been associated with HIV infection, oral cancer, cellular hyperplasia, smoking, or denture wearing. However, the various definitions are not consistently used in the literature. The role of smoking as a separate cofactor was raised by Arendorf et al., but this was not supported by other studies (4, 75, 154).

HIV-infected individuals

Oral candidiasis is seen in nearly 10 to 30% of asymptomatic HIV-1-infected patients in the United States and Europe, in 40 to 60% of patients with symptomatic HIV infection (formerly described as

AIDS-related complex), and in 50 to 90% of AIDS patients (125). Oral candidiasis is not only the most common fungal infection in HIV-infected individuals but is by far the most common opportunistic infection observed in this patient group, affecting nearly 90% of subjects at some stage during the course of HIV disease progression. The reports from the early 1980s have identified OPC as a clinical predictor of progression to AIDS (102, 162, 207). Other host factors besides advanced HIV disease alone have been claimed to contribute to OPC: low CD4 lymphocyte count, xerostomia, age >35 years, intravenous drug use, and certain racial populations, such as black intravenous drug users compared to white subjects (62, 135, 158). More recently, Gootfredsson et al. concluded that the amount of asymptomatic oropharyngeal yeast carriage in persons with HIV infection is more significantly correlated with HIV viremia than with CD4 cell count (71). It was discussed by several authors that HIV viral load suppression induced by highly active antiretroviral therapy may further contribute to the clinically observed reductions of oral and esophageal candidiasis and other opportunistic infections (71, 101, 116, 145, 158). It may be argued that highly active antiretroviral therapy can induce recovery of CD4 T-cell reactivity against *C. albicans* similar to other opportunistic pathogens, and therefore reconstitute immune defense mechanisms (120). *C. albicans* is the most commonly isolated species from samples taken from the oral cavity. However, from molecular epidemiological studies, we now understand that several strains of *C. albicans* can colonize the mucous membranes. Colonization with up to three genotypically different strains of *C. albicans* may occur either in parallel or sequentially, but in most cases one "dominant" strain (better described as genotype) persists and is associated with recurrent infections. For a patient, intrastrain variation may occur (3, 11, 13, 140, 168, 180). These persistent strains may be transferred via intimate contact between sexual partners (144). However, even when the genotype of *C. albicans* persists, the phenotypical expression of the strains may change (138). Although strains from patients with AIDS were genetically less diverse than either control strains or oral commensal strains, the majority did not form a genetically distinct group, nor was a more virulent strain demonstrated by molecular typing or invasiveness in murine models (205, 215). In a study with clinical isolates from patients with AIDS in Leicester, United Kingdom, it was observed that the majority of the original commensal strains were replaced early in AIDS and replacement occurred only once (190). The genetic similarities of isolates within and between groups were assessed by fingerprinting using Southern blot hybridization with the Ca^3 probe. Results were analyzed by computer-assisted, automated Dendron system, but several other DNA probes or typing techniques have been successfully applied such as randomly amplified polymorphic DNA, pulsed-field gel electrophoresis, and others (18, 52, 201).

Non-HIV-infected individuals

In non-HIV-infected individuals, the epidemiological data are not as intensively studied as in HIV-infected individuals. Predisposing factors, either local or systemic, are given in Table 1. Patients with hematological malignancies and solid tumors often are affected by OPC as well as other fungal infections. Natural physical barriers to colonization and invasion are lost during anticancer therapy. It is believed that oral candidiasis is frequent (>75%) and that good oral hygiene and dental care, together with antifungal agents either given prophylactically or therapeutically, are important components in the care of patients receiving chemotherapy, because colonization of the gastrointestinal tract may serve as a portal of entry for invasive candidiasis when mucositis occurs (61, 164, 170, 186). However, only colonization at multiple body sites has been found to be a risk factor for the development of invasive candidiasis and not OPC alone (73, 131). It is not known whether OPC may be regarded as a marker of uncontrolled or progressive disease as seen in patients with progressive HIV infection or is due to concomitant treatments such as corticosteroids, antibiotics, or immunosuppressive drugs that have been associated with oral thrush (21). The most important local factor for OPC is the presence of a denture in the oral cavity. Unclean dentures and insufficient hygiene care are important predisposing factors. Removal of the denture alone may eliminate the infection (25).

Treatment

Recommendations for therapy of various forms of candidiasis have been recently outlined as practice guidelines by Rex et al. (178). A number of options, either local or systemic, are available for the treatment of OPC. Most of these data were obtained from HIV-infected individuals (Table 2). Prior to 1980, the compound most commonly used for treatment of oral thrush was gentian crystal violet, but this approach became unpopular due to local necrosis and staining of the oral mucosa (85). Oral polyenes and azoles have finally replaced this compound. Several studies have been conducted comparing local (topical) and systemic therapy. Clinical response rates were similar, but signs and symptoms were more rapidly resolved

Table 2. Therapy of oropharyngeal candidiasis in HIV-infected and non-HIV-infected individuals (summarized from published trials)

Reference	No. of patients	Therapy, dosage[a]	Duration (days)	Clinical cure (%)	Mycological cure (%)
HIV-infected adults					
De Wit, 1989 (50)	18	Fluco, 50 mg	28	100	87
	19	Keto, 200 mg		62.5	69
Chave, 1989 (38)	23	Fluco, 150 mg	1	96 (day7)	87 (day7)
Just-Nübling, 1990 (94)	106	Fluco, 50–300 mg	4–23	93	70
Koletar, 1990 (106)	19	Fluco, 100 mg	14	100	75
	20	Clotrim, 5 × 10 mg		65	20
Smith, 1991 (195)	45	Itra, 200 mg	28	93	85
	40	Keto, 2 × 200 mg		93	83
Pons, 1993 (165)	176	Fluco, 100 mg	14	98	65
	158	Clotrim, 5 × 10 mg		94	48
De Wit, 1993 (49)	28	Fluco, 150 mg	1	87.5	35
	28	Fluco, 50 mg	7	96	62
Plettenberg, 1994 (163)	103	Fluco, 100 mg	7–21	87	57
Sangeorzan, 1994 (189)	23	Fluco, 100 mg	14	96	49
	22	Clotrim, 5 × 10 mg		91	27
De Repentigny, 1996 (47)	51	Itra, 200 mg	14	71	63
	55	Keto, 200 mg		60	62
Pons, 1997[b] (166)	83	Fluco, 100 mg[c]	14	87	60
	84	Nystatin, 4 × 5 × 10[6c]		52	6
Murray, 1997[d] (147)	75	Itra, 200 mg[c]	14	77	60
	74	Clotrim, 5 × 10 mg		70	32
Moshi, 1998 (146)	75	Nystatin, 3 × 1 × 10[6c]	14	63.5	No data
	75	2% sodium benzoate, 3 × 10 ml		55.6	
Graybill, 1998[b] (72)	60	Itra, 2 × 100 mg[c]	7	86	52
	59	Itra, 2 × 100 mg[c]	14	97	88
	60	Fluco, 100 mg	14	87	77
Phillips, 1998 (160)	72	Fluco, 100 mg	14	90	53
	60	Itra, 2 × 100 mg[c]	7	82	44
	62	Itra, 100 mg[c]	14	90	57
Linpiyawan, 2000 (122)	14	Itra, 2 × 100 mg[c]	7	66.7	No data
	15	Clotrim, 5 × 10 mg		73.3	
HIV-infected children					
Hernández, 1994 (80)	24	Fluco, 3 mg/kg/day[c]	5–49	88	71
	22	Keto, 7 mg/kg/day[c]		81	57
Flynn, 1995[d] (67)	94	Fluco, 2–3 mg/kg/day[c]	14	91	76
	88	Nystatin, 4 × 4 × 10[6] U/day[c]		51	11
Non-HIV-infected adults					
Meunier, 1990[e] (141)	19	Fluco, 2 × 50 mg/day	4–27	78	50
	18	Keto, 2 × 20 mg/day		78	50
De Bock, 1998[e] (45)	126	Fluco, 100 mg/day	10	86	80
	126	Itra, 200 mg/day	15	80	68

[a]Fluco, fluconazole; Keto, ketoconazole; Clotrim, clotrimoxazole; Itra, itraconazole.
[b]Day 1 double dose as loading dose.
[c]Oral suspension.
[d]Mixed population with more than 80% HIV-infected individuals.
[e]Cancer patients.

with systemic treatment. Most patients will respond to topical therapy with clotrimazole troches (one 10-mg troche 5 times daily), or nystatin (as a suspension of 100,000 U/ml 4 times daily) for 7 to 14 days, but longer treatment for up to 28 days may be needed in some cases due to the lower clinical response rate compared to that with azoles. In Europe amphotericin B suspension (100 mg 4 to 6 times per day) is used frequently instead of clotrimazole because clotrimazole is marketed for vaginal candidiasis only (24). However, information on efficacy is derived from studies with antifungal prophylaxis and not from comparative trials for OPC (17, 48, 139). Oral fluconazole (100 mg per day for up to 14 days) has become the drug of choice in many patients, because the clinical response is usually apparent within 1 to 2 days and side effects due to therapy are minimal (70). The early studies have shown that 50 mg of fluconazole daily is effective for most cases of OPC, but more recently a 100 mg dosage was advocated and used in most studies to prolong the disease-free interval in severely immunocompromised patients (76). Itraconazole as a solution (100 mg 2 times per day up to 14 days) is regarded as efficacious as fluconazole. Absorption of ketoconazole and itraconazole capsules depends on gastric acidity and may be, therefore, regarded only as second choice treatment in patients with hypochlorhydria. Mycological responses are not as high as clinical response rates (Table 2), and *Candida* spp. can still be cultured from the oropharynx in many patients. Single-dose treatment has been shown to be effective in HIV-infected individuals, but prolonged therapy for 14 days and longer has shown somewhat higher mycological responses. However, clinical evidence of relapse and recurrence is a common finding irrespective of treatment, as seen in the majority of studies. Thus, mycological cure may not be achieved and perhaps should not be regarded as an important parameter for response to treatment. In HIV-infected individuals who suffer from recurrent OPC, a possible progression of HIV infection should be considered, and HIV viral load and $CD4^+$ lymphocyte counts should be determined. Using a scoring system to assess a clinical response, Hood et al. summarized the evaluation of their findings, that resolution of dysphagia and oral pain correlated best with response to therapy, unlike retrosternal pain and throat pain (87). The superiority of the itraconazole solution over the itraconazole capsules was not demonstrated in other patient groups such as those with *Candida*-associated denture stomatitis. Cross et al. found that in patients who are not immunocompromised, the absorption of liquid preparation was no greater than that of the capsules, and serum concentrations were lower than described in AIDS patients (35, 42). In *Candida*-associated denture stomatitis, the most important therapeutic measure is institution of effective oral and denture hygiene; administration of antifungal agents should be combined with these basic measures (24). In a study by Bissell et al. in 59 patients with denture-related disease, 50 mg of fluconazole daily for 14 days compared with amphotericin lozenges, and a cream preparation for 28 days showed similar clinical response rates in both treatment groups (17). Further effective options may include miconazole lacquer, which is applied to the fitting surface of the dentures (23). Although properly studied, it is assumed that the therapeutic guidelines for AIDS patients do not differ from those for other risk groups (e.g., oncology patients) (164).

Recurrences of oral or esophageal candidiasis can be prevented in HIV-infected individuals with low CD4 cell counts ($<200/\mu l$) when a maintenance suppressive treatment is given either daily (50 to 200 mg/day) or once weekly (150 to 200 mg), and continuous therapy is associated with a lower annual relapse rate than intermittent therapy (60, 95, 117, 128, 130, 167, 175, 191, 202). Because of the potential for the development of resistance in vitro and refractory disease in patients (as shown for fluconazole), as well as other arguments, such as high costs, drug interactions with antiretroviral drugs, and low mortality associated with mucosal candidiasis, prophylaxis is only recommended when recurrences are frequent or severe (210).

ESOPHAGEAL CANDIDIASIS

Epidemiology

Candida esophagitis occurs in patients with chronic diseases, most of whom have been previously treated with antibiotics, steroids, or omeprazole, but the disease most frequently occurs in those with advanced HIV infection (40). Although a variety of both opportunistic and nonopportunistic disorders result in esophageal disease in the HIV population, candidal esophagitis is the most common cause of symptomatic disease. In 1993, esophageal candidiasis (21.3%) was among the four most common AIDS-defining opportunistic infections in patients taking prophylaxis against *Pneumocystis carinii* pneumonia (88). In the era of combination antiretroviral therapy, the incidence of esophageal candidiasis (EC) was lower than 4 years earlier (in 1994, 8.0%; in 1998, 5.4%, respectively) but was ranked as number one of all opportunistic illnesses (145). Women appeared to be even more susceptible to EC, because in the era before *Pneumocystis* prophylaxis, *Candida* esophagitis was observed even more commonly than PCP (33).

Clinical Presentation

Patients with *Candida* esophagitis may present with either dysphagia or odynophagia and develop ulcers and erosions on the esophagus (Color plate 10). Oral candidiasis is usually present at the time of diagnosis. However, while about 25% do not have OPC and as many as 40% of patients may have no symptoms, the absence of OPC does not exclude esophageal involvement, nor does the presence of dysphagia and OPC indicate that the patient has *Candida* esophagitis (74). According to Wilcox et al., the positive and negative predictive values of OPC for EC were 90% and 82%, respectively (15). It is still controversial whether routine endoscopy (esophagogastroduodenoscopy [EGD]) is needed to establish the diagnosis; but a presumptive diagnosis on clinical grounds should be established and empirical antifungal therapy should be started. This approach is supported by a decision analysis to assess cost-effectiveness done by Rabeneck and Laine in HIV-infected individuals (172). In this analysis, empirical therapy with fluconazole was the most cost-effective strategy for all probabilities of EC. In a more recent study by Bashir and Wilcox, EGD influenced patient management in 78% of cases (total 156 patients), and the authors concluded that selective symptom-specific use of EGD, particularly in patients with esophageal symptoms refractory to antifungal therapy or gastrointestinal bleeding, usually identifies specific treatable abnormalities. It should be kept in mind that in patients who do not improve clinically after 3 weeks of therapy, resistant *Candida* esophagitis or ulcerations of either viral (cytomegalovirus infection) or idiopathic origin may be the cause (157, 219).

In patient populations at risk for EC but without HIV infection, establishing the diagnosis by endoscopy and biopsy for histology may be still more appropriate, because confirmation of a diagnosis rests on histological evidence of tissue invasion by the fungus. Endoscopy is the most definitive of the available diagnostic procedures and is preferable to barium swallow radiography (Fig. 1) (214).

In 1976 Kodsi et al. proposed a grading scale of I to IV of severity based on endoscopic appearance of candidal esophageal lesions in 27 patients (105). Barbaro et al. have used a modified classification (scale 0 to III) for clinical studies with antifungal agents: grade 0, normal esophageal mucosa; grade I, individual raised plaques, each <2 mm in size; grade II, individual raised plaques >2 mm in size; grade III, confluent plaques combined or not combined with ulceration and/or increased friability of mucosa (7–10). Furthermore, this group in their studies used the following clinical classification: grade 0, absence of symptoms; grade I, symptoms of mild entity not compromising the capability to swallow both solid and liquid substances; grade II, symptoms of moderate entity not compromising (grade IIa) or compromising (grade IIb) the capability to swallow liquid substances; grade III, symptoms of severe entity compromising either the capability to swallow solid substances only (grade IIIa) or compromising the capability to swallow both solid and liquid substances (grade IIIb).

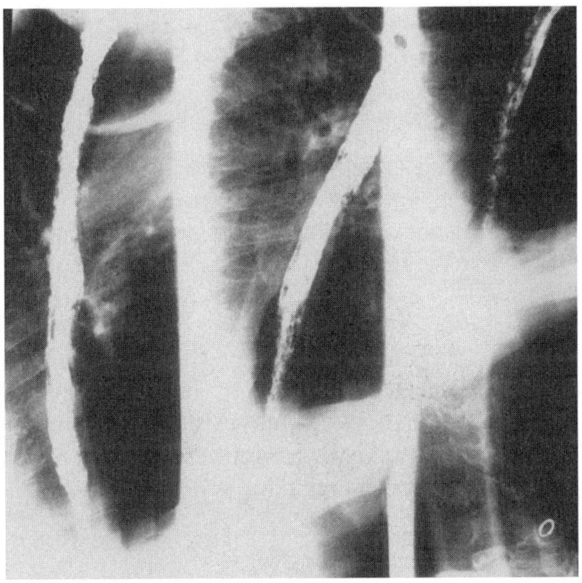

Figure 1. *Candida* esophagitis, as demonstrated by barium swallow radiography in a patient with AIDS.

Treatment

Treatment for EC is essentially the same as for oral candidiasis. However, systemic therapy is recommended over local therapy by most authorities and all patients should be treated with a systemic antifungal agent (178). Fluconazole, which is equally effective in oral and esophageal candidiasis, has become the standard agent (200 mg loading followed by 100 mg/day for 14 to 21 days) (Table 3). Ketoconazole oral tablets and itraconazole oral capsules are effective and may be alternatives but are less effective than fluconazole capsules. As mentioned above, their use is limited because of problems with drug absorption. Itraconazole absorption was increased by >30% with an oral solution in hydroxypropyl-β-cyclodextrin and efficacy may be even improved because of a topical effect of the solution (14, 72, 133). Bioavailability of the itraconazole oral solution appeared not to be modified by the severity of HIV disease (179). Clinical response to itraconazole solution (200 mg/day) may be observed within a few days and therapy may be considered as effective as with fluconazole capsules (218). This is in contrast to the capsule formulation, which may take even weeks to build up steady-state concentrations unless a loading dose is given as recommended for invasive aspergillosis (46).

Almost all patients with AIDS who are successfully treated for EC develop recurrent disease, usually within 2 to 3 months. Two-thirds of patients are symptomatic and one-third is associated with oral thrush (111).

VULVOVAGINAL CANDIDIASIS

Genital candidiasis may affect the vulva and vaginal area, as well as the perianal and crural folds, caus-

Table 3. Therapy of esophageal candidiasis in HIV-infected and non-HIV-infected individuals (summarized from published trials; adults only)

Reference	No. of patients	Therapy, dosage[a]	Duration (days)	Endoscopic cure (%)	Cure of symptoms (%)
HIV-infected patients					
Chave, 1990 (39)	33	Fluco, 400 mg	1	94	96
Brockmeyer, 1991 (19)	10	Fluco, 400 mg	8	100	100
	10	AmB, 0.4 mg/kg + 5-FC, 150 mg/kg		100	100
Laine, 1992 (112)	87	Fluco, 100 mg	14	91	85
	82	Keto, 200 mg	Up to 64	52	65
Barchiesi, 1992[b] (12)	38	Fluco, 200 mg	6–46	No data	76.3
	39	Keto, 400 mg	6–33		79.4
Laine, 1995 (113)	42	Fluco, 100 mg[c]	14 + after resolution	95	100
Barbaro, 1995 (8)	62	Fluco, 2 × 100 mg	21	74	75.5
	61	Itra, 2 × 100 mg		47.2	74.5
Barbaro, 1995 (9)	20	Fluco, 3 mg/kg/day	35	65	80
	20	5-FC, 100 mg/kg/day		15	60
	20	Placebo		0	0
De Repentigny, 1996 (47)	18	Itra, 200 mg	28	No data	100
	19	Keto, 200 mg			91
Barbaro, 1996 (7)	1,105	Fluco, 200 mg	14+	81	82
	1,108	Itra, 200 mg		66	75
Barbaro, 1996 (10)	30	Fluco, 3 mg/kg/day	14	69	76
	30	Itra, 3 mg/kg/day + 5-FC, 100 mg/kg/day		72	72
	25	Placebo		23 (partial)	27 (partial)
Wilcox, 1997[d] (218)	57	Fluco, 100 mg	21+	94	94
	53	Itra, 100 mg[c]	Up to 64	94	91
Non-HIV-infected patients					
Lake, 1996[e] (114)	13	Fluco, 2 × 100 mg	7–28	4/6	11/13
	12	Ampho B, 0.3 mg/kg/day		2/5	6/12
Péter, 1996[f] (159)	9	Fluco, 150 mg	1	8/9	No data
	11	Fluco, 50 mg	7	9/11	

[a] Fluco, fluconazole; AmB, amphotericin B; Keto, ketoconazole; Itra, itraconazole; 5-FC, 5-fluorocytosine.
[b] Mixed population with oral (27 of 31) and esophageal candidiasis (7 of 13).
[c] Oral suspension.
[d] Day 1 double dose as loading dose.
[e] Cancer patients.
[f] Patients with alcoholic liver disease.

ing candidal intertrigo. Vulvovaginal candidiasis (VVC) is a mucosal infection caused by several *Candida* spp., with *C. albicans* as the most common yeast obtained from vaginal fungal cultures (197). The emergence of *C. glabrata* vaginal colonization has been described as a significant problem in HIV-infected women receiving fluconazole prophylaxis (212).

Epidemiology

C. albicans is responsible for more than 80% of episodes of VVC (197). It is estimated that 75% of all women will experience at least one episode of VVC in their lifetime. Approximately 10 to 20% of healthy women usually harbor *Candida* spp. and other yeasts in their vagina (149). Subgroups at higher risk for VVC are pregnant, HIV-infected women with a 40 to 60% prevalence of vaginitis and colonization, and to a lesser extent, HIV-negative, pregnant women with a 20 to 40% colonization rate (26, 192). In HIV-infected women, a strong correlation between CD4 cell count and appearance of recurrent VVC was observed, involving 20 to 30% of women with CD4 counts of less than 350/μl (43). VVC can occur concomitantly with sexually transmitted diseases or following antibacterial vaginal or systemic therapy.

Pathogenesis

The pathogenesis of VVC is not completely understood and much information on the immunopathogenesis is derived from animal studies (65, 183). As in OPC, multiple factors are involved, including various *Candida* virulence factors, antibiotic usage, reproductive hormone levels, and other factors that alter the normal vaginal flora or change the avidity of epithelial cells for *Candida* species. Cantorna et al. have shown that mice deficient in phagocytic cells and/or T cells showed no increase in susceptibility to vaginitis (32). Data from Imam et al. in HIV-positive women demonstrated that *Candida* often infected the vaginal mucosa when there was no significant reduction in CD4 lymphocyte counts (91). *Candida* mucosal infections in HIV-infected women appear to occur in a hierarchical pattern starting with VVC, followed by OPC, and finally EC when CD4 cell counts fall below 100/μl (43). However, in pregnant, HIV-infected women, a CD4 cell count of >200/μl was significantly associated with increased vaginal colonization and VVC during pregnancy and postpartum (26). A mechanism that may be responsible for the increased rates of candidiasis during pregnancy is hormone-enhanced binding to vaginal epithelial cells resulting in mycelial formation (169). Vaginal candidiasis is not considered a sexually transmitted disease, but an increase in frequency has been observed in women who begin regular sexual activity (197). As demonstrated by molecular typing studies, in patients with recurrent VVC, a single strain of *C. albicans* usually dominates in both the patient and the male partner that is maintained through sequential infections (124).

Clinical Presentation

Clinical signs and symptoms are not highly specific and misdiagnosing may occur, but the prominent symptoms include vulvovaginal itching and irritation as reported by McCormack et al. in 67% of healthy female college students whose cultures contained yeasts in contrast to 22% of women who were not colonized (136). Other symptoms may be burning and dyspareuria. A diagnosis of VVC is suggested clinically by pruritus and erythema in the vulvovaginal area. On examination, vulvular erythema and mucosal edema may be seen together with white patches analogous to those seen in oral thrush that can be removed by gentle scraping. The diagnosis is established by the finding of normal vaginal pH (4 to 4.5) and positive microscopy results of saline or 10% potassium hydroxide preparations of lesions. In patients with symptoms compatible with vaginitis but negative microscopy, a fungal culture is recommended (136). Recurrent VVC, which affects up to 5% of HIV-negative women, is defined as at least three or four episodes in a 12-month period (196). Complicated VVC is defined as severe and recurrent vaginitis with predominantly non-*C. albicans Candida* spp. in an immunocompromised host (178).

Treatment

Current treatment recommendations (Table 4) for uncomplicated vaginal candidiasis were published in 1998 by the Centers for Disease Control and Prevention and apply to both HIV-positive and HIV-negative women (37). Intravaginal formulations effectively treat VVC. Therapy with azole antifungal agents is more effective than with topical nystatin. Clinical cure may be achieved in 80 to 90% of patients

Table 4. Treatment options for uncomplicated VVC[a]

Agent	Dosage
Intravaginal agents	
Butoconazole	2% cream 5 g intravaginally for 3 days[b,c]
Clotrimazole	1% cream 5 g intravaginally for 7 to 14 days[b,c]
Clotrimazole	100-mg vaginal tablet for 7 days[b]
Clotrimazole	100-mg vaginal tablet, two tablets for 3 days[b]
Clotrimazole	500-mg vaginal tablet, one tablet in a single application[b]
Miconazole	2% cream 5 g intravaginally for 7 days[b,c]
Miconazole	200-mg vaginal suppository, one suppository for 3 days[b,c]
Miconazole	100-mg vaginal suppository, one suppository for 7 days[b,c]
Nystatin	100,000-unit vaginal tablet, one tablet for 14 days
Tioconazole	6.5% ointment 5 g intravaginally in a single application[b,c]
Terconazole	0.4% cream 5 g intravaginally for 7 days[b]
Terconazole	0.8% cream 5 g intravaginally for 3 days[b]
Terconazole	80-mg vaginal suppository, one suppository for 3 days[b]
Boric acid	600-mg in a gelatine capsule, once daily for 14 days
Oral agents	
Fluconazole	150-mg oral tablet, one tablet in single dose
Itraconazole	2 × 200 mg on a single day *or* 200-mg oral tablet daily for 3 days

[a]Adapted from the recommendations by the Centers for Disease Control and Prevention and Rex et al. (37, 178).
[b]These creams and suppositories are oil-based and might weaken latex condoms and diaphragms. Refer to condom product labeling for additional information.
[c]Over-the-counter preparations.

Table 5. Therapy of VVC in non-HIV-infected females with oral azoles (selected studies)

Reference	No. of patients	Therapy, dosage[a]	Duration (days)	Clinical cure (%)	Mycological cure (%)
Comparative studies with oral azoles					
Kutzer, 1988 (109)	183	Fluco, 150 mg	1	92	77
		Keto, 2 × 200 mg	5	89	77
Rees, 1992 (174)	176	Fluco, 150 mg	1	94	82
	178	Itra, 2 × 200 mg	1	93	72
Wooley, 1995 (221)	72	Fluco, 150 mg	1	92	83
	82	Clotrimazole, 200 mg v.t.[b]	1	93	95
	75	Itra, 2 × 200 mg	1	92	96
Mikamo, 1998 (142)	50	Fluco, 150 mg	1	76	70
	50	Itra, 200 mg	3	88	74
	50	Clotrimazole, 100 mg	6	58	60
Fluconazole single-dose efficacy					
Sobel, 1995 (198)	218	Fluco, 150 mg	1	94	77
	214	Clotrimazole, 100 mg v.t.[b]	7	97	72
O-Prasertsawat, 1995 (155)	53	Fluco, 150 mg	1	89	79
	50	Clotrimazole, 200 mg v.t.[b]	3	90	80
Kaplan, 1997 (96)	428	Fluco, 150 mg	1	72	78
Edelman, 1999 (56)	213	Fluco, 150 mg (pooled data)	1	95	93

[a] Fluco, fluconazole; Keto, ketoconazole; Itra, itraconazole.
[b] v.t., vaginal treatment.

who complete a full course of therapy. Most intravaginal regimens require 3 or 7 days of therapy, but a single application of either a 500-mg clotrimazole vaginal tablet or 6.5% tioconazole ointment has proven to be effective in more than 10 comparative studies (56). Oral azoles require only a single oral application either of 150 mg fluconazole or single day application of itraconazole 200 mg twice a day (178). Clinical efficacy of fluconazole and itraconazole seems to be very similar, and long-term mycologic cure rates were higher compared to intravaginal clotrimazole; however, fluconazole was studied much more intensively (14) (Table 5). There were few significant differences in either the clinical or mycologic cure rates of single-dose therapy as outlined in a review on single-dose therapy for VVC by Edelman and Grant (56). However, complicated or recurrent infection (e.g., VVC in a patient who has uncontrolled diabetes or infection caused by a less susceptible fungal pathogen such as *C. glabrata*) requires a longer duration of therapy (i.e., 10 to 14 days) (37).

RESISTANT MUCOSAL CANDIDIASIS

Resistant Oral and Esophageal Candidiasis

Oral and esophageal candidiasis, refractory to systemic therapy with antifungal agents resulting in treatment failure as well as development of resistance in *C. albicans* to antifungal agents in vitro, has been associated with the repeated or continuous use of azole antifungal agents in general, but fluconazole in particular (177). Common factors that led to the presence of a resistant *Candida* strain in patients may be due to replacement by a more resistant species (e.g., *C. krusei, C. glabrata*) or replacement with a more resistant strain of *C. albicans.* Azole drug resistance did not become a significant problem until this group of compounds began to be used in patients with HIV infection. A correlation of in vitro susceptibility testing of *C. albicans* with in vivo response to antifungal therapy has been observed for oral and esophageal candidal infections in HIV-infected patients, but not for other forms of candidiasis (e.g., candidemia) (176). Various definitions of clinical drug failure in patients with mucosal candidiasis have been proposed. Fichtenbaum and Powderly have summarized data from recent studies and defined fluconazole-refractory mucosal candidiasis as a progressive disease with lack of improvement after treatment with fluconazole 200 mg orally or intravenously daily for at least 7 days (63). Clinical, cellular, and molecular factors that contribute to azole resistance have been reviewed by White et al. and will not be discussed here (217). It appears that development of resistance occurred in a single previously sensitive *C. albicans* strain even if several other *C. albicans* genotypes may be detected in a single patient throughout the course of HIV disease (143, 172). Several different molecular mechanisms of drug resistance have been described in

C. albicans isolates from unrelated patients (69, 217). Clinical patterns that were associated with fluconazole refractory mucosal disease include very advanced HIV disease with a CD4 cell count of <50/μl, a history of recurrent candidiasis, extensive previous fluconazole exposure, history of opportunistic infections (e.g., tuberculosis or toxoplasmosis), and treatment with antituberculosis drugs (110, 127, 134, 181, 208). Rarely, the development of secondary resistance in *C. albicans* has been reported in non-HIV-infected patients, such as patients with cancer or undergoing bone marrow transplantation (129, 188). Patients who are unresponsive to fluconazole at a dose of 200 mg daily may still respond to higher doses of fluconazole (400 to 800 mg) but will ultimately fail therapy with fluconazole. An early report on therapy of "resistant" oral candidiasis recommended that surgical excision of affected areas of oral mucosa was found to be the most effective therapy (126). Today, this may not be the appropriate approach, but there are a number of options for treatment that may be derived from noncomparative trials (Table 6). Switching to another azole such as itraconazole cyclodextrin oral solution may be the best alternative, but oral polyenes may have some effect as well. Parenteral amphotericin B is regarded as the drug of choice in patients with severe disease. However, data from small studies gave conflicting results on the success of amphotericin B for this particular indication since patients showed either clinical improvement or no response at a dose ranging from 0.5 to 0.7 mg/kg of body weight per day intravenously (6, 213). In a report by Swindells et al., adjunctive therapy with granulocyte-macrophage colony-stimulating factor (125 μg/m^2 subcutaneously for 14 days) led to improvement in the signs and symptoms of OPC in three patients (204). More interestingly, recent reports described the resolution of fluconazole-refractory OPC as well as a decreasing incidence of OPC after the initiation of potent combination antiretroviral therapy, including protease inhibitors (5, 159, 211, 222).

Resistant Vulvovaginal Candidiasis

Most studies indicate that up to 95% of clinical *Candida* isolates responsible for VVC are *C. albicans*.

Table 6. Antifungal treatment options for fluconazole-refractory oral/esophageal candidiasis

Reference	No. of patients	Therapy	Dosage	Clinical response[a]	Mycological data[b]
Dewsnup, 1994 (51)	2	Oral amphotericin B suspension (homemade preparation)	AmB-D,[c] 4 × 1 mg/day	1 CR, 1 PR	Both *C. glabrata*; MIC of FLU >100[d]
Cartledge, 1994 (36)	27	Itraconazole oral suspension	1 or 2 × 200 mg for 14 days	18/25 CR	No data
Philips, 1996 (161)	34	Itraconazole oral suspension	200 mg/day for 14 days	22/34 CR	*C. albicans* MIC of FLU 4 to ≥64[d]
Eichel, 1996 (58)	20	Itraconazole oral suspension	200–800 mg/day for 7 days	19/20 CR or PR	Reduction in *Candida* CFU/ml in 20 patients/no MICs
Nguyen, 1996 (148)	8	Oral amphotericin B suspension (homemade preparation)	AmB-D 5 × 0.2–1 mg/day	6/8 PR	4 of 5 *C. albicans* MIC of FLU ≥25[d]
Martins, 1997 (132)	2	Fluconazole oral suspension	2 × 100 mg/day	1 CR + 1 PR	*C. albicans* MIC of FLU 0.5 + 64[d]
Hood, 1998 (86)	11	Oral amphotericin B suspension	4 × 200 mg/day for 10 days	6/11 CR	3/11 *C. albicans* MIC of FLU ≥16[d]
Cartledge, 1998 (34)	26	D0870 capsules	150 mg loading + 25 mg/day for 7 days	1 CR, 16 PR	Correlation between higher D0870 MICs and clinical failure
Jandourek, 1998 (92)	13	Melaleuca oral solution	4 × 15 ml for 2–4 weeks	7/12 PR at 2 weeks, 2 CR at 4 weeks	Mycological response 7 of 12; all MICs for *C. albicans* >20[d]
Hegener, 1998 (78)	12	Voriconazole capsules	2 × 200 mg/day	7 CR + 3 PR after 7 days	All MICs for *C. albicans* ≥12.5[d]
Fichtenbaum, 2000 (64)	54	Oral amphotericin B suspension	4 × 100 mg/day for 14–28 days	5 CR + 18 PR at 4 weeks	45/56 MICs for *C. albicans* ≥64[d]

[a]CR, complete response; PR, partial response.
[b]FLU, fluconazole.
[c]AmB-D, amphotericin B deoxycholate suspension.
[d]Concentration in μg/ml.

Reports of clinical and in vitro resistance to azoles occurring in women with symptomatic or recurrent VVC due to *C. albicans* are very rare in contrast to reports on oral and esophageal *Candida* infections (68, 200). The reasons for this difference are not clear, but differences in microbiology, virulence factors, and host-predisposing factors may be attributed. Treatment failures with azoles and azole-resistant VVC are more often linked with the detection of *C. glabrata* in fungal cultures. According to results from the HIV Epidemiology Research Study group, vaginal colonization (24%) with *C. glabrata* is more frequent in HIV-positive women than oral colonization (13%) (192). This difference was less clear in women with active disease (15% *C. glabrata* in the oral cavity versus 18% in the vagina). The emergence of *C. glabrata* in the vaginal flora was associated with fluconazole prophylaxis. In a study of the effect of fluconazole prophylaxis on the vaginal flora of 323 HIV-infected women by the Terry Beirn Community Programs for Clinical Research in AIDS, *C. glabrata* was recovered from 40 women assigned to fluconazole prophylaxis and 29 with placebo (212). The clinical picture of *C. glabrata* vaginitis tends to be more indolent chronic with more burning than itching, often accompanied by a watery discharge compared to VVC caused by *C. albicans*. Treatment of *C. glabrata* vaginitis may be effective in up to 81% of symptomatic women with local application of boric acid 600 mg/day in a gelatin capsule for 14 days as described by Sobel and Chaim and others (194, 199, 216).

CHRONIC MUCOCUTANEOUS CANDIDIASIS

CMC is a collection of syndromes in which patients have chronic and/or recurrent infections of the skin, nails, and mucous membranes with *Candida* species (151). Four subtypes of CMC have been described: CMC with familial susceptibility, CMC with endocrinopathy, CMC with both familial susceptibility and endocrinopathy, and CMC with onset later than 10 years of age (81). Several disorders may coexist or accompany patients with CMC, such as infectious diseases other than HIV infection, autoimmune diseases, endocrinopathies, thymoma, dental enamel dysplasia, vitiligo, and alopecia totalis (100). The central defect in patients with CMC is their inability to develop effective cell-mediated immune responses against *Candida* (119). Characteristically, patients with CMC have negative delayed hypersensitive skin reactions against *C. albicans* and decreased lymphokine production after stimulation by *Candida* antigens. Most CMC patients have normal serum and saliva immunoglobulin concentrations and normal or elevated concentrations of *Candida* serum antibodies (22). The importance of Th1 cytokines in resistance and Th2 in susceptibility to *Candida* infections has been demonstrated in murine models. Investigations by Kobrynski et al. showed that a decrease in $CD4^+$/$CD29^+$, T-helper inducer cells along with T-helper cell dysregulation could lead to defective memory responses to antigens in CMC patients and a decrease in cell-mediated immunity due to inhibition of Th1 cells by increased levels of IL-4 (104). These findings were supported by Lilic et al. who found that *Candida* antigens trigger a predominantly Th2 instead of a Th1 cytokine response in patients with CMC (121). Treatment strategies should combine treatment with antifungal agents and immunologic reconstitution. Prolonged antifungal treatment is required and is temporarily effective with azole antifungal agents (fluconazole, ketoconazole, or itraconazole), but relapses are frequently seen when therapy is stopped (178). As in OPC in HIV-infected patients, development of resistance is of concern with long-term suppressive therapy as shown for ketoconazole (77, 89). Successful reconstitution of the immune function has been described with either transplantation of cultured thymus tissue, infusions of blood leukocytes from donors with cell-mediated immunity against *Candida*, allogeneic bone marrow transplantation, and use of *Candida*-specific transfer factor (84, 100).

SKIN MANIFESTATIONS

Candida species, mostly *C. albicans*, but others such as *C. tropicalis*, *C. guilliermondii*, and *C. parapsilosis* as well, can cause superficial infections in both the skin and the nails (150). The organism has a predilection for warm and moist areas (intertriginous areas) which are created by maceration and occlusion. In HIV-infected patients, candidal skin infections have been frequently observed together with other superficial mycotic infections (2). Candidal skin infection is a common cause of diaper rash in infants. The macular erythematous rash is most marked in the intertriginous areas of the gluteal crease, perineum, and inguinal fold. A similar distribution of intertrigo occurs in the elderly and obese and diabetic, adult patients. The infection may begin in adults with vesicopustules that enlarge and progress to maceration and finally erythema. In women, inframammary areas may be affected, and frequent exposure of the hands to water may result in candidiasis of the digital folds of the hands. Itching and burning are the common symptoms. Diagnosis of cutaneous candidal skin infections is made by scraping the infected areas and examining the material with 10 to 15% potassium hydroxide (54). The most important aspect of treatment is keeping the infected areas dry and exposed to the air. Second, topical antifungal agents are the therapy of choice for uncomplicated cutaneous candidiasis. Topical azoles and clotrimazole, miconazole, and nystatin are effective when applied as creams or powder combined with or without a corticosteroid several times a day.

REFERENCES

1. **Adams, F.** 1939. Hippocrates, ca. 460-377 BC. *In Epidemics,* vol. 3. Williams and Wilkins, Baltimore, Md.
2. **Aly, R., and T. Berger.** 1996. Common superficial fungal infections in patients with AIDS. *Clin. Infect. Dis.* **22**(Suppl. 2):S128–S132.
3. **Anthony, R. M., J. Midgley, S. P. Sweet, and S. A. Howell.** 1995. Multiple strains of *Candida albicans* in the oral cavity of HIV positive and HIV negative patients. *Microb. Ecol. Health Dis.* **8**:23–30.
4. **Arendorf, T. M., and D. M. Walker.** 1980. The prevalence and intra-oral distribution of *Candida albicans* in man. *Arch. Oral Biol.* **25**:1–10.
5. **Arribas, J. R., S. Hernandez-Albujar, J. J. Gonzalez-Garcia, J. M. Pena, A. Gonzalez, T. Canedo, R. Madero, J. J. Vazquez, and W. G. Powderly.** 2000. Impact of protease inhibitor therapy on HIV-related oropharyngeal candidiasis. *AIDS* **14**: 979–985.
6. **Baily, G. G., F. M. Perry, D. W. Denning, and B. K. Mandal.** 1994. Fluconazole-resistant candidosis in an HIV cohort. *AIDS* **8**:787–792.
7. **Barbaro, G., G. Barbarini, W. Calderon, B. Grisorio, P. Alcini, and G. Di Lorenzo.** 1996. Fluconazole versus itraconazole for candida esophagitis in acquired immunodeficiency syndrome. *Candida* Esophagitis. *Gastroenterology* **111**: 1169–1177.
8. **Barbaro, G., G. Barbarini, and G. Di Lorenzo.** 1995. Fluconazole compared with itraconazole in the treatment of esophageal candidiasis in AIDS patients: a double-blind, randomized, controlled clinical study. *Scand. J. Infect. Dis.* **27**: 613–617.
9. **Barbaro, G., G. Barbarini, and G. Di Lorenzo.** 1995. Fluconazole vs. flucytosine in the treatment of esophageal candidiasis in AIDS patients: a double-blind, placebo-controlled study. *Endoscopy* **27**:377–383.
10. **Barbaro, G., G. Barbarini, and G. Di Lorenzo.** 1996. Fluconazole vs itraconazole-flucytosine association in the treatment of esophageal candidiasis in AIDS patients. A double-blind, multicenter placebo-controlled study. The *Candida* Esophagitis Multicenter Italian Study (CEMIS) Group. *Chest* **110**:1507–1514.
11. **Barchiesi, F., L. F. Di Francesco, P. Compagnucci, D. Arzeni, O. Cirioni, and G. Scalise.** 1997. Genotypic identification of sequential *Candida albicans* isolates from AIDS patients by polymerase chain reaction techniques. *Eur. J. Clin. Microbiol. Infect. Dis.* **16**:601–605.
12. **Barchiesi, F., A. Giacometti, D. Arzeni, P. Branchesi, G. Crescenzi, F. Ancarani, and G. Scalise.** 1992. Fluconazole and ketoconazole in the treatment of oral and esophageal candidiasis in AIDS patients. *J. Chemother.* **4**:381–386.
13. **Barchiesi, F., R. J. Hollis, D. A. McGough, G. Scalise, M. G. Rinaldi, and M. A. Pfaller.** 1995. DNA subtypes and fluconazole susceptibilities of *Candida albicans* isolates from the oral cavities of patients with AIDS. *Clin. Infect. Dis.* **20**:634–640.
14. **Barone, J. A., B. L. Moskovitz, J. Guarnieri, A. E. Hassell, J. L. Colaizzi, R. H. Bierman, and L. Jessen.** 1998. Enhanced bioavailability of itraconazole in hydroxypropyl-beta-cyclodextrin solution versus capsules in healthy volunteers. *Antimicrob. Agents Chemother.* **42**:1862–1865.
15. **Bashir, R. M., and C. M. Wilcox.** 1996. Symptom-specific use of upper gastrointestinal endoscopy in human immunodeficiency virus-infected patients yields high dividends. *J. Clin. Gastroenterol.* **23**:292–298.
16. **Berg, F. T.** 1846. *Om Torsk Hos Barn.* LJ Hierta, Stockholm, Sweden.
17. **Bissell, V., D. H. Felix, and D. Wray.** 1993. Comparative trial of fluconazole and amphotericin in the treatment of denture stomatitis. *Oral Surg. Oral Med. Oral Pathol.* **76**:35–39.
18. **Bostock, A., M. N. Khattak, R. Matthews, and J. Burnie.** 1993. Comparison of PCR fingerprinting, by random amplification of polymorphic DNA, with other molecular typing methods for *Candida albicans. J. Gen. Microbiol.* **139**(Sep. Pt. 9):2179–2184.
19. **Brockmeyer, N. H., D. Hantschke, T. Olbricht, U. A. Hengge, and M. Goos.** 1991. Comparative study of the therapy of *Candida* esophagitis in HIV-1-infected patients with fluconazole or amphotericin B and flucytosine. *Mycoses* **34**(Suppl. 1):83–86.
20. **Budtz-Jorgensen, E.** 1974. The significance of *Candida albicans* in denture stomatitis. *Scand. J. Dent. Res.* **82**:151–190.
21. **Budtz-Jorgensen, E.** 1990. Etiology, pathogenesis, therapy, and prophylaxis of oral yeast infections. *Acta Odontol. Scand.* **48**:61–69.
22. **Budtz-Jorgensen, E.** 1990. Histopathology, immunology, and serology of oral yeast infections. Diagnosis of oral candidosis. *Acta Odontol. Scand.* **48**:37–43.
23. **Budtz-Jorgensen, E., and P. Carlino.** 1994. A miconazole lacquer in the treatment of *Candida*-associated denture stomatitis. *Mycoses* **37**:131–135.
24. **Budtz-Jorgensen, E., and T. Lombardi.** 2000. Antifungal therapy in the oral cavity. *Periodontol.* **10**:89–106.
25. **Budtz-Jorgensen, E., P. Mojon, A. Rentsch, and N. Deslauriers.** 2000. Effects of an oral health program on the occurrence of oral candidosis in a long-term care facility. *Comm. Dent. Oral Epidemiol.* **28**:141–149.
26. **Burns, D. N., R. Tuomala, B.-H. Chang, R. Hershow, H. Minkoff, E. Rodriguez, C. Zorrilla, H. Hammill, J. Regan, and for the Woman and Infants Transmission Study Group.** 1997. Vaginal colonization or infection with *Candida albicans* in human immunodeficiency virus-infected women during pregnancy and during the postpartum period. *Clin. Infect. Dis.* **24**:201–210.
27. **Calderone, R. A., and P. C. Braun.** 1991. Adherence and receptor relationships of *Candida albicans. Microbiol. Rev.* **55**:1–20.
28. **Calderone, R., R. Diamond, J. M. Senet, J. Warmington, S. Filler, and J. E. Edwards.** 1994. Host cell-fungal cell interactions. *J. Med. Vet. Mycol.* **32**(Suppl. 1):151–168.
29. **Cannon, R. D., A. R. Holmes, A. B. Mason, and B. C. Monk.** 1995. Oral *Candida:* clearance, colonization, or candidiasis? *J. Dent. Res.* **74**:1152–1161.
30. **Cantorna, M. T., and E. Balish.** 1991. Acquired immunity to systemic candidiasis in immunodeficient mice. *J. Infect. Dis.* **164**:936–943.
31. **Cantorna, M. T., and E. Balish.** 1991. Role of CD4+ lymphocytes in resistance to mucosal candidiasis. *Infect. Immun.* **59**:2447–2455.
32. **Cantorna, M., D. Mook, and E. Balish.** 1990. Resistance of congenitally immunodeficient gnotobiotic mice to vaginal candidiasis. *Infect. Immun.* **58**:3813–3815.

33. **Carpenter, C. C., K. H. Mayer, A. Fisher, M. B. Desai, and L. Durand.** 1989. Natural history of acquired immunodeficiency syndrome in women in Rhode Island. *Am. J. Med.* **86**(6 Pt. 2):771–775.
34. **Cartledge, J. D., D. W. Denning, B. Dupont, N. Clumeck, S. De Wit, J. Midgley, D. A. Hawkins, and B. G. Gazzard.** 1998. Treatment of HIV-related fluconazole-resistant oral candidosis with D0870, a new triazole antifungal. *AIDS* **12:** 411–416.
35. **Cartledge, J. D., J. Midgely, and B. G. Gazzard.** 1997. Itraconazole solution: higher serum drug concentrations and better clinical response rates than the capsule formulation in acquired immunodeficiency syndrome patients with candidosis. *J. Clin. Pathol.* **50:**477–480.
36. **Cartledge, J. D., J. Midgley, M. Youle, and B. G. Gazzard.** 1994. Itraconazole cyclodextrin solution—effective treatment for HIV-related candidosis unresponsive to other azole therapy. *J. Antimicrob. Chemother.* **33:**1071–1073. (Letter.)
37. **Centers for Disease Control and Prevention.** 1998. 1998 guidelines for treatment of sexually transmitted diseases. *Morb. Mortal. Wkly. Rep.* **47:**1–111.
38. **Chave, J. P., A. Cajot, J. Bille, and M. P. Glauser.** 1989. Single-dose therapy for oral candidiasis with fluconazole in HIV-infected adults: a pilot study. *J. Infect. Dis.* **159:** 806–807. (Letter.)
39. **Chave, J. P., P. Francioli, B. Hirschel, and M. P. Glauser.** 1990. Single-dose therapy for esophageal candidiasis with fluconazole [letter]. *AIDS* **4:**1034–1035.
40. **Chocarro Martinez, A., F. Galindo Tobal, G. Ruiz-Irastorza, A. Gonzalez Lopez, F. Alvarez Navia, C. Ochoa Sangrador, and M. I. Martin Arribas.** 2000. Risk factors for esophageal candidiasis. *Eur. J. Clin. Microbiol. Infect. Dis.* **19:**96–100.
41. **Coleman, D. C., D. J. Sullivan, D. E. Bennett, G. P. Moran, H. J. Barry, and D. B. Shanley.** 1997. Candidiasis: the emergence of a novel species, *Candida dubliniensis. AIDS* **11:** 557–567.
42. **Cross, L. J., J. Bagg, D. Oliver, and D. Warnock.** 2000. Serum itraconazole concentrations and clinical responses in *Candida*-associated denture stomatitis patients treated with itraconazole solution and itraconazole capsules. *J. Antimicrob. Chemother.* **45:**95–99.
43. **Cu-Uvin, S., T. P. Flanigan, J. D. Rich, M. D. Mileno, K. H. Mayer, and C. C. Carpenter.** 1996. Human immunodeficiency virus infection and acquired immunodeficiency syndrome among North American women. *Am. J. Med.* **101:** 316–322.
44. **Darouiche, R. O.** 1998. Oropharyngeal and esophageal candidiasis in immunocompromised patients: treatment issues. *Clin. Infect. Dis.* **26:**259–274.
45. **De Bock, R., V. Krcmery, M. Aoun, A. Marinus, R. Sylvester, and B. De Pauw.** An EORTC IFICG phase II randomized study comparing fluconazole to itraconazole in nonneutropenic cancer patients with oropharyngeal candidiasis, abstr. MN-21. *In 38th Intersci. Conf. Antimicrob. Agents Chemother.* American Society for Microbiology, Washington, D.C.
46. **Denning, D. W.** 1998. Invasive aspergillosis. *Clin. Infect. Dis.* **26:**781–803.
47. **de Repentigny, L., and J. Ratelle.** 1996. Comparison of itraconazole and ketoconazole in HIV-positive patients with oropharyngeal or esophageal candidiasis. Human Immunodeficiency Virus Itraconazole Ketoconazole Project Group. *Chemotherapy* **42:**374–383.
48. **de Vries-Hospers, H. G., N. H. Mulder, D. T. Sleijfer, and H. K. van-Saene.** 1982. The effect of amphotericin B lozenges on the presence and number of *Candida* cells in the oropharynx of neutropenic leukemia patients. *Infection* **10:**71–75.
49. **De Wit, S., H. Goossens, and N. Clumeck.** 1993. Single-dose versus 7 days of fluconazole treatment for oral candidiasis in human immunodeficiency virus-infected patients: a prospective, randomized pilot study [letter]. *J. Infect. Dis.* **168:** 1332–1333.
50. **De Wit, S., D. Weerts, H. Goossens, and N. Clumeck.** 1989. Comparison of fluconazole and ketoconazole for oropharyngeal candidiasis in AIDS. *Lancet* **i:**746–748.
51. **Dewsnup, D. H., and D. A. Stevens.** 1994. Efficacy of oral amphotericin B in AIDS patients with thrush clinically resistant to fluconazole. *J. Med. Vet. Mycol.* **32:**389–393.
52. **Diaz-Guerra, T. M., J. V. Martinez-Suarez, F. Laguna, and J. L. Rodriguez-Tudela.** 1997. Comparison of four molecular typing methods for evaluating genetic diversity among *Candida albicans* isolates from human immunodeficiency virus-positive patients with oral candidiasis. *J. Clin. Microbiol.* **35:** 856–861.
53. **Dodd, C. L., D. Greenspan, M. H. Katz, J. L. Westenhouse, D. W. Feigal, and J. S. Greenspan.** 1991. Oral candidiasis in HIV infection: pseudomembranous and erythematous candidiasis show similar rates of progression to AIDS. *AIDS* **5:** 1339–1343.
54. **Drake, L. A., S. M. Dinehart, E. R. Farmer, R. W. Goltz, G. F. Graham, M. K. Hordinsky, C. W. Lewis, D. M. Pariser, J. W. Skouge, S. B. Webster, D. C. Whitaker, B. Butler, B. J. Lowery, B. E. Elewski, M. L. Elgart, P. H. Jacobs, J. L. Lesher, Jr., and R. K. Scher.** 1996. Guidelines of care for superficial mycotic infections of the skin: onychomycosis. *J. Am. Acad. Dermatol.* **34**(2 Pt. 1):116–121.
55. **Dronda, F., M. Alonso-Sanz, F. Laguna, F. Chaves, J. V. Martinez-Suarez, J. L. Rodriguez-Tudela, A. Gonzalez-Lopez, and E. Valencia.** 1996. Mixed oropharyngeal candidiasis due to *Candida albicans* and non-*albicans Candida* strains in HIV-infected patients. *Eur. J. Clin. Microbiol. Infect. Dis.* **15:**446–452.
56. **Edelman, D. A., and S. Grant.** 1999. One-day therapy for vaginal candidiasis. A review. *J. Reprod. Med.* **44:**543–547.
57. **EEC-Clearinghouse on Oral Problems Related to HIV Infection and WHO Collaborating Centre on Oral Manifestations of the Human Immunodeficiency Virus.** 1991. An update of the classification and diagnostic criteria of oral lesions in HIV infection. *J. Oral Pathol. Med.* **20:**97–100.
58. **Eichel, M., G. Just-Nübling, E. B. Helm, and W. Stille.** 1996. Itraconazole suspension in the treatment of HIV-infected patients with fluconazole-resistant oropharyngeal candidiasis and esophagitis. *Mycoses.* **39**(Suppl. 1):102–106.
59. **Epstein, J. B., and A. W. Chow.** 1999. Oral complications associated with immunosuppression and cancer therapies. *Infect. Dis. Clin. N. Am.* **13:**901–923.
60. **Esposito, R., A. Castagna, and C. Uberti-Foppa.** 1990. Maintenance therapy of oropharyngeal candidiasis in HIV-infected patients with fluconazole [letter]. *AIDS* **4:**1033–1034.
61. **Feld, R.** 1997. The role of surveillance cultures in patients likely to develop chemotherapy-induced mucositis. *Support Care Cancer* **5:**371–375.
62. **Fetter, A., M. Partisani, H. Koenig, M. Kremer, and J. M. Lang.** 1993. Asymptomatic oral *Candida albicans* carriage in HIV-infection: frequency and predisposing factors. *J. Oral. Pathol. Med.* **22:**57–59.
63. **Fichtenbaum, C. J., and W. G. Powderly.** 1998. Refractory mucosal candidiasis in patients with human immunodeficiency virus infection. *Clin. Infect. Dis.* **26:**556–565.
64. **Fichtenbaum, C. J., R. Zackin, N. Rajicic, W. G. Powderly, L. J. Wheat, and B. S. Zingman.** 2000. Amphotericin B oral suspension for fluconazole-refractory oral candidiasis in per-

sons with HIV infection. Adult AIDS Clinical Trials Group Study Team 295. *AIDS* **14**:845–852.

65. **Fidel, P. L., Jr., J. Cutright, and C. Steele.** 2000. Effects of reproductive hormones on experimental vaginal candidiasis. *Infect. Immun.* **68**:651–657.
66. **Fidel, P. L., Jr., and J. D. Sobel.** 1994. The role of cell-mediated immunity in candidiasis. *Trends Microbiol* **2**: 202–206.
67. **Flynn, P. M., C. K. Cunningham, T. Kerkering, A. R. San-Jorge, V. B. Peters, P. A. Pitel, J. Harris, G. Gilbert, L. Castagnaro, and P. Robinson.** 1995. Oropharyngeal candidiasis in immunocompromised children: a randomized, multicenter study of orally administered fluconazole suspension versus nystatin. The Multicenter Fluconazole Study Group. *J. Pediatr.* **127**:322–328.
68. **Fong, I. W., R. M. Bannatyne, and P. Wong.** 1993. Lack of in vitro resistance of *Candida albicans* to ketoconazole, itraconazole and clotrimazole in women treated for recurrent vaginal candidiasis. *Genitourin. Med.* **69**:44–46.
69. **Franz, R., S. L. Kelly, D. C. Lamb, D. E. Kelly, M. Ruhnke, and J. Morschhäuser.** 1998. Multiple molecular mechanism contribute to a stepwise development of fluconazole resistance in clinical *Candida albicans* strains. *Antimicrob. Agents Chemother.* **42**:3065–3072.
70. **Goa, K. L., and L. B. Barradell.** 1995. Fluconazole. An update of its pharmacodynamic and pharmacokinetic properties and therapeutic use in major superficial and systemic mycoses in immunocompromised patients. *Drugs* **50**:658–690.
71. **Gottfredsson, M., G. M. Cox, O. S. Indridason, G. M. de Almeida, A. E. Heald, and J. R. Perfect.** 1999. Association of plasma levels of human immunodeficiency virus type 1 RNA and oropharyngeal *Candida* colonization. *J. Infect. Dis.* **180**:534–537.
72. **Graybill, J. R., F. Vazquez, R. O. Darouiche, R. Morhart, D. Greenspan, C. Tuazon, L. J. Wheat, J. Carey, I. Leviton, R. G. Hewitt, R. R. MacGregor, W. Valenti, M. Restrepo, and B. L. Moskovitz.** 1998. Randomized trial of itraconazole oral solution for oropharyngeal candidiasis in HIV/AIDS patients. *Am. J. Med.* **104**:33–39.
73. **Guiot, H. F., W. E. Fibbe, and J. W. van-'t-Wout.** 1994. Risk factors for fungal infection in patients with malignant hematologic disorders: implications for empirical therapy and prophylaxis. *Clin. Infect. Dis.* **18**:525–532.
74. **Haulk, A. A., and A. M. Sugar.** 1991. *Candida* esophagitis. *Adv. Intern. Med.* **36**:307–318.
75. **Hauman, C. H., I. O. Thompson, F. Theunissen, and P. Wolfaardt.** 1993. Oral carriage of *Candida* in healthy and HIV-seropositive persons. *Oral Surg. Oral Med. Oral Pathol.* **76**: 570–572.
76. **Hay, R. J.** 1990. Overview of studies of fluconazole in oropharyngeal candidiasis. *Rev. Infect. Dis.* **12**(Suppl. 3): S334–S337.
77. **Hay, R. J., and Y. M. Clayton.** 1988. Fluconazole in the management of patients with chronic mucocutaneous candidosis [letter]. *Br. J. Dermatol.* **119**:683–684.
78. **Hegener, P., P. F. Troke, G. Fätkenheuer, V. Diehl, and M. Ruhnke.** 1998. Treatment of fluconazole resistant candidosis with voriconazole in patients with AIDS. *AIDS* **12**: 2227–2241.
79. **Hermans, P. E., J. A. Ulrich, and H. Markowitz.** 1969. Chronic mucocutaneous candidiasis as a surface expression of deep-seated abnormalities. Report of a syndrome of superficial candidiasis, absence of delayed hypersensitivity and aminoaciduria. *Am. J. Med.* **47**:503–519.
80. **Hernandez-Sampelayo, T.** 1994. Fluconazole versus ketoconazole in the treatment of oropharyngeal candidiasis in HIV-infected children. Multicentre Study Group. *Eur. J. Clin. Microbiol. Infect. Dis.* **13**:340–344.
81. **Higgs, J. M., and R. S. Wells.** 1974. Classification of chronic mucocutaneous candidiasis with observations on the clinical picture and its therapy. *Hautarzt.* **25**:159–165.
82. **Hoegl, L., G. Schoenian, M. Ollert, and H. C. Korting.** 1998. *Candida sake:* a relevant species in the context of HIV-associated oropharyngeal candidosis? *J. Mol. Med.* **76**:70–73.
83. **Hoegl, L., E. Thoma-Greber, M. Rocken, and H. C. Korting.** 1998. Persistent oral candidosis by non-*albicans Candida* strains including *Candida glabrata* in a human immunodeficiency virus-infected patient observed over a period of 6 years. *Mycoses* **41**:335–338.
84. **Hoh, M. C., H. P. Lin, L. L. Chan, and S. K. Lam.** 1996. Successful allogeneic bone marrow transplantation in severe chronic mucocutaneous candidiasis syndrome. *Bone Marrow Transplant.* **18**:797–800.
85. **Holmberg, K.** 1980. Oral mycoses and antifungal agents. *Swed. Dent. J.* **4**:53–61.
86. **Hood, S., J. Evans, J. Bond, E. Wilkins, and D. W. Denning.** 1998. The treatment of oropharyngeal candidiasis in HIV-infected patients with oral amphotericin B suspension *A.P.C.S.* **12**:625–627.
87. **Hood, S. V., S. Hollis, M. Percy, G. Atkinson, K. Williams, and D. W. Denning.** 1999. Assessment of therapeutic response of oropharyngeal and esophageal candidiasis in AIDS with use of a new clinical scoring system: studies with D0870. *Clin. Infect. Dis.* **28**:587–596.
88. **Hoover, D. R., A. J. Saah, H. Bacellar, J. Phair, R. Detels, R. Anderson, and R. A. Kaslow.** 1993. Clinical manifestations of AIDS in the era of pneumocystis prophylaxis. Multicenter AIDS Cohort Study. *N. Engl. J. Med.* **329**:1922–1926.
89. **Horsburgh, C. R., Jr., and C. H. Kirkpatrick.** 1983. Long-term therapy of chronic mucocutaneous candidiasis with ketoconazole: experience with twenty-one patients. *Am. J. Med.* **74**:23–29.
90. **Hostetter, M. K.** 1994. Adhesins and ligands involved in the interaction of *Candida* spp. with epithelial and endothelial surfaces. *Clin. Microbiol. Rev.* **7**:29–42.
91. **Imam, N., C. C. Carpenter, K. H. Mayer, A. Fisher, M. Stein, and S. B. Danforth.** 1990. Hierarchical pattern of mucosal candida infections in HIV-seropositive women. *Am. J. Med.* **89**:142–146.
92. **Jandourek, A., J. K. Vaishampayan, and J. A. Vazquez.** 1998. Efficacy of melaleuca oral solution for the treatment of fluconazole refractory oral candidiasis in AIDS patients. *AIDS* **12**: 1033–1037.
93. **Jones-Carson, J., A. Vazquez-Torres, T. Warner, and E. Balish.** 2000. Disparate requirement for T cells in resistance to mucosal and acute systemic candidiasis. *Infect. Immun.* **68**: 2363–2365.
94. **Just-Nübling, G., G. Gentschew, M. Dohle, C. Bottinger, E. B. Helm, and W. Stille.** 1990. Fluconazole in the treatment of oropharyngeal candidosis in HIV-positive patients. *Mycoses* **33**:435–440.
95. **Just-Nübling, G., G. Gentschew, K. Meissner, J. Odewald, S. Staszewski, E. B. Helm, and W. Stille.** 1991. Fluconazole prophylaxis of recurrent oral candidiasis in HIV-positive patients. *Eur. J. Clin. Microbiol. Infect. Dis.* **10**:917–921.
96. **Kaplan, B., D. Rabinerson, and Y. Gibor.** 1997. Single-dose systemic oral fluconazole for the treatment of vaginal candidiasis. *Int. J. Gynaecol. Obstet.* **57**:281–286.
97. **Kennedy, M. J., R. A. Calderone, J. E. Cutler, T. Kanabe, M. H. Riesselman, R. Robert, J. M. Senet, V. Annaix, A. Bouali, C. Mahaza, G. Tronchin, J. P. Bouchara, M. Miegeville, A. Marot-Leblond, and E. Segal.** 1992. Molecular basis

of *Candida albicans* adhesion. *J. Med. Vet. Mycol.* **30**(Suppl 1):95–122.

98. **Kimura, L. H., and N. N. Pearsall.** 1978. Adherence of *Candida albicans* to human buccal epithelial cells. *Infect. Immun.* **21**:64–68.
99. **King, R. D., J. C. Lee, and A. L. Morris.** 1980. Adherence of *Candida albicans* and other *Candida* species to mucosal epithelial cells. *Infect. Immun.* **27**:667–674.
100. **Kirkpatrick, C. H.** 1994. Chronic mucocutaneous candidiasis. *J. Am. Acad. Dermatol.* **31**(3 Pt. 2):S14–S17.
101. **Klein, R. S., J. H. Arnsten, and J. D. Sobel.** 2000. Oropharyngeal *Candida* colonization and human immunodeficiency virus type 1 infection [letter]. *J. Infect. Dis.* **181**:812–813.
102. **Klein, R. S., C. A. Harris, C. B. Small, B. Moll, M. Lesser, and G. H. Friedland.** 1984. Oral candidiasis in high-risk patients as the initial manifestation of the acquired immunodeficiency syndrome. *N. Engl. J. Med.* **311**:354–358.
103. **Kleinegger, C. L., S. R. Lockhart, K. Vargas, and D. R. Soll.** 1996. Frequency, intensity, species, and strains of oral *Candida* vary as a function of host age. *J. Clin. Microbiol.* **34**: 2246–2254.
104. **Kobrynski, L. J., L. Tanimune, L. Kilpatrick, D. E. Campbell, and S. D. Douglas.** 1996. Production of T-helper cell subsets and cytokines by lymphocytes from patients with chronic mucocutaneous candidiasis. *Clin. Diagn. Lab. Immunol.* **3**: 740–745.
105. **Kodsi, B. E., C. Wickremesinghe, P. J. Kozinn, K. Iswara, and P. K. Goldberg.** 1976. *Candida* esophagitis: a prospective study of 27 cases. *Gastroenterology* **71**:715–719.
106. **Koletar, S. L., J. A. Russell, R. J. Fass, and J. F. Plouffe.** 1990. Comparison of oral fluconazole and clotrimazole troches as treatment for oral candidiasis in patients infected with human immunodeficiency virus. *Antimicrob. Agents Chemother.* **34**: 2267–2268.
107. **Kraehenbuhl, J. P., and M. R. Neutra.** 1992. Molecular and cellular basis of immune protection of mucosal surfaces. *Physiol. Rev.* **72**:853–879.
108. **Krause, W., H. Matheis, and K. Wulf.** 1969. Fungaemia and funguria after oral administration of *Candida albicans*. *Lancet* **i**:598–599.
109. **Kutzer, E., R. Oittner, S. Leodolter, and K. W. Brammer.** 1988. A comparison of fluconazole and ketoconazole in the oral treatment of vaginal candidiasis; report of a double-blind multicentre trial. *Eur. J. Obstet. Gynecol. Reprod. Biol.* **29**: 305–313.
110. **Laguna, F., J. L. Rodriguez-Tudela, J. V. Martinez-Suarez, R. Polo, E. Valencia, T. M. Diaz-Guerra, F. Dronda, and F. Pulido.** 1997. Patterns of fluconazole susceptibility in isolates from human immunodeficiency virus-infected patients with oropharyngeal candidiasis due to *Candida albicans*. *Clin. Infect. Dis.* **24**:124–130.
111. **Laine, L.** 1994. The natural history of esophageal candidiasis after successful treatment in patients with AIDS. *Gastroenterology* **107**:744–746.
112. **Laine, L., R. H. Dretler, C. N. Conteas, C. Tuazon, F. M. Koster, F. Sattler, K. Squires, and M. Z. Islam.** 1992. Fluconazole compared with ketoconazole for the treatment of *Candida* esophagitis in AIDS. A randomized trial. *Ann. Intern. Med.* **117**:655–660.
113. **Laine, L., and L. Rabeneck.** 1995. Prospective study of fluconazole suspension for the treatment of oesophageal candidiasis in patients with AIDS. *Aliment. Pharmacol. Ther.* **9**: 553–556.
114. **Lake, D. E., J. Kunzweiler, M. Beer, D. N. Buell, and M. Z. Islam.** 1996. Fluconazole versus amphotericin B in the treatment of esophageal candidiasis in cancer patients. *Chemotherapy* **42**:308–314.
115. **Langenbeck, B.** 1839. Auffindung von Pilzen aus der Schleimhaut der Speiseröhre einer Typhus-Leiche. *Neue Not. Geb. Natur-u-Heilkunde (Froriep.)* **12**:145–147.
116. **Ledergerber, B., M. Egger, V. Erard, R. Weber, B. Hirschel, H. Furrer, M. Battegay, P. Vernazza, E. Bernasconi, M. Opravil, D. Kaufmann, P. Sudre, P. Francioli, and A. Telenti.** 1999. AIDS-related opportunistic illnesses occurring after initiation of potent antiretroviral therapy: the Swiss HIV Cohort Study. *JAMA* **282**:2220–2226.
117. **Leen, C. L., E. M. Dunbar, M. E. Ellis, and B. K. Mandal.** 1990. Once-weekly fluconazole to prevent recurrence of oropharyngeal candidiasis in patients with AIDS and AIDS-related complex: a double-blind placebo-controlled study. *J. Infect.* **21**:55–60. (Erratum, **21**:183.)
118. **Lehner, T.** 1972. Cell-mediated immune responses in oral disease: a review. *J. Oral. Pathol.* **1**:39–58.
119. **Lehner, T., J. M. Wilton, and L. Ivanyi.** 1972. Immunodeficiencies in chronic muco-cutaneous candidosis. *Immunology* **22**:775–787.
120. **Li, T. S., R. Tubiana, C. Katlama, V. Calvez, H. Ait-Mohand, and B. Autran.** 1998. Long-lasting recovery in CD4 T-cell function and viral-load reduction after highly active antiretroviral therapy in advanced HIV-1 disease. *Lancet* **351**: 1682–1686.
121. **Lilic, D., A. J. Cant, M. Abinun, J. E. Calvert, and G. P. Spickett.** 1996. Chronic mucocutaneous candidiasis. I. Altered antigen-stimulated IL-2, IL-4, IL-6 and interferon-gamma (IFN-gamma) production. *Clin. Exp. Immunol.* **105**: 205–212.
122. **Linpiyawan, R., K. Jittreprasert, and A. Sivayathorn.** 2000. Clinical trial: clotrimazole troche vs. itraconazole oral solution in the treatment of oral candidosis in AIDS patients. *Int. J. Dermatol.* **39**:859–861.
123. **Lipperheide, V., L. Andraka, J. Ponton, and G. Quindos.** 1993. Evaluation of the albicans IDR plate method for the rapid identification of *Candida albicans*. *Mycoses* **36**: 417–420.
124. **Lockhart, S. R., B. D. Reed, C. L. Pierson, and D. R. Soll.** 1996. Most frequent scenario for recurrent *Candida* vaginitis is strain maintenance with "substrain shuffling": demonstration by sequential DNA fingerprinting with probes Ca3, C1, and CARE2. *J. Clin. Microbiol.* **34**:767–777.
125. **Lucht, E., and C. E. Nord.** 1996. Opportunistic oral infections in patients infected with HIV-1. *Rev. Med. Microbiol.* **7**:151–163.
126. **Mackie, R. M., D. Parratt, and W. M. Jenkins.** 1978. The relationship between immunological parameters and response to therapy in resistant oral candidosis. *Br. J. Dermatol.* **98**:344–348.
127. **Maenza, J. R., W. G. Merz, M. J. Romagnoli, J. C. Keruly, R. D. Moore, and J. E. Gallant.** 1997. Infection due to fluconazole-resistant *Candida* in patients with AIDS: prevalence and microbiology. *Clin. Infect. Dis.* **24**:28–34.
128. **Manfredi, R., A. Mastroianni, O. V. Coronado, and F. Chiodo.** 1997. Fluconazole as prophylaxis against fungal infection in patients with advanced HIV infection. *Arch. Intern. Med.* **157**:64–69.
129. **Marr, K. A., T. C. White, J. A. van-Burik, and R. A. Bowden.** 1997. Development of fluconazole resistance in *Candida albicans* causing disseminated infection in a patient undergoing marrow transplantation. *Clin. Infect. Dis.* **25**:908–910.
130. **Marriott, D. J., P. D. Jones, J. F. Hoy, B. R. Speed, and J. L. Harkness.** 1993. Fluconazole once a week as secondary prophylaxis against oropharyngeal candidiasis in HIV-in-

fected patients. A double-blind placebo-controlled study. *Med. J. Aust.* **158**:312–316.

131. **Martino, P., C. Girmenia, A. Micozzi, F. De-Bernardis, M. Boccanera, and A. Cassone.** 1994. Prospective study of *Candida* colonization, use of empiric amphotericin B and development of invasive mycosis in neutropenic patients. *Eur. J. Clin. Microbiol. Infect. Dis.* **13**:797–804.
132. **Martins, M. D., and J. H. Rex.** 1997. Fluconazole suspension for oropharyngeal candidiasis unresponsive to tablets. *Ann. Intern. Med.* **126**:332–333.
133. **Mascarenas, C. A., T. C. Hardin, G. J. Pennick, M. G. Rinaldi, and J. R. Graybill.** 1998. Treatment of thrush with itraconazole solution: evidence for topical effect. *Clin. Infect. Dis.* **26**:1242–1243.
134. **Masia Canuto, M., F. Gutierrez Rodero, V. Ortiz de la Tabla Ducasse, I. Hernandez Aguado, C. Martin Gonzalez, A. Sanchez Sevillano, and A. Martin Hidalgo.** 2000. Determinants for the development of oropharyngeal colonization or infection by fluconazole-resistant *Candida* strains in HIV-infected patients. *Eur. J. Clin. Microbiol. Infect. Dis.* **19**:593–601.
135. **McCarthy, G. M.** 1992. Host factors associated with HIV-related oral candidiasis. A review. *Oral Surg. Oral Med. Oral Pathol.* **73**:181–186.
136. **McCormack, W. M., K. M. Starko, and S. H. Zinner.** 1988. Symptoms associated with vaginal colonization with yeast. *Am. J. Obstet. Gynecol.* **158**:31–33.
137. **McCourtie, J., and L. J. Douglas.** 1984. Relationship between cell surface composition, adherence, and virulence of *Candida albicans*. *Infect. Immun.* **45**:6–12.
138. **McCullough, M. J., B. C. Ross, B. D. Dwyer, and P. C. Reade.** 1994. Genotype and phenotype of oral *Candida albicans* from patients infected with the human immunodeficiency virus. *Microbiology* **140**:1195–1202.
139. **Menichetti, F., A. Del-Favero, P. Martino, G. Bucaneve, A. Micozzi, D. D'Antonio, P. Ricci, M. Carotenuto, V. Liso, A. M. Nosari, et al.** 1994. Preventing fungal infection in neutropenic patients with acute leukemia: fluconazole compared with oral amphotericin B. The GIMEMA Infection Program. *Ann. Intern. Med.* **120**:913–918.
140. **Metzgar, D., A. van Belkum, D. Field, R. Haubrich, and C. Wills.** 1998. Random amplification of polymorphic DNA and microsatellite genotyping of pre- and posttreatment isolates of *Candida* spp. from human immunodeficiency virus-infected patients on different fluconazole regimens. *J. Clin. Microbiol.* **36**:2308–2313.
141. **Meunier, F., M. Aoun, and M. Gerard.** 1990. Therapy for oropharyngeal candidiasis in the immunocompromised host: a randomized double-blind study of fluconazole vs. ketoconazole. *Rev. Infect. Dis.* **12**(Suppl. 3):S364–S368.
142. **Mikamo, H., K. Kawazoe, Y. Sato, Y. Hayasaki, and T. Tamaya.** 1998. Comparative study on the effectiveness of antifungal agents in different regimens against vaginal candidiasis. *Chemotherapy* **44**:364–368.
143. **Millon, L., A. Manteaux, G. Reboux, C. Drobacheff, M. Monod, T. Barale, and Y. Michel-Briand.** 1994. Fluconazole-resistant recurrent oral candidiasis in human immunodeficiency virus-positive patients: persistence of *Candida albicans* strains with the same genotype. *J. Clin. Microbiol.* **32**:1115–1118.
144. **Miyasaki, S. H., J. B. Hicks, D. Greenspan, I. Polacheck, L. A. MacPhail, T. C. White, N. Agabian, and J. S. Greenspan.** 1992. The identification and tracking of *Candida albicans* isolates from oral lesions in HIV-seropositive individuals. *J. Acquir. Immune Defic. Syndr.* **5**:1039–1046.
145. **Moore, R. D., and R. E. Chaisson.** 1999. Natural history of HIV infection in the era of combination antiretroviral therapy. *AIDS* **13**:1933–1942.
146. **Moshi, A. H., A. F. Jorgensen, and K. Pallangyo.** 1998. Treatment of oral candidiasis: a study to determine the clinical response of sodium benzoate compared with nystatin suspension. *AIDS* **12**:2237–2238.
147. **Murray, P. A., S. L. Koletar, I. Mallegol, J. Wu, and B. L. Moskovitz.** 1997. Itraconazole oral solution versus clotrimazole troches for the treatment of oropharyngeal candidiasis in immunocompromised patients. *Clin. Ther.* **19**:471–480.
148. **Nguyen, M. T., P. J. Weiss, R. C. LaBarre, L. K. Miller, E. C. Oldfield, and M. R. Wallace.** 1996. Orally administered amphotericin B in the treatment of oral candidiasis in HIV-infected patients caused by azole-resistant Candida albicans [letter]. *AIDS* **10**:1745–1747.
149. **Odds, F. C.** 1988. *Candida and Candidosis. A Review and Bibliography*, 2nd ed., p. 124–135. Baillière Tindall, London, United Kingdom.
150. **Odds, F. C.** 1988. Candidosis of the skin, nails and other external sites, p. 136–142. *In Candida and Candidosis. A Review and Bibliography*, 2nd ed. Baillière Tindall, London, United Kingdom.
151. **Odds, F. C.** 1988. Chronic mucocutaneous candidosis, p. 143–152. *In Candida and Candidosis. A Review and Bibliography,* 2nd ed. Baillière Tindall, London, United Kingdom.
152. **Odds, F. C.** 1988. Ecology of *Candida* and epidemiology of candidosis, p. 68–92. *In Candida and Candidosis. A Review and Bibliography,* 2nd ed. Baillière Tindall, London, United Kingdom.
153. **Odds, F. C., and R. Bernaerts.** 1994. CHROMagar Candida, a new differential isolation medium for presumptive identification of clinically important *Candida* species. *J. Clin. Microbiol.* **32**:1923–1929.
154. **Oliver, D. E., and E. J. Shillitoe.** 1984. Effects of smoking on the prevalence and intraoral distribution of *Candida albicans*. *J. Oral. Pathol.* **13**:265–270.
155. **O-Prasertsawat, P., and A. Bourlert.** 1995. Comparative study of fluconazole and clotrimazole for the treatment of vulvovaginal candidiasis. *Sex. Transm. Dis.* **22**:228–230.
156. **Palmer, G. D., P. G. Robinson, S. J. Challacombe, W. Birnbaum, D. Croser, P. L. Erridge, T. Hodgson, D. Lewis, A. McLaren, and J. M. Zakrzewska.** 1996. Aetiological factors for oral manifestations of HIV. *Oral Dis.* **2**:193–197.
157. **Parente, F., M. Cernuschi, G. Rizzardini, A. Lazzarin, L. Valsecchi, and G. Bianchi-Porro.** 1991. Opportunistic infections of the esophagus not responding to oral systemic antifungals in patients with AIDS: their frequency and treatment. *Am. J. Gastroenterol.* **86**:1729–1734.
158. **Patton, L. L., R. McKaig, R. Strauss, D. Rogers, and J. J. Eron, Jr.** 2000. Changing prevalence of oral manifestations of human immuno-deficiency virus in the era of protease inhibitor therapy. *Oral Surg. Oral Med. Oral Pathol. Oral Radiol. Endod.* **89**:299–304.
159. **Péter, Z., Z. Horvath, M. Makara, L. Telegdy, J. Zala, and T. Zagoni.** 1996. Comparison of single-dose and 7-day fluconazole treatment of fungal esophagitis in alcoholic liver disease. *Z. Gastroenterol.* **34**:361–364.
160. **Phillips, P., K. De-Beule, G. Frechette, S. Tchamouroff, B. Vandercam, L. Weitner, A. Hoepelman, G. Stingl, and B. Clotet.** 1998. A double-blind comparison of itraconazole oral solution and fluconazole capsules for the treatment of oropharyngeal candidiasis in patients with AIDS. *Clin. Infect. Dis.* **26**:1368–1373.
161. **Phillips, P., J. Zemcov, W. Mahmood, J. S. Montaner, K. Craib, and A. M. Clarke.** 1996. Itraconazole cyclodextrin solution for fluconazole-refractory oropharyngeal candidia-

sis in AIDS: correlation of clinical response with in vitro susceptibility. *AIDS* **10:**1369–1376.

162. **Plettenberg, A., E. Reisinger, U. Lenzner, H. Listemann, M. Ernst, P. Kern, M. Dietrich, and W. Meigel.** 1990. Oral candidosis in HIV-infected patients. Prognostic value and correlation with immunological parameters. *Mycoses* **33:** 421–425.
163. **Plettenberg, A., A. Stoehr, G. Hoffken, C. Bergs, B. Tschechne, M. Ruhnke, W. Heise, S. Dieckmann, and W. Meigel.** 1994. Fluconazole therapy of oral candidiasis in HIV-infected patients: results of a multicentre study. *Infection* **22:** 118–123.
164. **Polsky, B.** 1996. Treatment of trush in oncology patients. *J. Mycol. Méd.* **6**(Suppl. 2):20–23.
165. **Pons, V., D. Greenspan, and M. Debruin.** 1993. Therapy for oropharyngeal candidiasis in HIV-infected patients: a randomized, prospective multicenter study of oral fluconazole versus clotrimazole troches. The Multicenter Study Group. *J. Acquir. Immune Defic. Syndr.* **6:**1311–1316.
166. **Pons, V., D. Greenspan, F. Lozada-Nur, L. McPhail, J. E. Gallant, A. Tunkel, C. C. Johnson, J. McCarty, H. Panzer, M. Levenstein, A. Barranco, and S. Green.** 1997. Oropharyngeal candidiasis in patients with AIDS: randomized comparison of fluconazole versus nystatin oral suspensions. *Clin. Infect. Dis.* **24:**1204–1207.
167. **Powderly, W. G., D. Finkelstein, J. Feinberg, P. Frame, W. He, C. van-der-Horst, S. L. Koletar, M. E. Eyster, J. Carey, H. Waskin, T. M. Hooton, N. Hyslop, S. A. Spector, S. A. Bozzette, and for the NIAID AIDS Clinical Trials Group.** 1995. A randomized trial comparing fluconazole with clotrimazole troches for the prevention of fungal infections in patients with advanced human immunodeficiency virus infection. NIAID AIDS Clinical Trials Group. *N. Engl. J. Med.* **332:**700–705.
168. **Powderly, W. G., K. Robinson, and E. J. Keath.** 1992. Molecular typing of *Candida albicans* isolated from oral lesions of HIV-infected individuals. *AIDS* **6:**81–84.
169. **Powell, B. L., and D. J. Drutz.** 1983. Confirmation of corticosterone and progesterone binding activity in *Candida albicans*. *J. Infect. Dis.* **147:**359.
170. **Prentice, A. G.** 1989. Oral and gastrointestinal candidosis: prophylaxis during immunosuppressive therapy. *Mycoses* **32**(Suppl. 2):42–46.
171. **Rabeneck, L., and L. Laine.** 1994. Esophageal candidiasis in patients infected with the human immunodeficiency virus. A decision analysis to assess cost-effectiveness of alternative management strategies. *Arch. Intern. Med.* **154:**2705–2710.
172. **Redding, S., J. Smith, G. Farinacci, M. Rinaldi, A. Fothergill, J. Rhine-Chalberg, and M. Pfaller.** 1994. Resistance of *Candida albicans* to fluconazole during treatment of oropharyngeal candidiasis in a patient with AIDS: documentation by in vitro susceptibility testing and DNA subtype analysis. *Clin. Infect. Dis.* **18:**240–242.
173. **Redding, S. W., R. C. Zellars, W. R. Kirkpatrick, R. K. McAtee, M. A. Caceres, A. W. Fothergill, J. L. Lopez-Ribot, C. W. Bailey, M. G. Rinaldi, and T. F. Patterson.** 1999. Epidemiology of oropharyngeal *Candida* colonization and infection in patients receiving radiation for head and neck cancer. *J. Clin. Microbiol.* **37:**3896–3900.
174. **Rees, T., and R. Phillips.** 1992. Multicenter comparison of one-day oral therapy with fluconazole or itraconazole in vaginal candidiasis. *Int. J. Gynaecol. Obstet.* **37**(Suppl. 1):33–38.
175. **Revankar, S. G., W. R. Kirkpatrick, R. K. McAtee, O. P. Dib, A. W. Fothergill, S. W. Redding, M. G. Rinaldi, S. G. Hilsenbeck, and T. F. Patterson.** 1998. A randomized trial of continuous or intermittent therapy with fluconazole for oropharyngeal candidiasis in HIV-infected patients: clinical outcomes and development of fluconazole resistance. *Am. J. Med.* **105:**7–11.
176. **Rex, J. H., M. A. Pfaller, A. L. Barry, P. W. Nelson, and C. D. Webb.** 1995. Antifungal susceptibility testing of isolates from a randomized, multicenter trial of fluconazole versus amphotericin B as treatment of nonneutropenic patients with candidemia. NIAID Mycoses Study Group and the Candidemia Study Group. *Antimicrob. Agents Chemother.* **39:**40–44.
177. **Rex, J. H., M. G. Rinaldi, and M. A. Pfaller.** 1995. Resistance of *Candida* species to fluconazole. *Antimicrob. Agents Chemother.* **39:**1–8.
178. **Rex, J. H., T. J. Walsh, J. D. Sobel, S. G. Filler, P. G. Pappas, W. E. Dismukes, and J. E. Edwards.** 2000. Practice guidelines for the treatment of candidiasis. *Clin. Infect. Dis.* **30:** 662–678.
179. **Reynes, J., C. Bazin, F. Ajana, A. Datry, J. P. Le-Moing, E. Chwetzoff, and J. C. Levron.** 1997. Pharmacokinetics of itraconazole (oral solution) in two groups of human immunodeficiency virus-infected adults with oral candidiasis. *Antimicrob. Agents Chemother.* **41:**2554–2558.
180. **Reynes, J., C. Pujol, C. Moreau, M. Mallie, F. Renaud, F. Janbon, and J. M. Bastide.** 1996. Simultaneous carriage of *Candida albicans* strains from HIV-infected patients with oral candidiasis: multilocus enzyme electrophoresis analysis. *FEMS Microbiol. Lett.* **137:**269–273.
181. **Ruhnke, M., A. Eigler, I. Tennagen, B. Geiseler, E. Engelmann, and M. Trautmann.** 1994. Emergence of fluconazole-resistant strains of *Candida albicans* in patients with recurrent oropharyngeal candidosis and human immunodeficiency virus infection. *J. Clin. Microbiol.* **32:**2092–2098.
182. **Russell, C., and K. M. Lay.** 1973. Natural history of *Candida* species and yeasts in the oral cavities of infants. *Arch. Oral. Biol.* **18:**957–962.
183. **Saavedra, M., B. Taylor, N. Lukacs, and P. L. Fidel, Jr.** 1999. Local production of chemokines during experimental vaginal candidiasis. *Infect. Immun.* **67:**5820–5826.
184. **Samaranayake, L. P.** 1992. Oral mycoses in HIV infection. *Oral Surg. Oral Med. Oral Pathol.* **73:**171–180.
185. **Samaranayake, L. P., C. A. Wilkieson, P. J. Lamey, and T. W. MacFarlane.** 1995. Oral disease in the elderly in long-term hospital care. *Oral Dis.* **1:**147–151.
186. **Sandford, G. R., W. G. Merz, J. R. Wingard, P. Charache, and R. Saral.** 1980. The value of fungal surveillance cultures as predictors of systemic fungal infections. *J. Infect. Dis.* **142:** 503–509.
187. **Sangeorzan, J. A., S. F. Bradley, X. He, L. T. Zarins, G. L. Ridenour, R. N. Tiballi, and C. A. Kauffman.** 1994. Epidemiology of oral candidiasis in HIV-infected patients: colonization, infection, treatment, and emergence of fluconazole resistance. *Am. J. Med.* **97:**339–346.
188. **Sanguinetti, A., K. Carmichael, and K. Campbell.** 1993. Fluconazole resistant *Candida albicans* after long-term suppressive therapy. *Arch. Intern. Med.* **153:**1122–1124.
189. **San-Millán, R., L. Ribacoba, J. Ponton, and G. Quindos.** 1996. Evaluation of a commercial medium for identification of *Candida* species. *Eur. J. Clin. Microbiol. Infect. Dis.* **15:** 153–158.
190. **Schmid, J., F. C. Odds, M. J. Wiselka, K. G. Nicholson, and D. R. Soll.** 1992. Genetic similarity and maintenance of *Candida albicans* strains from a group of AIDS patients, demonstrated by DNA fingerprinting. *J. Clin. Microbiol.* **30:** 935–941.
191. **Schuman, P., L. Capps, G. Peng, J. Vazquez, W. el-Sadr, A. I. Goldman, B. Alston, C. L. Besch, A. Vaughn, M. A. Thompson, M. N. Cobb, T. Kerkering, and J. D. Sobel.** 1997.

Weekly fluconazole for the prevention of mucosal candidiasis in women with HIV infection. A randomized, double-blind, placebo-controlled trial. Terry Beirn Community Programs for Clinical Research on AIDS. *Ann. Intern. Med.* **126:** 689–696.

192. **Schuman, P., J. D. Sobel, S. E. Ohmit, K. H. Mayer, C. C. Carpenter, A. Rompalo, A. Duerr, D. K. Smith, D. Warren, and R. S. Klein.** 1998. Mucosal candidal colonization and candidiasis in women with or at risk for human immunodeficiency virus infection. HIV Epidemiology Research Study (HERS) Group. *Clin. Infect. Dis.* **27:**1161–1167.
193. **Scully, C., M. el-Kabir, and L. P. Samaranayake.** 1994. *Candida* and oral candidosis: a review. *Crit. Rev. Oral Biol. Med.* **5:**125–157.
194. **Shinohara, Y. T., and S. A. Tasker.** 1997. Successful use of boric acid to control azole-refractory *Candida* vaginitis in a woman with AIDS [letter]. *J. Acquir. Immune. Defic. Syndr. Hum. Retrovirol.* **16:**219–220.
195. **Smith, D. E., J. Midgley, M. Allan, G. M. Connolly, and B. G. Gazzard.** 1991. Itraconazole versus ketoconazole in the treatment of oral and oesophageal candidosis in patients infected with HIV. *AIDS* **5:**1367–1371.
196. **Sobel, J. D.** 1990. Vaginal infections in adult women. *Med. Clin. N. Am.* **74:**1573–1602.
197. **Sobel, J. D.** 1997. Vaginitis. *N. Engl. J. Med.* **337:** 1896–1903.
198. **Sobel, J. D., D. Brooker, G. E. Stein, J. L. Thomason, D. P. Wermeling, B. Bradley, and L. Weinstein.** 1995. Single oral dose fluconazole compared with conventional clotrimazole topical therapy of *Candida vaginitis.* Fluconazole Vaginitis Study Group. *Am. J. Obstet. Gynecol.* **172:**1263–1268.
199. **Sobel, J. D., and W. Chaim.** 1997. Treatment of *Torulopsis glabrata* vaginitis: retrospective review of boric acid therapy. *Clin. Infect. Dis.* **24:**649–652.
200. **Sobel, J. D., and J. A. Vazquez.** 1996. Symptomatic vulvovaginitis due to fluconazole-resistant *Candida albicans* in a female who was not infected with human immunodeficiency virus. *Clin. Infect. Dis.* **22:**726–727.
201. **Soll, D. R.** 2000. The ins and outs of DNA fingerprinting the infectious fungi. *Clin. Microbiol. Rev.* **13:**332–370.
202. **Stevens, D. A., S. I. Greene, and O. S. Lang.** 1991. Thrush can be prevented in patients with acquired immunodeficiency syndrome and the acquired immunodeficiency syndrome-related complex. Randomized, double-blind, placebo-controlled study of 100-mg oral fluconazole daily. *Arch. Intern. Med.* **151:**2458–2464.
203. **Sullivan, D. J., T. J. Westerneng, K. A. Haynes, D. E. Bennett, and D. C. Coleman.** 1995. *Candida dubliniensis* sp. nov.: phenotypic and molecular characterization of a novel species associated with oral candidosis in HIV-infected individuals. *Microbiology* **141**(Pt. 7):1507–1521.
204. **Swindells, S., D. R. Kleinschmidt, and F. A. Hayes.** 1997. Pilot study of adjunctive GM-CSF (yeast-derived) for fluconazole-resistant oral candidiasis in HIV-1 infection. *Infect. Dis. Clin. Pract.* **6:**278–279.
205. **Taylor, B. N., C. Fichtenbaum, M. Saavedra, M. Slavinsky, R. Swoboda, K. Wozniak, A. Arribas, W. Powderly, and P. L. Fidel, Jr.** 2000. In vivo virulence of *Candida albicans* isolates causing mucosal infections in people infected with the human immunodeficiency virus. *J. Infect. Dis.* **182:**955–959.
206. **Tom, W., and J. S. Aaron.** 1987. Esophageal ulcers caused by *Torulopsis glabrata* in a patient with acquired immune deficiency syndrome. *Am. J. Gastroenterol.* **82:**766–768.
207. **Torssander, J., L. Morfeldt-Manson, G. Biberfeld, A. Karlsson, P. O. Putkonen, and J. Wasserman.** 1987. Oral *Candida albicans* in HIV infection. *Scand. J. Infect. Dis.* **19:**291–295.
208. **Troillet, N., C. Durussel, J. Bille, M. P. Glauser, and J. P. Chave.** 1993. Correlation between in vitro susceptibility of *Candida albicans* and fluconazole-resistant oropharyngeal candidiasis in HIV-infected patients. *Eur. J. Clin. Microbiol. Infect. Dis.* **12:**911–915.
209. **Umazume, M., E. Ueta, and T. Osaki.** 1995. Reduced inhibition of *Candida albicans* adhesion by saliva from patients receiving oral cancer therapy. *J. Clin. Microbiol.* **33:** 432–439.
210. **USPHS/IDSA.** 2000. 1999 USPHS/IDSA guidelines for the prevention of opportunistic infections in persons infected with human immunodeficiency virus. *Clin. Infect. Dis.* **30**(Suppl. 1):S29–S65.
211. **Valdez, H., B. M. Gripshover, R. A. Salata, and M. M. Lederman.** 1998. Resolution of azole-resistant oropharyngeal candidiasis after initiation of potent combination antiretroviral therapy [letter]. *AIDS* **12:**538.
212. **Vazquez, J. A., J. D. Sobel, G. Peng, L. Steele-Moore, P. Schuman, W. Holloway, and J. D. Neaton.** 1999. Evolution of vaginal *Candida* species recovered from human immunodeficiency virus-infected women receiving fluconazole prophylaxis: the emergence of *Candida glabrata*? Terry Beirn Community Programs for Clinical Research in AIDS (CPCRA). *Clin. Infect. Dis.* **28:**1025–1031.
213. **Vuffray, A., C. Durussel, P. Boerlin, F. Boerlin-Petzold, J. Bille, M. P. Glauser, and J. P. Chave.** 1994. Oropharyngeal candidiasis resistant to single-dose therapy with fluconazole in HIV-infected patients [letter]. *AIDS* **8**(5):708–709.
214. **Wheeler, R. R., J. E. Peacock, Jr., J. M. Cruz, and J. E. Richter.** 1987. Esophagitis in the immunocompromised host: role of esophagoscopy in diagnosis. *Rev. Infect. Dis.* **9:**88–96.
215. **Whelan, W. L., D. R. Kirsch, K. J. Kwon-Chung, S. M. Wahl, and P. D. Smith.** 1990. *Candida albicans* in patients with the acquired immunodeficiency syndrome: absence of a novel of hypervirulent strain. *J. Infect. Dis.* **162:**513–518.
216. **White, D. J., E. M. Johnson, and D. W. Warnock.** 1993. Management of persistent vulvo vaginal candidosis due to azole-resistant *Candida glabrata. Genitourin. Med.* **69:** 112–114.
217. **White, T. C., K. A. Marr, and R. A. Bowden.** 1998. Clinical, cellular, and molecular factors that contribute to antifungal drug resistance. *Clin. Microbiol. Rev.* **11:**382–402.
218. **Wilcox, C. M., R. O. Darouiche, L. Laine, B. L. Moskovitz, I. Mallegol, and J. Wu.** 1997. A randomized, double-blind comparison of itraconazole oral solution and fluconazole tablets in the treatment of esophageal candidiasis. *J. Infect. Dis.* **176:**227–232.
219. **Wilcox, C. M., R. F. Straub, L. N. Alexander, and W. S. Clark.** 1996. Etiology of esophageal disease in human immunodeficiency virus-infected patients who fail antifungal therapy. *Am. J. Med.* **101:**599–604.
220. **Wilkieson, C., L. P. Samaranayake, T. W. MacFarlane, P. J. Lamey, and D. MacKenzie.** 1991. Oral candidosis in the elderly in long term hospital care. *J. Oral Pathol. Med.* **20:** 13–16.
221. **Woolley, P. D., and S. P. Higgins.** 1995. Comparison of clotrimazole, fluconazole and itraconazole in vaginal candidiasis. *Br. J. Clin. Pract.* **49:**65–66.
222. **Zingman, B. S.** 1996. Resolution of refractory AIDS-related mucosal candidiasis after initiation of didanosine plus saquinavir *N. Engl. J. Med.* **334:**1674–1675. (Letter.)

Candida and Candidiasis
Edited by Richard A. Calderone
© 2002 ASM Press, Washington, D.C.

Chapter 23

Candidemia

BART JAN KULLBERG AND SCOTT G. FILLER

Invasive candidiasis exists in various forms, and the terminology used to describe these divergent manifestations has been confusing. *Candida* infections other than those on the skin and mucous membranes are referred to as invasive candidiasis. Invasive candidiasis includes candidemia, acute or chronic hematogenously disseminated candidiasis, and infection of a single deep organ, either by hematogenous seeding or direct inoculation. The vast majority of cases of invasive candidiasis are the result of bloodstream invasion and hematogenous spread of the organism. Candidemia is defined as the isolation of *Candida* spp. from at least one blood culture specimen. Candidemia may or may not be accompanied by clinical signs of infection, e.g., fever, chills, or the sepsis syndrome. Candidemia may give rise to hematogenous spread of *Candida* to one or multiple organs. The term acute disseminated candidiasis refers to this entity, regardless of whether the preceding candidemia has been documented by positive blood cultures or not. For example, patients with multiple noncontiguous organ infections due to *Candida* spp. or those with candidal endophthalmitis are diagnosed as having acute disseminated candidiasis, acquired through hematogenous spread. The presence of multiple nodular candidal skin lesions is also diagnostic of disseminated candidiasis, even without documentation of candidemia.

Chronic disseminated candidiasis is a form of disseminated infection also known as hepatosplenic candidiasis. This syndrome occurs in patients with hematologic malignancies, who develop signs of invasive candidiasis in multiple organs over a period of several weeks to months. The syndrome is the result from a candidemia during the episode of neutropenia, which may or may not have been documented by positive blood cultures. It is discussed more fully in chapter 24.

Nonhematogenous *Candida* infection of a single deep organ occurs infrequently. It is likely that most cases of localized, deep-seated candidiasis that are described in the literature as primary infections are in fact cases of disseminated candidiasis in which the manifestations of infection are most prominent in a single organ. Primary, localized infections occur most frequently after abdominal surgery, with perforation of the gut leading to contamination of the peritoneal cavity with *Candida* colonizing the intestinal tract. Candiduria is also common in hospitalized patients. However, in the vast majority of cases, the presence of candiduria represents colonization rather than a true infection.

This chapter focuses on candidemia and the systemic aspects of acute disseminated candidiasis. *Candida* infections of specific organs, whether or not caused by hematogenous spread, are discussed in chapter 24, as are the manifestations of chronic disseminated candidiasis.

EPIDEMIOLOGY

Candidemia has become increasingly important in the hospital setting for a number of reasons. The frequency of candidemia among hospitalized patients has doubled during the 1980s and 1990s, and *Candida* spp. have now become as common as enteric gram-negative bacilli as a cause of sepsis (1, 5). In the United States, candidemia currently ranks as the fourth most common cause of bloodstream infections (5, 25). Although the incidence of candidemia in Europe is lower than that in the United States, the incidence in Europe has also been increasing. Whereas the incidence of candidemia in U.S. university hospitals was 2 episodes per 10,000 patient days, it was

Bart Jan Kullberg • Department of Medicine, Nijmegen University Medical Center St. Radboud, Geert Grooteplein 8, Mailstop 541, 6525 GA Nijmegen, The Netherlands. **Scott G. Filler** • Harbor-UCLA Research and Education Institute, 1124 W. Carson St., RB-2, Torrance, CA 90509.

only 0.5 per 10,000 patient days in The Netherlands. The increasing incidence of candidemia is largely attributed to the proportional increase in immunocompromised and intensive care patients (94). During the past decade, this trend of increasing incidence may at least in part have been slowed down by the development of strategies for antifungal prophylaxis and preemptive therapy. As a result of increased use of antifungal drugs, the now decreasing incidence of infections caused by fluconazole-susceptible *Candida* strains is accompanied by an increase in the incidence of infections due to azole-resistant *Candida* spp., such as *Candida krusei* and *Candida glabrata* (66).

Candidemia has always been considered to be a nosocomial infection that is strongly associated with neutropenia, recent surgery, or the presence of intravascular lines. Nevertheless, recent data suggest that community-acquired candidemia may occur with increasing frequency (50, 118). This finding underscores how changing patterns of health care delivery are resulting in increasing numbers of nonhospitalized persons who are at risk for *Candida* bloodstream infection.

PORTAL OF ENTRY

It is assumed that the majority of disseminated *Candida* infections originate from the gastrointestinal tract. This assumption is supported by the observation of Krause et al., who reported that a healthy person with a normal gastrointestinal tract who drank a suspension containing a large amount of *Candida albicans* developed candidemia and candiduria (54). The high incidence of candidemia after gastrointestinal surgery is likely due to the interruption of the integrity of the gastrointestinal tract mucosa (20). Furthermore, gastrointestinal surgery, especially when there is intra-abdominal sepsis, may lead to neutrophil dysfunction that also contributes to susceptibility to candidemia (108). Likewise, patients with leukemia or lymphoma receive chemotherapeutic regimens that cause serious damage to the intestinal mucosa, leading to *Candida* colonization and subsequent bloodstream invasion (16). Animal experiments have underscored the effects of cytostatic drugs such as cytosine-arabinoside on promoting invasion of *Candida* spp. (127).

The notion that candidemia originates from *Candida* spp. colonizing the gastrointestinal tract implies that candidemia is preceded by colonization. Indeed, previous colonization is an independent risk factor for candidemia (16, 43, 51, 67, 131), and molecular typing of strains has shown that infecting *Candida* strains were identical to those previously colonizing the same patients (95, 119). In several studies performed in two different settings, i.e., in neutropenic cancer patients (43, 67) and in surgical intensive care patients (88), no case of invasive candidiasis was documented in noncolonized subjects, whereas there was a strong correlation between colonization at multiple sites and the subsequent development of candidemia.

In cancer patients, sequential relationships between risk factors have been demonstrated by Bow et al. (16). Antibacterial prophylaxis is linked to an increased incidence of infections with gram-positive organisms and, in turn, to prolonged fever during neutropenia. Persistent fever is associated with prolonged antibiotic therapy and increased numbers of second-line antibiotic regimens. Modifications of antibiotic regimens are, in turn, correlated with *Candida* colonization, which is strongly linked to the development of disseminated candidiasis (16). Alternatively, there is a growing body of evidence that *Candida* spp. may use the skin rather than the gastrointestinal tract as a portal of entry, especially in the case of intravascular catheter-related infections. Mechanisms of transmission include cross-infection among patients in intensive care units (ICU) attributed to hand carriage by health care workers (19, 47, 122), contaminated medications, parenteral nutrition, and medical devices (107, 128). Between 17 and 75% of nurses were found to carry *Candida* spp. on their hands (112, 122). Notably, the most common species isolated from the hands of these nurses was *Candida parapsilosis,* a species frequently implicated in outbreaks of candidiasis involving an exogenous source (83).

RISK FACTORS FOR CANDIDEMIA

Many studies have identified risk factors that predispose to candidemia and disseminated candidiasis (35, 45, 50, 53, 91, 131). A population-based survey for candidemia in the 1990s identified underlying conditions including cancer in 26%, abdominal surgery in 14%, diabetes mellitus in 13%, and human immunodeficiency virus (HIV) in 10% (50). Using multivariate analysis to correct for confounding variables, it emerges that the important independent predictors include the number of antibiotics used prior to infection, the presence of central venous catheters, neutropenia, prior colonization with *Candida* spp., and hemodialysis or azotemia. Protracted severe neutropenia has been well recognized as a major risk factor for development of disseminated candidiasis. Bodey et al. have described the quantitative relationship between the depth and duration of neutropenia and the frequency of candidemia (12, 14). These studies point to the central role of neutrophils in the host defense against disseminated candidiasis.

Probably the most important risk factors are the use of antibiotics and the use of indwelling intravenous catheters (131). Broad-spectrum antibiotics eliminate the endogenous bacterial flora in the gastrointestinal tract to permit the growth of *Candida* spp. and other yeasts (104). In their seminal case-control study, Wey et al. have found an odds ratio for development of candidemia of 12.5 for patients who received three to five antibiotics compared with those who received none to two antibiotics, and an odds ratio of 30.5 for those who received more than five antibiotics (131). This correlation has been found in both the general hospital population (95, 129, 131) and in neutropenic cancer patients (16, 41). Some studies have suggested a specifically increased risk when vancomycin (49, 101) or quinolones (66, 134) are used in the latter population. In surgical patients, interruption of the integrity of the gastrointestinal mucosa is the single most important route of candidal infection (20). This is the reason that patients undergoing intra-abdominal surgery are at significantly greater risk for disseminated candidiasis than are patients who have other types of major surgery, such as cardiothoracic procedures.

CANDIDEMIA IN CANCER PATIENTS

Disseminated candidiasis is one of the main causes of death in neutropenic cancer patients (10, 11, 43, 118). In autopsy surveys, the prevalence of disseminated candidiasis among cancer patients found postmortem ranged from 2% in western Europe to 26% in Japan (10). A prospective, multicenter surveillance study by the Invasive Fungal Infection Group of the European Organization for Research and Treatment of Cancer (EORTC) found a crude 30-day mortality of 39% among candidemic cancer patients (118). From this study, it appears that candidemia is not limited to patients with advanced, terminal disease. Half of the patients with candidemia had nonadvanced disease, and candidemia developed relatively shortly after the diagnosis of cancer (118).

The type of underlying neoplastic disease, the duration of neutropenia, and the antineoplastic chemotherapy regimen contribute to the risk for infection, and the incidence of candidemia is significantly linked to remission-inducing regimens for leukemia that lead to gut epithelial damage (16, 43, 66, 134). However, the level of candidal colonization appears to be the most important determinant of infection (16, 43, 67). In recent years, a shift has occurred in the etiology of candidemia. Although in most studies *C. albicans* is still the most frequent cause of candidemia in patients with solid tumors, there is an increase in the prevalence of non-*C. albicans* species of *Candida,* predominantly among patients with hematologic malignancies (66, 118, 134). Whether this is a direct result of the widespread use of fluconazole is controversial, since a similar shift in causative organisms has been found before the introduction of fluconazole (71) and in patients with no prior antifungal exposure (48). Clearly, in centers that use fluconazole prophylaxis as standard practice for bone marrow transplant patients, a reduction in incidence of *C. albicans* and *Candida tropicalis* infections is accompanied by an increased incidence of *C. krusei* and *C. glabrata* (1, 66). In patients on fluconazole prophylaxis, colonizing and invasive strains of *C. albicans* often are azole resistant (66).

CANDIDEMIA IN SOLID-ORGAN TRANSPLANT RECIPIENTS

The combination of prolonged immunosuppressive therapy with specific surgical procedures renders solid-organ transplant recipients at high risk for developing disseminated candidiasis. Although suppression of cell-mediated immunity as such is not associated with increased incidence of candidemia, it enhances the susceptibility to colonization of mucosal surfaces with *Candida* spp., which, in turn, may lead to invasion of the bloodstream either at the site of surgery or elsewhere. Renal transplantation is associated with the lowest incidence of fungal infection of all solid-organ transplants. Candidiasis is a major problem in liver transplant patients, accounting for 15 to 30% of the life-threatening infections in this population (22, 80). Intra-abdominal candidiasis results from the sequence of opening the colonized upper small bowel and extensive intraoperative bleeding. Specific risk factors for development of candidemia in liver transplant recipients are renal failure, length of the transplant operation, retransplantation or reoperation, and cytomegalovirus (CMV) infection (22). Candidemia occurs relatively early in the posttransplant period and appears to be unrelated to the level of immunosuppression or antirejection therapy (22).

A substantial percentage of candidal infections in transplant recipients may originate from the donor organ. For example, heart-lung transplant recipients have a high incidence of airway colonization with *Candida,* probably originating from the donor trachea (59). Likewise, the donor duodenal segment used in liver or pancreas transplant procedures is frequently colonized with *Candida* spp. and may be a source of infection (89). The defective killing of *Candida* spp. by granulocytes in diabetic pancreas transplant recipients aggravates the problem (93). Infection with CMV has been recognized as a risk factor for fungal infection in renal or liver transplant patients (81, 106, 111). CMV infection may predispose to disseminated candidiasis through a variety of mechanisms, including inhibition of granulocyte function (22, 111).

CANDIDEMIA IN THE ICU

The combination of intravascular catheters, broad-spectrum antibiotic use, mechanical ventilation, and abdominal surgery renders ICU patients at a high risk of candidemia (116, 121). In Europe, a point prevalence study identified *Candida* spp. as the fifth most common pathogen in the ICU, being identified in 17% of the patients (117). Although this rate may reflect misdiagnosis of candidal colonization as infection in many cases, more than half of these patients were receiving antifungal agents. Invasive candidiasis in ICU patients is almost always preceded by colonization (20, 88). In a small prospective study, half of the surgical ICU patients colonized with *Candida* spp. at two or more body sites subsequently developed invasive disease (88). In contrast, in a series of 37 consecutive ICU patients colonized with *Candida* spp. in bronchial lavage samples, none developed candidemia or invasive candidiasis (96), indicating the immense difference between the incidences of colonization and infection in this patient group. Likewise, in a prospective multicenter study in Germany, only 1% of long-stay ICU patients developed candidemia (82).

CANDIDEMIA IN AIDS PATIENTS

Despite the frequent occurrence of mucocutaneous candidiasis in HIV-infected patients, the incidence of candidemia in this patient group is low. In several series, the annual incidence of candidemia among AIDS patients is between 0.2 and 1%. This observation underscores the notion that host defense mechanisms required for resistance to mucocutaneous and invasive candidiasis are divergent. Whereas intact cell-mediated immunity is required for the host defense against mucocutaneous candidiasis, functional phagocytes are critical for the host defense against disseminated candidiasis. Although HIV-infected patients have impaired cell-mediated immunity, the anticandidal activity of their neutrophils is largely intact (21). Thus, patients with HIV infection who develop disseminated candidiasis almost always have important additional risk factors for *Candida* infection, such as indwelling central catheters, parenteral nutrition, use of broad-spectrum antibiotics, or neutropenia due to HIV-related lymphoma or cytotoxic therapy (34, 37, 123).

CANDIDEMIA IN OTHER HIGH-RISK POPULATIONS

Other patients at high risk for disseminated candidiasis include patients with extensive burns (28, 91) and low-birth-weight infants (61, 103). Both burn patients and neonates have neutrophil dysfunction, which increases their susceptibility to disseminated candidiasis. Additional risk factors for candidemia in burn patients include the presence of large burns and prior bacterial infection (28), which may be a marker for increased antibiotic use. In neonates, the predisposing factors for candidemia are gestational age of less than 32 weeks, shock, disseminated intravascular coagulopathy, use of parenteral nutrition, presence of central venous catheters, and use of H_2 blockers (103).

CANDIDA SPP. CAUSING CANDIDEMIA

Many reports indicate that shifts have occurred in the distribution of infections caused by species other than *C. albicans*. Although *C. albicans* remains the most important cause of invasive and disseminated candidiasis, the incidence of other species, such as *C. tropicalis*, *C. glabrata*, and *C. krusei*, has been increasing (86, 94, 118). On the basis of various multicenter surveys performed the United States in the 1990s, *C. albicans* accounts for 50 to 55% of bloodstream isolates, *C. tropicalis* and *C. glabrata* for 10 to 20% each, *C. parapsilosis* for 10 to 15%, and *C. krusei* for 2 to 4% (75, 85, 86, 94, 99). In Europe, the distribution of species appears highly similar. In two surveys of candidemia in Europe, 49 to 53% were *C. albicans*, followed by *C. parapsilosis* (11 to 21%), *C. glabrata* (10 to 12%), *C. tropicalis* (6 to 11%), *C. krusei* (1 to 9%), and other *Candida* spp. (1 to 10%) (84, 118). In university hospitals in The Netherlands, the percentage of candidemia caused by species other than *C. albicans* has risen from 26 to 40% between 1987 and 1995. The most prevalent non-*C. albicans* species is *C. glabrata*, which accounts for 10 to 16% of all cases of candidemia (120). The increasing incidence of non-*C. albicans* species has been noted particularly among patients with hematologic malignancies (66, 118). It has been suggested that one explanation for the emergence of *C. glabrata* and *C. krusei* is the selection of less susceptible species by the pressure of antifungal agents such as fluconazole (66, 99, 132). However, this association has not been confirmed in large prospective studies (38, 70, 135). Whether *C. glabrata* may be more virulent than *C. albicans* is a matter of debate (8, 53, 132). Its variable susceptibility to both amphotericin B and fluconazole, as well as its predominance in patients with end-stage cancer, may contribute to the high mortality of patients with *C. glabrata* candidemia (118).

C. tropicalis appears to be more virulent than *C. albicans,* as there is a much higher frequency of invasive infections among immunocompromised hosts who are colonized with *C. tropicalis* (132). The increased incidence of *C. tropicalis,* particularly in patients with cancer, may be due to the increased invasiveness of the organism when the gastrointestinal mucosa is damaged and the intestinal flora is suppressed by antibiotics (118, 133).

Candidemia due to *C. parapsilosis* is generally associated with catheters, hyperalimentation, or prosthetic devices. The propensity of *C. parapsilosis* for intravenous catheters is due to its specific properties: in vitro, *C. parapsilosis* proliferates better on and is more adherent to acrylic than other *Candida* spp. in a glucose-rich solution (128). Also, *C. parapsilosis* is the most common species of *Candida* to be isolated from the hands of health care workers in the ICU, especially those who wear gloves (94). Thus, it is likely that contamination of prosthetic devices with this organism occurs via the hands of health care workers. In contrast to other *Candida* spp., colonization with *C. parapsilosis* rarely occurs before the onset of candidemia, suggesting an exogenous source of infection. This organism is an especially common cause of disseminated candidiasis in neonates (23, 61). It is less virulent than other species of *Candida*; several studies have shown lower morbidity and mortality among patients infected with *C. parapsilosis* than those infected with other *Candida* species (46, 118).

C. krusei is intrinsically resistant to fluconazole, and increased colonization and infection with this organism have been reported in some bone marrow transplant units when fluconazole prophylaxis has been used (66, 134). Independent of antifungal prophylaxis, *C. krusei* infections are found predominantly in patients with hematologic malignancies, whereas the incidence *C. krusei* infections in patients with solid tumors and ICU patients is low (36, 118). A recently described species, *Candida dubliniensis,* was initially thought to only cause oropharyngeal infections in HIV-positive patients. However, a number of cases of candidemia caused by *C. dubliniensis* have been reported both from the United States and Europe (17, 68). Since standard laboratory identification methods do not discriminate between *C. dubliniensis* and *C. albicans,* it is likely that some percentage of blood isolates that are identified as *C. albicans* are actually *C. dubliniensis* (17, 68).

OUTCOME AND MORTALITY

Of all nosocomial bloodstream infections, those caused by *Candida* spp. are associated with the highest crude mortality (25). Even in nonneutropenic patients with candidemia, the crude mortality of candidemia exceeds 50% in many studies (2, 45, 53, 60, 72, 98, 130). In a carefully conducted case-control study, the mortality directly attributable to candidemia was 38% (130). Mortality rates differ depending on the patient's underlying disease and other factors (43). The results of therapy in cancer patients have generally been discouraging. In several studies the mortality associated with candidemia has been very high in persistently neutropenic patients, whereas among patients with neutrophil recovery, survival rates have been 40 to 60% (39, 46, 64, 118). *C. glabrata* as the causative organism, advanced age, progressive underlying disease, and retention of intravascular catheters are independent risk factors for mortality (74, 78, 118).

SIGNS AND SYMPTOMS

There is no specific configuration of signs and symptoms that is characteristic for candidemia or disseminated candidiasis. The usual presentation is a seriously ill patient with persistent fever despite antibacterial antibiotics. Fever is present in most but not all patients with candidemia. The onset of fever may be either insidious or sudden, and its course may be continuous or spiking (12, 62).

Some patients present with the sepsis syndrome, including fever, hypotension, tachycardia, and tachypnea. Sepsis due to *Candida* spp. cannot be distinguished from gram-negative septicemia on clinical grounds. Occasional patients have a single spike of fever, leading to blood sampling for cultures. After several days, the blood cultures grow *Candida* spp.; however, the patient shows no further sign of infection after the initial temperature spike. Although it is tempting to assume that the candidemia has been transient in such cases, dissemination of *Candida* spp. has been documented despite the absence of pertinent clinical signs (9, 60).

All high-risk patients should be carefully examined for any signs suggestive of disseminated *Candida* infection. Characteristic skin lesions have been recognized in about 10% of patients, primarily those who are neutropenic. The lesions may be localized to the extremities or may be generalized and numerous. Mostly, the lesions present as pink to red nontender, firm, raised nodules, with discrete borders. *Candida* spp. can be visualized in the tissue with skin biopsy but are isolated from only 50% of cultures. Some patients with skin lesions have an associated myositis, which is tender on palpation.

Eye involvement has been reported in 10 to 30% of patients, although these lesions are usually absent in neutropenic patients (18, 24). All patients who are suspected to have disseminated candidiasis should have a thorough fundoscopic examination. The finding of candidal endophthalmitis, even in the absence of detectable candidemia, is diagnostic of a disseminated infection. In candidemic patients who receive prompt antifungal treatment, the lesions are usually limited to candidal chorioretinitis, whereas endophthalmitis may be encountered in patients who have had occult candidemia with delayed treatment (24). Some patients with ocular involvement complain of blurred vision or scotomas, whereas others report no visual disturbances.

DIAGNOSIS

The diagnosis of disseminated candidiasis may be difficult to establish, and therapy must often be initiated on the presumption of this infection. In several autopsy studies, *Candida* was isolated from antemortem blood cultures in only 10 to 50% of the autopsy-proven cases (10, 40), although modern blood culture techniques may be somewhat more sensitive (7, 124). Although sampling of blood for cultures is preferably done by peripheral venipuncture, positive blood cultures obtained through intravascular catheters do usually reflect true candidemia rather than colonization of the line. For example, in a series of cancer patients, the risk of disseminated infection or death from candidiasis was comparable regardless of whether positive cultures were obtained from both the intravenous catheter and a peripheral site or from the catheter only (60). The interpretation of the significance of recovery of *Candida* spp. from sites such as sputum, urine, and skin is difficult, because the organisms can frequently be recovered from these sites without causing infection. It has been suggested that urine cultures may have a role in identifying patients with candidemia, as a result of hematogenous dissemination of *Candida* spp. to the kidneys. However, the predictive value of candiduria for bloodstream infection is very low (105), except possibly for neonates. In a recent prospective multicenter survey of candiduria in hospitalized adults, only 1.3% of patients developed candidemia (52).

The role of surveillance cultures for the diagnosis of candidemia is controversial. Many patients at risk are colonized with *Candida* spp. but do not develop candidemia. Therefore, the positive predictive value of this finding is low. However, the absence of prior *Candida* colonization in neutropenic patients strongly reduces the chance of candidemia, and the negative predictive value is high in this setting (16, 43). Likewise, all patients in the surgical ICU with subsequent candidemia were found to be heavily colonized with *Candida* spp. in two surveys (82, 88). In view of the increasing incidence of *Candida* spp. other than *C. albicans,* and the impact of isolating species with altered susceptibility on the choice of antifungal therapy, it is required that a reasonable attempt should be made at fully speciating all isolates. Thus, just reporting the isolation of "*Candida* species" is no longer adequate.

THERAPY

During the past 30 years, there has been a nearly complete reversal of the approach to a positive blood culture for *Candida* spp. On the basis of literature dating from the 1960s, physicians considered a positive blood culture merely as colonization of a vascular catheter or a "benign, transient candidemia," not necessitating treatment. It was thought that skin *Candida* infection could easily contaminate blood cultures or might be a laboratory contaminant, and the organism was believed to have low virulence. Nowadays, it is clear that the mortality rate is alarming (50 to 75%) in patients with candidemia who have not been treated because their infection was considered to be benign (53, 60). Moreover, hematogenous dissemination occurred in 25 to 35% of patients who had been treated with catheter removal only and withholding of antifungal agents (9, 60). Unquestionably, some patients have transient, self-limited candidemias, especially those associated with an indwelling catheter and resolving upon removal of the catheter. However, clinical judgment has failed to differentiate those patients with self-limited candidemia from those who will develop progressive disease with dissemination or mortality (9, 60), and interpretation of presumed resolution of the candidemia should be made with recognition that half of the patients with disseminated candidiasis have not had a positive blood culture. These factors have resulted in a consensus among experts to treat patients with candidemia, regardless of whether it occurs in a compromised host and regardless of whether it is associated with an indwelling intravenous catheter (26, 100).

To treat the disseminated candidiasis, we have relied heavily on amphotericin B since its introduction in the 1950s. However, therapy with this drug has been limited by its acute and chronic toxicities, creating a need for effective and less toxic alternatives. The fact that amphotericin B has been (and by many still is) considered the "gold standard" of antifungal therapy is not by virtue of its effectiveness, which is at best moderate, but rather due to the lack of alternatives available until recently. The development of fluconazole and itraconazole, as well as of lipid-associated formulations of amphotericin B, has dramatically changed the therapeutic picture.

Despite the use of amphotericin B for many years, the optimum dosage schedule and duration of therapy have not been definitively determined. For susceptible *Candida* strains, a dose of 0.5 to 0.7 mg/kg of body weight/day seems to be appropriate (100). Importantly, a considerable proportion of *C. glabrata* and *C. krusei* isolates may be relatively resistant to amphotericin B (33, 100), although the frequency and the clinical relevance of these observations are uncertain. Awareness of potential resistance and judicious susceptibility testing of these species are warranted. Doses of approximately 1 mg/kg/day of amphotericin B may be needed to treat infections with *C. glabrata* or *C. krusei,* especially in the neutropenic host (100).

Depending on the severity of the candidemia, 5-fluorocytosine (5-FC) can be added to the regimen to provide rapid attainment of therapeutic blood levels. However, bone marrow suppression or diarrhea may be complications of simultaneous use of these agents. If 5-FC is used, serum levels should be monitored. Also, this drug is only available in an oral formulation. A number of studies have shown that fluconazole is efficacious for the treatment of invasive or disseminated candidiasis (4, 74, 115). The results of three prospective randomized trials comparing fluconazole with amphotericin B have shown that fluconazole at 400 mg/kg/day is as effective as amphotericin B in the management of candidemia in nonneutropenic patients (3, 87, 98). Given the markedly lower number of side effects of fluconazole, the latter is considered the drug of first choice for the treatment of *C. albicans* candidemia in nonneutropenic patients. For neutropenic patients with candidemia, the choice may be very similar to that in nonneutropenic patients, although no comparative trials have addressed the choice of therapy in this patient group. The outcomes of a matched-pair cohort study (4) and of the small neutropenic subgroup in a randomized comparative trial of fluconazole versus amphotericin B (3) suggest that fluconazole has similar or greater efficacy than amphotericin B for the treatment of candidemia in these patients. Thus, fluconazole may be the drug of choice in neutropenic patients as well. Unfortunately, all studies of candidemia have only included small numbers of infections caused by non-*C. albicans* species. Although the results associated with fluconazole in a small series patients infected with non-*albicans* species of *Candida* appear to be favorable (3, 114), knowledge of the species and/or susceptibility of the isolate should guide the choice of the antifungal agent. It would be rational to institute empiric therapy with amphotericin B for those patients who are known to be colonized with *C. krusei* or *C. glabrata,* or who have received fluconazole prophylaxis either immediately prior to or at the time of infection, and in settings where fluconazole-resistant isolates are frequent. In the clinically unstable patient infected with an isolate of unknown species, amphotericin B is also preferred by many authorities (100). For all others, fluconazole would be the drug of choice.

After culture results have become available, continuation of therapy with fluconazole is appropriate for most *Candida* spp. Because *C. glabrata* may have reduced susceptibility to both amphotericin B and azoles, the choice of therapy is difficult and antifungal susceptibility testing by an experienced laboratory should be considered (98). In cases of proven or suspected intermediate (dose-dependent) susceptibility to fluconazole, it may be warranted to increase the dose of fluconazole to 800 mg/day. Therapy should be switched to amphotericin B when the clinical response is poor (100). For *C. krusei,* amphotericin B is the drug of choice, whereas for *C. lusitaniae,* which is often resistant to amphotericin B, fluconazole is preferred (100). Randomized studies are presently under way to assess the optimal dose of fluconazole, which is likely to be more than 400 mg/day, and the efficacy of combination therapy with fluconazole and amphotericin B.

Ketoconazole is unreliable for the treatment of invasive or disseminated candidiasis due to uncertain oral bioavailability, and this drug should not be used. For the same reason, itraconazole capsules are also inadequate for treating this infection. Recently, an intravenous formulation of itraconazole has been licensed. The efficacy of this formulation for the treatment of disseminated candidiasis is currently under investigation.

Three lipid formulations of amphotericin B have been developed: liposomal amphotericin B (AmBisome), amphotericin B lipid complex (ABLC; Abelcet), and amphotericin B colloidal dispersion (ABCD; Amphocil, Amphotec). Until now, only ABLC and liposomal amphotericin B have been approved for use in proven candidiasis as a second-line treatment for patients who are intolerant or refractory to therapy with conventional amphotericin B. The preparations differ in their specific composition, distribution, and clearance, but they are similar in that they permit administration of higher doses of amphotericin B (3 to 7 mg/kg/day) with reduced toxicity. Although studies aiming at defining the optimal dose of liposomal amphotericin B have failed to show a clear dose-effect relationship (29, 92), subgroup analyses suggest that higher doses (4 to 8 mg/kg) may be more effective. In spite of the approval of these drugs in many countries, randomized trials establishing their efficacy for the treatment of invasive or disseminated candidiasis have been lacking. Thus, conventional amphotericin B deoxycholate remains the standard amphotericin B formulation for candidemia. A lipid-associated amphotericin B would be appropriate in patients who are refractory or intolerant to amphotericin B deoxycholate, or at a high risk for nephrotoxicity, for example, a renal transplant recipient receiving cyclosporine (100).

DURATION OF TREATMENT

The optimal duration of therapy for candidemia has not been well defined. Because *Candida* sp. tends to disseminate and cause metastatic infections, treatment for longer periods of time (3 to 6 weeks) has been advocated. However, several retrospective studies have revealed that late complications of candidemia are rare in patients with a favorable initial response to treatment, even after therapy of short duration (23, 32, 79). This suggests that treatment may be limited to 10 to 14 days after the last positive blood culture and disappearance of all signs and symptoms of infection in patients who have no risk factors for complicated disease (i.e., unremoved intravascular catheters, persistent neutropenia, or proven dissemination of infection [79, 100]).

CATHETER MANAGEMENT

Whether removal of central venous catheters is mandatory for patients with candidemia has been controversial. Although there is strong evidence that vascular catheters are not the primary site of candidemia in the majority of cases, and rather, that the gastrointestinal tract usually is the source (67, 88), removal of the catheter would eliminate a potential site of persistent infection. Although no studies have been specifically designed to address this particular question, several retrospective analyses have suggested that removal of central venous catheters reduces the incidence of complications of candidemia (31, 60, 78). In a post hoc analysis of one of the seminal therapeutic trials, it was shown that replacement of all (peripheral as well as central) vascular catheters before institution of therapy was associated with a reduction in the duration of candidemia (97). Therefore, it is recommended that all vascular catheters be exchanged in patients with candidemia (100). Given the difficulty in maintaining vital venous access in some settings, a decision to keep a central venous catheter in place may be made on an individual basis. However, if the patient's condition deteriorates or blood cultures remain positive, the catheter should still be removed.

IMMUNOTHERAPY

Resolution of candidemia is often dependent on recovery from granulocytopenia, indicating that host defense mechanisms are extremely important in the clearance of this opportunistic pathogen. Therefore, immunotherapy aimed at enhancing host defense mechanisms may prove extremely productive, although there are few clinical data on this subject (55). Case reports have described patients with progressive chronic disseminated candidiasis who responded to recombinant gamma interferon (rIFN-γ) therapy, which had initially been combined with recombinant granulocyte-macrophage colony-stimulating factor (rGM-CSF) (90). It was suggested that the rIFN-γ was largely responsible for the observed effect, rather than the rGM-CSF. This is in agreement with the finding of others, who found no beneficial effect of rGM-CSF in an open study of 17 patients with invasive fungal infections, of whom 8 had candidemia (63). In an earlier pilot trial, four of five patients with candidiasis responded to GM-CSF at a very high and toxic dose plus amphotericin B (13). A series of 30 cancer patients with invasive candidiasis were given M-CSF combined with an antifungal agent. These patients had improved survival compared with historical controls (73). Given the limited nature of these studies and the lack of a comparison group, no conclusions about the actual efficacy of these cytokines can be drawn. In the first randomized study on immunotherapy for candidemia, fluconazole alone was compared with fluconazole with recombinant granulocyte colony-stimulating factor in nonneutropenic patients with disseminated candidiasis. It was demonstrated that increasing the numbers of circulating neutrophils strongly correlates with accelerated clearance of *Candida* sp. from the bloodstream and reduced mortality, even in this nonneutropenic study population (57). Although this observation is to be confirmed in larger studies, on the basis of the current knowledge it may be reasonable to administer recombinant granulocyte colony-stimulating factor in patients with severe or refractory disseminated candidiasis, especially when the neutrophil count is low.

PREVENTION

Based on the risk factors for candidemia and disseminated candidiasis, it is clear that reduction of the use of broad-spectrum antibiotics is a key factor in preventing *Candida* infection. Despite the strong association of the depth and duration of neutropenia with the occurrence of disseminated candidiasis, the use of hematopoietic growth factors to shorten the duration of chemotherapy-induced granulocytopenia has not led to a reduction of disseminated candidiasis in any study performed to date (56). This may be due in part to the fact that the numbers of patients enrolled in these studies have been insufficient to detect such a difference. The use of antifungal agents for the prophylaxis of disseminated candidiasis has been highly controversial. No studies have clearly demonstrated a benefit of topical agents such as clotrimazole, miconazole, nystatin, or oral amphotericin B on the occurrence of invasive infections (126). Also, ketoconazole has not unequivocally been shown to reduce the incidence of disseminated candidiasis in cancer patients (126).

The erratic bioavailability of itraconazole capsules in neutropenic patients has limited their use, and a protective effect of itraconazole capsules on disseminated candidiasis in neutropenic patients has not been convincingly shown (15, 77). An oral solution with an improved pharmacokinetic profile is now available. Prophylaxis with itraconazole oral solution in neutropenic patients with hematologic malignancies significantly reduced the incidence of invasive candidiasis in one placebo-controlled study (69), whereas a similar study failed to demonstrate this protective effect (44).

Prospective, placebo-controlled trials have demonstrated that prophylactic fluconazole in allogeneic bone marrow transplant patients prevents both superficial and invasive candidal infections in these patients (38, 109). As a result, fluconazole prophylaxis is standard therapy in many transplant centers (66). An 8-year follow-up of one of these trials showed a significantly better long-term survival in fluconazole recipients compared with placebo recipients. Also, there was a lower incidence of severe graft-versus-host disease in the fluconazole arm (65). It has been suggested that the prolonged use of fluconazole for 75 days during the time of both neutropenia and acute graft-versus-host disease in this particular study may have contributed to the beneficial effect (65, 109). However, comparative studies on the optimal dose and duration of fluconazole prophylaxis are lacking.

In contrast to these favorable results in allogeneic bone marrow transplant patients, several large controlled trials in neutropenic leukemic patients have failed to show benefit from fluconazole prophylaxis in invasive candidiasis (70, 76, 135). More recently, others have demonstrated a beneficial effect of fluconazole in patients with acute myeloid leukemia and autologous bone marrow transplant recipients (102).

An increasing incidence of fluconazole-resistant isolates may be the price to be paid for the widespread prophylactic use of the drug, although this association has not been confirmed in large prospective studies (38, 70, 135). Also, it should be noted that fluconazole prophylaxis does not provide protection against molds.

It is likely that the divergent results of prophylaxis trials are due to differences in the incidence of disseminated candidiasis in the study populations: those with high basal incidence rates have demonstrated a benefit of fluconazole prophylaxis (30, 38, 76), whereas those in low incidence settings cannot detect a further reduction in disseminated candidiasis (43, 70). Also, patients on specific types of cytotoxic chemotherapy (e.g., cytarabine plus anthracycline-based regimens) and patients not receiving hematopoietic growth factors may benefit most from prophylaxis (102). Therefore, strategies for preventive antifungal therapy should be based on recognition of these differences in risk factors (100, 125), and (meta)analyses that simply combine data from multiple, diverse populations of neutropenic patients are of little value. The strong correlation between the level of candidal colonization and the risk for disseminated candidiasis has led to studies in which the decision to initiate prophylaxis in an individual patient is based on the finding of a high grade of colonization. This strategy may lead to a high level of protection at the lowest possible environmental exposure to azoles (42, 43, 125).

Similar strategies have been proposed for patients undergoing liver transplantation (22). Those transplant recipients who have specific risk factors (renal insufficiency, long operative time, retransplantation, massive blood transfusion, or early *Candida* colonization posttransplant) benefit from prophylaxis (100). In prospective randomized studies, both fluconazole and liposomal amphotericin B have been shown effective in preventing disseminated candidiasis (58, 113). In pancreas transplant recipients, no prospective studies have been performed, but the risk of developing invasive candidiasis appears to be similar to that following liver transplantation, and a large retrospective study has suggested a protective effect of fluconazole prophylaxis (6, 89). Following transplantation of other solid organs, the risk of disseminated candidiasis appears to be too low to warrant antifungal prophylaxis (100).

For surgical ICU patients, there is no general consensus regarding prophylaxis, and most experts do not recommend it (100). It is likely that there are subpopulations of patients who are at high risk for deep candidiasis and may benefit from antifungal prophylaxis (110). Prophylaxis with fluconazole was successful in highly selected critically ill patients who had recently undergone abdominal surgery and experienced recurrent gastrointestinal perforations or anastomotic leakage (27).

Irrespective of whether oncology patients, solid-organ transplant recipients, or ICU patients are addressed, fluconazole prophylaxis is a double-edged sword, and selection of resistance may well occur if it is used injudiciously. Careful selection of subpopulations at the highest risk of candidiasis will yield an optimal benefit from targeted prophylaxis.

REFERENCES

1. **Abi-Said, D., E. Anaissie, O. Uzun, I. Raad, H. Pinzcowski, and S. Vartivarian.** 1997. The epidemiology of hematogenous candidiasis caused by different *Candida* species. *Clin. Infect. Dis.* **24:**1122–1128.
2. **Anaissie, E., G. P. Bodey, H. Kantarjian, J. Ro, S. E. Vartivarian, R. Hopfer, J. Hoy, and K. Rolston.** 1989. New spectrum of fungal infections in patients with cancer. *Rev. Infect. Dis.* **11:**369–378.
3. **Anaissie, E. J., D. Abi-Said, O. Uzun, J. Mera, L. O. Gentry, T. Williams, D. P. Kontoyiannis, C. L. Karl, and G. P. Bodey.** 1996. Management of invasive candidal infections: results of a prospective, randomized, multicenter study of fluconazole versus amphotericin B and review of the literature. *Clin. Infect. Dis.* **23:**974–972.
4. **Anaissie, E. J., S. E. Vartivarian, D. Abi-Said, O. Uzun, H. Pinczowski, D. P. Kontoyiannis, P. Khoury, K. Papadakis, A. Gardner, I. I. Raad, J. Gilbreath, and G. P. Bodey.** 1996. Fluconazole versus amphotericin B in the treatment of hematogenous candidiasis: A matched cohort study. *Am. J. Med.* **101:**170–176.
5. **Beck-Sagué, C. M., and W. R. Jarvis.** 1993. Secular trends in the epidemiology of nosocomial fungal infections in the United States, 1980–1990. *J. Infect. Dis.* **167:**1247–1251.
6. **Benedetti, E., A. C. Gruessner, C. Troppmann, B. E. Papalois, D. E. Sutherland, D. L. Dunn, and R. W. Gruessner.** 1996. Intra-abdominal fungal infections after pancreatic transplantation: incidence, treatment, and outcome. *J. Am. Coll. Surg.* **183:**307–316.
7. **Berenguer, J., M. Buck, F. Witebsky, F. Stock, P. A. Pizzo, and T. J. Walsh.** 1993. Lysis-centrifugation blood cultures in the detection of tissue-proven invasive candidiasis. Disseminated versus single-organ infection. *Diagn. Microbiol. Infect. Dis.* **17:**103–109.
8. **Berkowitz, I. D., S. J. Robboy, A. W. Karchmer, and L. J. Kunz.** 1979. *Torulopsis glabrata* fungemia—a clinical pathological study. *Medicine* (Baltimore) **58:**430–440.
9. **Beutler, S. M., L. S. Young, L. A. Lindquist, J. Z. Montgomerie, and J. E. Edwards, Jr.** 1982. Delayed complications of candidemia, p. 154. *In Progr. Abstr. 22nd Intersci. Conf. Antimicrob. Agents Chemother.* American Society for Microbiology, Washington, D.C.
10. **Bodey, G., B. Bueltmann, W. Duguid, D. Gibbs, H. Hanak, M. Hotchi, G. Mall, P. Martino, F. Meunier, S. Milliken, S. Naoe, M. Okudaira, D. Scevola, and J. Van't Wout.** 1992. Fungal infections in cancer patients: an international autopsy survey. *Eur. J. Clin. Microbiol. Infect. Dis.* **11:**99–109.
11. **Bodey, G. P.** 1984. Candidiasis in cancer patients. *Am. J. Med.* 77(4D):13–19.
12. **Bodey, G. P.** 1966. Fungal infections complicating acute leukemia. *J. Chron. Dis.* **19:**667–687.
13. **Bodey, G. P., E. Anaissie, J. Gutterman, and S. Vadhan-Raj.** 1993. Role of granulocyte-macrophage colony-stimulating factor as adjuvant therapy for fungal infection in patients with cancer. *Clin. Infect. Dis.* **17:**705–707.
14. **Bodey, G. P., M. Buckley, Y. S. Sathe, and E. J. Freireich.** 1966. Quantitative relationships between circulating leukocytes and infections in patients with leukemia. *Ann. Intern. Med.* **64:**328–340.
15. **Boogaerts, M. A., B. E. Verhoef, P. Zachee, H. Demnyck, L. Verbist, and K. De Beule.** 1989. Antifungal prophylaxis with itraconazole in prolonged neutropenia: correlation with plasma levels. *Mycoses.* **32**(Suppl. 1)**:**103–108.
16. **Bow, E. J., R. Loewen, M. S. Cheang, and B. Schacter.** 1995. Invasive fungal disease in adults undergoing remission-induction therapy for acute myeloid leukemia: the pathogenetic role of the antileukemic regimen. *Clin. Infect. Dis.* **21:**361–369.
17. **Brandt, M. E., L. H. Harrison, M. Pass, A. N. Sofair, S. Huie, R. K. Li, C. J. Morrison, D. W. Warnock, and R. A. Hajjeh.** 2000. *Candida dubliniensis* fungemia: the first four cases in North America. *Emerg. Infect. Dis.* **6:**46–49.
18. **Brooks, R. G.** 1989. Prospective study of *Candida* endophthalmitis in hospitalized patients with candidemia. *Arch. Intern. Med.* **149:**2226–2228.
19. **Burnie, J. P., F. C. Odds, W. Lee, C. Webster, and J. D. Williams.** 1985. Outbreak of systemic *Candida albicans* in intensive care unit caused by cross infection. *Br. Med. J.* **290:**746–748.
20. **Calandra, T., J. Bille, R. Schneider, F. Mosimann, and P. Francioli.** 1989. Clinical significance of *Candida* isolated from peritoneum in surgical patients. *Lancet* **ii:**1437–1440.
21. **Cassone, A., P. Chiani, I. Quinti, and A. Torosantucci.** 1997. Possible participation of polymorphonuclear cells stimulated by microbial immunomodulators in the dysregulated cytokine patterns of AIDS patients. *J. Leukoc. Biol.* **62:**60–66.
22. **Collins, L. A., M. H. Samore, M. S. Roberts, R. Luzzati, R. L. Jenkins, W. D. Lewis, and A. W. Karchmer.** 1994. Risk factors for invasive fungal infections complicating orthotopic liver transplantation. *J. Infect. Dis.* **170:**644–652.
23. **Debusk, C. H., R. Daoud, M. C. Thirumoorthi, F. M. Wilson, and R. Khatib.** 1994. Candidemia: current epidemiologic characteristics and a long-term follow-up of the survivors. *Scand. J. Infect. Dis.* **26:**697–703.
24. **Donahue, S. P., C. M. Greven, J. J. Zuravleff, A. W. Eller, M. H. Nguyen, J. E. Peacock, M. W. Wagener, and V. L. Yu.** 1994. Intraocular candidiasis in patients with candidemia. Clinical implications derived from a prospective multicenter study. *Ophthalmology* **101:**1302–1309.
25. **Edmond, M. B., S. E. Wallace, D. K. McClish, M. A. Pfaller, R. N. Jones, and R. P. Wenzel.** 1999. Nosocomial bloodstream infections in United States hospitals: a three-year analysis. *Clin. Infect. Dis.* **29:**239–244.

26. **Edwards, J. E., Jr.** 1992. Should all patients with candidemia be treated with antifungal agents? *Clin. Infect. Dis.* **15:** 422–423.
27. **Eggimann, P., P. Francioli, J. Bille, R. Schneider, M. M. Wu, G. Chapuis, R. Chiolero, A. Pannatier, J. Schilling, S. Geroulanos, M. P. Glauser, and T. Calandra.** 1999. Fluconazole prophylaxis prevents intra-abdominal candidiasis in high-risk surgical patients. *Crit. Care Med.* **27:**1066–1072.
28. **Ekenna, O., R. J. Sherertz, and H. Bingham.** 1993. Natural history of bloodstream infections in a burn patient population: the importance of candidemia. *Am. J. Infect. Control* **21:**189–195.
29. **Ellis, M., D. Spence, B. E. De Pauw, F. Meunier, A. Marinus, L. Collette, R. Sylvester, J. F. G. M. Meis, M. Bogaerts, D. Selleslag, V. Krcmery, W. Von Sinner, P. MacDonald, C. Doyen, and B. Vandercam.** 1998. An EORTC international multicenter randomized trial (EORTC number 19923) comparing two dosages of liposomal amphotericin B for treatment of invasive aspergillosis. *Clin. Infect. Dis.* **27:** 1406–1412.
30. **Ellis, M. E., H. Clink, P. Ernst, M. A. Halim, D. Spence, M. Kalin, S. M. Hussain Qadri, J. Burnie, and W. Greer.** 1994. Controlled study of fluconazole in the prevention of fungal infections in neutropenic patients with haematological malignancies and bone marrow transplant recipients. *Eur. J. Clin. Microb. Infect. Dis.* **13:**3–11.
31. **Eppes, S. C., J. L. Troutman, and L. T. Gutman.** 1989. Outcome of treatment of candidemia in children whose central catheters were removed or retained. *Pediatr. Infect. Dis. J.* **8:**99–104.
32. **Fichtenbaum, C. J., M. German, W. C. Dunagan, V. J. Fraser, G. Medoff, J. Diego, and W. G. Powderly.** 1999. A pilot study of the management of uncomplicated candidemia with a standardized protocol of amphotericin B. *Clin. Infect. Dis.* **29:** 1551–1556.
33. **Fisher, M. A., S. H. Shen, J. Haddad, and W. F. Tarry.** 1989. Comparison of in vitro activity of fluconazole with that of amphotericin B against *Candida tropicalis, Candida glabrata,* and *Candida krusei. Antimicrob. Agents Chemother.* **33:** 1443–1446.
34. **Fisher-Hoch, S. P., and L. Hutwagner.** 1995. Opportunistic candidiasis: an epidemic of the 1980s. *Clin. Infect. Dis.* **21:** 897–904.
35. **Fraser, V. J., M. Jones, J. Dunkel, S. Storfer, G. Medoff, and W. C. Dunagan.** 1992. Candidemia in a tertiary care hospital: epidemiology, risk factors, and predictors of mortality. *Clin. Infect. Dis.* **15:**414–421.
36. **Goldman, M., J. C. Pottage, Jr., and D. C. Weaver.** 1993. *Candida krusei* fungemia. Report of 4 cases and review of the literature. *Medicine* (Baltimore) **72:**143–150.
37. **Gonzalez, C. E., D. Venzon, S. Lee, B. U. Mueller, P. A. Pizzo, and T. J. Walsh.** 1996. Risk factors for fungemia in children infected with human immunodeficiency virus: a case-control study. *Clin. Infect. Dis.* **23:**515–521.
38. **Goodman, J. L., D. J. Winston, R. A. Greenfield, P. H. Chandrasekar, B. Fox, H. Kaizer, R. K. Shadduck, T. C. Shea, P. Stiff, D. J. Friedman, W. G. Powderly, J. L. Silber, H. Horowitz, A. Lichtin, S. N. Wolff, K. F. Mangan, S. M. Silver, D. Weisdorf, W. G. Ho, G. Gilbert, and D. Buell.** 1992. A controlled trial of fluconazole to prevent fungal infections in patients undergoing bone marrow transplantation. *N. Engl. J. Med.* **326:**845–851.
39. **Goodrich, J. M., E. C. Reed, M. Mori, L. D. Fisher, S. Skerrett, P. S. Dandliker, B. Klis, G. W. Counts, and J. D. Meyers.** 1991. Clinical features and analysis of risk factors for invasive candidal infection after marrow transplantation. *J. Infect. Dis.* **164:**731–740.
40. **Groll, A. H., P. M. Shah, C. Mentzel, M. Schneider, G. Just-Nuebling, and K. Huebner.** 1996. Trends in the postmortem epidemiology of invasive fungal infections at a university hospital. *J. Infect.* **33:**23–32.
41. **Gualtieri, R. J., G. R. Donowitz, D. L. Kaiser, C. E. Hess, and M. A. Sande.** 1983. Double-blind randomized study of prophylactic trimethoprim/sulfamethoxazole in granulocytopenic patients with hematologic malignancies. *Am. J. Med.* **74:**934–940.
42. **Guiot, H. F. L., W. E. Fibbe, and J. W. Van't Wout.** 1996. Prevention of invasive candidiasis by fluconazole in patients with malignant hematological disorders and a high grade of *Candida* colonization, abstr. L033. *In 36th Intersci. Conf. Antimicrob. Agents and Chemother.* American Society for Microbiology, Washington, D.C.
43. **Guiot, H. F. L., W. E. Fibbe, and J. W. Van't Wout.** 1994. Risk factors for fungal infection in patients with malignant hematologic disorders—implications for empirical therapy and prophylaxis. *Clin. Infect. Dis.* **18:**525–532.
44. **Harousseau, J. L., A. W. Dekker, A. Stamatoullas-Bastard, A. Fassas, W. Linkesch, J. Gouveia, R. De Bock, M. Rovira, W. F. Seifert, H. Joosen, M. Peeters, and K. De Beule.** 2000. Itraconazole oral solution for primary prophylaxis of fungal infections in patients with hematological malignancy and profound neutropenia: a randomized, double-blind, double-placebo, multicenter trial comparing itraconazole and amphotericin B. *Antimicrob. Agents Chemother.* **44:**1887–1893.
45. **Harvey, R. L., and J. P. Myers.** 1987. Nosocomial fungemia in a large community teaching hospital. *Arch. Intern. Med.* **147:**2117–2120.
46. **Horn, R., B. Wong, T. E. Kiehn, and D. Armstrong.** 1985. Fungemia in a cancer hospital: changing frequency, earlier onset, and results of therapy. *Rev. Infect. Dis.* **7:**646–655.
47. **Isenberg, H. D., V. Tucci, F. Cintron, C. Singer, G. S. Weinstein, and D. H. Tyras.** 1989. Single-source outbreak of *Candida tropicalis* complicating coronary bypass surgery. *J. Clin. Microbiol.* **27:**2426–2428.
48. **Iwen, P. C., D. M. Kelly, E. C. Reed, and S. H. Hinrichs.** 1995. Invasive infection due to *Candida krusei* in immunocompromised patients not treated with fluconazole. *Clin. Infect. Dis.* **20:**342–347.
49. **Jarvis, W. R.** 1995. Epidemiology of nosocomial fungal infections, with emphasis on *Candida* species. *Clin. Infect. Dis.* **20:**1526–1530.
50. **Kao, A. S., M. E. Brandt, W. R. Pruitt, L. A. Conn, B. A. Perkins, D. S. Stephens, W. S. Baughman, A. L. Reingold, G. A. Rothrock, M. A. Pfaller, R. W. Pinner, and R. A. Hajjeh.** 1999. The epidemiology of candidemia in two United States cities: results of a population-based active surveillance. *Clin. Infect. Dis.* **29:**1164–1170.
51. **Karabinis, A., C. Hill, and B. Leclercq.** 1988. Risk factors for candidemia in cancer patients. A case-control study. *J. Clin. Microbiol.* **26:**129–132.
52. **Kauffman, C. A., J. A. Vazquez, J. D. Sobel, H. A. Gallis, D. S. McKinsey, A. W. Karchmer, A. M. Sugar, P. K. Sharkey, G. J. Wise, R. Mangi, A. Mosher, J. Y. Lee, and W. E. Dismukes.** 2000. Prospective multicenter surveillance study of funguria in hospitalized patients. *Clin. Infect. Dis.* **30:**14–18.
53. **Komshian, S. V., A. K. Uwaydah, J. D. Sobel, and L. R. Crane.** 1989. Fungemia caused by *Candida* species and *Torulopsis glabrata* in the hospitalized patient: frequency, characteristics, and evaluation of factors influencing outcome. *Rev. Infect. Dis.* **11:**379–390.
54. **Krause, W., H. Matheis, and K. Wulf.** 1969. Fungaemia and

funguria after oral administration of *Candida albicans*. *Lancet* i:598–599.

55. **Kullberg, B. J.** 1997. Trends in immunotherapy of fungal infections. *Eur. J. Clin. Microbiol. Infect. Dis.* **16**:51–55.
56. **Kullberg, B. J., and E. J. Anaissie.** 1998. Cytokines as therapy for opportunistic fungal infections. *Res. Immunol.* **149**: 478–488.
57. **Kullberg, B. J., K. Vandewoude, R. Herbrecht, F. Jacobs, M. Aoun, and P. Kujath.** 1998. A double-blind, randomized, placebo-controlled phase II study of filgrastim (recombinant granulocyte colony-stimulating factor) in combination with fluconazole for treatment of invasive candidiasis and candidemia in nonneutropenic patients, abstr. J-700, p. 479. *In 38th Intersci. Conf. Antimicrob. Agents Chemother.* American Society for Microbiology, Washington, D.C.
58. **Kung, N., N. Fisher, B. Gunson, M. Hastings, and D. Mutimer.** 1995. Fluconazole prophylaxis for high-risk liver transplant recipients. *Lancet* **345**:1234–1235.
59. **Kusne, S., J. S. Dummer, N. Singh, S. Iwatsuki, L. Makowka, C. Esquivel, A. G. Tzakis, T. E. Starzl, and M. Ho.** 1988. Infections after liver transplantation. An analysis of 101 consecutive cases. *Medicine* (Baltimore) **67**:132–143.
60. **Lecciones, J. A., J. W. Lee, E. E. Navarro, F. G. Witebsky, D. Marshall, S. M. Steinberg, P. A. Pizzo, and T. J. Walsh.** 1992. Vascular catheter-associated fungemia in patients with cancer: analysis of 155 episodes. *Clin. Infect. Dis.* **14**: 875–883.
61. **Levy, I., L. G. Rubin, S. Vasishtha, V. Tucci, and S. K. Sood.** 1998. Emergence of *Candida parapsilosis* as the predominant species causing candidemia in children. *Clin. Infect. Dis.* **26**: 1086–1088.
62. **Louria, D. B., D. P. Stiff, and B. Bennett.** 1962. Disseminated moniliasis in adults. *Medicine* **42**:307–333.
63. **Maertens, J., H. Demuynck, G. Verhoef, P. Vendenberghe, P. Zachée, and M. Boogaerts.** 1997. Granulocyte-macrophage colony-stimulating factor (GM-CSF) fails to improve outcome in invasive fungal infections in neutropenic cancer patients, abstr. P560. *In Abstr. 13th Congr. Int. Soc. Human Anim. Mycol.* International Society for Human and Animal Mycology, Adelaide, Australia.
64. **Maksymiuk, A. W., S. Thongprasert, R. Hopfer, M. Luna, V. Fainstein, and G. P. Bodey.** 1984. Systemic candidiasis in cancer patients. *Am. J. Med.* 77 (Suppl. 4D):20–27.
65. **Marr, K. A., K. Seidel, M. A. Slavin, R. A. Bowden, H. G. Schoch, M. E. Flowers, L. Corey, and M. Boeckh.** 2000. Prolonged fluconazole prophylaxis is associated with persistent protection against candidiasis-related death in allogeneic marrow transplant recipients: long-term follow-up of a randomized, placebo-controlled trial. *Blood* **96**:2055–2061.
66. **Marr, K. A., K. Seidel, T. C. White, and R. A. Bowden.** 2000. Candidemia in allogeneic blood and marrow transplant recipients: evolution of risk factors after the adoption of prophylactic fluconazole. *J. Infect. Dis.* **181**:309–316.
67. **Martino, P., C. Girmenia, A. Micozzi, F. De Bernardis, M. Boccanera, and A. Cassone.** 1994. Prospective study of *Candidia* colonization, use of empiric amphotericin B and development of invasive mycosis in neutropenic patients. *Eur. J. Clin. Microbiol. Infect. Dis.* **13**:797–804.
68. **Meis, J. F., M. Ruhnke, B. E. De Pauw, F. C. Odds, W. Siegert, and P. E. Verweij.** 1999. *Candida dubliniensis* candidemia in patients with chemotherapy-induced neutropenia and bone marrow transplantation. *Emerg. Infect. Dis.* **5**: 150–153.
69. **Menichetti, F., A. Del Favero, P. Martino, G. Bucaneve, A. Micozzi, C. Girmenia, G. Barbabietola, L. Pagano, P. Leoni, G. Specchia, A. Caiozzo, R. Raimondi, F. Mandelli, and GIMEMA Infection Program. Gruppo Italiano Malattie Ematologiche dell' Adulto.** 1999. Itraconazole oral solution as prophylaxis for fungal infections in neutropenic patients with hematologic malignancies: a randomized, placebo-controlled, double-blind, multicenter trial. *Clin. Infect. Dis.* **28**: 250–255.
70. **Menichetti, F., A. Delfavero, P. Martino, G. Bucaneve, A. Micozzi, D. Dantonio, P. Ricci, M. Carotenuto, V. Liso, A. M. Nosari, T. Barbui, G. Fasola, F. Mandelli, M. Montillo, G. Barbabietola, A. Dinota, L. Pagano, P. Jacopino, N. Isabella, R. Fontana, G. Landonio, G. Broccia, L. Cudillo, S. Difazio, L. Pacilli, M. Monaco, A. M. Carella, A. Chierichini, G. Quintini, A. Gabbas, P. Citarella, A. Dallasta, F. Ronconi, F. Dore, and P. Galieni.** 1994. Preventing fungal infection in neutropenic patients with acute leukemia: fluconazole compared with oral amphotericin B. *Ann. Intern. Med.* **120**: 913–918.
71. **Merz, W. G., J. E. Karp, D. Schron, and R. Saral.** 1986. Increased incidence of fungemia caused by *Candida krusei*. *J. Clin. Microbiol.* **24**:581–584.
72. **Miller, P. J., and R. P. Wenzel.** 1987. Etiologic organisms as independent predictors of death and morbidity associated with bloodstream infections. *J. Infect. Dis.* **156**:471–477.
73. **Nemunaitis, J., K. Shannon-Dorcy, F. R. Appelbaum, J. Meyers, A. Owens, R. Day, D. Ando, C. O'Neill, D. Buckner, and J. Singer.** 1993. Long-term follow-up of patients with invasive fungal disease who received adjunctive therapy with recombinant human macrophage colony-stimulating factor. *Blood* **82**:1422–1427.
74. **Nguyen, M. H., J. E. Peacock, Jr., D. C. Tanner, A. J. Morris, M. L. Nguyen, D. R. Snydman, M. M. Wagener, and V. L. Yu.** 1995. Therapeutic approaches in patients with candidemia. Evaluation in a multicenter, prospective, observational study. *Arch. Intern. Med.* **155**:2429–2435.
75. **Nguyen, M. H., J. E. Peacock, A. J. Morris, D. C. Tanner, M. L. Nguyen, D. R. Snydman, M. M. Wagener, M. G. Rinaldi, and V. L. Yu.** 1996. The changing face of candidemia: emergence of non-*Candida albicans* species and antifungal resistance. *Am. J. Med.* **100**:617–623.
76. **Ninane, J., and a Multicentre Study Group.** 1994. A multicentre study of fluconazole versus oral polyenes in the prevention of fungal infection in children with hematological or oncological malignancies. *Eur. J. Clin. Microbiol. Infect. Dis.* **13**:330–337.
77. **Nucci, M., I. Biasoli, T. Akiti, F. Silveira, C. Solza, G. Barreiros, N. Spector, A. Derossi, and W. Pulcheri.** 2000. A double-blind, randomized, placebo-controlled trial of intraconazole capsules as antifungal prophylaxis for neutropenic patients. *Clin. Infect. Dis.* **30**:300–305.
78. **Nucci, M., A. L. Colombo, F. Silveira, R. Richtmann, R. Salomao, M. L. Branchini, and N. Spector.** 1998. Risk factors for death in patients with candidemia. *Infect. Control Hosp. Epidemiol.* **19**:846–850.
79. **Oude Lashof, A. M. L., J. P. Donnelly, J. F. G. M. Meis, J. W. M. Van der Meer, and B. J. Kullberg.** 1998. Duration of antifungal treatment and development of delayed complications in patients with candidemia, p. 478, abstr. J97. *In Program Abstr. 38th Intersci. Conf. Antimicrob. Agents Chemother.* American Society for Microbiology, Washington, D.C.
80. **Paya, C. V.** 1993. Fungal infections in solid-organ transplantation. *Clin. Infect. Dis.* **16**:677–688.
81. **Peterson, P. K., H. H. Balfour, Jr., S. C. Marker, D. S. Fryd, R. J. Howard, and R. L. Simmons.** 1980. Cytomegalovirus disease in renal allograft recipients: a prospective study of the clinical features, risk factors and impact on renal transplantation. *Medicine* (Baltimore) **59**:283–300.

82. **Petri, M. G., J. Konig, H. P. Moecke, H. J. Gramm, H. Barkow, P. Kujath, R. Dennhart, H. Schafer, N. Meyer, P. Kalmar, P. Thulig, J. Muller, and H. Lode.** 1997. Epidemiology of invasive mycosis in ICU patients: a prospective multicenter study in 435 non-neutropenic patients. *Intensive Care Med.* **23:**317–325.
83. **Pfaller, M. A.** 1996. Nosocomial candidiasis: emerging species, reservoirs, and modes of transmission. *Clin. Infect. Dis.* 22(Suppl. 2):S73–S88.
84. **Pfaller, M. A., R. N. Jones, G. V. Doern, A. C. Fluit, J. Verhoef, H. S. Sader, S. A. Messer, A. Houston, S. Coffman, and R. J. Hollis.** 1999. International surveillance of blood stream infections due to *Candida* species in the European SENTRY Program: species distribution and antifungal susceptibility including the investigational triazole and echinocandin agents. SENTRY Participant Group (Europe). *Diagn. Microbiol. Infect. Dis.* **35:**19–25.
85. **Pfaller, M. A., R. N. Jones, S. A. Messer, M. B. Edmond, R. P. Wenzel, and The SCOPE Participant Group.** 1998. National surveillance of nosocomial blood stream infection due to species of *Candida* other than *Candida albicans:* frequency of occurrence and antifungal susceptibility in the SCOPE Program. *Diagn. Microbiol. Infect. Dis.* **30:**121–129.
86. **Pfaller, M. A., S. A. Messer, R. J. Hollis, R. N. Jones, G. V. Doern, M. E. Brandt, and R. A. Hajjeh.** 1999. Trends in species distribution and susceptibility to fluconazole among blood stream isolates of *Candida* species in the United States. *Diagn. Microbiol. Infect. Dis.* **33:**217–222.
87. **Phillips, P., S. Shafran, G. Garber, C. Rotstein, F. Smaill, I. Fong, I. Salit, M. Miller, K. Williams, J. M. Conly, J. Singer, S. Ioannou, and Canadian Candidemia Study Group.** 1997. Multicenter randomized trial of fluconazole versus amphotericin B for treatment of candidemia in non-neutropenic patients. *Eur. J. Clin. Microbiol. Infect. Dis.* **16:**337–345.
88. **Pittet, D., M. Monod, P. M. Suter, E. Frenk, and R. Auckenthaler.** 1994. *Candida* colonization and subsequent infections in critically ill surgical patients. *Ann. Surg.* **220:**751–758.
89. **Potter van Loon, B. J., A. T. Lichtendahl, S. S. Mulder, H. Van Houten, H. G. Gooszen, and P. J. Van den Broek.** 1989. Microbial contamination of donor duodenum in whole-pancreas transplantation. *Diabetes* 38(Suppl. 1):242–243.
90. **Poynton, C. H., R. A. Barnes, and J. Rees.** 1998. Interferon γ and granulocyte-macrophage colony-stimulating factor for the treatment of hepatosplenic candidosis in patients with acute leukemia. *Clin. Infect. Dis.* **26:**239–240.
91. **Prasad, J. K., I. Feller, and P. D. Thomson.** 1987. A ten-year review of *Candida* sepsis and mortality in burn patients. *Surgery* **101:**213–216.
92. **Prentice, H. G., I. M. Hann, R. Herbrecht, M. Aoun, S. Kvaloy, D. Catovsky, C. R. Pinkerton, S. A. Schey, F. Jacobs, A. Oakhill, R. F. Stevens, P. J. Darbyshire, and B. E. Gibson.** 1997. A randomized comparison of liposomal versus conventional amphotericin B for the treatment of pyrexia of unknown origin in neutropenic patients. *Br. J. Haematol.* **98:** 711–718.
93. **Raith, L., M. Csato, and A. Dobozy.** 1983. Decreased *Candida albicans* killing activity of granulocytes from patients with diabetes mellitus. *Mykosen* **26:**557–564.
94. **Rangel-Frausto, M. S., T. Wiblin, H. M. Blumberg, L. Saiman, J. Patterson, M. Rinaldi, M. Pfaller, J. E. Edwards, Jr., W. Jarvis, J. Dawson, and R. P. Wenzel.** 1999. National epidemiology of mycoses survey (NEMIS): variations in rates of bloodstream infections due to *Candida* species in seven surgical intensive care units and six neonatal intensive care units. *Clin. Infect. Dis.* **29:**253–258.
95. **Reagan, D. R., M. A. Pfaller, R. J. Hollis, and R. P. Wenzel.** 1990. Characterization of the sequence of colonization and nosocomial candidemia using DNA fingerprinting and a DNA probe. *J. Clin. Microbiol.* **28:**2733–2738.
96. **Rello, J., M. E. Esandi, E. Diaz, D. Mariscal, M. Gallego, and J. Valles.** 1998. The role of *Candida* sp. isolated from bronchoscopic samples in nonneutropenic patients. *Chest* **114:**146–149.
97. **Rex, J. H., J. E. Bennett, A. M. Sugar, P. G. Pappas, J. Serody, J. E. Edwards, and R. G. Washburn, for the NIAID Mycoses Study Group and the Candidemia Study Group.** 1995. Intravascular catheter exchange and duration of candidemia. *Clin. Infect. Dis.* **21:**994–996.
98. **Rex, J. H., J. E. Bennett, A. M. Sugar, P. G. Pappas, C. M. Van der Horst, J. E. Edwards, R. G. Washburn, W. M. Scheld, A. W. Karchmer, A. P. Dine, M. J. Levenstein, and C. D. Webb, for the Candidemia Study Group and the National Institute of Allergy and Infectious Diseases Mycoses Study Group.** 1994. A randomized trial comparing fluconazole with amphotericin B for the treatment of candidemia in patients without neutropenia. *N. Engl. J. Med.* **331:**1325–1330.
99. **Rex, J. H., M. A. Pfaller, A. L. Barry, P. W. Nelson, C. D. Webb, and the NIAID Study Group and the Candidemia Study Group.** 1995. Antifungal susceptibility testing of isolates from a randomized, multicenter trial of fluconazole versus amphotericin B as treatment of nonneutropenic patients with candidemia. *Antimicrob. Agents Chemother.* **39:**40–44.
100. **Rex, J. H., T. J. Walsh, J. D. Sobel, S. G. Filler, P. G. Pappas, W. E. Dismukes, and J. E. Edwards.** 2000. Practice guidelines for the treatment of candidiasis. *Clin. Infect. Dis.* **30:** 662–678.
101. **Richet, H. M., A. Andremont, C. Tancrede, J. L. Pico, and W. R. Jarvis.** 1991. Risk factors for candidemia in patients with acute lymphocytic leukemia. *Rev. Infect. Dis.* **13:** 211–215.
102. **Rotstein, C., E. J. Bow, M. Laverdiere, S. Ioannou, D. Carr, N. Moghaddam, and The Canadian Fluconazole Prophylaxis Study Group.** 1999. Randomized placebo-controlled trial of fluconazole prophylaxis for neutropenic cancer patients: benefit based on purpose and intensity of cytotoxic therapy. *Clin. Infect. Dis.* **28:**331–340.
103. **Saiman, L., E. Ludington, M. Pfaller, S. Rangel-Frausto, R. T. Wiblin, J. Dawson, H. M. Blumberg, J. E. Patterson, M. Rinaldi, J. E. Edwards, R. P. Wenzel, W. Jarvis, and The National Epidemiology of Mycosis Survey Study Group.** 2000. Risk factors for candidemia in neonatal intensive care unit patients. *Pediatr. Infect. Dis. J.* **19:**319–324.
104. **Samonis, G., H. Anastassiadou, M. Dassiou, Y. Tselentis, and G. P. Bodey.** 1994. Effects of broad-spectrum antibiotics on colonization of gastrointestinal tracts of mice by *Candida albicans. Antimicrob. Agents Chemother.* **38:**602–603.
105. **Sandord, G. R., W. G. Merz, J. R. Wingard, P. Charache, and R. Saral.** 1980. The value of fungal surveillance cultures as predictors of systemic fungal infections. *J. Infect. Dis.* **142:** 503–509.
106. **Schooley, R. T., M. S. Hirsch, R. B. Colvin, A. B. Cosimi, N. E. Tolkoff-Rubin, R. T. McCluskey, R. C. Burton, P. S. Russell, J. T. Herrin, F. L. Delmonico, J. V. Giorgi, W. Henle, and R. H. Rubin.** 1983. Association of herpesvirus infections with T-lymphocyte-subset alterations, glomerulopathy, and opportunistic infections after renal transplantation. *N. Engl. J. Med.* **308:**307–313.
107. **Sherertz, R. J., K. S. Gledhill, K. D. Hampton, M. A. Pfaller, L. B. Givner, J. S. Abramson, and R. G. Dillard.** 1992. Outbreak of *Candida* bloodstream infections associated with retrograde medication administration in a neonatal intensive care unit. *J. Pediatr.* **120:**455–461.

108. **Simms, H. H., and R. D'Amico.** 1992. Intra-abdominal sepsis alters tumor necrosis factor-alpha and interleukin-1 beta binding to human neutrophils. *Crit. Care Med.* **20:**11–16.
109. **Slavin, M. A., B. Osborne, R. Adams, M. J. Levenstein, H. G. Schoch, A. R. Feldman, J. D. Meyers, and R. A. Bowden.** 1995. Efficacy and safety of fluconazole prophylaxis for fungal infections after marrow transplantation—a prospective, randomized, double-blind study. *J. Infect. Dis.* **171:** 1545–1552.
110. **Slotman, G. J., and K. W. Burchard.** 1987. Ketoconazole prevents *Candida* sepsis in critically ill surgical patients. *Arch. Surg.* **122:**147–151.
111. **Snydman, D. R., B. G. Werner, B. Heinze-Lacey, V. P. Berardi, N. L. Tilney, R. L. Kirkman, E. L. Milford, S. I. Cho, H. L. Bush, Jr., A. S. Levey, and et al.** 1987. Use of cytomegalovirus immune globulin to prevent cytomegalovirus disease in renal-transplant recipients. *N. Engl. J. Med.* **317:** 1049–1054.
112. **Strausbaugh, L. J., D. L. Sewell, T. T. Ward, M. A. Pfaller, T. Heitzman, and R. Tjoelker.** 1994. High frequency of yeast carriage on hands of hospital personnel. *J. Clin. Microbiol.* **32:**2299–2300.
113. **Tollemar, J., K. Hockerstedt, B. G. Ericzon, H. Jalanko, and O. Ringden.** 1995. Liposomal amphotericin B prevents invasive fungal infections in liver transplant recipients. A randomized, placebo-controlled study. *Transplantation* **59:**45–50.
114. **Van't Wout, J. W.** 1996. Fluconazole treatment of candidal infections caused by non-*albicans Candida* species. *Eur. J. Clin. Microbiol. Infect. Dis.* **15:**238–242.
115. **Van't Wout, J. W., H. Mattie, and R. Van Furth.** 1988. A prospective study of the efficacy of fluconazole (UK 49,858) against deep-seated fungal infections. *Antimicrob. Agents Chemother.* **31:**665–672.
116. **Vincent, J. L., E. Anaissie, H. Bruining, W. Demajo, M. el-Ebiary, J. Haber, Y. Hiramatsu, G. Nitenberg, P. O. Nystrom, D. Pittet, T. Rogers, P. Sandven, G. Sganga, M. D. Schaller, and J. Solomkin.** 1998. Epidemiology, diagnosis and treatment of systemic *Candida* infection in surgical patients under intensive care. *Intensive Care Med.* **24:**206–216.
117. **Vincent, J. L., D. J. Bihari, P. M. Suter, H. A. Bruining, J. White, M. H. Nicolas-Chanoin, M. Wolff, R. C. Spencer, M. Hemmer, and EPIC International Advisory Committee.** 1995. The prevalence of nosocomial infection in intensive care units in Europe. Results of the European Prevalence of Infection in Intensive Care (EPIC) Study. *JAMA* **274:**639–644.
118. **Viscoli, C., C. Girmenia, A. Marinus, L. Collette, P. Martino, B. Lebau, D. Spence, V. Krcmery, B. E. De Pauw, F. Meunier, and The Invasive Fungal Infection Group of the EORTC.** 1999. Candidemia in cancer patients. A prospective, multicenter surveillance study in Europe by the the Invasive Fungal Infection Group (IFIG) of the European Organization for Research and Treatment of Cancer (EORTC). *Clin. Infect. Dis.* **28:**1071–1079.
119. **Voss, A., R. J. Hollis, R. P. Wenzel, and B. N. Doebbeling.** 1994. Investigation of the sequence of colonization and candidemia in non-neutropenic patients. *J. Clin. Microbiol.* **32:** 975–980.
120. **Voss, A., J. A. J. W. Kluytmans, J. G. M. Koeleman, L. Spanjaard, C. M. J. E. Vandenbroucke-Grauls, H. A. Verbrugh, M. C. Vos, A. Y. L. Weersink, J. A. A. Hoogkamp-Korstanje, and J. F. G. M. Meis.** 1996. Occurrence of yeast bloodstream infections between 1987 and 1995 in five Dutch university hospitals. *Eur. J. Clin. Microbiol. Infect. Dis.* **15:**909–912.
121. **Voss, A., J. L. M. L. Le Noble, F. M. Verduyn Lunel, N. A. Foudraine, and J. F. G. M. Meis.** 1997. Candidemia in intensive care unit patients: risk factors for mortality. *Infection* **25:**9–11.
122. **Voss, A., M. A. Pfaller, R. J. Hollis, J. Rhine-Chalberg, and B. N. Doebbeling.** 1995. Investigation of *Candida albicans* transmission in a surgical intensive care unit cluster by using genomic DNA typing methods. *J. Clin. Microbiol.* **33:** 576–580.
123. **Walsh, T. J., C. Gonzalez, E. Roilides, B. U. Mueller, N. Ali, L. L. Lewis, T. O. Whitcomb, D. J. Marshall, and P. A. Pizzo.** 1995. Fungemia in children infected with the human immunodeficiency virus: new epidemiologic patterns, emerging pathogens, and improved outcome with antifungal therapy. *Clin. Infect. Dis.* **20:**900–906.
124. **Walsh, T. J., J. W. Hathorn, J. D. Sobel, W. G. Merz, V. Sanchez, S. M. Maret, H. R. Buckley, M. A. Pfaller, R. Schaufele, C. Sliva, E. Navarro, J. Lecciones, P. Chandrasekar, J. Lee, and P. A. Pizzo.** 1991. Detection of circulating *Candida* enolase by immunoassay in patients with cancer and invasive candidiasis. *N. Engl. J. Med.* **324:**1026–1031.
125. **Walsh, T. J., J. Hiemenz, and P. A. Pizzo.** 1994. Evolving risk factors for invasive fungal infections—all neutropenic patients are not the same. *Clin. Infect. Dis.* **18:**793–798.
126. **Walsh, T. J., and J. W. Lee.** 1993. Prevention of invasive fungal infections in patients with neoplastic disease. *Clin. Infect. Dis.* **17:**S468–S480.
127. **Walsh, T. J., and P. A. Pizzo.** 1992. Experimental gastrointestinal and disseminated candidiasis in immunocompromised animals. *Eur. J. Epidemiol.* **8:**477–483.
128. **Weems, J. J., Jr., M. E. Chamberland, J. Ward, M. Willy, A. A. Padhye, and S. L. Solomon.** 1987. *Candida parapsilosis* fungemia associated with parenteral nutrition and contaminated blood pressure transducers. *J. Clin. Microbiol.* **25:** 1029–1032.
129. **Wenzel, R.** 1995. Nosocomial candidemia: risk factors and attributable mortality. *Clin. Infect. Dis.* **20:**1531–1534.
130. **Wey, S. B., M. Mori, M. A. Pfaller, R. F. Woolson, and R. P. Wenzel.** 1988. Hospital-acquired candidemia. The attributable mortality and excess length of stay. *Arch. Intern. Med.* **148:**2642–2645.
131. **Wey, S. B., M. Mori, M. A. Pfaller, R. F. Woolson, and R. P. Wenzel.** 1989. Risk factors for hospital-acquired candidemia. A matched case-control study. *Arch. Intern. Med.* **149:** 2349–2353.
132. **Wingard, J. R.** 1995. Importance of *Candida* species other than *C. albicans* as pathogens in oncology patients. *Clin. Infect. Dis.* **20:**115–125.
133. **Wingard, J. R., J. D. Dick, W. G. Merz, G. R. Sandford, R. Saral, and W. H. Burns.** 1980. Pathogenecity of *Candida tropicalis* and *Candida albicans* after gastrointestinal inoculation in mice. *Infect. Immun.* **29:**808–813.
134. **Wingard, J. R., W. G. Merz, M. G. Rinaldi, T. R. Johnson, J. E. Karp, and R. Saral.** 1991. Increase in *Candida krusei* infection among patients with bone marrow transplantation and neutropenia treated prophylactically with fluconazole. *N. Engl. J. Med.* **325:**1274–1277.
135. **Winston, D. J., P. H. Chandrasekar, H. M. Lazarus, J. L. Goodman, J. L. Silber, H. Horowitz, R. K. Shadduck, C. S. Rosenfeld, W. G. Ho, M. Z. Islam, and D. N. Buell.** 1993. Fluconazole prophylaxis of fungal infections in patients with acute leukemia—results of a randomized placebo-controlled, double-blind, multicenter trial. *Ann. Intern. Med.* **118:** 495–503.

Candida and Candidiasis
Edited by Richard A. Calderone

Chapter 24

Deep-Seated Candidal Infections

SCOTT G. FILLER AND BART JAN KULLBERG

Deep-seated candidal infections can arise either from direct inoculation or as a result of hematogenous seeding. In general, the majority of these infections are caused by *Candida albicans*. With the exception of candiduria, none of the deep-seated candidal infections have been studied in large, prospective randomized multicenter trials. Thus, the diagnosis and treatment of these infections are based mainly on case series and anecdotal reports.

CANDIDURIA

Candiduria occurs very frequently; *Candida* species now represent the most common organism to be isolated from the urine of patients hospitalized in the United States. In patients in medical intensive care units, *Candida* species account for 31% of urinary isolates (61). When candiduria is present, *C. albicans* is the causative organism in 50 to 68% of cases (38, 61). Interestingly, approximately 25% of patients with candiduria have concomitant bacteriuria. Risk factors for candiduria include the presence of a urinary catheter or other urinary tract abnormality, advanced age, prior use of antimicrobial agents, and diabetes mellitus (38). In a large, prospective, multicenter study of funguria, 85% of patients with funguria had a nonfungal infection in the month preceding funguria (38). These infections were mainly bacterial urinary tract infections or pneumonia. These findings underscore the importance of antibacterial agents in predisposing patients to developing candiduria.

In the majority of patients, candiduria represents colonization of the lower urinary tract. However, in neonates, candiduria is associated with either a renal abscess or renal fungus ball in up to 40% of cases (10). Also, in a few patients, candiduria may result from hematogenous seeding of the kidneys during disseminated candidiasis and may be one of the first manifestations of this infection. Candiduria should be suspected as a marker of a disseminated candidal infection in high-risk patients, such as those with neutropenia and low-birth-weight infants (19).

Patients with candiduria are frequently asymptomatic. Only a few percent of patients have typical symptoms of a urinary tract infection such as dysuria, urgency, frequency, or flank pain. Although a significant percentage of patients with candiduria may have a fever, it is probable that in many cases the fever is due to another source of infection, rather than the candiduria. The urinary sediment in patients with candiduria is nonspecific. Approximately 50% of patients with candiduria have pyuria, and 35% have hematuria. Budding yeasts are seen in the urinalysis of 60% of patients with *Candida* organisms growing in their urine (38).

The decision to treat candiduria depends on the clinical situation. Symptomatic patients, those with neutropenia or renal allografts, and low-birth-weight infants should be treated with antifungal therapy (60). Also, as there is a high incidence of candidemia in patients who have candiduria and either urinary obstruction or a urologic manipulation (4), these patients should receive antifungal therapy. If possible, any prosthetic material in the urinary tract, such as a ureteral stent or Foley catheter, should be removed or at least replaced. Fluconazole, 200 mg per day, is the treatment of choice for susceptible organisms, and therapy should be for 7 to 14 days. The dose of fluconazole should be reduced in patients with significant impairment of renal function. However, there is some evidence that candiduria in these patients may not respond as well to fluconazole, possibly due to a lower concentration of the drug in the urine (69). Continuous bladder irrigation with 50 to 200 μg of amphotericin B per ml of sterile water for 3 days may be some-

Scott G. Filler • Harbor UCLA Medical Center, 1000 W. Carson St., RB-2, Torrance, CA 90509. **Bart Jan Kullberg** • Department of Medicine (541), University Medical Center, Geert Grooteplein 8, Mailstop 541, 6525 GA Nijmegen, The Netherlands.

what effective in treating candiduria (60). Amphotericin B bladder irrigation should not be used in patients who are at high risk for either renal or hematogenously disseminated candidiasis, because this therapy does not result in significant systemic concentrations of the drug.

The vast majority of individuals with candiduria are asymptomatic and are at low risk for hematogenously disseminated candidiasis. These patients should rarely be treated. This recommendation is based on the results of a recently completed prospective, multicenter study of adults with asymptomatic or minimally symptomatic candiduria (69). This study compared the efficacy of 200 mg of fluconazole for 14 days versus placebo. At the end of treatment, candiduria resolved in 50% of patients receiving fluconazole and 29% of patients receiving placebo. However, 14 days after therapy was completed, the rates of candiduria were similar (~67%) in both the treated and untreated patients. Furthermore, there were no cases of hematogenously disseminated candidiasis in either group. Thus, in the absence of significant risk factors for hematogenously disseminated candidiasis, there is minimal benefit of treating asymptomatic candiduria (60).

INTRA-ABDOMINAL CANDIDAL INFECTIONS

Candidal peritonitis usually occurs in one of two clinical settings. The first is a patie
nt on chronic ambulatory peritoneal dialysis (CAPD). *Candida* species cause approximately 75% of cases of fungal peritonitis in patients on CAPD (29, 76). Children on CAPD have a higher incidence of candidal peritonitis, especially due to *Candida parapsilosis,* than do adults (79). Risk factors for *Candida* peritonitis in patients on CAPD include prior antibiotic use and previous episodes of peritonitis (29). Candidal peritonitis is frequently diagnosed in CAPD patients by observing fungal elements on a Gram stain of the peritoneal dialysate (49). In cases where no organism is seen on the Gram stain, *Candida* spp. usually can be cultured from the dialysate.

The second type of patient in whom candidal peritonitis develops is one who has had a liver or pancreas transplant or surgery for gastrointestinal perforation or pancreatitis (3, 12, 14, 33, 70). In such a patient, additional risk factors for candidal peritonitis include prolonged antibiotics, a second unplanned abdominal operation, and hospital-acquired gastrointestinal perforation (3, 14, 22, 57). Candidal peritonitis should usually be treated when the organism is isolated from the peritoneal cavity, either in pure culture or in conjunction with bacteria. As *Candida* frequently colonizes peritoneal drains, isolation of this organism from a drain should not be considered diagnostic of candidal peritonitis.

Patients with candidal peritonitis should be treated with fluconazole when the organism is likely susceptible to this drug. The dose should be adjusted for renal function and hemodialysis. Amphotericin B is also effective for treatment of candidal peritonitis and should be used especially when *Candida krusei* or other fluconazole-resistant organisms are either isolated or suspected (60). Intraperitoneal instillation of amphotericin B should be avoided as it causes a painful chemical peritonitis. Although an intravenous formulation of itraconazole is available, there is very little experience with this agent for the treatment of candidal peritonitis. When a peritoneal catheter is present, it should be removed to cure the infection and prevent relapse (16, 49). A small placebo-controlled trial suggested that prophylaxis with fluconazole may reduce the incidence of candidal peritonitis in very high-risk patients who have recurrent gastrointestinal perforation or anastomotic leakage (23).

Candida sp. can also infect the biliary tree and is a rare cause of acalculous cholecystitis (21, 34). It is frequently isolated as part of mixed flora. Most patients are debilitated and have been treated with broad-spectrum antibiotics in the intensive care unit for a prolonged period. Although the majority of patients with candidal cholecystitis are colonized with *Candida* spp., detectable candidemia occurs infrequently. Nevertheless, acalculous cholecystitis due to *Candida* spp. is associated with a high mortality. The mainstays of treatment include antifungal therapy and decompression of the biliary tree. As both fluconazole and amphotericin B achieve therapeutic concentrations in the bile, local instillation into the bile tract is unnecessary (60).

HEPATOSPLENIC CANDIDIASIS (CHRONIC DISSEMINATED CANDIDIASIS)

Hepatosplenic candidiasis (also called chronic disseminated candidiasis) is predominantly an infection of neutropenic patients, especially those with leukemia. Although the infection is initiated while neutropenia is present, it is frequently not detected until after neutropenia has resolved. Presenting signs and symptoms include fever, abdominal pain, hepatomegaly, and splenomegaly. Liver function tests and C-reactive protein levels are frequently elevated. Imaging of the abdomen usually reveals multiple focal lesions in the liver, spleen, and kidney. Ultrasonography is less sensitive than either computed tomography scanning or magnetic resonance imaging for detecting these lesions (7, 63). Although finding multiple lesions in the liver and spleen in a patient with leukemia who has recently recovered from neutropenia is suggestive of hepatosplenic candidiasis, it is important to make a microbiologic diagnosis to guide the choice of therapy. For example, fungi such as *Aspergillus* spp. and *Blastoschizomyces* spp. can also cause hepatosplenic infections (45). The infecting microorganism can sometimes be isolated by blood culture. In the remaining patients, a lesion should be aspirated either percutaneously or by laparoscopy. The aspiration has the highest chance of being diagnostic if it is performed within 3 weeks of recovery from neutropenia and a specific lesion is targeted (as opposed to performing a blind biopsy) (6).

Treatment of hepatosplenic candidiasis requires long-term antifungal therapy; however, the optimal treatment regimen remains controversial and should be individualized to the patient (22, 60). Fluconazole is a reasonable choice for a patient who is clinically stable and likely infected with a susceptible organism. Some mycologists recommend treating all patients with amphotericin B for 1 to 2 weeks before switching to fluconazole. Amphotericin B is also appropriate for patients who are likely infected with an organism that is likely resistant to fluconazole. Lipid formulations of amphotericin B are attractive for the treatment of hepatosplenic candidiasis because they have a reduced chance of causing nephrotoxicity. Amphotericin B lipid complex has been used to treat hepatosplenic candidiasis in both adults and children (64, 74). However, the efficacies of the various lipid formulations of amphotericin B for the treatment of any hematogenously disseminated candidal infection have never been directly compared with amphotericin B deoxycholate.

Once antifungal therapy is initiated, it should be continued until the lesions either resolve or calcify. In one retrospective study of patients with hepatosplenic candidiasis who were treated with amphotericin B, the patients remained febrile for a median of 19 days after therapy was initiated and required a median of 112 days of therapy (65). The long-term outcome in patients with hepatosplenic candidiasis is dependent mainly on the success of treatment for their underlying malignancy (5). Thus, it is important to continue the anticancer therapy, even if it entails ablative chemotherapy for bone marrow transplantation, during treatment for hepatosplenic candidiasis (36, 75).

ENDOCARDITIS

Candida species are the most common cause of fungal endocarditis (24, 62). Risk factors for candidal endocarditis include prosthetic valve surgery, preexisting valvular heart disease, intravenous catheters, broad-spectrum antibiotics, intravenous drug abuse, and immunosuppression (24, 52, 62). Prosthetic valve surgery is the greatest risk factor for candidal endocarditis, and over 50% of patients with this infection have had such surgery (24). Endocarditis usually occurs within the first year of surgery but may occur years later (48, 51, 52).

Patients with candidal endocarditis have a clinical presentation similar to bacterial endocarditis. However, there appears to be a higher incidence of large thrombi that may embolize to the major blood vessels. In addition, it has been reported that endophthalmitis occurs more frequently (62). Blood cultures grow *Candida* species in approximately 85% of the patients; in the remaining cases the mycologic diagnosis is made by either culture or histology of the infected valve (24). The majority of patients are symptomatic for approximately 1 month before the diagnosis of endocarditis is made. As with bacterial endocarditis, transesophageal echocardiography is more sensitive than transthoracic echocardiography for detecting vegetations (53). Vegetations occur most frequently on the aortic valve, followed by the mitral and tricuspid valves (24). Multivalvular involvement is relatively common, and vegetations may also form on nonvalvular structures, such as pacemaker wires, atrial myxomas, or the ventricular wall.

The standard treatment of candidal endocarditis is amphotericin B for at least 6 weeks combined with valve replacement and debridement of all infected tissue (51–53). In patients who are not surgical candidates, chronic suppressive therapy with fluconazole has been successful (53), and a few patients with native valve endocarditis have even been cured with fluconazole alone (78). Even when antifungal therapy is combined with valve replacement, there is approximately a 30% chance of relapse (24, 51). Most relapses occur within the first 3 years after therapy; however, late relapses occurring as long as 9 years after initial therapy have been reported (48). Because of the significant relapse rate, it has been suggested that all patients with candidal prosthetic valve endocarditis should be placed on lifelong suppressive therapy with fluconazole (48, 51).

PERICARDITIS AND MYOCARDITIS

Purulent pericarditis due to *Candida* species is a rare, life-threatening infection. Risk factors include immunosuppression, cardiac surgery, and broad-spectrum antibiotics. The signs and symptoms of candidal pericarditis are nonspecific, and the diagnosis is made by either culture of the pericardial fluid or histologic examination of the pericardial tissue. Treatment usually requires pericardiectomy combined with antifungal therapy, usually amphotericin B (40, 56).

Candidal myocarditis is also rare. It is seen most commonly in patients who are immunocompromised due to neutropenia or corticosteroids (8). Intravenous drug abuse and broad-spectrum antibiotics are also predisposing factors for this infection (15, 55). In some cases, myocarditis occurs concomitantly with endocarditis. Myocarditis may also be a manifestation of hematogenously candidiasis. Arrhythmias due to abnormalities of the conduction system are common (55). The majority of cases of candidal myocarditis are diagnosed at autopsy. However, this infection should be suspected in patients with candidemia and cardiac conduction abnormalities. These patients should receive aggressive antifungal therapy.

THROMBOPHLEBITIS

Although *Candida* species are the fourth most common cause of intravenous catheter infections in intensive care unit patients in the United States (61), candidal septic thrombophlebitis is relatively rare. Colonization with *Candida* species and therapy with broad-spectrum antibiotics are major risk factors for this infection (32, 73). Patients with candidal thrombophlebitis are almost always febrile and frequently have edema of the extremity that is drained by the involved vein. When a peripheral vein is involved, local signs of inflammation may be minimal or absent (32). Candidemia is usually present and often persists despite apparently adequate antifungal therapy. Cultures of the catheter tip may also grow *Candida* species. Excision of the infected vein should be performed whenever possible. Antifungal therapy should be continued for 2 weeks after the infected vein has been removed (60).

ENDOPHTHALMITIS

Candida species are the leading cause of fungal endophthalmitis (25, 68). Although candidal endophthalmitis is most commonly caused by *C. albicans*, other species of *Candida* can also cause this infection (35). Approximately 15 to 28% of nonneutropenic patients with candidemia have evidence of endophthalmitis when a thorough funduscopic examination is performed (9, 59). Because the white, cotton ball-like lesions that are seen on funduscopy are composed predominantly of neutrophils, candidal endophthalmitis is less commonly detected in patients who are neutropenic. In the vast majority of cases, endophthalmitis develops as a result of hematogenous seeding. Thus, the risk factors for this infection are similar to those for hematogenously disseminated candidiasis, and the presence of a disseminated infection should be strongly suspected in all patients with candidal endophthalmitis. Intravenous heroin addicts (44) and patients who have had either an intraocular lens implant (37) or a corneal transplant (39) can also develop candidal endophthalmitis. In patients who have had eye surgery, the infection develops as a result of direct inoculation of the organism into the eye at the time of surgery.

The diagnosis of candidal endophthalmitis can be made presumptively in patients with candidemia and typical eye findings. However, blood cultures may fail to grow *Candida* organisms in approximately 50% of the cases. In these patients, a vitreous aspirate should be performed to determine the microbial etiology of the infection. Aspiration of the anterior chamber of the eye is rarely diagnostic. The treatment for candidal endophthalmitis depends on the severity of the infection and the location of the lesion(s). Even a small lesion in the macula can result in severe impairment of visual acuity and thus should be treated aggressively. Although amphotericin B has long been considered the gold standard for treatment of candidal endophthalmitis, there are increasing numbers of reports of successful therapy with fluconazole (2, 18, 59). This agent is a logical choice for patients with small lesions that are located away from the macula (22). In addition, fluconazole is frequently used as follow-up therapy because candidal endophthalmitis usually requires 6 to 8 weeks of treatment (60). Many clinical mycologists would use amphotericin B plus flucytosine as the initial therapy when there is either extensive infection or a lesion that is located in or adjacent to the macula. Pars plana vitrectomy should be performed in patients who have vitritis that is extensive or progressive while on antifungal therapy. This procedure aids in clearing the infection and minimizes loss of visual acuity (18, 25, 44). If a foreign body, such as an intraocular lens implant is present, it should be removed whenever possible to prevent relapse (37).

MENINGITIS

Candidal meningitis most frequently occurs in premature infants and in patients who have had a recent neurosurgical procedure (26, 54). It is seen less commonly in patients who are immunocompromised due to neutropenia, AIDS, or hereditary neutrophil function defects (1, 13, 43, 47). In premature infants, meningitis arises via hematogenous seeding. Thus, the risk factors for meningitis in neonates are similar to those for hematogenously disseminated candidiasis: low birth weight, broad-spectrum antibiotics, total parenteral nutrition, and an indwelling central venous catheter (26). Meningitis in neurosurgical patients arises from direct inoculation of the organism into the central nervous system around the time of surgery. The majority of these patients have had either a craniotomy or cerebiospinal fluid (CSF) shunt (28, 50). Additional risk factors include broad-spectrum antibiotics and antecedent bacterial meningitis (54).

The clinical presentation of candidal meningitis depends on the host. In neonates, there is frequently metabolic acidosis and respiratory decompensation, which is manifested by an increase in oxygen requirement and apnea. On CSF examination, pleocytosis is inconsistent and the predominant leukocyte type can range from mononuclear cells to neutrophils. Although hypoglycorrhachia is common, it is sometimes absent. CSF Gram stain is usually negative; however, the culture grows *Candida* species in about 75% of cases. *Candida* species can also be cultured from the blood in the majority of neonates (26). Adults with candidal meningitis usually have a subacute onset of symptoms, which include fever, headache, and altered mental status. Neck stiffness occurs infrequently. CSF leukocytosis is very common in these patients, and as in neonates, either mononuclear cells or neutrophils can predominate. Hypoglycorrhachia and an elevated CSF protein are common. The organism can be seen on CSF Gram stain in approximately 40% of the cases, and it grows in culture approximately 80% of the time (54). Culturing multiple large-volume samples of the CSF can enhance recovery of the organism (28). Detectable candidemia is rare in patients who develop candidal meningitis after a neurosurgical procedure.

Candidal meningitis should be treated initially with amphotericin B (54, 60). Flucytosine should be added when feasible. However, many low-birth-weight infants are unable to take oral medications safely. In these patients, the use of amphotericin B alone is curative approximately 90% of the time (26). Because relapses can occur, therapy should be continued for 4 weeks after clinical resolution of the infection (60). There is much less experience with fluconazole; it should be reserved for follow-up or suppressive therapy. Liposomal amphotericin B has been used successfully to treat a small number of neonates with candidal meningitis (66). In the rabbit model of candidal meningitis, liposomal amphotericin B is equivalent in efficacy to amphotericin B deoxycholate and superior to both amphotericin B lipid complex and amphotericin B colloidal dispersion (30). If prosthetic material is present in the central nervous system, it should be replaced or removed whenever possible.

PNEUMONIA

Candidal pneumonia is a rare infection that is frequently overdiagnosed. When the infection occurs, it develops either as a result of hematogenous seeding or by aspiration of infected secretions (31, 46). Risk factors include neutropenia, candidal esophagitis, use of broad-spectrum antibiotics, and hematologic malignancy. When the pneumonia arises from hematogenous seeding, a miliary pattern may be seen on chest radiograph. These patients may also have candidemia or evidence of infection in other organs. Patients who develop candidal pneumonia from aspiration of infected secretions usually have nonspecific patchy or lobar infiltrates that may be either unilateral or bilateral (11, 31). In these patients, the infection usually remains localized to the lung.

To diagnose candidal pneumonia, it is essential to obtain histological evidence of fungal invasion of the lung tissue (31, 46). Because *Candida* species commonly colonize the oropharynx and tracheobronchial tree of hospitalized patients, the diagnosis of candidal pneumonia cannot be made by sputum Gram stain or culture. Furthermore, even the isolation of a large number of organisms from bronchial brushings or bronchoalveolar lavage specimens in nonneutropenic patients is almost always indicative of colonization rather than true infection (58).

This infection should only be treated when the diagnosis has been confirmed by histology. Primary candidal pneumonia is usually treated with amphotericin B. When pneumonia is a manifestation of hematogenously disseminated candidiasis, then therapy should be directed at the disseminated infection (60).

OSTEOMYELITIS AND ARTHRITIS

The usual route of infection in both candidal osteomyelitis and arthritis is hematogenous seeding. Both types of infection have been reported to occur either during or following hematogenously disseminated candidiasis. Thus, the risk factors for such infections are typical for hematogenously disseminated candidiasis (20, 27, 77). In addition, there can be hematogenous seeding of a bone or a joint in the absence of other organ involvement. This situation has been reported most frequently in intravenous drug users (41). The vertebrae are the most common site of infection when osteomyelitis arises from hematogenous infection; candidal arthritis most frequently involves the knees (67). Candidal osteomyelitis can also develop as a result of direct inoculation during a wound infection (27). Candidal arthritis has developed as complication of intra-articular injections. In these cases, *C. parapsilosis* is the most common infecting organism (17, 20). Finally, *Candida* species are a rare cause of prosthetic joint infection (42, 71).

Candidal osteomyelitis has been treated successfully with prolonged courses of either amphotericin B or fluconazole (27, 41, 72). Because of significant nephrotoxicity associated with long-term amphotericin B, a reasonable approach is to treat the patient with amphotericin B for 2 to 3 weeks, followed by fluconazole for 6 to 12 months (60). As with osteomyelitis caused by other microorganisms, it is important to debride any devitalized bone and remove all infected hardware, if feasible.

Treatment of candidal arthritis requires adequate drainage of the infected joint, which usually requires surgery. A synovectomy should be performed when the infection is severe or does not resolve rapidly with drainage and antifungal therapy alone (17, 20, 67). The principles of antifungal therapy for candidal arthritis are similar to those for osteomyelitis. Both fluconazole and amphotericin B achieve therapeutic levels in the synovial fluid. Therefore, intra-articular antifungal therapy is unnecessary (60). Candidal infection of a prosthetic joint is rarely cured with antifungal therapy alone; all prosthetic material should be removed whenever possible (42, 71).

REFERENCES

1. **Agus, S., S. Spektor, and Z. Israel.** 2000. CNS granulomatosis in a child with chronic granulomatous disease. *Br. J. Neurosurg.* **14:**59–61.
2. **Akler, M. E., H. Vellend, D. M. McNeely, S. L. Walmsley, and W. L. Gold.** 1995. Use of fluconazole in the treatment of candidal endophthalmitis. *Clin. Infect. Dis.* **20:**657–664.
3. **Alden, S. M., E. Frank, and L. Flancbaum.** 1989. Abdominal candidiasis in surgical patients. *Am. Surg.* **55:**45–49.
4. **Ang, B. S., A. Telenti, B. King, J. M. Steckelberg, and W. R. Wilson.** 1993. Candidemia from a urinary tract source: microbiological aspects and clinical significance. *Clin. Infect. Dis.* **17:**662–666.
5. **Anttila, V. J., E. Elonen, S. Nordling, A. Sivonen, T. Ruutu, and P. Ruutu.** 1997. Hepatosplenic candidiasis in patients with acute leukemia: incidence and prognostic implications. *Clin. Infect. Dis.* **24:**375–380.
6. **Anttila, V. J., M. Farkkila, S. E. Jansson, M. Taavitsainen, S. S. Kaukoranta-Tolvanen, S. Nordling, P. Koukila-Kahkola, T. Ruutu, and P. Ruutu.** 1997. Diagnostic laparoscopy in patients with acute leukemia and suspected hepatic candidiasis. *Eur. J. Clin. Microbiol. Infect. Dis.* **16:**637–643.
7. **Anttila, V. J., P. Ruutu, S. Bondestam, S. E. Jansson, S. Nordling, M. Farkkila, A. Sivonen, M. Castren, and T. Ruutu.** 1994. Hepatosplenic yeast infection in patients with acute leukemia: a diagnostic problem. *Clin. Infect. Dis.* **18:**979–981.
8. **Atkinson, J. B., D. H. Connor, M. Robinowitz, H. A. McAllister, and R. Virmani.** 1984. Cardiac fungal infections: review of autopsy findings in 60 patients. *Hum. Pathol.* **15:**935–942.
9. **Brooks, R. G.** 1989. Prospective study of *Candida* endophthalmitis in hospitalized patients with candidemia. *Arch. Intern. Med.* **149:**2226–2228.
10. **Bryant, K., C. Maxfield, and G. Rabalais.** 1999. Renal candidiasis in neonates with candiduria. *Pediatr. Infect. Dis. J.* **18:** 959–963.
11. **Buff, S. J., R. McLelland, H. A. Gallis, R. Matthay, and C. E. Putman.** 1982. *Candida albicans* pneumonia: radiographic appearance. *Am. J. Roentgenol.* **138:**645–648.
12. **Calandra, T., J. Bille, R. Schneider, F. Mosimann, and P. Francioli.** 1989. Clinical significance of *Candida* isolated from peritoneum in surgical patients. *Lancet* **ii:**1437–1440.
13. **Casado, J. L., C. Quereda, J. Oliva, E. Navas, A. Moreno, V. Pintado, J. Cobo, and I. Corral.** 1997. Candidal meningitis in HIV-infected patients: analysis of 14 cases. *Clin. Infect. Dis.* **25:**673–676.
14. **Castaldo, P., R. J. Stratta, R. P. Wood, R. S. Markin, K. D. Patil, M. S. Shaefer, A. N. Langnas, E. C. Reed, S. J. Li, T. J. Pillen, and B. W. Shaw, Jr.** 1991. Clinical spectrum of fungal infections after orthotopic liver transplantation. *Arch. Surg.* **126:**149–156.
15. **Cavaliere, A.** 1980. *Candida* myocarditis in a young heroin addict. *Pathol. Res. Pract.* **168:**224–228.
16. **Chan, T. M., C. Y. Chan, S. W. Cheng, W. K. Lo, C. Y. Lo, and I. K. Cheng.** 1994. Treatment of fungal peritonitis complicating continuous ambulatory peritoneal dialysis with oral fluconazole: a series of 21 patients. *Nephrol. Dial. Transplant.* **9:**539–542.
17. **Christensson, B., L. Ryd, L. Dahlberg, and S. Lohmander.** 1993. *Candida albicans* arthritis in a nonimmunocompromised patient. Complication of placebo intraarticular injections. *Acta Orthop. Scand.* **64:**695–698.
18. **Christmas, N. J., and W. E. Smiddy.** 1996. Vitrectomy and systemic fluconazole for treatment of endogenous fungal endophthalmitis. *Ophthalmic. Surg. Lasers* **27:**1012–1018.
19. **Chun, C. S., and R. B. Turner.** 1991. The outcome of candiduria in pediatric patients. *Diagn. Microbiol. Infect. Dis.* **14:** 119–123.
20. **Cuende, E., C. Barbadillo, E. M. R., C. Isasi, A. Trujillo, and J. L. Andreu.** 1993. *Candida* arthritis in adult patients who are not intravenous drug addicts: report of three cases and review of the literature. *Semin. Arthritis Rheum.* **22:**224–241.
21. **Diebel, L. N., A. M. Raafat, S. A. Dulchavsky, and W. J. Brown.** 1996. Gallbladder and biliary tract candidiasis. *Surgery* **120:**760–765.
22. **Edwards, J. E., Jr., G. P. Bodey, R. A. Bowden, T. Buchner, B. E. de Pauw, S. G. Filler, M. A. Ghannoum, M. Glauser, R. Herbrecht, C. A. Kauffman, S. Kohno, P. Martino, F. Meunier, T. Mori, M. A. Pfaller, J. H. Rex, T. R. Rogers, R. H. Rubin, J. Solomkin, C. Viscoli, T. J. Walsh, and M. White.** 1997. International conference for the development of a consensus on the management and prevention of severe candidal infections. *Clin. Infect. Dis.* **25:**43–59.
23. **Eggimann, P., P. Francioli, J. Bille, R. Schneider, M. M. Wu, G. Chapuis, R. Chiolero, A. Pannatier, J. Schilling, S. Geroulanos, M. P. Glauser, and T. Calandra.** 1999. Fluconazole prophylaxis prevents intra-abdominal candidiasis in high-risk surgical patients. *Crit. Care. Med.* **27:**1066–1072.
24. **Ellis, M. E., H. Al-Abdely, A. Sandridge, W. Greer, and W. Ventura.** 2001. Fungal endocarditis: evidence in the world literature, 1965–1995. *Clin. Infect. Dis.* **32:**50–62.
25. **Essman, T. F., H. W. Flynn, Jr., W. E. Smiddy, R. D. Brod, T. G. Murray, J. L. Davis, and P. E. Rubsamen.** 1997. Treatment

outcomes in a 10-year study of endogenous fungal endophthalmitis. *Ophthalmic. Surg. Lasers* **28**:185–194.

26. **Fernandez, M., E. H. Moylett, D. E. Noyola, and C. J. Baker.** 2000. Candidal meningitis in neonates: a 10-year review. *Clin. Infect. Dis.* **31**:458–463.
27. **Gathe, J. C., Jr., R. L. Harris, B. Garland, M. W. Bradshaw, and T. W. Williams, Jr.** 1987. Candida osteomyelitis. Report of five cases and review of the literature. *Am. J. Med.* **82**: 927–937.
28. **Geers, T. A., and S. M. Gordon.** 1999. Clinical significance of *Candida* species isolated from cerebrospinal fluid following neurosurgery. *Clin. Infect. Dis.* **28**:1139–1147.
29. **Goldie, S. J., L. Kiernan-Tridle, C. Torres, N. Gorban-Brennan, D. Dunne, A. S. Kliger, and F. O. Finkelstein.** 1996. Fungal peritonitis in a large chronic peritoneal dialysis population: a report of 55 episodes. *Am. J. Kidney Dis.* **28**:86–91.
30. **Groll, A. H., N. Giri, V. Petraitis, R. Petraitiene, M. Candelario, J. S. Bacher, S. C. Piscitelli, and T. J. Walsh.** 2000. Comparative efficacy and distribution of lipid formulations of amphotericin B in experimental *Candida albicans* infection of the central nervous system. *J. Infect. Dis.* **182**:274–282.
31. **Haron, E., S. Vartivarian, E. Anaissie, R. Dekmezian, and G. P. Bodey.** 1993. Primary *Candida* pneumonia. Experience at a large cancer center and review of the literature. *Medicine* (Baltimore) 72:137–142.
32. **Hauser, C. J., P. Bosco, M. Davenport, D. Ehrensaft, M. Latif, and B. T. McNamara.** 1989. Surgical management of fungal peripheral thrombophlebitis. *Surgery* **105**:510–514.
33. **Hesse, U. J., D. E. Sutherland, R. L. Simmons, and J. S. Najarian.** 1986. Intraabdominal infections in pancreas transplant recipients. *Ann. Surg.* **203**:153–162.
34. **Hiatt, J. R., M. R. Kobayashi, J. E. Doty, and K. P. Ramming.** 1991. Acalculous *Candida* cholecystitis: a complication of critical surgical illness. *Am. Surg.* 57:825–829.
35. **Joshi, N., and B. H. Hamory.** 1991. Endophthalmitis caused by non-*albicans* species of *Candida. Rev. Infect. Dis.* **13**: 281–287.
36. **Katayama, K., S. Koizumi, M. Yamagami, Y. Tamaru, T. Ichihara, M. Konishi, S. Maekawa, H. Seki, and N. Taniguchi.** 1994. Successful peritransplant therapy in children with active hepatosplenic candidiasis. *Int. J. Hematol.* **59**:125–130.
37. **Kauffman, C. A., S. F. Bradley, and A. K. Vine.** 1993. *Candida* endophthalmitis associated with intraocular lens implantation: efficacy of fluconazole therapy. *Mycoses* 36:13–17.
38. **Kauffman, C. A., J. A. Vazquez, J. D. Sobel, H. A. Gallis, D. S. McKinsey, A. W. Karchmer, A. M. Sugar, P. K. Sharkey, G. J. Wise, R. Mangi, A. Mosher, J. Y. Lee, and W. E. Dismukes.** 2000. Prospective multicenter surveillance study of funguria in hospitalized patients. The National Institute of Allergy and Infectious Diseases (NIAID) Mycoses Study Group. *Clin. Infect. Dis.* **30**:14–18.
39. **Kloess, P. M., R. D. Stulting, G. O. D. Waring, and L. A. Wilson.** 1993. Bacterial and fungal endophthalmitis after penetrating keratoplasty. *Am. J. Ophthalmol.* **115**:309–316.
40. **Kraus, W. E., P. N. Valenstein, and G. R. Corey.** 1988. Purulent pericarditis caused by *Candida:* report of three cases and identification of high-risk populations as an aid to early diagnosis. *Rev. Infect. Dis.* **10**:34–41.
41. **Lafont, A., A. Olive, M. Gelman, J. Roca-Burniols, R. Cots, and J. Carbonell.** 1994. *Candida albicans* spondylodiscitis and vertebral osteomyelitis in patients with intravenous heroin drug addiction. Report of 3 new cases. *J. Rheumatol.* **21**: 953–956.
42. **Lambertus, M., D. Thordarson, and M. B. Goetz.** 1988. Fungal prosthetic arthritis: presentation of two cases and review of the literature. *Rev. Infect. Dis.* **10**:1038–1043.
43. **Ludviksson, B. R., O. Thorarensen, T. Gudnason, and S. Halldorsson.** 1993. *Candida albicans* meningitis in a child with myeloperoxidase deficiency. *Pediatr. Infect. Dis. J.* **12**: 162–164.
44. **Martinez-Vazquez, C., J. Fernandez-Ulloa, J. Bordon, B. Sopena, J. de la Fuente, A. Ocampo, and M. Rubianes.** 1998. *Candida albicans* endophthalmitis in brown heroin addicts: response to early vitrectomy preceded and followed by antifungal therapy. *Clin. Infect. Dis.* **27**:1130–1133.
45. **Martino, P., M. Venditti, A. Micozzi, G. Morace, L. Polonelli, M. P. Mantovani, M. C. Petti, V. L. Burgio, C. Santini, P. Serra, and F. Mandelli.** 1990. *Blastoschizomyces capitatus:* an emerging cause of invasive fungal disease in leukemia patients. *Rev. Infect. Dis.* **12**:570–582.
46. **Masur, H., P. P. Rosen, and D. Armstrong.** 1977. Pulmonary disease caused by *Candida* species. *Am. J. Med.* **63**:914–925.
47. **McCullers, J. A., S. L. Vargas, P. M. Flynn, B. I. Razzouk, and J. L. Shenep.** 2000. Candidal meningitis in children with cancer. *Clin. Infect. Dis.* **31**:451–457.
48. **Melgar, G. R., R. M. Nasser, S. M. Gordon, B. W. Lytle, T. F. Keys, and D. L. Longworth.** 1997. Fungal prosthetic valve endocarditis in 16 patients. An 11-year experience in a tertiary care hospital. *Medicine* (Baltimore) **76**:94–103.
49. **Montenegro, J., R. Aguirre, O. Gonzalez, I. Martinez, and R. Saracho.** 1995. Fluconazole treatment of *Candida* peritonitis with delayed removal of the peritoneal dialysis catheter. *Clin. Nephrol.* **44**:60–63.
50. **Montero, A., J. Romero, J. A. Vargas, C. A. Regueiro, G. Sanchez-Aloz, F. De Prados, A. De la Torre, and G. Aragon.** 2000. *Candida* infection of cerebrospinal fluid shunt devices: report of two cases and review of the literature. *Acta Neurochir.* **142**: 67–74.
51. Muehrcke, D. D., **B. W. Lytle, and D. M. Cosgrove, 3rd.** 1995. Surgical and long-term antifungal therapy for fungal prosthetic valve endocarditis. *Ann. Thorac. Surg.* **60**:538–543.
52. **Nasser, R. M., G. R. Melgar, D. L. Longworth, and S. M. Gordon.** 1997. Incidence and risk of developing fungal prosthetic valve endocarditis after nosocomial candidemia. *Am. J. Med.* **103**:25–32.
53. **Nguyen, M. H., M. L. Nguyen, V. L. Yu, D. McMahon, T. F. Keys, and M. Amidi.** 1996. *Candida* prosthetic valve endocarditis: prospective study of six cases and review of the literature. *Clin. Infect. Dis.* **22**:262–267.
54. **Nguyen, M. H., and V. L. Yu.** 1995. Meningitis caused by *Candida* species: an emerging problem in neurosurgical patients. *Clin. Infect. Dis.* **21**:323–327.
55. **Parker, J. C., Jr.** 1980. The potentially lethal problem of cardiac candidosis. *Am. J. Clin. Pathol.* **73**:356–361.
56. **Rabinovici, R., D. Szewczyk, P. Ovadia, J. R. Greenspan, and J. J. Sivalingam.** 1997. *Candida pericarditis: clinical profile and treatment. Ann. Thorac. Surg.* **63**:1200–1204.
57. **Rantala, A., O. P. Lehtonen, K. Kuttila, T. Havia, and J. Niinikoski.** 1991. Diagnostic factors for postoperative candidosis in abdominal surgery. *Ann. Chir. Gynaecol.* **80**:323–328.
58. **Rello, J., M. E. Esandi, E. Diaz, D. Mariscal, M. Gallego, and J. Valles.** 1998. The role of *Candida* sp. isolated from bronchoscopic samples in nonneutropenic patients. *Chest* **114**: 146–149.
59. **Rex, J. H., J. E. Bennett, A. M. Sugar, P. G. Pappas, C. M. van der Horst, J. E. Edwards, R. G. Washburn, W. M. Scheld, A. W. Karchmer, A. P. Dine, M. J. Levenstein, and C. D. Webb.** 1994. A randomized trial comparing fluconazole with amphotericin B for the treatment of candidemia in patients without neutropenia. Candidemia Study Group and the National Institute of Allergy and Infectious Diseases (NIAID) Mycoses Study Group. *N. Engl. J. Med.* **331**:1325–1330.

60. **Rex, J. H., T. J. Walsh, J. D. Sobel, S. G. Filler, P. G. Pappas, W. E. Dismukes, and J. E. Edwards.** 2000. Practice guidelines for the treatment of candidiasis. Infectious Diseases Society of America. *Clin. Infect. Dis.* **30:**662–678.
61. **Richards, M. J., J. R. Edwards, D. H. Culver, and R. P. Gaynes.** 1999. Nosocomial infections in medical intensive care units in the United States. National Nosocomial Infections Surveillance System. *Crit. Care Med.* **27:**887–892.
62. **Rubinstein, E., and R. Lang.** 1995. Fungal endocarditis. *Eur. Heart J.* **16**(Suppl. B)**:**84–89.
63. **Sallah, S., R. Semelka, N. Kelekis, S. Worawattanakul, and W. Sallah.** 1998. Diagnosis and monitoring response to treatment of hepatosplenic candidiasis in patients with acute leukemia using magnetic resonance imaging. *Acta Haematol.* **100:** 77–81.
64. **Sallah, S., R. C. Semelka, W. Sallah, J. R. Vainright, and D. L. Philips.** 1999. Amphotericin B lipid complex for the treatment of patients with acute leukemia and hepatosplenic candidiasis. *Leuk. Res.* **23:**995–999.
65. **Sallah, S., R. C. Semelka, R. Wehbie, W. Sallah, N. P. Nguyen, and P. Vos.** 1999. Hepatosplenic candidiasis in patients with acute leukaemia. *Br. J. Haematol.* **106:**697–701.
66. **Scarcella, A., M. B. Pasquariello, B. Giugliano, M. Vendemmia, and A. de Lucia.** 1998. Liposomal amphotericin B treatment for neonatal fungal infections. *Pediatr. Infect. Dis. J.* **17:** 146–148.
67. **Silveira, L. H., M. L. Cuellar, G. Citera, G. E. Cabrera, E. Scopelitis, and L. R. Espinoza.** 1993. *Candida* arthritis. *Rheum. Dis. Clin. N. Am.* **19:**427–437.
68. **Smiddy, W. E.** 1998. Treatment outcomes of endogenous fungal endophthalmitis. *Curr. Opin. Ophthalmol.* **9:**66–70.
69. **Sobel, J. D., C. A. Kauffman, D. McKinsey, M. Zervos, J. A. Vazquez, A. W. Karchmer, J. Lee, C. Thomas, H. Panzer, and W. E. Dismukes.** 2000. Candiduria: a randomized, double-blind study of treatment with fluconazole and placebo. The National Institute of Allergy and Infectious Diseases (NIAID) Mycoses Study Group. *Clin. Infect. Dis.* **30:**19–24.
70. **Solomkin, J. S., A. B. Flohr, P. G. Quie, and R. L. Simmons.** 1980. The role of *Candida* in intraperitoneal infections. *Surgery* **88:**524–530.
71. **Tunkel, A. R., C. Y. Thomas, and B. Wispelwey.** 1993. *Candida* prosthetic arthritis: report of a case treated with fluconazole and review of the literature. *Am. J. Med.* **94:**100–103.
72. **Turner, D. L., S. A. Johnson, and S. A. Rule.** 1999. Successful treatment of candidal osteomyelitis with fluconazole following failure with liposomal amphotericin B. *J. Infect.* **38:**51–53.
73. **Walsh, T. J., C. I. Bustamente, D. Vlahov, and H. C. Standiford.** 1986. Candidal suppurative peripheral thrombophlebitis: recognition, prevention, and management. *Infect. Control* **7:**16–22.
74. **Walsh, T. J., P. Whitcomb, S. Piscitelli, W. D. Figg, S. Hill, S. J. Chanock, P. Jarosinski, R. Gupta, and P. A. Pizzo.** 1997. Safety, tolerance, and pharmacokinetics of amphotericin B lipid complex in children with hepatosplenic candidiasis. *Antimicrob. Agents Chemother.* **41:**1944–1948.
75. **Walsh, T. J., P. O. Whitcomb, S. G. Revankar, and P. A. Pizzo.** 1995. Successful treatment of hepatosplenic candidiasis through repeated cycles of chemotherapy and neutropenia. *Cancer* **76:**2357–2362.
76. **Warady, B. A., M. Bashir, and L. A. Donaldson.** 2000. Fungal peritonitis in children receiving peritoneal dialysis: a report of the NAPRTCS. *Kidney Int.* **58:**384–389.
77. **Weisse, M. E., D. A. Person, and J. T. Berkenbaugh, Jr.** 1993. Treatment of *Candida* arthritis with flucytosine and amphotericin B. *J. Perinatol.* **13:**402–404.
78. **Wells, C. J., G. J. Leech, A. M. Lever, and M. H. Wansbrough-Jones.** 1995. Treatment of native valve *Candida* endocarditis with fluconazole. *J. Infect.* **31:**233–235.
79. **Yinnon, A. M., D. Gabay, D. Raveh, Y. Schlesinger, I. Slotki, D. Attias, and B. Rudensky.** 1999. Comparison of peritoneal fluid culture results from adults and children undergoing CAPD. *Perit. Dial. Int.* **19:**51–55.

Candida and Candidiasis
Edited by Richard A. Calderone

Chapter 25

Current Understanding of the Modes of Action of and Resistance Mechanisms to Conventional and Emerging Antifungal Agents for Treatment of *Candida* Infections

DOMINIQUE SANGLARD AND JACQUES BILLE

Candida infections in humans are favored by various alterations in immune defenses such as those associated with the AIDS epidemic, cancer chemotherapy, and solid-organ and bone marrow transplantations. Their rising incidence has paralleled the increasing number of immunocompromised patients. Antifungal treatments against *Candida* infections are hampered by several factors, including the limited number of active agents, the emergence of refractory fungal species, and the development of resistance. This situation has triggered the search for new antifungal agents with novel modes of action. Different cellular processes involved in the biosynthesis of components required for the growth of fungal cells have been targeted by antifungal agents. Figure 1 gives a schematic overview of the pathways and targets of the most relevant antifungal agents, which will be discussed in the following sections. These sections will integrate in a concise manner for each class of antifungals the current knowledge on their mode of action (Table 1) and their spectrum of activity mainly against *Candida* species (Table 2) and summarize their clinical use for *Candida* infections. Because the use of antifungal agents is associated with possible resistance problems, the current understanding of resistance mechanisms to these agents will be presented (Table 1). Finally, the characteristics of new agents (Tables 1 and 2) and innovative approaches for the treatment of *Candida* infections will be discussed. The reader is also referred to excellent reviews detailing the mode of action and the pharmacodynamic properties of classic and currently developed agents that will not be covered here (57, 60, 82, 84, 89, 90).

Activities of antifungal agents are determined by in vitro susceptibility tests and, therefore, the experimental conditions used in these tests constitute key parameters in the evaluation of these activities. The development of standardized antifungal drug susceptibility tests, as outlined by the National Committee for Clinical Laboratory Standards (NCCLS), has unified the efforts of several reference laboratories. The introduction of NCCLS document M27-A has permitted interlaboratory reproducibility and comparisons of antifungal activities among yeast pathogens (187). In the following sections, the reported MIC of a given antifungal agent will be mostly those obtained by the use of NCCLS standard protocols.

ANTIFUNGAL DRUGS IN CURRENT USE: MODES OF ACTION, SPECTRUM OF ACTIVITY, AND CLINICAL USE

Given that ergosterol biosynthesis is specific to fungi and is necessary for their growth, this feature has been largely exploited by scientists responsible for the design and isolation of antifungal agents. As a result, most of the antifungal agents used in medicine target the ergosterol biosynthetic pathway and include polyenes, azoles, allylamines, or morpholine derivatives (Fig. 2). Among currently used antifungal agents, 5-fluorocytosine (5-FC) is one of the few that does not directly interfere with the ergosterol biosynthetic pathway.

Polyenes

Polyenes belong to a class of natural antifungal compounds discovered in the early 1950s. One of the most successful polyene derivatives, amphotericin B

Dominique Sanglard and Jacques Bille • Institute of Microbiology, University Hospital of Lausanne (CHUV), 1011 Lausanne, Switzerland.

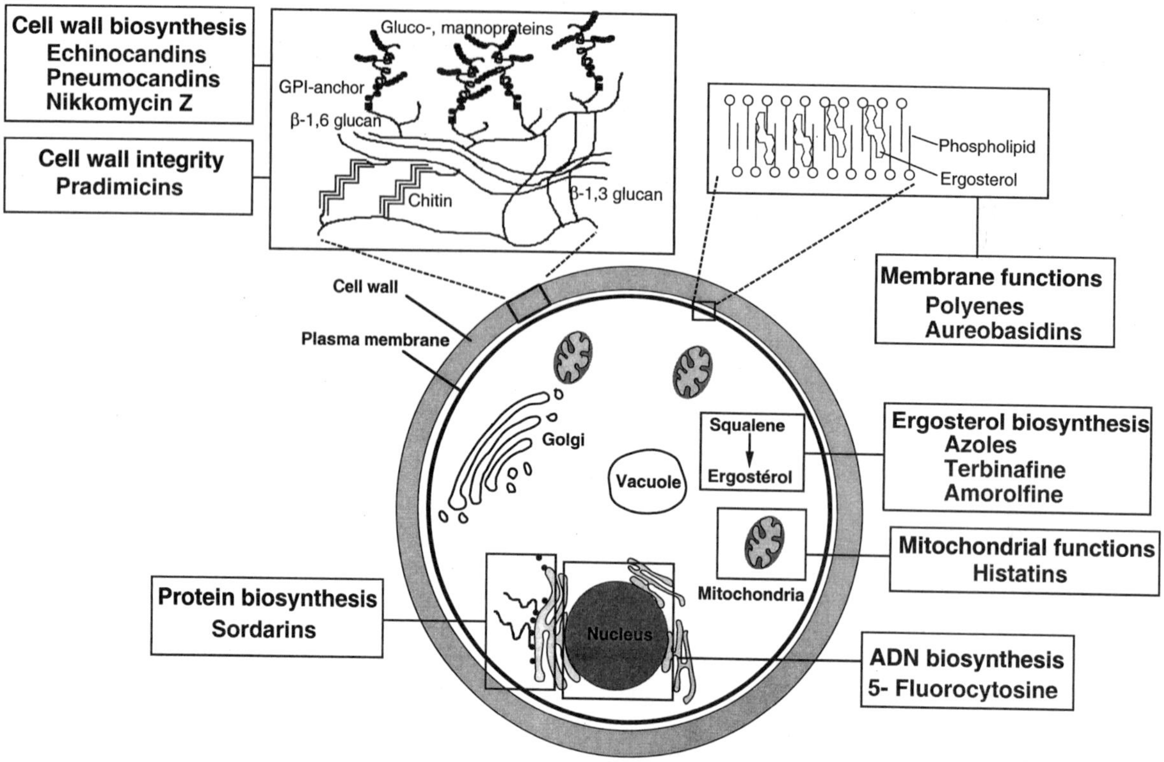

Figure 1. Schematic view of a fungal cell and of the principal targets of antifungal agents.

Table 1. Overview of the mode of action and resistance mechanisms of current and emerging antifungal agents active against *Candida* species

Antifungal agent(s)	Mode(s) of action	Mechanism(s) of resistance in clinical and laboratory isolates
Amphotericin B (AmB)	Binding to ergosterol	Absence of ergosterol or decrease of ergosterol content in cells
		Increased catalase activity
5-Fluorocytosine (5-FC)	Inhibition of DNA synthesis	Defect in cytosine permease
		Deficiency or lack of enzymes implicated in the metabolism of 5-FC
		Deregulation of the pyrimidine biosynthetic pathway
Azoles (ketoconazole, itraconazole, fluconazole, voriconazole, posaconzole, rauconazole)	Inhibition of 14α-lanosterol demethylase (*ERG11*)	Enhanced efflux mediated by multidrug transporters
		Decrease of affinity in Erg 11p by mutations
		Upregulation of *ERG11*
		Alterations in the ergosterol biosynthetic pathway
Allylamines (terbinafine)	Inhibition of squalene epoxidase	N.R.[a]
Morpholines (amorolfine)	Inhibition of sterol Δ^{14} reductase (*ERG24*) and the Δ^{7-8} isomerase (*ERG2*)	N.R.
Griseofulvin	Binding to tubulin	N.R.
Cyclic lipopeptides (caspofungin, micafungin, V-echinocandin)	Inhibition of β-1,3 glucan synthase (*CaFKSI*)	Loss of β-1,3 glucan synthase function
Nikkomycin Z	Inhibition of chitin synthase	N.R.
Pradimicins	Calcium-dependent binding to mannan	N.R.
Sordarins	Inhibition of elongation factor 2 (*EFT2*)	N.R.
Cationic antimicrobial peptides	Formation of pores at the site of cellular membranes	Loss of mitochondrial function

[a] N.R., not reported.

Table 2. Activities of current and emerging antifungal agents against *Candida* species

Antifungal agent	MIC$_{90}$[a] (μg/ml)					Reference(s)
	C. albicans	*C. glabrata*	*C. krusei*	*C. parapsilosis*	*C. tropicalis*	
Amphotericin B (AmB)	0.5	1	0.5	0.5	0.5	42
5-Fluorocytosine (5-FC)	4	0.5	16–32	1	4	42
Azoles						
Fluconazole	1	64	64	2.0	2.0	
Itraconazole	0.25	4.0	2.0	0.5	0.5	212, 213
Voriconazole	0.06	2.0	1.0	0.12	0.25	
Posaconazole	0.06	4.0	0.5	0.12	0.25	
Ravuconazole	0.03	4.0	0.5	0.12	0.25	
Terbinafine	4	>128	>128	0.125	>128	240
Amorolfine	10	N.A.[b]	1	1	1	53
Cyclic lipopeptides						
Caspofungin (MK-0991)	0.5	0.5	1	0.5	1	21
Micafungin (FK-463)	0.0156	0.0156	0.125	1	0.0313	174
V-Echinocandin (LY-303366)	0.125	0.5	0.25	4 (210)	0.125	37
Sordarin						
GM 222712	0.004	0.5	>32	1	0.06	112
GM 237354	0.015	4	>32	16	0.12	
Pradimicin (BMS-181184)	8	4	4	8	16	77

[a] MIC$_{90}$ is defined as the MIC to which 90% of a study population belongs.
[b] N.A., not available.

(AmB) (Fig. 3), is produced by *Streptomyces nodosus* (80). AmB can form soluble salts in both basic and acidic environments, is not orally nor intramuscularly absorbed, and is virtually insoluble in water. AmB has been solubilized in a micellar preparation with deoxycholate for its clinical use for more than 3 decades (28). Although AmB is an effective antifungal drug, it possesses several drawbacks limiting its clinical utility. Systemic and renal problems are often encountered with AmB (10). To reduce its unwanted side effects, AmB has been formulated in liposomes (Ambisome) (5), lipid complexes (Abelcet) (223), and colloidal suspensions (Amphotec) (119, 288) to allow the use of higher doses of AmB against fungal patho-

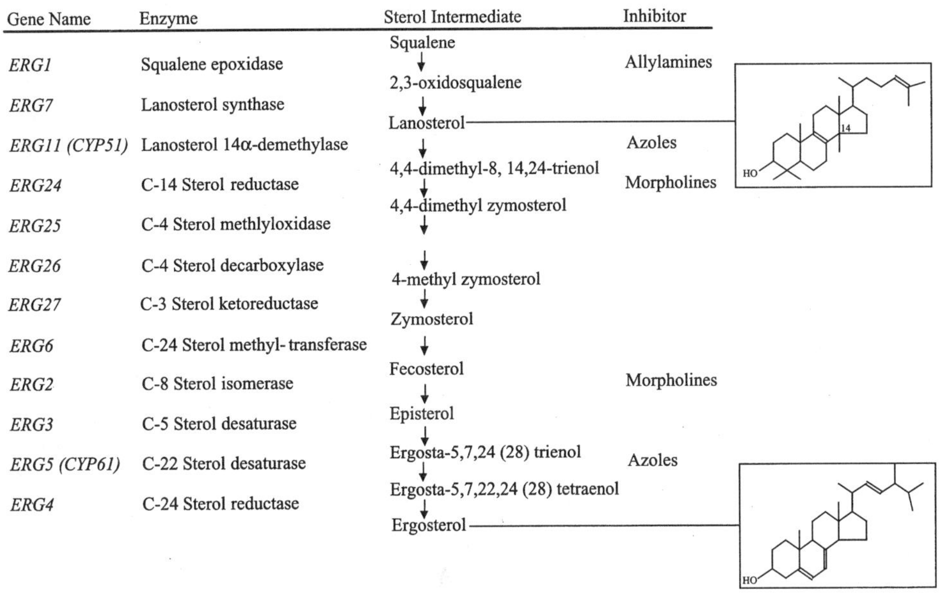

Figure 2. The ergosterol biosynthesis pathway as a target of current antifungal agents.

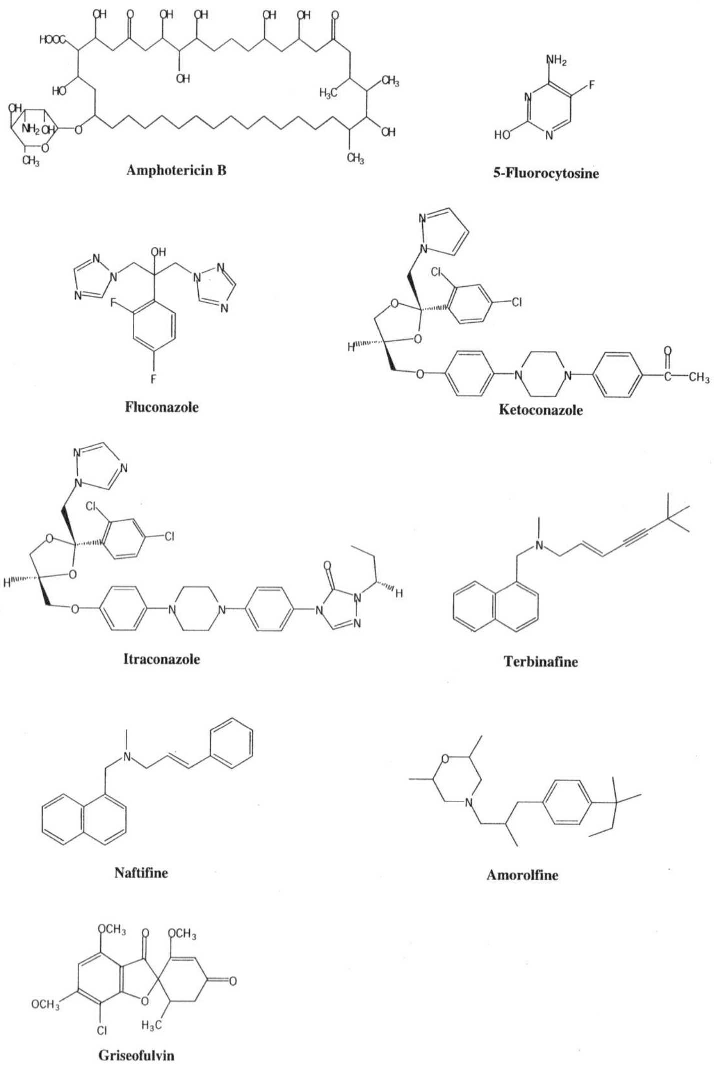

Figure 3. Chemical structures of antifungal agents in current use.

gens and at the same time reduce its toxic effects to mammalian cells. AmB incorporated into liposomes may participate in a selective transfer mechanism from the "donor" liposome to the ergosterol-containing "target" in the fungal cell membrane or with the help of the fungal and/or host phospholipases (101). A liposomal preparation of nystatin, another polyene antifungal agent (Nyotran), is currently undergoing preclinical and clinical evaluation (153).

Mode of action

The primary mode of action of polyenes including AmB or nystatin is to bind ergosterol in the membrane bilayer of susceptible fungi. This interaction is thought to result in the production of aqueous pores consisting of polyene molecules linked to the membrane sterols. This configuration gives rise to a pore-like structure in which the polyene hydroxyl residues face inward, leading to altered permeability, leakage of vital cytoplasmic components (mono- or divalent cations), and death of the organism (25). Some lines of evidence also suggest that AmB exerts oxidative damage to the cell, contributing to its toxic effect (254). Polyenes can bind also other sterols such as cholesterol, which accounts for much of their human toxicity (27). The advantage of AmB, however, is its much higher affinity for ergosterol-containing membranes than for cholesterol-containing membranes. Bolard and Milhaud (26) have discussed in details the interaction of polyenes with lipids.

Antifungal activity

AmB has a strong fungicidal effect on most important yeast and fungal pathogens. Time-kill curves have been reported in several studies and showed that AmB induces a 3- to 4-log decrease in viable counts in a time span of 2 to 4 h at supra-MIC concentrations (66). The killing potency of AmB against fungal pathogens questions the validity of the methods used to measure its activity. AmB MICs are dependent on several factors and among them the composition of the testing medium is important. Rex et al. (226) and Arikan et al. (11) recommend the use of a special broth medium (AM3) to determine AmB MICs in *Candida* and *Aspergillus* species. Presently, a standard protocol using AM3 medium has been recommended by the NCCLS in protocol M-27A. Recently, Peron et al. (208) evaluated an agar diffusion method using an E-test with RPMI or AM3 as media to discriminate AmB-resistant from AmB-susceptible *Candida* isolates. The MICs at which 90% of the isolates tested are inhibited (MIC_{90}) for AmB against various *Candida* species including *C. albicans, C. glabrata, C. parapsilosis,* or *C. tropicalis* ranged from 0.25 to 1 μg/ml. AmB fungicidal concentrations are usually 0.5 to 2 times the MIC in *Candida* species. The MIC_{90} for *Aspergillus* species, especially *A. fumigatus,* tends to be higher and is about 4 μg/ml (257).

Clinical indications

Due to its high in vitro efficacy and its fungicidal effect, AmB is still used as initial treatment in a large variety of severe or life-threatening fungal diseases including endemic and opportunistic mycoses. Recommendations of dosage, duration, and combination with other antifungals depend on the fungal agent, the type of infection, and the status of the host. For treating *Candida* infections, AmB is recommended for systemic candidiasis, particularly in neutropenic and/or unstable patients as well as for *Candida* meningitis and ophthalmitis. Another indication consists of infections due to *Candida* species either intrinsically resistant to azoles (*C. krusei, C. glabrata*) or after development of resistance under azole therapy, which is common in cases of oropharyngeal and esophageal candidiasis in AIDS patients (59, 65, 231).

5-FC

5-FC (Fig. 3) belongs to the class of pyrimidine analogs that was developed in the 1950s as a potential antineoplastic agent. Abandoned as an anticancer drug due to its lack of activity against tumors, it showed, however, good in vitro and in vivo antifungal activity. Because it is highly water soluble, it can be administered by oral and intravenous (i.v.) routes (215).

Mode of action

5-FC is taken up by fungal cells by a cytosine permease and is deaminated by a cytosine deaminase to 5-fluorouracil (5-FU), a potent antimetabolite. 5-FU can be converted to a nucleoside triphosphate and, when incorporated into RNA, causes miscoding. In addition, 5-FU can be converted to a deoxynucleoside, which inhibits thymidylate synthase and, thereby, DNA synthesis. 5-FC shows little toxicity in mammalian cells, since cytosine deaminase is absent or poorly active in these cells. 5-FU is, however, a potent anticancer agent but is impermeable to fungal cells (54, 218). The conversion of 5-FC to 5-FU is possible by intestinal bacteria, and, therefore, 5-FC can show toxicity in oral formulations (55).

Antifungal activity

5-FC is fungicidal in susceptible yeasts and fungi. The spectrum of activity is, however, limited since its in vitro activity in filamentous fungi is inoculum dependent, with MICs well beyond achievable serum concentrations at high inocula. A high variability in 5-FC MICs is observed in fungal species, because of the occurrence of intrinsic resistance, which is high in *Aspergillus* species followed by *Candida* species and *Cryptococcus neoformans.* MIC_{90} of 5-FC are in the range of 0.5 to 4 μg/ml for *Candida* species, including *C. albicans, C. parapsilosis, C. tropicalis, C. glabrata,* or *C. neoformans* (42).

Clinical indications

5-FC is usually not administered as a single agent because of the rapid development of resistance (256). It is, therefore, mainly used in combination with other agents and particularly with AmB. In vitro data regarding the combination of both drugs against *Candida* species and *C. neoformans* are numerous and are contradictory, showing antagonistic, indifferent, or synergistic effects (90). However, the combination of AmB with 5-FC had superior effects in animal models of invasive candidiasis or cryptococcosis than single agents. In patients, the combination of AmB with 5-FC was superior to AmB or fluconazole in cryptococcal meningitis (23, 151, 152) and superior to fluconazole in intensive-care unit (ICU) patients with *Candida* peritonitis (1). It is currently recommended to associate AmB with 5-FC for *Candida* meningitis (231).

Azoles

Azole antifungal agents discovered in the late 1960s are synthetic compounds belonging to the largest group of antifungal agents. Azole antifungal agents used in medicine are categorized into N-1 substituted imidazoles (ketoconazole, miconazole, clotrimazole) and triazoles (fluconazole, itraconazole) (Fig. 3). The new generation of azole antifungal agents under development (posaconazole, ravuconazole, voriconazole) (see "Antifungals in Development with Established Mode of Action") belongs also to triazoles.

Mode of action

Azoles have a cytochrome P450 as a common cellular target in yeast or fungi (Fig. 2). This cytochrome P450 is named CYP51A1, according to an internationally recognized nomenclature (189), and is involved in the 14α-demethylation of lanosterol (268). CYP51A1 is also now referred to as Erg11p, the product of the *ERG11* gene. The unhindered nitrogen of the imidazole or triazole ring of azole antifungal agents binds to the heme iron of the cytochrome P450 as a sixth ligand, thus inhibiting the enzymatic reaction. The affinity of imidazole and triazole derivatives is not only dependent on this interaction, but is also determined by the N-1 substituent, which is actually responsible for the high affinity of azole antifungal agents to their target (267). Each of these agents has distinct pharmacokinetics, and antifungal efficacy is quite different between yeast and fungal species of medical relevance (159). Recently, another target for azole antifungal agents was described as sterol Δ^{22}-desaturase, which is a cytochrome P450 enzyme involved in the last step of ergosterol biosynthesis, i.e., the desaturation of ergosta-5,7-dienol into ergosterol (Fig. 2) (129). Another report from Vanden Bossche et al. (266) suggests an additional target of azole antifungal agents, which is an NADPH-dependent 3-ketosteroid reductase that catalyzes the last step of demethylation at the C-4 methyl group of yeast sterols. Accumulation of 3-ketosteroids (obtusifolione or 14α-methlylfecosterone) has been detected in *Histoplasma capsulatum* and *C. neoformans* upon incubation of cells with itraconazole as a result of NADPH-dependent 3-ketosteroid reductase inhibition and provides until now only indirect evidence that azole antifungal agents inhibit this enzyme (264).

Antifungal activity

Azole antifungal agents have a broad spectrum of activity. They are active against dermatophytes, filamentous fungi, *Candida* species (Table 2), *C. neoformans,* and dimorphic fungi such as *H. capsulatum* or *Coccidioides immitis.* Some azole derivatives are, however, more active than others. For example, fluconazole is relatively inactive against *A. fumigatus* or *C. krusei,* as opposed to itraconazole. Azole antifungal agents are only fungistatic against most yeast and fungal species, with the exception of *C. neoformans, H. capsulatum, Aspergillus* spp., and dermatophytes. A recurrent problem with azole antifungal agents is their poor water solubility, except for fluconazole. Azole antifungal agents are, therefore, mostly administered as oral preparations. Fluconazole, due to its favorable pharmacokinetics, is found both as oral and i.v. formulations.

Clinical indications

Clinical indications of azole antifungal agents depend largely on the type of derivatives. Itraconazole has excellent activity against dermatophytes. Itraconazole is used as second-line agent in patients with *Aspergillus* infections who are refractory or intolerant to AmB. Itraconazole is also effective in the treatment of superficial candidiasis (vaginal candidiasis or oropharyngeal candidiasis in AIDS patients and some fluconazole-resistant superficial candidiasis in AIDS patients). Against *Candida* infections, fluconazole has demonstrated the broadest clinical efficacy for mucosal candidiasis (both vaginal and oropharyngeal) as well as chronic mucocutaneous candidiasis. Fluconazole is also recommended as a first choice in the treatment of invasive *Candida* infections in nonneutropenic patients such as solid-organ transplant patients, surgical and ICU patients, or those with urinary tract infections due to susceptible *Candida* spp. (225). Even in neutropenic patients, candidemia can be successfully treated with fluconazole, as long as the patients are stable and the infection is not due to *Candida* species less susceptible to fluconazole (for example, *C. glabrata*) or intrinsically resistant to this agent (for example, *C. krusei*). High doses of fluconazole (600 to 800 mg/day) have been shown to be safe and afford a better response rate than lower doses in surgical patients with *Candida* deep-seated infections (86, 273).

Allylamines

The allylamines are synthetic compounds discovered in the 1970s. Terbinafine and naftifine (Fig. 3) belong to this class of antifungal agents. Other compounds structurally related to allylamines have been described (butenafine, a benzylamine; tolnaftate, a thiocarbamate). Historically, the antifungal activity of allylamines began by accident, when it was discovered that naftifine, the first allylamine synthesized by Sandoz Research, had antifungal activity although it was first identified by a central nervous system discovery program (N. Ryder, personal communication).

Mode of action

Allylamines, as well as benzylamines and thiocarbamates, target squalene epoxidase, which is the first postsqualene enzyme of the ergosterol biosynthetic pathway (Fig. 2). This enzyme is encoded by *ERG1*, an essential gene in *Saccharomyces cerevisiae* (123). *ERG1* has been isolated in *C. albicans* (72). Squalene epoxidase is a membrane-bound microsomal enzyme and requires molecular oxygen, NADPH, and flavin adenine dinucleotide for activity. Allylamines are reversible, noncompetitive inhibitors of squalene epoxidase. The inhibitory effect of allylamines in yeast and fungi is thought to be due to ergosterol depletion and squalene accumulation. Among allylamines, benzylamines, and thiocarbamates, only terbinafine is used as a systemic agent. Other agents are used topically.

Antifungal activity

Terbinafine is fungicidal against dermatophytes and filamentous fungi (12) but is only fungistatic against the majority of *Candida* spp. Typical terbinafine MICs are in the range of 0.001 μg/ml to 0.5 μg/ml for dermatophytes. High MICs are found in *Mucor* spp. (>16 μg/ml) and *Fusarium* spp. (range, 0.13 to >16 μg/ml) (124, 239). Higher variations in MICs have been measured in terbinafine MICs for yeast species of clinical interest. For example, the MIC_{90} for terbinafine of 259 *C. albicans* clinical isolates is 4 μg/ml (240). Terbinafine is, however, inactive against *C. glabrata, C. krusei,* and *C. tropicalis* (MIC >128 μg/ml) (240) but highly active against *C. parapsilosis* (MIC_{90}, 0.125 μg/ml) and *C. neoformans* (MIC range, 0.06 to 0.125 μg/ml) (240).

Clinical indications

Because of its high efficacy against dermatophytes, terbinafine is the antifungal drug of choice for the treatment of superficial mycoses or nail infections caused by these molds (239, 240). Although some investigators suggest that terbinafine alone or in combination with other antifungal agents could be used for the treatment of susceptible yeast infections (18, 19, 124), no clinical studies have been conducted with *Candida* infections.

Morpholines

The morpholines (amorolfine, fenpropimorph, tridemorph) (Fig. 3) are totally synthetic compounds and, with the exception of amorolfine, are mostly used in agricultural fungicide preparations.

Mode of action

Amorolfine inhibits two enzymes in a single biosynthetic pathway. The enzymes involved are the sterol Δ^{14} reductase and the Δ^{7-8} isomerase, which reside downstream of the azole target enzyme (Fig. 2). These enzymes are encoded by the *ERG24* and *ERG2* genes, respectively (100). Current data suggest that the primary target of amorolfine is the sterol Δ^{14} reductase, because of the earlier position of this enzyme in the ergosterol biosynthetic pathway, even if the sterol Δ^{14} reductase exhibits IC_{50}s much higher than measured for the sterol Δ^{7-8} isomerase (173). Inhibition of yeast growth by morpholine derivatives results in the formation of ignosterol, a sterol by-product occurring when the *ERG24* gene is deleted in *S. cerevisiae* (45).

Antifungal activity

Amorolfine has strong fungicidal activities against dermatophytes and filamentous fungi but only fungistatic activities in yeast pathogens (216). A study showed that the growth of 80% of 138 *Candida* spp. and of 100 *C. neoformans* isolates was completely inhibited by ≤1 μg/ml of amorolfine. In general, dermatophytes show higher susceptibilities (MIC range, 0.01 to 1 μg/ml amorolfine) than do yeast pathogens (53).

Clinical indications

Amorolfine is used as topical treatment of dermatophytes and vulvovaginal candidiasis (98). It showed, however, no activity in a model of experimental invasive candidiasis (216).

Griseofulvin

Griseofulvin (Fig. 3) is the unique representative of a class of drugs produced by the molds *Penicillium griseofulvum* and *Penicillium janczewski.* Griseofulvin is one of the first antifungal agents discovered, as early as 1939 (202). Its use as an orally active antifungal agent against ringworm in humans was first described by Williams et al. (285).

Mode of action

Griseofulvin inhibits mitosis by interfering with microtubule function. It does not bind directly to tubulin but instead interacts with microtubule-associated proteins (30, 136).

Antifungal activity

Griseofulvin is a systemic agent mainly active against dermatophytes and to a lesser extent against filamentous fungi but without activity against yeast pathogens. A mean MIC of 0.36 μg of griseofulvin per ml was measured in a recent study comprising 173 dermatophytes (284); the MIC_{90} was 3.13 μg/ml. These values were confirmed in different studies and are lower than the drug levels reached in skin and nails (125, 194).

Clinical indications

Given its high activity against dermatophytes, griseofulvin is a drug mainly used to treat skin infections and onychomycosis. Griseofulvin is still considered as a valuable antifungal agent for the treatment of tinea capitis in children (24). The trend in the treatment of mycoses caused by dermatophytes is, however, to replace this old agent by other more efficacious antifungal agents (i.e., terbinafine, itraconazole, or voriconazole) (38, 192).

ANTIFUNGALS IN DEVELOPMENT WITH ESTABLISHED MODE OF ACTION

Among the antifungal agents in development with an established mode of action, azole antifungal agents have a preponderant position. In an attempt

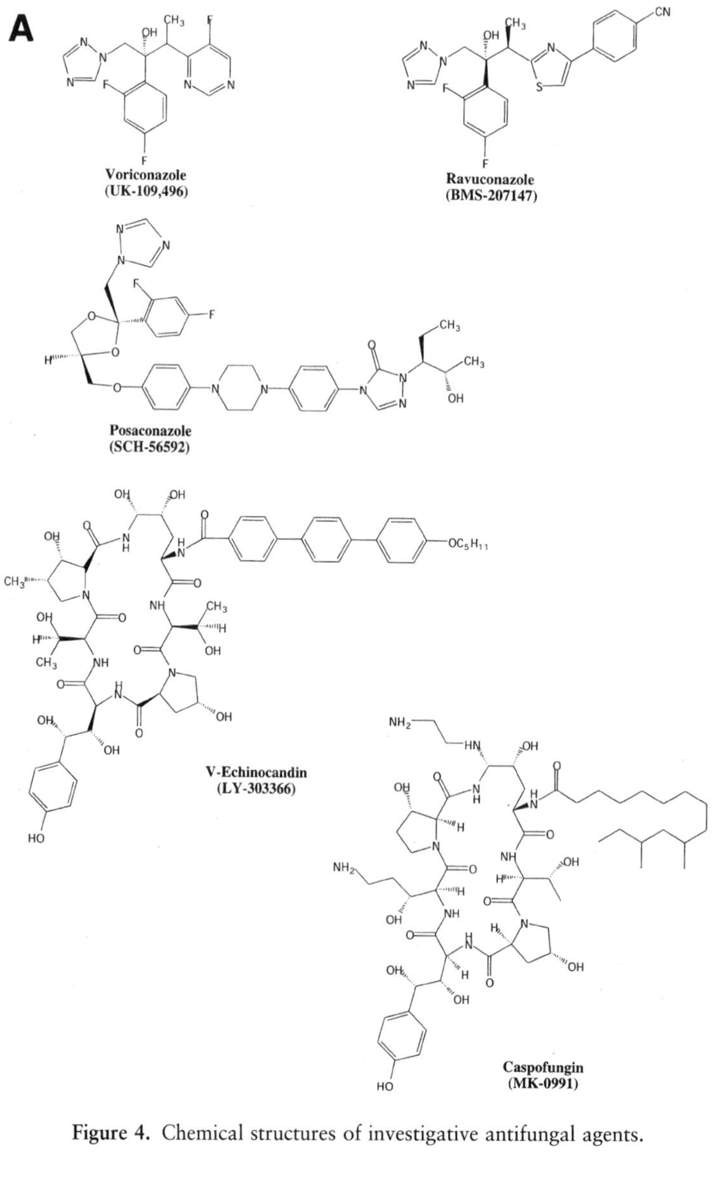

Figure 4. Chemical structures of investigative antifungal agents.

to increase the efficacy of azoles, several new derivatives are currently being developed and they exhibit enhanced spectra of activity and improved pharmacokinetics. The agents at the front of the developmental process are three azole derivatives, i.e., voriconazole, posaconazole, and ravuconazole (Fig. 4A). Although limited published data are available on these new azoles, some of their properties are summarized here and are compared to each other whenever possible.

Voriconazole

Voriconazole (Fig. 4A) is the most advanced investigational new azole agent. It is structurally related to fluconazole; it is, however, more potent in inhibiting in vitro ergosterol biosynthesis in *C. albicans, C. krusei,* or *A. fumigatus* than its companion compound (115, 242). The in vitro activity of voriconazole against *Candida* species is excellent with an MIC_{90} in the range of 0.5 μg/ml. Voriconazole is most active against *C. albicans* (MIC_{90}, 0.06 μg/ml) and is least active against *C. glabrata* (MIC_{90}, 2.0 μg/ml). Voriconazole is active against dimorphic fungi (*Blastomyces dermatitidis, C. immitis,* and *H. capsulatum*) (154) and against a wide range of filamentous fungi and dermatophytes, especially *A. fumigatus* (68). Voriconazole is available as i.v. and oral administrations. Following oral administration, voriconazole is rapidly

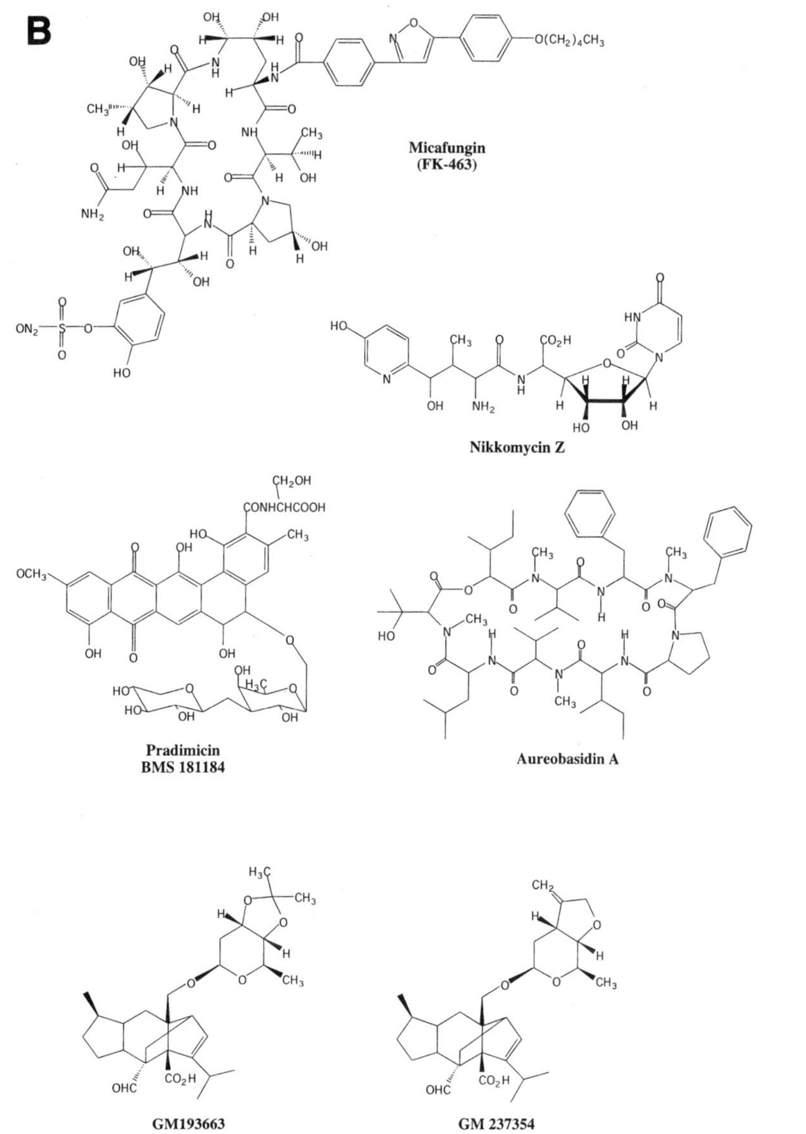

Figure 4. *Continued.*

and extensively absorbed, with a bioavailability of 90%, a time to maximum concentration of drug in serum (T_{max}) of less than 2 h, and a half-life of about 6 h. Voriconazole is generally well tolerated by patients, although reversible side effects such as visual disturbance or elevated liver transaminases have been reported. Phase II and phase III clinical trials have been recently completed, and they showed comparable or higher efficacy of voriconazole as compared to other standard antifungal drug treatments such as AmB, fluconazole, or itraconazole (138, 252). Voriconazole has shown similar efficacy as fluconazole in the treatment of esophageal candidiasis in immunocompromised adults (64). Voriconazole was at least equal to liposomal AmB as empirical treatment in febrile neutropenic adults (277).

Posaconazole

Posaconazole (UK-109496) (Fig. 4A) is structurally related to itraconazole. It is developed as an oral agent and for i.v. use as a water-soluble prodrug derivative (SCH-59884). SCH-59884 is dephosphorylated in vivo to an active intermediate ester, which is in turn hydrolyzed to posaconazole (SCH-56592). Posaconazole has comparable activity to voriconazole against several yeast (*Candida* spp. in particular) and fungal pathogens in term of MIC_{90} but is more active than itraconazole, especially against *Aspergillus* spp., with geometric mean MICs 3 to 4 times lower than those of itraconazole (31). The long half-life of posaconazole after oral administration in animal models (18 to 22 h) constitutes a major difference from voriconazole. Posaconazole has been found equally effective as fluconazole in the treatment of esophageal candidiasis in human immunodeficiency virus (HIV)-infected patients in two studies (191, 269). In a small open study of fungal infections refractory to classic antifungal drugs, the response rate of *Candida* infections with posaconazole was 75% (92).

Ravuconazole

Ravuconazole (BMS-2077147) (Fig. 4A) is the latest investigated azole agent undergoing clinical development. It is less structurally related to other azole derivatives. Like voriconazole and posaconazole, ravuconazole exhibits high in vitro activity against most *Candida* and *Aspergillus* spp. with comparable MIC_{90} (MIC_{90}, 0.5 μg/ml) for *Candida* spp. (209). No clinical trial data have been yet published with ravuconazole.

Among the few in vitro studies comparing the activities of the three new investigative agents against a high number of fungal pathogens, the general trend is that their antifungal activity is decreased in yeast species displaying high MICs for conventional azole derivatives such as fluconazole or itraconazole. The resistance that developed following the use of these agents seems, therefore, to have an impact on MICs of the new agents. When MICs of yeast species are elevated for both fluconazole and itraconazole, the MICs for the new investigative agents are usually higher than those observed for most susceptible isolates (58, 78, 212).

ANTIFUNGAL AGENTS IN DEVELOPMENT WITH NOVEL MODES OF ACTION

The treatment of invasive fungal diseases has been limited to AmB with or without combination of 5-FC for many years. Therapeutic options have not improved much until the introduction in the 1980s of azole derivatives (fluconazole and itraconazole). Because the occurrence of fungal infections tends to increase and because the current antifungal agents do not meet all desirable criteria, antifungal drug research has been very active in the discovery of new potential agents. One of the key factors in the development of new drugs is the identification and characterization of new cellular targets. Drug screening programs now include, beside classical screenings of natural products, the design of active compounds directed against essential targets and the use of genomic information. These approaches were recently reported for the search of *C. albicans* genes necessary for growth and their use as targets in classical screening of active compounds (48). With the help of molecular biology and information about fungal and human genomes, valuable fungal targets for the development of antifungal drugs are now considered as those being essential for survival but unique to this class of eukaryotes. In this section the current status of antifungal drug discovery will be summarized.

Antifungal Drugs Acting at the Level of the Cell Wall Composition

The fungal cell wall is an essential component for the maintenance of turgor pressure of the cell and is absent from mamalian cells (see chapter 12). The fundamental components of the cell wall of most fungi comprise chitin, α- and β-linked glucans, mannoproteins, and glycosylphosphatidylinositol (GPI)-anchored proteins (Fig. 1). Enzymes responsible for the structural organization of the cell wall or for the biosynthesis of individual components are, therefore, attractive targets for developing novel antifungal drugs.

Cyclic lipopeptides

Cyclic lipopeptide antifungal agents of the echinocandin class are natural products discovered in the 1970s. Echinocandins are fatty acid derivatives of cyclic hexapeptides. They are noncompetitive inhibitors of β-1,3 glucan synthase, which is part of an enzyme complex that forms the major glucan polymers of most pathogenic fungi. β-1,3 glucan synthases in *S. cerevisiae* are encoded by two separate genes, *FKS1* and *FKS2* (147), whose simultaneous deletion is lethal. *FKS*-like genes have been cloned from other fungal pathogens, including *C. albicans, C. neoformans,* and *Paracoccidioides brasiliensis* (62, 175, 204, 260). Synthetic variations on the echinocandin moiety have produced several molecules with improved water solubility, antifungal potency, and efficacy in animal models. The compounds that are currently being developed include L-743872 (also known as MK-0991 or caspofungin), LY303366 (V-echinocandin), and FK463 (micafungin).

MK-0991 (caspofungin). Caspofungin (Fig. 4A) is a semisynthetic analog of pneumocandin Bo and the first commercialized echinocandin derivative (201). It is water soluble and is only available in parenteral form. It has high fungicidal activity against a large number of *Candida* spp., *Aspergillus* spp., and dimorphic molds (*H. capsulatum, C. immitis, B. dermatitidis*). MICs for these pathogens are in a range between 0.12 and 2 μg/ml. Caspofungin shows, however, no or little activity against *C. neoformans, Trichosporon beigelii,* and *Rhizopus* and *Fusarium* spp. In murine models of superficial or invasive candidiasis, disseminated or pulmonary aspergillosis, caspofungin has shown comparable activity to that of AmB (3, 4). Caspofungin shows also good activity in animal models of infections due to *C. glabrata* and *Pneumocystis carinii* (87, 221). One major drawback of caspofungin is its poor oral bioavailability (<1%) (3). The first clinical trials with invasive *Aspergillosis* sp. and candidemia are currently under way.

LY303366 (V-echinocandin). V-Echinocandin (Fig. 4A) is a water-soluble echinocandin B derivative that is both orally and parenterally administrable. Like caspofungin, it has broad fungicidal activity against yeast and fungal pathogens with approximately the same limitations. The MIC_{90} in a collection of 219 *Candida* spp. was 0.25 μg/ml (37). V-Echinocandin is less active against *C. parapsilosis* than it is against other *Candida* species (210). In animal models of infections with *C. albicans* and *A. fumigatus*, V-echinocandin showed excellent activity (46, 206, 207). V-Echinocandin is now being evaluated in a phase II clinical trial.

FK463 (micafungin). Micafungin (Fig. 4B) is a semisynthetic, water-soluble echinocandin-like lipopeptide with a sulfonate moiety, isolated from the culture broth of *Coleophoma empedri* (259). Micafungin is fungicidal to susceptible yeast species. The MIC range for *Candida* spp. is between 0.0039 and 2 μg/ml and from 0.0039 to 0.0313 μg/ml for *Aspergillus* spp. Micafungin, however, is only fungistatic against *Aspergillus* spp. Micafungin had no activity against *C. neoformans, Trichosporon* spp., or *Fusarium solani* (259). Animal models of infection with *C. albicans* and *A. fumigatus* have demonstrated that micafungin is as active as fluconazole or AmB (121, 171). In humans, micafungin has been used with success for esophageal candidiasis in HIV-infected persons. In a study under way, micafungin is given in disseminated candidiasis (188).

Nikkomycin Z

Nikkomycin Z (Fig. 4B) belongs to a class of nucleoside peptide antibiotics produced by *Streptomyces* species. Nikkomycin Z inhibits chitin synthesis by competing with the substrate of chitin synthase, UDP-*N*-acetylglucosamine. Chitin is a linear polymer of β-(1,4)-linked *N*-acetylglucosamine and is an essential component of the cell wall. Chitin synthesis is catalyzed by multiple chitin synthase isoenzymes. At least three chitin synthase genes (CHS) have been cloned in *S. cerevisiae* (29). Deletion of chitin synthase 3 (*CHS3*) in *C. albicans* resulted in reduction of virulence in an animal model of infection. Nikkomycin Z has modest activity against *Candida* spp. It is more active against fungi with high chitin content such as *C. immitis* and *B. dermatitidis.* Nikkomycin Z showed good activity in murine models of pulmonary blastomycosis, coccidioidomycosis, and histoplasmosis (41, 88, 104). The future of nikkomycin Z is still uncertain, even though it has potential for the treatment of endemic fungi. Besides the redundancy of chitin synthase genes, permeability of nikkomycin Z in fungal cells can be a serious limitation to the development of this compound since peptides in the bloodstream may alter the dipeptide permease-dependent entry of this compound into cells.

Pradimicins

Pradimicins belong to a unique class of benzonaphtacene quinones conjugated with a D-amino acid and a disaccharide side chain. Pradimicins are natural products produced by *Actinomadura* spp. that were discovered in the 1980s (197). Pradimicins have been derivatized to a large number of compounds; however, only BMS 181184 (Fig. 4B) was targeted for further clinical development (79, 196). The MIC_{90} of yeast pathogens was ≤ 8 μg/ml, and similar values were found for filamentous fungi and dermatophytes, with the exception of *Fusarium* spp. (MIC, >64 μg/ml) (249, 250). Pradimicins are fungicidal, and their mode of action involves the formation of a calcium-dependent complex with the sugar moiety of mannoproteins. The pradimicin-mannoprotein complex is thought to perturb cell wall organization, leading to leakage of intracellular components and, ultimately, cell death (249, 250, 263). BMS 181184 (Fig. 3) had excellent activity in the treatment of experimental invasive pulmonary aspergillosis in persistently neutropenic rabbits (85), thus underscoring the potential of pradimicin derivatives for therapy of invasive aspergillosis in the neutropenic host. BMS 181184 was also tested in a murine model of invasive candidiasis due to *C. tropicalis* and showed good activity (224). Further development of pradimicin as an antifungal drug was, however, stopped because of hepatoxicity problems in clinical trials. In addition, it was found recently that pradimicin could induce apoptosis in mammalian cells, compounding the problems in the development of this drug as an antifungal agent (198–200).

Antifungal Drugs Acting at the Level of Protein Synthesis

Protein synthesis is an attractive target in the development of antimicrobial agents. One major problem, however, is the high similarity of both fungal and mammalian protein synthesis. At the level of ribosome protein biosynthesis, the structural and sequence similarity between fungal and mammalian ribosomal RNAs, subunits, and soluble factors is remarkable, with the exception of elongation factor 3 (EF3). Sordarins were found as successful compounds targeting fungal protein biosynthesis. Sordarins are natural fungal products from *Graphium putredinis* (61) and were found as highly specific inhibitors of translation elongation factor 2 (EF2) in yeasts. EF2 in *S. cerevisiae* is expressed from the *EFT1* and *EFT2* genes (34). Several sordarin derivatives were obtained, and some of them, such as GM 222712 and GM 237354 (Fig. 4B), showed excellent in vitro activities against a variety of pathogenic fungi, including *Candida* spp., *C. neoformans, P. carinii,* and some filamentous fungi (*Aspergillus flavus* and *A. fumigatus*). For example, the MIC_{90} of GM 222712 and GM 237354 was 0.004 and 0.015 μg/ml, respectively, for *C. albicans*. However, their activities against *C. glabrata* and *C. parapsilosis* are poor and absent for *C. krusei* (34). The in vivo activity of GM193663 and GM237354 was studied recently in mouse models of disseminated candidiasis and aspergillosis and in a rat model of pneumocystosis. The sordarin derivatives were successful in the treatment of candidiasis and pneumocystosis but gave less satisfactory results for pulmonary aspergillosis (168). *C. immitis* was susceptible both in vitro and in vivo to the GM compounds, which were found to be equivalent to or superior than fluconazole in a murine model of systemic coccidioidomycosis (40). Although their development in clinical trials has not been undertaken yet, sordarins showed that protein synthesis is a valuable target for the design of future antifungal agents.

Antifungal Drugs Acting at the Level of the Plasma Membrane

Aureobasidins

Sphingolipids are essential components of the cytoplasmic membrane in both mammalian and fungal cells but differ in their biosynthesis and structure. The early biosynthetic steps leading to ceramide formation are shared by both mammalian and fungal cells. Inhibitors such as sphingofungin, fumonisins, and australifungins target these early steps and, even though they have antifungal activity, show host toxicity (82). Biosynthetic reactions beyond ceramide formation are unique to fungal cells. One of these steps is the addition of phosphatidylinositol to ceramide by the enzyme inositol phosphoceramide synthase (IPC) to form inositolphosphoceramide. This step is essential for sphingolipid biosynthesis in *S. cerevisiae*. The deletion of the gene encoding IPC synthase in *S. cerevisiae* (*AUR1*) is lethal (186). Aureobasidin A (Fig. 4B) is the target of IPC synthase and competes this enzyme at nanomolar concentrations. Aureobasidin A is a natural compound produced by the black yeast *Aureobasidium pullulans* and belongs to the class of cyclic desipeptide antifungal agents. This compound possesses fungicidal activity against most *Candida* spp., with MICs in the range of 0.5 to 2.0 μg/ml. Aureobasidin A, however, has no activity against *A. fumigatus, A. flavus* (MIC, >50 μg/ml), or *C. neoformans* (144, 293). Aureobasidin A showed good efficacy in the treatment of murine systemic candidiasis when given orally or subcutaneously. Aureobasidin A fungicidal action in mice with candidiasis was more effective than that of fluconazole and AmB (258). Other nanomolar inhibitors of IPC synthase are khafrefungin and the macrolide rustimicin (99, 160–162).

Proton ATPase inhibitors

The fungal plasma-membrane proton pump is a high-abundance, essential enzyme with a number of well-understood molecular properties that should facilitate the development of new antifungal agents. The proton pump is important for intracellular pH regulation and the maintenance of electrochemical proton gradients needed for nutrient uptake. It is a member of the P-type class of ion-transport enzymes, which are present in nearly all external cellular membranes. Typical P-type enzymes such as the Na+,K(+)-ATPase and H+,K(+)-ATPase are well established as specific targets for surface-active cardiac glycosides and antiulcer therapeutics. The fungal plasma membrane H(+)-ATPase possesses important attributes that make it desirable as a target for antifungal drug discovery. First, the enzyme is essential for fungal cell physiology. Secondly, the well-characterized biochemistry and genetics of the H(+)-ATPase (encoded by the *PMA1* gene of *S. cerevisiae*) facilitate the detailed analysis of the interaction of lead or model compounds with the enzyme. Studies with omeprazole, which is not suitable as an antifungal agent but can be used under selective conditions to target H(+)-ATPase, indicate that the enzyme can be inhibited from its extramembrane surface. Finally, a number of primary and secondary screens are available to identify compounds that are targeted to the H(+)-ATPase and affect one or more functional properties. These screens have already yielded promising H(+)-ATPase-directed antagonists (205). The cloning of the *C. albicans PMA1* gene will facilitate the discovery of specific inhibitors (170).

Efflux pump inhibitors

Multidrug transporters of different families have been reported in *C. albicans*. These proteins are responsible for the active efflux of a large variety of compounds, including antifungal agents. ABC-transporters genes (*CDR1, CDR2, CgCDR1*) or major facilitator genes (*CaMDR1*) are, in fact, upregulated in azole-resistant *Candida* spp. and are responsible not only for azole resistance but also for cross-resistance to other agents (see "Resistance to Antifungal Agents" below). The inhibition of multidrug efflux transporters is, therefore, attractive not only for reversing resistance, but also for potentiating the activity of already active agents by inhibiting their efflux from the cell. This strategy has been used for some time in cancer cells. Specific inhibitors of efflux pumps, particularly of Cdr1p, have been identified recently (157, 176). The use of these inhibitors resulted in the decrease of fluconazole MICs in *C. albicans* and *C. glabrata* (36). Efflux pump inhibitors were also used in a murine model of invasive candidiasis simultaneously with fluconazole; this combination increased the efficacy of fluconazole (255). Efflux pump inhibitors are, therefore, attractive molecules that could be used not only with fluconazole but also with other antifungal agents that are substrates for these pumps.

Cationic Antimicrobial Peptides as Antifungal Agents

Cationic antimicrobial peptides have been the focus of intensive research over the past years. Their activities have been documented in bacteria and are now being investigated in fungi. Cationic antimicrobial peptides are peptides of 12 to 50 amino acids with a net positive charge of +2 to +7 due to an excess of basic amino acids (arginine, lysine, and histidine) compared to acidic amino acids. These naturally occurring or synthetic peptides belong to four major structural classes: (i) β-sheet stabilized by disulfide bridges, (ii) α-helices, (iii) extended helices with a predominance of one or more amino acids, and (iv) loop structures (95–97, 251). Cationic peptides with antifungal activity are thought to act by causing cell lysis caused by an unknown mechanism. Electrostatic interactions with negatively charged cell surfaces followed by insertion into cell membranes, which then permeabilize and kill cells, seem to be the most likely scenario. Cationic peptides with antifungal activity originate from different sources.

Mammalian peptides

Neutrophils are an important source of cationic antifungal peptides. Antifungal activities were demonstrated for bactericidal/permeability-increasing proteins (BPI), α-, β-defensins, and lactoferrin, which are granule-associated and reside in neutrophils (185). Peptides derived from domain III of BPI proteins have potent activities against *Candida* spp., *C. neoformans*, and *A. fumigatus* (155). These peptides were effective not only in a model of pulmonary aspergillosis but prevented death in a murine model of invasive candidiasis and produced a dose-dependent reduction in *C. albicans* CFU in infected kidneys (9). Defensins from rabbit (NP-1, NP-2, NP-3) or from human origin (HNP-1, HNP-2, HNP-3) have different potencies against *C. albicans, C. neoformans,* or *A. fumigatus*. MICs in the range of 3.75 to 15 μg/ml were measured for NP-1 against *C. neoformans*. MICs for *A. fumigatus* or *C. albicans* are in the 50 to 100 μg/ml range (52). Lactoferrin, an iron-binding peptide, is found in secondary granules of polymorphonuclear leukocytes (PMN) and in different biological fluids, including milk, saliva, tears, or vaginal secretions. The fungicidal effect of lactoferrin in *C. albicans* is only observed with the iron-free protein.

The cleavage of lactoferrin to smaller peptides can produce lactoferricin, an 18-amino acid-long peptide with enhanced antifungal activity (MIC for *C. albicans* can be as low as 0.8 μg/ml). In addition to its antimicrobial effect, lactoferricin has immune-stimulating activities (290). Lactoferricin can increase the activity of natural killer cells; exposure of polymorphonuclear leukocytes to lactoferrin results in increased superoxide release, increases their chemokinesis, and enhances their adherence to endothelium (14, 145). Another source of cationic antimicrobial peptides is the salivary histatins. They are present in multiple forms and are identified as histatins 1, 3, and 5, all of which are histidine-rich proteins containing 38, 32, and 24 amino acids, respectively. Histatin 5 is the most active and is fungicidal against *C. albicans*, histatin 3 has moderate activity, and histatin 1 exhibits the lowest level of activity (289). Histatin 5 has IC_{50}s ranging from 2 to 8 μM in *C. albicans*, depending on the strain tested, but shows the lowest activity against *C. glabrata* (108, 262). Histatin 5 also exerts strong fungicidal activity against *C. neoformans* and *A. fumigatus* (108, 261). Rather than affecting plasma membrane structures by pore formation, histatins seem to target mitochondria in yeasts, as suggested by recent studies, and provoke ATP release from intact cells (107, 140). This mode of action in yeast could be probably valid for other cationic, antimicrobial peptides. Extracellular ATP acts as a cytotoxic mediator by possibly binding to P2X(7)-like membrane receptors to cause cell death (139).

Amphibian and insect peptides

Skin from African frogs contains at least two types of antimicrobial peptides with antifungal activity (magainins and dermaseptins). Magainin 1 and 2 have amphipathic α-helices structures that, by binding to membranes, cause cell lysis (122, 292). Dermaseptins are a family of cationic (lysine-rich), amphipathic antifungal peptides of 28 to 34 residues consisting of 5 antifungal peptides (dermaseptins s1, s2, s3, s4, and s5) (181, 182). Dermaseptins are believed to act by forming amphipathic alpha-helices, which associate with the cell membrane, leading to increased cell permeability and disruption (43). Dermaseptins are active against *C. albicans, C. neoformans,* or *A. fumigatus* in the range of 5 to 60 μg/ml (50, 52). Antimicrobial peptides from insects with antifungal activity have been discovered from the silk moth *Hyalophora ceprocia* and were named cecropins A and B. These peptides are not lethal against mammalian cells at microbicidal concentrations and have been safely administered to animals. Both cecropins A and B were fungicidal in acidic medium (pH 5 to 6), but only cecropin A retained lethality in neutral pH medium (51). D-isomers of cecropin have also antimicrobial activities and are more resistant to proteolysis than the naturally occurring L-form (274). D-cecropin B was shown recently to be fungicidal from 3 to 25 μg/ml to *A. fumigatus, F. oxysporum,* and *C. albicans* (51).

NEW THERAPEUTIC APPROACHES BY STIMULATION OF THE IMMUNE SYSTEM

Chemotherapy is probably the best way to fight fungal infections. However, chemotherapy by antifungal agents still has limitations, even though new agents with a broad spectrum of activity and novel modes of action have been discovered and will be discovered. With the recent progress made in the understanding of host immunity to fungi, it is possible to implement some of the discoveries to improve antifungal treatments (219). This subject is covered extensively in chapters 13 to 17 but is briefly described below. The availability of recombinant cytokines, some of which increase host defense responses, offers new perspectives for the prevention and treatment of invasive fungal diseases (83). The outcome of mucosal and systemic *C. albicans* infections is largely dependent on whether the CD4 Th1 or Th2 subset predominates. Th1 cell development leads to resistance and onset of protective immunity, whereas Th2 cell responses are associated with susceptibility. The Th cell paradigm in candidiasis can provide a potential to induce a proper response to infection if one could control the emerging Th cell phenotype. Cytokines act as growth factors for $CD4^+$ Th cells and mediate most of their action in vivo. To induce a proper Th1 protective antifungal response, administration of exogenous Th1-promoting cytokines and neutralization of endogenously produced Th2 cytokines are possible strategies. Several studies have shown, however, in a murine model of invasive candidiasis that (i) blockade of Th2 cytokines, interleukin (IL)-4 and IL-10, was sufficient and required for a Th1-protective response in mice susceptible to infection (235, 238); and (ii) exogenous administration of Th1-promoting cytokines such as IL-12 did not induce Th1-protective cells in susceptible mice (236, 237). Th2 cytokines might, therefore, have a dominant effect over Th1 cytokines, and thus, removal of Th2 cytokines rather than an exogenous supply of Th1 cytokines might be beneficial in the onset of protective immunity. Neutrophils play an important immunoregulatory role in candidiasis. Neutrophils can produce cytokines such as IL-12 and IL-10. It is known that IL-12 is released early in response to *C. albicans*, thus inducing Th1 development in vivo, whereas IL-10 is released in response to a virulent strain, inducing Th2 development (232–234). IL-12 release and the resulting Th1 response require the presence of IL-4, however, thus demonstrating that cytokines might have paradoxically opposite effects in the immune response to *C. albicans* (172). IL-12 remains a strong candidate for the development of an anti-*Candida* response (219). The potential of IL-12 for the treatment of candidiasis is dependent, however, on the type of disease and the underlying host conditions. IL-12 might be ineffective in reversing the pathological state. Romani and collaborators suggest that IL-12 may be beneficial only in the neutropenic patient as its effect would be otherwise opposed to the counterregulatory effect of IL-10 (234). Administration of hematopoietic human cytokines such as granulocyte colony-stimulating factor (G-CSF), granulocyte-macrophage colony-stimulating factor (GM-CSF), or macrophage colony-stimulating factor (M-CSF) may decrease the duration of neutropenia under chemotherapy or increase the fungicidal functions of macrophages or neutrophils. Active and passive immunization might be also a promising strategy for the treatment of prevention of fungal infections. Several reports document protection against *C. albicans* infections by antibodies raised against diverse cell components, i.e., a β-oligomannoside epitope of an adhesin (93), or antimannan and antiproteinase antibody (49) or by direct vaccination with a liposome-mannan vaccine (94). Another example of the potential of antibodies to combat fungal infections comes from the use of yeast-killer toxin-internal image antibodies. In a recent report, the ability to kill *C. albicans* in vitro and in vivo was obtained by anti-idiotypic antibodies mimicking the activity of a *Pichia anomala* killer toxin that was obtained by immunizing with a killer-toxin-neutralizing monoclonal antibody (KT4). This strategy was further implemented by expression of the *P. anomala* yeast-killer anti-idiotypic single chain format antibody (scFvH6) in the human commensal *Streptococcus gordonii,* for which vaginal colonization and effectiveness in heterologous protein production are known. The bacterium was able to release the therapeutic antibody locally to protect effectively against experimental vaginitis with *C. albicans* (22). There are currently diverse examples of immunological approaches to treat fungal infections (83, 219). Importantly, these approaches might have their greatest impact in combination with antifungal therapy.

RESISTANCE TO ANTIFUNGAL AGENTS

Microbiological Resistance and Clinical Resistance

Resistance to antifungal drugs has clinical and microbiological components. Clinical resistance can be understood as a failure of treatment and persistance of fungal infection despite appropriate antifungal drug therapy. A successful clinical response to therapy typically not only depends on the susceptibility of the pathogenic organism but also relies heavily on the host immune system, drug penetration and distribution, patient compliance, and absence of a protected or persistent focus of infection (e.g., a catheter or abscess). Microbiological resistance of a given pathogen must be regarded as a quantifiable variable, determined by measurement of drug susceptibility (for example, MICs), and must be defined with respect to a reference population. A fungal pathogen resistant to a given antifungal drug is, therefore, a microorganism having an MIC higher than the average value measured in the total population. Microbiological or in vitro resistance of a given fungal pathogen relies on measurement of MICs. The introduction of standardized methods approved by the NCCLS for measuring MICs of a number of antifungal agents in selected fungal pathogens (i.e., *Candida* spp., *C. neoformans*) has been essential for interlaboratory comparisons and use in clinical and research laboratories. Recently proposed protocols are now being developed for dermatophytes and filamentous fungi (69). Ideally, microbiological resistance will be predictive of clinical resistance, meaning that, above a given MIC for a fungal pathogen, the so-called breakpoint MIC, the infection caused by this pathogen will not be cured. MIC breakpoints have been proposed that separate susceptible from resistant *Candida* spp. strains for 5-FC and two azole compounds (fluconazole, itraconazole) (229) (Table 3). A third category, named DDS (for dose dependent susceptible), has been created for azoles to categorize strains with intermediate MICs, allowing a higher dosage to be efficacious. It should be noted, however, that these breakpoints have been established on the basis of results of clinical trials mostly from cases of oropharyngeal and esophageal candidiasis in HIV-infected patients before the introduction of highly active antiretroviral therapy (HAART). Thus, these breakpoints have been largely validated only for fluconazole or itraconazole usage

Table 3. NCCLS interpretive breakpoints against *C. albicans*

Antifungal agent	MIC breakpoint (μg/ml) for the following category:		
	Susceptible	Dose-dependent susceptible	Resistant
Fluconazole	8	16–32	64
Itraconazole	0.125	0.25–0.5	1
5-Fluorocytosine	4		32

for *C. albicans* infections. For other *Candida* species and other drugs, the data are still sparse.

The clinical relevance of antifungal resistance is still limited to a few situations. For AmB, the lack of an in vitro method that clearly separates susceptible from resistant strains does not help to establish an in vitro–in vivo correlation. Animal models show a good correlation between MICs and clinical outcome (8). In humans, cases of in vitro AmB resistance associated with clinical failure have been rarely observed during the past 20 years (67, 220). Recently, some degree of in vitro–in vivo correlation has been found in an observational study of *Candida* bloodstream infections: treatment of cases due to a *Candida* isolate with an AmB MIC of ≥0.38 μg/ml had a success rate of 11%, compared to 62% when the MIC was <0.38 μg/ml (39). For 5-FC, to which in vitro resistance (defined as an MIC of >32 μg/ml) of *Candida* spp. isolates is frequent, both of intrinsic or acquired origins, a mouse model of systemic candidiasis has shown a good in vitro–in vivo correlation (256). There are no clinical studies available where 5-FC has been administered as a single agent. For azole derivatives, in particular for fluconazole, much more data are available. Three different situations should be distinguished:

(i) Intrinsic resistance to fluconazole that varies greatly from species to species within the genus *Candida,* with *C. albicans* and *C. parapsilosis* being the most susceptible species, and *C. krusei, C. glabrata,* and *C. norvegensis* being the least susceptible. It is, therefore, important to identify all clinically significant non-*C. albicans* species to the species level for initial information regarding the level of susceptibility.

(ii) The setting of oropharyngeal and esophageal candidiasis in HIV-infected patients, particularly before HAART. Esophageal candidiasis creates a special situation with chronic disease, multiple treatments, often an extremely high inoculum, and defect in host immunity. In this setting, in vitro acquired resistance of *Candida* species, mainly *C. albicans,* to azoles is almost systematic, and many studies have shown a good correlation between the incremental increase of azole MICs and the development of clinical resistance. Both the duration of treatment and the total doses have been correlated with failure (for review, see reference 230).

(iii) Other clinical settings, for example, systemic and deep-seated *Candida* infections, for which the correlation between in vitro resistance and clinical failure is far from clearly established. Most cases of documented failure either during prophylaxis or treatment can be linked to the use of low doses of azoles, to a less susceptible non-*C. albicans Candida* species (*C. krusei, C. glabrata*), or to some host factors (severe immunosuppression, undrained focus of infection).

In the largest prospective study published so far, comparing AmB to fluconazole for the treatment of candidemia episodes in nonneutropenic patients, no correlation could be established between in vitro susceptibility or resistance to the drug administered and clinical success or failure (228). This was certainly due to the complexity of medical problems presented by candidemia patients, in particular the role of intravascular devices in the clearing of this infection. A handful of cases of severe *Candida* infections have been published so far, in which documented acquired in vitro resistance during azole therapy led to clinical failure or death. The patients, all severely immunocompromised, developed resistance after 2 to 3 weeks of fluconazole treatment (142, 167).

A major change observed during the past decade in the area of antifungal resistance has been the so-called shift toward more resistant *Candida* species. In many countries, *C. albicans,* which was the overwhelming dominant species involved in significant infection such as candidemia or other deep-seated infection, is now decreasing in proportion, whereas other species, especially *C. glabrata,* are increasing. Among the incriminated risk factors for this shift, one finds the administration of azoles, particularly when used as prophylactic agents (2, 190). However, if this seems true for *C. glabrata,* no significant increase of *C. krusei* infection has been demonstrated.

The epidemiology of *Candida* resistance is largely not yet established; it is documented in AIDS patients with oropharyngeal candidiasis but to a lesser extent in bloodstream infections (209). In the ICU, hemato-oncology and surgical patients, representing now the majority of candidemic patients, the data are largely incomplete, but the percentage of resistance to azoles in susceptible species is still low. This is also the case in vaginal candidiasis, where azole-resistant *C. albicans* strains are exceedingly rare (253), despite the chronic course of the disease and repeated use of azole preparations. Population-based studies are needed to establish the true proportion of resistant clinical *Candida* isolates in various clinical settings.

Mechanisms of Resistance to Antifungal Drugs

The problem of antifungal drug resistance observed during the past decade has stimulated studies to understand the molecular mechanisms of resistance to these agents. The understanding of mechanisms of resistance to current antifungal drugs is also important to the design of new compounds. It is, therefore, important to present the current knowledge of this specific subject. In principle, when microbiological resistance to an antifungal drug in a fungal pathogen is detected by the measurement of MICs, it can be further categorized into primary or secondary resistance. Primary resistance, also called intrinsic resistance, is observed usually prior to in vivo or in vitro drug exposure. Secondary resistance (or acquired resistance) develops, however, upon exposure to an antifungal agent and can be either reversible or stably acquired. Several examples of transient adaptation to azole antifungal agents measured by increasing MICs have been documented, which could be reversed more or less rapidly by several subcultures in azole-free media (33, 166, 227). In vitro acquisition of antifungal resistance is, however, mostly stable, since it is maintained over several generations in drug-free media. The stable resistance phenotype is thought to be the result of genetic alterations, and their identification is the focus of different molecular studies.

Mechanisms of resistance to polyenes

Microbiological resistance to AmB can be intrinsic or acquired. Intrinsic resistance to AmB is common for some *C. lusitaniae* (211) and *Trichosporon* species (276), while acquired resistance during antifungal treatments with AmB is still rarely reported among fungal and yeast isolates. Some *C. lusitaniae* isolates are also able to develop in vitro rapid switches to AmB resistance when exposed to the drug (291). Acquired resistance to AmB is often associated with alteration of membrane lipids and especially sterols. Recently, clinical *C. albicans* isolates resistant to AmB were described lacking ergosterol and accumulating other sterols (3β-ergosta-7,22-dienol and 3β-ergosta-8-enol) typical for a defect in the sterol $\Delta^{5,6}$ desaturase system (132, 193). Such a defect is known in *S. cerevisiae* harboring a defect of the $\Delta^{5,6}$ desaturase gene *ERG3* (130). A defect in Δ^{8-7} isomerase in a clinical *C. neoformans* isolate from an AIDS patient was linked also with AmB resistance (134). A decrease in the content of cell membrane-associated ergosterol can also cause AmB resistance, since AmB requires the presence of ergosterol to cause damage to fungal cells. Different investigators supported this possibility by demonstrating that (i) development of inducible resistance (induced by adaptation mechanism) in a strain of *C. albicans* was accompanied by a decrease in the ergosterol content of the cells (35) and (ii) clinical polyene-resistant *C. albicans* isolates obtained from neutropenic patients had a 74 to 85% decrease in their ergosterol content (56). Another mechanism accounting for the resistance of yeast to AmB is thought to be mediated by increased catalase activity, which can contribute to diminish oxidative damage caused by this agent (254).

Mechanisms of resistance to 5-FC

5-FC is also an antifungal agent against which resistance can be intrinsic or acquired. Resistance may occur due to the deficiency or lack of enzymes implicated in the metabolism of 5-FC or may be due to the deregulation of the pyrimidine biosynthetic pathway, whose products can compete with the fluorinated metabolites of 5-FC (280). Detailed investigations on the molecular mechanisms of resistance to 5-FC have shown that intrinsic resistance to 5-FC in fungi can be due to a defect in the cytosine permease (as observed in *S. cerevisiae* and *C. glabrata* but not in *C. albicans* and *C. neoformans*), whereas acquired resistance results from a failure to metabolize 5-FC to 5-FUTP and 5-FdUMP or from the loss of a feedback control of pyrimidine biosynthesis (135). Due to the high prevalence of intrinsic resistance to 5-FC, this compound is best utilized in combination with other antifungal agents, for example, with AmB (217).

Mechanisms of resistance to azole antifungal agents

Reports on resistance to azole antifungal agents have been rare until the late 1980s. The first cases of resistance were reported in *C. albicans* after prolonged therapy with miconazole and ketoconazole (117, 118, 126). Following the use of fluconazole for a wide variety of clinical settings, antifungal resistance to this agent has been more frequently reported (283). There are several mechanisms by which yeasts can become resistant to azole antifungal agents. These mechanisms are summarized in Fig. 5. In clinical isolates resistance to azole antifungal agents can be the result of the following phenomena: (i) cells can fail to accumulate these agents; (ii) the cellular content of Erg11p can be elevated; (iii) the affinity of Erg11p to these agents can be decreased; (iv) the ergosterol biosynthetic pathway can be altered by inactivation of the sterol $\Delta^{5,6}$ desaturase. The following sections will develop each of these distinct mechanisms.

Resistance by altered drug transport. Failure to accumulate azole antifungal agents has been identified as a cause of azole resistance in several posttreatment clinical yeast species, including *C. albicans* (114, 241, 248, 271), *C. glabrata* (116, 203, 244), *C. krusei* (270), *C. dubliniensis* (183), or *C. neoformans* (272). In theory, failure to accumulate azole antifungal agents can be the consequence of impaired drug import or enhanced drug efflux. So far, since several

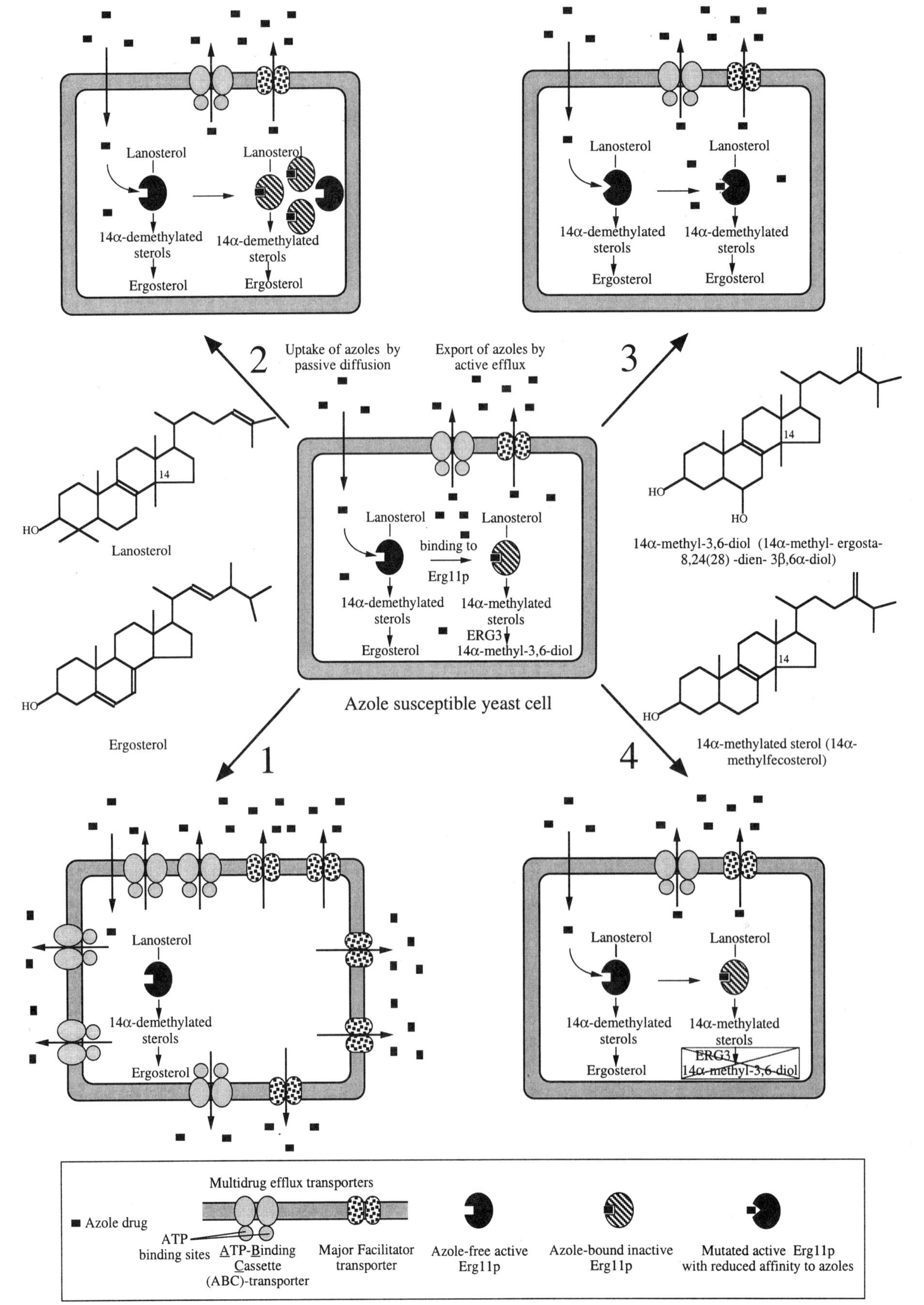

Uptake of azoles by passive diffusion
Export of azoles by active efflux
2
3
1
4
Lanosterol
14α-demethylated sterols
Ergosterol
binding to Erg11p
14α-methylated sterols
ERG3
14α-methyl-3,6-diol
Azole susceptible yeast cell
14α-methyl-3,6-diol (14α-methyl- ergosta-8,24(28) -dien- 3β,6α-diol)
14α-methylated sterol (14α-methylfecosterol)
14
HO
Multidrug efflux transporters
Azole drug
ATP binding sites
ATP-Binding Cassette (ABC)-transporter
Major Facilitator transporter
Azole-free active Erg11p
Azole-bound inactive Erg11p
Mutated active Erg11p with reduced affinity to azoles

studies conclude that azole import is mediated by passive diffusion, enhanced drug efflux has been the most likely drug transport mechanism for explaining reduced accumulation of azole antifungal agents in resistant isolates (244, 248). However, definitive evidence for passive diffusion of azole antifungal agents into cells remains to be established. An understanding of the molecular mechanisms responsible for the failure of accumulation of azole antifungal agents in resistant yeasts has progressed recently. In azole-resistant *C. albicans* isolates from AIDS patients with oropharyngeal candidiasis, multidrug efflux transporters of the ATP-binding cassette (ABC) superfamily and of the class of major facilitators (MF) have been reported to be responsible for the low level of accumulation of azole antifungal agents. Two genes for these transporters, the ABC-transporter gene *CDR1* and the MF gene *BEN*^{r} (also named *MDR1*), were shown to be upregulated in resistant isolates (248). The upregulation of both transporters in azole-resistant *C. albicans* species has now been confirmed by several other laboratories (7, 73, 75, 158, 281). The upregulation of ABC-transporter genes functionally similar to *CDR1* was also further established in non-*C. albicans* species. Thus, in *C. glabrata,* the *CgCDR1* and *PDH1* genes and, in *C. dubliniensis,* the *CdCDR1* genes were shown to be upregulated in azole-resistant isolates (178, 183, 244).

Other multidrug efflux transporter genes of both classes exist in *C. albicans* and some of them were cloned recently. These are the ABC-transporter genes *CDR2* (246), *CDR3* (15), and *CDR4* (74). There are also a number of other partial nucleotide sequences of ABC-transporters reported by Walsh et al. (275) and of other sequences accessible from the *C. albicans* sequencing project. For some of these new ABC-transporters, their participation in the resistance to azole antifungal agents is known: *CDR2* is upregulated to the levels reached by *CDR1* in *C. albicans* isolates cross resistant to azole derivatives (246). *CDR3* is expressed at very low levels in *C. albicans,* and its expression is dependent on the white-opaque transition in this yeast. However, *CDR3* expression does not appear to be linked to the resistance of *C. albicans* to azole derivatives (15). The levels of *CDR4* expression are generally higher than those of *CDR3* (243a) but are not related to the resistance of clinical yeasts to azole derivatives investigated so far (74). An additional MF gene has been recently cloned and was named *FLU1* since it conferred, among different azole antifungal agents tested, specific resistance to fluconazole in a *S. cerevisiae* strain in which the ABC-transporter gene *PDR5* was deleted (32). The expression of *FLU1* did not correlate with the development of azole resistance in *C. albicans* isolates investigated so far, suggesting that this gene is not involved in resistance to these agents (32).

Although upregulation of multidrug transporter genes has been linked with azole resistance in several cases, there are still few studies that support this correlation by genetic experiments. In one study both alleles of *MDR1* were disrupted in a clinical strain upregulating this transporter. The deletion of both *MDR1* alleles resulted in a decrease in fluconazole susceptibility, thus confirming the role of this transporter in azole resistance (287). The deletion of *CDR1* and *CDR2* has up to now been realized only in laboratory strains. Deletion of both genes resulted also in decreased azole susceptibility, thus establishing by genetic evidence a role of these transporters in azole resistance (246, 247). Genetic evidence for supporting the role of multidrug transporter in azole resistance was also given in *C. glabrata.* The deletion of *CgCDR1* in a clinical azole-resistant strain resulted in a dramatic decrease of fluconazole MICs to levels obtained for most of azole-susceptible isolates (244).

Azole resistance can be obtained by the exposure in vitro of diverse yeast species with different azoles. Examples reported up to now have described upregulation of multidrug transporters as being responsible for azole resistance. Cowen and collaborators (44) have investigated adaptation in *C. albicans* to inhibitory concentrations of fluconazole in replicated experimental populations isolated from a single azole-susceptible cell. Replicate populations grown with fluconazole adapted to the presence of drug as indicated by an increase in MIC. In distinct populations with higher fluconazole MIC than the azole-susceptible parent, *CDR1, CDR2,* and *MDR1* expression was upregulated and stably maintained over 50 generations in drug-free medium. *MDR1* upregulation could also be demonstrated in *C. dubliniensis* exposed in vitro to fluconazole (183, 184). Marr and collaborators (166) obtained from bone marrow transplant patients under fluconazole treatment *C. albicans* isolates developing azole resistance. Increase in fluconazole

Figure 5. Schematic view of resistance mechanisms to azole antifungal agents. The mechanisms are numbered from 1 to 4. (1) Failure in accumulation of azoles due to upregulation of multidrug transporter genes; (2) elevation of Erg11p cellular content; (3) decrease in Erg11p affinity; (4) alteration of the ergosterol biosynthetic pathway by inactivation of the sterol $\Delta^{5,6}$ desaturase.

MIC was coupled with upregulation of *CDR1* but was decreased with paralleled decrease in *CDR1* expression in drug-free subculture. Azole-susceptible isolates from this type of patient, when exposed in vitro to fluconazole, developed reversible azole resistance by the same *CDR1* upregulation mechanism. Interestingly, only a portion of individually exposed colonies were rendered less susceptible to fluconazole, thus indicating that heteroresistance, which was already described in azole-exposed *C. neoformans* isolates (180), could occur in specific *C. albicans* isolates (165). In vitro acquisition of azole resistance was also described in *C. tropicalis.* In this case also, azole resistance was reversible after subculture in drug-free medium. Azole resistance was paralleled with simultaneous upregulation of two different multidrug transporter genes (*CtMDR1* and a *CDR1*-like gene) from both the ABC-transporter and the MF families (17). Last, it was shown that *C. glabrata* could be converted in vitro to azole resistance at high frequency by mitochondrial loss. The phenomenon was called HFAR (for high frequency azole resistance) and occurred at frequencies ranging from 2 to 4 $\times$ 10^{-4}. Azole resistance obtained in this case could be maintained over several generations in drug-free medium and was coupled with upregulation of *CgCDR1* and the novel ABC-transporter gene *CgCDR2* (243).

Regulation of multidrug transporter genes in fungal pathogens. Currently, it is not clear how multidrug transporter genes are regulated in fungal pathogens. Multidrug transporter genes are regulated in *S. cerevisiae* by a network of transcription factors with leucine zipper dimerization domains (*YAP1* and *YAP2*) or "zinc 2-cysteine 6" DNA binding motifs (*PDR1, PDR3*). Alteration of the transcription factor *PDR1* is associated with increased transcription of the ABC-transporter gene *PDR5* (16). *YAP1* and *YAP2* are implicated in the transcription regulation of *PDR5* and another ABC-transporter *YCF1* (177, 279). It is possible, therefore, that similar transcription factors are operative in the regulation of ABC-transporter genes in *C. albicans* or *C. glabrata* isolates. The fact that both *CDR1* and *CDR2* are coordinately upregulated in azole-resistant *C. albicans* cells supports the hypothesis that the same factors can act in *trans* on the structural elements of these genes.

Recently, a few reports have emerged on the regulation of the *C. albicans* ABC-transporter gene *CDR1.* In a first study, the protein encoded by the *CDR1* gene, Cdr1p, was fused to the green fluorescent protein (GFP) (111). The expression of the resulting fusion protein was visualized by fluorescence microscopy and quantified by fluorescence flow cytometry. It was found that not only fluconazole but also cycloheximide, when incubated with cells at a concentration higher than their MIC, could induce the production of the Cdr1p-GFP fusion protein. In another study, *CDR1* expression could be induced by several other agents (miconazole, nystatin, vinblastin) and, among them, human steroid hormones (progesterone, β-estradiol) (141). However, in this study, fluconazole did not induce *CDR1,* opposite of the results from the first study.

In a separate study, upregulation of *CDR1* and *CDR2* in *C. albicans* was obtained by exposure to fluphenazine, albendazole, and sulfadiazine (109). Transient upregulation of *CDR1/CDR2* by these substances antagonized azole antifungals and thus substantially increased MICs to these agents (109). The functional dissection of the *CDR1* promoter has demonstrated the presence of multiple activating and repressing regulatory domains, thus suggesting a complex network of regulatory elements on this promoter (222).

MDR1 can be induced transiently by benomyl and other unrelated drugs (91). Recently, Alarco et al. (6) cloned a gene, *CAP1,* similar to the *S. cerevisiae YAP1* gene. Alarco et al. (6) showed that the expression of *CAP1* in *S. cerevisiae* could activate the transcription of an MF gene called *FLR1,* which has functional similarity to the *C. albicans MDR1* gene. Therefore, a possible role of *CAP1* in regulating *MDR1* is possible. The role of *CAP1* in mediating the expression of *MDR1* in *C. albicans* remains to be established. However, this possibility is likely since there is now genetic evidence for attributing upregulation of *MDR1* in *C. albicans* by a still uncharacterized transcription factor (286).

Substrates of multidrug transporters. A major implication of the involvement of multidrug efflux transporters in resistance to azole antifungal agents is that these transporters have the ability to mediate cross-resistance to unrelated antifungal agents or metabolic inhibitors. To determine whether a given substance is a potential substrate for multidrug efflux transporters, different approaches have been taken. One consists of functional expression of the *C. albicans* multidrug efflux transporters in *S. cerevisiae* carrying a deletion of the *PDR5* gene (246, 247). Depending on the acquisition of resistance of *S. cerevisiae* mutants expressing these specific transporters against a given compound, the substance can be considered as a potential substrate for the expressed multidrug transporter. Another approach consists of exposing *C. albicans* mutants for specific transporters to different substances. If a given substance is a substrate for the deleted multidrug transporter, then cells become hypersusceptible to this substance (247).

Table 4. Substrates of multidrug transporters from *C. albicans*

Multidrug transporter	Substrate(s)	Transporter specificity for the given substrate
Cdr1p, Cdr2p, Mdr1p, Flu1p	Fluconazole, terbinafine, cerulenin, brefeldin A, cycloheximide, β-estradiol	Low
Cdr1p, Mdr1p, Flu1p	Sulfomethuron methyl	Low
Cdr1p, Cdr2p, Mdr1p	Amorolfine, fluphenazine	Medium
Cdr1p, Cdr2p	Ketoconazole, itraconazole, rhodamine 6G	Medium
Mdr1p	Benomyl, 1-10 phenantroline, 4-nitroquinolone-*N*-oxide	High
Flu1p	Mycophenolic acid	High

Using both approaches, potential substrates for the multidrug efflux transporters encoded by *CDR1, CDR2, MDR1,* and *FLU1* could be identified (Table 4). The list of substrates for efflux multidrug transporters given in Table 4 is not exhaustive. In fact, it was shown recently that the steroid hormone β-estradiol could be transported by the *CDR1* gene product (Cdr1p) when expressed in *S. cerevisiae* (141). Several antifungal agents could not be assigned as substrates (AmB, pradimicin, 5-FC, nikkomycin Z). Table 4 shows that not only fluconazole but other antifungal agents such as terbinafine and amorolfine can be used simultaneously as substrates by several multidrug efflux transporters. This implies that multidrug efflux transporter genes, when overexpressed in yeast clinical isolates, have the potential of mediating cross-resistance to different antifungal agents. Several data, in fact, suggest that the upregulation of *MDR1* is responsible for the specific resistance to fluconazole in *Candida* isolates (183, 184, 287), thus correlating with the observation that *MDR1* overexpression in *S. cerevisiae* was only conferring resistance to fluconazole in this species (246). Recently, Albertson et al. (7) reported the characterization of a *C. albicans* spontaneous mutant specifically resistant to fluconazole, but not to other azole derivatives, in which the *MDR1* gene was upregulated. Oppositely, *CDR1* overexpression in *S. cerevisiae* was conferring cross-resistance to different azole derivatives, including fluconazole, itraconazole, and ketoconazole (246).

Resistance to azole antifungal agents involving alterations of the cellular target. Alterations of affinity of azole derivatives to Erg11p is another important mechanism of resistance that has been described in different posttreatment yeast species, namely *C. albicans* (265) and recently in *C. neoformans* (149). Affinity alterations are thought to be due to mutations in the gene encoding Erg11p (*ERG11*), which, by conformational changes, can affect the binding of azole derivatives. When comparing *ERG11* sequences from matched pairs of azole-susceptible and azole-resistant *C. albicans* isolates, several laboratories have described nucleotide substitutions in *ERG11* alleles from azole-resistant *C. albicans* isolates resulting in amino acid changes. In Table 5 a list of mutations in *ERG11* is presented. A total of 83 amino acid substitutions have been reported by these studies. This illustrates the high allelic variability for *ERG11,* unlike most other genes in lower eukaryotes. The effect of amino substitutions on azole resistance has not been yet determined systematically. In vitro binding assays of azoles with mutant Erg11p protein variants have been carried out for the substitutions R467K, G464S, and Y132H, which are found in *ERG11* alleles of azole-resistant isolates (131, 133, 150). Functional expression of PCR-amplified *ERG11* alleles in *S. cerevisiae* followed by azole susceptibility assays have also been performed as a convenient alternative to the first assay to reveal mutations coupled with the development of azole resistance (245). While some *ERG11* alleles contain a single mutation responsible for azole resistance, other *ERG11* alleles were found to contain several mutations with potential additive effects. The recently reported crystal structure of a cytochrome P450 from *Mycobacterium tuberculosis,* while a soluble ortholog of Erg11p, will help determine the effect of mutations on the protein conformation and interferences with azole binding (214).

Upregulation of *ERG11* has been mentioned as a possible cause of azole resistance in a few clinical isolates of *C. albicans* and *C. glabrata.* Upregulation of *ERG11* did not exceed a factor of 3 to 5 in azole-resistant isolates when compared with *ERG11* expression in related azole-susceptible strains (158, 164, 248, 281). Upregulation of *ERG11* can be achieved in principle by deregulating the gene transcription or by gene amplification. The latter possibility has been demonstrated in a *C. glabrata* isolate re-

Table 5. Amino substitutions in *ERGII* alleles recovered from *C. albicans* clinical isolates

Amino acid substitution	Reference(s)	Amino acid substitution	Reference(s)
F14L	D. Sanglard, unpublished	H310R	D. Sanglard, unpublished
V19A	D. Sanglard, unpublished	Y334C	D. Sanglard, unpublished
L35S	D. Sanglard, unpublished	K344R	D. Sanglard, unpublished
R44G	D. Sanglard, unpublished	P360S	D. Sanglard, unpublished
W57K	D. Sanglard, unpublished	I366T	D. Sanglard, unpublished
F72L	71	H373L	D. Sanglard, unpublished
K90E	D. Sanglard, unpublished	L376V	D. Sanglard, unpublished
G100S	D. Sanglard, unpublished	F380L	D. Sanglard, unpublished
F105L	156	K398N	D. Sanglard, unpublished
K108E	D. Sanglard, unpublished	S405P	D. Sanglard, unpublished
S110P	D. Sanglard, unpublished	S405F	71, 245
A114V	D. Sanglard, unpublished	G421D	D. Sanglard, unpublished
D116E	71, 128, 163, 166, 245	R426K	D. Sanglard, unpublished
F126L	71, 282	A432T	D. Sanglard, unpublished
K128T	128, 156, 163, 245	V437I	71, 245
Y132H	13, 128, 245	F439L	D. Sanglard, unpublished
R138K	D. Sanglard, unpublished	S442F	D. Sanglard, unpublished
T140M	D. Sanglard, unpublished	G443E	D. Sanglard, unpublished
K143E	71	D446G	D. Sanglard, unpublished
F145L	13	Y447G	D. Sanglard, unpublished
K147R	156	G448E	156
A149V	163	F449L	71
D153	163	G450R	D. Sanglard, unpublished
R157K	D. Sanglard, unpublished	G450E	71, 163
V159I	D. Sanglard, unpublished	V452A	163
E165Y	163	V456I	D. Sanglard, unpublished
T172A	163	Y460H	D. Sanglard, unpublished
S175G	163	G464S	156, 163, 166, 245
F205L	163	G465S	163
S203F	163	R467K	163, 245, 282
T229A	71	H468Y	D. Sanglard, unpublished
P230A	71	I471V	D. Sanglard, unpublished
N237Y	71	I471T	128
E266D	71, 156, 163	Y477H	D. Sanglard, unpublished
K274H	D. Sanglard, unpublished	L480S	D. Sanglard, unpublished
S279F	163	V488I	166
K287R	156	R492G	D. Sanglard, unpublished
A298T	D. Sanglard, unpublished	T494I	D. Sanglard, unpublished
A298V	D. Sanglard, unpublished	T513P	D. Sanglard, unpublished
I304N	D. Sanglard, unpublished	W520G	D. Sanglard, unpublished
I304T	D. Sanglard, unpublished	W520R	D. Sanglard, unpublished
		E521D	D. Sanglard, unpublished

sistant to azole derivatives (164). Upregulation of *ERG11* can also be obtained by exposure of *C. albicans* to ergosterol biosynthesis inhibitors, especially to azole antifungal agents (110). Exposure of *C. albicans* to this type of drug affects the expression of other *ERG* genes, as recently confirmed by genomewide expression studies performed in *C. albicans* (47).

Resistance mechanisms involving alterations in the ergosterol biosynthetic pathway. An analysis of the sterol composition of azole-resistant yeasts has provided several hypotheses on specific alterations of enzymes involved in the complex ergosterol biosynthetic pathway. Accumulation of ergosta-7,22-dienol-3β-ol was observed in two distinct azole-resistant *C. albicans* clinical isolates, which is a feature consistent with an absence of sterol $\Delta^{5,6}$ desaturase activity encoded by *ERG3* (132, 193). Interestingly, azole resistance in these two isolates was coupled with resistance to AmB, which was expected because of the absence of ergosterol in these cells. Some controversy still exists on the role of *ERG3* in development of azole resistance. For example, it has been reported in *C. glabrata* that null mutations in both *ERG3* and *ERG11* were required to establish azole resistance, while a null mutation in the *ERG3* gene alone was not sufficient for the acquisition of azole resistance but was compatible with AmB resistance only (81). The *ERG3* defect in *S. cerevisiae* suppresses the lethality resulting from the inactivation of *ERG11* and is linked to the acquisition of resistance to azole derivatives (20, 130). The role of *ERG3* in azole resistance originates also from the observation that treatment of a normal yeast cell with azoles inhibits Erg11p and thus results in the accumulation of 14α-methylated sterols and 14α-methylergosta-8,24(28)-dien-3β,6α-diol. Formation of this latter sterol metabolite is thought to be catalyzed by the *ERG3* gene product (the sterol $\Delta^{5,6}$ desaturase) and thus inactivation of this gene suppresses toxicity and causes azole resistance (see Fig. 5, part 4). This specific mechanism of resistance to azole derivatives seems to mimic azole resistance obtained in laboratory conditions in *S. cerevisiae* by mutations of the *ERG3* gene (278). Loss of function mutations in *ERG3* alleles from the *C. albicans* azole-resistant Darlington strain were characterized recently (179). Unfortunately, the effects of these mutations on azole resistance were masked by other azole resistance mechanisms in this strain (179).

Combination of mechanisms. The multiplicity of mechanisms of resistance to azole antifungal agents enables yeast cells to develop a stepwise increase in resistance to these agents. There are still few clinical isolates that have been analyzed at the molecular level for the presence and the combination of these different mechanisms. The combination of resistance mechanisms is a common feature in the stepwise development of azole resistance in *C. albicans* (73, 158, 245, 281). Azole resistance in *C. glabrata* isolates investigated thus far seems, however, to be caused by a single mechanism (i.e., upregulation of multidrug transporters) (244). In Table 6, an overview of the mechanisms of azole resistance found in sequential *C. albicans* isolates from four different patients is presented (245). Development of resistance is based on a unique combination of mechanisms, which enables not only a stepwise increase in resistance to azole derivatives but also an increase in resistance to specific azoles.

Resistance Mechanisms to Allylamines and Morphololines

Resistance to allylamines in yeast and fungi has been rarely reported (70). However, the potential of developing resistance by the action of multidrug efflux transporters exists. For example, the overexpression in *S. cerevisiae* of the *C. albicans CDR1* and *CDR2* genes and of the *CaMDR1* gene can confer resistance to terbinafine (246), showing that this compound is a substrate for these transporters. Consistent with these results is the observation that several *C. albicans* isolates resistant to azole antifungal agents by multidrug transporter gene upregulation are also less susceptible to terbinafine (240).

Acquired resistance to morpholine derivatives has not been reported so far in yeast pathogens, and this is probably due to the limited use of this antifungal agent for the treatment of superficial fungal infections. However, resistance to morpholine derivatives can be obtained in *S. cerevisiae* by the overexpression of the *ERG24* gene, among those involved in sterol

Table 6. Combination of resistance mechanism and stepwise increase of azole resistance (245)

Patient no.	*C. albicans* isolates[a]	Relative MIC increase			Resistance mechanism linked to MIC increase
		Fluconazole	Ketoconazole	Itraconazole	
I	C23	1	1	1	S405F mutation on one *ERG11* allele
	C39	32	8	2	S405F mutation on both *ERG11* alleles Increase of mRNA for *CDRI* and *CDR2*
III	C33	1	1	1	
	C34	8	1	2	S405F mutation on both *ERG11* alleles
	C82	128	32	32	Increase of mRNA for *CDR1* and *CDR2*
	C26	512	256	64	Y132H mutation on both *ERG11* alleles
IV	C27	1	1	1	
	C37	8	2	2	G464S, R467K mutations on both *ERG11* alleles
	C40	128	128	32	Y132H mutation on one *ERG11* allele Increase of *MDR1* mRNA
V	C43	1	1	1	G129A mutation on one *ERG11* allele
	C56	512	256	64	G129A, G464S mutations on both ERG11 alleles Increase of mRNA for *CDR1* and *CDR2*

[a] Sequential isolates from each patient.

biosynthesis (148). Moreover, recent work has pointed out that amorolfine, as in the case of terbinafine, could be a substrate of *C. albicans* multidrug efflux transporters encoded by the *CDR1* and *CDR2* genes (246). *C. albicans* clinical isolates resistant to azole antifungal agents are also less susceptible to amorolfine (113). A potential exists, therefore, for developing resistance to this agent.

Resistance Mechanisms to Other Antifungal Agents

The search for potential resistance of fungi to investigative antifungal drugs is a standard process in the development of antifungal drugs. The isolation of drug-resistant mutants is not only often necessary for dissecting the mode of action of antifungal drugs but also to evaluate the risk of development of resistance in clinical situations. Below, we discuss resistance mechanisms of antifungal agents at the investigative stage and those with novel modes of action.

Pneumocandin/echinocandins

Pneumocandin resistance was first investigated in the model yeast *S. cerevisiae* with a mutant R560-1C resistant to the semisynthetic pneumocandin derivative L-733,560. Glucan synthesis catalyzed by a crude membrane fraction prepared from the *S. cerevisiae* was resistant to inhibition by L-733,560. The nearly 50-fold increase in the 50% inhibitory concentration against glucan synthase was paralleled with an increase in whole-cell resistance (63). Pneumocandin resistance has been established in *C. albicans* either by mutagenesis or by spontaneous selection at a low frequency of resistant mutants on pneumocandin-containing medium. Resistant mutants increased their MICs to pneumocandin derivatives by 50- to 100-fold. The IC_{50} of glucan synthase activity was affected to variable degrees from 4- to over 5,000-fold in these mutants, suggesting that alterations in this enzyme were responsible for resistance. With the cloning of the *CaFKS1* gene encoding a subunit of the β-1,3 glucan synthase, genetic evidence was provided for this possibility since disruption of *CaFKS1* echinocandin-resistant alleles in *C. albicans*-resistant mutants resulted in loss of resistance (62, 175). These experiments also show that echinocandin derivatives were targeting the product of the *CaFKS1* gene in *C. albicans.* Not only was the development of echinocandin resistance a rare event in *C. albicans,* but it was coupled with reduced virulence of a resistant strain in animal models (76). Other echinocandin-resistant mutants have been produced without significant loss of virulence; these mutants were more refractory but still susceptible to treatment with the echinocandin L-733,560 than fully susceptible wild types (146). Resistance was not paralleled with changes in susceptibility to other agents and thus enables the use of alternative agents in the case of development of resistance.

Sordarins

To identify targets of sordarins, spontaneous resistant mutants in *S. cerevisiae* were selected at frequencies of 10^{-7} to 10^{-8} on YPD medium plates containing a sordarin derivative (GM193663). The observation that eukaryotic elongation factor 2 (eEF2) was the major determinant of sordarin specificity was confirmed by the identification of unique sordarin-resistant alleles mainly in *EFT2* that encodes eEF2 in *S. cerevisiae* (34). Mutations in *EFT2* were clustered, forming a possible drug-binding pocket on a three-dimensional model of *eEF2,* and mutant cell extracts lost the capacity to bind to the inhibitors (34). Additional mutants not affecting *EFT2* were recently mapped to the essential ribosomal protein L10e (127). Five unique L10e alleles were characterized and sequenced, and several nucleotide changes that differ from the wild-type sequence were identified. Changes that result in the resistance phenotype mapped to 4 amino acid substitutions and 1 amino acid deletion clustered in a conserved 10-amino-acid region of L10e. Like the previously identified eEF2 mutations, the mutant ribosomes showed reduced sordarin-conferred stabilization of the eEF2-nucleotide-ribosome complex. The results suggest a functional linkage between L10e and eEF2, which is consistent with the function of ribosome as a critical partner in forming the stabilized posttranslocational complex (127).

Aureobasidin (AbA)

Analysis of AbA-resistant mutants in *S. cerevisiae* has helped identify the target enzyme of this antifungal agent. Resistance was induced by in vitro exposure of *S. cerevisiae* to AbA and was found to reside in a dominant mutation of a single gene, which was named *AUR1* (for aureobasidin resistance) (105). This gene was identified as encoding a phosphatidylinositol ceramide phosphoinositol transferase (IPC synthase) (186). Subsequently, other mutations in *AUR1* alleles were described in *S. cerevisiae* and also in *AUR1*-related genes of other yeasts and fungi (102, 103, 106, 143). Further analysis of AbA-resistant isolates revealed *YOR1* as another *S. cerevisiae* resistance gene, which is an ABC-transporter known to contribute to oligomycin, reveromycin, and organic anion resistance (195). A recessive mutation (*aur3*^{R}) was also responsible for AbA resistance in *S. cerevisiae.* Genetic studies showed that the *aur3*^{R} mutation was localized to the *PDR1* gene, which encodes a transcriptional regulator of *PDR5* and *YOR1*. The activated *PDR1* allele in the *aur3*^{R} mutant was responsible for an increased expression of *YOR1* and thus probably enhanced efflux of AbA (195). Interaction of AbA with multidrug resistance protein is not restricted to yeast, since this substance interacted with human MDR1/Pgp or MDR2/Pgp (137).

Impact of Mechanisms of Resistance in the Design of New Antifungal Agents

The discovery of mechanisms of resistance to established or investigative antifungal agents has several potential impacts on the design of new antifungal drugs. A major advance in the understanding of antifungal drug resistance mechanisms was the involvement of multidrug transporters in the development of resistance. It is highly desirable to avoid interference of new antifungal drugs with multidrug transporters, because these transporters, when expressed in cells to high levels, can cause resistance to multiple unrelated substances. Molecular tools are now available to exclude potential new antifungal agents as substrates of multidrug efflux transporters.

The availability of mutated enzymes that confer resistance to their target antifungal agents can also assist in improving existing agents by chemical derivatization. For example, when using the different mutant *ERG11* alleles as described in "Mechanisms of resistance to azole antifungal agents" in affinity assays with new azole derivatives, it is possible to estimate their performance with respect to their binding efficiency and design their structures to become insensitive to *ERG11* mutations.

FUTURE DIRECTIONS AND CONCLUSIONS

Antifungal drug discovery is now exploring the use of genomic information as an additional exploration tool in drug target screening. No doubt future agents will emerge from the use of this important source of information in conjunction with traditional drug screening procedures. Genomic information is now being extended to a significant number of yeast and fungal pathogens including *C. albicans, C. neoformans*, and *A. fumigatus*. Genomic information is likely to assist in the future identification of the mode of actions of antifungal drugs with unknown targets. Several examples of drug target identification have been reported with the help of the *S. cerevisiae* genome and even "off-targets" of several classical antifungal agents have been now characterized (120, 169). A genomewide expression study of *C. albicans* genes performed for the first time by de Backer et al. (47) has confirmed the validity of this approach by investigating the effect of itraconazole on gene expression.

Before the introduction of new antifungal agents will be seen in clinical practice, treatment options will remain with the few existing agents. To extend the range of activities of these agents when needed, it will be important to explore their possible potentation by combination with each other or by combination with companion drugs or with immunomodulators.

REFERENCES

1. **Abele-Horn, M., A. Kopp, U. Sternberg, A. Ohly, A. Dauber, W. Russwurm, W. Buchinger, O. Nagengast, and P. Emmerling.** 1996. A randomized study comparing fluconazole with amphotericin B/5-flucytosine for the treatment of systemic *Candida* infections in intensive care patients. *Infection* **24:**426–432.
2. **Abi-Said, D., E. Anaissie, O. Uzun, I. Raad, H. Pinzcowski, and S. Vartivarian.** 1997. The epidemiology of hematogenous candidiasis caused by different *Candida* species. *Clin. Infect. Dis.* **24:**1122–1128.
3. **Abruzzo, G. K., A. M. Flattery, C. J. Gill, L. Kong, J. G. Smith, V. B. Pikounis, J. M. Balkovec, A. F. Bouffard, J. F. Dropinski, H. Rosen, H. Kropp, and K. Bartizal.** 1997. Evaluation of the echinocandin antifungal MK-0991 (L-743,872): efficacies in mouse models of disseminated aspergillosis, candidiasis, and cryptococcosis. *Antimicrob. Agents Chemother.* **41:**2333–2338.
4. **Abruzzo, G. K., C. J. Gill, A. M. Flattery, L. Kong, C. Leighton, J. G. Smith, V. B. Pikounis, K. Bartizal, and H. Rosen.** 2000. Efficacy of the echinocandin caspofungin against disseminated aspergillosis and candidiasis in cyclophosphamide-induced immunosuppressed mice. *Antimicrob. Agents Chemother.* **44:**2310–2318.
5. **Adler-Moore, J.** 1994. AmBisome targeting to fungal infections. *Bone Marrow Transpl.* **14:**S3–S7.
6. **Alarco, A. M., and M. Raymond.** 1999. The bZip transcription factor Cap1p is involved in multidrug resistance and oxidative stress response in *Candida albicans. J. Bacteriol.* **181:**700–708.
7. **Albertson, G. D., M. Niimi, R. D. Cannon, and H. F. Jenkinson.** 1996. Multiple efflux mechanisms are involved in *Candida albicans* fluconazole resistance. *Antimicrob. Agents Chemother.* **40:**2835–2841.
8. **Anaissie, E. J., N. C. Karyotakis, R. Hachem, M. C. Dignani, J. H. Rex, and V. Paetznick.** 1994. Correlation between in vitro and in vivo activity of antifungal agents against *Candida* species. *J. Infect. Dis.* **170:**384–389.
9. **Appenzeller, L., E. Lim, P. Wong, M. Fadem, P. Motchnik, B. M., and R. Little.** 1996. In vivo fungicidal activity of optimized domain III peptides derived from bactericidal/permeability-increasing protein (BPI), abstr. F-187, p. 132. *In Program Abstr. 36th Intersci. Conf. Antimicrob. Agents Chemother.* American Society for Microbiology, Washington, D.C.
10. **Aramwit, P., B. G. Yu, A. Lavasanifar, J. Samuel, and G. S. Kwon.** 2000. The effect of serum albumin on the aggregation state and toxicity of amphotericin B. *J. Pharm. Sci.* **89:**1589–1593.

11. **Arikan, S., M. Lozano-Chiu, V. Paetznick, S. Nangia, and J. H. Rex.** 1999. Microdilution susceptibility testing of amphotericin B, itraconazole, and voriconazole against clinical isolates of *Aspergillus* and *Fusarium* species. *J. Clin. Microbiol.* **37:**3946–3951.
12. **Arzeni, D., F. Barchiesi, P. Compagnucci, A. Cellini, O. Simonetti, A. M. Offidani, and G. Scalise.** 1998. In vitro activity of terbinafine against clinical isolates of dermatophytes. *Med. Mycol.* **36:**235–237.
13. **Asai, K., N. Tsuchimori, K. Okonogi, J. R. Perfect, O. Gotoh, and Y. Yoshida.** 1999. Formation of azole-resistant *Candida albicans* by mutation of sterol 14α—demethylase P450. *Antimicrob. Agents Chemother.* **43:**1163–1169.
14. **Asako, H., I. Kurose, R. E. Wolf, and D. N. Granger.** 1994. Mechanisms of lactoferrin-induced leukocyte-endothelial cell adhesion in postcapillary venules. *Microcirculation* **1:**27–34.
15. **Balan, I., A. M. Alarco, and M. Raymond.** 1997. The *Candida albicans* CDR3 gene codes for an opaque-phase ABC transporter. *J. Bacteriol.* **179:**7210–7218.
16. **Balzi, E., and A. Goffeau.** 1994. Genetics and biochemistry of yeast multidrug resistance. *Biochim. Biophys. Acta* **1187:** 152–162.
17. **Barchiesi, F., D. Calabrese, D. Sanglard, L. Falconi Di Francesco, F. Caselli, D. Giannini, A. Giacometti, S. Gavaudan, and G. Scalise.** 2000. Experimental induction of fluconazole resistance in *Candida tropicalis* ATCC 750. *Antimicrob. Agents Chemother.* **44:**1578–1584.
18. **Barchiesi, F., L. F. Di Francesco, P. Compagnucci, D. Arzeni, A. Giacometti, and G. Scalise.** 1998. In-vitro interaction of terbinafine with amphotericin B, fluconazole and itraconazole against clinical isolates of *Candida albicans. J. Antimicrob. Chemother.* **41:**59–65.
19. **Barchiesi, F., L. Falconi Di Francesco, and G. Scalise.** 1997. In vitro activities of terbinafine in combination with fluconazole and itraconazole against isolates of *Candida albicans* with reduced susceptibility to azoles. *Antimicrob. Agents Chemother.* **41:**1812–1814.
20. **Bard, M., N. D. Lees, T. Turi, D. Craft, L. Cofrin, R. Barbuch, C. Koegel, and J. C. Loper.** 1993. Sterol synthesis and viability of *ERG11* (cytochrome P450 lanosterol demethylase) mutations in *Saccharomyces cerevisiae* and *Candida albicans. Lipids* **28:**963–967.
21. **Bartizal, K., C. J. Gill, G. K. Abruzzo, A. M. Flattery, L. Kong, P. M. Scott, J. G. Smith, C. E. Leighton, A. Bouffard, J. F. Dropinski, and J. Balkovec.** 1997. In vitro preclinical evaluation studies with the echinocandin antifungal MK-0991 (L-743,872). *Antimicrob. Agents Chemother.* **41:** 2326–2332.
22. **Beninati, C., M. R. Oggioni, M. Boccanera, M. R. Spinosa, T. Maggi, S. Conti, W. Magliani, F. De Bernardis, G. Teti, A. Cassone, G. Pozzi, and L. Polonelli.** 2000. Therapy of mucosal candidiasis by expression of an anti-idiotype in human commensal bacteria. *Nat. Biotechnol.* **18:** 1060–1064.
23. **Bennett, J. E., W. E. Dismukes, R. J. Duma, G. Medoff, M. A. Sande, H. Gallis, J. Leonard, B. T. Fields, M. Bradshaw, H. Haywood, Z. A. McGee, T. R. Cate, C. G. Cobbs, J. F. Warner, and D. W. Alling.** 1979. A comparison of amphotericin B alone and combined with flucytosine in the treatment of cryptoccal meningitis. *N. Engl. J. Med.* **301:**126–131.
24. **Bennett, M. L., A. B. Fleischer, J. W. Loveless, and S. R. Feldman.** 2000. Oral griseofulvin remains the treatment of choice for tinea capitis in children. *Pediatr. Dermatol.* **17:** 304–309.
25. **Bolard, J.** 1991. Mechanisms of action of anti-candida drug: amphotericin B and its derivatives, p. 213–238. *In* R. Prasad (ed.), *Candida albicans. Cellular and Molecular Biology.* Springer-Verlag, Berlin, Germany.
26. **Bolard, J., and J. Milhaud.** 1996. Interaction of the anti-*Candida* amphotericin B (and other polyene antibiotics) with lipids, p. 253–274. *In* R. Prasad and M. Ghannoum (ed.), *Lipids of Pathogenic Fungi.* CRC Press, Inc., Boca Raton, Fla.
27. **Bolard, J., M. Seigneuret, and G. Boudet.** 1980. Interaction between phospholipid bilayer membranes and the polyene antibiotic amphotericin B: lipid state and cholesterol content dependence. *Biochim. Biophys. Acta* **599:**280–293.
28. **Brajtburg, J., W. G. Powderly, G. S. Kobayashi, and G. Medoff.** 1990. Amphotericin B: current understanding of mechanisms of action. *Antimicrob. Agents Chemother.* **34:** 183–188.
29. **Bullawa, C. E.** 1993. Genetics and molecular biology of chitin synthesis in fungi. *Ann. Rev. Microbiol.* **47:**505–534.
30. **Butters, J. A., S. J. Kendall, I. E. Wheeler, and D. W. Hollomon.** 1995. Tubulins: lessons from existing products that can be applied to targets new antifungals, p. 131–142. *In* G. K. Dixon, L. G. Copping, and D. W. Hollomon (ed.), *Antifungal Agents: Discovery and Mode of Action.* BIOS Scientific Publishers, Oxford, United Kingdom.
31. **Cacciapuoti, A., D. Loebenberg, E. Corcoran, F. Menzel, Jr., E. L. Moss, Jr., C. Norris, M. Michalski, K. Raynor, J. Halpern, C. Mendrick, B. Arnold, B. Antonacci, R. Parmegiani, T. Yarosh-Tomaine, G. H. Miller, and R. S. Hare.** 2000. In vitro and in vivo activities of SCH 56592 (posaconazole), a new triazole antifungal agent, against *Aspergillus* and *Candida. Antimicrob. Agents Chemother.* **44:**2017–2022.
32. **Calabrese, D., J. Bille, and D. Sanglard.** 2000. A novel multidrug efflux transporter gene of the major facilitator superfamily from *Candida albicans* (*FLU1*) conferring resistance to fluconazole. *Microbiology* **146:**2743–2754.
33. **Calvet, H. M., M. R. Yeaman, and S. G. Filler.** 1997. Reversible fluconazole resistance in *Candida albicans:* a potential in vitro model. *Antimicrob. Agents Chemother.* **41:**535–539.
34. **Capa, L., A. Mendoza, J. L. Lavandera, F. Gomez de las Heras, and J. F. Garcia-Bustos.** 1998. Translation elongation factor 2 is part of the target for a new family of antifungals. *Antimicrob. Agents Chemother.* **42:**2694–2699.
35. **Capek, A., A. Simek, L. Bruna, A. Svab, and Z. Budesinsky.** 1974. Antimicrobial agents. XX. Ergosterol content of *Candida albicans* cells during adaptation to antimycotics. *Folia Microbiol.* **19:**79–80.
36. **Chamberland, S., J. Blais, D. P. Cotter, M. K. Hoang, J. Galazzo, A. Staley, M. Lee, and G. H. Miller.** 1999. Impact of MC-510,027, a fungal efflux pump inhibitor, on the susceptibility of clinical isolates of *Candida* spp. to antifungal agents, abstr. 1270, p. 328. *In Program Abstr. 39th Intersci. Conf. Antimicrob. Agents Chemother.* American Society for Microbiology, Washington, D.C.
37. **Chavez, M., S. Bernal, A. Valverde, M. J. Gutierrez, G. Quindos, and E. M. Mazuelos.** 1999. In-vitro activity of voriconazole (UK-109,496), LY303366 and other antifungal agents against oral *Candida* spp. isolates from HIV-infected patients. *J. Antimicrob. Chemother.* **44:**697–700.
38. **Chiritescu, M. M., M. E. Chiritescu, and R. K. Scher.** 1996. Newer systemic antifungal drugs for the treatment of onychomycosis. *Clin. Podiatr. Med. Surg.* **13:**741–758.
39. **Clancy, C. J., and M. H. Nguyen.** 1999. Correlation between in vitro susceptibility determined by E test and response to therapy with amphotericin B: results from a multicenter prospective study of candidemia. *Antimicrob. Agents Chemother.* **43:**1289–1290.
40. **Clemons, K. V., and D. A. Stevens.** 2000. Efficacies of sordarin derivatives GM193663, GM211676, and GM237354 in

a murine model of systemic coccidioidomycosis. *Antimicrob. Agents Chemother.* **44**:1874–1877.

41. **Clemons, K. V., and D. A. Stevens.** 1997. Efficacy of nikkomycin Z against experimental pulmonary blastomycosis. *Antimicrob. Agents Chemother.* **41**:2026–2028.
42. **Coleman, D. C., M. G. Rinaldi, K. A. Haynes, J. H. Rex, R. C. Summerbell, E. J. Anaissie, A. Li, and D. J. Sullivan.** 1998. Importance of *Candida* species other than *Candida albicans* as opportunistic pathogens. *Med. Mycol.* **36**:156–165.
43. **Coote, P. J., C. D. Holyoak, D. Bracey, D. P. Ferdinando, and J. A. Pearce.** 1998. Inhibitory action of a truncated derivative of the amphibian skin peptide dermaseptin S3 on *Saccharomyces cerevisiae. Antimicrob. Agents Chemother.* **42**: 2160–2170.
44. **Cowen, L. E., D. Sanglard, D. Calabrese, C. Sirjusingh, J. B. Anderson, and L. M. Kohn.** 2000. Evolution of drug resistance in experimental populations of *Candida albicans. J. Bacteriol.* **182**:1515–1522.
45. **Crowley, J. H., S. J. Smith, F. W. Leak, and L. W. Parks.** 1996. Aerobic isolation of an *ERG24* null mutant of *Saccharomyces cerevisiae. J. Bacteriol.* **178**:2991–2993.
46. **Current, W. L., J. Tang, C. Boylan, W. P., D. Zeckner, W. Turner, M. Rodriguez, C. Dixon, D. Ma, and J. A. Radding.** 1995. Glucan biosynthesis as a target for antifungals: the echinocandin class of antifungal agents, p. 143–160. *In* G. K. Dixon, L. G. Copping, and D. W. Hollomon (ed.), *Antifungal Agents: Discovery and Mode of Action.* BIOS Scientific Publishers, Oxford, United Kingdom.
47. **De Backer, M. D., T. Ilyina, X. J. Ma, S. Vandoninck, W. H. Luyten, and H. Vanden Bossche.** 2001. Genomic profiling of the response of *Candida albicans* to itraconazole treatment using a DNA microarray. *Antimicrob. Agents Chemother.* **45**:1660–1670.
48. **De Backer, M. D., B. Nelissen, M. Logghe, J. Viaene, I. Loonen, S. Vandoninck, R. de Hoogt, S. Dewaele, F. A. Simons, P. Verhasselt, G. Vanhoof, R. Contreras, and W. H. Luyten.** 2001. An antisense-based functional genomics approach for identification of genes critical for growth of *Candida albicans. Nat. Biotechnol.* **19**:235–241.
49. **De Bernardis, F., M. Boccanera, D. Adriani, E. Spreghini, G. Santoni, and A. Cassone.** 1997. Protective role of antimannan and anti-aspartyl proteinase antibodies in an experimental model of *Candida albicans* vaginitis in rats. *Infect. Immun.* **65**:3399–3405.
50. **De Lucca, A. J., J. M. Bland, T. J. Jacks, C. Grimm, and T. J. Walsh.** 1998. Fungicidal and binding properties of the natural peptides cecropin B and dermaseptin. *Med. Mycol.* **36**:291–298.
51. **De Lucca, A. J., J. M. Bland, C. B. Vigo, T. J. Jacks, J. Peter, and T. J. Walsh.** 2000. D-cecropin B: proteolytic resistance, lethality for pathogenic fungi and binding properties. *Med. Mycol.* **38**:301–308.
52. **De Lucca, A. J., and T. J. Walsh.** 1999. Antifungal peptides: novel therapeutic compounds against emerging pathogens. *Antimicrob. Agents Chemother.* **43**:1–11.
53. **De Vroey, C., P. Desmet, Z. Q. Li, P. Mukamurangwa, and C. Raes-Wuytack.** 1996. Further studies on the in vitro antifungal activity of amorolfine. *Mycoses* **39**:41–44.
54. **Diasio, R. B., J. E. Bennett, and C. E. Myers.** 1978. Mode of action of 5-fluorocytosine. *Biochem. Pharmacol.* **27**: 703–707.
55. **Diasio, R. B., D. E. Lakings, and J. E. Bennett.** 1978. Evidence for conversion of 5-fluorocytosine to 5-fluorouracil in humans: possible factor in 5-fluorocytosine clinical toxicity. *Antimicrob. Agents Chemother.* **14**:903–908.
56. **Dick, J. D., W. G. Merz, and R. Saral.** 1980. Incidence of polyene-resistant yeasts recovered from clinical specimens. *Antimicrob. Agents Chemother.* **18**:158–163.
57. **DiDomenico, B.** 1999. Novel antifungal drugs. *Curr. Opin. Microbiol.* **2**:509–515.
58. **Diekema, D. J., M. A. Pfaller, S. A. Messer, A. Houston, R. J. Hollis, G. V. Doern, and R. N. Jones.** 1999. In vitro activities of BMS-207147 against over 600 contemporary clinical bloodstream isolates of *Candida* species from the SENTRY Antimicrobial Surveillance Program in North America and Latin America. *Antimicrob. Agents Chemother.* **43**: 2236–2239.
59. **Dismukes, W. E.** 2000. Introduction to antifungal drugs. *Clin. Infect. Dis.* **30**:653–657.
60. **Dodds, E. S., R. H. Drew, and J. R. Perfect.** 2000. Antifungal pharmacodynamics: review of the literature and clinical applications. *Pharmacotherapy* **20**:1335–1355.
61. **Dominguez, J. M., V. A. Kelly, O. S. Kinsman, M. S. Marriott, F. Gomez de las Heras, and J. J. Martin.** 1998. Sordarins: a new class of antifungals with selective inhibition of the protein synthesis elongation cycle in yeasts. *Antimicrob. Agents Chemother.* **42**:2274–2278.
62. **Douglas, C. M., J. A. D'Ippolito, G. J. Shei, M. Meinz, J. Onishi, J. A. Marrinan, W. Li, G. K. Abruzzo, A. Flattery, K. Bartizal, A. Mitchell, and M. B. Kurtz.** 1997. Identification of the *FKS1* gene of *Candida albicans* as the essential target of 1,3-beta-D-glucan synthase inhibitors. *Antimicrob. Agents Chemother.* **41**:2471–2479.
63. **Douglas, C. M., J. A. Marrinan, W. Li, and M. B. Kurtz.** 1994. A *Saccharomyces cerevisiae* mutant with echinocandin-resistant 1,3-beta-D-glucan synthase. *J. Bacteriol.* **176**: 5686–5696.
64. **Dupont, B., R. Ally, J. Burke, M. R. Hodges, and A. J. Romero.** 2000. A double-blind, randomized, multicenter trial of voriconazole (VORI) vs. fluconazole (FLU) for the treatment of esophageal candidiasis (EC) in immunocompromised adults, abstr. 706, p. 365. *In Abstr. 40th Intersci. Conf. Antimicrob. Agents Chemother.* American Society for Microbiology, Washington, D.C.
65. **Edwards, J. E., Jr., G. P. Bodey, R. A. Bowden, T. Buchner, B. E. de Pauw, S. G. Filler, M. A. Ghannoum, M. Glauser, R. Herbrecht, C. A. Kauffman, S. Kohno, P. Martino, F. Meunier, T. Mori, M. A. Pfaller, J. H. Rex, T. R. Rogers, R. H. Rubin, J. Solomkin, C. Viscoli, T. J. Walsh, and M. White.** 1997. International conference for the development of a consensus on the management and prevention of severe candidal infections. *Clin. Infect. Dis.* **25**:43–59.
66. **Ernst, E. J., M. E. Klepser, and M. A. Pfaller.** 2000. Postantifungal effects of echinocandin, azole, and polyene antifungal agents against *Candida albicans* and *Cryptococcus neoformans. Antimicrob. Agents Chemother.* **44**:1108–1111.
67. **Espinel-Ingroff, A.** 1997. Clinical relevance of antifungal resistance. *Infect. Dis. Clin. N. Am.* **11**:929–944.
68. **Espinel-Ingroff, A.** 1998. In vitro activity of the new triazole voriconazole (UK-109,496) against opportunistic filamentous and dimorphic fungi and common and emerging yeast pathogens. *J. Clin. Microbiol.* **36**:198–202.
69. **Espinel-Ingroff, A., F. Barchiesi, K. C. Hazen, J. V. Martinez-Suarez, and G. Scalise.** 1998. Standardization of antifungal susceptibility testing and clinical relevance. *Med. Mycol.* **36**: 68–78.
70. **Evans, E. G.** 1999. Resistance of *Candida* species to antifungal agents used in the treatment of onychomycosis: a review of current problems. *Br. J. Dermatol.* **141**:33–35.
71. **Favre, B., M. Didmon, and N. S. Ryder.** 1999. Multiple amino acid substitutions in lanosterol 14α-demethylase con-

tribute to azole resistance in *Candida albicans*. *Microbiology* **145**:2715–2725.

72. **Favre, B., and N. S. Ryder.** 1997. Cloning and expression of squalene epoxidase from the pathogenic yeast *Candida albicans*. *Gene* **189**:119–126.
73. **Franz, R., S. L. Kelly, D. C. Lamb, D. E. Kelly, M. Ruhnke, and J. Morschhauser.** 1998. Multiple molecular mechanisms contribute to a stepwise development of fluconazole resistance in clinical *Candida albicans* strains. *Antimicrob. Agents Chemother.* **42**:3065–3072.
74. **Franz, R., S. Michel, and J. Morschhauser.** 1998. A fourth gene from the *Candida albicans* CDR family of ABC transporters. *Gene* **220**:91–98.
75. **Franz, R., M. Ruhnke, and J. Morschhauser.** 1999. Molecular aspects of fluconazole resistance development in *Candida albicans*. *Mycoses* **42**:453–458.
76. **Frost, D. J., M. Knapp, K. Brandt, A. Shadron, and R. C. Goldman.** 1997. Characterization of a lipopeptide-resistant strain of *Candida albicans*. *Can. J. Microbiol.* **43**:122–128.
77. **Fung-Tomc, J. C., B. Minassian, E. Huczko, B. Kolek, D. P. Bonner, and R. E. Kessler.** 1995. In vitro antifungal and fungicidal spectra of a new pradimicin derivative, BMS-181184. *Antimicrob. Agents Chemother.* **39**:295–300.
78. **Fung-Tomc, J. C., T. C. White, B. Minassian, E. Huczko, and D. P. Bonner.** 1999. In vitro antifungal activity of BMS-207147 and itraconazole against yeast strains that are non-susceptible to fluconazole. *Diagn. Microbiol. Infect. Dis.* **35**: 163–167.
79. **Furumai, T., K. Saitoh, M. Kakushima, S. Yamamoto, K. Suzuki, C. Ikeda, S. Kobaru, M. Hatori, and T. Oki.** 1993. BMS-181184, a new pradimicin derivative. Screening, taxonomy, directed biosynthesis, isolation and characterization. *J. Antibiot.* **46**:265–274.
80. **Gallis, H. A., R. H. Drew, and W. W. Pickard.** 1990. Amphotericin B: 30 years of clinical experience. *Rev. Infect. Dis.* **12**: 308–329.
81. **Geber, A., C. A. Hitchcock, J. E. Swartz, F. S. Pullen, K. E. Marsden, K. J. Kwon-Chung, and J. E. Bennett.** 1995. Deletion of the *Candida glabrata ERG3* and *ERG11* genes: effect on cell viability, cell growth, sterol composition, and antifungal susceptibility. *Antimicrob. Agents Chemother.* **39**: 2708–2717.
82. **Georgopapadakou, N. H.** 1998. Antifungals: mechanism of action and resistance, established and novel drugs. *Curr. Opin. Microbiol.* **1**:547–557.
83. **Georgopapadakou, N. H., and T. J. Walsh.** 1996. Antifungal agents: chemotherapeutic targets and immunologic strategies. *Antimicrob. Agents Chemother.* **40**:279–291.
84. **Ghannoum, M. A., and L. B. Rice.** 1999. Antifungal agents: mode of action, mechanisms of resistance, and correlation of these mechanisms with bacterial resistance. *Clin. Microbiol. Rev.* **12**:501–517.
85. **Gonzalez, C. E., A. H. Groll, N. Giri, D. Shetty, I. Al-Mohsen, T. Sein, E. Feuerstein, J. Bacher, S. Piscitelli, and T. J. Walsh.** 1998. Antifungal activity of the pradimicin derivative BMS 181184 in the treatment of experimental pulmonary aspergillosis in persistently neutropenic rabbits. *Antimicrob. Agents Chemother.* **42**:2399–2404.
86. **Graninger, W., E. Presteril, B. Schneeweiss, B. Teleky, and A. Georgopoulos.** 1993. Treatment of *Candida albicans* fungaemia with fluconazole. *J. Infect.* **26**:133–146.
87. **Graybill, J. R., R. Bocanegra, M. Luther, A. Fothergill, and M. J. Rinaldi.** 1997. Treatment of murine *Candida krusei* or *Candida glabrata* infection with L-743,872. *Antimicrob. Agents Chemother.* **41**:1937–1939.
88. **Graybill, J. R., L. K. Najvar, R. Bocanegra, R. F. Hector, and M. F. Luther.** 1998. Efficacy of nikkomycin Z in the treatment of murine histoplasmosis. *Antimicrob. Agents Chemother.* **42**:2371–2374.
89. **Groll, A. H., A. J. De Lucca, and T. J. Walsh.** 1998. Emerging targets for the development of novel antifungal therapeutics. *Trends Microbiol.* **6**:117–124.
90. **Groll, A. H., S. C. Piscitelli, and T. J. Walsh.** 1998. Clinical pharmacology of systemic antifungal agents: a comprehensive review of agents in clinical use, current investigational compounds, and putative targets for antifungal drug development. *Adv. Pharmacol.* **44**:343–500.
91. **Gupta, V., A. Kohli, S. Krishnamurthy, N. Puri, S. A. Aalamgeer, S. Panwar, and R. Prasad.** 1998. Identification of polymorphic mutant alleles of *CaMDR1*, a major facilitator of *Candida albicans* which confers multidrug resistance, and its in vitro transcriptional activation. *Curr. Genet.* **34**:192–199.
92. **Hachem, R. Y., I. I. Raad, C. M. Afif, R. Negroni, J. Graybill, S. Hadley, H. Kantarjian, S. Adams, and G. Mukwaya.** 2000. An open, non-comparative multicenter study to evaluate efficacy and safety of posaconazole (SCH 56592) in the treatment of invasive fungal infections (IFI) refractory (R) to or intolerant (I) to standard therapy (ST), abstr. 232, p. 372. *In Abstr. 40th Intersci. Conf. Antimicrob. Agents Chemother.*, American Society for Microbiology, Washington, D.C.
93. **Han, Y., and J. E. Cutler.** 1997. Assessment of a mouse model of neutropenia and the effect of an anti-candidiasis monoclonal antibody in these animals. *J. Infect. Dis.* **175**: 1169–1175.
94. **Han, Y., M. H. Riesselman, and J. E. Cutler.** 2000. Protection against candidiasis by an immunoglobulin G3 (IgG3) monoclonal antibody specific for the same mannotriose as an IgM protective antibody. *Infect. Immun.* **68**:1649–1654.
95. **Hancock, R. E.** 1999. Host defence (cationic) peptides: what is their future clinical potential? *Drugs* **57**:469–473.
96. **Hancock, R. E., and G. Diamond.** 2000. The role of cationic antimicrobial peptides in innate host defences. *Trends Microbiol.* **8**:402–410.
97. **Hancock, R. E., and M. G. Scott.** 2000. The role of antimicrobial peptides in animal defenses. *Proc. Natl. Acad. Sci. USA* **97**:8856–8861.
98. **Haria, M., and H. M. Bryson.** 1995. Amorolfine. A review of its pharmacological properties and therapeutic potential in the treatment of onychomycosis and other superficial fungal infections. *Drugs* **49**:103–120.
99. **Harris, G. H., A. Shafiee, M. A. Cabello, J. E. Curotto, O. Genilloud, K. E. Goklen, M. B. Kurtz, M. Rosenbach, P. M. Salmon, R. A. Thornton, D. L. Zink, and S. M. Mandala.** 1998. Inhibition of fungal sphingolipid biosynthesis by rustmicin, galbonolide B and their new 21-hydroxy analogs. *J. Antibiot.* **51**:837–844.
100. **Hartman, P. G., and D. Sanglard.** 1997. Inhibitors of ergostrol biosynthesis as antifungal agents. *Curr. Pharmaceutic. Design* **3**:177–208.
101. **Hartsel, S., and J. Bolard.** 1996. Amphotericin B: new life for an old drug. *Trends Pharmacol. Sci.* **17**:445–449.
102. **Hashida-Okado, T., A. Ogawa, I. Kato, and K. Takesako.** 1998. Transformation system for prototrophic industrial yeasts using the *AUR1* gene as a dominant selection marker. *FEBS Lett.* **425**:117–122.
103. **Hashida-Okado, T., R. Yasumoto, M. Endo, K. Takesako, and I. Kato.** 1998. Isolation and characterization of the aureobasidin A-resistant gene, *aur1R*, on *Schizosaccharomyces pombe*: roles of Aur1p+ in cell morphogenesis. *Curr. Genet.* **33**:38–45.
104. **Hector, R. F., B. L. Zimmer, and D. Pappagianis.** 1990. Evaluation of nikkomycin X and Z in murine model of coccidioi-

domycosis, histoplasmosis and blastomycosis. *Antimicrob. Agents Chemother.* **34:**587–593.

105. **Heidler, S. A., and J. A. Radding.** 1995. The *AUR1* gene in *Saccharomyces cerevisiae* encodes dominant resistance to the antifungal agent aureobasidin A (LY295337). *Antimicrob. Agents Chemother.* **39:**2765–2769.
106. **Heidler, S. A., and J. A. Radding.** 2000. Inositol phosphoryl transferases from human pathogenic fungi. *Biochim. Biophys. Acta* **1500:**147–152.
107. **Helmerhorst, E. J., P. Breeuwer, W. van't Hof, E. Walgreen-Weterings, L. C. Oomen, E. C. Veerman, A. V. Amerongen, and T. Abee.** 1999. The cellular target of histatin 5 on *Candida albicans* is the energized mitochondrion. *J. Biol. Chem.* **274:**7286–7291.
108. **Helmerhorst, E. J., I. M. Reijnders, W. van't Hof, I. Simoons-Smit, E. C. Veerman, and A. V. Amerongen.** 1999. Amphotericin B- and fluconazole-resistant *Candida* spp., *Aspergillus fumigatus,* and other newly emerging pathogenic fungi are susceptible to basic antifungal peptides. *Antimicrob. Agents Chemother.* **43:**702–704.
109. **Henry, K. W., M. C. Cruz, S. K. Katiyar, and T. D. Edlind.** 1999. Antagonism of azole activity against *Candida albicans* following induction of multidrug resistance genes by selected antimicrobial agents. *Antimicrob. Agents Chemother.* **43:**1968–1974.
110. **Henry, K. W., J. T. Nickels, and T. D. Edlind.** 2000. Upregulation of *ERG* genes in *Candida* species by azoles and other sterol biosynthesis inhibitors. *Antimicrob. Agents Chemother.* **44:**2693–2700.
111. **Hernaez, M. L., C. Gil, J. Pla, and C. Nombela.** 1998. Induced expression of the *Candida albicans* multidrug resistance gene *CDR1* in response to fluconazole and other antifungals. *Yeast* **14:**517–526.
112. **Herreros, E., C. M. Martinez, M. J. Almela, M. S. Marriott, F. G. De Las Heras, and D. Gargallo-Viola.** 1998. Sordarins: in vitro activities of new antifungal derivatives against pathogenic yeasts, *Pneumocystis carinii,* and filamentous fungi. *Antimicrob. Agents Chemother.* **42:**2863–2869.
113. **Hiratani, T., and H. Yamaguchi.** 1994. Cross-resistance of *Candida albicans* to several different families of antifungals with ergosterol biosynthesis-inhibiting activity. *Jpn. J. Antibiot.* **47:**125–128.
114. **Hitchcock, C. A., B. K. Barrett, and N. J. Russell.** 1986. The lipid composition of azole-sensitive and azole-resistant strains of *Candida albicans. J. Gen. Microbiol.* **132:**2421–2431.
115. **Hitchcock, C. A., G. W. Pye, G. P. Oliver, and P. F. Troke.** 1995. UK-109,496, a novel, wide-spectrum triazole derivative for the treatment of fungal infections: antifungal activity and selectivity in vitro, abstr. F72, p. 125. *In Abstr. 35th Intersci. Conf. Antimicrob. Agents Chemother.* American Society for Microbiology, Washington, D.C.
116. **Hitchcock, C. A., G. W. Pye, P. F. Troke, E. M. Johnson, and D. W. Warnock.** 1993. Fluconazole resistance in *Candida glabrata. Antimicrob. Agents Chemother.* **37:**1962–1965.
117. **Holt, R. J., and A. Azmi.** 1978. Miconazole-resistant *Candida. Lancet* **i:**50–51.
118. **Horsburgh, C. R., and C. H. Kirkpatrick.** 1983. Long-term therapy of chronic mucocutaneous candidiasis with ketoconazole: experience with twenty-one patients. *Am. J. Med.* **74**(Suppl. 1B)**:**23–29.
119. **Hostetler, J. S., K. V. Clemons, L. H. Hanson, and D. A. Stevens.** 1992. Efficacy and safety of amphotericin B colloidal dispersion compared with those of amphotericin B deoxycholate suspension for treatment of disseminated murine cryptococcosis. *Antimicrob. Agents Chemother.* **36:**2656–2660.
120. **Hughes, T. R., M. J. Marton, A. R. Jones, C. J. Roberts, R. Stoughton, C. D. Armour, H. A. Bennett, E. Coffey, H. Dai, Y. D. He, M. J. Kidd, A. M. King, M. R. Meyer, D. Slade, P. Y. Lum, S. B. Stepaniants, D. D. Shoemaker, D. Gachotte, K. Chakraburtty, J. Simon, M. Bard, and S. H. Friend.** 2000. Functional discovery via a compendium of expression profiles. *Cell* **102:**109–126.
121. **Ikeda, F., Y. Wakai, S. Matsumoto, K. Maki, E. Watabe, S. Tawara, T. Goto, Y. Watanabe, F. Matsumoto, and S. Kuwahara.** 2000. Efficacy of FK463, a new lipopeptide antifungal agent, in mouse models of disseminated candidiasis and aspergillosis. *Antimicrob. Agents Chemother.* **44:**614–618.
122. **Jacob, L., and M. Zasloff.** 1994. Potential therapeutic applications of magainins and other antimicrobial agents of animal origin. *Ciba Found. Symp.* **186:**197–216.
123. **Jandrositz, A., F. Turnowsky, and G. Hogenauer.** 1991. The gene encoding squalene epoxidase from *Saccharomyces cerevisiae:* cloning and characterization. *Gene* **107:**155–160.
124. **Jessup, C. J., N. S. Ryder, and M. A. Ghannoum.** 2000. An evaluation of the in vitro activity of terbinafine. *Med. Mycol.* **38:**155–159.
125. **Jessup, C. J., J. Warner, N. Isham, I. Hasan, and M. A. Ghannoum.** 2000. Antifungal susceptibility testing of dermatophytes: establishing a medium for inducing conidial growth and evaluation of susceptibility of clinical isolates. *J. Clin. Microbiol.* **38:**341–344.
126. **Johnson, E. M., M. D. Richardson, and D. W. Warnock.** 1984. In vitro resistance with imidazole antifungals in *Candida albicans. J. Antimicrob. Chemother.* **13:**541–558.
127. **Justice, M. C., T. Ku, M. J. Hsu, K. Carniol, D. Schmatz, and J. Nielsen.** 1999. Mutations in ribosomal protein L10e confer resistance to the fungal-specific eukaryotic elongation factor 2 inhibitor sordarin. *J. Biol. Chem.* **274:**4869–4875.
128. **Kakeya, H., Y. Miyazaki, H. Miyazaki, K. Nyswaner, B. Grimberg, and J. E. Bennett.** 2000. Genetic analysis of azole resistance in the Darlington strain of *Candida albicans. Antimicrob. Agents Chemother.* **44:**2985–2990.
129. **Kelly, S. L., D. C. Lamb, B. C. Baldwin, A. J. Corran, and D. E. Kelly.** 1997. Characterization of *Saccharomyces cerevisiae* CYP61, sterol delta22-desaturase, and inhibition by azole antifungal agents. *J. Biol. Chem.* **272:**9986–9988.
130. **Kelly, S. L., D. C. Lamb, A. J. Corran, B. C. Baldwin, and D. E. Kelly.** 1995. Mode of action and resistance to azole antifungals associated with the formation of 14α-methylergosta-8,24(28)-dien-3β,6α-diol. *Biochem. Biophys. Res. Commun.* **207:**910–915.
131. **Kelly, S. L., D. C. Lamb, and D. E. Kelly.** 1999. Y132H substitution in *Candida albicans* sterol 14alpha-demethylase confers fluconazole resistance by preventing binding to haem. *FEMS Microbiol. Lett.* **180:**171–175.
132. **Kelly, S. L., D. C. Lamb, D. E. Kelly, J. Loeffler, and H. Einsele.** 1996. Resistance to fluconazole and amphotericin in *Candida albicans* from AIDS patients. *Lancet* **348:**1523–1524.
133. **Kelly, S. L., D. C. Lamb, J. Loeffler, H. Einsele, and D. E. Kelly.** 1999. The G464S amino acid substitution in *Candida albicans* sterol 14alpha-demethylase causes fluconazole resistance in the clinic through reduced affinity. *Biochem. Biophys. Res. Commun.* **262:**174–179.
134. **Kelly, S. L., D. C. Lamb, M. Taylor, A. J. Corran, B. C. Baldwin, and W. G. Powderly.** 1994. Resistance to amphotericin B associated with defective sterol delta 8-7 isomerase in a *Cryptococcus neoformans* strain from an AIDS patient. *FEMS Microbiol. Lett.* **122:**39–42.
135. **Kerridge, D., M. Fasoli, and J. F. Wayman.** 1988. Drug resis-

tance in *Candida albicans* and *Candida glabrata*. *Ann. N. Y. Acad. Sci.* **544:**245–259.

136. **Kerridge, D., and H. Vanden Bossche.** 1990. Drug discovery: a biochemist's approach. *Handbook Exp. Pharmacol.* **96:** 31–76.
137. **Kino, K., Y. Taguchi, K. Yamada, T. Komano, and K. Ueda.** 1996. Aureobasidin A, an antifungal cyclic depsipeptide antibiotic, is a substrate for both human MDR1 and MDR2/P-glycoproteins. *FEBS Lett.* **399:**29–32.
138. **Klepser, M. E., H. L. Hoffman, and E. J. Ernst.** 2000. Novel triazole antifungal agents. *Exp. Opin. Investig. Drugs* **9:** 593–605.
139. **Koshlukova, S. E., M. W. Araujo, D. Baev, and M. Edgerton.** 2000. Released ATP is an extracellular cytotoxic mediator in salivary histatin 5-induced killing of *Candida albicans*. *Infect. Immun.* **68:**6848–6856.
140. **Koshlukova, S. E., T. L. Lloyd, M. W. Araujo, and M. Edgerton.** 1999. Salivary histatin 5 induces non-lytic release of ATP from *Candida albicans* leading to cell death. *J. Biol. Chem.* **274:**18872–18879.
141. **Krishnamurthy, S., V. Gupta, R. Prasad, S. L. Panwar, and R. Prasad.** 1998. Expression of *CDR1*, a multidrug resistance gene of *Candida albicans*—transcriptional activation by heat shock, drugs and human steroid hormones. *FEMS Microbiol. Lett.* **160:**191–197.
142. **Kuehnert, M. J., E. Clark, S. R. Lockhart, D. R. Soll, J. Chia, and W. R. Jarvis.** 1998. *Candida albicans* endocarditis associated with a contaminated aortic valve allograft: implications for regulation of allograft processing. *Clin. Infect. Dis.* **27:** 688–691.
143. **Kuroda, M., T. Hashida-Okado, R. Yasumoto, K. Gomi, I. Kato, and K. Takesako.** 1999. An aureobasidin A resistance gene isolated from *Aspergillus* is a homolog of yeast *AUR1*, a gene responsible for inositol phosphorylceramide (IPC) synthase activity. *Mol. Gen. Genet.* **261:**290–296.
144. **Kurome, T., T. Inoue, K. Takesako, and I. Kato.** 1998. Syntheses of antifungal aureobasidin A analogs with alkyl chains for structure-activity relationship. *J. Antibiot.* **51:**359–367.
145. **Kurose, I., T. Yamada, R. Wolf, and D. N. Granger.** 1994. P-selectin-dependent leukocyte recruitment and intestinal mucosal injury induced by lactoferrin. *J. Leukoc. Biol.* **55:** 771–777.
146. **Kurtz, M. B., G. Abruzzo, A. Flattery, K. Bartizal, J. A. Marrinan, W. Li, J. Milligan, K. Nollstadt, and C. M. Douglas.** 1996. Characterization of echinocandin-resistant mutants of *Candida albicans:* genetic, biochemical, and virulence studies. *Infect. Immun.* **64:**3244–32451.
147. **Kurtz, M. B., and C. M. Douglas.** 1997. Lipopeptide inhibitors of fungal glucan synthase. *J. Med. Vet. Mycol.* **35:**79–86.
148. **Lai, M. H., M. Bard, C. A. Pierson, J. F. Alexander, M. Goebl, G. T. Carter, and D. R. Kirsch.** 1994. The identification of a gene family in the *Saccharomyces cerevisiae* ergosterol biosynthesis pathway. *Gene* **140:**41–49.
149. **Lamb, D. C., A. Corran, B. C. Baldwin, J. Kwon-Chung, and S. L. Kelly.** 1995. Resistant P450A1 activity in azole antifungal tolerant *Cryptococcus neoformans* from AIDS patients. *FEBS Lett.* **368:**326–330.
150. **Lamb, D. C., D. E. Kelly, T. C. White, and S. L. Kelly.** 2000. The R467K amino acid substitution in *Candida albicans* sterol 14alpha-demethylase causes drug resistance through reduced affinity. *Antimicrob. Agents Chemother.* **44:**63–67.
151. **Larsen, R. A., S. A. Bozzette, B. E. Jones, D. Haghighat, M. A. Leal, D. Forthal, M. Bauer, J. G. Tilles, J. A. McCutchan, and J. M. Leedom.** 1994. Fluconazole combined with flucytosine for treatment of cryptococcal meningitis in patients with AIDS. *Clin. Infect. Dis.* **19:**741–745.
152. **Larsen, R. A., M. A. Leal, and L. S. Chan.** 1990. Fluconazole compared with amphotericin B plus flucytosine for cryptococcal meningitis in AIDS. A randomized trial. *Ann. Intern. Med.* **113:**183–187.
153. **Larson, J. L., T. L. Wallace, R. W. Tyl, M. C. Marr, C. B. Myers, and P. A. Cossum.** 2000. The reproductive and developmental toxicity of the antifungal drug Nyotran (liposomal nystatin) in rats and rabbits. *Toxicol. Sci.* **53:**421–429.
154. **Li, R. K., M. A. Ciblak, N. Nordoff, L. Pasarell, D. W. Warnock, and M. R. McGinnis.** 2000. In vitro activities of voriconazole, itraconazole, and amphotericin B against *Blastomyces dermatitidis, Coccidioides immitis,* and *Histoplasma capsulatum*. *Antimicrob. Agents Chemother.* **44:**1734–1736.
155. **Lim, E., P. Wong, M. Fadem, P. Motchnik, B. M., and R. Little.** 1996. Fungicidal activity of synthetic peptides derived from bactericidal/permeability-increasing protein (BPI), abstr. F-185, p. 132. *In Abstr. 36th Intersci. Conf. Antimicrob. Agents Chemother.* American Society for Microbiology, Washington, D.C.
156. **Loffler, J., S. L. Kelly, H. Hebart, U. Schumacher, C. Lass-Florl, and H. Einsele.** 1997. Molecular analysis of CYP51 from fluconazole-resistant *Candida albicans* strains. *FEMS Microbiol. Lett.* **151:**263–268.
157. **Lomovskaya, O., M. Warren, A. Mistry, A. Staley, J. Galazzo, H. Fuernkranz, M. Lee, G. H. Miller, and D. Sanglard.** 1999. Inhibitors of fungal efflux pumps, abstr. 1269, p. 328. *In Abstr. 39th Intersci. Conf. Antimicrob. Agents Chemother.* American Society for Microbiology, Washington, D.C.
158. **Lopez-Ribot, J., R. K. McAtee, L. Lee, W. R. Kirkpatrick, T. C. White, D. Sanglard, and T. F. Patterson.** 1998. Distinct patterns of gene expression associated with the development of fluconazole resistance in serial *Candida albicans* isolates from HIV-infected patients with oropharyngeal candidiasis. *Antimicrob. Agents Chemother.* **42:**2932–2937.
159. **Lyman, C. A., and T. J. Walsh.** 1992. Systemically administered antifungal agents. A review of their clinical pharmacology and therapeutic applications. *Drugs* **44:**9–35.
160. **Mandala, S. M., and G. H. Harris.** 2000. Isolation and characterization of novel inhibitors of sphingolipid synthesis: australifungin, viridiofungins, rustmicin, and khafrefungin. *Methods Enzymol.* **311:**335–348.
161. **Mandala, S. M., R. A. Thornton, J. Milligan, M. Rosenbach, M. Garcia-Calvo, H. G. Bull, G. Harris, G. K. Abruzzo, A. M. Flattery, C. J. Gill, K. Bartizal, S. Dreikorn, and M. B. Kurtz.** 1998. Rustmicin, a potent antifungal agent, inhibits sphingolipid synthesis at inositol phosphoceramide synthase. *J. Biol. Chem.* **273:**14942–14949.
162. **Mandala, S. M., R. A. Thornton, M. Rosenbach, J. Milligan, M. Garcia-Calvo, H. G. Bull, and M. B. Kurtz.** 1997. Khafrefungin, a novel inhibitor of sphingolipid synthesis. *J. Biol. Chem.* **272:**32709–32714.
163. **Marichal, P., L. Koymans, S. Willemsens, D. Bellens, P. Verhasselt, W. Luyten, M. Borgers, F. C. Ramaekers, F. C. Odds, and H. V. Bossche.** 1999. Contribution of mutations in the cytochrome P450 14α-demethylase (Erg11p, Cyp51p) to azole resistance in *Candida albicans*. *Microbiology* **145:** 2701–2713.
164. **Marichal, P., H. Vanden Bossche, F. C. Odds, G. Nobels, D. W. Warnock, V. Timmerman, C. Van Broeckhoven, S. Fay, and P. Mose-Larsen.** 1997. Molecular biological characterization of an azole-resistant *Candida glabrata* isolate. *Antimicrob. Agents Chemother.* **41:**2229–2237.
165. **Marr, K. A., C. N. Lyons, K. Ha, T. R. Rustad, and T. C. White.** 2001. Inducible azole resistance associated with a heterogeneous phenotype in *Candida albicans*. *Antimicrob. Agents Chemother.* **45:**52–59.

166. **Marr, K. A., C. N. Lyons, T. R. Rustad, R. A. Bowden, T. C. White, and T. Rustad.** 1998. Rapid, transient fluconazole resistance in *Candida albicans* is associated with increased mRNA levels of *CDR*. *Antimicrob. Agents Chemother.* **42:**2584–2589.
167. **Marr, K. A., T. C. White, J. A. van Burik, and R. A. Bowden.** 1997. Development of fluconazole resistance in *Candida albicans* causing disseminated infection in a patient undergoing marrow transplantation. *Clin. Infect. Dis.* **25:**908–910.
168. **Martinez, A., P. Aviles, E. Jimenez, J. Caballero, and D. Gargallo-Viola.** 2000. Activities of sordarins in experimental models of candidiasis, aspergillosis, and pneumocystosis. *Antimicrob. Agents Chemother.* **44:**3389–3394.
169. **Marton, M. J., J. L. DeRisi, H. A. Bennett, V. R. Iyer, M. R. Meyer, C. J. Roberts, R. Stoughton, J. Burchard, D. Slade, H. Dai, D. E. Bassett, Jr., L. H. Hartwell, P. O. Brown, and S. H. Friend.** 1998. Drug target validation and identification of secondary drug target effects using DNA microarrays. *Nat. Med.* **4:**1293–1301.
170. **Mason, A. B., T. B. Kardos, D. S. Perlin, and B. C. Monk.** 1996. Functional complementation between transmembrane loops of *Saccharomyces cerevisiae* and *Candida albicans* plasma membrane H(+)-ATPases. *Biochim. Biophys. Acta* **1284:**181–190.
171. **Matsumoto, S., Y. Wakai, T. Nakai, K. Hatano, T. Ushitani, F. Ikeda, S. Tawara, T. Goto, F. Matsumoto, and S. Kuwahara.** 2000. Efficacy of FK463, a new lipopeptide antifungal agent, in mouse models of pulmonary aspergillosis. *Antimicrob. Agents Chemother.* **44:**619–621.
172. **Mencacci, A., G. Del Soro, E. Cenci, C. Fè d'Ostani, A. Bacci, C. Motagnoli, M. Kopf, and L. Romani.** 1998. Endogenous interleukin 4 is required for development of protective CD4+ T helper type 1 cell response to *Candida albicans*. *J. Exp. Med.* **1877:**307–317.
173. **Mercer, E. I.** 1991. Morpholine antifungals and their mode of action. *Biochem. Soc. Trans.* **19:**788–793.
174. **Mikamo, H., Y. Sato, and T. Tamaya.** 2000. In vitro antifungal activity of FK463, a new water-soluble echinocandin-like lipopeptide. *J. Antimicrob. Chemother.* **46:**485–487.
175. **Mio, T., M. Adachi-Shimizu, Y. Tachibana, H. Tabuchi, S. B. Inoue, T. Yabe, T. Yamada-Okabe, M. Arisawa, T. Watanabe, and H. Yamada-Okabe.** 1997. Cloning of the *Candida albicans* homolog of *Saccharomyces cerevisiae GSC1/FKS1* and its involvement in beta-1,3-glucan synthesis. *J. Bacteriol.* **179:**4096–4105.
176. **Mistry, A., M. S. Warren, J. Blais, A. L. Staley, J. L. Galazzo, H. Fuernkranz, S. Chamberland, M. D. Lee, W. J. Watkins, O. Lomovskaya, G. H. Miller, and D. Sanglard.** 2000. More inhibitors of fungal efflux pumps, abstr. 1500, p. 208. *In Abstr. 40th Intersci. Conf. Antimicrob. Agents Chemother.* American Society for Microbiology, Washington, D.C.
177. **Miyahara, K., D. Hirata, and T. Miyakawa.** 1996. yAP-1- and yAP-2-mediated, heat shock-induced transcriptional activation of the multidrug resistance ABC transporter genes in *Saccharomyces cerevisiae*. *Curr. Genet.* **29:**103–105.
178. **Miyazaki, H., Y. Miyazaki, A. Geber, T. Parkinson, C. Hitchcock, D. J. Falconer, D. J. Ward, K. Marsden, and J. E. Bennett.** 1998. Fluconazole resistance associated with drug efflux and increased transcription of a drug transporter gene, *PDH1*, in *Candida glabrata*. *Antimicrob. Agents Chemother.* **42:**1695–1701.
179. **Miyazaki, Y., A. Geber, H. Miyazaki, D. Falconer, T. Parkinson, C. Hitchcock, B. Grimberg, K. Nyswaner, and J. E. Bennett.** 1999. Cloning, sequencing, expression and allelic sequence diversity of *ERG3* (C-5 sterol desaturase gene) in *Candida albicans*. *Gene* **236:**43–51.
180. **Mondon, P., R. Petter, G. Amalfitano, R. Luzzati, E. Concia, I. Polacheck, and K. J. Kwon-Chung.** 1999. Heteroresistance to fluconazole and voriconazole in *Cryptococcus neoformans*. *Antimicrob. Agents Chemother.* **43:**1856–1861.
181. **Mor, A., M. Amiche, and P. Nicolas.** 1994. Structure, synthesis, and activity of dermaseptin b, a novel vertebrate defensive peptide from frog skin: relationship with adenoregulin. *Biochemistry* **33:**6642–6650.
182. **Mor, A., K. Hani, and P. Nicolas.** 1994. The vertebrate peptide antibiotics dermaseptins have overlapping structural features but target specific microorganisms. *J. Biol. Chem.* **269:**31635–31641.
183. **Moran, G. P., D. Sanglard, S. Donnelly, D. B. Shanley, D. J. Sullivan, and D. C. Coleman.** 1998. Identification and expression of multidrug transporters responsible for fluconazole resistance in *Candida dubliniensis*. *Antimicrob. Agents Chemother.* **42:**1819–1830.
184. **Moran, G. P., D. J. Sullivan, M. C. Henman, C. E. McCreary, B. J. Harrington, D. B. Shanley, and D. C. Coleman.** 1997. Antifungal drug susceptibilities of oral *Candida dubliniensis* isolates from human immunodeficiency virus (HIV)-infected and non-HIV-infected subjects and generation of stable fluconazole-resistant derivatives in vitro. *Antimicrob. Agents Chemother.* **41:**617–623.
185. **Muller, F. M., C. A. Lyman, and T. J. Walsh.** 1999. Antimicrobial peptides as potential new antifungals. *Mycoses* **42:**77–82.
186. **Nagiec, M. M., E. E. Nagiec, J. A. Baltisberger, G. B. Wells, R. L. Lester, and R. C. Dickson.** 1997. Sphingolipid synthesis as a target for antifungal drugs. Complementation of the inositol phosphorylceramide synthase defect in a mutant strain of *Saccharomyces cerevisiae* by the *AUR1* gene. *J. Biol. Chem.* **272:**9809–9817.
187. **National Committee for Clinical Laboratory Standards.** 1995. Reference method for broth dilution antifungal susceptibility testing of yeast. Tentative standard M27-A, Vol. 12. National Committee for Clinical Laboratory Standards, Villanova, Pa.
188. **Neely, M. N., and M. A. Ghannoum.** 2000. The exciting future of antifungal therapy. *Eur. J. Clin. Microbiol. Infect. Dis.* **19:**897–914.
189. **Nelson, D. R., L. Koymans, T. Kamataki, J. J. Stegeman, R. Feyereisen, D. J. Waxman, M. R. Waterman, O. Gotoh, M. J. Coon, R. W. Estabrook, I. C. Gunsalus, and D. W. Nebert.** 1996. P450 superfamily: update on new sequences, gene mapping, accession numbers and nomenclature. *Pharmacogenetics* **6:**1–42.
190. **Nguyen, M. H., J. E. Peacock, Jr., A. J. Morris, D. C. Tanner, M. L. Nguyen, D. R. Snydman, M. M. Wagener, M. G. Rinaldi, and V. L. Yu.** 1996. The changing face of candidemia: emergence of non-*Candida albicans* species and antifungal resistance. *Am. J. Med.* **100:**617–623.
191. **Nieto, L., R. Northland, P. Pittisuttithum, C. Firnhaber, S. Jacobson, W. Greaves, R. T. Plott, and M. Taglietti.** 2000. Posaconazole equivalent to fluconazole in the treatment of oropharyngeal candidiasis, abstr. 1108, p. 372. *In Abstr. 40th Intersci. Conf. Antimicrob. Agents Chemother.* American Society for Microbiology, Washington, D.C.
192. **Niewerth, M., and H. C. Korting.** 2000. The use of systemic antimycotics in dermatotherapy. *Eur. J. Dermatol.* **10:**155–160.
193. **Nolte, F. S., T. Parkinson, D. J. Falconer, S. Dix, J. Williams, C. Gilmore, R. Geller, and J. R. Wingard.** 1997. Isolation and characterization of fluconazole- and amphotericin B-resistant *Candida albicans* from blood of two patients with leukemia. *Antimicrob. Agents Chemother.* **44:**196–199.

194. **Norris, H. A., B. E. Elewski, and M. A. Ghannoum.** 1999. Optimal growth conditions for the determination of the antifungal susceptibility of three species of dermatophytes with the use of microdilution method. *J. Am. Acad. Dermatol.* **40:** S9–S13.
195. **Ogawa, A., T. Hashida-Okado, M. Endo, H. Yoshioka, T. Tsuruo, K. Takesako, and I. Kato.** 1998. Role of ABC transporters in aureobasidin A resistance. *Antimicrob. Agents Chemother.* **42:**755–761.
196. **Oki, T., M. Kakushima, M. Hirano, A. Takahashi, A. Ohta, S. Masuyoshi, M. Hatori, and H. Kamei.** 1992. In vitro and in vivo antifungal activities of BMS-181184. *J. Antibiot.* **45:** 1512–1517.
197. **Oki, T., K. Saitoh, K. Tomatsu, K. Tomita, M. Konishi, and H. Kawaguchi.** 1988. Novel antifungal antibiotic BMY-28567. Structural study and biological activities. *Ann. N. Y. Acad. Sci.* **544:**184–187.
198. **Oki, T., Y. Yamazaki, T. Furumai, and Y. Igarashi.** 1997. Pradimicin, a mannose-binding antibiotic, induced carbohydrate-mediated apoptosis in U937 cells. *Biosci. Biotechnol. Biochem.* **61:**1408–1410.
199. **Oki, T., Y. Yamazaki, N. Nomura, T. Furumai, and Y. Igarashi.** 1999. High-mannose type oligosaccharide-dependent apoptosis in U937 cells induced by pradimicin, a mannose-binding antibiotic. *J. Antibiot.* **52:**449–454.
200. **Oki, T., Y. Yamazaki, N. Nomura, T. Furumai, and Y. Igarashi.** 1999. Involvement of Ca2+ ion and reactive oxygen species as a mediator in pradimicin-induced apoptosis. *J. Antibiot.* **52:**455–459.
201. **Onishi, J., M. Meinz, J. Thompson, J. Curotto, S. Dreikorn, M. Rosenbach, C. Douglas, G. Abruzzo, A. Flattery, L. Kong, A. Cabello, F. Vicente, F. Pelaez, M. T. Diez, I. Martin, G. Bills, R. Giacobbe, A. Dombrowski, R. Schwartz, S. Morris, G. Harris, A. Tsipouras, K. Wilson, and M. B. Kurtz.** 2000. Discovery of novel antifungal (1,3)-beta-D-glucan synthase inhibitors. *Antimicrob. Agents Chemother.* **44:**368–377.
202. **Oxford, A. E., M. Raistrick, and P. Simonart.** 1939. Studies in biochemistry of microorganisms LX griseofulvin $C_{17}H_{16}O_6Cl$ metabolic product of *Penicillium griseoulvin. Biochem. J.* **33:**240–248.
203. **Parkinson, T., D. J. Falconer, and C. A. Hitchcock.** 1995. Fluconazole resistance due to energy-dependent drug efflux in *Candida glabrata. Antimicrob. Agents Chemother.* **39:** 1696–1699.
204. **Pereira, M., M. S. Felipe, M. M. Brigido, C. M. Soares, and M. O. Azevedo.** 2000. Molecular cloning and characterization of a glucan synthase gene from the human pathogenic fungus *Paracoccidioides brasiliensis. Yeast* **16:**451–462.
205. **Perlin, D. S., D. Seto-Young, and B. C. Monk.** 1997. The plasma membrane H(+)-ATPase of fungi. A candidate drug target? *Ann. N. Y. Acad. Sci.* **834:**609–617.
206. **Petraitiene, R., V. Petraitis, A. H. Groll, M. Candelario, T. Sein, A. Bell, C. A. Lyman, C. L. McMillian, J. Bacher, and T. J. Walsh.** 1999. Antifungal activity of LY303366, a novel echinocandin B, in experimental disseminated candidiasis in rabbits. *Antimicrob. Agents Chemother.* **43:**2148–2155.
207. **Petraitis, V., R. Petraitiene, A. H. Groll, A. Bell, D. P. Callender, T. Sein, R. L. Schaufele, C. L. McMillian, J. Bacher, and T. J. Walsh.** 1998. Antifungal efficacy, safety, and single-dose pharmacokinetics of LY303366, a novel echinocandin B, in experimental pulmonary aspergillosis in persistently neutropenic rabbits. *Antimicrob. Agents Chemother.* **42:**2898–2905.
208. **Peyron, F., A. Favel, A. Michel-Nguyen, M. Gilly, P. Regli, and A. Bolmstrom.** 2001. Improved detection of amphotericin B-resistant isolates of *Candida lusitaniae* by Etest. *J. Clin. Microbiol.* **39:**339–342.
209. **Pfaller, M. A., R. N. Jones, G. V. Doern, A. C. Fluit, J. Verhoef, H. S. Sader, S. A. Messer, A. Houston, S. Coffman, and R. J. Hollis.** 1999. International surveillance of blood stream infections due to *Candida* species in the European SENTRY program: species distribution and antifungal susceptibility including the investigational triazole and echinocandin agents. SENTRY Participant Group (Europe). *Diagn. Microbiol. Infect. Dis.* **35:**19–25.
210. **Pfaller, M. A., S. A. Messer, and S. Coffman.** 1997. In vitro susceptibilities of clinical yeast isolates to a new echinocandin derivative, LY303366, and other antifungal agents. *Antimicrob. Agents Chemother.* **41:**763–766.
211. **Pfaller, M. A., S. A. Messer, and R. J. Hollis.** 1994. Strain delineation an antifungal susceptibilities of epidemiologically releated and unrelated isolates of *Candida lusitaniae. Diagn. Microbiol. Infect. Dis.* **20:**127–133.
212. **Pfaller, M. A., S. A. Messer, R. J. Hollis, R. N. Jones, G. V. Doern, M. E. Brandt, and R. A. Hajjeh.** 1998. In vitro susceptibilities of *Candida* bloodstream isolates to the new triazole antifungal agents BMS-207147, SCH 56592, and voriconazole. *Antimicrob. Agents Chemother.* **42:** 3242–3244.
213. **Pfaller, M. A., S. A. Messer, R. J. Hollis, R. N. Jones, G. V. Doern, M. E. Brandt, and R. A. Hajjeh.** 1999. Trends in species distribution and susceptibility to fluconazole among blood stream isolates of *Candida* species in the United States. *Diagn. Microbiol. Infect. Dis.* **33:**217–222.
214. **Podust, L. M., T. L. Poulos, and M. R. Waterman.** 2001. Crystal structure of cytochrome P450 14α-sterol demethylase (CYP51) from *Mycobacterium tuberculosis* in complex with azole inhibitors. *Proc. Natl. Acad. Sci. USA* **98:**3068–3073.
215. **Polak, A.** 1990. Mode of action studies, p. 153–182. *In* J. F. Ryley (ed.), *Chemotherapy of Fungal Diseases.* Springer-Verlag, Berlin, Germany.
216. **Polak, A.** 1992. Preclinical data and mode of action of amorolfine. *Dermatology* **184:**3–7.
217. **Polak, A., and P. G. Hartman.** 1991. Antifungal chemotherapy. *Progr. Drug Res.* **37:**181–269.
218. **Polak, A., and H. J. Scholer.** 1975. Mode of action of 5-fluorocytosine and mechanisms of resistance. *Chemotherapy* **21:**113–130.
219. **Polonelli, L., and A. Cassone.** 1999. Novel strategies for treating candidiasis. *Curr. Opin. Infect. Dis.* **12:**61–66.
220. **Powderly, W. G., G. S. Kobayashi, G. P. Herzig, and G. Medoff.** 1988. Amphotericin B-resistant yeast infection in severely immunocompromised patients. *Am. J. Med.* **84:**826–832.
221. **Powles, M. A., P. Liberator, J. Anderson, Y. Karkhanis, J. F. Dropinski, F. A. Bouffard, J. M. Balkovec, H. Fujioka, M. Aikawa, D. McFadden, and D. Schmatz.** 1998. Efficacy of MK-991 (L-743,872), a semisynthetic pneumocandin, in murine models of *Pneumocystis carinii. Antimicrob. Agents Chemother.* **42:**1985–1989.
222. **Puri, N., S. Krishnamurthy, S. Habib, S. E. Hasnain, S. K. Goswami, and R. Prasad.** 1999. *CDR1*, a multidrug resistance gene from *Candida albicans*, contains multiple regulatory domains in its promoter and the distal AP-1 element mediates its induction by miconazole. *FEMS Microbiol. Lett.* **180:**213–219.
223. **Rapp, R. P., P. O. Gubbins, and M. E. Evans.** 1997. Amphotericin B lipid complex. *Ann. Pharmacother.* **31:**1174–1186.
224. **Restrepo, M. I., L. K. Najvar, A. W. Fothergill, and J. R. Graybill.** 1998. Pradimicin therapy of disseminated *Candida tropicalis* infection in the mouse. *Med. Mycol.* **36:**181–184.
225. **Rex, J. H., J. E. Bennett, A. M. Sugar, P. G. Pappas, C. M.**

van der Horst, J. E. Edwards, R. G. Washburn, W. M. Scheld, A. W. Karchmer, A. P. Dine, M. J. Levenstein, and C. D. Webb. 1994. A randomized trial comparing fluconazole with amphotericin B for the treatment of candidemia in patients without neutropenia. Candidemia Study Group and the National Institute. *N. Engl. J. Med.* **331:**1325–1330.

226. **Rex, J. H., C. R. Cooper, Jr., W. G. Merz, J. N. Galgiani, and E. J. Anaissie.** 1995. Detection of amphotericin B-resistant *Candida* isolates in a broth-based system. *Antimicrob. Agents Chemother.* **39:**906–909.

227. **Rex, J. H., P. W. Nelson, V. L. Paetznick, M. Lozano-Chiu, A. Espinel-Ingroff, and E. J. Anaissie.** 1998. Optimizing the correlation between results of testing in vitro and therapeutic outcome in vivo for fluconazole by testing critical isolates in a murine model of invasive candidiasis. *Antimicrob. Agents Chemother.* **42:**129–134.

228. **Rex, J. H., M. A. Pfaller, A. L. Barry, P. W. Nelson, and C. D. Webb.** 1995. Antifungal susceptibility testing of isolates from a randomized, multicenter trial of fluconazole versus amphotericin B as treatment of nonneutropenic patients with candidemia. NIAID Mycoses Study Group and the Candidemia Study Group. *Antimicrob. Agents Chemother.* **39:**40–44.

229. **Rex, J. H., M. A. Pfaller, J. N. Galgiani, M. S. Bartlett, A. Espinel-Ingroff, M. A. Ghannoum, M. Lancaster, F. C. Odds, M. G. Rinaldi, T. J. Walsh, and A. L. Barry.** 1997. Development of interpretive breakpoints for antifungal susceptibility testing: conceptual framework and analysis of in vitro-in vivo correlation data for fluconazole, itraconazole, and *Candida* infections. Subcommittee on Antifungal Susceptibility Testing of the National Committee for Clinical Laboratory Standards. *Clin. Infect. Dis.* **24:**235–247.

230. **Rex, J. H., M. G. Rinaldi, and M. A. Pfaller.** 1995. Resistance of *Candida* species to fluconazole. *Antimicrob. Agents Chemother.* **39:**1–8.

231. **Rex, J. H., T. J. Walsh, J. D. Sobel, S. G. Filler, P. G. Pappas, W. E. Dismukes, and J. E. Edwards.** 2000. Practice guidelines for the treatment of candidiasis. Infectious Diseases Society of America. *Clin. Infect. Dis.* **30:**662–678.

232. **Romani, L., F. Bistoni, and P. Puccetti.** 1997. Initiation of T-helper cell immunity to *Candida albicans* by IL-12: the role of neutrophils. *Chem. Immunol.* **68:**110–135.

233. **Romani, L., A. Mencacci, E. Cenci, G. Del Sero, F. Bistoni, and P. Puccetti.** 1997. An immunoregulatory role for neutrophils in CD4+ T helper subset selection in mice with candidiasis. *J. Immunol.* **158:**2356–2362.

234. **Romani, L., A. Mencacci, E. Cenci, R. Spaccapelo, G. Del Sero, I. Nicoletti, G. Trinchieri, F. Bistoni, and P. Puccetti.** 1997. Neutrophil production of IL-12 and IL-10 in candidiasis and efficacy of IL-12 therapy in neutropenic mice. *J. Immunol.* **158:**5349–5356.

235. **Romani, L., A. Mencacci, U. Grohmann, S. Mocci, P. Mosci, P. Puccetti, and F. Bistoni.** 1992. Neutralizing antibody to interleukin 4 induces systemic protection and T helper type 1-associated immunity in murine candidiasis. *J. Exp. Med.* **176:**19–25.

236. **Romani, L., A. Mencacci, L. Tonnetti, R. Spaccapelo, E. Cenci, P. Puccetti, S. F. Wolf, and F. Bistoni.** 1994. IL-12 is both required and prognostic in vivo for T helper type 1 differentiation in murine candidiasis. *J. Immunol.* **153:**5167–5175.

237. **Romani, L., A. Mencacci, L. Tonnetti, R. Spaccapelo, E. Cenci, S. Wolf, P. Puccetti, and F. Bistoni.** 1994. Interleukin-12 but not interferon-gamma production correlates with induction of T helper type-1 phenotype in murine candidiasis. *Eur. J. Immunol.* **24:**909–915.

238. **Romani, L., P. Puccetti, A. Mencacci, E. Cenci, R. Spaccapelo, L. Tonnetti, U. Grohmann, and F. Bistoni.** 1994. Neutralization of IL-10 up-regulates nitric oxide production and protects susceptible mice from challenge with *Candida albicans. J. Immunol.* **152:**3514–3521.

239. **Ryder, N. S.** 1999. Activity of terbinafine against serious fungal pathogens. *Mycoses* **42:**115–119.

240. **Ryder, N. S., S. Wagner, and I. Leitner.** 1998. In vitro activities of terbinafine against cutaneous isolates of *Candida albicans* and other pathogenic yeasts. *Antimicrob. Agents Chemother.* **42:**1057–1061.

241. **Ryley, J. F., G. Wilson, and K. J. Barrett-Bee.** 1984. Azole resistance in *Candida albicans. J. Med. Vet. Mycol.* **22:**53–63.

242. **Sanati, H., P. Belanger, R. Fratti, and M. Ghannoum.** 1997. A new triazole, voriconazole (UK-109,496), blocks sterol biosynthesis in *Candida albicans* and *Candida krusei. Antimicrob. Agents Chemother.* **41:**2492–2496.

242a. **Sanglard, D.** Unpublished data.

243. **Sanglard, D., F. Ischer, and J. Bille.** 2001. Role of ATP-binding-cassette transporter genes in high-frequency acquisition of resistance to azole antifungals in *Candida glabrata. Antimicrob. Agents Chemother.* **45:**1174–1183.

244. **Sanglard, D., F. Ischer, D. Calabrese, P. A. Majcherczyk, and J. Bille.** 1999. The ATP binding cassette transporter gene *CgCDR1* from *Candida glabrata* is involved in the resistance of clinical isolates to azole antifungal agents. *Antimicrob. Agents Chemother.* **43:**2753–2765.

245. **Sanglard, D., F. Ischer, L. Koymans, and J. Bille.** 1998. Amino acid substitutions in the cytochrome P450 lanosterol 14α-demethylase (CYP51A1) from azole-resistant *Candida albicans* clinical isolates contributing to the resistance to azole antifungal agents. *Antimicrob. Agents Chemother.* **42:**241–253.

246. **Sanglard, D., F. Ischer, M. Monod, and J. Bille.** 1997. Cloning of *Candida albicans* genes conferring resistance to azole antifungal agents: characterization of *CDR2*, a new multidrug ABC-transporter gene. *Microbiology* **143:**405–416.

247. **Sanglard, D., F. Ischer, M. Monod, and J. Bille.** 1996. Susceptibilities of *Candida albicans* multidrug transporter mutants to various antifungal agents and other metabolic inhibitors. *Antimicrob. Agents Chemother.* **40:**2300–2305.

248. **Sanglard, D., K. Kuchler, F. Ischer, J. L. Pagani, M. Monod, and J. Bille.** 1995. Mechanisms of resistance to azole antifungal agents in *Candida albicans* isolates from AIDS patients involve specific multidrug transporters. *Antimicrob. Agents Chemother.* **39:**2378–2386.

249. **Sawada, Y., T. Murakami, T. Ueki, Y. Fukagawa, and T. Oki.** 1991. Mannan-mediated anticandidal activity of BMY-28864, a new water-soluble pradimicin derivative. *J. Antibiot.* **44:**119–121.

250. **Sawada, Y., K. Numata, T. Murakami, H. Tanimichi, S. Yamamoto, and T. Oki.** 1990. Calcium-dependent anticandidal action of pradimicin A. *J. Antibiot.* **43:**715–721.

251. **Scott, M. G., H. Yan, and R. E. Hancock.** 1999. Biological properties of structurally related alpha-helical cationic antimicrobial peptides. *Infect. Immun.* **67:**2005–2009.

252. **Sheehan, D. J., C. A. Hitchcock, and C. M. Sibley.** 1999. Current and emerging azole antifungal agents. *Clin. Microbiol. Rev.* **12:**40–79.

253. **Sobel, J. D., S. E. Ohmit, P. Schuman, R. S. Klein, K. Mayer, A. Duerr, J. A. Vazquez, and A. Rompalo.** 2000. The evolution of *Candida* species and fluconazole susceptibility among oral and vaginal isolates recovered from human immunodeficiency virus (HIV)-seropositive and at-risk HIV-seronegative women. *J. Infect. Dis.* **183:**286–293.

254. **Sokol-Anderson, M. L., J. Brajtburg, and G. Medoff.** 1986.

Amphotericin B-induced oxidative damage and killing of *Candida albicans. J. Infect. Dis.* **154**:76–83.

255. **Sorensen, K., E. Corcoran, D. Clark, K. Huie, S. Chen, V. Tembe, D. Griffith, O. Lomovskaya, W. Watkins, and N. M. Dudley.** 2000. In vivo potentiation of fluconazole by the fungal efflux pump inhibitor MC-510,011 in a mouse model of pyelonephritis due to fluconazole-susceptible and resistant *Candida albicans,* p. 209. *In Abstr. 40th Intersci. Conf. Antimicrob. Agents Chemother.* American Society for Microbiology, Washington, D.C.
256. **Stiller, R. L., J. E. Bennett, H. J. Scholer, M. Wall, A. Polak, and D. A. Stevens.** 1983. Correlation of in vitro susceptibility test results with in vivo response: flucytosine therapy in a systemic candidiasis model. *J. Infect. Dis.* **147**:1070–1077.
257. **Sutton, D. A., S. E. Sanche, S. G. Revankar, A. W. Fothergill, and M. G. Rinaldi.** 1999. In vitro amphotericin B resistance in clinical isolates of *Aspergillus terreus,* with a head-to-head comparison to voriconazole. *J. Clin. Microbiol.* **37**: 2343–2345.
258. **Takesako, K., H. Kuroda, T. Inoue, F. Haruna, Y. Yoshikawa, I. Kato, K. Uchida, T. Hiratani, and H. Yamaguchi.** 1993. Biological properties of aureobasidin A, a cyclic depsipeptide antifungal antibiotic. *J. Antibiot.* **46**:1414–1420.
259. **Tawara, S., F. Ikeda, K. Maki, Y. Morishita, K. Otomo, N. Teratani, T. Goto, M. Tomishima, H. Ohki, A. Yamada, K. Kawabata, H. Takasugi, K. Sakane, H. Tanaka, F. Matsumoto, and S. Kuwahara.** 2000. In vitro activities of a new lipopeptide antifungal agent, FK463, against a variety of clinically important fungi. *Antimicrob. Agents Chemother.* **44**: 57–62.
260. **Thompson, J. R., C. M. Douglas, W. Li, C. K. Jue, B. Pramanik, X. Yuan, T. H. Rude, D. L. Toffaletti, J. R. Perfect, and M. Kurtz.** 1999. A glucan synthase *FKS1* homolog in *Cryptococcus neoformans* is single copy and encodes an essential function. *J. Bacteriol.* **181**:444–453.
261. **Tsai, H., and L. A. Bobek.** 1997. Human salivary histatin-5 exerts potent fungicidal activity against *Cryptococcus neoformans. Biochim. Biophys. Acta* **1336**:367–369.
262. **Tsai, H., and L. A. Bobek.** 1997. Studies of the mechanism of human salivary histatin-5 candidacidal activity with histatin-5 variants and azole-sensitive and -resistant *Candida* species. *Antimicrob. Agents Chemother.* **41**:2224–2228.
263. **Ueki, T., K. Numata, Y. Sawada, T. Nakajima, Y. Fukagawa, and T. Oki.** 1993. Studies on the mode of antifungal action of pradimicin antibiotics. I. Lectin-mimic binding of BMY-28864 to yeast mannan in the presence of calcium. *J. Antibiot.* **46**:149–161.
264. **Vanden Bossche, H., P. Marichal, J. Gorrens, D. Bellens, M. C. Coene, W. Lauwers, L. Le Jeune, H. Moereels, and P. A. J. Janssen.** 1990. Mode of action of antifungals of use in immunocompromised patients. Focus on *Candida glabrata* and *Histoplasma capsulatum,* p. 223–243. *In* H. Vanden Bossche, D. W. R. Mackenzie, G. Cauwenbergh, J. Van Custem, E. Drouhet, and B. Dupont (ed.), *Mycoses in AIDS Patients.* Plenum Press, New York, N.Y.
265. **Vanden Bossche, H., P. Marichal, J. Gorrens, D. Bellens, H. Moereels, and P. A. J. Janssen.** 1990. Mutation in cytochrome P450-dependent 14α-demethylase results in decreased affinity for azole antifungals. *Biochem. Soc. Trans.* **18**:56–59.
266. **Vanden Bossche, H., P. Marichal, L. J. L., M. C. Coene, J. Gorrens, and W. Cools.** 1993. Effects of itraconazole on cytochrome P-450-dependent sterol 14α-demethylation and reduction of 3-ketosteroids in *Cryptococcus neoformans. Antimicrob. Agents Chemother.* **37**:2101–2105.
267. **Vanden Bossche, H., P. Marichal, and H. Moereels.** 1993. Molecular mechanisms of antifungal activity and fungal resistance: focus on inhibitors of ergosterol biosynthesis, p. 179–197. *In* B. Maresca, G. S. Kobayashi, and H. Yamaguchi (ed.), *Molecular Biology and Its Application to Medical Mycology.* Springer-Verlag, Berlin, Germany.
268. **Vanden Bossche, H., P. Marichal, and F. C. Odds.** 1994. Molecular mechanisms of drug resistance in fungi. *Trends Microbiol.* **2**:393–400.
269. **Vazquez, J. A., R. Northland, S. Miller, G. Dickinson, and G. Wright.** 2000. Posaconazole compared to fluconazole for oral candidiasis in HIV-positive patients, abstr. 1107, p. 372. *In Abstr. 40th Intersci. Conf. Antimicrob. Agents Chemother.* American Society for Microbiology, Washington, D.C.
270. **Venkateswarlu, K., D. W. Denning, N. J. Manning, and S. L. Kelly.** 1996. Reduced accumulation of drug in *Candida krusei* accounts for itraconazole resistance. *Antimicrob. Agents Chemother.* **40**:2443–2446.
271. **Venkateswarlu, K., D. W. Denning, N. J. Manning, and S. L. Kelly.** 1995. Resistance to fluconazole in *Candida albicans* from aids patients correlated with reduced intracellular accumulation of drug. *FEMS Microbiol. Lett.* **131**:337–341.
272. **Venkateswarlu, K., M. Taylor, N. J. Manning, M. G. Rinaldi, and S. L. Kelly.** 1997. Fluconazole tolerance in clinical isolates of *Cryptococcus neoformans. Antimicrob. Agents Chemother.* **41**:748–751.
273. **Voss, A., and B. E. de Pauw.** 1999. High-dose fluconazole therapy in patients with severe fungal infections. *Eur. J. Clin. Microbiol. Infect. Dis.* **18**:165–174.
274. **Wade, D., A. Boman, B. Wahlin, C. M. Drain, D. Andreu, H. G. Boman, and R. B. Merrifield.** 1990. All-D amino acid-containing channel-forming antibiotic peptides. *Proc. Natl. Acad. Sci. USA* **87**:4761–4765.
275. **Walsh, T. J., M. Kasai, A. Francesconi, D. Landsman, and S. J. Chanock.** 1997. New evidence that *Candida albicans* possesses additional ATP-binding cassette MDR-like genes—implications for antifungal azole resistance. *J. Med. Vet. Mycol.* **35**:133–137.
276. **Walsh, T. J., G. P. Melcher, M. G. Rinaldi, J. Lecciones, D. A. McGough, P. Kelly, J. Lee, D. Callender, M. Rubin, and P. A. Pizzo.** 1990. *Trichosporon beigelii,* an emerging pathogen resistant to amphotericin B. *J. Clin. Microbiol.* **28**: 1616–1622.
277. **Walsh, T. J., P. Pappas, D. Winston, J. Blumer, F. Peterson, S. Yanovich, S. Raffalli, P. Stiff, R. Greenberg, G. Donowitz, M. Schuster, C. Arndt, J. Reinhardt, A. Reboli, E. Anaissie, S. Hadley, G. Garber, J. Wingard, G. Fioritoni, and J. Lee.** 2000. Voriconazole versus liposomal amphotericin B for empirical antifungal therapy of persistently febrile neutropenic patients: a randomized, international, multicenter trial, abstr. L-1. *In Late Breaker 40th Intersci. Conf. Antimicrob. Agents Chemother.* American Society for Microbiology, Washington, D.C.
278. **Watson, P. F., M. E. Rose, and S. L. Kelly.** 1988. Isolation and analysis of ketoconazole resistant mutants of *Saccharomyces cerevisiae. J. Med. Vet. Mycol.* **26**:153–162.
279. **Wemmie, J. A., M. S. Szczypka, D. J. Thiele, and W. S. Moye Rowley.** 1994. Cadmium tolerance mediated by the yeast AP-1 protein requires the presence of an ATP-binding cassette transporter-encoding gene, *YCF1. J. Biol. Chem.* **269**: 32592–32597.
280. **Whelan, W. L.** 1988. The genetic basis of resistance to 5-fluorocytosine in *Candida* species and *Cryptococcus neoformans. Crit. Rev. Microbiol.* **15**:45–56.
281. **White, T. C.** 1997. Increased mRNA levels of *ERG16, CDR,* and *MDR1* correlate with increases in azole resistance in *Candida albicans* isolates from a patient infected with human

immunodeficiency virus. *Antimicrob. Agents Chemother.* **41:** 1482–1487.

282. **White, T. C.** 1997. The presence of an R467K amino acid substitution and loss of allelic variation correlate with an azole-resistant lanosterol 14-alpha-demethylase in *Candida albicans. Antimicrob. Agents Chemother.* **41:**1488–1494.
283. **White, T. C., K. A. Marr, and R. A. Bowden.** 1998. Clinical, cellular, and molecular factors that contribute to antifungal drug resistance. *Clin. Microbiol. Rev.* **11:**382–402.
284. **Wildfeuer, A., H. P. Seidl, I. Paule, and A. Haberreiter.** 1998. In vitro evaluation of voriconazole against clinical isolates of yeasts, moulds and dermatophytes in comparison with itraconazole, amphotericin B and griseofulvin. *Mycoses* **41:** 309–319.
285. **Williams, D. J., R. M. Marten, and I. Sarkany.** 1958. Oral treatment of ringworm by griseofulvin. *Lancet* **ii:**1212.
286. **Wirsching, S., S. Michel, G. Kohler, and J. Morschhauser.** 2000. Activation of the multiple drug resistance gene *MDR1* in fluconazole-resistant, clinical *Candida albicans* strains is caused by mutations in a trans-regulatory factor. *J. Bacteriol.* **182:**400–404.
287. **Wirsching, S., S. Michel, and J. Morschhauser.** 2000. Targeted gene disruption in *Candida albicans* wild-type strains: the role of the *MDR1* gene in fluconazole resistance of clinical *Candida albicans* isolates. *Mol. Microbiol.* **36:**856–865.
288. **Wong-Beringer, A., R. A. Jacobs, and B. J. Guglielmo.** 1998. Lipid formulations of amphotericin B: clinical efficacy and toxicities. *Clin. Infect. Dis.* **27:**603–618.
289. **Xu, T., S. M. Levitz, R. D. Diamond, and F. G. Oppenheim.** 1991. Anticandidal activity of major human salivary histatins. *Infect. Immun.* **59:**2549–2554.
290. **Xu, Y. Y., Y. H. Samaranayake, L. P. Samaranayake, and H. Nikawa.** 1999. In vitro susceptibility of *Candida* species to lactoferrin. *Med. Mycol.* **37:**35–41.
291. **Yoon, S. A., J. A. Vazquez, P. E. Steffan, J. D. Sobel, and R. A. Akins.** 1999. High-frequency, in vitro reversible switching of *Candida lusitaniae* clinical isolates from amphotericin B susceptibility to resistance. *Antimicrob. Agents Chemother.* **43:**836–845.
292. **Zasloff, M., B. Martin, and H. C. Chen.** 1988. Antimicrobial activity of synthetic magainin peptides and several analogues. *Proc. Natl. Acad. Sci. USA.* **85:**910–913.
293. **Zhong, W., M. W. Jeffries, and N. H. Georgopapadakou.** 2000. Inhibition of inositol phosphorylceramide synthase by aureobasidin A in *Candida* and *Aspergillus* species. *Antimicrob. Agents Chemother.* **44:**651–653.

VII. LABORATORY WORK UP OF CANDIDIASIS

Candida and Candidiasis
Edited by Richard A. Calderone

Chapter 26

Culture- and Non-Culture-Based Diagnostics for *Candida* Species

MALCOLM D. RICHARDSON AND PETTERI CARLSON

CULTURE-BASED AND NON-CULTURE-BASED DIAGNOSTICS FOR *CANDIDA* SPECIES

The clinical manifestations of superficial, mucosal, or deep invasive *Candida* infections are not specific for *Candida* species only and can be caused by other organisms. The laboratory identification of *Candida* species is, therefore, essential for establishing a definitive diagnosis of candidiasis. The purpose of this chapter is to outline the typical laboratory techniques used to process clinical specimens and to describe the methods used to visualize and detect *Candida* species in tissue, the methods used to recover *Candida* spp. using a variety of culture techniques, and those tests used to identify these organisms. Standard approaches to the laboratory diagnosis of candidiasis depend on:

- direct microscopy of clinical specimens
- recovery of *Candida* species in cultures of blood, body fluids, tissues, or specimens from other sites
- identification of organisms to species level: this has both prognostic and therapeutic significance
- identification of organisms morphologically consistent with *Candida* species in tissue

Numerous reviews and guidelines concerning the isolation and identification of *Candida* species have been published in the literature (2, 3, 6, 20, 24, 26, 27).

Taking and Transport of Specimens

Yeasts can be isolated from many body sites, including skin, mucocutaneous areas, nails, sputum, bronchoalveolar lavage fluid, urine, cerebrospinal fluid, and blood, and from biopsy or necropsy tissue (20, 22, 26, 27). It is essential that specimens taken with swabs are not allowed to dry out before culture. Fluid specimens should be processed as quickly as possible.

Clinical Manifestations of Candidiasis and Essential Investigations

Detailed descriptions of the clinical manifestations of superficial and systemic candidiasis can be found in Dupont (5), Richardson and Elewski (21), Richardson and Warnock (23) and in chapters 22 through 24 in this book.

Skin and mucous membrane infections

The initial investigation is direct microscopy (15). The thinner a preparation is made for direct microscopy, the more chance there is of finding fungal elements in a specimen. Keratinous and epithelial tissue and sputum samples are digested and "cleared" before viewing. Potassium hydroxide (KOH) in concentrations varying from 10 to 30% is normally used for this purpose (15). Random samples should be taken from several pieces of the material provided.

Skin scrapings immersed in KOH solution show typical budding yeast cells and pseudohyphae with lateral blastoconidia, often in small groups at intervals along the pseudohyphae (15). Pseudohyphae branch only at septa. Positive KOH preparations from skin and mucous membranes are more significant than cultures, especially when hyphae and pseudohyphae are present.

The sensitivity of direct microscopy of clinical specimens can be enhanced by the use of fluorescent optical brighteners (15), such as Calcofluor white (Sigma Chemical Company). Calcofluor white binds

Malcolm D. Richardson • Mycology Unit, Department of Bacteriology and Immunology, University of Helsinki, Haartman Institute, PO Box 21, Haartmaninkatu 3, 00014 Helsinki, Finland. **Petteri Carlson** • Department of Bacteriology, Helsinki University Central Hospital Laboratory Diagnostics, Haartmaninkatu 3, PO Box 400, 00029 HUS, Finland.

to the chitin components in fungal cells walls (15). This is a very simple technique that is used extensively by diagnostic laboratories and is particularly suitable when scanty fungus is present.

Intertriginous candidiasis is often difficult to diagnose if the lesions are other than typical in appearance. Isolation of *Candida albicans* from swabs or scrapings is of dubious significance because the organism is a frequent colonizer of a range of cutaneous lesions, whereas microscopic demonstration of the organism in scrapings of lesions is much more significant. The diagnosis of nail-fold infections (paronychia) caused by *Candida* spp. rests in part on the characteristic clinical appearance. However, microscopic examination and culture are needed to confirm the diagnosis. Material can be taken from the swollen periungual nail wall or from under the nail fold using a disposable microbiological loop or moistened swab. Pus can be obtained from under the nail fold by applying light pressure. Microscopic demonstration of the typical morphology of *Candida* species or isolation of the fungus from nail can be difficult with proximal lesions, but material from a distal or lateral lesion, together with subungual debris, will often confirm the diagnosis.

Respiratory secretions

Candida species tend to be present in small numbers in sputum and bronchial secretions, and so it is often necessary to concentrate the fungal elements in the sample to be examined by centrifugation. Before this can take place, the specimen first has to be homogenized to break down the mucin. Although KOH could be used to prepare a specimen for microscopy, it would preclude attempts to culture. A sample suitable for microscopy and culture can be obtained by using pancreatic enzymes or *N*-acetyl cysteine available commercially (15). Sputum and other respiratory secretions usually show only budding yeast cells.

Particular care must be taken in interpreting the results of sputum culture as this material is often contaminated with organisms from the mouth. Culture of bronchial secretions (obtained through a bronchoscope) provides more reliable evidence of lung colonization or infection.

Detection of candidemia

Detection of *Candida* species in the bloodstream is a key clinical laboratory strategy for establishing a diagnosis of invasive candidiasis (5, 23). Blood cultures should be performed in all cases of suspected deep-seated candidiasis. However, it is not unusual for numerous attempts to be required before the organism is successfully isolated. Blood should be drawn through intravenous catheters and from peripheral veins. Blood cultures are positive in no more than 50% of neutropenic patients with disseminated candidiasis (5). The significance of the isolation of *Candida* spp. from the blood has been interpreted in many different ways. During the past decade, there has been increasing appreciation of the significance of candidemia (8). Dismissing the isolation of *Candida* species from a single blood culture as a skin contaminant has long been questioned as a potentially hazardous interpretation (8). The dogma that two consecutive positive blood cultures are required to affirm the significance of the first blood culture is no longer tenable. Waiting for a second *Candida*-positive blood culture may lead to delay in administering potentially lifesaving therapy. Virtually all blood cultures that yield *Candida* species are considered to be significant until proved otherwise (8). Indeed, even blood cultures growing *Candida* species from a vascular catheter should not be considered as colonization since vascular catheters may be the target of fungemia from a distal site or the portal of entry of *Candida* species.

The detection of candidemia requires a good blood culture system complemented by good laboratory practice and communication. Blood culture systems for *Candida* spp. should utilize as rich a culture medium as possible to allow the recovery of very small numbers of yeasts and should aim to achieve the following:

- neutralization or removal of antimicrobial substances, such as serum fungicidal factors, either natural blood components or antimicrobial agents
- minimization of contamination
- the earliest possible detection of yeasts

Blood culture systems for yeasts range from "in-house" and commercial manual systems to fully automated commercial systems. These systems rely on a variety of detection principles and culture environments to detect microorganisms. Many systems and their respective media have been compared, each system having its own limitations and advantages. Fully automated continuous monitoring systems are simple to use in comparison with manual and semiautomated systems. In addition, fully automated systems have the advantage that positive cultures may be detected earlier.

Traditional biphasic systems have the advantage of simple closed subculture, achieved by tilting of the culture bottle, but colony recognition may be impaired by the glass. The most sensitive method for isolating fungi from blood specimens is lysis centrifugation, commercially available as the Isolator system.

Table 1. Commercial systems for detection of *Candida* spp. in blood

System	Manufacturer	Detection principle
Automated		
BacT/Alert	Organon Teknika	Colorimetric detection of CO_2
Bactec 9240	Becton Dickinson	Fluorescent detection of CO_2
VitalMicroscan	bioMerieux	Fluorescent detection of charged radicals
Sentinel	Difco Laboratories	Detection of changes in redox potential
Bactec NR660, 730, 860	Becton Dickinson	Detection of CO_2 production by infrared spectrophotometry
Manual		
Conventional bottles	Many	Detection of macroscopic evidence of microbial growth and blind subculture
Signal	Oxoid	Gas production displaces culture medium to an indicator device
Septi-Chek	Becton Dickinson	Macroscopic detection of growth in diphasic media system
Isolator	Oxoid	Detection of growth on solid media following lysis centrifugation of blood sample

However, these systems are technically demanding and are not widely used. The Isolator tube contains saponin, which lyses leukocytes and erythrocytes, releasing intracellular fungi, which are then concentrated by centrifugation. The sediment should be streaked onto enriched media such as brain heart infusion agar or sheep blood agar. Optimally, the Isolator tube should be processed within 16 h of blood collection; until processing, the tube should be maintained at room temperature.

Examples of other commercial blood systems used for the detection of *Candida* species in blood are given in Table 1 (19).

Factors affecting isolation of *Candida* species from blood. A number of clinical and technical factors may affect the isolation of yeasts from blood samples, regardless of the system employed (19).

Clinical factors

- Method of collection
- Number and timing of samples
- Previous antimicrobial therapy

Technical factors

- Volume of sample
- Culture media used
- Neutralization of antifungals
- Incubation time and temperature
- Agitation of media
- Headspace atmosphere

A number of specific points relating to the optimal recovery of *Candida* species from blood can be made. Arterial blood has been reported to be apparently superior in detecting disseminated *Candida* infection compared to venous blood (20). The volume of blood cultured is the most critical factor in the detection of bloodstream infection, and it is recommended that 20 to 30 ml of blood be cultured (20). A volume of 1 to 2 ml is recommended for neonates (20). A variety of blood culture media are commercially available. They differ in the types and proportions of various supplements and anticoagulants, volumes of broth, headspace atmospheres, and the presence of antimicrobial-neutralizing agents. The aerobic bottle may require transient venting to increase the oxygen content in the headspace for aerobic organisms such as *C. albicans*. All positive specimens and blind subcultures, depending on the system used, should be subcultured on glucose-peptone (Sabouraud) agar and incubated at 28 to 30°C for up to 5 days. Cultures should be read at 1 to 2 days and at 5 days.

Methods for detection of *Candida* species in blood are many; controlled comparisons are few (14). The vented FAN aerobic blood culture medium has been shown to be superior to the standard BacT/ALERT aerobic medium for the detection of fungemia as well as bacteremia (29). The BACTEC selective fungal medium (FM) (BD Biosciences, Sparks, Md.) allowed detection of more episodes of fungemia than did a resin-containing medium with equal volumes of blood cultured (14). A comparison between vented FAN and FM for the ability to recover fungi from the blood of patients who were at increased risk of having fungemia has also been reported (14). From 5,109 cultures processed for which both FAN and FM bottles were adequately filled, fungi were recovered from 87 cultures. Of these, 47 were detected with both bottles, 12 were detected with FAN only, and 28 were detected with FM only ($P < 0.05$). FAN was the first bottle positive for 36 of the 47 cultures for which both bottles yielded the same fungus, whereas the FM bottle was the first bottle positive for 11 cultures ($P < 0.001$). A total of 54 episodes of fungemia were identified, with 40 detected by both media, 4 detected only by FAN, and 10 detected only by FM (*P*, not significant). It was concluded that the vented FAN aerobic bottle is comparable to the FM bottle for detecting episodes of yeast infection but has the added benefit of detecting bacteria (14).

Intravascular catheters. Intravascular catheters are an important source of candidemia (5, 23). The intravascular catheter may serve as the portal of entry or as the target of *Candida* species circulating from another site of entry, most commonly the gastrointestinal (GI) tract. When the catheter is removed from the patient, a 5 cm long portion of the catheter tip is often submitted to the microbiology laboratory for investigation. The tip should be rolled over the surface of a glucose-peptone agar plate, after which the catheter tip may be cultured in broth medium. The plate should be incubated at 37°C for 48 h and the amount of growth subsequently should be recorded. The presence of 15 CFU has been suggested to be significant in implicating bacteria as the cause of bacteremia involving a catheter (5, 23). However, a similar significance threshold for *Candida* species CFUs recovered has not been established. Indeed, the recovery of any quantity of *Candida* species from a vascular catheter tip should prompt a thorough clinical reevaluation for systemic candidiasis. Quantification of *Candida* species following broth culture of the catheter tip also carries no quantitative significance other than to indicate contamination or colonization of the vascular catheter by *Candida* species.

Oral candidiasis

The clinical manifestations of oral candidiasis are often characteristic but can be confused with other disorders. For this reason, the diagnosis should be confirmed by demonstration of the various morphological forms of the fungus in smears prepared from swabs or scrapings of lesions and its isolation in culture. As *C. albicans* is a normal commensal in the mouth in a significant proportion of the human population (16), its isolation alone cannot be considered diagnostic of infection.

Methods. Swabs should be moistened with sterile water or saline prior to taking the specimen or sent to the laboratory in transport medium. Swabs should be inoculated onto glucose-peptone agar or the chromogenic medium CHROMagar Candida (Becton Dickinson) (17) and incubated for 48 h at 37°C. Imprint cultures using a small square of polystyrene foam can also be used. Commercial systems include Dentocult CA and Oricult-N (Orion Diagnostics, Espoo, Finland) (4).

Vaginal candidiasis

The diagnosis of vaginal candidiasis depends on a combination of typical symptoms and signs and the demonstration of the fungus in smears or its isolation in culture. The latter is much more sensitive and reliable (about 90%) than the former (about 40%) (16). Swabs should be taken from discharge in the vagina and from the lateral vaginal wall and sent to the laboratory in transport medium. Culture should be performed on glucose-peptone agar or CHROMagar and incubated for 48 h at 37°C. Alternatively, broth media or dipslides have been used in vaginal yeast cultures. Substantial controversy exists about the interpretation of a positive culture result (16). Traditionally, any growth of *Candida* organisms from a vaginal specimen has been considered a pathological finding (16). More recently, however, it has been shown that symptomatic candidiasis is usually associated with higher numbers of vaginal yeasts than those found in asymptomatic carriers (7, 11, 18). Unfortunately, conventional mycological laboratory techniques for yeast quantitation involve serial dilutions (11), and dipslides or broth media do not allow for quantitation. More recently, the Oricult-N semiquantitative dipslide method (Orion Diagnostics) has been evaluated for the laboratory diagnosis of vaginal candidiasis (4). It was compared with microscopy and broth culture with specimens from both symptomatic women and a group of healthy volunteers. Oricult-N was positive for 14.5% of 124 symptomatic patients and 12% of 50 asymptomatic controls. The results for broth cultures were 17 and 22%, respectively. Thus, the test group and the control group did not differ significantly by either method. High vaginal yeast counts (10^5 CFU/ml) were detected by Oricult-N in 7% of patients and in 0% of controls, but both groups harbored low numbers of yeasts. An accurate quantitative cutoff point separating levels of yeasts associated with infection from that associated with vaginal yeast carriage could not be defined in the study. Nevertheless, the easy semiquantitation allowed by the Oricult-N method could be helpful, especially in low-level carriers of *Candida* spp. because other potential causes of vaginal symptoms should be considered. The Oricult-N method is technically simple and could be applied in primary health care. Further studies are required, however, before Oricult-N can be recommended as a routine diagnostic tool.

Urinary tract candidiasis

Isolation of *Candida* spp. from urine is often indicative of serious infection, provided the patient does not have an indwelling urethral catheter. In noncatheterized patients, care must be taken to ensure that vaginal or perineal infection does not lead to contamination of urine specimens. In infants, suprapubic aspiration is the best method of urine collection. Isolation of *Candida tropicalis* from urine is more often indicative of disseminated candidiasis than isolation of *C. albicans* (23). It has been suggested that counts of more than 1×10^4 CFU/ml of urine in a noncatheterized patient should be regarded as significant (23), but this has never been validated. High counts in a patient with an indwelling catheter are seldom significant.

Central nervous system infections

Isolation of *Candida* spp. from cerebrospinal fluid provides reliable evidence for the diagnosis of meningitis but often requires repeated culture of large amounts of fluid. All specimens obtained from ventricular shunts or reservoirs should be cultured for *Candida* species.

LABORATORY IDENTIFICATION OF *CANDIDA* SPECIES

There is no doubt that yeasts isolated from normally sterile sites such as blood, cerebrospinal fluid, and synovial fluid should be identified in the laboratory or be sent to a reference laboratory. Approximately 70 to 80% of yeasts isolated in a clinical microbiology laboratory are *C. albicans.* If the germ tube test is positive, further testing is not normally required. Traditionally, methods for the identification of *Candida* species rely on a combination of morphological and biochemical characteristics (2, 3).

The principal morphological and biochemical tests include:

- appearance and color of colonies on primary isolation media (Sabourauds, CHROMagar)
- size and shape of cells
- production of hyphae and/or pseudohyphae
- ability to produce germ tubes
- ability to produce chlamydoconidia (chlamydospores)
- assimilation of carbohydrates
- assimilation of nitrate
- fermentation of sugars

Some of the traditional identification methods, particularly the biochemical tests, are cumbersome and time-consuming to perform. Consequently, a number of rapid tests and commercial identification systems have been developed and introduced into microbiology laboratories.

Candida species generally grow well on common mycological and bacteriological media, including Sabouraud glucose agar, sheep blood agar, and horse blood agar. Some species of *Candida,* such as *C. albicans* and *C. dubliniensis,* grow in the presence of cycloheximide. Colonies of *Candida* species grown at temperatures between 25 and 37°C have a smooth to wrinkled textured colony of white to beige color when grown on glucose-peptone agar (Saborauds). Different *Candida* species in a mixed specimen may be distinguished on media containing chromogenic compounds such as CHROMagar Candida medium (17). However, CHROMagar is only useful for the presumptive identification of certain medically important species, including *C. albicans, C. tropicalis, C. glabrata, C. krusei, C. dubliniensis,* and to an extent, *C. parapsilosis* (17, 24). Following 48 h of growth at 37°C on this medium, *C. albicans* appears light blue-green. Other pathogenic species of *Candida* appear as purple or pink. The recently described chlamydospore- and germ-positive yeast *C. dubliniensis* that has been recovered primarily from the oral cavities of human immunodeficiency virus (HIV)-infected individuals usually appears as dark green colonies on this medium and can be easily distinguished from other *Candida* species (24). However, it must be emphasized that CHROMagar Candida agar is useful only for identifying colonies of *C. dubliniensis* following primary plating from clinical specimens as isolates can lose their dark green coloration on this medium following subculture or storage (24). On Czapek Dox agar using the Dalmau (or similar) technique *Candida* species (with the exception of *C. glabrata*) usually produce abundant hyphae growing from the edge of the original inoculum. Clusters of oval to spherical blastospores (blastoconidia) may be seen along the length of hyphae. The arrangement of hyphae and blastospores is often characteristic of a particular species.

Chlamydospore Production

With the Dalmau techniques, large, highly refractile, thick-walled chlamydoconidia may be seen terminally or on short lateral branches in *C. albicans* isolates. Approximately 60% of clinical isolates of *C. albicans* produce chlamydoconidia (3). The test provides a rapid presumptive identification step for *C. albicans* and *C. dubliniensis*. Alternative media to Czapek Dox for inducing chlamydospore production include cornmeal agar and rice-agar-Tween (3).

Germ Tube Production

The germ tube test provides a rapid identification test for *C. albicans* that can be carried out on primary or purified cultures. The formation of germ tubes in serum or similar media is characteristic of 95 to 97% of clinical isolates of *C. albicans* and *C. dubliniensis*.

Commercial Kits for Identifying Medically Important *Candida* Species

For laboratories where the identification of yeasts constitutes a small part of the routine workload, the use of commercially produced auxanographic kits is particularly attractive. All of these kits will identify *Candida* species within 24 to 36 h, and many of them will provide an identification profile that can be used for epidemiological strain typing purposes.

The following products have found a useful place in the routine laboratory, although the list is not exhaustive: API ID 32C, API 20C AUX (commonly used in the United States), Fungicrom, Auxacolor, Candifast, and Fungitest.

The development of commercial kits has provided the routine laboratory with the opportunity to standardize the identification of *Candida* species. However, for many laboratories, the costs involved may exclude the use of kits, but this decision must be weighed against the efforts in preparing media and reagents.

HISTOPATHOLOGICAL APPEARANCE OF *CANDIDA* SPECIES IN TISSUE

Candida species can appear as yeasts and pseudohyphae, or as yeast cells alone, in tissues from superficial and systemic sites (9) (Fig. 1). *C. albicans* can usually be distinguished from other yeasts by the presence of yeasts plus hyphae and/or pseudohyphae. Yeasts are round to ovoid (4 to 8 μm in diameter) with single or multiple buds. In some sections hyphae are numerous. It is important to ensure that yeast-like structures accompanying hyphae are budding, as

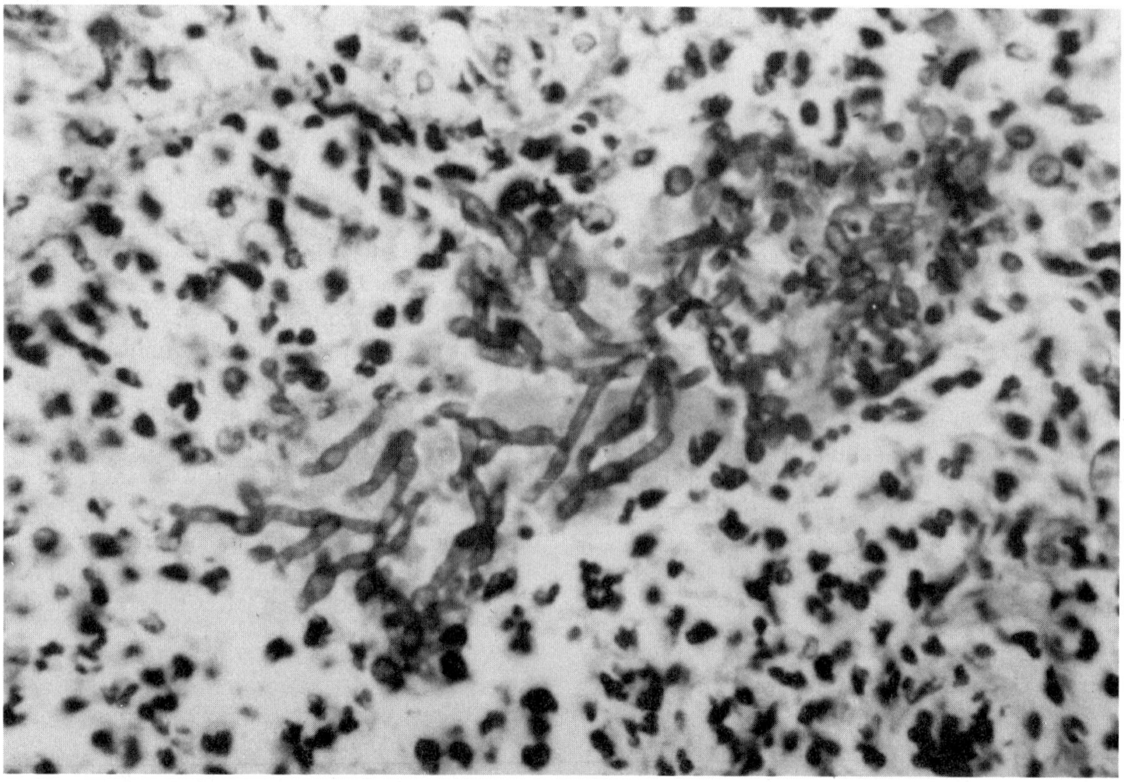

Figure 1. Histopathological appearance of renal candidiasis. Note that both pseudohyphae and blastoconidia can be seen. Reprinted from reference 23a with permission.

hyphae cut in cross section may appear as yeasts on cursory examination. Some non-*C. albicans* species such as *C. glabrata* are usually small or ovoid yeasts (2 to 5 μm). Hyphae are absent.

Immunohistochemical Identification of *Candida* spp. in Tissue

Although it is usually possible to identify some members of the genus *Candida* in tissue on the basis of their morphology by using special stains such as periodic acid-Schiff or methenamine silver (Grocott's modification), this is not always the case (9). For instance, if the fungal elements do not show their characteristic features or are atypical in shape or in size, the true identity of the fungus may be in doubt. This often occurs in biopsy material from which only a small amount of tissue is taken. In this situation further methods of identification are useful.

There are many examples in which fungal elements suggestive of *Candida* pseudohyphae are seen in conventionally stained tissue sections but culture of the tissue specimen is negative, e.g., in chronic hepatosplenic candidiasis (1). As an illustrative example, in 26 leukemia patients with hepatosplenic yeast infection, 17 diagnoses were based on the findings from microscopy of samples obtained invasively, whereas a positive fungal culture was the basis of diagnosis for only 5 patients (1). Here the application of immunohistochemical methods using specific monoclonal antibodies to particular epitopes of *Candida* sp. would be very helpful (9, 12). One such monoclonal antibody is 3H8 (Societé de Recherche et de Réalisations Biotechnologies, Paris, France), which is specific for *C. albicans* and *C. dubliniensis* (13). The antibody has been characterized as an immunoglobulin G1, which recognizes mannoproteins of high molecular mass present in the *C. albicans* cell wall. Enzyme-linked immunosorbent assays have shown that the presence of the epitope recognized by the monoclonal antibody 3H8 was similar in both yeast and mycelial cell walls of *C. albicans* (13). Immunohistochemical studies using this antibody demonstrated that it specifically recognized *C. albicans* in tissue, detecting mycelial forms and, to a lesser extent, blastospores, suggesting that it could be a powerful tool in the evaluation of fungal infections in paraffin-embedded tissue.

IDENTIFICATION OF *CANDIDA* SPP. IN TISSUE BY MOLECULAR METHODS

Candida species have been identified in tissue by PCR following amplification of fungal nucleic acid from tissue specimens (25, 28). For example, the identification of *Candida* spp. in keratinous tissue using PCR has recently been reported (25). In this study, three primer pairs, which amplify specific fragments of the highly conserved gene encoding for the small ribosomal unit (18S rRNA) and the adjacent internal transcribed spacer (ITS) region, were first tested with template DNA extracted from pure cultures of clinically significant human and animal fungal species and were found to be fungus specific. Subsequently, these primer pairs, in single amplification or double-rounded PCR assays, allowed specific amplification when applied to a wide variety of fungal DNAs from human and animal tissue specimens, including tissue containing dermatophytes (genera *Trichophyton* and *Microsporum*), several yeast species (genera *Candida, Saccharomyces, Cryptococcus,* and *Malassezia*), and molds (genera *Aspergillus* and *Penicillium*). The PCR assay was able to detect as little as 10 pg of fungal DNA, corresponding to approximately 25 fungal genomes per sample specimen. The procedure was used in conjunction with a small-scale DNA extraction method and was successfully applied to 40 human and veterinary specimens. In each case, results obtained by PCR were confirmed by culture. This simple, time-saving, and sensitive procedure allows early recognition of fungal pathogens in keratinous samples (25).

In another study, fungi were detected in tissue samples by amplifying the fungal ITS region (ITS1-5.8S rRNA-ITS2) by PCR followed by multiplex liquid hybridization (10). With this approach where lung biopsy specimens were positive in culture for *C. albicans,* hybridization also identified *C. albicans.* As part of the same study, liver biopsy specimens, which were histopathology positive for *C. albicans* but culture negative, were also found to be positive for *C. albicans* following hybridization using probes for *C. albicans, C. glabrata, C. parapsilosis, C. krusei,* and *C. tropicalis* (10).

These studies demonstrate the potential of molecular approaches for the detection and identification of fungal species in tissue specimens.

REFERENCES

1. **Anttila, V.-J., P. Ruutu, S. Bondestam, S.-E. Jansson, S. Nordling, M. Färkkilä, A. Sivonen, M. Castren, and T. Ruutu.** 1994. Hepatosplenic yeast infection in patients with acute leukemia: a diagnostic problem. *Clin. Infect. Dis.* **18:**979–981.
2. **Barnett, J. A., R. W. Payne, and D. Yarrow.** 2000. *Yeast: Characteristics and Identification,* 3rd ed. Cambridge University Press, Cambridge, United Kingdom.
3. **Buckely, H. R.** 1989. Identification of yeasts, p. 97–109. *In* E. G. V. Evans and M. D. Richardson (ed.), *Medical Mycology—A Practical Approach.* IRL Press at Oxford University Press, Oxford, United Kingdom.

4. **Carlson, P., M. Richardson, and J. Paavonen.** 2000. Evaluation of the Oricult-N dipslide for laboratory diagnosis of vaginal candidosis. *J. Clin. Microbiol.* **38:**1063–1065.
5. **Dupont, B.** 1991. Clinical manifestations and management of candidosis in the compromised patient, p. 55–83. *In* D. W. Warnock and M. D. Richardson (ed.), *Fungal Infection in the Compromised Patient,* 2nd ed. John Wiley & Sons, Ltd., Chichester, United Kingdom.
6. **Evans, E. G. V., and M. D. Richardson.** 1989. *Medical Mycology—A Practical Approach.* IRL Press at Oxford University Press, Oxford, United Kingdom.
7. **Evans, E. G. V., C. J. N. Lacey, and J. A. Carney.** 1986. Criteria for the diagnosis of vaginal candidosis: evaluation of a new latex agglutination test. *Eur. J. Obstet. Gynecol. Reprod. Biol.* **22:**365–371.
8. **Flanagan, P. G., and R. A. Barnes.** 1998. Fungal infection in the intensive care unit. *J. Hosp. Infect.* **38:**163–177.
9. **Hay, R. J.** 1989. Histopathology, p. 261–281. *In* E. G. V. Evans and M. D. Richardson (ed.), *Medical Mycology—A Practical Approach.* IRL Press at Oxford University Press, Oxford, United Kingdom.
10. **Hendolin, P. H., L. Paulin, P. Koukila-Kähkölä, V.-J. Anttila, H. Malmberg, M. Richardson, and J. Ylikoski.** 2000. Panfungal PCR and multiplex liquid hybridization for detection of fungi in tissue specimens. *J. Clin. Microbiol.* **38:**4186–4192.
11. **Hopwood, V., T. Crowley, C. T. Horrocks, J. D. Milne, P. K. Taylor, and D. W. Warnock.** 1988. Vaginal candidosis relation between yeast counts and symptoms and clinical signs in non-pregnant women. *Genitourin. Med.* **64:**331–334.
12. **Jensen, H. E., H. C. Schonheyder, M. Hotchi, and L. Kaufman.** 1996. Diagnosis of systemic mycoses by specific immunohistochemical tests. *APMIS* **104:**241–258.
13. **Marcilla, A., C. Monteagudo, S. Mormeneo, and R. Sentandreu.** 1999. Monoclonal antibody 3H8: a useful tool in the diagnosis of candidiasis. *Microbiology* **145:**695–701.
14. **McDonald, L. C., M. P. Weinstein, J. Fune, S. Mirrett, L. G. Reimer, and L. B. Reller.** 2001. Controlled comparison of BacT/ALERT FAN aerobic medium and BACTEC fungal blood culture medium for detection of fungemia. *J. Clin. Microbiol.* **39:**622–624.
15. **Milne, L. J. R.** 1989. Direct microscopy, p. 17–45. *In* E. G. V. Evans and M. D. Richardson (ed.), *Medical Mycology—A Practical Approach.* IRL Press at Oxford University Press, Oxford, United Kingdom.
16. **Odds, F. C.** 1988. *Candida and Candidosis,* 3rd ed. Baillière Tindall, London, United Kingdom.
17. **Odds, F. C., and R. Bernaert.** 1994. CHROMagar Candida, a new differential isolation medium for presumptive identification of clinically important *Candida* species. *J. Clin. Microbiol.* **32:**1923–1929.
18. **Odds, F. C., C. E. Webster, P. Mayuranathan, and P. D. Simmons.** 1988. *Candida* concentrations in the vagina and their association with signs and symptoms of vaginal candidosis. *J. Med. Vet. Mycol.* **26:**277–283.
19. **Public Health Laboratory Service.** 1998. *Public Health Laboratory Service Standard Operating Procedure—Investigation of Blood Cultures. Reference no. B.SOP 37, issue no. 1.* Public Health Laboratory Service, London, United Kingdom.
20. **Reisner, B. S., G. L. Woods, R. B. Thomson, D. H. Larone, L. S. Garcia, and R. Y. Shimizu.** 1999. Specimen processing, p. 64–104. *In* P. R. Murray, E. J. Baron, M. A. Pfaller, F. C. Tenover, and R. H. Yolken (ed.), *Manual of Clinical Microbiology,* 7th ed. ASM Press, Washington, D.C.
21. **Richardson, M. D., and B. Elewski.** 2000. *Fast Facts: Superficial Fungal Infections.* Health Press, Oxford, United Kingdom.
22. **Richardson, M. D., and E. G. V. Evans.** 1989. Culture and isolation of fungi, p. 47–63. *In* E. G. V. Evans and M. D. Richardson (ed.), *Medical Mycology—A Practical Approach.* IRL Press at Oxford University Press, Oxford, United Kingdom.
23. **Richardson, M. D., and D. W. Warnock.** 1997. *Fungal Infection: Diagnosis and Management,* 2nd ed. Blackwell Science, Oxford, United Kingdom.

23a. **Richardson, M. D., D. W. Warnock, and C. K. Campbell.** 1995. *Slide Atlas of Fungal Infection: Systemic Fungal Infections.* Blackwell Science Ltd., Oxford, United Kingdom.

24. **Sullivan, D., and D. Coleman.** 1998. *Candida dubliniensis:* characteristics and identification. *J. Clin. Microbiol.* **36:** 329–334.
25. **Turin, L., F. Riva, G. Galviati, and T. Cainelli.** 2000. Fast, simple and highly sensitive double-rounded polymerase chain reaction assay to detect medically relevant fungi in dermatological specimens. *Eur. J. Clin. Invest.* **30:**511–518.
26. **Walsh, T. J., and P. A. Pizzo.** 1993. Laboratory diagnosis of candidiasis, p. 109–135. *In* G. P. Bodey (ed.), *Candidiasis: Pathogenesis, Diagnosis and Treatment.* Raven Press Ltd., New York, N. Y.
27. **Warren, N. G., and K. C. Hazen.** 1999. *Candida, Cryptococcus,* and other yeasts of medical importance, p. 1184–1199. *In* P. R. Murray, E. J. Baron, M. A. Pfaller, F. C. Tenover, and R. H. Yolken (ed.), *Manual of Clinical Microbiology,* 7th ed. ASM Press, Washington, D.C.
28. **Werner, J. A., T. Gorogh, B. M. Lippert, and H. Rudert.** 1995. DNA amplification for the in vitro detection of *Candida albicans* in head and neck squamous cell carcinomas. *Eur. Arch. Otorhinolaryngol.* **252:**417–421.
29. **Wilson, M. L., M. P. Weinstein, L. G. Reimer, S. Mirrett, and L. B. Reller.** 1992. Controlled comparison of the BacT/Alert and BACTEC 660/730 non-radiometric blood culture systems. *J. Clin. Microbiol.* **30:**323–329.

Candida and Candidiasis
Edited by Richard A. Calderone
© 2002 ASM Press, Washington, D.C.

Chapter 27

Non-Culture-Based Diagnostics

José Pontón, María D. Moragues, and Guillermo Quindós

The multiple problems associated with the clinical and microbiological diagnosis of invasive candidiasis (described in chapters 23, 24, and 26) have prompted the development of non-culture-based laboratory methods. These methods must accomplish the difficult task of differentiating normal colonization of human mucous membranes by *Candida* species, particularly *Candida albicans,* from tissue invasion and candidemia requiring antifungal therapy. At present, non-culture-based laboratory methods for the diagnosis of invasive candidiasis rely on the detection of antibodies against *Candida* antigens, detection of *Candida* antigens, and detection of nonantigenic *Candida* components, such as the metabolites D-arabinitol and mannose, the cell wall component (1→3)-β-D-glucan, or *Candida* nucleic acids (Fig. 1). Detection of *Candida* DNA is described in chapter 28.

Early studies of non-culture-based laboratory methods for the diagnosis of invasive candidiasis date to the 1950s when techniques to detect anti-*Candida* antibodies were first used. At that time, blood culture detection techniques often failed to recover *Candida* organisms (19, 180, 287, 290) and only serological techniques could provide useful information for the clinician (274). During the following years, other techniques for the detection of anti-*Candida* antibodies, *Candida* antigens, and metabolites were developed. However, despite the numerous methods and techniques devised, none of them have found widespread clinical use. Currently, the situation has changed; blood culture methods have substantially increased our ability to detect *Candida* fungemia (186, 227, 288), and new and sensitive tests based on the amplification of *Candida* DNA are being developed for the laboratory diagnosis of invasive candidiasis (176). Despite these advances, the problems associated with the laboratory diagnosis of invasive candidiasis are far from solved. Detection of *Candida* antigens, metabolites, and cell wall components, as well as detection of anti-*Candida* antibodies, is useful for confirming fungemia, especially in particular patient populations. For instance, blood culture seems to be more effective in detecting candidemia in intensive care patients than in patients with hematological malignancies (108). Thus, febrile patients with hematological malignancies could benefit more from the use of non-culture methods for the diagnosis of invasive candidiasis than intensive care patients.

Detection of *Candida* DNA by PCR has an important advantage in that it is exquisitely sensitive, but at present it is technically cumbersome, and it has yet to be demonstrated conclusively that this approach is able to overcome the limitations of serological assays. A comparison of the performance of several non-culture methods for the diagnosis of invasive candidiasis in allogeneic bone marrow and solid-organ transplant recipients has been reported by Chryssanthou et al. (41). In this study, detection of *C. albicans* DNA by PCR, (1→3)-β-D-glucan, mannan, and the antigen detected by the Cand-Tec test in serum was compared with detection of D-arabinitol in urine. Although the tests were positive in some patients, no single test was sufficient to establish a diagnosis of invasive candidiasis. These results confirm data obtained from different studies, suggesting that it will be difficult to develop a single test with sufficient sensitivity and specificity to make a definitive diagnosis in a patient with invasive candidiasis (126, 287, 289). Physicians may need to rely on cumulative information from serial specimens and diagnostic techniques to have sufficient confidence to begin antifungal therapy for invasive candidiasis (108, 130, 290). Non-culture-based laboratory methods may also be used as markers of complete eradication of invasive

José Pontón and Guillermo Quindós • Departamento de Inmunología, Microbiología y Parasitología, Facultad de Medicina y Odontología, Universidad del País Vasco, Barrio Sarriena s/n, 48940 Leioa, Vizcaya, Spain. **María D. Moragues** • Departamento de Enfermería I, Universidad del País Vasco, Barrio Sarriena s/n, 48940 Leioa, Vizcaya, Spain.

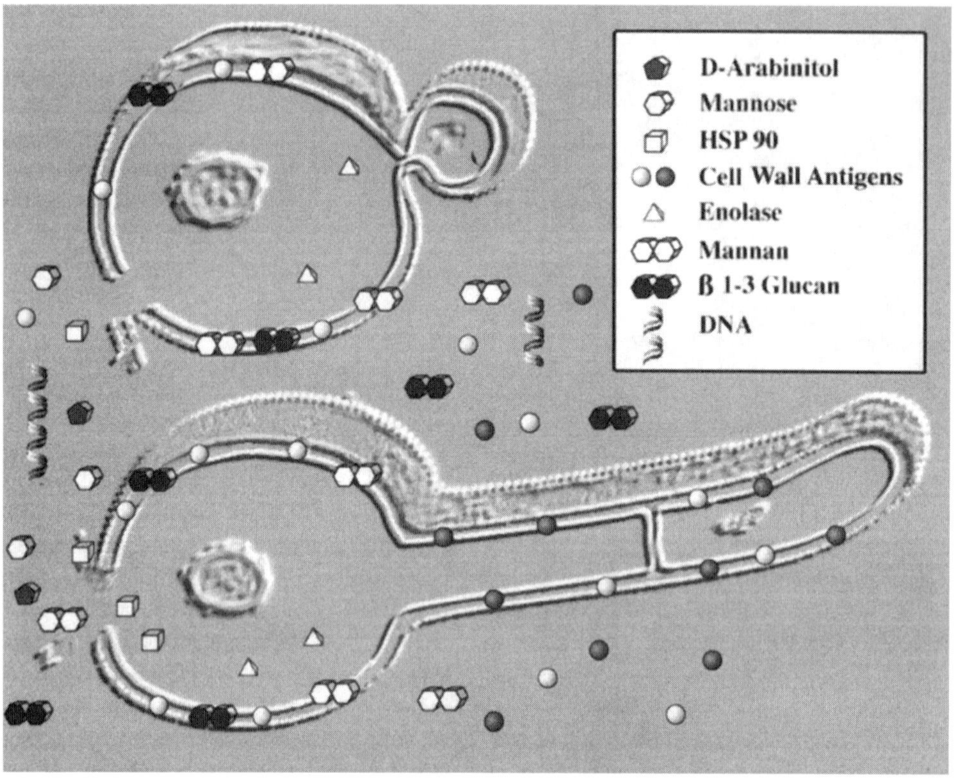

Figure 1. Schematic diagram showing the main antigenic and nonantigenic components of *C. albicans* used in non-culture-based diagnostic tests for invasive candidiasis. The upper part of the figure depicts a budding *C. albicans* blastospore and the lower part depicts a *C. albicans* cell with a hyphal extrusion. Cytoplasmic components are released in broken cells.

candidiasis when monitoring the efficacy of antifungal therapy (18, 28, 99, 126, 159, 253).

DETECTION OF ANTIBODIES

As mentioned earlier, techniques for the detection of an antibody response by patients with invasive candidiasis were the first to be developed. After almost 50 years of experience in this field, two main limitations are evident for the detection of antibodies in patients with invasive candidiasis: (i) the specificity of the tests may be low because antibody titers can be high in patients who are only colonized with *Candida* spp. (50) and (ii) the tests may present a low sensitivity because the antibody response may be delayed, reduced, or absent in immunocompromised patients (23). However, it may be possible to overcome these limitations because the specificity of the tests for antibody detection can be increased by selecting the appropriate antigens and an increase in the sensitivity of the tests can be obtained by using techniques such as the enzyme-linked immunosorbent assay (ELISA). A useful test must combine improvements in both sensitivity and specificity, since nothing is gained from a more sensitive test unless a more specific antigen is also used (52).

Assays for the detection of antibodies against *Candida* antigens have changed over the years. Initial studies used whole cells, or very complex antigenic extracts, to detect antibodies to *C. albicans* by techniques such as complement fixation (195, 252), agglutination (61, 63, 76, 86, 130, 137, 155, 188, 263, 273, 296), double immunodiffusion (45, 61, 63, 76, 86, 130, 137, 188, 261, 263, 270, 272, 273), counterimmunoelectrophoresis (CIE) (45, 84, 86, 94, 130, 147, 192, 230), crossed immunoelectrophoresis (76), germ tube dispersion (188), and indirect immunofluorescence (3, 91, 135–137, 155, 273). As an example of these studies, Harding et al. (86) compared antibody detection by whole cell agglutination, double immunodiffusion, and CIE for the diagnosis of invasive candidiasis primarily in an immunocompetent patient population. An agglutination titer of 1:160 or greater was invariably found when either or both precipitin tests were positive. However, 17% of patients without evidence of invasive candidiasis also had agglutination titers ≥1:160. Specificities for double immunodiffusion and CIE tests were 97% and 96%, respectively. The sensitivity of the tests ranged from 75% for double immunodiffusion, 83% for whole cell agglutination, and 92% for CIE. Because of the crossreactivity shown by *C. tropicalis* and *C. glabrata* with *C. albicans,* the tests were also useful for the diagnosis of infection caused by these non-*C. albicans* species. Interestingly, in some patients, the agglutination titer rose with the progression of the disease and fell as a result of successful antifungal therapy, stressing the value of serial antibody determinations in the management of patients with invasive candidiasis. Unfortunately, when double immunodiffusion and CIE tests have been used for the diagnosis of invasive candidiasis in immunocompromised patients, their sensitivity was low and they were found to be of limited diagnostic value (63, 84, 179, 215, 216). A summary of these early studies is presented in Table 1.

In general, early studies on antibody detection for the diagnosis of invasive candidiasis were limited in several ways: (i) the crude antigen preparations used in different laboratories could not be standardized to enable good test reproducibility among laboratories; (ii) because most of the antigenic extracts contained cell wall mannan and antimannan antibodies have been detected in healthy human sera (38, 196), the antigens used could not distinguish antibodies formed during mucosal colonization from those produced during invasive infection; (iii) the techniques used in most studies showed a low sensitivity for the diagnosis of invasive candidiasis in immunocompromised patients; and (iv) there was a bias in most of these studies because sera from patients with invasive candidiasis were often used to assess the sensitivity of the assays whereas their specificity was determined with sera from healthy volunteers as controls (108). Several authors have reviewed the early diagnostic tests used for detecting antibodies in patients with invasive candidiasis (52, 93, 96, 118, 129, 131, 189, 247, 274).

Studies performed after 1980 attempted to improve the results obtained in the previous decades by using purified antigens and more sensitive techniques such as the ELISA (11, 56, 67, 82, 87, 122, 124, 128, 168, 182, 184, 194, 241, 246, 254), radioimmunoassay (RIA) (82, 106, 117, 154, 166), and immunoblotting (6, 89, 204, 245, 293) (Table 2). Initially, these antigens were purified mainly from the cell wall and the cytoplasm from both blastoconidia and germ tubes of *C. albicans*. However, differentiation between cell wall and cytoplasmic antigens may be difficult since most of the cytoplasmic antigens relevant for antibody detection have also been recently detected in the cell wall (36, 151). Enolase can be used to illustrate this point; this enzyme was initially described in cytoplasmic extracts (264), but there is recent experimental evidence indicating that enolase is also an integral component of the cell wall of *C. albicans* and is associated with glucan (2). The usefulness of antibody detection in the diagnosis of invasive candidiasis has been extensively reviewed in the literature (48, 107, 108, 141, 151, 203, 209, 239).

The antigenic composition of the cell wall of *C. albicans* has been extensively studied in an attempt to identify antigens of diagnostic relevance (151, 189, 212). Six different types of antigens have been described in the *C. albicans* cell wall (206). Type I antigens are truly germ tube-specific and are expressed on the germ tube cell wall surface only. Type II antigens are expressed on both the germ tube cell surface and within the blastoconidium cell wall. These antigens would appear as germ tube-specific if tested by indirect immunofluorescence, but they can be extracted from the blastoconidium cell wall with treatments that remove the outermost layers. Presence of type II antigens within the blastoconidium cell wall would explain the induction of antibodies to germ tubes in rabbits immunized with dithiothreitol extracts from blastoconidia, heat-killed blastoconidia, and formalin-killed blastoconidia (225), or in both patients (221) and rabbits (16) infected with *Candida* species that are unable to produce germ tubes in serum. Type III antigens are expressed on both the blastoconidium and germ tube surface. Type IV antigens are expressed within the cell wall of both blastoconidia and germ tubes. Type V antigens are expressed on the blastoconidium cell surface and within the germ tube cell wall, and type VI antigens are expressed on the blastoconidium surface only. A summary of the different types of antigens described in the cell wall of *C. albicans* is shown in Table 3.

Mannan is an abundant type III antigen located on the *Candida* cell wall surface. This antigen is highly immunogenic for humans, who usually respond with a rise in the antimannan antibody titers when large numbers of *Candida* cells enter the bloodstream (105). Antimannan antibodies have been detected in many studies (5, 6, 67, 85–87, 113, 122, 130, 137, 182, 194, 241, 249, 273, 281, 286, 296) (Table 2). Detailed information about the kinetics of antimannan antibodies during invasive candidiasis was obtained in the studies performed by Jones and associates (79, 105, 106). By using a carefully standardized ELISA to measure antimannan antibody levels in sequential serum samples from patients with acute leukemia, Greenfield et al. (79) reported a sensitivity of 64.3% and a specificity of 97.2% in the diagnosis of invasive candidiasis. A positive test for antimannan antibodies increased the chances that an episode was complicated by invasive candidiasis to 86.7 to 90.0%.

Table 1. Early studies (until 1980) on antibody detection for the diagnosis of invasive candidiasis

Year	Method(s)[a]	Antigen[b]	No. of patients with invasive candidiasis			No. of controls			Sensitivity (%)	Specificity (%)	Efficiency (%)	Reference
			Neutrop.	Nonneutrop.	Total	Neutrop.	Nonneutrop.	Total				
1978	CIE	BC	–	–	6	–	–	34	83.3	85.3	85	78
1978	LA	BC	–	–	53	–	–	170	81	89	87	130[c]
1972	ID	BCW	–	–	3	–	–	14	100	42.9	52.9	137
1968	IFA	WB	–	–	47	–	–	122	70.2	96	88.8	59
1972	IFA	WB	7	17	24	–	–	9	67	11.1	51.5	273
1972	IFA	WB	–	–	3	–	–	14	100	64.3	70.6	137
1977	IFA (IgM)	WB	–	–	16	–	–	81	75	95.1	91.8	3
1977	IFA (IgA)	WB	–	–	16	–	–	81	75	76.5	76.3	3
1977	IFA (IgG)	WB	–	–	16	–	–	81	100	82.7	85.6	3
1978	WCA	WB	–	–	53	–	–	170	55	84	77	130[c]
1969	WCA	WB	23	–	23	10	–	10	60.9	100	72.7	216
1972	WCA	WB	–	–	3	–	–	14	100	71.4	76.5	137
1972	WCA	WB	7	17	24	–	–	9	89	100	90.1	273
1976	WCA	WB	–	–	24	–	–	76	83	83	83	86
1977	WCA	WB	–	–	12	–	–	31	50	41.9	44.2	63
1978	WCA	WB	–	–	5	–	–	196	60	67	67	76
1978	CIE	BH	–	–	53	–	–	170	89	88	88	130[c]
1979	CIE	BH	–	–	15	–	–	42	33.3	95.2	78.9	291
1978	ID	BH	–	–	53	–	–	170	89	90	90	130[a]
1976	HA	MAN	–	–	19	–	–	286	94.7	0.7	6.6	292
1972	ID	CY (S Ag)	7	17	24	–	–	9	70	100	78.8	273
1980	CIE	MC	–	–	17	–	–	47	41.2	100	82.5	178
1979	ID	ME	–	17	17	–	41	41	70.6	97.6	89.7	90[c]
1978	IFA	POL	–	–	6	–	–	34	100	79.4	82.5	78
1980	CIE	P	–	–	12	–	–	50	75	90	87.1	144
1977	HA	WCE	–	–	8	–	287	287	100	43.9	45.4	155
1976	CIE	WCE	–	–	24	–	–	76	92	96	95	86
1977	CIE	WCE	–	–	24	–	–	140	70.8	97.9	93.9	46
1979	CIE	WCE	2	–	2	37	–	37	100	89	89.7	179
1980	CIE	WCE	–	–	17	–	–	47	94	40	56	178
1969	ID	WCE	23	–	23	10	–	10	17.4	100	42.4	216
1976	ID	WCE	–	–	24	–	–	76	75	97	92	86
1976	ID	WCE (S Ag)	–	–	19	–	–	286	52.6	96.9	94.1	292
1977	ID	WCE	–	–	24	–	–	140	87.5	98.6	97	46
1978	ID	WCE	–	–	5	–	–	196	100	76	76.5	76
1977	ID	WCE	–	–	12	–	–	31	50	22.6	30.2	63
1978	XIE	WCE	–	–	5	–	–	196	100	98	98	76

[a]Methods: CIE, counterimmunoelectrophoresis; HA, hemagglutination; ID, immunodiffusion; IFA, immunofluorescence assay; LA, latex agglutination; WCA, whole cell agglutination; XIE, cross-immunoelectrophoresis.
[b]Antigens: BC, blastospore cytoplasm; BCW, blastospore cell wall; WB, whole blastospores; BH, blastosphore homogenate; MAN, mannan; CY, cytoplasmic; MC, mycelium cytoplasm; ME, mycelium extract; POL, polysaccharidic; P, proteinase; WCE, whole cell extract.
[c]Not including patients with superficial candidiasis among the controls.

Table 2. Studies performed after 1980 on antibody detection for the diagnosis of invasive candidiasis

Year	Method(s)[a]	Antigen[b]	No. of patients with invasive candidiasis			No. of controls			Sensitivity (%)	Specificity (%)	Efficiency (%)	Reference
			Neutrop.	Nonneutrop.	Total	Neutrop.	Nonneutrop.	Total				
1997	IB	29 kDa	1	7	8	–	–	383	100	63	63.7	293
1998	ELISA	52 kDa METAL	–	–	40	–	–	36	83	97	89.5	56[c]
1993	CIE	BC	–	–	30	–	–	14	80	28.6	63.6	283
1994	CIE (IgG)	BC	–	7	7	–	277	277	71.4	98.9	98.3	122
1983	ELISA	BC (54.3 kDa)	20	–	20	80	–	80	25	98.8	83	82
1992	ELISA (IgM)	BC	–	–	28	–	–	92	35.7	90.1	74.2	254
1993	ELISA	BC	9	19	28	13	113	126	46.4	100	90.3	184
1988	IB	BC (47 kDa)	55	37	92	–	21	21	73.9	61.9	67.3	159
1994	IB	BC (47 kDa)	–	–	17	–	–	47	82.4	86.7	85.1	37
1997	IB	BC (47 kDa)	1	7	8	–	–	383	100	30	31.5	293
1994	ID	BC	–	–	17	–	–	47	23.5	93.3	68.1	37
1987	IFA	BC	–	–	14	–	–	46	68	75	69.2	210[c]
1988	IFA	BC	–	36	36	–	80	80	91	50	62.9	17[c]
1989	IFA	BC	–	36	36	–	96	96	91	50	61.4	18[c]
1993	CIE	BC+MAN	–	–	30	–	–	14	70	78.6	72.7	283
1996	CIE	BC+MAN	9	27	36	8	6	14	64	89	70	281
1983	ELISA	BC+MAN	20	–	20	80	–	80	70	97.4	92	82
1993	IFA (IgM)	BC+MAN	–	–	10	–	–	70	100	100	100	85
1993	IFA (IgG)	BC+MAN	–	–	10	–	–	70	80	81.4	81.3	85
1988	HA	BCW	–	36	36	–	80	80	75	87	83.6	17[c]
1989	HA	BCW	–	36	36	–	96	96	97	60	70.5	18[c]
1994	HA (IgM)	BCW	–	7	7	–	277	277	100	90	90.6	122
1990	IFA	BCW (SER A)	5	17	22	10	32	42	45.5	60.9	69	20
1990	IFA	BCW (SER B)	5	17	22	10	32	42	50	62.5	69	20
1990	IFA	BCW	13	14	27	35	119	154	100	2.6	17.1	221
1995	IFA	BCW	8	20	28	14	20	34	57	85	73	226
1997	IFA (IgA)	BCW	–	22	22	–	24	24	77.3	75	76.1	279
1997	IFA (IgG)	BCW	–	22	22	–	24	24	81.8	54.2	67.4	279
1997	IFA (IgM)	BCW	–	22	22	–	24	24	59.1	75	65.2	279
1994	TA	BCW	–	–	17	–	–	47	76.5	40	53.2	37
1996	CoCIE	BCW+S	–	–	56	–	–	833	58.9	96.4	94	5
1996	IFA	BCW+S	–	–	56	–	–	833	48.2	96.4	93.4	5
1981	HA	WB	–	–	24	–	–	33	78	64	70.2	128[c]
1981	IFA	WB	–	–	24	–	–	33	67	79	73.7	128[c]
1988	CIE	CY	13	10	23	26	7	33	43.5	78.8	64.3	201
1989	CIE-XIE	CY	7	–	7	12	–	12	14	100	68.4	278
1984	ELISA	CY	–	–	12	–	–	36	100	100	100	116[c]
1986	ELISA	CY	13	1	14	–	–	162	64	90	88.1	67
1989	ELISA	CY	–	–	23	–	–	30	78	100	90.1	167
1986	HA	CY	13	1	14	–	–	162	86	80	80.7	67
1987	HA	CY	13	10	23	26	7	33	39.1	81.8	64.3	202

Continued on following page

Table 2. *Continued*

Year	Method(s)[a]	Antigen[b]	No. of patients with invasive candidiasis			No. of controls			Sensitivity (%)	Specificity (%)	Efficiency (%)	Reference
			Neutrop.	Nonneutrop.	Total	Neutrop.	Nonneutrop.	Total				
1986	ID	CY	13	1	14	–	–	162	29	94	88.6	67
1989	MIA	CY	–	–	23	–	–	30	100	100	100	167
1994	ELISA	ENO	–	30	30	–	18	18	50	100	82.5	282
1994	ELISA	ENO	46	–	46	14	–	14	53	95	61.7	282
1995	ELISA	ENO	–	–	37	–	–	43	73	95	85	11
1994	IB	ENO	–	27	27	–	30	30	92.5	95	94	170
1986	CIE	GC	–	–	14	–	–	22	86	77	80.6	153
1986	ELISA	GC	–	–	14	–	–	22	73	91	83.3	153
1989	CIE–XIE	MAN	7	–	7	12	–	12	43	83	68.4	278
1981	ELISA	MAN	10	–	10	82	–	82	100	0	1.1	168
1983	ELISA	MAN	20	–	20	80	–	80	64.3	97.2	91	83
1986	ELISA	MAN	23	–	23	64	–	64	60.9	93.8	85.1	109
1986	ELISA	MAN	–	–	45	–	–	105	55.6	88.6	78.7	109
1989	ELISA	MAN	–	–	23	–	–	30	83	100	92.5	167
1989	ELISA (IgA)	MAN	7	–	7	12	–	12	100	50	68.4	278
1989	ELISA (IgM)	MAN	7	–	7	12	–	12	57.1	75	63.2	278
1994	ELISA (IgA)	MAN	–	6	6	–	277	277	100	83.6	83.9	122
1999	ELISA	MAN	–	43	43	–	–	230	40	98	88.6	249[c]
1996	HA	MAN	9	27	36	8	6	14	64	86	72	281
1996	IB (IgE)	MAN	–	–	14	–	–	30	85.7	80	81.8	244
1981	LA	MAN	10	–	10	82	–	82	14	86.6	78.3	168
1989	MIA	MAN	–	–	23	–	–	30	100	100	100	167
1996	RAST (IgE)	MAN	–	–	14	–	–	30	71.4	90	84.1	244
1995	ELISA	MANP	–	–	37	–	–	43	78	82	80	11
1993	ELISA	MCW	9	19	28	13	113	126	89.2	98.6	96.8	184
1987	IFA (IgA)	MCW	–	11	11	–	98	98	81.8	100	98.2	220
1987	IFA (IgG)	MCW	–	11	11	–	98	98	72.7	100	97.2	220
1987	IFA (IgG+IgA)	MCW	–	11	11	–	98	98	100	100	100	220
1988	IFA (IgG+IgA)	MCW	–	11	11	–	40	40	100	100	100	219
1990	IFA	MCW	13	14	27	35	119	154	77.8	96.8	94.4	221
1993	IFA	MCW	5	–	5	23	20	43	100	97.7	97.9	285

1994	IFA	MCW	–	–	26	12	46	58	84.6	87.9	86.9	208
1995	IFA	MCW	8	20	28	14	20	34	82	94	89	226
1997	IFA	MCW	7	1	8	71	–	71	87.5	95.2	92.4	70
1997	IFA (IgA)	MCW	–	22	22	–	24	24	40.9	100	71.7	279
1997	IFA (IgG)	MCW	–	22	22	–	24	24	40.9	100	71.7	279
1997	IFA (IgM)	MCW	–	22	22	–	24	24	9.1	100	56.5	279
1981	CIE	M	–	–	24	–	–	33	78	64	70.2	128[c]
1992	ELISA (IgG)	M	–	–	68	–	–	89	67.6	77.3	73.2	31
1981	CIE	S	–	–	24	–	–	33	100	52	71.9	128[c]
1986	CoCIE	S	–	–	40	–	–	994	69	100	98.8	211
1987	CoCIE	S	–	–	14	–	–	46	76	91	88.3	210
1990	CoCIE	S	–	–	10	–	–	30	50	76.7	70	20
1991	ELISA (IgG)	S	8	19	27	–	201	201	81.5	97	95.2	301
1992	ELISA (IgG)	S	–	–	68	–	–	89	58.8	83.3	72.6	31
1990	IP	S	5	17	22	10	32	42	50	62.5	69	20
1996	MIA	S	–	–	56	–	–	833	80.4	90.2	89.5	5
1988	CIE	S+M	–	36	36	–	80	80	58	97	85.3	17[c]
1989	CIE	S+M	–	36	36	–	96	96	58	96	85.6	18[c]
1988	WCA	WC	13	10	23	26	7	33	34.8	84.8	64.3	201
1981	CIE	WCE	–	–	18	–	–	70	77.8	97.1	93.2	44
1981	ELISA (IgA)	WCE	–	–	24	–	–	33	78	70	73.7	128[c]
1981	ELISA (IgG)	WCE	–	–	24	–	–	33	89	76	80.7	128[c]
1981	ELISA (IgM)	WCE	–	–	24	–	–	33	67	88	78.9	128[c]
1985	ELISA	WCE	–	–	13	–	–	72	92	89	90	64
1989	ELISA	WCE	–	–	23	–	–	30	83	100	92.5	167
1981	ID	WCE	–	–	24	–	–	33	100	67	80.7	128[c]
1981	ID	WCE	10	–	10	82	–	82	14	76.8	69.6	168
1981	LA	WCE	–	–	18	–	–	70	94.4	50	59.1	44
1989	MIA	WCE	–	–	23	–	–	30	100	100	100	167

[a]Methods: CIE, counterimmunoelectrophoresis; CoCIE, cocounterimmunoelectrophoresis; ELISA, enzyme-linked immunosorbent assay; HA, hemagglutination; IB, immunoblotting; ID, immunodiffusion; IFA, immunofluorescence assay; IP, immunoprecipitation; MIA, micro-immunocapture assay; RAST, radio allergo sorbent test; TA, tube agglutination; CF, complement fixation; GTD, germ tube dispersion; WCA, whole cell agglutination; XIE, cross-immunoelectrophoresis.

[b]Antigens: METAL, metallopeptidase; BC, blastospore cytoplasm; MAN, mannan; BCW, blastospore cell wall; SER A, serotype A; SER B, serotype B; WB, whole blastospores; CY, cytoplasmic; ENO, enolase; GC, germling cytoplasm; MANP, mannoprotein; MCW, mycelium cell wall; S, somatic; M, metabolic; WCE, whole cell extract.

[c]Not including patients with superficial candidiasis among the controls.

Table 3. Examples of type I–IV cell wall antigens of *C. albicans*

Antigen type	Antigens described	Reference
I	200 and 155 kDa	266
	260 and 180 kDa	33
	3D9[a]	206
	2G8 and 4E1	53
	Hwp1	258
	16B1F10[a]	149
	12B12[a]	149
II	Ag 1.183[a]	190
	C3d receptor	111
	15C9[a]	206
	PA10F[a]	206
	11C11[a]	206
III	Mp58	34
	B9E[a]	206
	N3B[a]	206
	Mannans	206
	3H8[a]	146
IV	C6[a]	21
	AF-1[a]	35
	3B7[a]	65
	3G6[a]	65
	G3B[a]	206
	21E6[a]	206
	D9F[a]	206
	14.8[a]	206
	Enolase	2

[a]These antigens have been described using a monoclonal antibody.

However, if serial tests for antibody to mannan remained negative, this likelihood decreased to 8.6 to 12.5% (79). Interestingly, serodiagnosis was achieved before clinical diagnosis in 67% of the patients tested. In contrast to this study, Meckstroth et al. (168) were not able to discriminate leukemic patients with invasive candidiasis from those without invasive candidiasis on the basis of the detection of antibodies to cell wall mannan by ELISA. By using a hemagglutination assay to detect antibodies against mannan in immunocompromised patients, van Deventer et al. (281) reported a sensitivity of 64% and a specificity of 86%. Similar results (sensitivity 53% and specificity 94%) were obtained by Sendid et al. (249) in a mainly immunocompetent patient population using a commercially available test to detect antibodies to cell wall mannan by ELISA (Platelia *Candida* Ab, Sanofi Diagnostics Pasteur, Marnes-la-Coquette, France). Interestingly, detection of mannan seemed to complement antimannan antibody detection for the diagnosis of invasive candidiasis, since patients positive for mannan antigenemia did not have significant levels of antimannan antibodies or vice versa. In a small group of patients in whom both mannan and antimannan antibodies were detected, kinetic studies showed that detection of antimannan antibodies was inversely correlated to the presence of mannan antigenemia (Fig. 2). Combining results obtained with each test allowed the diagnosis of invasive candidiasis with a sensitivity of 80% and a specificity of 93%. Other studies reported that detection of antimannan antibodies was a valuable marker of invasive candidiasis (5, 85, 113), or useful for confirming the diagnosis in immunocompetent patients (241).

In the *Candida* cell wall, mannan is covalently associated with proteins to form mannoproteins (36). Among the complex array of mannoproteins described in the *C. albicans* cell wall, Pontón and Jones (204, 205) identified a component of 230 to 250 kDa from the germ-tube cell wall surface, which was recognized by sera from patients with invasive candidia-

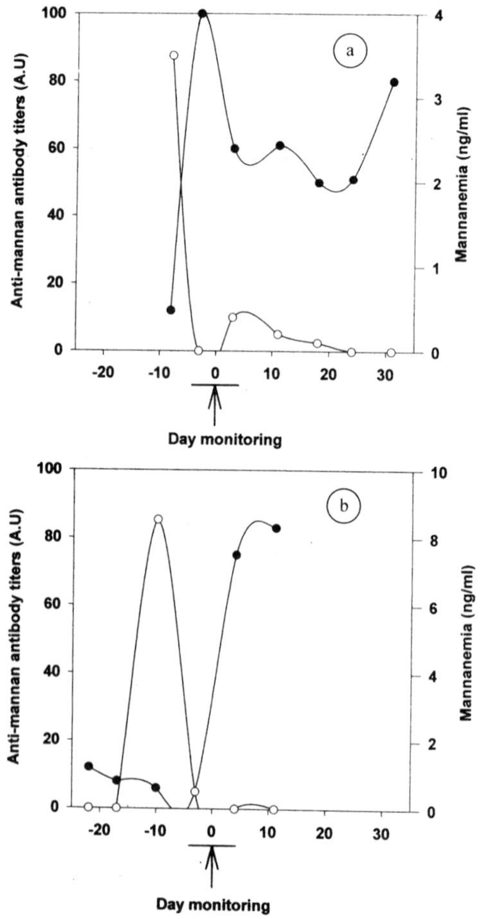

Figure 2. Kinetics of mannan (○) and antimannan antibodies (●) in two patients (a and b) with invasive candidiasis. The arrow marks the date of the isolation of *C. albicans* from blood and a drain. Reprinted from the *Journal of Clinical Microbiology* (249) with permission of the authors and the publisher.

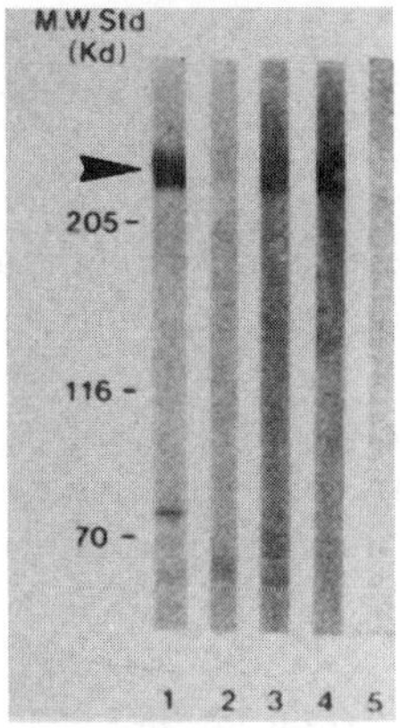

Figure 3. Western immunoblots of proteins separated by electrophoresis in a sodium dodecyl sulfate–6% polyacrylamide gel electrophoresis gel. The gel was loaded with a dithiothreitol germ tube extract (lanes 1, 3, and 4) and a dithiothreitol blastospore extract (lanes 2 and 5) and stained with either sera from a rabbit immunized with *C. albicans* germ tubes (lanes 1 and 2) or with sera from two patients with invasive candidiasis (lanes 3 through 5) that had been adsorbed with heat-killed blastospores. The arrow indicates the 230 to 250-kDa germ tube-specific cell wall component. Reprinted from *Infection and Immunity* (205) with permission of the authors and the publisher.

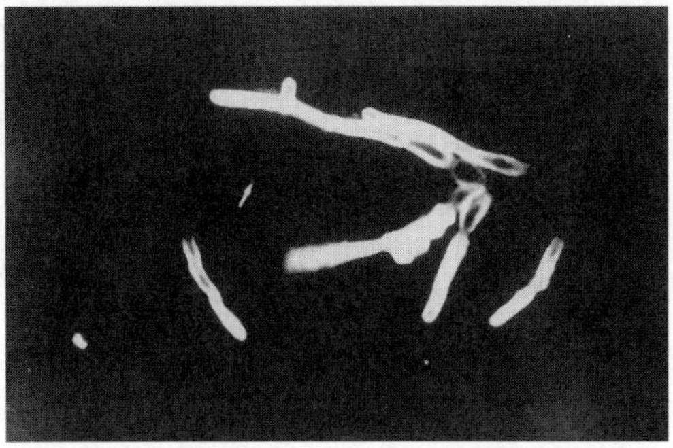

Figure 4. Detection of antibodies to *C. albicans* germ tubes by indirect immunofluorescence. Only germ tubes are stained. Arrow points to one of the many blastospores not visible under fluorescence. Reprinted from the *European Journal of Clinical Microbiology* (221) with permission of the authors and the publisher.

sis (Fig. 3). Identification of *C. albicans* germ tube-specific antigens was considered to be important since the filamentous phase of *C. albicans* is found in infected tissues (212) and, therefore, detection of antibodies against antigens expressed during tissue invasion may increase the specificity of tests based on the detection of antibodies (60). Several germ tube-specific antigens have also been described by other groups (1, 22, 30, 32, 33, 140, 143, 150, 258, 266–268) (Table 3).

Taking advantage of the location of the 230 to 250-kDa antigen on the germ tube cell wall surface, Quindós et al. (220) developed an indirect immunofluorescence assay to detect antibodies against this antigen in sera from patients with invasive candidiasis (Fig. 4). Detection of antibodies to *C. albicans* germ tubes (CAGT) was useful in the diagnosis of invasive candidiasis in different groups of patients, including heroin addicts and hematological and intensive care patients (70, 99, 208, 219–222, 226, 279). The test showed an overall sensitivity of 77 to 89% and a specificity of 91 to 100% (208, 219–221). These results are in contrast to those obtained when antibodies to *C. albicans* blastoconidia were detected, since detection of antibodies to *C. albicans* blastoconidia, which are mainly directed against mannans, is more sensitive than detection of antibodies to CAGT, but less specific (208, 219–221, 279, 285). Sera sequentially drawn from patients at risk of developing invasive candidiasis showed antibodies to CAGT before the microbiological diagnosis was made, especially in patients with tissue-proven invasive candidiasis (70). Since antibodies to CAGT were detected in sera from all patients with tissue-proven invasive candidiasis but negative by blood culture, detection of antibodies to CAGT seemed to complement blood culture for the diagnosis of patients with hematological malignancies and invasive candidiasis (70). The kinetics of the antibody response to CAGT in a patient with invasive candidiasis is shown in Fig. 5. One interesting feature concerning the detection of antibodies to CAGT is that patients with infections caused by *Candida* species other than *C. albicans* may also be positive, although they usually yield lower titers than patients infected by *C. albicans*. In addition to infections caused by both serotypes of *C. albicans*, antibodies to CAGT have been detected in patients infected with *C. tropicalis*, *C. parapsilosis*, *C. glabrata*, *C. dubliniensis*, and *C. krusei* (70, 208, 221, 226, 242). Antibodies to CAGT have also been detected in rabbits infected with *C. guilliermondii* (16). Initial studies showed encouraging results, both in sensitivity and specificity, when detection of antibodies to CAGT was performed in sera from immunocompromised patients with invasive candidiasis, since immunocompromised patients presented lower but detectable antibody titers (221). These results have been confirmed by other studies, which included bone marrow transplant recipients and patients with hematological disorders (70, 295). In addition to its diagnostic potential, detection of antibodies to CAGT may be useful for the therapeutic monitoring of patients with invasive candidiasis, since the administration of antifungal therapy usually results in decreasing titers of antibodies to CAGT in sera from patients who survive the infection (70, 222). The kinetics of the antibody re-

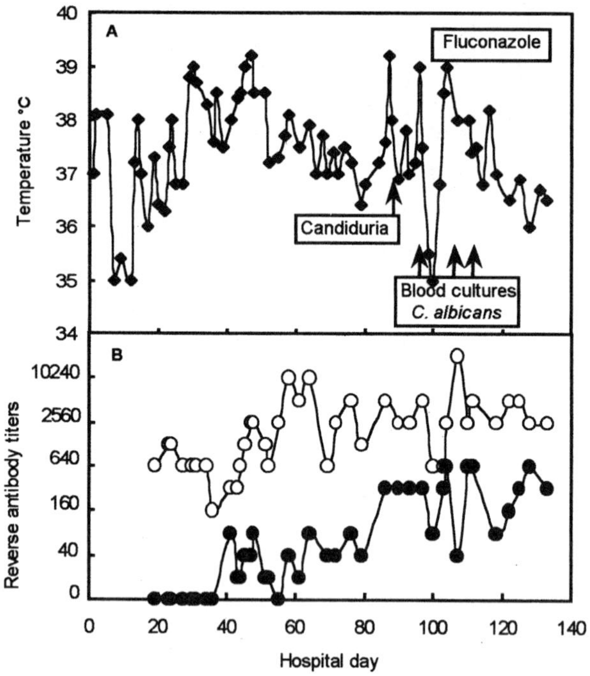

Figure 5. Kinetics of body temperature (◆), antibodies to *C. albicans* germ tubes (●), and blastospores (○) in a patient with invasive candidiasis. This case is representative of the usefulness of detection of antibodies to CAGT in sequentially drawn sera for the diagnosis of invasive candidiasis. Reprinted from the *Revista Iberoamericana de Micología* (99) with permission of the authors and the publisher.

sponse to CAGT in a patient with invasive candidiasis who responded to antifungal treatment is shown in Fig. 6.

By using an ELISA to detect antibodies raised against a β-mercaptoethanol extract from *C. albicans* germ tubes in sera depleted of antimannan antibodies, Navarro et al. (184) reported a sensitivity of 89.2% and a specificity of 98.6% for the diagnosis of invasive candidiasis in a population of patients, including bone marrow transplant patients. Poulain et al. (213) devised a method to detect antibodies against a *C. albicans* somatic antigen, which showed a common precipitin line with antibodies present in a rabbit anti-*C. albicans* germ tube antiserum. The test showed a specificity and a sensitivity ranging from 100 to 69% for the diagnosis of invasive candidiasis (211). However, Bougnoux et al. (20) were not able to differentiate patients with invasive candidiasis from patients colonized by *Candida* spp. using this test (Table 2).

Antibodies to CAGT present in patients with invasive candidiasis are likely to be directed against both *C. albicans* type I and II antigens (206), and they can be detected by indirect immunofluorescence using *C. albicans* germ tubes. Since the germ tube cell wall also contains mannan, to detect antibodies to CAGT, the sera have to be adsorbed, a process that is time-consuming and requires large amounts of heat-killed blastoconidia (206). A test based on the detection of antibodies against type I antigens may not require the adsorption of the sera and would therefore facilitate serodiagnosis of invasive candidiasis. In this regard, by using an ELISA and purified *C. albicans* type I and II antigens, Bikandi et al. (14) detected antibodies in sera from patients with invasive candidiasis with a sensitivity of 78% and a specificity of 68% without removing the antimannan antibodies from the sera. In a similar study, Berdin et al. (11) developed an ELISA to detect IgG antibodies against a *C. albicans* type I antigen in patients with invasive candidiasis and reported a sensitivity of 78% and a specificity of 82%.

Although cytoplasmic extracts were used early in the development of serological tests for the diagnosis of invasive candidiasis (274), it was necessary to develop techniques to fractionate or resolve complex antigenic mixtures to identify immunodominant antigens in these extracts. By using polyacrylamide gel electrophoresis and ammonium sulfate precipitation of cytoplasmic extracts, Jones (105, 106) described a major *C. albicans* antigen that was recognized by

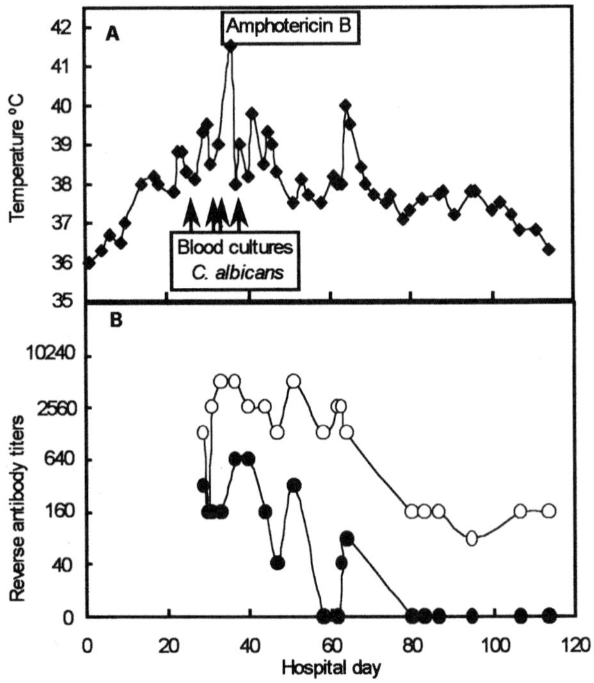

Figure 6. Kinetics of body temperature (◆), antibodies to *C. albicans* germ tubes (●), and blastospores (○) in a patient with invasive candidiasis. This case is representative of the role of detection of antibodies to CAGT in sequentially drawn sera for monitoring the efficacy of antifungal therapy in patients with invasive candidiasis. Reprinted from the *Revista Iberoamericana de Micología* (99) with permission of the authors and the publisher.

antibodies present in sera from patients with invasive candidiasis. The antigen had a molecular mass of 54.3 kDa and was also present in *C. tropicalis* and *C. guilliermondii* (80, 81). Antibodies to this antigen were detected by ELISA in sequential serum samples from patients with acute leukemia by Greenfield et al. (79), who reported a sensitivity of 21.4% and a specificity of 100% for the diagnosis of invasive candidiasis. Other studies have also demonstrated the usefulness of finding antibodies to the 54.3-kDa antigen in patients with invasive candidiasis (67, 116). In general, an improvement in the specificity of the tests was observed when crude cytoplasmic antigens were replaced by purified cytoplasmic antigens (301) (Table 2). Antigens having similar molecular masses to that identified by Jones (106) were also described by other groups, including antigens of 44 to 52 kDa (264), 47 kDa (164, 185, 300), 45 kDa (6, 301), and 43 kDa (71). Given the similarities in the molecular masses of these antigens, it is likely that some of them were equivalent or closely related; two of them have been extensively characterized. The 47-kDa antigen has been shown to be a breakdown product of the heat shock protein (HSP) 90 (161), and the 44- to 52-kDa antigen has been shown to be a monomeric subunit of the glycolytic enzyme enolase (66, 152). Antibodies to the 47-kDa antigen were detected by immunoblotting in sera from 71 to 74% of patients with invasive candidiasis, in sera from 38% of patients with superficial candidiasis or *Candida* colonization (164, 165), as well as in 70% of long-term intensive care patients without evidence of invasive candidiasis (293). When the antibody response to the 47-kDa antigen was studied in hematological and nonhematological patients, hematological patients were more likely not to have any detectable antibody or to produce mainly IgM antibodies whereas nonhematological patients mounted a predominantly immunoglobulin (Ig) G response or produced IgG and IgM (165). Since all patients who recovered from invasive candidiasis produced strong antibody responses to the 47-kDa antigen and fatal cases produced none or minor responses to this antigen, detection of antibodies to the 47-kDa antigen of *C. albicans* may be of prognostic value (164, 165).

Candida antigens with enzymatic activity have also been used as targets for antibody detection. Using an ELISA to detect the IgG antibody response against enolase, van Deventer et al. (282) reported a sensitivity of 50% and a specificity of 86% for the diagnosis of invasive candidiasis in immunocompetent patients and a sensitivity of 53% and a specificity of 78% in immunodeficient patients. Mitsutake et al. (170) detected antibodies to enolase by immunoblotting with sera from primarily an immunocompetent patient population with a sensitivity of 92.5% and a specificity of 95%. In addition to patients infected by *C. albicans,* antibodies to *C. albicans* enolase were also detected in patients infected by *C. parapsilosis, C. tropicalis, C. guilliermondii,* and *C. glabrata* (170). Staib et al. (259, 260) showed that patients with invasive candidiasis and patients colonized with *Candida* spp. had antibodies to culture filtrate-containing proteolytic enzymes of *C. albicans.* Macdonald and Odds (144) detected antibodies to a purified *C. albicans* proteinase by CIE and observed that patients with invasive candidiasis had higher titers than patients without candidiasis. However, using an ELISA and a purified *C. albicans* proteinase, Rüchel et al. (241) reported that monitoring of antiproteinase antibodies alone was not useful for the diagnosis of invasive candidiasis. Na and Song (181) have recently reported that detection of antibodies against a *C. albicans*-secreted aspartyl proteinase in patients with invasive candidiasis had a sensitivity of 69.7% and a specificity of 76%. The low specificity of detection of *C. albicans* antiproteinase antibodies may be related to its induction in mucosal infections such as vulvovaginal candidiasis or to cross-reactivity between *C. albicans* and *Aspergillus* proteinases (100, 181). El Moudni et al. (56) detected antibodies against a *C. albicans* metallopeptidase by ELISA with a sensitivity of 83% and a specificity of 97% in the diagnosis of invasive candidiasis (Table 2).

Although in most studies only anti-*Candida* IgG antibodies were detected, other immunoglobulin classes have been found in other studies. Aubert et al. (5) used an immunocapture technique to detect IgM, IgA, and IgE anti-*Candida* antibodies against somatic antigens in immunocompetent patients and found that IgA was a particularly valuable marker of invasive candidiasis. Detection of IgA antibodies to CAGT showed a higher sensitivity than IgG or IgM detection in the diagnosis of invasive candidiasis (220). Gutierrez et al. (85) detected IgM antibodies to *C. albicans* whole cells by indirect immunofluorescence in patients with first-time candidemia and reported a 100% sensitivity and specificity. Kostiala et al. (128) detected rises in titers of IgG and IgA antibodies by ELISA in sera sequentially drawn from patients with candidemia. Elevated levels of IgE antibodies to *C. albicans* surface antigens have been detected in patients with invasive candidiasis and patients with vaginal candidiasis (154). IgE antibodies to *C. albicans* phosphomannan, enolase, alcohol dehydrogenase, aldolase, and phosphoglycerate kinase, respectively, have also been detected in allergic patients (atopic dermatitis or bronchial asthma) (101–103, 112, 245, 251).

The specificity of the antigen-antibody reaction

can be exploited in the diagnosis of infections by *Candida* species that express specific antigens when blood culture or other diagnostic techniques are negative. Taking advantage of the antigenic differences between *C. dubliniensis* and *C. albicans* (15), Salesa et al. (242) showed that it is possible to differentiate candidemia caused by *C. dubliniensis* from that caused by *C. albicans*. In this study a *C. dubliniensis*-infected patient presented a characteristic and specific antibody response against a cell wall component of 170 to 160 kDa. Antibodies to this antigen have also been detected in an animal model of infection with *C. dubliniensis* (207).

Although during the past 20 years there has been a decline in the use of antibody tests for the diagnosis of invasive candidiasis because there is a general belief that they are both insensitive and nonspecific (48, 49, 108, 197), there is evidence in the literature suggesting that detection of antibodies in highly immunocompromised patients, such as neutropenic bone marrow transplant recipients or liver transplant recipients, is possible and useful for the diagnosis of invasive candidiasis (95, 124, 184, 278, 285). Since the main limitations of antibody detection (low sensitivity and specificity) are especially manifested when only a single serum sample is studied, detection of antibodies using commercially available test kits with multiple sequential sera from the patient at risk for developing invasive candidiasis should be performed. This will allow a kinetic study of the antibody response in the patient to be performed, which will provide a more reliable reflection of the development of the infection (99, 105, 128, 129, 166, 249, 281). Detection of antibodies to enolase and germ tube mannoproteins may be useful in the diagnosis of patients with invasive candidiasis, provided that standardized and easy-to-perform tests are commercialized in the future. An ELISA will be particularly suitable to detect these antibodies since it permits quantitation, which may be useful since antibodies to these antigens may occasionally be detected in colonized patients.

DETECTION OF ANTIGENS

In an attempt to overcome the sensitivity and specificity problems reported in some studies designed for antibody detection in immunocompromised patients with invasive candidiasis, many investigators turned to the detection of circulating *Candida* antigens. A wide variety of assays have been developed for the detection of circulating *Candida* antigens, including CIE (120, 134), hemagglutination inhibition (292), latex agglutination (8, 18, 20, 24, 28, 29, 47, 58, 69, 72, 85, 88, 109, 113, 119, 126, 127, 139, 158–160, 171, 186, 191, 199, 202, 210, 214, 217, 232, 236–239, 243, 254, 275), ELISA (4, 20, 51, 67, 68, 134, 139, 142, 168, 171, 177, 181, 183, 198, 240, 241, 248, 249, 276), immunoblotting (62), dot immunoassay (43, 159, 162, 163, 224), liposomal immunoassay (85, 288), and RIA (262, 291) (Table 4). Antigens detected by these assays include mannan and mannoproteins (7, 18, 20, 43, 51, 67–69, 74, 75, 85, 88, 98, 109, 113, 120, 139, 142, 171, 177, 183, 198, 199, 214, 232, 248, 249, 276, 291, 292), the noncharacterized Cand-Tec antigen (8, 20, 28, 29, 47, 58, 69, 72, 109, 113, 119, 126, 127, 139, 171, 186, 191, 199, 202, 210, 217, 236–239, 243, 254, 275), HSP90 (62, 159, 163), enolase (85, 171, 288), and other immunodominant cytoplasmic antigens (4, 24, 158–160, 162, 181, 224, 240, 241, 262) (Table 4). The subject area has been intensively reviewed (9, 10, 25–27, 48, 49, 52, 96, 108, 110, 118, 125, 129, 141, 156, 157, 160, 189, 197, 203, 228, 239, 284, 287, 290).

Mannan is the major circulating antigen in patients with invasive candidiasis (108, 189), and it was first detected in 1973 in the serum from a patient with chronic mucocutaneous candidiasis (7). Due to the universal presence of antimannan antibodies, mannan usually circulates in the form of immune complexes that are rapidly cleared by the liver and kidneys (142, 229). Kappe and Muller (114) showed that the half-life of mannan in a rabbit model is 2 h. Mannan is a very complex mixture of different oligomannosidic epitopes (151, 212), and their clearance from blood may not follow the same kinetics. By using two monoclonal antibodies to prepare two different latex assays, it has been demonstrated that levels of α and β mannose residues were different in patients with invasive candidiasis and that detection of both epitopes by latex agglutination improved the diagnosis because detection of both epitopes showed complementary kinetics (214, 284). Since the rapid clearance of mannan from blood and its binding by antimannan antibodies make its detection difficult by serological assays, dissociation of the complexes by heat, protease, acid, or NaOH treatments and testing of sequential serum samples are two strategies that have been used in most studies to improve the sensitivity of assays (48, 108).

Early tests devised for mannan detection showed high specificity but poor sensitivity (Table 4). Using a hemagglutination inhibition assay, Weiner and Yount (292) detected mannan in sera of patients with invasive candidiasis with a sensitivity of 31.5% and a specificity of 100%. In a subsequent study, Weiner and Coats-Stephen (291) dissociated immune complexes by acid and heat treatments and were able to detect mannan in sera by RIA with a sensitivity of 46.7%

and a specificity of 100%. Kerkering et al. (120) reported a 100% sensitivity and a 93.3% specificity in the diagnosis of invasive candidiasis in a mixed patient population by CIE. However, Lehmann and Reiss (134), using a similar technique, were not able to detect mannan in six leukemic patients with invasive candidiasis.

Mannan concentrations in serum from patients with invasive candidiasis are found in the low nanogram per milliliter range (108, 228). When a sensitive assay such as the ELISA was developed, the sensitivity increased in some studies but not in others (Table 4). Mannan antigenemia preceded a significant rise in antibodies against mannan and cytoplasmic antigens by 6 to 23 days (67), and it has been found to complement blood cultures for the diagnosis of invasive candidiasis in immunocompromised patients (51). Detection of mannan in serum by a biotin-streptavidin ELISA may be useful for the diagnosis of *Candida* pyelonephritis (276). De Bernardis et al. (43) developed a dot immunobinding assay to detect a β-1,2-oligomannosidic epitope of a mannoprotein expressed by *C. albicans, C. tropicalis, C. parapsilosis, C. guilliermondii,* and *C. glabrata,* but not by *C. krusei* and *C. famata.* Detection of *Candida* mannoproteinemia was useful to differentiate central venous catheter-related candidemia from invasive candidiasis and in the diagnosis of neutropenic enterocolitis, a disease in which *Candida* species have been implicated (74, 75). Detection of protein and mannoprotein antigens in sequentially drawn sera has also been useful in the diagnosis of invasive candidiasis in neutropenic cancer patients (177).

Due to the antigenic differences between the mannans of *C. albicans* and *C. krusei* (193), a test devised to detect *C. albicans* mannan may not be appropriate to detect mannan from *C. krusei* or *C. glabrata* (183). By using an ELISA to detect *C. albicans* and *C. krusei* mannans, Fujita and Hasimoto (68) reported a sensitivity of 74% and a specificity of 100% for the diagnosis of invasive candidiasis in patients infected by *C. albicans, C. guilliermondii, C. krusei, C. parapsilosis,* and *C. tropicalis* but not by *C. glabrata.*

Although ELISAs are usually more sensitive than those based on the agglutination of latex particles (68), the latter are simpler to perform in a clinical setting. Kahn and Jones (109) developed a latex agglutination assay to detect mannan in sera sequentially collected from leukemic patients after dissociation of immune complexes with protease and heat treatment. The test showed a sensitivity of 78% and a specificity of 92.5%. Lower diagnostic sensitivities were observed in patients from whom only one or two serum samples were assayed at the time the infection was suspected (109).

In addition to serum, mannan has been detected in other clinical specimens. Since circulating mannan is cleared by the kidneys, an increase in sensitivity may be obtained by detecting the antigen in urine. Robert et al. (232) reported the detection of mannan in the urine of 10 out of 16 patients with invasive candidiasis and in none from blood donors. Immunohistochemical detection of mannan facilitated the diagnosis of candidal pneumonia and distinguished clinically significant pulmonary candidiasis from colonization (98).

Although most of the earlier tests were developed and tested in research laboratories, some tests for mannan detection have been commercialized, thus making possible a broad evaluation (239). The LA-*Candida* Antigen Detection System (Immuno Mycologics, Inc., Norman, Okla.) was based on latex particles coated by polyclonal antimannan antibodies to detect the antigen in sera pretreated with heat and protease. However, when the system was evaluated by different groups, it was found to be insensitive (18, 69, 113, 199).

Pfaller et al. (198) evaluated the ICON *Candida* Assay system (Hybritec Inc., San Diego, Calif.), which detects mannan with polyclonal antibodies in an ELISA format. After dissociation of immune complexes with protease and heat treatment, it yielded a sensitivity of 86% and a specificity of 92% for the diagnosis of invasive candidiasis in a mainly immunocompetent patient population. The test was positive in patients infected by *C. albicans, C. glabrata,* or *C. lusitaniae* but not in a patient infected by *C. krusei.* Although the test was positive with sera taken within 3 days of the first positive blood culture or biopsy in 79% of patients with invasive candidiasis, detectable mannanemia preceded diagnosis by these other methods in only 36% of patients. However, the test tended to complement the diagnosis made on the basis of a positive blood culture.

Monoclonal antibody EBCA1, which reacts with mannans from *C. albicans, C. tropicalis, C. glabrata, C. guilliermondii, C. parapsilosis,* and *C. pseudotropicalis,* but not with mannan from *C. krusei* (73), coated on latex beads in the Pastorex *Candida* test (Sanofi Diagnostics Pasteur), has been used to detect systemic candidiasis. When evaluating the test, Herent et al. (88) reported a sensitivity of 52.6% and a specificity of 100% for the diagnosis of invasive candidiasis in a mainly immunocompetent patient population. Although sera were treated to dissociate the immunocomplexes with EDTA and heat, the test showed a low sensitivity in patients who had high titers of antimannan antibodies. However, the test detected man-

Table 4. Studies on antigen detection tests for the diagnosis of invasive candidiasis

Year	Method[a]	Antigen[b]	No. of patients with invasive candidiasis			No. of controls			Sensitivity (%)	Specificity (%)	Efficiency (%)	Reference
			Neutrop.	Nonneutrop.	Total	Neutrop.	Nonneutrop.	Total				
1988	DIA	47 kDa	35	52	87	75	82	157	77	97	80.3	159
1989	DIA	60 kDa	52	–	52	–	–	557	69	97	94.6	162
1989	DIA	60 kDa	–	40	40	–	–	557	80	97	95.8	162
1982	ELISA	CY	–	–	20	–	–	70	80	92.8	90	4
1994	ELISA	CY	5	–	5	26	–	26	67	100	93.5	177
1987	HIA	CY	13	10	23	26	7	33	54	88	69.6	202
1993	IB	CY	8	11	19	–	–	69	84.2	94.4	92	224
1985	LA	CY	30	61	91	4	765	769	96.7	98.8	98.5	24
1988	LA	CY (1:8)	36	18	54	85	48	133	88.9	97	94.7	158
1988	LA	CY (1:10)	36	18	54	85	48	133	46.3	99.2	83.95	158
1988	LA	CY	55	37	92	–	21	21	89.1	100	91.2	160
1989	LA	CY (1:10)	52	–	52	–	–	557	33	97	91.5	162
1989	LA	CY (1:10)	–	40	40	–	–	557	68	97	95	162
1980	RIA	CY	–	–	19	–	–	26	63.2	100	84.4	162
1996	DIA	ENO	–	–	39	–	–	40	71.8	100	86.1	171
1991	IF	ENO	24	–	24	146	–	146	75	96	92.9	288
1993	IF	ENO	–	–	10	–	–	70	70	97	93.8	85
1991	DIA	HSP90	–	–	65	–	–	15	70	100	76.3	163
1979	CIE	MAN	–	–	8	–	–	75	100	93.3	93.9	120
1979	ELISA	MAN	–	–	7	–	–	20	100	100	100	248[c]
1981	ELISA	MAN	10	–	10	82	–	82	70	91	89.1	168
1982	ELISA	MAN	8	7	15	–	–	126	53.3	93.7	89.4	142
1985	ELISA	MAN	19	4	23	8	57	65	65	100	90.9	51
1986	ELISA	MAN	–	–	10	–	–	70	90	96	91.3	67
1990	ELISA	MAN	–	–	14	–	–	32	29	96.9	76.1	20
1990	ELISA	MAN	6	26	32	1	16	17	33	100	57.1	139
1991	ELISA	MAN	8	11	19	–	–	117	84.2	99.1	97.1	183
1992	ELISA	MAN	–	–	78	–	–	161	74	100	91.6	68
1993	ELISA	MAN	–	–	14	–	–	100	86	92	91.2	198

1993	ELISA	MAN	–	–	41	–	–	20	43.9	100	62.3	276[c]
1995	ELISA	MAN	–	–	11	–	–	52	55.6	83.7	77.8	277[c]
1999	ELISA	MAN	–	43	43	–	–	230	53	94	87.5	249
1976	HIA	MAN	–	–	19	–	–	286	31.5	100	95.7	292
1987	IGSS	MAN	–	–	14	–	–	46	76	91	88.3	210[c]
1985	LA	MAN	–	–	21	–	–	68	80.9	88.2	86.5	8
1986	LA	MAN	23	–	23	64	–	64	78	92.5	80.5	109
1986	LA	MAN	–	–	45	–	–	105	19	96.2	73.3	109
1988	LA	MAN	–	36	36	–	90	90	0	100	71.4	17[c]
1989	LA	MAN	–	36	36	–	96	96	0	100	72.7	18[c]
1989	LA	MAN	7	–	7	12	–	12	57.1	100	84.2	278
1990	LA	MAN	–	–	16	–	–	49	44	43	43.1	199
1992	LA	MAN	–	–	78	–	–	161	38	100	79.9	68
1993	LA	MAN	–	–	10	–	–	70	0	100	87.5	85
1993	LA	MAN	–	–	10	–	–	23	60	95.7	85	126
1995	LA	MAN	1	10	11	–	36	36	27.3	100	83	174[a]
1996	LA	MAN	–	–	39	–	–	40	25.6	100	63.3	171
1997	LA	MAN	2	18	20	–	–	35	35	100	76.4	214[c]
1999	LA	MAN	–	–	4	–	–	36	25	100	92.5	41
1979	RIA	MAN	–	–	15	–	–	42	46.7	100	86	291
1997	LA	MAN+PLM	2	18	20	–	–	35	50	100	81.8	214[c]
1993	DIA	MANP	15	–	15	57	–	57	66.7	93	87.5	43
1997	DIA	MANP	–	–	17	–	–	14	76.5	92.9	83.9	74
1992	LA	MANP	–	–	19	–	–	60	52.6	100	88.6	88
1997	LA	PLM	2	18	20	–	–	35	35	100	76.4	214[c]
1999	ELISA	P	13	20	33	–	–	25	93.9	96	94.8	181[c]
1985	CIE	WCE	–	–	13	–	–	72	15	100	87.1	64
1985	ELISA	WCE	–	–	13	–	–	72	61	61	61	64

[a] Methods: CIE, counterimmunoelectrophoresis; DIA, dot immunobinding assay; ELISA, enzyme–linked immunosorbent assay; HIA, hemagglutination inhibition assay; IB, immunoblotting; ID, immunodiffusion; IF, immunofiltration; IGSS, immuno/gold-silver staining; LA, latex agglutination; RIA, radioimmunoassay.

[b] Antigens: CY, cytoplasmic; ENO, enolase; MAN, mannan; PLM, phospholipomannan; MANP, mannoprotein; P, proteinase; WCE, whole cell extract.

[c] Not including patients with superficial candidiasis among the controls.

nan before other diagnostic methods in 6 out of 10 patients tested. Differences in sensitivity have been observed in other studies with the Pastorex *Candida* system. Mitsutake et al. (171) demonstrated a sensitivity of 25.6% and a specificity of 100% in patients with candidemia. However, in contrast, Gutiérrez et al. (85) found the test insensitive for the diagnosis of candidemia. In an attempt to increase the sensitivity of mannan detection, an ELISA was developed using monoclonal antibody EBCA1 (Platelia *Candida* Ag, Sanofi Diagnostics Pasteur). Although it was more sensitive than the Pastorex *Candida* system, an increase in the sensitivity of the detection of mannanemia was not observed in comparison with previous studies (Table 4) (249). Mannanemia was detected, on average, at 6.2 days before isolation of *C. albicans*. As mentioned previously, kinetic studies showed that detection of mannanemia was inversely correlated to the presence of antimannan antibodies (Fig. 1). Although this system has not yet been thoroughly assessed, a false-positive reaction has been observed in intensive care patients treated with hydroxyethyl starch. Due to the antigenic differences presented by mannans from different *Candida* species, a test for detecting mannan should include a mixture of monoclonal antibodies directed against epitopes expressed by the clinically relevant *Candida* species to increase its sensitivity.

After the identification of major *Candida* cytoplasmic antigens, researchers developed assays to detect them in the sera from patients with invasive candidiasis. Stevens et al. (262) detected a *Candida* cytoplasmic protein antigen in sera of 12 of 19 patients with invasive candidiasis and in none of the 26 controls. Araj et al. (4) found elevated levels of a cytoplasmic heat-stable protein antigen by ELISA in all of seven cancer patients tested with invasive candidiasis. Reboli (224) reported a sensitivity of 84.2% and a specificity of 94.4% in the diagnosis of invasive candidiasis caused by *C. albicans, C. tropicalis, C. krusei, C. parapsilosis,* and *C. glabrata* in a mixed patient population using a dot immunobinding assay to detect *Candida* cytoplasmic antigens. Comparable sensitivities were found for neutropenic and nonneutropenic patients. By using a latex agglutination assay to detect an undefined *Candida* antigen, Matthews and Burnie (24, 158–160) reported differences in sensitivity and in the maximum antigen titers detected between neutropenic and nonneutropenic patients with invasive candidiasis. Neutropenic patients tended to have lower antigen titers than nonneutropenic patients, a situation that it is likely to be related to the presence of IgM antibodies with high affinity for the antigen. When serial sera from a patient were examined, the kinetics of the antigen titers were found to have clinical significance, since antigen titers fell in response to antifungal therapy and remained high in patients who died. In addition to infections caused by *C. albicans,* the latex test yielded positive agglutination reactions with sera from patients infected with *C. parapsilosis, C. tropicalis,* and *C. guilliermondii,* but not with sera from patients infected with *C. glabrata* (24). Similar differences in sensitivity were observed when the immunodominant 47-kDa antigen of *C. albicans,* a product of HSP90 broken down in vivo by host neutrophils or released by amphotericin B treatment (25), was detected in sera from patients with invasive candidiasis (165). By using a dot immunobinding assay and a 47-kDa-antigen-specific antibody, the antigen has been detected in 77% of neutropenic patients and in 87.5% of nonneutropenic patients with invasive candidiasis (159). The main limitations of the 47-kDa-antigen-specific antibody are its poor specificity to detect infections caused by *Candida* species other than *C. albicans* and the need to obtain the antibody by affinity chromatography, which yields small amounts of relatively low-affinity antibody (159, 162). The 47-kDa antigen has also been detected by immunoblotting the urine of patients with invasive candidiasis (62). To increase the sensitivity of the dot immunobinding assay, the 47-kDa-antigen-specific antibody was replaced by an antibody to an epitope of *C. albicans* HSP90 (LKVIRK), which was recognized by all patients who had antibodies to the 47-kDa antigen. The epitope-specific antibody was less sensitive but more specific than the 47-kDa-antigen-specific antibody, which recognized multiple epitopes (163). Detection of a cytoplasmic antigen of 60 kDa by a dot immunobinding assay showed a sensitivity of 69% and 80% in neutropenic patients and nonneutropenic patients with invasive candidiasis, respectively (162). However, 25% of patients with superficial candidiasis and colonized patients were also positive by the assay.

The Cand-Tec test (Ramco Laboratories Inc., Houston, Tex.) is based on the work described in 1983 by Gentry et al. (72), who developed an agglutination assay with latex particles sensitized with sera from rabbits immunized with whole heat-killed *C. albicans* blastoconidia to detect an uncharacterized heat-labile antigen of *C. albicans*. The antigen does not contain mannan, and it is detected without immune complex dissociation steps. The antigen may need processing by human host cells to be detected (54, 83, 108), and it has been suggested that it may be a host component that is cross-reactive with an antigen of *C. albicans* (10, 108). Mitsuya et al. (172) have identified a component of ≥4,000 kDa in sera from guinea pigs intraperitoneally infected with *C. albicans* and a component of 3,000 to 4,000 kDa in sera from patients with invasive candidiasis that react with the Cand-Tec test. In contrast to the guinea pig antigen, which contained mannan and complement component C3, the antigen detected by the Cand-Tec test in humans seemed to consist of immune complexes formed by IgM and a component of 200 kDa that reacts with concanavalin A. Although there is a vast literature on the performance of the Cand-Tec test, there is no consensus about its value for the diagnosis of invasive candidiasis because variable results have been reported in different studies (Table 5). In general, evaluations performed during the 1980s tended to consider the test useful for the diagnosis of invasive candidiasis (28, 29, 47, 69, 72, 113, 210, 217), for excluding severe candidiasis (237), for the evaluation of critically ill hospitalized patients with candiduria (265), and for monitoring the response to antifungal therapy (28). However, it was considered to be of little benefit for the diagnosis of invasive candidiasis in some studies with immunocompromised patients (58, 186). The situation is the opposite with evaluations performed during the 1990s, which usually considered that the test was not acceptable for the diagnosis of invasive candidiasis (119, 243, 254) or candidemia (126, 171, 199). However, Kono et al. (127) and Tokunaga et al. (275) concluded that the test was useful for the diagnosis of invasive candidiasis. The Cand-Tec test has been reported to be helpful for differentiating between peripheral colonization and invasive candidiasis (20) and for differentiating between candidemia resulting from invasive candidiasis and catheter-related candidemia (239). Rosemurgy et al. (236) documented the relationship between an increase in Cand-Tec titers and death in severely injured patients, and Iwasaki et al. (104) have recently reported that serial antigen detection by the Cand-Tec assay is a very useful method for the early diagnosis of invasive candidiasis in febrile neutropenic patients and for determining the timing of the initiation of early antifungal therapy.

The reasons for the variability in the results obtained in these different studies are not clear, but they may be related to several factors, including (i) the definition of invasive candidiasis, (ii) the patient population studied, (iii) the timing of collection of sera and the number of sera, (iv) interference by rheumatoid factor and a thermostable antigen, (v) the titer used as cutoff, and (vi) the infecting *Candida* species and the cross-reactivity with antigens from other fungi. The criteria for diagnosing invasive candidiasis are different in some studies. For example, patients with *Candida* esophagitis were included among the patients with invasive candidiasis in one study (58) but not in another (69). Some authors have observed lower titers in leukemic patients and in sera obtained late in the course of infection (28, 109, 237). It has also been reported that antigenemia occurs only transiently during the course of infection (8, 28, 109) and that it may be influenced by the renal function of the patients studied, although an association between Cand-Tec titers and creatinine levels reported in some studies (20, 186) has not been demonstrated in others (29, 199, 217, 243). Gentry et al. (72) reported that nonspecific agglutination reactions with the Cand-Tec system could be due to the presence of rheumatoid factor, and Rüchel (238) has reported the presence of a thermostable antigen in the sera of patients with false-positive results. Positive results have been obtained with the test with sera from patients infected by *C. albicans, C. tropicalis, C. parapsilosis, C. glabrata, C. lusitaniae, C. rugosa,* and *C. krusei* (29, 72, 186, 243), but also in patients with aspergillosis or cryptococcosis (139, 186, 199, 239). However, patients infected by *C. albicans* have been shown to have higher titers than those infected by non-*C. albicans Candida* (29). It is possible that some of the problems listed above can be solved if the antigen detected by the Cand-Tec system is fully characterized. Walsh et al. (288) evaluated a liposomal immunoassay (Directigen, Becton Dickinson, Baltimore, Md.) to detect enolase antigenemia in cancer patients with invasive candidiasis. The assay was positive in patients infected by *C. albicans* and *C. tropicalis.* The sensitivity of the assay in serum seeded with antigen was 0.5 to 1.0 μg/liter. The assay detected antigenemia in 85% of patients with deep tissue infection and in 64% of patients with fungemia, and showed a specificity of 96%. Since enolase antigenemia was detected in the absence of fungemia in five patients with tissue-proven candidiasis, but not in six patients with fungemia alone, the assay complemented blood culture. The study documented the transient nature of enolase antigenemia, and daily sampling was proposed in febrile patients with neutropenia. Similar values of both sensitivity and specificity were reported by Gutierrez et al. (88) in patients with candidemia using the Directigen assay. By using an in-house ELISA to detect enolase, Mitsutake et al. (171) reported a sensitivity of 71.8% and a specificity of 100% in the diagnosis of candidemia.

In addition to enolase, detection of other *Candida* enzymes has been used for the serodiagnosis of invasive candidiasis (Table 4). An ELISA was developed by Rüchel and associates (240, 241) to detect *C. albicans* proteinases, which reach serum concentrations of 0.13 μg/ml and have a half-life of approximately 60 min. However, the assay showed a low sensitivity and specificity for the diagnosis of invasive candidiasis (241). The low sensitivity may be related to the presence of antiproteinase antibodies in pa-

Table 5. Studies on Cand-Tec antigen detection test for the diagnosis of invasive candidiasis

Year	No. of patients with invasive candidiasis			No. of controls			Sensitivity (%)	Specificity (%)	Efficiency (%)	Reference
	Neutrop.	Nonneutrop.	Total	Neutrop.	Nonneutrop.	Total				
1983	6	27	33	–	100	100	90.9	100	97.7	72
1985	–	–	18	–	–	31	27.8	96.8	71.4	8
1986	–	–	8	–	–	40	100	85	87.5	69
1986	23	–	23	64	–	64	48	73.4	66.7	109
1986	–	–	45	–	–	105	22	89.5	69.3	109
1986	–	–	80	–	–	248	90	87.9	88.4	217
1987	–	–	36	–	–	16	94.4	100	96.2	47
1987	5	8	13	27	84	111	66.7	85.6	80.5	200
1987	13	10	23	26	7	33	52.2	66.7	60.7	202
1987	–	–	14	–	–	46	40	100	85	210
1988	–	–	32	–	–	179	21.9	99.4	87.7	250
1989	23	14	37	98	60	158	46	80	73.3	29
1989	26	3	29	110	3	113	38	90	79.6	58
1989	11	–	11	206	–	206	54.5	29	30.4	186
1990	5	17	22	10	32	42	86.4	50	62.5	20
1990	11	31	42	6	28	34	49	43	47.4	199
1990	6	26	32	1	16	17	57	100	71.4	139
1992	–	–	19	–	–	60	47.5	100	87.3	88
1992	–	1	1	–	70	70	100	77.1	80.3	119
1992	4	19	23	118	61	179	87	36	42	243
1992	–	–	28	–	–	92	81.5	80.4	83.3	254
1992	–	–	28	–	–	92	59.3	92.9	83.3	254
1992	–	–	29	–	–	44	31	100	69.9	275
1993	–	–	30	–	–	14	26.7	85.7	45.5	283
1993	–	–	10	–	–	24	70	79.2	61.8	126
1994	5	–	5	26	–	26	33	92	80.6	177
1995	1	10	11	–	36	36	73	100	93.6	174[a]
1995	–	–	11	–	–	52	11.1	97.7	82.5	277[a]
1996	–	–	39	–	–	40	76.9	87.5	82.3	171
1996	9	27	36	8	6	14	69	64.3	68	281
1999	–	–	4	–	–	36	25	86.1	80	41

[a] Not including patients with superficial candidiasis among the controls.

tient's sera, since immunodominant protein antigens induce large quantities of antibodies that bind the antigen and facilitate clearance. The proteinaceous nature of the antigen precluded a simple disassociation of immune complexes, as can be achieved with mannan (239). However, Na and Song (181) developed a monoclonal antibody-based ELISA inhibition technique to detect a *C. albicans*-secreted aspartyl proteinase and reported a sensitivity of 93.9% and a specificity of 96% for the diagnosis of invasive candidiasis.

There is a wide consensus that antigen detection may be useful for the diagnosis of invasive candidiasis in immunocompromised patients since, theoretically, monitoring antigen levels is independent of the immunological status of the patient and may give an early indication of infection. However, antigen detection may not automatically be the serological test of choice in immunocompromised patients as it may depend on the type of antigen and the mechanisms needed for its release in infected tissues. For instance, the antigen detected by the Cand-Tec test seems to require processing of *C. albicans* by human host cells for detection (54, 83, 108), and it has been reported that leukemic patients with invasive candidiasis may have low antigen titers (28, 109, 159, 237). A similar feature has been reported for other antigens (160). However, it is not clear if this is also the case with mannan and enolase. Common features of antigen detection observed with all antigen detection assays are the low levels of circulating antigens and the transient nature of antigenemia (74, 224, 249, 287). Therefore, antigen detection tests for the diagnosis of invasive candidiasis would require the use of sensitive assays and frequent sampling, possibly on a daily basis in patients at high risk.

DETECTION OF NONANTIGENIC COMPONENTS

Several nonantigenic components released by *Candida* species during infection can also be used in the diagnosis of invasive candidiasis. This topic has been the subject of a large number of reviews (39, 52, 96, 108, 110, 125, 129, 133, 141, 189, 197, 228, 231, 287).

When studying the gas-liquid chromatography profiles of sera from patients with candidemia, Miller et al. (169) observed two peaks that were identified as isomers of mannose. Detection of these peaks allowed candidemia and superficial colonization to be differentiated. Using the same technique, Monson and Wilkinson (175) detected mannose in sera from six nondiabetic patients with invasive candidiasis. However, diabetic patients with blood glucose levels ≥300 mg/dl but not patients with renal insufficiency showed mannose concentrations in serum similar to those observed in patients with invasive candidiasis. Increased mannose concentrations were also found in cerebrospinal fluid from two of the patients with invasive candidiasis. After treating sera to release all mannose present in specimens, including that present in glycoproteins, Marier et al. (148) detected increased concentrations of mannose (>453.49 μg/ml) by gas-liquid chromatography in five of seven patients with disseminated candidiasis and in two patients with candidemia tested. Increased levels were also found in 6 of 15 patients with localized candidiasis, including patients with chronic mucocutaneous candidiasis, infected wounds, and gastrointestinal and urinary tract infections (Table 6). De Repentigny et al. (51) detected nonspecific increases in mannose concentrations in the sera of control patients without candidiasis, which were not explained by diabetic ketoacidosis, *Candida* colonization, or corticosteroid administration. Soyama (255) developed an enzymatic assay to detect D-mannose in sera from four patients with invasive candidiasis. All four patients presented increased D-mannose concentrations, but diabetic patients with uncontrolled hyperglycemia showed D-mannose concentrations that overlapped values found in the patients with invasive candidiasis.

D-arabinitol is a metabolite produced by *C. albicans, C. tropicalis, C. parapsilosis,* and *C. kefyr* (12), whereas *C. glabrata* and *C. krusei* produce trace amounts (12, 132). It was first detected by Kiehn et al. (121) in sera from 15 of 20 patients with invasive candidiasis and in 3 colonized patients with renal failure using gas-liquid chromatography. Roboz et al. (234) reported similar results using gas chromatography-mass spectrometry (Table 6). Colonized patients and six cases of superficial candidiasis had D-arabinitol levels within the normal range. Monitoring of D-arabinitol levels for a period of 1 year in a patient with leukemia showed a good correlation with the clinical course of the patient since maximum levels coincided with the diagnosis of invasive candidiasis and a decrease was observed in response to the antifungal treatment (234). Another group has also found that detection of D-arabinitol was useful in the diagnosis of invasive candidiasis (42). However, in other studies the serum arabinitol concentration was not a reliable indicator of candidiasis (57, 92, 294). Elevated D-arabinitol levels have been detected in patients with renal failure (42, 77, 121, 234, 256, 294, 298, 299), with sarcoidosis (115), or receiving corticosteroids (51). Since D-arabinitol is cleared by the kidneys at the same rate as creatinine (57, 298), the arabinitol/creatinine ratio corrects for variations in serum D-arabinitol concentrations that are due to dif-

Table 6. Studies on metabolite detection tests for the diagnosis of invasive candidiasis

Year	Method(s)[a]	Metabolite[b]	No. of patients with invasive candidiasis			No. of patients without invasive candidiasis			Sensitivity (%)	Specificity (%)	Efficiency (%)	Reference
			Neutrop.	Nonneutrop.	Total	Neutrop.	Nonneutrop.	Total				
1985	E	ARA	47	–	47	91	42	133	50–74	86–91	76.6–86.7	256
1993	E	ARA	–	–	9	–	–	22	78	95.5	74.2	126
1988	GC	ARA	–	–	4	–	–	27	100	100	100	299[c]
1989	GC	ARA	–	–	4	–	–	69	100	100	100	297[c]
1980	GC-MS	ARA	–	–	11	–	–	6	81.8	100	88.2	234
1979	GLC	ARA	–	–	20	–	–	93	75	96.8	92.9	121
1981	GLC	ARA	1	15	16	–	35	35	56.3	60	58.8	57
1983	GLC	ARA	–	–	34	–	–	111	59	70.3	67.6	294
1983	GLC	ARA	12	13	25	15	58	73	84	93.2	90.8	77
1985	GLC	ARA	19	4	23	8	45	53	26	87	68.4	51
1986	GLC	ARA	–	–	27	–	–	78	92.6	87.2	88.6	42[c]
1987	GLC	ARA	13	10	23	26	7	33	39.1	87.9	67.9	202
1990	SFC	ARA	5	17	22	10	32	42	45.5	76.2	65.6	20
1990	GC-MS	D/L ARA ratio	–	–	12	–	–	31	83.3	100	93.2	233[c]
1997	GC	D/L ARA ratio	33	–	33	67	56	123	100	94	94.9	40
1996	GC-MS	D/L ARA ratio	17	–	17	44	50	94	88	91	91	138
1999	GC-MS	D/L ARA ratio	–	–	3	–	–	35	66.7	60	60.5	41
2000	GC-MS	D/L ARA ratio	–	–	6	–	–	111	100	93.7	94	253
1995	E	ARA/C	–	–	68	–	–	610	61.8	95.2	91.9	289
1983	GLC	ARA/C	12	13	25	15	58	73	64	96	87.8	77
1985	GLC	ARA/C	19	4	23	8	57	65	13	93	68.4	51
1992	SFC	D-ARA/C	–	–	78	–	–	161	50	91	77.8	68
1995	SFC	D-ARA/C	–	–	11	–	–	52	77.8	88.4	85.7	277[c]
1974	GLC	FA	–	–	12	–	–	51	100	100	100	169
1993	E	(1→3)-β-D-G	–	–	9	–	–	22	78	95.5	90.3	126
1995	E	(1→3)-β-D-G	1	10	11	–	36	36	100	100	100	174[c]
1995	E	(1→3)-β-D-G	–	–	41	–	–	59	90	100	96	187[d]
1996	E	(1→3)-β-D-G	–	–	39	–	–	40	84.4	87.5	86.1	171
1999	E	(1→3)-β-D-G	–	–	4	–	–	36	50	58.3	57.5	41
1992	E	MANS	–	–	22	–	49	49	68.2	91.8	77.5	218[c]
1981	GLC	MANS	–	–	6	–	–	242	100	97.1	97.2	175
1982	GLC	MANS	–	–	23	–	–	31	56.5	100	83.3	148
1985	GLC	MANS	19	4	23	8	57	65	39	87	71.1	51
1988	HPLC	MANS	–	–	5	–	–	13	60	100	88.9	223
1984	GLC	MANS+ARA	–	–	21	–	–	68	100	75	80.9	145

[a]Methods: E, enzymatic; GC-MS, gas chromatography-mass spectrometry; GLC, gas-liquid chromatography; HPLC, high-performance liquid chromatography; MS, mass spectrometry; SFC, spectrofluorometry chromatography.
[b]Metabolite: ARA, Arabinitol; C, Creatinine; FA, fatty acids; G, glucan; MANS, Mannose.
[c]Not including patients with superficial candidiasis among the controls.
[d]Calculated on invasive mycoses (candidiasis is not specified).

ferences in the renal function (77, 294). Elevated arabinitol/creatinine ratios have been detected in 69% of patients with candidemia but also in 36% of patients colonized by *Candida* spp. (294). The arabinitol/creatinine ratio may not be useful in patients on continuous ambulatory peritoneal dialysis or hemodialysis, since serum concentrations of creatinine fall more quickly than that of arabinitol during dialysis (42). It has been shown that it is possible to differentiate the arabinitol produced by *Candida* spp. from the arabinitol usually found in humans since *Candida* species produce only D-arabinitol (13), whereas humans produce only L-arabinitol (280). Elevated D-arabinitol levels were observed in four patients with invasive candidiasis (299) but not in patients with sarcoidosis treated with steroids (297), and the D-arabinitol/L-arabinitol ratio was useful for differentiating patients with invasive candidiasis from those with renal failure (233).

Since D-arabinitol is excreted by the kidneys, and D-arabinitol/L-arabinitol ratios in urine are similar to those found in sera from patients with invasive candidiasis and healthy individuals (233, 235), there have been several reports on the detection of D-arabinitol in urine. The D-arabinitol/L-arabinitol ratio in urine has been shown to be a useful early marker of invasive candidiasis (40, 55, 132, 138) (Fig. 7), and two groups have reported sensitivities ranging from 88 to 100% and specificities ranging from 91 to 94% in the diagnosis of invasive candidiasis in patients with cancer

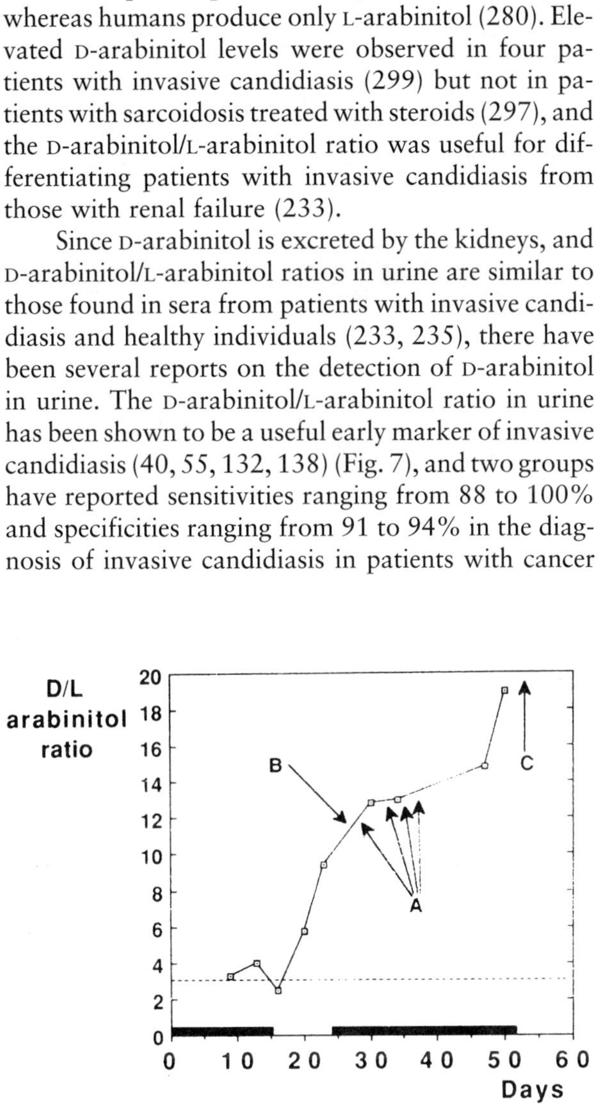

Figure 7. D/L-arabinitol ratios in urine from a 13-year-old girl with disseminated candidiasis. (A) Blood cultures positive for *C. albicans*; (B) onset of antifungal chemotherapy; (C) death of the patient. The horizontal black bar indicates a body temperature of >38.3°C. The interrupted line at 3.0 corresponds to the mean plus 3 standard deviations D/L-arabinitol ratio of hospitalized adult controls without disseminated *Candida* infection. Reprinted from the *Journal of Clinical Microbiology* (132) with permission of the authors and the publisher.

(40, 138) (Table 6). Furthermore, the D-arabinitol/L-arabinitol ratio seems to be useful for monitoring the effect of the antifungal treatment (253).

The detection of D-arabinitol in clinical laboratories may be hampered by the need for sophisticated gas chromatography-mass spectrometry equipment. However, D-arabinitol can also be detected in serum by an enzymatic method, which has been found suitable for the diagnosis of invasive candidiasis (256, 269). By using this assay and the D-arabinitol/creatinine ratio, sensitivities ranging from 50 to 74% and specificities ranging from 86 to 91% have been reported for the diagnosis of invasive candidiasis (68, 289). The assay shows a good correlation with gas chromatography results (269) and has been shown to be positive earlier than blood culture and to be useful for the therapeutic monitoring of patients with invasive candidiasis (257, 269, 289). The enzymatic detection of D-arabinitol has also been used for the diagnosis of candidemia (300) and *Candida* pyelonephritis (275, 277).

In addition to mannan, glucan is a major component of the fungal cell wall that is also released during infection (173). An assay to detect (1→3)-β-D-glucan in plasma, although not specific for *Candida* infections, has been used in the diagnosis of mycoses, including invasive candidiasis (126, 171, 174, 187, 271). The usefulness of (1→3)-β-D-glucan detection in the diagnosis of fungal infections has been reviewed by Verweij et al. (284). Humans lack glucanases that can digest (1→3)-β-D-glucan, and the elimination of this metabolite is slow (125). The preliminary evaluation of the assay has shown a sensitivity greater than 78% and a specificity greater than 87.5% in the diagnosis of candidemia (Table 6). However, low sensitivity and specificity have been reported in a recent study (41). False-positive results have been detected in patients on hemodialysis with apparatus incorporating cellulose membranes, as well as those under treatment with albumin or globulin products, anticancer agents (lentinan, crestin, and sizofuran), and sulfonamides (125). There are two commercially available tests to detect (1→3)-β-D-glucan: the Fungitec G test (Seikagaku Kogyo Corporation, Tokyo, Japan) and the Wako WB003 test (Wako Pure Chemical Industries, Osaka, Japan) (97), but the performance of both assays in the diagnosis of invasive candidiasis needs more extensive evaluation.

COMBINATIONS OF TESTS

Although certain assays have been reported to have a high sensitivity for the diagnosis of invasive candidiasis (Tables 1, 2, 4–6), in general, combinations of tests may be useful to overcome the deficiencies of individual tests. Combinations of tests, including detection of antibodies and antigens (64, 123, 249, 254), antigens and nonantigenic components (41, 126, 171), and antibodies, antigens, and nonantigenic components (20, 202) have all been studied. Different combinations of tests used in individual studies make comparisons between studies difficult, but combinations of tests that detect antibodies and antigens have been found to improve diagnosis of invasive candidiasis (64, 249, 254). The need for a combination of tests is particularly evident when a specific antigen and antibodies to this antigen are detected in the same patient, since the antibodies may facilitate the clearance of the antigen. Detection of mannan and antimannan antibodies has been shown to be complementary in patients with invasive candidiasis (Fig. 1) (249). The accuracy of diagnosis of candidemia was increased when several combinations of tests were used, including (1→3)-β-D-glucan and mannan detection (126, 171) and enolase and (1→3)-β-D-glucan detection (171). Platenkamp et al. (202) reported a sensitivity of 77% and a specificity of 100% when a combination of antibody, antigen, and D-arabinitol detection was used to differentiate invasive candidiasis from *Candida* colonization in immunocompromised patients. However, Bougnoux et al. (20) did not find the combination of antibody, antigen, and D-arabinitol assays useful to differentiate disseminated from peripheral candidiasis.

CONCLUSION

Substantial progress has been made in non-culture-based diagnosis of invasive candidiasis with the development of a variety of methods for the detection of antibodies, antigens, and nonantigenic components. However, no single test has found widespread clinical use due to the difficulties in obtaining consistently reliable serological diagnosis in all patients with invasive candidiasis and due to the limited number of commercial assays available. There is a consensus in the literature that diagnosis based on a single specimen lacks sensitivity. Therefore, it is necessary to test sequential samples taken while the patient is at greatest risk for developing invasive candidiasis to optimize the diagnosis. Testing of serum samples should begin at patient admission to obtain baseline data, and consideration should be given to the fact that different assays may be needed for the diagnosis of invasive candidiasis in immunocompetent and immunocompromised patients. Furthermore, patients should be screened taking into account the different expected kinetics of each assay (weekly for antibody and [1→3]-β-D-glucan detection, and at least twice a week for antigen and D-arabinitol detection). Results obtained from a panel of diagnostic tests, in association with blood culture findings and clinical aspects of the patient, will likely be the most useful strategy for early diagnosis of patients with invasive candidiasis and monitoring of therapeutic response.

Acknowledgments. We thank David C. Coleman for his invaluable comments about the manuscript. The assistance of Elena González Miranda in preparing Fig. 1 is gratefully acknowledged.

REFERENCES

1. **Alloush, H. M., J. L. Lopez-Ribot, and W. L. Chaffin.** 1996. Dynamic expression of cell wall proteins of *Candida albicans* revealed by probes from cDNA clones. *J. Med. Vet. Mycol.* **34:**91–97.
2. **Angiolella, L., M. Facchin, A. Stringaro, B. Maras, N. Simonetti, and A. Cassone.** 1996. Identification of a glucan-associated enolase as a main cell wall protein of *Candida albicans* and an indirect target of lipopeptide antimycotics. *J. Infect. Dis.* **173:**684–690.
3. **Ansorg, R., D. Gunesch, B. Bandelow, and R. Thomssen.** 1977. Differentiation and diagnostic significance of immunoglobulin classes of antibodies against cell wall antigens of yeast and mycelial phase of *Candida albicans. Mykosen* **20:** 167–177.
4. **Araj, G. F., R. L. Hopfer, S. Chesnut, V. Fainstein, and G. P. Bodey, Sr.** 1982. Diagnostic value of the enzyme-linked immunosorbent assay for detection of *Candida albicans* cytoplasmic antigen in sera of cancer patients. *J. Clin. Microbiol.* **16:**46–52.
5. **Aubert, D., D. Puygauthier-Toubas, P. Leon, B. Pignon, F. Foudrinier, F. Marnef, J. Boulant, and J. M. Pinon.** 1996. Characterization of specific anti-*Candida* IgM, IgA and IgE: diagnostic value in deep-seated infections. *Mycoses* **39:** 169–176.
6. **Au-Young, J. K., F. A. Troy, and E. Goldstein.** 1985. Serologic analysis of antigen-specific reactivity in patients with systemic candidiasis. *Diagn. Microbiol. Infect. Dis.* **3:** 419–432.
7. **Axelsen, N. H., and C. H. Kirkpatrick.** 1973. Simultaneous characterization of free *Candida* antigens and *Candida* precipitins in a patient's serum by means of crossed immunoelectrophoresis with intermediate gel. *J. Immunol. Methods* **2:** 245–249.
8. **Bailey, J. W., E. Sada, C. Brass, and J. E. Bennett.** 1985. Diagnosis of systemic candidiasis by latex agglutination for serum antigen. *J. Clin. Microbiol.* **21:**749–752.
9. **Barnes, R. A.** 1990. Immunological diagnosis of fungal infection in the immunocompromised host. *Rev. Med. Microbiol.* **1:**58–65.
10. **Bennett, J. E.** 1987. Rapid diagnosis of candidiasis and aspergillosis. *Rev. Infect. Dis.* **9:**398–402.
11. **Berdin, B., F. Boux de Casson-Raimbeau, A. Marot-Leblond, R. Robert, and J. M. Senet.** 1995. Etude préliminaire évaluant l'intérêt de l'utilisation d'antigène purifié (Ag3D9, Ag48) pour le sérodiagnostic des candidoses profondes par méthode immunoenzymatique ELISA (enzyme linked immunosorbent assay). *J. Mycol. Méd.* **5:**140–144.
12. **Bernard, E. M., K. J. Christiansen, S.-F. Tsang, T. E. Kiehn, and D. Armstrong.** 1981. Rate of arabinitol production by pathogenic yeast species. *J. Clin. Microbiol.* **14:**189–194.

13. **Bernard, E. M., B. Wong, and D. Armstrong.** 1985. Stereoisomeric configuration of arabinitol in serum, urine, and tissues in invasive candidiasis. *J. Infect. Dis.* **151:**711–715.
14. **Bikandi, J., M. C. Arilla, P. Regúlez, M. D. Moragues, G. Quindós, and J. Pontón.** 1993. Serodiagnosis of invasive candidiasis detecting antibodies against purified *Candida albicans* germ tube antigens. *XXIX Ann. Meet. Br. Soc. Mycopathol.* British Society for Mycopathology, Manchester, United Kingdom.
15. **Bikandi, J., R. San Millán, M. D. Moragues, G. Cebas, M. Clarke, D. C. Coleman, D. J. Sullivan, G. Quindós, and J. Pontón.** 1998. Rapid identification of *Candida dubliniensis* by indirect immunofluorescence based on differential localization of antigens on *C. dubliniensis* blastospores and *Candida albicans* germ tubes. *J. Clin. Microbiol.* **36:**2428–2433.
16. **Bikandi, J., R. San Millán, P. Regúlez, M. D. Moragues, G. Quindós, and J. Pontón.** 1998. Detection of antibodies to *Candida albicans* germ tubes during experimental infections by different *Candida* species. *Clin. Diagn. Lab. Immunol.* **5:** 369–374.
17. **Bisbe, J., J. M. Miró, J. M. Torres, C. Alia, J. Mallolas, and M. Amaral.** 1988. Diagnóstico serológico de la candidiasis diseminada en heroinómanos. *Enf. Infec. Microbiol. Clin.* **6:** 279–280.
18. **Bisbe, J., J. M. Miró, J. M. Torres, X. Latorre, C. Alia, M. Amaral, D. Estivill, J. Mallolas, A. Trilla, and E. Soriano.** 1989. Diagnostic value of serum antibody and antigen detection in heroin addicts with systemic candidiasis. *Rev. Infect. Dis.* **11:**310–315.
19. **Bodey, G. P.** 1966. Fungal infections complicating acute leukemia. *J. Chronic Dis.* **19:**667–687.
20. **Bougnoux, M.-E., C. Hill, D. Moissenet, M. F. de Chauvin, M. Bonnay, I. Vicens-Sprauel, F. Pietri, M. McNeil, L. Kaufman, J. Dupouy-Camet, C. Bohuon, and A. Andremont.** 1990. Comparison of antibody, antigen, and metabolite assays for hospitalized patients with disseminated or peripheral candidiasis. *J. Clin. Microbiol.* **28:**905–909.
21. **Brawner, D. L., and J. E. Cutler.** 1986. Variability in expression of cell wall surface antigens of *Candida albicans* during morphogenesis. *Infect. Immun.* **51:**337–343.
22. **Broom, M. F., M. G. Shepherd, and P. A. Sullivan.** 1991. Changes in cell envelope glycoproteins during germ tube formation of *Candida albicans. Microbios* **67:**7–21.
23. **Buckley, H. R., M. D. Richardson, E. G. V. Evans, and L. J. Wheat.** 1992. Immunodiagnosis of invasive fungal infection. *J. Med. Vet. Mycol.* **30**(Suppl. 1)**:**249–260.
24. **Burnie, J. P.** 1985. A reverse passive latex agglutination test for the diagnosis of systemic candidosis. *J. Immunol. Methods* **82:**267–280.
25. **Burnie, J. P.** 1987. Latex tests in the early diagnosis of systemic candidosis. *Serodiagn. Immunother.* **1:**3–5.
26. **Burnie, J. P.** 1991. Developments in the serological diagnosis of opportunistic fungal infections. *J. Antimicrob. Chemother.* **28**(Suppl. A)**:**23–33.
27. **Burnie, J. P.** 1995. Early diagnosis of systemic fungal infection. *Curr. Opin. Infect. Dis.* **8:**258–260.
28. **Burnie, J. P., and J. D. Williams.** 1985. Evaluation of the Ramco latex agglutination test in the early diagnosis of systemic candidiasis. *Eur. J. Clin. Microbiol.* **4:**98–101.
29. **Cabezudo, I., M. Pfaller, T. Gerarden, F. Koontz, R. Wenzel, R. Gingrich, K. Heckman, and C. P. Burns.** 1989. Value of Cand-Tec candida antigen assay in the diagnosis and therapy of systemic candidiasis in high-risk patients. *Eur. J. Clin. Microbiol. Infect. Dis.* **8:**770–777.
30. **Calderone, R. A., and E. Wadsworth.** 1988. Characterization of mannoproteins from a virulent *Candida albicans* strain and its derived, avirulent strain. *Rev. Infect. Dis.* **10:**423–427.
31. **Carceller, A., J. M. Torres-Rodríguez, M. Lowinger, and C. Alía.** 1992. Enzimoinmunoanálisis estandarizado para la detección de anticuerpos IgG frente a *Candida albicans* en la candidiasis sistémica. *Enf. Infec. Microbiol. Clin.* **10:** 195–199.
32. **Casanova, M., and W. L. Chaffin.** 1991. Cell wall glycoproteins of *Candida albicans* as released by different methods. *J. Gen. Microbiol.* **137:**1045–1051.
33. **Casanova, M., M. L. Gil, L. Cardeñoso, J. P. Martínez, and R. Sentandreu.** 1989. Identification of wall-specific antigens synthesized during germ tube formation by *Candida albicans. Infect. Immun.* **57:**262–271.
34. **Casanova, M., J. L. López-Ribot, C. Monteagudo, A. Llombart-Bosch, R. Sentandreu, and J. P. Martínez.** 1992. Identification of a 58-kilodalton cell surface fibrinogen-binding mannoprotein from *Candida albicans. Infect. Immun.* **60:** 4221–4229.
35. **Cassone, A., A. Torosantucci, M. Boccanera, G. Pellegrini, C. Palma, and F. Malavasi.** 1988. Production and characterisation of a monoclonal antibody to a cell-surface glucomannoprotein constituent of *Candida albicans* and other pathogenic *Candida* species. *J. Med. Microbiol.* **27:**233–238.
36. **Chaffin, W. L., J. L. López-Ribot, M. Casanova, D. Gozalbo, and J. P. Martínez.** 1998. Cell wall and associated proteins of *Candida albicans:* identification, function, and expression. *Microbiol. Mol. Biol. Rev.* **62:**130–180.
37. **Chakrabarti, A., P. Roy, D. Kumar, B. K. Sharma, K. S. Chugh, and D. Panigrahi.** 1994. Evaluation of three serological tests for detection of anti-candidal antibodies in diagnosis of invasive candidiasis. *Mycopathologia* **126:**3–7.
38. **Chew, W. H., and T. L. Theus.** 1967. *Candida* precipitins. *J. Immunol.* **98:**220–224.
39. **Christensson, B., G. Sigmundsdottir, and L. Larsson.** 1999. D-arabinitol—a marker for invasive candidiasis. *Med. Mycol.* **37:**391–396.
40. **Christensson, B., T. Wiebe, C. Pehrson, and L. Larsson.** 1997. Diagnosis of invasive candidiasis in neutropenic children with cancer by determination of D-arabinitol/L-arabinitol ratios in urine. *J. Clin. Microbiol.* **35:**636–640.
41. **Chryssanthou, E., L. Klingspor, J. Tollemar, B. Petrini, L. Larsson, B. Christensson, and O. Ringdén.** 1999. PCR and other non-culture methods for diagnosis of invasive *Candida*-infections in allogenic bone marrow and solid organ transplant recipients. *Mycoses* **42:**239–247.
42. **Deacon, A. G.** 1986. Estimations of serum arabinitol for diagnosing invasive candidosis. *J. Clin. Pathol.* **39:**842–850.
43. **De Bernardis, F., C. Girmenia, M. Boccanera, D. Adriani, P. Martino, and A. Cassone.** 1993. Use of a monoclonal antibody in a dot immunobiending assay for detection of circulating mannoprotein of *Candida* spp. in neutropenic patients with invasive candidiasis. *J. Clin. Microbiol.* **31:**3142–3146.
44. **Dee, T. H., G. M. Johnson, and C. S. Berger.** 1981. Sensitivity, specificity and predictive value of anti-*Candida* serum precipitin and agglutinin quantification: comparison of counterimmunoelectrophoresis and latex agglutination. *J. Clin. Microbiol.* **13:**750–753.
45. **Dee, T. H., and M. W. Rytel.** 1975. Clinical application of counterimmunoelectrophoresis in detection of *Candida* serum precipitins. *J. Lab. Clin. Med.* **85:**161–166.
46. **Dee, T. H., and M. W. Rytel.** 1977. Detection of *Candida* serum precipitins by counterimmunoelectrophoresis: an adjunct in determining significant candidiasis. *J. Clin. Microbiol.* **5:**453–457.
47. **DeLozier, J. B., III, C. W. Stratton, and J. R. Potts III.** 1987.

Rapid diagnosis of *Candida* sepsis in surgical patients. *Am. Surg.* **53**:600–602.

48. **De Repentigny, L.** 1989. Serological techniques for diagnosis of fungal infection. *Eur. J. Clin. Microbiol. Infect. Dis.* **8**: 362–375.
49. **De Repentigny, L.** 1992. Serodiagnosis of candidiasis, aspergillosis, and cryptococcosis. *Clin. Infect. Dis.* **14**(Suppl. 1): S11–S22.
50. **De Repentigny, L., L. Kaufman, G. T. Cole, D. Kruse, J.-P. Latgé, and R. C. Matthews.** 1994. Immunodiagnosis of invasive fungal infections. *J. Med. Vet. Mycol.* **32**(Suppl. 1): 239–252.
51. **De Repentigny, L., L. D. Marr, J. W. Keller, A. W. Carter, R. J. Kuykendall, L. Kaufman, and E. Reiss.** 1985. Comparison of enzyme immunoassay and gas-liquid chromatography for the rapid diagnosis of invasive candidiasis in cancer patients. *J. Clin. Microbiol.* **21**:972–979.
52. **De Repentigny, L., and E. Reiss.** 1984. Current trends in immunodiagnosis of candidiasis and aspergillosis. *Rev. Infect. Dis.* **6**:301–312.
53. **Deslauriers, N., J. Michaud, B. Carré, and C. Léveillée.** 1996. Dynamic expression of cell-surface antigens probed with *Candida albicans*-specific monoclonal antibodies. *Microbiology* **142**:1239–1248.
54. **Drutz, D. J.** 1987. Controversies in the diagnosis and management of infectious diseases. Session V. Fungal infections. Summary and discussion. *Rev. Infect. Dis.* **9**:417–420.
55. **Eisen, D. P., R. MacGinley, B. Christensson, L. Larsson, and M. L. Woods.** 2000. *Candida tropicalis* vertebral osteomyelitis complicating epidural catheterisation with disease paralleled by elevated D-arabinitol/L-arabinitol ratios. *Eur. J. Clin. Microbiol. Infect. Dis.* **19**:61–63.
56. **El Moudni, B., M.-H. Rodier, G. Daniault, and J. L. Jacquemin.** 1998. Improved immunodiagnosis of human candidiasis by enzyme-linked immunosorbent assay using a *Candida albicans* 52-kilodalton metallopeptidase. *Clin. Diagn. Lab. Immunol.* **5**:823–825.
57. **Eng, R. H. K., H. Chmel, and M. Buse.** 1981. Serum levels of arabinitol in the detection of invasive candidiasis in animals and humans. *J. Infect. Dis.* **143**:677–683.
58. **Escuro, R. S., M. Jacobs, S. L. Gerson, A. R. Machicao, and H. M. Lazarus.** 1989. Prospective evaluation of a *Candida* antigen detection test for invasive candidiasis in immunocompromised adult patients with cancer. *Am. J. Med.* **87**: 621–627.
59. **Esterly, N. B.** 1968. Serum antibody titers to *Candida albicans* utilizing an immunofluorescence technique. *Am. J. Clin. Pathol.* **50**:291–296.
60. **Evans, E. G. V., M. D. Richardson, F. C. Odds, and K. T. Holland.** 1973. Relevance of antigenicity of *Candida albicans* growth phases to diagnosis of systemic candidiasis. *Br. Med. J.* **4**:86–87.
61. **Everett, E. D., F. M. LaForce, and T. C. Eickhoff.** 1975. Serologic studies in suspected visceral candidiasis. *Arch. Intern. Med.* **135**:1075–1078.
62. **Ferreira, R. P., B. Yu, Y. Niki, and D. Armstrong.** 1990. Detection of *Candida* antigenuria in disseminated candidiasis by immunoblotting. *J. Clin. Microbiol.* **28**:1075–1078.
63. **Filice, G., B. Yu, and D. Armstrong.** 1977. Immunodiffusion and agglutination tests for *Candida* in patients with neoplastic disease: inconsistent correlation of results with invasive infections. *J. Infect. Dis.* **135**:349–357.
64. **Fisher, J. F., R. C. Trincher, J. F. Agel, T. B. Buxton, C. A. Walker, D. H. Johnson, R. E. Cormier, W. H. Chew, and J. P. Rissing.** 1985. Disseminated candidiasis: a comparison of two immunologic techniques in the diagnosis. *Am. J. Med. Sci.* **290**:135–142.
65. **Fortier, B., V. Hopwood, and D. Poulain.** 1988. Electric and chemical fusions for the production of monoclonal antibodies reacting with the in-vivo growth phase of *Candida albicans*. *J. Med. Microbiol.* **27**:239–245.
66. **Franklyn, K. M., J. R. Warmington, A. K. Ott, and R. B. Ashman.** 1990. An immunodominant antigen of *Candida albicans* shows homology to the enzyme enolase. *Immunol. Cell Biol.* **68**:173–178.
67. **Fujita, S., F. Matsubara, and T. Matsuda.** 1986. Enzyme-linked immunosorbent assay measurement of fluctuations in antibody titer and antigenemia in cancer patients with and without candidiasis. *J. Clin. Microbiol.* **23**:568–575.
68. **Fujita, S.-I., and T. Hashimoto.** 1992. Detection of serum *Candida* antigens by enzyme-linked immunosorbent assay and a latex agglutination test with anti-*Candida albicans* and anti-*Candida krusei* antibodies. *J. Clin. Microbiol.* **30**: 3132–3137.
69. **Fung, J. C., S. T. Donta, and R. C. Tilton.** 1986. *Candida* detection system (CAND-TEC) to differentiate between *Candida albicans* colonization and disease. *J. Clin. Microbiol.* **24**: 542–547.
70. **García-Ruiz, J. C., M. C. Arilla, P. Regúlez, G. Quindós, A. Alvarez, and J. Pontón.** 1997. Detection of antibodies to *Candida albicans* germ tubes for the diagnosis and therapeutic monitoring of invasive candidiasis in patients with hematologic malignancies. *J. Clin. Microbiol.* **35**:3284–3287.
71. **Gatermann, S., J. Heesemann, and R. Laufs.** 1986. Identification of *Candida albicans* antigens recognized by sera of patients with candidiasis. *Mykosen* **29**:343–354.
72. **Gentry, L. O., I. D. Wilkinson, A. S. Lea, and M. F. Price.** 1983. Latex agglutination test for detection of *Candida* antigen in patients with disseminated disease. *Eur. J. Clin. Microbiol.* **2**:122–128.
73. **George, E., M. L. Garrigues, J. L. Poirot, J. P. Masini, and M. C. Meyohas.** 1991. Diagnostic des candidoses systémiques par un test au latex. Résultats d'une année de suivi sérologique chez des patients à risque. *J. Mycol. Med.* **1**: 25–28.
74. **Girmenia, C., P. Martino, F. De Bernardis, and A. Cassone.** 1997. Assessment of detection of *Candida* mannoproteinemia as a method to differentiate central venous catheter-related candidemia from invasive disease. *J. Clin. Microbiol.* **35**: 903–906.
75. **Girmenia, C., A. Micozzi, C. Cartoni, F. De Bernardis, A. Cassone, and P. Martino.** 1999. Detection of *Candida* mannoproteinemia in patients with neutropenic enterocolitis. *Eur. J. Clin. Microbiol. Infect. Dis.* **18**:55–58.
76. **Glew, R. H., H. R. Buckley, H. M. Rosen, R. C. Moellering, and J. E. Fischer.** 1978. Serologic tests in the diagnosis of systemic candidiasis. *Am. J. Med.* **64**:586–591.
77. **Gold, J. W. M., B. Wong, E. M. Bernard, T. E. Kiehn, and D. Armstrong.** 1983. Serum arabinitol concentrations and arabinitol/creatinine ratios in invasive candidiasis. *J. Infect. Dis.* **147**:504–513.
78. **Goudswaard, J., and G. Virella.** 1978. New immunofluorescent antibody test for diagnosis of candidiasis using macrophage-engulfed antigens as substrate. *J. Immunol. Methods* **20**:357–363.
79. **Greenfield, R. A., M. J. Bussey, J. L. Stephens, and J. M. Jones.** 1983. Serial enzyme-linked immunosorbent assays for antibody to *Candida* antigens during induction chemotherapy for acute leukemia. *J. Infect. Dis.* **148**:275–283.
80. **Greenfield, R. A., and J. M. Jones.** 1981. Purification and

characterization of a major cytoplasmic antigen of *Candida albicans*. *Infect. Immun.* 34:469–477.

81. **Greenfield, R. A., and J. M. Jones.** 1982. Comparison of cytoplasmic extracts of eight *Candida* species and *Saccharomyces cerevisiae*. *Infect. Immun.* 35:1157–1161.
82. **Greenfield, R. A., J. L. Stephens, M. J. Bussey, and J. M. Jones.** 1983. Quantitation of antibody to *Candida* mannan by enzyme-linked immunosorbent assay. *J. Lab. Clin. Med.* 101:758–771.
83. **Greenfield, R. A., D. L. Troutt, R. C. Rickard, and D. H. Altmiller.** 1988. Comparison of antibody, antigen, and metabolite assays in rat models of systemic and gastrointestinal candidiasis. *J. Clin. Microbiol.* 26:409–417.
84. **Guinan, M. E., M. R. Portas, and H. R. Hill.** 1979. The *Candida* precipitin test in an immunosuppressed population. *Cancer* 43:299–302.
85. **Gutiérrez, J., C. Maroto, G. Piédrola, E. Martín, and J. A. Pérez.** 1993. Circulating *Candida* antigens and antibodies: useful markers of candidemia. *J. Clin. Microbiol.* 31: 2550–2552.
86. **Harding, S. A., G. R. Sandford, and W. G. Merz.** 1976. Three serologic tests for candidiasis. Diagnostic value in distinguishing deep or disseminated infection from superficial infection or colonization. *Am. J. Clin. Pathol.* 65:1001–1009.
87. **Hayette, M. P., G. Strecker, C. Faille, D. Dive, D. Camus, D. W. R. Mackenzie, and D. Poulain.** 1992. Presence of human antibodies reacting with *Candida albicans* O-linked oligomannosides revealed by using an enzyme-linked immunosorbent assay and neoglycolipids. *J. Clin. Microbiol.* 30: 411–417.
88. **Herent, P., D. Stynen, F. Hernando, J. Fruit, and D. Poulain.** 1992. Retrospective evaluation of two latex agglutination tests for detection of circulating antigen during invasive candidosis. *J. Clin. Microbiol.* 30:2158–2164.
89. **Hernando, F. L., J. C. Cailliez, P. A. Trinel, C. Faille, D. W. R. Mackenzie, and D. Poulain.** 1993. Qualitative and quantitative differences in recognition patterns of *Candida albicans* protein and polysaccharide antigens by human sera. *J. Med. Vet. Mycol.* 31:219–226.
90. **Ho, Y. M., M. H. Ng, and C. T. Huang.** 1979. Antibodies to germinating and yeast cells of *Candida albicans* in human and rabbit sera. *J. Clin. Pathol.* 32:399–405.
91. **Ho, Y. M., M. H. Ng, C. H. Teoh-Chan, P. C. K. Yue, and C. T. Huang.** 1976. Indirect immunofluorescence assay for antibody to germ tube of *Candida albicans*—a new diagnostic test. *J. Clin. Pathol.* 29:1007–1010.
92. **Holak, E. J., J. Wu, and S. L. Spruance.** 1986. Value of serum arabinitol for the management of *Candida* infections in clinical practice. *Mycopathologia* 93:99–104.
93. **Holmberg, K.** 1978. Serological diagnosis of systemic candidiasis and invasive aspergillosis. *Scand. J. Infect. Dis.* Suppl. 16:26–32.
94. **Hopfer, R. L., and D. Gröschel.** 1979. Detection by counterimmunoelectrophoresis of anti-*Candida* precipitins in sera from cancer patients. *Am. J. Clin. Pathol.* 72:215–218.
95. **Hoppe, J. E., D. Friess, and D. Niethammer.** 1995. Orointestinal yeast colonization of paediatric oncologic patients during antifungal prophylaxis: results of quantitative culture and *Candida* serology and comparison of three polyenes. *Mycoses* 38:41–49.
96. **Hopwood, V., and D. W. Warnock.** 1986. New developments in the diagnosis of opportunistic fungal infection. *Eur. J. Clin. Microbiol.* 5:379–388.
97. **Hossain, M. A., T. Miyazaki, K. Mitsutake, H. Kakeya, Y. Yamamoto, K. Yanagihara, S. Kawamura, T. Otsubo, Y. Hirakata, T. Tashiro, and S. Kohno.** 1997. Comparison between Wako-WB003 and Fungitec G tests for detection of (1→3)-beta-D-glucan in systemic mycosis. *J. Clin. Lab. Anal.* 11: 73–77.
98. **Humphrey, D. M., and M. H. Weiner.** 1983. Candidal antigen detection in pulmonary candidiasis. *Am. J. Med.* 74: 630–640.
99. **Iruretagoyena, J. R., P. Regúlez, G. Quindós, and J. Pontón.** 2000. Antibodies to *Candida albicans* germ tubes in two intensive care patients with invasive candidiasis. *Rev. Iberoam. Micol.* 17:93–96.
100. **Ishiguro, A., M. Homma, T. Sukai, K. Higashide, S. Torii, and K. Tanaka.** 1992. Immunoblotting analysis of sera from patients with candidal vaginitis and healthy females. *J. Med. Vet. Micol.* 30:281–292.
101. **Ishiguro, A., M. Homma, S. Torii, and K. Tanaka.** 1992. Identification of *Candida albicans* antigens reactive with immunoglobulin E antibody of human sera. *Infect. Immun.* 60: 1550–1557.
102. **Ito, K., A. Ishiguro, T. Kanbe, K. Tanaka, and S. Torii.** 1995. Detection of IgE antibody against *Candida albicans* enolase and its crossreactivity to *Saccharomyces cerevisiae* enolase. *Clin. Exp. Allergy* 25:522–528.
103. **Ito, K., A. Ishiguro, T. Kanbe, K. Tanaka, and S. Torii.** 1995. Characterization of IgE-binding epitopes on *Candida albicans* enolase. *Clin. Exp. Allergy* 25:529–535.
104. **Iwasaki, H., H. Misaki, T. Nakamura, and T. Ueda.** 2000. Surveillance of the serum *Candida* antigen titer for initiation of antifungal therapy after postremission chemotherapy in patients with acute leukemia. *Int. J. Hematol.* 71:266–272.
105. **Jones, J. M.** 1980. Kinetics of antibody responses to cell wall mannan and a major cytoplasmic antigen of *Candida albicans* in rabbits and humans. *J. Lab. Clin. Med.* 96:845–860.
106. **Jones, J. M.** 1980. Quantitation of antibody against cell wall mannan and a major cytoplasmic antigen of *Candida* in rabbits, mice and humans. *Infect. Immun.* 30:78–89.
107. **Jones, J. M.** 1989. Humoral immune response to *Candida albicans*, p. 375–400. *In* E. Kurstak (ed.), *Immunology of Fungal Diseases.* Marcel Dekker, Inc., New York, N.Y.
108. **Jones, J. M.** 1990. Laboratory diagnosis of invasive candidiasis. *Clin. Microbiol. Rev.* 3:32–45.
109. **Kahn, F. W., and J. M. Jones.** 1986. Latex agglutination tests for detection of *Candida* antigens in sera of patients with invasive candidiasis. *J. Infect. Dis.* 153:579–585.
110. **Kalin, M., and B. Petrini.** 1996. Clinical and laboratory diagnosis of invasive *Candida* infection in neutropenic patients. *Med. Oncol.* 13:223–231.
111. **Kanbe, T., R. K. Li, E. Wadsworth, R. A. Calderone, and J. E. Cutler.** 1991. Evidence for expression of the C3d receptor of *Candida albicans* in vitro and in vivo obtained by immunofluorescence and immunoelectron microscopy. *Infect. Immun.* 59:1832–1838.
112. **Kanbe, T., M. Morishita, K. Ito, K. Tomita, K. Utsunomiya, and A. Ishiguro.** 1996. Evidence for the presence of immunoglobulin E antibodies specific to the cell wall phosphomannoproteins of *Candida albicans* in patients with allergies. *Clin. Diagn. Lab. Immunol.* 3:645–650.
113. **Kappe, R.** 1989. Coexistence of free antigens, free antibodies and immune complexes in sera from patients with suspected deep-seated candidiasis. *Mycoses* 32:24–32.
114. **Kappe, R., and J. Müller.** 1991. Rapid clearance of *Candida albicans* mannan antigens by liver and spleen in contrast to prolonged circulation of *Cryptococcus neoformans* antigens. *J. Clin. Microbiol.* 29:1665–1669.
115. **Karam, G. H., A. M. Elliot, S. Polt, and C. G. Cobbs.** 1984. Elevated serum D-arabinitol levels in patients with sarcoidosis. *J. Clin. Microbiol.* 19:26–29.

116. **Karwowska, W., and B. Lisowska-Grospierre.** 1984. Diagnostic significance of the human antibody response to a major cytoplasmic antigen of *Candida albicans*. *Immunol. Lett.* **8:** 127–129.
117. **Karwowska, W., G. de Saint Basile, and B. Lisowska-Grospierre.** 1984. Antibody levels to *Candida albicans* carbohydrate and major cytoplasmic antigens isolated from standard and patient strains. *Ann. Immunol.* **135D:**145–159.
118. **Kaufman, L.** 1983. Mycoserology: its vital role in diagnosing systemic mycotic infections. *Jpn. J. Med. Mycol.* **24:**1–8.
119. **Kealey, G. P., J. A. Heinle, R. W. Lewis II, M. A. Pfaller, and M. D. Rosenquist.** 1992. Value of the *Candida* antigen assay in diagnosis of systemic candidiasis in burn patients. *J. Trauma* **32:**285–288.
120. **Kerkering, T. M., A. Espinel-Ingroff, and S. Shadomy.** 1979. Detection of *Candida* antigenemia by counterimmunoelectrophoresis in patients with invasive candidiasis. *J. Infect. Dis.* **140:**659–664.
121. **Kiehn, T. E., E. M. Bernard, J. W. M. Gold, and D. Armstrong.** 1979. Candidiasis: detection by gas-liquid chromatography of D-arabinitol, a fungal metabolite, in human serum. *Science* **206:**577–580.
122. **Klingspor, L., T. H. Eberhard, G. Stintzing, and J. Tollemar.** 1994. Antibody response to *Candida* and its use in clinical practice. *Mycoses* **37:**199–204.
123. **Klingspor, L., G. Stintzing, A. Fasth, and J. Tollemar.** 1996. Deep *Candida* infection in children receiving allogeneic bone marrow transplants: incidence, risk factors and diagnosis. *Bone Marrow Transplant.* **17:**1043–1049.
124. **Klingspor, L., G. Stintzing, and J. Tollemar.** 1995. Deep *Candida* infection in child liver transplant recipients: serological diagnosis and incidence. *Acta Paediatr.* **84:**424–428.
125. **Kohno, S.** 1991. Serological diagnosis of deep-seated mycoses. *Asian Med. J.* **34:**460–466.
126. **Kohno, S., K. Mitsutake, S. Maesaki, A. Yasuoka, T. Miyazaki, M. Kaku, H. Koga, and K. Hara.** 1993. An evaluation of serodiagnostic tests in patients with candidemia: beta-glucan, mannan, *Candida* antigen by Cand-Tec and D-arabinitol. *Microbiol. Immunol.* **37:**207–212.
127. **Kono, K., T. Tamaki, M. Tanaka, N. Matsuno, M. Uchiyama, H. Ito, N. Kaji, N. Ioya, M. Kawaguchi, M. Yoshida, and M. Kozaki.** 1992. A *Candida* antigen detection system for fungus infection in renal transplant patients. *Transplant. Proc.* **24:**1554–1555.
128. **Kostiala, I., A. A. I. Kostiala, U. Larinkari, V. V. Valtonen, and A. Miettinen.** 1981. Antibodies against antigens of *Candida albicans* in patients with fungaemia and bacteraemia, studied by ELISA, precipitation, passive haemagglutination and immunofluorescence techniques. *J. Med. Microbiol.* **14:** 483–492.
129. **Kozinn, P. J., and C. L. Taschdjian.** 1985. Laboratory diagnosis of candidiasis, p. 85–110. *In* G. P. Bodey and V. Fainstein (ed.), *Candidiasis,* 1st ed. Raven Press, New York, N.Y.
130. **Kozinn, P. J., C. L. Taschdjian, P. K. Goldberg, W. P. Protzman, D. W. R. Mackenzie, J. S. Remington, S. Anderson, and M. S. Seelig.** 1978. Efficiency of serologic tests in the diagnosis of systemic candidiasis. *Am. J. Clin. Pathol.* **70:** 893–898.
131. **Kozinn, P. J., C. L. Taschdjian, B. E. Kodsi, G. J. Wise, M. S. Seelig, and P. K. Goldberg.** 1982. Diagnosis of systemic or visceral candidosis. *Can. Med. Assoc. J.* **126:**1386–1390.
132. **Larsson, L., C. Pehrson, T. Wiebe, and B. Christensson.** 1994. Gas chromatographic determination of D-arabinitol/L-arabinitol ratios in urine: a potential method for diagnosis of disseminated candidiasis. *J. Clin. Microbiol.* **32:**1855–1859.
133. **Lehmann, P. F.** 1983. The detection of fungal metabolites including antigens in body fluids, p. 303–324. *In* D. H. Howard (ed.), *Fungi Pathogenic for Humans and Animals.* Marcel Dekker, Inc., New York, N.Y.
134. **Lehmann, P. F., and E. Reiss.** 1980. Detection of *Candida albicans* mannan by immunodiffusion, counterimmunoelectrophoresis and enzyme-linked immunoassay. *Mycopathologia* **70:**83–88.
135. **Lehner, T.** 1966. Immunofluorescence study of *Candida albicans* in candidiasis carriers and controls. *J. Pathol. Bacteriol.* **91:**97–104.
136. **Lehner, T.** 1970. Serum fluorescent antibody and immunoglobulin estimations in candidosis. *J. Med. Microbiol.* **3:** 475–481.
137. **Lehner, T., H. R. Buckley, and I. G. Murray.** 1972. The relationship between fluorescent, agglutinating and precipitating antibodies to *Candida albicans* and their immunoglobulin classes. *J. Clin. Pathol.* **25:**344–348.
138. **Lehtonen, L., V.-J. Anttila, T. Ruutu, J. Salonen, J. Nikoskelainen, E. Eerola, and P. Ruutu.** 1996. Diagnosis of disseminated candidiasis by measurement of urine D-arabinitol/L-arabinitol ratio. *J. Clin. Microbiol.* **34:**2175–2179.
139. **Lemieux, C., G. St.-Germain, J. Vincelette, L. Kaufman, and L. de Repentigny.** 1990. Collaborative evaluation of antigen detection by a commercial latex agglutination test and enzyme immunoassay in the diagnosis of invasive candidiasis. *J. Clin. Microbiol.* **28:**249–253.
140. **Leusch, H. G.** 1989. Detection and characterization of two antigens specific for cell walls of *Candida albicans* mycelial growth phase. *Curr. Microbiol.* **19:**193–198.
141. **Lew, M. A.** 1989. Diagnosis of systemic *Candida* infections. *Annu. Rev. Med.* **40:**87–97.
142. **Lew, M. A., G. R. Siber, D. M. Donahue, and F. Maiorca.** 1982. Enhanced detection with an enzyme-linked immunosorbent assay of candida mannan in antibody-containing serum after heat extraction. *J. Infect. Dis.* **145:**45–56.
143. **López-Ribot, J. L., M. Casanova, J. P. Martínez, and R. Sentandreu.** 1991. Characterization of cell wall proteins of yeast and hydrophobic mycelial cells of *Candida albicans. Infect. Immun.* **59:**2324–2332.
144. **Macdonald, F., and F. C. Odds.** 1980. Purified *Candida albicans* proteinase in the serological diagnosis of systemic candidosis. *JAMA* **243:**2409–2411.
145. **Maliwan, N., R. W. Reid, and R. B. Katzen.** 1984. Gas-liquid chromatography for rapid diagnosis and monitoring of invasive candidal infections and candidemia. *Arch. Pathol. Lab. Med.* **108:**108–111.
146. **Marcilla, A., C. Monteagudo, S. Mormeneo, and R. Sentandreu.** 1999. Monoclonal antibody 3H8: a useful tool in the diagnosis of candidiasis. *Microbiology* **145:**695–701.
147. **Marier, R., and V. T. Andriole.** 1978. Usefulness of serial antibody determinations in diagnosis of candidiasis as measured by discontinuous counterimmunoelectrophoresis using HS antigen. *J. Clin. Microbiol.* **8:**15–22.
148. **Marier, R., E. Milligan, and Y.-D. Fan.** 1982. Elevated mannose levels detected by gas-liquid chromatography in hydrolysates of serum from rats and humans with candidiasis. *J. Clin. Microbiol.* **16:**123–128.
149. **Marot-Leblond, A., L. Grimaud, S. Nail, S. Bouterige, V. Apaire-Marchais, D. J. Sullivan, and R. Robert.** 2000. New monoclonal antibody specific for *Candida albicans* germ tube. *J. Clin. Microbiol.* **38:**61–67.
150. **Marot-Leblond, A., R. Robert, J. Aubry, P. Ezcurra, and J. M. Senet.** 1993. Identification and immunochemical characterization of a germ tube specific antigen of *Candida albicans. FEMS Immunol. Med. Microbiol.* **7:**175–186.
151. **Martínez, J. P., M. L. Gil, J. L. López-Ribot, and W. L. J.**

Chaffin. 1998. Serologic response to cell wall mannoproteins and proteins of *Candida albicans. Clin. Microbiol. Rev.* **11:** 121–141.

152. **Mason, A. B., M. E. Brandt, and H. R. Buckley.** 1989. Enolase activity associated with a *Candida albicans* cytoplasmic antigen. *Yeast* **5:**S231–S240.
153. **Mason, A. B., and J. M. B. Smith.** 1986. Germling protoplast antigens of *Candida albicans* in the serodiagnosis of invasive candidiasis. *J. Infect. Dis.* **153:**146–150.
154. **Mathur, S., J. M. Goust, E. O. Horger III, and H. H. Fudenberg.** 1977. Immunoglobulin E anti-*Candida* antibodies and candidiasis. *Infect. Immun.* **18:**257–259.
155. **Mathur, S., J. Koistinen, C. U. Kyong, E. O. Horger III, G. Virella, and H. H. Fudenberg.** 1977. Antibodies to *Candida albicans* in IgA-deficient humans. *J. Infect. Dis.* **136:** 436–438.
156. **Matthews, R. C.** 1993. Early diagnosis of systemic candidal infection. *J. Antimicrob. Chemother.* **31:**809–812.
157. **Matthews, R. C.** 1996. Comparative assessment of the detection of candidal antigens as a diagnostic tool. *J. Med. Vet. Mycol.* **34:**1–10.
158. **Matthews, R. C., and J. P. Burnie.** 1988. A prospective assessment of a reverse passive latex agglutination test in the serodiagnosis of systemic candidosis. *Serodiagn. Immunother. Infect. Dis.* **2:**95–101.
159. **Matthews, R. C., and J. P. Burnie.** 1988. Diagnosis of systemic candidosis by an enzyme-linked dot immunobinding assay for a circulating immunodominant 47-kilodalton antigen. *J. Clin. Microbiol.* **26:**459–463.
160. **Matthews, R. C., and J. P. Burnie.** 1988. New developments in the serological diagnosis of *Candida* infection. *Mycoses* **31**(Suppl. 2):34–38.
161. **Matthews, R. C., and J. P. Burnie.** 1989. Cloning of a cDNA sequence encoding a major fragment of the 47 kilodalton stress protein homologue of *Candida albicans. FEMS Microbiol. Lett.* **60:**25–30.
162. **Matthews, R. C., J. P. Burnie, A. Fox, A. Baskerville, C. Wells, S. Strachan, and I. Clark.** 1989. The diagnostic and therapeutic potential of a monoclonal antibody to the 60-kilodalton nuclear antigen of *Candida albicans. Serodiagn. Immunother. Infect. Dis.* **3:**75–86.
163. **Matthews, R. C., J. P. Burnie, and W. Lee.** 1991. The application of epitope mapping to the development of a new serological test for systemic candidosis. *J. Immunol. Methods* **143:** 73–79.
164. **Matthews, R. C., J. P. Burnie, and S. Tabaqchali.** 1984. Immunoblot analysis of the serological response in systemic candidosis. *Lancet* **ii:**1415–1418.
165. **Matthews, R. C., J. P. Burnie, and S. Tabaqchali.** 1987. Isolation of immunodominant antigens from the sera of patients with systemic candidosis and characterization of the serological response to *Candida albicans. J. Clin. Microbiol.* **25:** 230–237.
166. **Mauch, H.** 1983. Diagnostic value of monitoring kinetics of antibody responses in candidiasis by a solid-phase radioimmunoassay. *Am. J. Clin. Pathol.* **79:**200–205.
167. **McHugh, T. M., Y. J. Wang, H. O. Chong, L. L. Blackwood, and D. P. Stites.** 1989. Development of a microsphere-based fluorescent immunoassay and its comparison to an enzyme immunoassay for the detection of antibodies to three antigen preparations from *Candida albicans. J. Immunol. Methods* **116:**213–219.
168. **Meckstroth, K. L., E. Reiss, J. W. Keller, and L. Kaufman.** 1981. Detection of antibodies and antigenemia in leukemic patients with candidiasis by enzyme-linked immunosorbent assay. *J. Infect. Dis.* **144:**24–32.
169. **Miller, G. C., M. W. Witwer, A. I. Braude, and C. E. Davis.** 1974. Rapid identification of *Candida albicans* septicaemia in man by gas-liquid chromatography. *J. Clin. Invest.* **54:** 1235–1240.
170. **Mitsutake, K., S. Kohno, T. Miyazaki, H. Miyazaki, S. Maesaki, and H. Koga.** 1994. Detection of *Candida* enolase antibody in patients with candidiasis. *J. Clin. Lab. Anal.* **8:** 207–210.
171. **Mitsutake, K., T. Miyazaki, T. Tashiro, Y. Yamamoto, H. Kakeya, T. Otsubo, S. Kawamura, M. A. Hossain, T. Noda, Y. Hirakata, and S. Kohno.** 1996. Enolase antigen, mannan antigen, Cand-Tec antigen, and β-glucan in patients with candidemia. *J. Clin. Microbiol.* **34:**1918–1921.
172. **Mitsuya, M., K. Wada, K. Makimura, and H. Yamaguchi.** 1996. The antigen (CANDTEC antigen) detected by CAND TEC test for diagnosis of candidiasis. *Rinsho Byori.* **44:** 512–517.
173. **Miyazaki, T., S. Kohno, H. Koga, M. Kaku, K. Mitsutake, S. Maesaki, A. Yasuoka, K. Hara, S. Tanaka, and H. Tamura.** 1992. G test, a new direct method for diagnosis of candida infection: comparison with assays for beta-glucan and mannan antigen in a rabbit model of systemic candidiasis. *J. Clin. Lab. Anal.* **6:**315–318.
174. **Miyazaki, T., S. Kohno, K. Mitsutake, S. Maesaki, K.-I. Tanaka, N. Ishikawa, and K. Hara.** 1995. Plasma (1→3)-β-D-glucan and fungal antigenemia in patients with candidemia, aspergillosis, and cryptococcosis. *J. Clin. Microbiol.* **33:** 3115–3118.
175. **Monson, T. P., and K. P. Wilkinson.** 1981. Mannose in body fluids as an indicator of invasive candidiasis. *J. Clin. Microbiol.* **14:**557–562.
176. **Morace, G., L. Pagano, M. Sanguinetti, B. Posteraro, L. Mele, F. Equitani, G. D'Amore, G. Leone, and G. Fadda.** 1999. PCR-restriction enzyme analysis for detection of *Candida* DNA in blood from febrile patients with hematological malignancies. *J. Clin. Microbiol.* **37:**1871–1875.
177. **Morhart, M., R. Rennie, B. Ziola, E. Bow, and T. J. Louie.** 1994. Evaluation of enzyme immunoassay for *Candida* cytoplasmic antigens in neutropenic cancer patients. *J. Clin. Microbiol.* **32:**766–776.
178. **Munoz, M., G. Estes, M. Kilpatrick, A. Di Salvo, and G. Virella.** 1980. Purification of cytoplasmic antigens from the mycelial phase of *Candida albicans:* possible advantages of its use in *Candida* serology. *Mycopathologia* **72:**47–53.
179. **Myerowitz, R. L., H. Layman, S. Petursson, and R. B. Yee.** 1979. Diagnostic value of *Candida* precipitins determined by counterimmunoelectrophoresis in patients with acute leukemia: a prospective study. *Am. J. Clin. Pathol.* **72:**963–967.
180. **Myerowitz, R. L., G. J. Pazin, and C. M. Allen.** 1977. Disseminated candidiasis. Changes in incidence, underlying diseases and pathology. *Am. J. Clin. Pathol.* **68:**29–38.
181. **Na, B. K., and C. Y. Song.** 1999. Use of monoclonal antibody in diagnosis of candidiasis caused by *Candida albicans:* detection of circulating aspartyl proteinase antigen. *Clin. Diagn. Lab. Immunol.* **6:**924–929.
182. **Nagy, F., Z. Szènàsi, E. Szöllösy, I. Kiss, and V. Varrò.** 1989. Determination and kinetics of antibody response to *Candida albicans* in ulcerative colitis. *Hepato-Gastroenterol.* **36:** 182–184.
183. **Nakamura, A., N. Ishikawa, and H. Suzuki.** 1991. Diagnosis of invasive candidiasis by detection of mannan antigen by using the avidin-biotin enzyme immunoassay. *J. Clin. Microbiol.* **29:**2363–2367.
184. **Navarro, D., E. Monzonis, J. L. López-Ribot, P. Sepúlveda, M. Casanova, J. M. Nogueira, and J. P. Martínez.** 1993. Diagnosis of systemic candidiasis by enzyme immunoassay de-

tection of specific antibodies to mycelial phase cell wall and cytoplasmic candidal antigens. *Eur. J. Clin. Microbiol. Infect. Dis.* **12:**839–846.

185. **Neale, T. J., J. C. Muir, and B. Drake.** 1987. The immunochemical characterization of circulating immune complex constituents in *Candida albicans* osteomyelitis by isoelectric focusing, immunoblot, and immunoprint. *Aust. N. Z. J. Med.* **17:**201–209.
186. **Ness, M. J., W. P. Vaughan, and G. L. Woods.** 1989. *Candida* antigen latex test for detection of invasive candidiasis in immunocompromised patients. *J. Infect. Dis.* **159:**495–502.
187. **Obayashi, T., M. Yoshida, T. Mori, H. Goto, A. Yasuoka, H. Iwasaki, H. Teshima, S. Kohno, A. Horiuchi, A. Ito, H. Yamaguchi, K. Shimada, and T. Kawai.** 1995. Plasma (1→3)-β-D-glucan measurement in diagnosis of invasive deep mycosis and fungal febrile episodes. *Lancet* **345:**17–20.
188. **Oblack, D., J. Schwarz, and I. A. Holder.** 1976. Comparative evaluation of the *Candida* agglutinin test, precipitin test, and germ tube dispersion test in the diagnosis of candidiasis. *J. Clin. Microbiol.* **3:**175–179.
189. **Odds, F. C.** 1988. *Candida and Candidosis,* 2nd ed. Baillière Tindall, London, United Kingdom.
190. **Ollert, M. K., and R. A. Calderone.** 1990. A monoclonal antibody that defines a surface antigen on *Candida albicans* hyphae cross-reacts with yeast cell protoplasts. *Infect. Immun.* **58:**625–631.
191. **Örmälä, T., M. Korppi, M.-L. Katila, T. Ojanen, and M. Perkkiö.** 1995. Prospective evaluation of *Candida* antigen and antibody assays for detection of *Candida* infections in children with malignant disease. *Acta Paediatr.* **84:**183–187.
192. **Parsons, E. R., and E. Nassau.** 1974. *Candida* serology in open-heart surgery. *J. Med. Microbiol.* **7:**415–423.
193. **Pavliak, V., and J. Sandula.** 1988. Cross-reactivity of pathogenic *Candida* mannans studied by enzyme-linked immunosorbent assay (ELISA) and precipitin methods. *Mycoses* **31:** 34–39.
194. **Pavliak, V., J. Sandula, A. Tomsikova, and J. Gallo.** 1988. Determination of antibodies to *Candida albicans* cell wall components by immunodiffusion, ELISA and its rapid modification. *Mycoses* **31:**426–432.
195. **Peck, S. M., R. Bergamini, L. C. Kelcec, and C. R. Rein.** 1955. The serodiagnosis of moniliasis: its value and limitations. *J. Invest. Dermatol.* **25:**301–310.
196. **Pepys, J., J. Faux, J. L. Longbottom, D. S. McCarthy, and F. E. Hargreave.** 1968. *Candida albicans* precipitins in respiratory disease in man. *J. Allergy* **41:**305–318.
197. **Pfaller, M. A.** 1992. Laboratory aids in the diagnosis of invasive candidiasis. *Mycopathologia* **120:**65–72.
198. **Pfaller, M. A., I. Cabezudo, B. Buschelman, M. Bale, T. Howe, M. Vitug, H. J. Linton, and M. Densel.** 1993. Value of the hybritech ICON *Candida* assay in the diagnosis of invasive candidiasis in high-risk patients. *Diagn. Microbiol. Infect. Dis.* **16:**53–60.
199. **Phillips, P., A. Dowd, P. Jewesson, G. Radigan, M. G. Tweeddale, A. Clarke, I. Geere, and M. Kelly.** 1990. Nonvalue of antigen detection immunoassays for diagnosis of candidemia. *J. Clin. Microbiol.* **28:**2320–2326.
200. **Piens, M. A., D. Guyotat, J. Pichot, and M. Mojon.** 1987. Intérêts et limites de la détection d'antigène *Candida* circulant (Cand-Tec) dans le diagnostic des candidoses profondes. *Ann. Biol. Clin.* **45:**579–581.
201. **Platenkamp, G.-J.** 1988. Application of serological tests in the diagnosis of invasive candidiasis. *Mycoses* **31**(Suppl. 2): 27–33.
202. **Platenkamp, G.-J., A. M. van Duin, J. C. Porsius, H. J. A. Schouten, P. E. Zondervan, and M. F. Michel.** 1987. Diagnosis of invasive candidiasis in patients with and without signs of immune deficiency: a comparison of six detection methods in human serum. *J. Clin. Pathol.* **40:**1162–1167.
203. **Pontón, J.** 1996. Avances en el diagnóstico de laboratorio de la candidiasis sistémica. *Rev. Iberoam. Micol.* **13**(Suppl. 1): S16–S19.
204. **Ponton, J., and J. M. Jones.** 1986. Analysis of cell wall extracts of *Candida albicans* by sodium dodecyl sulfate-polyacrilamide gel electrophoresis and Western blot techniques. *Infect. Immun.* **53:**565–572.
205. **Ponton, J., and J. M. Jones.** 1986. Identification of two germ tube specific cell wall antigens of *Candida albicans. Infect. Immun.* **54:**864–868.
206. **Pontón, J., A. Marot-Leblond, P. A. Ezkurra, B. Barturen, R. Robert, and J. M. Senet.** 1993. Characterization of *Candida albicans* cell wall antigens with monoclonal antibodies. *Infect. Immun.* **61:**4842–4847.
207. **Pontón, J., M. D. Moragues, M. J. Omaetxebarria, N. Elguezabal, and D. Coleman.** 2000. Serological differentiation of experimentally induced *Candida dubliniensis* and *Candida albicans* infections, abstr. 215. *In Abstr. 14th Congr. Int. Soc. Hum. Anim. Mycol.* International Society for Human and Animal Mycology, Buenos Aires, Argentina.
208. **Pontón, J., G. Quindós, M. C. Arilla, and D. W. R. Mackenzie.** 1994. Simplified adsorption method for detection of antibodies to *Candida albicans* germ tubes. *J. Clin. Microbiol.* **32:**217–219.
209. **Pontón, J., G. Quindós, and R. Cisterna.** 1991. Humoral responses of the host to fungi, p. 289–339. *In* D. K. Arora, L. Ajello, and K. G. Mukerji (ed.), *Handbook of Applied Mycology*, vol. 2. *Humans, Animals, and Insects.* Marcel Dekker, Inc., New York, N.Y.
210. **Poulain, D., A. Ayadi, and J. Fruit.** 1987. Détection d'un antigène témoin d'infection systémique à *Candida* à l'aide d'un anticorps monoclonal couplé à l'or colloïdal. *Ann. Biol. Clin.* **45:**565–572.
211. **Poulain, D., J. Fruit, L. Fournier, E. Dei Cas, and A. Vernes.** 1986. Diagnosis of systemic candidiasis: application of co-counterimmunoelectrophoresis. *Eur. J. Clin. Microbiol.* **5:** 427–434.
212. **Poulain, D., V. Hopwood, and A. Vernes.** 1985. Antigenic variability of *Candida albicans. Crit. Rev. Microbiol.* **12:** 223–270.
213. **Poulain, D., and J. M. Pinon.** 1986. Diagnosis of systemic candidiasis: development of co-counter immunoelectrophoresis. *Eur. J. Clin. Microbiol.* **5:**420–426.
214. **Poulain, D., R. Robert, F. Mesnard, B. Sendid, G. Lepage, and D. Camus.** 1997. Clearances of *Candida albicans* derived α- and β-linked mannose residues in sera from patients with candidiasis. *Eur. J. Clin. Microbiol. Infect. Dis.* **16:**16–20.
215. **Preisler, H. D., H. F. Hasenclever, and E. S. Henderson.** 1971. Anti-*Candida* antibodies in patients with acute leukemia. A prospective study. *Am. J. Med.* **51:**352–361.
216. **Preisler, H. D., H. F. Hasenclever, A. A. Levitan, and E. S. Henderson.** 1969. Serologic diagnosis of disseminated candidiasis in patients with acute leukemia. *Ann. Intern. Med.* **70:** 19–29.
217. **Price, M. F., and L. O. Gentry.** 1986. Incidence and significance of *Candida* antigen in low-risk and high-risk patient populations. *Eur. J. Clin. Microbiol.* **5:**416–419.
218. **Quindós, G.** 1992. Valoración diagnóstica de la detección enzimática de manosa sérica en la candidiasis invasiva. *Enf. Infec. Microbiol. Clin.* **10:**227–229.
219. **Quindós, G., M. Alvarez, P. Regúlez, J. Pontón, and R. Cisterna.** 1988. Diagnóstico de las candidiasis sistémicas en ad-

ictos a drogas por via parenteral mediante detección de anticuerpos antimicelio. *Med. Clin.* (Barcelona) **90:**451–455.

220. **Quindós, G., J. Pontón, and R. Cisterna.** 1987. Detection of antibodies to *Candida albicans* germ tube in the diagnosis of systemic candidiasis. *Eur. J. Clin. Microbiol.* **6:**142–146.
221. **Quindós, G., J. Pontón, R. Cisterna, and D. W. R. Mackenzie.** 1990. Value of detection of antibodies to *Candida albicans* germ tube in the diagnosis of systemic candidosis. *Eur. J. Clin. Microbiol. Infect. Dis.* **9:**178–183.
222. **Quindós, G., I. F. Rowe, C. S. Higgens, J. Pontón, R. Cisterna, and D. W. R. Mackenzie.** 1990. Candidal infection of the bone: assessment of serologic tests in diagnosis and management. *Diagn. Microbiol. Infect. Dis.* **13:**297–302.
223. **Quindós, G., A. Zatón, I. Gutiérrez, J. Pontón, and R. Cisterna.** 1988. Utilidad de la cromatografia líquida de alta presión en el diagnóstico de la candidiasis sistémica. *Enf. Infec. Microbiol. Clin.* **6:**203–207.
224. **Reboli, A. C.** 1993. Diagnosis of invasive candidiasis by a dot immunobinding assay for *Candida* antigen detection. *J. Clin. Microbiol.* **31:**518–523.
225. **Regúlez, P., M. C. Arilla, J. Bikandi, G. Quindós, R. Cisterna, and J. Pontón.** 1992. Identification of antigens reacting with anti-*Candida albicans* germ tube antibodies. *Eur. J. Epidermiol.* **8:**356–361.
226. **Regúlez, P., M. C. Arilla, J. C. García-Ruiz, M. D. Moragues, G. Quindós, and J. Pontón.** 1995. Estudio comparativo de dos técnicas para el diagnóstico serológico de la candidiasis invasiva. *Enf. Infec. Microbiol. Clin.* **13:**229–235.
227. **Reimer, L. G., M. L. Wilson, and M. P. Weinstein.** 1997. Update on detection of bacteremia and fungemia. *Clin. Microbiol. Rev.* **10:**444–465.
228. **Reiss, E., and C. Morrison.** 1993. Nonculture methods for diagnosis of disseminated candidiasis. *Clin. Microbiol. Rev.* **6:**311–323.
229. **Reiss, E., L. Stockman, R. J. Kuykendall, and S. J. Smith.** 1981. Dissociation of mannan-serum complexes and detection of *Candida albicans* mannan by enzyme immunoassay variations. *Clin. Chem.* **28:**306–310.
230. **Remington, J. S., J. D. Gaines, and M. A. Gilmer.** 1972. Demonstration of *Candida* precipitins in human sera by counterimmunoelectrophoresis. *Lancet* **i:**413.
231. **Richardson, M. D., and M. H. Kokki.** 1999. New perspectives in the diagnosis of systemic fungal infections. *Ann. Med.* **31:**327–335.
232. **Robert, R., G. Tronchin, V. Annaix, A. Bouali, and J.-M. Senet.** 1989. Use of coated latex particles for identification and localization of *Candida albicans* cell surface receptors and for detection of related circulating antigens and/or antibodies in patient sera and urine, p. 217–230. *In* G. A. Quash and J. D. Rodwell (ed.), *Covalently Modified Antigens and Antibodies in Diagnosis and Therapy.* Marcel Dekker, Inc., New York, N.Y.
233. **Roboz, J., E. Nieves, and J. F. Holland.** 1990. Separation and quantification by gas chromatography-mass spectrometry of arabinitol enantiomers to aid the differential diagnosis of disseminated candidiasis. *J. Chromatogr.* **500:**413–426.
234. **Roboz, J., R. Suzuki, and J. F. Holland.** 1980. Quantification of arabinitol in serum by selected ion monitoring as a diagnostic technique in invasive candidiasis. *J. Clin. Microbiol.* **12:**594–602.
235. **Roboz, J., Q. Yu, and J. F. Holland.** 1992. Filter paper sampling of whole blood and urine for the determination of D/L arabinitol ratios by mass spectrometry. *J. Microbiol. Methods* **15:**207–214.
236. **Rosemurgy, A. S. II, E. E. Zervos, J. F. Sweeney, and J. Y. Djeu.** 1997. *Candida* antigen titre dilution and death after injury. *Br. J. Surg.* **84:**771–774.
237. **Rüchel, R.** 1989. Candidosis: diagnostic tools in the laboratory. *Mycoses* **32**(Suppl. 1)**:**18–22.
238. **Rüchel, R.** 1989. Identification of certain false-positive results in the Cand-Tec test for candidal antigen. *Mycoses* **32:**627–630.
239. **Rüchel, R.** 1993. Diagnosis of invasive mycoses in severely immunosuppressed patients. *Ann. Hematol.* **67:**1–11.
240. **Rüchel, R., and B. Böning.** 1983. Detection of *Candida* proteinase by enzyme immunoassay and interaction of the enzyme with alpha-2-macroglobulin. *J. Immunol. Methods* **61:**107–116.
241. **Rüchel, R., B. Böning-Stutzer, and A. Mari.** 1988. A synoptical approach to the diagnosis of candidosis relying on serological antigen and antibody tests, on culture, and on evaluation of clinical data. *Mycoses* **31:**87–106.
242. **Salesa, R., M. D. Moragues, R. Sota, J. Pemán, G. Quindós, and J. Pontón.** 2001. Specific antibody response in a patient with *Candida dubliniensis* fungemia. *Rev. Iberoam. Micol.* **18:**42–44.
243. **Sánchez, M. L., M. A. Pfaller, I. Cabezudo, M. Bale, and B. Buschelman.** 1992. Diagnosis of disseminated candidiasis in hospitalized patients using the Cand-Tec latex agglutination assay. *Mycopathologia* **118:**153–162.
244. **Savolainen, J., A. Rantala, M. Nermes, L. Lehtonen, and M. Viander.** 1996. Enhanced IgE response to *Candida albicans* in postoperative invasive candidiasis. *Clin. Exp. Allergy* **26:**452–460.
245. **Savolainen, J., M. Viander, and A. Koivikko.** 1990. IgE-, IgA- and IgG-antibody responses to carbohydrate and protein antigens of *Candida albicans* in asthmatic children. *Allergy* **45:**54–63.
246. **Schønheyder, H., H. Brincker, H. Olsen, and A. Stenderup.** 1987. The serological response to *Candida albicans* in leukemic patients prophylactically treated with ketoconazole. *Mykosen* **30:**5–9.
247. **Seeliger, H. P. R.** 1982. Significance of immunological methods for diagnosis of fungal disease. *Chemotherapy* **28:**54–63.
248. **Segal, E., R. A. Berg, P. A. Pizzo, and J. E. Bennett.** 1979. Detection of *Candida* antigen in sera of patients with candidiasis by an enzyme-linked immunosorbent assay-inhibition technique. *J. Clin. Microbiol.* **10:**116–118.
249. **Sendid, B., M. Tabouret, J. L. Poirot, D. Mathieu, J. Fruit, and D. Poulain.** 1999. New enzyme immunoassays for sensitive detection of circulating *Candida albicans* mannan and antimannan antibodies: useful combined test for diagnosis of systemic candidiasis. *J. Clin. Microbiol.* **37:**1510–1517.
250. **Shah, P. M., V. Schäfer, M. Bungert, and H. Knothe.** 1988. Evaluation of the Cand-Tec latex agglutination Ramco in disseminated candidosis. *Mycoses* **31:**433–437.
251. **Shen, H. D., K. B. Choo, H. H. Lee, J. C. Hsieh, W. L. Lin, W. R. Lee, and S. H. Han.** 1991. The 40-kilodalton allergen of *Candida albicans* is an alcohol dehydrogenase: molecular cloning and immunological analysis using monoclonal antibodies. *Clin. Exp. Allergy* **21:**675–681.
252. **Shivananda, P. G., J. N. Sarvamangala, A. Elias, and K. N. A. Rao.** 1981. Complement fixation tests in systemic candidiasis. *Indian J. Med. Res.* **73:**720–724.
253. **Sigmundsdóttir, G., B. Christensson, L. J. Björklund, K. Håkansson, C. Pehrson, and L. Larsson.** 2000. Urine D-arabinitol/L-arabinitol ratio in diagnosis of invasive candidiasis in newborn infants. *J. Clin. Microbiol.* **38:**3039–3042.
254. **Smith, K. K., and S. M. H. Qadri.** 1992. Rapid diagnosis of systemic candidiasis using commercial antigen and/or antibody detection kits. *J. Microbiol. Methods* **16:**231–237.

255. **Soyama, K.** 1984. Enzymatic determination of D-mannose in serum. *Clin. Chem.* **30:**293–294.
256. **Soyama, K., and E. Ono.** 1985. Enzymatic fluorometric method for the determination of D-arabinitol in serum by initial rate analysis. *Clin. Chim. Acta* **149:**149–154.
257. **Soyama, K., C. Shimazaki, S. Misawa, and S. Imashuku.** 1986. Early diagnosis of invasive candidiasis in leukemia: evaluation of D-arabinitol in serum. *Jpn. J. Med. Mycol.* **27:** 165–169.
258. **Staab, J. F., C. A. Ferrer, and P. Sundstrom.** 1996. Developmental expression of a tandemly repeated, proline- and glutamine-rich amino acid motif on hyphal surfaces on *Candida albicans*. *J. Biol. Chem.* **271:**6298–6305.
259. **Staib, F., M. Focking, B. Fröhlich, and A. Blisse.** 1977. *Candida albicans*- Serumpräzipitine bei blutspendern: auffällige serologische und kulturelle *Candida albicans*-befunde bei alkoholikern. *Mykosen* **20:**423–430.
260. **Staib, F., S. K. Mishra, and T. L. Abel.** 1977. Serodiagnostic value of extracellular antigens of an actively proteolysing culture of *Candida albicans*. *Zbl. Bakt. Hyg. I. Abt. Orig. A.* **238:**284–287.
261. **Stallybrass, F. C.** 1964. *Candida* precipitins. *J. Pathol. Bacteriol.* **87:**89–97.
262. **Stevens, P., S. Huang, L. S. Young, and M. Berdischewsky.** 1980. Detection of *Candida* antigenemia in human invasive candidiasis by a new solid phase radioimmunoassay. *Infection* **8**(Suppl. 3):S334–S338.
263. **Stickle, D., L. Kaufman, S. O. Blumer, and D. W. Mclaughlin.** 1972. Comparison of a newly-developed latex agglutination test and an immunodiffusion test in the diagnosis of systemic candidiasis. *Appl. Microbiol.* **23:**490–499.
264. **Strockbine, N. A., M. T. Largen, S. M. Zweibel, and H. R. Buckley.** 1984. Identification and molecular weight characterization of antigens from *Candida albicans* that are recognized by human sera. *Infect. Immun.* **43:**715–721.
265. **Suits, T., G. J. Wise, and B. Walters.** 1989. Candidal antigenemia: a prognostic determinant. *J. Urol.* **141:**1381–1384.
266. **Sundstrom, P. M., and G. E. Kenny.** 1985. Enzymatic release of germ tube-specific antigens from cell walls of *Candida albicans*. *Infect. Immun.* **49:**609–614.
267. **Sundstrom, P. M., E. J. Nichols, and G. E. Kenny.** 1987. Antigenic differences between mannoproteins of germ tubes and blastospores of *Candida albicans*. *Infect. Immun.* **55:** 616–620.
268. **Sundstrom, P. M., M. R. Tam, E. J. Nichols, and G. E. Kenny.** 1988. Antigenic differences in the surface mannoproteins of *Candida albicans* as revealed by monoclonal antibodies. *Infect. Immun.* **56:**601–606.
269. **Switchenko, A. C., C. G. Miyada, T. C. Goodman, T. J. Walsh, B. Wong, M. J. Becker, and E. F. Ullman.** 1994. An automated enzymatic method for measurement of D-arabinitol, a metabolite of pathogenic *Candida* species. *J. Clin. Microbiol.* **32:**92–97.
270. **Syverson, R. E., H. R. Buckley, and J. R. Gibian.** 1978. Increasing the predictive value positive of the precipitin test for the diagnosis of deep-seated candidiasis. *Am. J. Clin. Pathol.* **70:**826–831.
271. **Tamura, H., S. Tanaka, T. Ikeda, T. Obayashi, and Y. Hashimoto.** 1997. Plasma (1→3)-β-D-glucan assay and immunohistochemical staining of (1→3)-β-D-glucan in the fungal cell walls using a novel horseshoe crab protein (T-GBP) that specifically binds to (1→3)-β-D-glucan. *J. Clin. Lab. Anal.* **11:** 104–109.
272. **Taschdjian, C. L., M. B. Cuesta, P. J. Kozinn, and L. Caroline.** 1969. A modified antigen for serodiagnosis of systemic candidiasis. *Am. J. Clin. Pathol.* **52:**468–472.
273. **Taschdjian, C. L., P. J. Kozinn, M. B. Cuesta, and E. F. Toni.** 1972. Serodiagnosis of candidal infections. *Am. J. Clin. Pathol.* **57:**195–205.
274. **Taschdjian, C. L., M. S. Seelig, and P. J. Kozinn.** 1973. Serological diagnosis of candidal infections. *Crit. Rev. Clin. Lab. Sci.* **4:**19–60.
275. **Tokunaga, S., M. Ohkawa, T. Nakashima, and H. Hisazumi.** 1992. *Candida* antigen detection by a latex agglutination test in candiduria patients. *Urol. Int.* **49:**163–166.
276. **Tokunaga, S., M. Ohkawa, and M. Takashima.** 1993. Diagnostic value of determination of serum mannan concentrations in patients with candiduria. *Eur. J. Clin. Microbiol. Infect. Dis.* **12:**542–545.
277. **Tokunaga, S., M. Ohkawa, M. Takashima, C. Seto, and S. Nakamura.** 1995. D-arabinitol versus mannan antigen and candidal protein antigen as a serum marker for *Candida* pyelonephritis. *Eur. J. Clin. Microbiol. Infect. Dis.* **14:**118–121.
278. **Tollemar, J., K. Holmberg, O. Ringdén, and B. Lönnqvist.** 1989. Surveillance tests for the diagnosis of invasive fungal infections in bone marrow transplant recipients. *Scand. J. Infect. Dis.* **21:**205–212.
279. **Torres-Rodríguez, J. M., N. Madrenys-Brunet, J. Nolla-Salas, A. Carceller, and C. Tur.** 1997. Candiduria in non-neutropenic critically-ill surgical patients. Detection of IgA, IgG and IgM antibodies to *Candida albicans* by germ tube immunofluorescence. *Mycoses* **40:**439–444.
280. **Touster, O., and D. R. D. Shaw.** 1962. Biochemistry of the acylic polyols. *Physiol. Rev.* **42:**181–225.
281. **van Deventer, A. J. M., W. H. F. Goessens, J. H. van Zeijl, J. W. Mouton, M. F. Michel, and H. A. Verbrugh.** 1996. Kinetics of anti-mannan antibodies useful in confirming invasive candidiasis in immunocompromissed patients. *Microbiol. Immunol.* **40:**125–131.
282. **van Deventer, A. J. M., H. J. A. van Vliet, W. C. J. Hop, and W. H. F. Goessens.** 1994. Diagnostic value of anti-*Candida* enolase antibodies. *J. Clin. Microbiol.* **32:**17–23.
283. **van Deventer, A. J. M., H. J. A. van Vliet, L. Voogd, W. C. J. Hop, and W. H. F. Goessens.** 1993. Increased specificity of antibody detection in surgical patients with invasive candidiasis with cytoplasmic antigens depleted of mannan residues. *J. Clin. Microbiol.* **31:**994–997.
284. **Verweij, P. E., D. Poulain, T. Obayashi, T. F. Patterson, D. W. Denning, and J. Ponton.** 1998. Current trends in the detection of antigenaemia, metabolites and cell wall markers for the diagnosis and therapeutic monitoring of fungal infections. *Med. Mycol.* **36**(Suppl. 1):146–155.
285. **Villalba, R., A. I. González, M. J. Linares, M. Casal, and A. Torres.** 1993. Detection of antibodies to *Candida albicans* germ tube as a possible aid in diagnosing systemic candidiasis in bone marrow transplant patients. *Eur. J. Clin. Microbiol. Infect. Dis.* **12:**347–349.
286. **Wain, W. H., L. Georgakopoulos, and D. W. R. Mackenzie.** 1981. *Candida* antibodies in heart surgery patients. *J. Infect.* **3:**237–245.
287. **Walsh, T. J., and S. J. Chanock.** 1998. Diagnosis of invasive fungal infections: advances in nonculture systems. *Curr. Clin. Top. Infect. Dis.* **18:**101–153.
288. **Walsh, T. J., J. W. Hathorn, J. D. Sobel, W. G. Merz, V. Sanchez, S. M. Maret, H. R. Buckley, M. A. Pfaller, R. Schaufele, C. Sliva, E. Navarro, J. Lecciones, P. Chandrasekar, J. Lee, and P. A. Pizzo.** 1991. Detection of circulating *Candida* enolase by immunoassay in patients with cancer and invasive candidiasis. *N. Engl. J. Med.* **324:**1026–1031.
289. **Walsh, T. J., W. G. Merz, J. W. Lee, R. Schaufele, T. Sein, P. O. Whitcomb, M. Ruddel, W. Burns, J. R. Wingard, A. C. Switchenko, T. Goodman, and P. A. Pizzo.** 1995. Diagno-

sis and therapeutic monitoring of invasive candidiasis by rapid enzymatic detection of serum D-arabinitol. *Am. J. Med.* **99**:164–172.

290. **Walsh, T. J., and P. A. Pizzo.** 1993. Laboratory diagnosis of candidiasis, p. 109–135. *In* G. P. Bodey (ed.), *Candidiasis. Pathogenesis, Diagnosis and Treatment,* (2nd ed.). Raven Press, New York, N.Y.
291. **Weiner, M. H., and M. Coats-Stephen.** 1979. Immunodiagnosis of systemic candidiasis: mannan antigenemia detected by radioimmunoassay in experimental and human infections. *J. Infect. Dis.* **140**:989–993.
292. **Weiner, M. H., and W. J. Yount.** 1976. Mannan antigenemia in the diagnosis of invasive *Candida* infections. *J. Clin. Invest.* **58**:1045–1053.
293. **Weis, C., R. Kappe, and H.-G. Sonntag.** 1997. Western blot analysis of the immune response to *Candida albicans* antigens in 391 long-term intensive care patients. *Mycoses* **40**: 153–157.
294. **Wells, C. L., M. S. Sirany, and D. J. Blazevic.** 1983. Evaluation of serum arabinitol as a diagnostic test for candidiasis. *J. Clin. Microbiol.* **18**:353–357.
295. **Wingard, J. R., W. G. Merz, and R. Saral.** 1979. *Candida tropicalis:* a major pathogen in immunocompromised patients. *Ann. Intern. Med.* **91**:539–543.
296. **Winner, H. I.** 1955. A study of *Candida albicans* agglutinins in human sera. *J. Hyg.* **53**:509–512.
297. **Wong, B., R. P. Baughman, and K. L. Brauer.** 1989. Levels of the *Candida* metabolite D-arabinitol in sera of steroid-treated and untreated patients with sarcoidosis. *J. Clin. Microbiol.* **27**:1859–1862.
298. **Wong, B., E. M. Bernard, J. W. M. Gold, D. Fong, and D. Armstrong.** 1982. The arabinitol appearance rate in laboratory animals and humans: estimation from the arabinitol/creatinine ratio and relevance to the diagnosis of candidiasis. *J. Infect. Dis.* **146**:353–359.
299. **Wong, B., and K. L. Brauer.** 1988. Enantioselective measurement of fungal D-arabinitol in the sera of normal adults and patients with candidiasis. *J. Clin. Microbiol.* **26**:1670–1674.
300. **Yeo, S. F., Y. Y. Zhang, D. Schafer, S. Campbell, and B. Wong.** 2000. A rapid, automated enzymatic fluorometric assay determination of D-arabinitol in serum. *J. Clin. Microbiol.* **38**:1439–1443.
301. **Zöller, L., I. Krämer, R. Kappe, and H.-G. Sonntag.** 1991. Enzyme immunoassays for invasive *Candida* infections: reactivity of somatic antigens of *Candida albicans*. *J. Clin. Microbiol.* **29**:1860–1867.

Candida and Candidiasis
Edited by Richard A. Calderone

Chapter 28

Molecular Approaches to Identification and Typing of *Candida* Species

DEREK J. SULLIVAN AND DAVID C. COLEMAN

The incidence of systemic candidiasis has increased steadily over the last two decades (3, 5, 33, 48, 83). There are many risk factors that can predispose individuals to systemic candidiasis, including antineoplastic therapy, immunosuppressive therapy for organ transplantation, hematologic malignancy, intubation, catheterization, and broad-spectrum antibacterial therapy. Consequently, as the number of patients with these risk factors continues to grow rapidly, it is to be expected that the incidence of systemic candidiasis will also continue to increase in parallel. In contrast, the introduction of highly active antiretroviral therapy for the treatment of human immunodeficiency virus (HIV) infection and AIDS in the late 1990s has had a significant effect on reducing the number of these individuals suffering from oral candidiasis (17, 24, 41, 52). However, there have been reports of treatment failure and lack of patient compliance, which could conceivably lead to an upturn in the incidence of this manifestation of *Candida* infection (7, 23, 136). Therefore, given the increasing incidence of systemic candidiasis and the uncertain future of the incidence of superficial candidiasis, there is a growing need for the development and implementation of laboratory techniques that allow the rapid diagnosis of these infections. In addition, the emergence of non-*Candida albicans* species as opportunistic pathogens (78, 84, 85), some of which exhibit reduced susceptibility to commonly used antifungal agents relative to *C. albicans* (e.g., *C. glabrata* and *C. krusei*), necessitates that the infecting organism should be identified to the species level so that the optimum antifungal therapy can be applied (118). In addition, to investigate the epidemiology of these infections and to monitor the emergence of strains with decreased susceptibility to antifungal drugs, it is essential that techniques that allow accurate strain discrimination be developed and applied. It is clear, therefore, that there is an urgent requirement for the application of accurate and rapid species and strain identification and differentiation techniques. Currently, there are a number of different strategies, including culture- and serology-based methods, used routinely to perform these tasks. These are described elsewhere in this volume. Another strategy that offers great potential in achieving the goal of rapid species and strain identification is based on the use of molecular biological methods. The purpose of this chapter is to describe in brief the molecular tools currently used and being developed to perform these tasks.

MOLECULAR-BASED METHODS OF IDENTIFICATION OF *CANDIDA* SPECIES

Systemic candidiasis is a very debilitating illness with an attributable mortality reported to be at least as high as 35% (131). However, if a confirmed diagnosis of candidiasis is obtained in the early stages of infection and antifungal therapy is administered promptly, the prognosis can be improved dramatically. Unfortunately, the sensitivity of currently used blood culture methods and histological analysis of biopsy material in detecting *Candida* species is relatively low, especially early in infection. This is due to the slow growth of many fungal species, with the result that it can take from 2 to 5 days (and often longer) for the species of the infecting organism to be cultured and identified correctly (51). In addition, in many cases the infecting organisms may be nonculturable or present in very low numbers. Consequently, many cases of systemic candidiasis are often diagnosed too late to save the patient and some cases are only diag-

Derek J. Sullivan and David C. Coleman • Microbiology Research Unit, Department of Oral Medicine and Pathology, School of Dental Science, University of Dublin, Trinity College, Dublin 2, Republic of Ireland.

nosed postmortem. Furthermore, in cases of a rapidly progressing disease, antifungal therapy is often given empirically, before a definitive diagnosis has been made. This approach is expensive, and more importantly, can contribute to the development of resistance in *C. albicans* and in other *Candida* species or to the selection of species, such as *C. glabrata* or *C. krusei,* which are inherently less susceptible than *C. albicans* to commonly used antifungal agents.

To decrease the time required to diagnose fungal infections and to identify the causative organisms, and therefore reduce the mortality associated with systemic candidiasis, a number of different strategies based on molecular tools have been adopted, each with its own specific advantages and disadvantages. Among the most promising of the techniques that have been adapted and applied to the rapid identification of *Candida* species in clinical samples are molecular biological techniques that allow the detection of microbial nucleic acid sequences directly in blood or biopsy material.

PCR-Based Methods

The molecular-based technology that has the greatest potential to revolutionize the clinical diagnosis of infectious diseases is that based on the use of PCR. PCR has been used extensively in forensic science and has been applied to the diagnosis of a broad range of diseases, including those caused by pathogenic bacteria and viruses. This technique can detect minuscule amounts of microbial nucleic acid in blood or tissue. During the last decade numerous studies have also been performed to investigate the effectiveness of PCR in the diagnosis of systemic infections caused by *C. albicans* (as well as other *Candida* species). In many trial studies as few as 1 to 5 *C. albicans* cells per ml of blood were detectable (34, 64, 132). These studies have resulted in the refinement of the technique to improve its sensitivity, specificity, and efficiency.

Target choice

In PCR a pair of synthetic oligonucleotides homologous to specific target sequences prime the amplification of the intervening DNA sequences using a thermostable DNA polymerase, usually *Taq*. A wide range of sequences have been chosen as targets for the development of fungal-specific PCR oligonucleotide primers. The most important feature of any pair of PCR primers to be used directly on clinical samples is that it does not prime the amplification of host DNA. Therefore, fungal-specific (e.g., sequences from the gene encoding the cytochrome P-450 lanosterol-α-demethylase [12, 13, 74]) or *Candida*-specific sequences (e.g., sequences encoding secretory aspartyl proteinase [34]) have been used effectively as PCR targets. To minimize the chances of false-positive reactions, extreme care must be taken in the original design of these primers. Prior to synthesis of the oligonucleotides it is essential to perform extensive homology searches with the nucleotide sequence databases, and once they have been synthesized, the primers should be tested in control experiments with host DNA and DNA from a variety of other microbial species. A variety of PCR primers have been developed that are species, genus, or fungus specific. In many cases pan-fungus or genus-specific primers have been used in combination with species-specific primers in nested PCR experiments, allowing species identification. To improve the sensitivity of PCR, many investigators have designed primers that amplify regions of DNA that are repeated in the fungal genome. The most commonly used target for diagnostic PCR primers is the ribosomal RNA gene operon, encoding the 18S, 5.8S, and 28S rRNA subunits of which there are 50 to 100 copies encoded on the largest *C. albicans* chromosome. Ribosomal RNA genes are also excellent targets because they have been studied extensively in phylogenetic analyses (32, 119) and have been shown to have conserved and divergent regions that are very amenable to the design of pan-fungal and species-specific primers (18, 38, 43, 69, 132, 134). The family of secretory aspartyl proteinases, which comprises at least nine related genes in the *C. albicans* genome, is another multicopy gene family that has been used as a target for PCR detection (34).

Sample preparation

Once the primers have been chosen, the next important step is the choice of sample and the methods used to extract the nucleic acid for use as a PCR template. In theory, PCR can be applied to almost any tissue; however, the overwhelming majority of studies on the diagnosis of systemic candidiasis have concentrated on the identification of *Candida* in blood samples. However, the treatment of blood samples to obtain sufficient quantities of yeast nucleic acid that is suitable for amplification is time-consuming and technically problematic. Firstly, blood and other tissue samples contain large amounts of host nucleic acid that has the potential to interfere with primer hybridization and amplification. Also, since many constituents of blood (especially hemaglobin) are inhibitors of *Taq* DNA polymerase, these must first be removed by lysing the erythrocytes and white blood cells (in water or with added detergents and DNase), followed by a centrifugation step. To release the nucleic acid from the *Candida* cells, the walls must first be disrupted to release the template nucleic acid. Conventional DNA preparation procedures rely on enzymatic degradation of the cell walls using incubation with Zymolyase and proteinase K, followed by purification steps involving phenol chloroform extraction and ethanol precipitation to remove contaminating proteins. These steps can take 3 or more hours to complete, use toxic and expensive materials, and are tedious to use with large numbers of samples. However, recent refinement of these techniques has led to greater time and cost efficiency. The application of commercially available spin columns, high-speed cell disrupters (incorporating chaotropic agents and lysing matrices), boiling steps, and the omission of the Zymolyase lytic step have led to reports of sample preparation being reduced to approximately 1 h (63, 71, 77, 106, 127). In one study, PCR was performed directly on samples taken from culture-positive BacT/Alert culture bottles (113). Due to the increased sample volume and increased number of target cells in each sample this allowed the use of less complex extraction methods and increased the sensitivity of species identification, while decreasing the time of species identification following culture from 2 to 4 days to 7 h. Another study has suggested that serum rather than whole blood may be a more suitable sample for the detection of infecting *Candida* species as it facilitates the detection of free candidal DNA (10).

Amplimer detection and species identification

In conventional PCR assays the amplified DNA is usually detected by agarose or polyacrylamide gel electrophoresis, a technique that is relatively easily performed but is unsuitable for large sample loads. As in other aspects of PCR design, many improvements are continually being developed to enhance the sensitivity and specificity of amplimer detection and species identification. In the cases when generic primers have been used, the species can be subsequently identified correctly by hybridization with species-specific oligonucleotide probes that are homologous to sequences within the amplimer. However, this step is often time-consuming and usually requires gel electrophoresis or slot blotting procedures, DNA transfer and hybridization, and signal detection (27, 71, 94, 106). An alternative method that has been introduced involves the use of oligonucleotides homologous to species-specific sequences in a subsequent nested PCR reaction (10, 39, 47, 92). Although this can improve the sensitivity and specificity of the original PCR, it sometimes necessitates a second electrophoresis step and has the potential to introduce contamination. Another simple method of species identification is to use restriction enzyme digestion analysis to identify restriction fragment length polymorphisms in each amplimer that are specific for individual species (74, 123). However, this requires the use of a range of different restriction enzymes and is likely to be too labor intensive for use in a routine clinical laboratory. In a number of studies species identification has been achieved on the basis of comparing amplimer size. However, the size differences observed in the amplified regions of different species are often very small and may only be detected by using sophisticated equipment, such as automated capillary electrophoresis sequencing machines in combination with fluorescently tagged amplimers (18, 40, 121). Thus, although this technique is very rapid and accurate, it is not readily available to many diagnostic laboratories. Single-strand conformational polymorphism analysis has also been used to identify specific *Candida* species (44, 128). In an attempt to avoid the necessity of electrophoresis and additional time-consuming techniques, several studies have developed methods of detecting species-specific amplimers using variations of microtitration plate enzyme immunoassay (EIA) technology (28, 34, 35). With this approach, PCR-amplified DNA fragments are hybridized in the liquid phase to specific digoxigenin-labeled probes as well as to a biotinylated capture probe. The hybridization mixture is then added to streptavidin-coated microtiter plate wells and positive reactions detected using peroxidase-conjugated anti-digoxigenin antibodies. In a recent study a matrix of DNA probes specific for 18 individual *Candida* species was described (28). In another adaptation, three *Candida* species were identifiable in a single reaction tube through the use of specific fluorescent probes (112). These methods show great promise for development and application with clinical samples and with automation; however, at present the techniques required are not readily available to most clinical laboratories.

Controls

The ability to detect very small amounts of DNA is one of the most important attributes of PCR. However, this extreme sensitivity can also lead to problems with false-positive results due to contamination with environmental microorganisms or cross-contamination with previously amplified products. It has been calculated that a typical aerosol droplet of 20 μm diameter can contain as many as 24,000 copies of an amplified product (80). Clearly, the potential for such false-positive results affects the suitability of PCR in the diagnosis of life-threatening diseases. However, even more important in clinical situations, PCR also has the potential to generate false-negative results due to the presence of inhibitors of *Taq* DNA polymerase. To circumvent these problems, a number of precautions can be adopted. Most important, to minimize cross-contamination with previously amplified DNA molecules, each stage of the PCR reaction should be performed in physically separated locations within the laboratory and with micropipettes dedicated for this purpose with tips designed to prevent the formation of aerosols. All solutions and reagents should be aliquoted into small volumes and discarded after a single use. Another method sometimes used involves the incorporation of dUTP in place of dTTP in the PCR mixture and incubation with uracil-DNA-glycosylase prior to amplification (34). Products amplified in this way cannot act as substrates in subsequent amplification reactions. Finally, the most efficient way of monitoring contamination is the judicious use of negative controls by including tests without added template or primers in each experiment. Similarly, false-negative results can also be controlled for by including suitable positive control reactions in each experiment. In samples where host DNA is also present with the target DNA, primers specific for a host gene can also be included (as long as the products of both primer pairs are easily differentiated) to ensure that the *Taq* DNA polymerase is not inhibited.

Comparison of PCR- and culture-based methods

Theoretically, PCR offers great potential for providing the basis of a rapid and sensitive diagnostic test for systemic candidiasis. However, has it lived up to this potential? Since the late 1980s there have been many studies investigating the efficacy of this technology in the diagnosis of a wide range of viral, bacterial, and fungal diseases. In conventional PCR tests in which human and rabbit blood samples have been deliberately inoculated or spiked with defined numbers of *Candida* cells, the sensitivity observed in most studies was in the region of 100 CFU per ml. In similar experiments using enhanced PCR product detection methods (e.g., nested PCR, hybridization, and EIA) the sensitivity can be increased by at least a factor of 10. In some studies as few as one to two cells or femtogram amounts of DNA per ml were detected (34, 35, 37, 47, 74, 127). In studies using animal infection models or clinical samples, PCR has been shown to be at least as efficient as culture at detecting circulating *Candida* cells (34, 64). In another study in which patients deemed to be at risk of candidemia were assessed, four out of nine patients who were culture-negative yielded positive PCR results. One of these PCR-positive patients subsequently became culture-positive 7 days later, thus indicating the potential of PCR to allow early diagnosis in individuals at risk (127). One complication, however, is that PCR also has the ability to detect *Candida* DNA or nonviable cells in blood, thus leading to positive test results that would prove negative on culture. Most studies have also demonstrated that PCR is an excellent means of correctly identifying particular species, with most studies reporting a specificity of 100%. Similar levels of specificity and sensitivity can be attained using conventional diagnostic methods; however, the main advantage of PCR over these methods is the speed with which results can be obtained. Most culture-based methods take a minimum of 48 h to allow detection of *Candida* in samples; however, species identification can take at least another 48 h (often longer in the case of slow-growing species). In contrast, PCR tests, even with additional adaptations to improve sensitivity and specificity, can be performed in as little as 8 h. Of course, this speed comes at a cost. Despite more than a decade of research, the necessary equipment is still relatively expensive and the techniques used involve complicated manipulations that are labor-intensive and are not amenable for use with large numbers of samples. Consequently, the majority of clinical diagnostic laboratories still rely on conventional nonmolecular procedures such as culture and serology.

New and future developments

There is a clear need for the development of improved methods to replace or complement currently used methods for the diagnosis of deep-seated fungal infections. The technique that has been investigated most extensively and that offers the greatest potential is PCR. Unfortunately, the current state of PCR technology is not sufficiently advanced to allow its widespread application for routine diagnosis. However, research into adapting PCR so that it is more applicable for use in diagnostic laboratories is continuing, and several developments suggest that rapid, user-friendly PCR-based technology will be applied to high-volume use in the routine diagnostic laboratory in the not too distant future. As discussed earlier, EIA-based methods using matrices of multiple species-specific oligonucleotides have great potential for automation. In addition, the development of novel real-time PCR methods in which products are detected in situ by fluorescent probes and molecular beacons (e.g., Taqman and Light Cycler) (11, 62, 81, 100) offers potential for even more rapid diagnosis. In addition, these techniques are able to quantify the amounts of fungal nucleic acid present in target samples, thus potentially allowing the microbial load to be measured. Finally, in this new era of genomics and microarray technology, it is only a matter of time before techniques involving microchips containing DNA arrays are applied to the automation and miniaturization of molecular methods for the diagnosis of infectious diseases, including systemic candidiasis. For the foreseeable future, routine diagnostic laboratories will have to rely on the conventional culture- and serology-based tests currently in use. However, even if rapid molecular tests are developed for routine diagnosis, it is likely that these will still have to be used in conjunction with nonmolecular methods.

Non-PCR-Based Molecular Diagnostic Methods

Although PCR is widely believed to be the molecular technique that offers the greatest potential for application to the diagnosis of fungal disease, attempts have also been made to adapt a number of other molecular methods to this purpose. One such method is fluorescent in situ hybridization. This involves the use of fluorescently labeled DNA probes to detect *Candida* cells in situ in histological samples, including deep tissue biopsies and blood. In pilot studies in which mice were infected with *C. albicans* or *C. parapsilosis,* cryosections of spleen, liver, and brain were hybridized directly with fluorescein-labeled oligonucleotides homologous to the respective 18S rRNA genes of each species. Epifluorescence microscopy subsequently revealed the presence of the organisms and identified each species correctly, although a separate sample had to be tested with each probe (57). Similar experiments in which human blood was spiked with *Candida* cells allowed the detection of 3 cells per 0.5 ml blood (approximately the same sensitivity as PCR-based methods) in the same time frame achievable by PCR (57). In a separate study, fluorescent in situ hybridization has been shown to be effective in the rapid identification of *Candida* cells in blood culture bottles within 2.5 h of the detection of growth within the bottle by an automated continuous reader (53).

Other molecular techniques that have been applied to identify *Candida* species are "whole-organism fingerprinting" methods such as pyrolysis-mass spectrometry and Fourier transform-infrared spectroscopy (120). The former relies on the mass-spectrometric analysis of the products of the organisms following pyrolysis, and the latter relies on the spectroscopic analysis of the bond strengths of molecules within the organisms. Both methods have been shown to be effective in discriminating between various closely related *Candida* species; however, these methods are not suitable for the direct analysis of infected primary tissue or blood samples. In addition, the equipment required is highly specialized and expensive and not likely to be available in routine diagnostic laboratories.

MOLECULAR-BASED METHODS OF STRAIN TYPING OF *CANDIDA* SPECIES

To understand fully how and why *Candida* species cause disease, we must first be able to identify particular strains and track them in outbreaks of infection. With such knowledge, it should be possible to determine the source of individual infections. Since *Candida* infections can either be acquired endogenously from the host's normal flora or exogenously from the environment, other infected patients, or health care workers, this information can be of great help in monitoring outbreaks of infection and in assessing the quality of cross-infection control measures. Similarly, strain identification can establish whether relapses in infection are due to a novel infecting organism or to persistence/reinfection by the original strain, thus potentially affecting the choice of therapy. Accurate techniques can also reveal whether more than one strain may be involved in an infection and can be used to determine the relative abundance of these strains during the course of the disease. Finally, molecular epidemiological methods can also allow the dynamics of yeast populations to be investigated and can help determine whether virulence or the development of drug resistance can be associated with specific clones or clusters of related strains.

The methods originally adopted to characterize and type specific *Candida* strains were based on the analysis of phenotypic traits, including colony morphology and color on indicator media, biochemical and serological tests, carbohydrate assimilation tests, and resistotyping. Although all of these tests are relatively easily performed, their specificity tends to be low since many unrelated strains of *Candida,* and sometimes even different *Candida* species, often share phenotypic characteristics. In addition, phenomena such as phenotypic switching can affect the reproducibility of results obtained with such tests. For these reasons, strain discrimination methods based on the analysis of genotypic differences have been developed. In particular, these methods rely most often on comparisons of the genomic content and organization or on the nucleotide sequence of specific loci of individual strains. To be useful in epidemiological studies each method must, above all, be very specific and allow the accurate identification of each strain reproducibly. Ideally, the same method should also be applicable to multiple species. In cases of large-scale studies, the method used should have the capacity for use with large sample numbers; it should also be rapid and inexpensive and ideally should not be labor-intensive. A wide variety of methods have been developed and adapted to detect genetic polymorphisms in yeast species. These methods vary in their resolution, and each has specific disadvantages and advantages that should be taken into account when choosing a method to investigate a particular clinical problem. Indeed, it is often recommended that more than one method be used to achieve optimal results. In tandem with the development and refinement of molecular epidemiological techniques, improved computer-assisted data analysis packages, such as DENDRON and GelCompar, have been developed and applied (114). These systems have the capacity to automatically correct gel electrophoresis anomalies, calculate fingerprint pattern relatedness, and draw dendrograms. Most important, these systems permit fingerprint patterns generated in different experiments to be validly compared by reference to the fingerprint patterns of control reference strains used in each experiment. This allows the accurate and quantitative comparison of strains from large data sets and the development of comprehensive databases with which new strains can be easily compared.

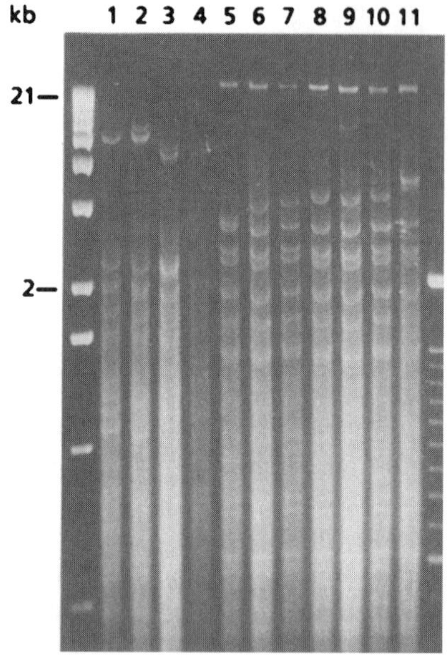

Figure 1. Agarose gel showing REA banding patterns of *Candida* species generated using the enzyme *Hin*F1. Lanes 1 and 2, *C. albicans*; lane 3, type II *C. stellatoidea*; lane 4, type I *C. stellatoidea*; lanes 5–11, *C. dubliniensis*. Molecular size markers are indicated on the left. Reprinted from *Microbiology* (119) with the permission of the publisher.

Restriction Enzyme Analysis (REA)

REA was the first method used to compare the genotypes of individual strains of *Candida* species and was used extensively in the earliest studies investigating the molecular epidemiology of *Candida* infections. It is a simple method that relies on the purification and subsequent digestion of total genomic DNA with specific restriction enzymes (e.g., *Eco*RI or *Hin*F1). Following digestion, the resulting DNA fragments are separated by electrophoresis on agarose gels and stained with ethidium bromide, and the resulting banding patterns compared visually. In most cases the restriction patterns obtained are very complex, often comprising thousands of bands, and are therefore very difficult to compare objectively, whether visually or using computer-assisted methods (Fig. 1). In some cases patterns of bands of above-average intensity, due to the presence of repeated sequences such as rDNA, can facilitate strain identification in species (4, 15, 66, 90, 107). However, despite the fact that REA is a simple and relatively inexpensive technique, its lack of discriminatory ability has largely led to it being replaced by other methods.

REA and Species-Specific DNA Fingerprinting Probes

The efficacy of DNA profiling of *Candida* strains has been greatly enhanced by the identification of species-specific repeat sequences that are distributed throughout the genome. To simplify the banding patterns obtained by restriction endonuclease digestion, usually with *Eco*RI, following electrophoresis (i.e., as in REA analysis), these can be transferred to nitrocellulose or nylon membranes using Southern blotting and subsequently hybridized with labeled fingerprinting probes corresponding to species-specific repetitive elements. In the case of *C. albicans,* among the first probes used were probes that corresponded to RNA genes (115) and mitochondrial DNA sequences (135). However, these probes yielded too few bands (e.g., three to five) for meaningful analysis. Currently, the most commonly used *C. albicans*-specific fingerprinting probes are the related probes 27A (108) and Ca3 (104), both of which contain the repetitive element RPS (19). These probes yield strain-specific fingerprint patterns composed of 10 to 20 bands of varying intensity. The effectiveness of these probes lies in the fact that some of these bands are highly polymorphic and others are nonvariable (Fig. 2). Another *C. albicans* probe that yields highly variable fingerprints is the CARE-2 probe (54); however, the extreme variability of the bands generated (e.g., the lack of monomorphic bands) decreases the efficacy of this probe for the analysis of distantly related isolates (114). Species-specific probes have since been developed for use in the epidemiological analysis of other clinically important *Candida* species, including *C. glabrata* (60), *C. tropicalis* (50), *C. krusei* (14), and *C. dubliniensis* (49) (Table 1). The simple and reproducible DNA fingerprints obtained with these probes greatly facilitate the

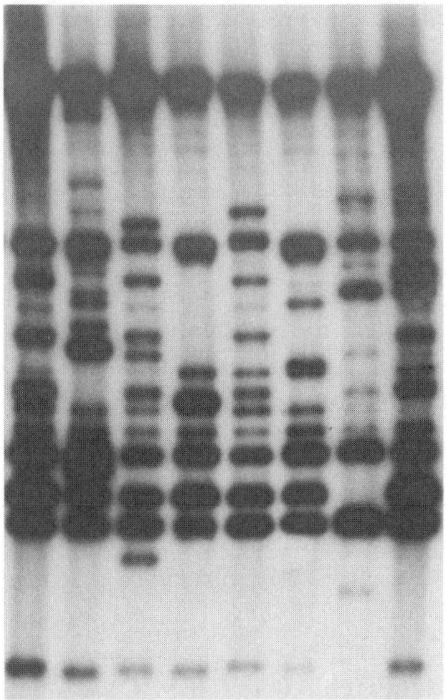

Figure 2. DNA fingerprint patterns of clinical *C. albicans* isolates generated using the *C. albicans*-specific probe 27A.

comparison of strains. The DNA patterns obtained with species-specific fingerprinting probes are amenable to computer-assisted analysis that can provide much more reliable and efficient quantitative comparison of large numbers of moderately related strains. Although this method is highly accurate and reproducible, Southern hybridization experiments are labor-intensive and time-consuming; therefore, this method is not particularly suitable for the rapid analysis of very large numbers of strains. Despite this, DNA fingerprinting using *Candida* species-specific semirepetitive probes is now the "gold standard" strain typing method for *Candida* species.

Oligonucleotide Fingerprinting

Rather than use species-specific probes, attempts have been made to develop probes that can be used to fingerprint strains from different species. The most commonly used of these probes correspond to microsatellite sequences, which are short repetitive sequences scattered throughout the genome. For use in fingerprinting experiments, short oligonucleotides, such as $(GT)_8$, $(GTG)_5$, $(GATA)_4$, $(GACA)_4$, and $(GGAT)_4$, are labeled with radionucleotides and hybridized to restriction enzyme-digested genomic DNA as described above. One advantage of this method is that multiple fingerprint patterns can be generated from the same DNA sample by performing sequential hybridizations with individual probes. Although used extensively with other eukaryotes (30, 37, 117), this method has been used infrequently with *Candida* species (116, 133). These oligonucleotides have also been used in strain typing studies using random amplified polymorphic DNA analysis (described below).

Table 1. *Candida* species-specific DNA fingerprinting probes

Candida species	Probe	Reference
C. albicans	Ca3	104
	27A	108
	CARE-2	54
	rDNA	115
	mDNA	135
C. dubliniensis	Cd25	49
C. glabrata	Cg6, Cg12	60
C. krusei	CkF1,2	14
C. tropicalis	Ct13-8	50

Pulsed-Field Gel Electrophoresis (PFGE)

PFGE is one of the techniques used most widely in *Candida* epidemiology. This technique is based on the separation of large chromosome-sized DNA molecules through agarose gels using an alternating electric field, which allows the separation of DNA fragments that are too large to be electrophoresed with conventional electrophoresis apparatus (111). This method can be used to discriminate between individual strains due to the fact that the sizes of individual chromosomes in different *Candida* strains can vary widely, resulting in different patterns of chromosome-sized bands known as karyotypes (Fig. 3). Although effective at strain typing in many *Candida* species (2, 16, 31, 67), karyotypes can vary as a result of phenotypic switching, a feature commonly found in *C. albicans* isolates in particular. In addition, the equipment re-

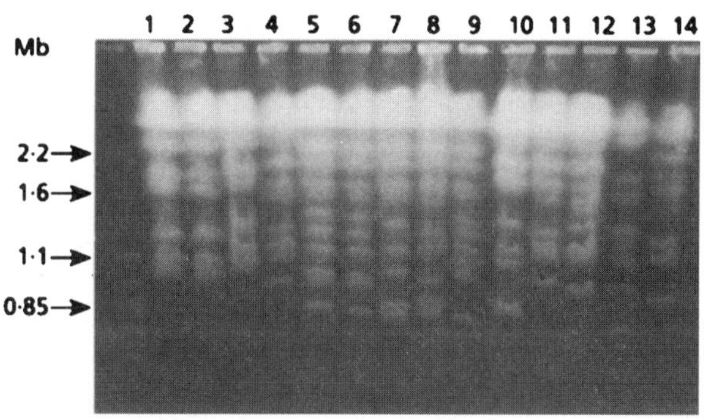

Figure 3. Electrophoretic karyotypes of *Candida* species generated using PFGE. Lanes 1 and 2, *C. albicans*; lane 3, type II *C. stellatoidea*; lane 4, type I *C. stellatoidea*; lanes 5–14, *C. dubliniensis*. Molecular size markers are indicated on the left. Reprinted from *Microbiology* (119) with the permission of the publisher.

quired is expensive, sample preparation is labor-intensive, and gels can take 72 h or more to run. Consequently, PFGE is not suitable for the analysis of large numbers of samples. In addition to the separation of chromosomes from *Candida* isolates, PFGE can also be used in REA in which restriction enzymes that cleave genomic DNA infrequently (e.g., *Sfi*I and *Not*I) generate large restriction fragments that are not resolvable by conventional agarose gel electrophoresis. The pattern of fragments thus obtained can be used to discriminate between strains (25, 90, 93, 101).

Randomly Amplified Polymorphic DNA (RAPD) Analysis

PCR technology, in addition to its application in the rapid identification of *Candida* species, has also been applied to the rapid differentiation of individual *Candida* strains belonging to particular species. However, RAPD differs from conventional PCR in that it is based on the use of a single oligonucleotide (usually 10 to 15 bp) of arbitrary sequence using low stringency amplification reaction conditions. Due to the low annealing temperatures used, primers can bind to many sites throughout the genome, thus allowing the amplification of products that vary in size. If the optimum amplification conditions and primer sequence have been determined empirically, these fragments, when separated by agarose gel electrophoresis and subsequently stained with ethidium bromide, can yield strain-specific fingerprint patterns comprising three to six bands. Differential banding patterns between strains occur as a result of nucleotide variation at the primer annealing sites (130). Amplimer profiles can be subjected to computer-assisted analysis, and it has been shown that the ability of RAPD to cluster moderately related isolates together is comparable to that of DNA fingerprinting with species-specific probes (95). The facts that so little sample DNA is required for RAPD and that PCR is rapid and easy to perform have led to the widespread use of this technique in the analysis of *Candida* populations (9, 42, 55, 56, 95, 102). However, extreme care must be taken to prevent variation in experimental conditions, as even subtle changes in temperature or magnesium concentration can lead to the appearance or disappearance of bands, thus affecting the reproducibility of the technique (29). To minimize these problems, it is advisable that only strongly amplified products should be used for analysis. In another attempt to improve reproducibility, a number of studies have investigated the use of primers homologous to microsatellite sequences (e.g., $[GTG]_5$ and $[AC]_{10}$) that have relatively high annealing temperatures (129).

Multilocus Enzyme Electrophoresis (MLEE)

Nucleic acids are not the only targets used to detect variation between strains. Nucleotide polymorphisms can result in amino acid substitutions in proteins that can lead to a change in the charge of the protein that can affect the proteins' mobility. Thus, when cell extracts are separated on starch gels and stained using specific enzyme stains, strain-specific staining profiles can be obtained. As with DNA fingerprinting methods, these protein-derived data can be analyzed by computer-assisted methods. MLEE is a powerful technique that has been widely applied to the analysis of *Candida* species and has proved particularly useful in population studies (1, 8, 95, 96, 103). However, despite its usefulness, MLEE is a time-consuming technique that requires specialized equipment.

MOLECULAR EPIDEMIOLOGY OF CANDIDIASIS

Before the early 1990s, approximately 70 to 80% of all yeasts associated with human disease were *C. albicans* (21, 48, 131). Because of this, there was little need to be able to identify other members of the genus *Candida.* However, the increased incidence of fungal diseases and the emergence of other *Candida* species as significant human pathogens, possibly as a result of the widespread introduction of antifungal drugs, have made the job of the clinical mycologist much more difficult. It is no longer sufficient to simply perform a germ tube test on yeasts isolated and cultured in the laboratory. For the clinician to prescribe the optimum drug therapy for a patient with suspected candidiasis, it is necessary that the infecting organism be identified to the species level in as short a time interval as possible. Despite the promise of molecular techniques to aid rapid identification of infecting organisms, this promise has yet to be fulfilled. In reality, routine clinical mycology laboratories still rely on culture-based detection and identification methods. Since the early 1990s several large-scale surveillance studies (e.g., NEMIS [90, 98], SCOPE [87, 88], and SENTRY [84, 86]) have been conducted to identify the trends in the epidemiology of nosocomial infections. These studies have been instrumental in cataloging the emergence of species such as *C. glabrata, C. krusei,* and *C. parapsilosis* as significant human pathogens. However, in all of these cases isolates belonging to each species were identified using routine methods, including culture on colorogenic media such as CHROMagar Candida medium (79) and carbohydrate assimilation tests using commercially available kits. Therefore, it is clear that although PCR-based species identification methods may prove useful in limited academic studies, the technology currently available is not yet sufficiently amenable to the large numbers of samples routinely processed in clinical laboratories. Despite this, research in the development of molecular-based diagnostic tests is continuing apace, and it is expected that within the foreseeable future, rapid and user-friendly molecular tests will become more widely available.

Although molecular techniques have yet to find their niche in the field of species identification and diagnostics, they have certainly played a major role in the analysis of strain identification and in epidemiological studies. The most obvious reason for this is that the alternative phenotypic-based methods used for discriminating strains are so uninformative and unreliable. Therefore, despite the fact that most molecular methods require specialized equipment, are expensive, and are relatively labor-intensive, they constitute an effective means of comparing individual isolates. As described earlier, each strain typing method has its own specific advantages and disadvantages. In most studies undertaken to compare the various molecular strain typing methods available, the results obtained have tended to be comparable. However, in many epidemiological studies it is recommended that more than one fingerprinting method should be used for confirmatory purposes (8, 9, 20, 95).

There have been numerous studies using DNA fingerprinting techniques to investigate the sources of nosocomial systemic *Candida* infections (6, 70, 90, 99, 105, 125). From these studies it has been revealed that the majority of infecting strains are acquired endogenously from the patient's own commensal flora (90, 124). Indeed, prior colonization with *Candida* species is a significant risk factor for the acquisition of candidemia (91, 131). In addition, the majority of cases appear to be caused by a single strain. In some cases, strains with identical genotype have been identified in separate patients, suggesting that outbreaks caused by a single clone can occur (70, 122). In addition, in other cases, strains identified in patients have also been identified in environmental samples, including in some cases the hands of health care workers (6, 70, 82, 126). Indeed, it has been suggested that in some cases certain strains or clusters of strains may be endemic within specific geographic regions and hospital wards (70, 89). These data confirm that although infections are mainly acquired endogenously, under certain circumstances infections can also be acquired exogenously. Clearly, DNA fingerprinting clinical isolates can prove helpful in determining the environmental sources of outbreaks and can highlight lapses in cross-infection control procedures. Similar studies investigating the origins of superficial candidiasis have revealed that the vast majority of these infections are acquired endogenously; however, transmission of strains between individuals (including vertical transmission between mother and child) has also been documented (26, 76, 126).

Patients with candidiasis often suffer from recurrent episodes of disease. DNA fingerprinting studies have shown that these are mainly caused by the persistence of the original infecting strain (8, 61). However, in some cases the original strain can be replaced by another strain from the same species or indeed from another *Candida* species (21, 58, 73, 110). Often these recurrent infections are due to the failure of antifungal therapy, for whatever reason, which has led to the development of resistance in the colonizing or infecting strain or to the selection of inherently less susceptible strains or species (58, 65). In the case of superficial infections, the situation is often particularly complex as anatomical sites such as the oral cavity and vagina can be colonized and/or infected by multiple species and strains. Thus, the dynamics of these populations can change over time or as a result of antifungal therapy. A characteristic of *C. albicans* (and its close relative *C. dubliniensis*) that went unrecognized until the development of sensitive DNA fingerprinting methods is its ability to exhibit the phenomenon of microevolution (49, 59, 61, 108, 116). This is manifested in minor variations in fingerprint profiles within a single clone. The significance of these microevolutionary events and the possible effects they may have on phenotype has yet to be established. However, in the case of *C. dubliniensis* the development of resistance to fluconazole has been associated with subtle changes in karyotype (75). Whether there is a correlation between these two phenomena has yet to be determined. However, in the absence of detectable sexual reproduction in vivo, microevolution might provide the means for *Candida* species to adapt to changing environmental conditions.

Strain typing methods, particularly MLEE, have also been used extensively in the analysis of the population biology of *C. albicans*. From these studies, it is abundantly clear that *C. albicans* is a heterogeneous species that reproduces clonally (1, 8, 97). However, data from recent fingerprinting studies (36), the identification in *C. albicans* of loci homologous to the *Saccharomyces cerevisiae* mating loci (45), and recent evidence that *C. albicans* can be forced to mate in vitro (46, 68) suggest that *C. albicans* may have the ability to reproduce sexually and therefore allow a limited degree of recombination. Large-scale fingerprinting studies have led to the suggestion that certain related groups of *C. albicans* clones may be endemic in specific hospitals and geographic areas (20, 72, 89,

109). However, there is no evidence to suggest that particular clones or clusters of strains are adapted to colonize specific anatomical sites or to cause infection in particular patient groups, such as HIV-infected individuals. In similar population studies investigating the development of fluconazole resistance, a correlation between resistance and specific genotypes was not detected, suggesting that fluconazole resistance arises mainly in strains independently and randomly and that the phenotype is acquired (and lost) relatively quickly (22). Interestingly, in a separate study a group of fluconazole-resistant *C. albicans* strains recovered from separate HIV-infected patients was found to form a discrete genetic cluster, suggesting that resistance arose independently in related strains or that a resistant strain was spread by horizontal transmission among patients (137).

When choosing to perform an epidemiological study using molecular techniques, a number of factors must be taken into account to ensure the validity of the data. First, the method (preferably two methods) to be used must be chosen carefully and have previously been validated and shown to be sensitive and reproducible. Second, when the original sampling is performed, to allow for the presence of multiple strains and for microevolution, it is also advisable that multiple colonies are chosen for analysis. Relevant control strains unrelated to those under study should also be included in the analysis. Finally, to quantify the relationships between related and unrelated strains, computer-assisted fingerprint comparison packages should be used. These systems also allow the storage of fingerprint data from separate experiments in databases that can subsequently be shared among laboratories participating in multicenter studies.

Studies using molecular fingerprinting techniques have already proved effective in investigating the epidemiology of *Candida* infections. It is anticipated that these methods will provide the basis for future studies investigating changes in the epidemiology of *Candida* infections, which will undoubtedly occur as patient populations change and continue to grow (e.g., as a result of highly active antiretroviral therapy, novel surgical procedures and cancer treatments) and as novel antifungal therapies are introduced to treat these infections.

REFERENCES

1. **Arnavielhe, S., T. De Meeus, A. Blancard, M. Mallie, F. Renaud, and J. M. Bastide.** 2000. Multicentric genetic study of *Candida albicans* isolates from non-neutropenic patients using MLEE typing: population structure and mode of reproduction. *Mycoses* **43:**109–117.
2. **Asakura, K., S.-I. Iwaguchi, M. Homma, T. Sukai, K. Higashide, and K. Tanaka.** 1991. Electrophoretic karyotypes of clinically isolated yeasts of *Candida albicans* and *C. glabrata. J. Gen. Microbiol.* **137:**2531–2538.
3. **Banerjee, S. N., T. G. Emori, D. H. Culver, R. P. Gaynes, W. R. Jarvis, T. Horan, J. R. Edwards, J. Tolson, T. Henderson, and W. J. Martone.** 1991. Secular trends in the epidemiology of nosocomial primary bloodstream infections in the United States, 1980–1989. *Am. J. Med.* **91**(Suppl. 3B): 86S–89S.
4. **Bart-Delabesse, E., P. Boiron, A. Carlotti, and B. Dupont.** 1993. *Candida albicans* genotyping in studies with patients with AIDS developing resistance to fluconazole. *J. Clin. Microbiol.* **31:**2933–2937.
5. **Beck-Sague, C., and W. R. Jarvis.** 1993. Secular trends in the epidemiology of nosocomial fungal infections in the United States, 1980–1990. National Nosocomial Infections Surveillance System. *J. Infect. Dis.* **167:**1247–1251.
6. **Betremieux, P., S. Chevrier, G. Quindos, D. Sullivan, L. Polonelli, and C. Guiguen.** 1994. Use of DNA fingerprinting and biotyping methods to study a *Candida albicans* outbreak in a neonatal intensive care unit. *Pediatr. Infect. Dis. J.* **13:** 899–905.
7. **Bini, T., L. Testa, E. Chiesa, F. Adorni, C. Abeli, B. Castelnuovo, S. Melzi, S. Sollima, M. Bongiovanni, and A. d'Arminio Monforte.** 2000. Outcome of a second-line protease inhibitor-containing regimen in patients failing or intolerant of a first highly active antiretroviral therapy. *J. Acquir. Immune Defic. Syndr.* **24:**115–122.
8. **Boerlin, P., F. Boerlin-Petzold, J. Goudet, C. Durussel, J. L. Pagani, J. P. Chave, and J. Bille.** 1996. Typing *Candida albicans* oral isolates from human immunodeficiency virus-infected patients by multilocus electrophoresis and DNA fingerprinting. *J. Clin. Microbiol.* **34:**1235–1248.
9. **Bostock, A., M. N. Khattak, R. Matthews, and J. Burnie.** 1993. Comparison of PCR fingerprinting, by random amplification of polymorphic DNA, with other molecular typing methods for *Candida albicans. J. Gen. Microbiol.* **139:** 2179–2184.
10. **Bougnoux, M., C. Dupont, J. Mateo, P. Saulnier, V. Faivre, D. Payen, and M. Nicolas-Chanoine.** 1999. Serum is more suitable than whole blood for diagnosis of systemic candidiasis by nested PCR. *J. Clin. Microbiol.* **37:**925–930.
11. **Brandt, M. E., A. A. Padhye, L. W. Mayer, and B. P. Holloway.** 1998. Utility of random amplified polymorphic DNA PCR and TaqMan automated detection in molecular identification of *Aspergillus fumigatus. J. Clin. Microbiol.* **36:** 2057–2062.
12. **Buchman, T. G., M. Rossier, W. G. Merz, and P. Charache.** 1990. Detection of surgical pathogens by in vitro DNA amplification. Part I. Rapid identification of *Candida albicans* by in vitro amplification of a fungus-specific gene. *Surgery* **108:** 338–346.
13. **Burgener-Kairuz, P., J. P. Zuber, P. Jaunin, T. G. Buchman, J. Bille, and M. Rossier.** 1994. Rapid detection and identification of *Candida albicans* and *Torulopsis (Candida) glabrata* in clinical specimens by species-specific nested PCR amplification of a cytochrome P-450 lanosterol-alpha-demethylase (L1A1) gene fragment. *J. Clin. Microbiol.* **32:**1902–1907.
14. **Carlotti, A., R. Grillot, A. Couble, and J. Villard.** 1994. Typing of *Candida krusei* clinical isolates by restriction endonuclease analysis and hybridization with the CkF1,2 DNA probe. *J. Clin. Microbiol.* **32:**1691–1699.
15. **Carlotti, A., G. Zambardi, A. Couble, N. Lefrancois, X. Martin, and J. Villard.** 1994. Nosocomial infection with *Candida*

albicans in a pancreatic transplant recipient investigated by means of restriction enzyme analysis. *J. Infect.* **29**:157–164.

16. **Carruba, G., E. Pontieri, F. De Bernardis, P. Martino, and A. Cassone.** 1991. DNA fingerprinting and electrophoretic karyotypes of environmental and clinical isolates of *Candida parapsilosis*. *J. Clin. Microbiol.* **29**:916–922.
17. **Cauda, R., E. Tacconelli, M. Tumbarello, G. Morace, F. De Bernardis, A. Torosantucci, and A. Cassone.** 1999. Role of protease inhibitors in preventing recurrent oral candidosis in patients with HIV infection: a prospective case-control study. *J. Acquir. Immune Defic. Syndr.* **21**:20–25.
18. **Chen, Y. C., J. D. Eisner, M. M. Kattar, S. L. Rassoulian-Barrett, K. LaFe, S. L. Yarfitz, A. P. Limaye, and B. T. Cookson.** 2000. Identification of medically important yeasts using PCR-based detection of DNA sequence polymorphisms in the internal transcribed spacer 2 region of the rRNA genes. *J. Clin. Microbiol.* **38**:2302–2310.
19. **Chindamporn, A., Y. Nakagawa, I. Mizuguchi, H. Chibana, M. Doi, and K. Tanaka.** 1998. Repetitive sequences (RPSs) in the chromosomes of *Candida albicans* are sandwiched between two novel stretches, HOK and RB2, common to each chromosome. *Microbiology* **144**:849–857.
20. **Clemons, K. V., F. Feroze, K. Holmberg, and D. A. Stevens.** 1997. Comparative analysis of genetic variability among *Candida albicans* isolates from different geographic locales by three genotypic methods. *J. Clin. Microbiol.* **35**: 1332–1336.
21. **Coleman, D. C., D. E. Bennett, P. J. Gallagher, S. R. Flint, A. Nolan, F. M. Mulcahy, D. J. Sullivan, M. C. Henman, R. J. Russell, and D. B. Shanley.** 1995. Oral candidiasis and HIV infection: antifungal drug resistance and changes in *Candida* population dynamics, p. 112–118. *In* J. S. Greenspan and D. Greenspan (ed.), *Oral Manifestations of HIV Infection.* Quintessence Publishing Co. Ltd., Chicago, Ill.
22. **Cowen, L. E., C. Sirjusingh, R. C. Summerbell, S. Walmsley, S. Richardson, L. M. Kohn, and J. B. Anderson.** 1999. Multilocus genotypes and DNA fingerprints do not predict variation in azole resistance among clinical isolates of *Candida albicans*. *Antimicrob. Agents Chemother.* **43**:2930–2938.
23. **d'Arminio Monforte, A., L. Testa, F. Adorni, E. Chiesa, T. Bini, G. C. Moscatelli, C. Abeli, S. Rusconi, S. Sollima, C. Balotta, M. Musicco, M. Galli, and M. Moroni.** 1998. Clinical outcome and predictive factors of failure of highly active antiretroviral therapy in antiretroviral-experienced patients in advanced stages of HIV-1 infection. *AIDS* **12**:1631–1637.
24. **Diz Dios, P., A. Ocampo, C. Miralles, I. Otero, I. Iglesias, and N. Rayo.** 1999. Frequency of oropharyngeal candidiasis in HIV-infected patients on protease inhibitor therapy. *Oral Surg. Oral Med. Oral Pathol. Oral Radiol. Endod.* **87**: 437–441.
25. **Doi, M., M. Homma, S. Iwaguchi, K. Horibe, and K. Tanaka.** 1994. Strain relatedness of *Candida albicans* strains isolated from children with leukemia and their bedside parents. *J. Clin. Microbiol.* **32**:2253–2259.
26. **Dromer, F., L. Improvisi, B. Dupont, M. Eliaszewicz, G. Pialoux, S. Fournier, and V. Feuillie.** 1997. Oral transmission of *Candida albicans* between partners in HIV-infected couples could contribute to dissemination of fluconazole-resistant isolates. *AIDS* **11**:1095–1101.
27. **Einsele, H., H. Hebart, G. Roller, J. Loffler, I. Rothenhofer, C. A. Muller, R. A. Bowden, J. van Burik, D. Engelhard, L. Kanz, and U. Schumacher.** 1997. Detection and identification of fungal pathogens in blood by using molecular probes. *J. Clin. Microbiol.* **35**:1353–1360.
28. **Elie, C. M., T. J. Lott, E. Reiss, and C. J. Morrison.** 1998. Rapid identification of *Candida* species with species-specific DNA probes. *J. Clin. Microbiol.* **36**:3260–3265.
29. **Ellsworth, D. L., K. D. Rittenhouse, and R. L. Honeycutt.** 1993. Artifactual variation in randomly amplified polymorphic DNA banding patterns. *BioTechniques* **14**:214–217.
30. **Epplen, C., G. Melmer, I. Siedlaczk, F.-W. Schwaiger, W. Mauler, and J. T. Epplen.** 1993. On the essence of "meaningless" simple repetitive DNA in eukaryotic genomes, p. 29–45. *In* S. D. J. Pena, R. Chakraborty, J. T. Epplen, and A. J. Jeffreys (ed.), *DNA Fingerprinting: State of the Science.* Birkauser Verlag, Basel, Switzerland.
31. **Espinel-Ingroff, A., A. Quart, L. Steele-Moore, I. Metcheva, G. A. Buck, V. L. Bruzzese, and D. Reich.** 1996. Molecular karyotyping of multiple yeast species isolated from nine patients with AIDS during prolonged fluconazole therapy. *J. Med. Vet. Mycol.* **34**:111–116.
32. **Fell, J. W., A. Statzell-Tallman, M. J. Lutz, and C. P. Kurtzman.** 1992. Partial rRNA sequences in marine yeasts; a model for identification of marine eukaryotes. *Mol. Mar. Biol. Biotechnol.* **1**:175–186.
33. **Fischer-Hoch, S. P., and L. Hutwagner.** 1995. Opportunistic candidiasis: an epidemic of the 1980s. *Clin. Infect. Dis.* **21**: 897–904.
34. **Flahaut, M., D. Sanglard, M. Monod, J. Bille, and M. Rossier.** 1998. Rapid detection of *Candida albicans* in clinical samples by DNA amplification of common regions from *C. albicans*-secreted aspartic proteinase genes. *J. Clin. Microbiol.* **36**: 395–401.
35. **Fujita, S., B. A. Lasker, T. J. Lott, E. Reiss, and C. J. Morrison.** 1995. Microtitration plate enzyme immunoassay to detect PCR-amplified DNA from *Candida* species in blood. *J. Clin. Microbiol.* **33**:962–967.
36. **Graser, Y., M. Volovsek, J. Arrington, G. Schonian, W. Presber, T. G. Mitchell, and R. Vilgalys.** 1996. Molecular markers reveal that population structure of the human pathogen *Candida albicans* exhibits both clonality and recombination. *Proc. Natl. Acad. Sci. USA* **93**:12473–1247.
37. **Haynes, K. A., D. J. Sullivan, D. C. Coleman, J. C. K. Clarke, R. Emilianus, C. Atkinson, and K. J. Cann.** 1995. Involvement of multiple *Cryptococcus neoformans* strains in a single episode of cryptococcosis and reinfection with novel strains in recurrent infection demonstrated by random amplication of polymorphic DNA and DNA fingerprinting. *J. Clin. Microbiol.* **33**:99–102.
38. **Haynes, K. A., and T. J. Westerneng.** 1996. Rapid identification of *Candida albicans, C. glabrata, C. parapsilosis* and *C. krusei* by species-specific PCR of large subunit ribosomal DNA. *J. Med. Microbiol.* **44**:390–396.
39. **Haynes, K. A., T. J. Westerneng, J. W. Fell, and W. Moens.** 1995. Rapid detection and identification of pathogenic fungi by polymerase chain reaction amplification of large subunit ribosomal DNA. *J. Med. Vet. Mycol.* **33**:319–325.
40. **Hendolin, P. H., L. Paulin, P. Koukila-Kahkola, V. J. Anttila, H. Malmberg, M. Richardson, and J. Ylikoski.** 2000. Panfungal PCR and multiplex liquid hybridization for detection of fungi in tissue specimens. *J. Clin. Microbiol.* **38**:4186–4192.
41. **Hoegl, L., E. Thoma-Greber, M. Rocken, and H. C. Korting.** 1998. HIV protease inhibitors influence the prevalence of oral candidosis in HIV-infected patients: a 2-year study. *Mycoses* **41**:321–325.
42. **Holmberg, K., and F. Feroze.** 1996. Evaluation of an optimised system for random amplified polumorphic DNA (RAPD)-analysis for genotypic mapping of *Candida albicans* strains. *J. Clin. Lab. Anal.* **10**:59–69.
43. **Holmes, A. R., R. D. Cannon, M. G. Shepherd, and H. F.**

Jenkinson. 1994. Detection of *Candida albicans* and other yeasts in blood by PCR. *J. Clin. Microbiol.* **32:**228–231.

44. **Hui, M., M. Ip, P. K. Chan, M. L. Chin, and A. F. Cheng.** 2000. Rapid identification of medically important *Candida* to species level by polymerase chain reaction and single-strand conformational polymorphism. *Diagn. Microbiol. Infect. Dis.* **38:**95–99.
45. **Hull, C. M., and A. D. Johnson.** 1999. Identification of a mating type-like locus in the asexual pathogenic yeast *Candida albicans. Science* **285:**1271–1275.
46. **Hull, C. M., R. M. Raisner, and A. D. Johnson.** 2000. Evidence for mating of the "asexual" yeast *Candida albicans* in a mammalian host. *Science* **289:**307–310.
47. **Jaeger, E. E., N. M. Carroll, S. Choudhury, A. A. Dunlop, H. M. Towler, M. M. Matheson, P. Adamson, N. Okhravi, and S. Lightman.** 2000. Rapid detection and identification of *Candida, Aspergillus,* and *Fusarium* species in ocular samples using nested PCR. *J. Clin. Microbiol.* **38:**2902–2908.
48. **Jarvis, W. R.** 1995. Epidemiology of nosocomial fungal infections, with emphasis on *Candida* species. *Clin. Infect. Dis.* **20:**1526–1530.
49. **Joly, S., C. Pujol, M. Rysz, K. Vargas, and D. R. Soll.** 1999. Development and characterization of complex DNA fingerprinting probes for the infectious yeast *Candida dubliniensis. J. Clin. Microbiol.* **37:**1035–1044.
50. **Joly, S., C. Pujol, K. Schroppel, and D. R. Soll.** 1996. Development and verification of two species fingerprinting probes for *Candida tropicalis* amenable for computer analysis. *J. Clin. Microbiol.* **34:**3063–3071.
51. **Jones, J. M.** 1990. Laboratory diagnosis of invasive candidiasis. *Clin. Microbiol. Rev.* **3:**779–783.
52. **Kaplan, J. E., D. Hanson, M. S. Dworkin, T. Frederick, J. Bertolli, M. L. Lindegren, S. Holmberg, and J. L. Jones.** 2000. Epidemiology of human immunodeficiency virus-associated opportunistic infections in the United States in the era of highly active antiretroviral therapy. *Clin. Infect. Dis.* **30**(Suppl. 1)**:**S5–S14.
53. **Kempf, V. A., K. Trebesius, and I. B. Autenrieth.** 2000. Fluorescent in situ hybridization allows rapid identification of microorganisms in blood cultures. *J. Clin. Microbiol.* **38:** 830–838.
54. **Lasker, B. A., L. S. Page, T. J. Lott, and G. S. Kobayashi.** 1992. Isolation, characterization, and sequencing of *Candida albicans* repetitive element 2. *Gene* **116:**51–57.
55. **Lehman, P. F., D. Lin, and B. A. Lasker.** 1992. Genotypic identification and characterization of species and strains within the genus *Candida* by using random amplified polymorphic DNA. *J. Clin. Microbiol.* **30:**3249–3254.
56. **Lin, D., and P. F. Lehmann.** 1995. Random amplified polymorphic DNA for strain delineation within *Candida tropicalis. J. Med. Vet. Mycol.* **33:**241–246.
57. **Lischewski, A., M. Kretschmar, H. Hof, R. Amann, J. Hacker, and J. Morschhauser.** 1997. Detection and identification of *Candida* species in experimentally infected tissue and human blood by rRNA-specific fluorescent in situ hybridization. *J. Clin. Microbiol.* **35:**2943–2948.
58. **Lischewski, A., M. Ruhnke, I. Tennagen, G. Schonian, J. Morschhäuser, and J. Hacker.** 1995. Molecular epidemiology of *Candida* isolates from AIDS patients showing different fluconazole resistance profiles. *J. Clin. Microbiol.* **33:**769–771.
59. **Lockhart, S. R., J. J. Fritch, A. S. Meier, K. Schroppel, T. Srikantha, R. Galask, and D. R. Soll.** 1995. Colonising populations of *Candida albicans* are clonal in origin but undergo microevolution through C1 fragment reorganisation as demonstrated by DNA fingerprinting and C1 sequencing. *J. Clin. Microbiol.* **33:**1501–1509.
60. **Lockhart, S. R., S. Joly, C. Pujol, J. D. Sobel, M. A. Pfaller, and D. R. Soll.** 1997. Development and verification of fingerprinting probes for *Candida glabrata. Microbiology* **143:** 3733–3746.
61. **Lockhart, S. R., B. D. Reed, C. L. Pierson, and D. R. Soll.** 1996. Most frequent scenario for recurrent *Candida* vaginitis is strain maintenance with "substrain shuffling": demonstration by sequential DNA fingerprinting with probes Ca3, C1, and CARE2. *J. Clin. Microbiol.* **34:**767–777.
62. **Loeffler, J., N. Henke, H. Hebart, D. Schmidt, L. Hagmeyer, U. Schumacher, and H. Einsele.** 2000. Quantification of fungal DNA by using fluorescence resonance energy transfer and the light cycler system. *J. Clin. Microbiol.* **38:**586–590.
63. **Löffler, J., H. Hebart, U. Schumacher, H. Reitze, and H. Einsele.** 1997. Comparison of different methods for extraction of DNA of fungal pathogens from cultures and blood. *J. Clin. Microbiol.* **35:**3311–3312.
64. **Löffler, J., H. Hebart, S. Sepe, U. Schumcher, T. Klingebiel, and H. Einsele.** 1998. Detection of PCR-amplified fungal DNA by using a PCR-ELISA system. *Med. Mycol.* **36:** 275–279.
65. **Lopez-Ribot, J., R. McAtee, L. Lee, W. Kirkpatrick, T. White, D. Sanglard, and T. Patterson.** 1998. Distinct patterns of gene expression associated with development of fluconazole resistance in serial *Candida albicans* isolates from human immunodeficiency virus-infected patients with oropharyngeal candidiasis. *Antimicrob. Agents Chemother.* **42:**2932–2937.
66. **Magee, B. B., T. M. D'Souza, and P. T. Magee.** 1987. Strain and species identification by restriction fragment length polymorphisms in the ribosomal DNA repeat of *Candida albicans. J. Bacteriol.* **169:**1639–1643.
67. **Magee, B. B., and P. T. Magee.** 1987. Electrophoretic karyotypes and chromosome numbers in *Candida* species. *J. Gen. Microbiol.* **133:**425–430.
68. **Magee, B. B., and P. T. Magee.** 2000. Induction of mating in *Candida albicans* by construction of MTLa and MTLalpha strains. *Science* **289:**310–313.
69. **Mannarelli, B. M., and C. P. Kurtzman.** 1998. Rapid identification of *Candida albicans* and other human pathogenic yeasts by using short oligonucleotides in a PCR. *J. Clin. Microbiol.* **36:**1634–1641.
70. **Marco, F., S. R. Lockhart, M. A. Pfaller, C. Pujol, M. S. Rangel-Frausto, T. Wiblin, H. M. Blumberg, J. E. Edwards, W. Jarvis, L. Saiman, J. E. Patterson, M. G. Rinaldi, R. P. Wenzel, and D. R. Soll.** 1999. Elucidating the origins of nosocomial infections with *Candida albicans* by DNA fingerprinting with the complex probe Ca3. *J. Clin. Microbiol.* **37:** 2817–2828.
71. **Martin, C., D. Roberts, M. van Der Weide, R. Rossau, G. Jannes, T. Smith, and M. Maher.** 2000. Development of a PCR-based line probe assay for identification of fungal pathogens. *J. Clin. Microbiol.* **38:**3735–3742.
72. **McCullough, M. J., K. V. Clemons, and D. A. Stevens.** 1999. Molecular epidemiology of the global and temporal diversity of *Candida albicans. Clin. Infect. Dis.* **29:**1220–1225.
73. **Metzgar, D., D. Field, R. Haubrich, and C. Wills.** 1998. Sequence analysis of a compound coding-region microsatellite in *Candida albicans* resolves homoplasies and provides a high-resolution tool for genotyping. *FEMS Immunol. Med. Microbiol.* **20:**103–109.
74. **Morace, G., M. Sanguinetti, B. Posteraro, G. Lo Cascio, and G. Fadda.** 1997. Identification of various medically important *Candida* species in clinical specimens by PCR-restriction enzyme analysis. *J. Clin. Microbiol.* **35:**667–672.
75. **Moran, G. P., D. J. Sullivan, M. C. Henman, C. E. McCreary, B. J. Harrington, D. B. Shanley, and D. C. Coleman.** 1997.

Antifungal drug susceptibilities of oral *Candida dubliniensis* isolates from human immunodeficiency virus (HIV)-infected and non-HIV-infected subjects and generation of stable fluconazole-resistant derivatives in vitro. *Antimicrob. Agents Chemother.* **41:**617–623.

76. **Müller, F. M., M. Kasai, A. Francesconi, B. Brillante, M. Roden, J. Peter, S. J. Chanock, and T. J. Walsh.** 1999. Transmission of an azole-resistant isogenic strain of *Candida albicans* among human immunodeficiency virus-infected family members with oropharyngeal candidiasis. *J. Clin. Microbiol.* **37:**3405–3408.
77. **Müller, F. M., K. E. Werner, M. Kasai, A. Francesconi, S. J. Chanock, and T. J. Walsh.** 1998. Rapid extraction of genomic DNA from medically important yeasts and filamentous fungi by high-speed cell disruption. *J. Clin. Microbiol.* **36:** 1625–1629.
78. **Nguyen, M. H., J. E. Peacock, A. J. Morris, D. C. Tanner, M. L. Nguyen, D. R. Snydman, M. M. Wagener, M. G. Rinaldi, and L. Y. Yu.** 1996. The changing face of candidemia: emergence of non-*Candida albicans* species and antifungal resistance. *Am. J. Med.* **100:**617–623.
79. **Odds, F. C., and R. Bernaerts.** 1994. CHROMagar Candida, a new differential isolation medium for presumptive identification of clinically important *Candida* species. *J. Clin. Microbiol.* **32:**1923–1929.
80. **Orrego, C.** 1990. Organizing a laboratory for PCR work, p. 447–454. *In* M. A. Innis, D. H. Gelfland, J. J. Sninsky, and T. J. White (ed.), *PCR Protocols: A Guide to Methods and Applications.* Academic Press, Inc., San Diego, Calif.
81. **Park, S., M. Wong, S. A. Marras, E. W. Cross, T. E. Kiehn, V. Chaturvedi, S. Tyagi, and D. S. Perlin.** 2000. Rapid identification of *Candida dubliniensis* using a species-specific molecular beacon. *J. Clin. Microbiol.* **38:**2829–2836.
82. **Pertowski, C. A., R. C. Baron, B. A. Lasker, S. B. Werner, and W. R. Jarvis.** 1995. Nosocomial outbreak of *Candida albicans* sternal wound infections following cardiac surgery traced to a scrub nurse. *J. Infect. Dis.* **172:**817–822.
83. **Pfaller, M. A.** 1995. Epidemiology of candidiasis. *J. Hosp. Infect.* **30:**329–338.
84. **Pfaller, M. A., R. N. Jones, G. V. Doern, A. C. Fluit, J. Verhoef, H. S. Sader, S. A. Messer, A. Houston, S. Coffman, and R. J. Hollis.** 1999. International surveillance of blood stream infections due to *Candida* species in the European SENTRY program: species distribution and antifungal susceptibility including the investigational triazole and echinocandin agents. *Diagn. Microbiol. Infect. Dis.* **35:**19–25.
85. **Pfaller, M. A., R. N. Jones, G. V. Doern, H. S. Sader, R. J. Hollis, S. A. Messer, and the Sentry Participant Group.** 1998. International surveillance of bloodstream infections due to *Candida* species: frequency of occurrence and antifungal susceptibilities of isolates collected in 1997 in the United States, Canada, and South America for the SENTRY program. *J. Clin. Microbiol.* **36:**1886–1889.
86. **Pfaller, M. A., R. N. Jones, G. V. Doern, H. S. Sader, S. A. Messer, A. Houston, S. Coffman, and R. J. Hollis.** 2000. Bloodstream infections due to *Candida* species: SENTRY antimicrobial surveillance program in North America and Latin America, 1997–1998. *Antimicrob. Agents Chemother.* **44:** 747–751.
87. **Pfaller, M. A., R. N. Jones, S. A. Messer, M. B. Edmond, and R. P. Wenzel.** 1998. National surveillance of nosocomial blood stream infection due to *Candida albicans:* frequency of occurrence and antifungal susceptibility in the SCOPE program. *Diagn. Microbiol. Infect. Dis.* **31:**327–332.
88. **Pfaller, M. A., R. N. Jones, S. A. Messer, M. B. Edmond, and R. P. Wenzel.** 1998. National surveillance of nosocomial blood stream infection due to species of *Candida* other than *Candida albicans:* frequency of occurrence and antifungal susceptibility in the SCOPE program. *Diagn. Microbiol. Infect. Dis.* **30:**121–129.
89. **Pfaller, M. A., S. R. Lockhart, C. Pujol, J. A. Swails-Wenger, S. A. Messer, M. B. Edmond, R. N. Jones, R. P. Wenzel, and D. R. Soll.** 1998. Hospital specificity, region specificity, and fluconazole resistance of *Candida albicans* bloodstream isolates. *J. Clin. Microbiol.* **36:**1518–1529.
90. **Pfaller, M. A., S. A. Messer, A. Houston, M. S. Rangel-Frausto, T. Wiblin, H. M. Blumberg, J. E. Edwards, W. Jarvis, M. A. Martin, H. C. Neu, L. Saiman, J. E. Patterson, J. C. Dibb, C. M. Roldsn, M. G. Rinaldi, and R. P. Wenzel.** 1998. National epidemiology of mycoses survey: a multicenter study of strain variation and antifungal susceptibility among isolates of *Candida* species. *Diagn. Microbiol. Infect. Dis.* **31:**289–296.
91. **Pittet, D., M. Monod, P. M. Suter, E. Frenk, and R. Auckenthaler.** 1994. *Candida* colonization and subsequent infections in critically ill surgical patients. *Ann. Surg.* **220:**751–758.
92. **Polanco, A., E. Mellado, C. Castilla, and J. L. Rodriguez-Tudela.** 1999. Detection of *Candida albicans* in blood by PCR in a rabbit animal model of disseminated candidiasis. *Diagn. Microbiol. Infect. Dis.* **34:**177–183.
93. **Pontieri, E., L. Gregori, M. Gennarelli, T. Ceddia, G. Novelli, B. Dallapiccola, F. De Bernardis, and G. Carruba.** 1996. Correlation of *Sfi*I macrorestriction endonuclease fingerprint analysis of *Candida parapsilosis* isolates with source of isolation. *J. Med. Microbiol.* **45:**173–178.
94. **Posteraro, B., M. Sanguinetti, L. Masucci, L. Romano, G. Morace, and G. Fadda.** 2000. Reverse cross blot hybridization assay for rapid detection of PCR-amplified DNA from *Candida* species, *Cryptococcus neoformans,* and *Saccharomyces cerevisiae* in clinical samples. *J. Clin. Microbiol.* **38:** 1609–1614.
95. **Pujol, C., S. Joly, S. R. Lockhart, S. Noel, M. Tibayrenc, and D. R. Soll.** 1997. Parity among the randomly amplified polymorphic DNA method, multilocus enzyme electrophoresis, and Southern blot hybridization with the moderately repetitive probe Ca3 for fingerprinting *C. albicans. J. Clin. Microbiol.* **35:**3248–3258.
96. **Pujol, C., F. Renaud, M. Mallie, T. de Meeus, and J.-M. Bastide.** 1997. Atypical strains of *Candida albicans* recovered from AIDS patients. *J. Med. Vet. Mycol.* **35:**115–121.
97. **Pujol, C., J. Reynes, F. Renaud, M. Raymond, M. Tibayrenc, F. J. Ayala, F. Janbon, M. Mallie, and J. M. Bastide.** 1993. The yeast *Candida albicans* has a clonal mode of reproduction in a population of infected human immunodeficiency virus-positive patients. *Proc. Natl. Acad. Sci. USA* **90:** 9456–9459.
98. **Rangel-Frausto, M. S., T. Wiblin, H. M. Blumberg, L. Saiman, J. Patterson, M. Rinaldi, M. Pfaller, J. E. Edwards, Jr., W. Jarvis, J. Dawson, and R. P. Wenzel.** 1999. National epidemiology of mycoses survey (NEMIS): variations in rates of bloodstream infections due to *Candida* species in seven surgical intensive care units and six neonatal intensive care units. *Clin. Infect. Dis.* **29:**253–258.
99. **Reagan, D. R., M. A. Pfaller, R. J. Hollis, and R. P. Wenzel.** 1995. Evidence of nosocomial spread of *Candida albicans* causing bloodstream infection in a neonatal intensive care unit. *Diagn. Microbiol. Infect. Dis.* **21:**191–194.
100. **Reiss, E., K. Tanaka, G. Bruker, V. Chazalet, D. Coleman, J. P. Debeaupuis, R. Hanazawa, J. P. Latge, J. Lortholary, K. Makimura, C. J. Morrison, S. Y. Murayama, S. Naoe, S. Paris, J. Sarfati, K. Shibuya, D. Sullivan, K. Uchida, and H.**

Yamaguchi. 1998. Molecular diagnosis and epidemiology of fungal infections. *Med. Mycol.* **36**(Suppl. 1):249–257.

101. **Riederer, K., P. Fozo, and R. Khatib.** 1998. Typing of *Candida albicans* and *Candida parapsilosis:* species-related limitations of electrophoretic karyotyping and restriction endonuclease analysis of genomic DNA. *Mycoses* **41:**397–402.
102. **Robert, F., F. Lebreton, M. E. Bougnoux, A. Paugam, D. Wassermann, M. Schlotterer, C. Tourte-Schaefer, and J. Dupouy-Camet.** 1995. Use of random amplified polymorphic DNA as a typing method for *Candida albicans* in epidemiological surveillance of a burns unit. *J. Clin. Microbiol.* **33:** 2366–2371.
103. **Rosa, E. A., C. V. Pereira, R. T. Rosa, and J. F. Hofling.** 2000. Grouping oral *Candida* species by multilocus enzyme electrophoresis. *Int. J. Evol. Microbiol.* **50:**1343–1349.
104. **Sadhu, C., M. J. McEachern, E. P. Rustchenko-Bulgac, J. Schmid, D. R. Soll, and J. B. Hicks.** 1991. Telomeric and dispersed repeat sequences in *Candida* yeasts and their use in strain identification. *J. Bacteriol.* **173:**842–850.
105. **Sanchez, V., J. A. Vasquez, D. Barth-Jones, L. Dembry, J. D. Sobel, and M. J. Zervos.** 1992. Epidemiology of nosocomial acquisition of *Candida lusitaniae. J. Clin. Microbiol.* **30:** 3005–3008.
106. **Sandhu, G. S., B. C. Kline, L. Stockman, and G. D. Roberts.** 1995. Molecular probes for diagnosis of fungal infections. *J. Clin. Microbiol.* **33:**2913–2919.
107. **Scherer, S., and D. A. Stevens.** 1987. Application of DNA typing methods to epidemiology and taxonomy of *Candida* species. *J. Clin. Microbiol.* **25:**675–679.
108. **Scherer, S., and D. A. Stevens.** 1988. A *Candida albicans* dispersed, repeated gene family and its epidemiologic applications. *Proc. Natl. Acad. Sci. USA* **85:**1542–1465.
109. **Schmid, J., S. Herd, P. R. Hunter, R. D. Cannon, M. S. Yasin, S. Samad, M. Carr, D. Parr, W. McKinney, M. Schousboe, B. Harris, R. Ikram, M. Harris, A. Restrepo, G. Hoyos, and K. P. Singh.** 1999. Evidence for a general-purpose genotype in *Candida albicans,* highly prevalent in multiple geographical regions, patient types and types of infection. *Microbiology* **145:**2405–2413.
110. **Schroppel, K., M. Rotman, R. Galask, K. Mac, and D. R. Soll.** 1994. Evolution and replacement of *Candida albicans* strains during recurrent vaginitis demonstrated by DNA fingerprinting. *J. Clin. Microbiol.* **32:**2646–2654.
111. **Schwartz, D. C., and C. R. Cantor.** 1984. Separation of yeast chromosome-sized DNAs by pulsed field gradient gel electrophoresis. *Cell* **37:**67–75.
112. **Shin, J. H., F. S. Nolte, B. P. Holloway, and C. J. Morrison.** 1999. Rapid identification of up to three *Candida* species in a single reaction tube by a 5′ exonuclease assay using fluorescent DNA probes. *J. Clin. Microbiol.* **37:**165–170.
113. **Shin, J. H., F. S. Nolte, and C. J. Morrison.** 1997. Rapid identification of *Candida* species in blood cultures by a clinically useful PCR method. *J. Clin. Microbiol.* **35:**1454–1459.
114. **Soll, D. R.** 2000. The ins and outs of DNA fingerprinting the infectious fungi. *Clin. Microbiol. Rev.* **13:**332–370.
115. **Stein, G. E., V. L. Sheridan, B. B. Magee, and P. T. Magee.** 1991. Use of rDNA restriction fragment length polymorphisms to differentiate strains of *Candida albicans* in women with vulvovaginal candidiasis. *Diagn. Microbiol. Infect. Dis.* **14:**459–464.
116. **Sullivan, D., D. Bennett, M. Henman, P. Harwood, S. Flint, F. Mulcahy, D. Shanley, and D. Coleman.** 1993. Oligonucleotide fingerprinting of isolates of *Candida* species other than *C. albicans* and of atypical *Candida* species from human immunodeficiency virus-positive and AIDS patients. *J. Clin. Microbiol.* **31:**2124–2133.
117. **Sullivan, D., K. Haynes, G. Moran, D. Shanley, and D. Coleman.** 1996. Persistence, replacement, and microevolution of *Cryptococcus neoformans* strains in recurrent meningitis in AIDS patients. *J. Clin. Microbiol.* **34:**1739–1744.
118. **Sullivan, D. J., M. C. Henman, G. P. Moran, L. C. O'Neill, D. E. Bennett, D. B. Shanley, and D. C. Coleman.** 1996. Molecular approaches to identification, epidemiology and taxonomy of non-*albicans Candida* species. *J. Med. Microbiol.* **44:**399–408.
119. **Sullivan, D. J., T. J. Westerneng, K. A. Haynes, D. E. Bennett, and D. C. Coleman.** 1995. *Candida dubliniensis* sp. nov.: phenotypic and molecular characterisation of a novel species associated with oral candidosis in HIV-infected individuals. *Microbiology* **141:**1507–1521.
120. **Timmins, E. M., S. A. Howell, B. K. Alsberg, W. C. Noble, and R. Goodacre.** 1998. Rapid differentiation of closely related *Candida* species and strains by pyrolysis-mass spectrometry and Fourier transform-infrared spectroscopy. *J. Clin. Microbiol.* **36:**367–374.
121. **Turenne, C. Y., S. E. Sanche, D. J. Hoban, J. A. Karlowsky, and A. M. Kabani.** 1999. Rapid identification of fungi by using the ITS2 genetic region and an automated fluorescent capillary electrophoresis system. *J. Clin. Microbiol.* **37:** 1846–1851.
122. **Vazquez, J. A., L. M. Dembry, V. Sanchez, M. A. Vazquez, J. D. Sobel, C. Dmuchowski, and M. J. Zervos.** 1998. Nosocomial *Candida glabrata* colonization: an epidemiologic study. *J. Clin. Microbiol.* **36:**421–426.
123. **Velegraki, A., M. E. Kambouris, G. Skiniotis, M. Savala, A. Mitroussia-Ziouva, and N. J. Legakis.** 1999. Identification of medically significant fungal genera by polymerase chain reaction followed by restriction enzyme analysis. *FEMS Immunol. Med. Microbiol.* **23:**303–312.
124. **Voss, A., R. J. Hollis, M. A. Pfaller, R. P. Wenzel, and B. N. Doebbeling.** 1994. Investigation of the sequence of colonization and candidemia in non-neutropenic patients. *J. Clin. Microbiol.* **32:**975–980.
125. **Voss, A., M. A. Pfaller, R. J. Hollis, J. Rhine-Chalberg, and B. N. Doebbeling.** 1995. Investigation of *Candida albicans* transmission in a surgical intensive care unit cluster by using genomic DNA typing methods. *J. Clin. Microbiol.* **33:** 576–580.
126. **Waggoner-Fountain, L. A., M. W. Walker, R. J. Hollis, M. A. Pfaller, J. E. Ferguson, 2nd, R. P. Wenzel, and L. G. Donowitz.** 1996. Vertical and horizontal transmission of unique *Candida* species to premature newborns. *Clin. Infect. Dis.* **22:**803–808.
127. **Wahyuningsih, R., H. J. Freisleben, H. G. Sonntag, and P. Schnitzler.** 2000. Simple and rapid detection of *Candida albicans* DNA in serum by PCR for diagnosis of invasive candidiasis. *J. Clin. Microbiol.* **38:**3016–3021.
128. **Walsh, T. J., A. Francesconi, M. Kasai, and S. J. Chanock.** 1995. PCR and single-strand conformational polymorphism for recognition of medically important opportunistic fungi. *J. Clin. Microbiol.* **33:**3216–3220.
129. **Weissing, K., R. Atkinson, and R. Gardner.** 1995. Genomic fingerprinting by microsatellite-primed PCR: a critical evaluation. *PCR Methods Applic.* **4:**249–255.
130. **Welsh, J., and M. McClelland.** 1990. Fingerprinting genomes using PCR with arbitrary primers. *Nucleic Acids Res.* **18:** 7213–7224.
131. **Wenzel, R. P.** 1995. Nosocomial candidemia: risk factors and attributable mortality. *Clin. Infect. Dis.* **20:**1531–1534.
132. **Widjojoatmodjo, M. N., A. Borst, R. A. Schukkink, A. T. Box, N. M. Tacken, B. Van Gemen, J. Verhoef, B. Top, and**

A. C. Fluit. 1999. Nucleic acid sequence-based amplification (NASBA) detection of medically important *Candida* species. *J. Microbiol. Methods* **38:**81–90.

133. **Wilkinson, B. M., L. Morris, D. J. Adams, E. G. Evans, C. J. Lacey, and R. M. Walmsley.** 1992. A new, sensitive polynucleotide probe for distinguishing *Candida albicans* strains and its use with computer assisted archiving and pattern comparison system. *J. Med. Vet. Mycol.* **30:**123–131.
134. **Williams, D. W., M. J. Wilson, M. A. Lewis, and A. J. Potts.** 1995. Identification of *Candida* species by PCR and restriction fragment length polymorphism analysis of intergenic spacer regions of ribosomal DNA. *J. Clin. Microbiol.* **33:** 2476–2479.
135. **Wills, J. W., B. A. Lasker, K. Sirotkin, and W. S. Riggsby.** 1984. Repetitive DNA of *Candida albicans:* nuclear and mitochondrial components. *J. Bacteriol.* **157:**918–924.
136. **Wit, F. W., R. van Leeuwen, G. J. Weverling, S. Jurriaans, K. Nauta, R. Steingrover, J. Schuijtemaker, X. Eyssen, D. Fortuin, M. Weeda, F. de Wolf, P. Reiss, S. A. Danner, and J. M. Lange.** 1999. Outcome and predictors of failure of highly active antiretroviral therapy: one-year follow-up of a cohort of human immunodeficiency virus type 1-infected persons. *J. Infect. Dis.* **179:**790–798.
137. **Xu, J., A. R. Ramos, R. Vilgalys, and T. G. Mitchell.** 2000. Clonal and spontaneous origins of fluconazole resistance in *Candida albicans. J. Clin. Microbiol.* **38:**1214–1220.

INDEX